Reversibility of Chronic Disease and Hypersensitivity, Volume 5
Treatment Options of Chemical Sensitivity

T0274207

Reversibility of Chronic Disease and Hypersensitivity, Volume 5

Treatment Options of Chemical Sensitivity

William J. Rea
Kalpana D. Patel

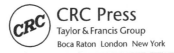

CRC Press
Taylor & Francis Group
Boca Raton London New York

CRC Press is an imprint of the
Taylor & Francis Group, an **informa** business

CRC Press
Taylor & Francis Group
6000 Broken Sound Parkway NW, Suite 300
Boca Raton, FL 33487-2742

First issued in paperback 2022

© 2018 by Taylor & Francis Group, LLC
CRC Press is an imprint of Taylor & Francis Group, an Informa business

No claim to original U.S. Government works

ISBN-13: 978-1-498-78136-7 (hbk)
ISBN-13: 978-1-03-233932-0 (pbk)
DOI: 10.1201/9781315155258

International Standard Book Number-978-1-4987-8136-7 (Hardback)

This book contains information obtained from authentic and highly regarded sources. Reasonable efforts have been made to publish reliable data and information, but the author and publisher cannot assume responsibility for the validity of all materials or the consequences of their use. The authors and publishers have attempted to trace the copyright holders of all material reproduced in this publication and apologize to copyright holders if permission to publish in this form has not been obtained. If any copyright material has not been acknowledged please write and let us know so we may rectify in any future reprint.

Except as permitted under U.S. Copyright Law, no part of this book may be reprinted, reproduced, transmitted, or utilized in any form by any electronic, mechanical, or other means, now known or hereafter invented, including pho-tocopying, microfilming, and recording, or in any information storage or retrieval system, without written permission from the publishers.

For permission to photocopy or use material electronically from this work, please access www.copyright.com (http://www.copyright.com/) or contact the Copyright Clearance Center, Inc. (CCC), 222 Rosewood Drive, Dan-vers, MA 01923, 978-750-8400. CCC is a not-for-profit organization that provides licenses and registration for a variety of users. For organizations that have been granted a photocopy license by the CCC, a separate system of payment has been arranged.

Trademark Notice: Product or corporate names may be trademarks or registered trademarks, and are used only for identification and explanation without intent to infringe.

Publisher's Note

The publisher has gone to great lengths to ensure the quality of this reprint but points out that some imperfections in the original copies may be apparent.

Visit the Taylor & Francis Web site at
http://www.taylorandfrancis.com

and the CRC Press Web site at
http://www.crcpress.com

Contents

Preface

The clinical aspects of the diagnosis and treatment of chemical sensitivity and chronic degenerative disease presented in this volume are now complete. This volume is for people interested in the origin of the clinical aspects of chemical sensitivity and chronic degenerative disease. The clinical aspects of chemical sensitivity are growing in leaps and bounds and need to be known and considered in every case of chronic degenerative disease.

In treating chronic degenerative disease, healthcare providers must consider every aspect of chemical sensitivity. In this way, they will be able to help more patients obtain health and prevent advanced disease. Also, considering the aspects of chemical sensitivity will help each clinician to direct research for the prevention of advanced irreversible end-stage disease. Modern technology has contributed to the advancement of chemical sensitivity, and it should be brought to bear on the solution of the problem.

Acknowledgments

Thanks to the great environmental clinicians and scientists who based their clinical findings on not only sound observations but also basic scientific facts of anatomy, physiology, and biochemistry. These astute physicians and surgeons include Drs. Theron Randolph, Laurence Dickey, Carlton Lee, Herbert Rinkle, Joseph Miller, Dor Brown, James Willoughby, French Hansel, Ed Binkley, Al Lieberman, Harris Husen, Marshal Mandel, Jean Monro, Sherry Rogers, Jonathan Maberly, Jonathan Wright, Joe Morgan, Klaus Runow, Clive Pyman, Colin Little Richard Travino, John Boyles, Wallace Rubin, Daniel Martinez, Jonathan Brostoff, Phyllis Saifer, Gary Oberg, Satosi Ishikawa and his group, and countless others.

Thanks to Chris Bishop and Dr. Yaqin Pan, whose help in analyzing the data and preparing the manuscript and illustrations was invaluable; their efforts were herculean, and the book could not have been completed without them. Thanks also to Drs. Alfred Johnson, Gerald Ross, Ralph Smiley, Thomas Buckley, Nancy Didriksen, Joel Butler, Ervin Fenyves, John Laseter, and Jon Pangborn, who supplied cases, data, reports, and critiques of what should and should not be done. Additional thanks to Drs. Sherry Rogers, Allan Lieberman, Bertie Griffiths, and Kalpana D. Patel, who proofread and helped compile sections of the book; to the staff at the EHC-Dallas for all of their support; to the members of the American Academy of Environmental Medicine and the Pan American Allergy Society for their contribution and support of the EHC-Dallas; to the American Environmental Health Foundation, who lent financial support to this effort; to Doris Rapp, Theron Randolph, Lawrence Dickey, John MaClennen, Dor Brown, Carlton Lee, James Willoughby Sr., George Kroker, Jean Monro, Jonathan Maberly, Klaus Runow, Colin Little, Marshall Mandell, Jozef Krop, Hongyu Zhang, Satoshi Ishikawa, Miko Miyata, Joseph Miller, and Ronald Finn for advice and for freely exchanging information.

We are especially indebted to Dr. Jonathan Pangborn, William B. Jakoby, Andrew L. Reeves, Thad Godish, Steve Levine, Alan Levin, Felix Gad Sulman, and Eduardo Gaitan, whose research, books, and papers provided an invaluable foundation for the preparation of this text.

William J. Rea, MD
Kalpana D. Patel, MD

Special Recognition

Special recognition goes to Yaqin Pan, MD, who constructed the tables in this volume, Alexis Plowden who did the majority of the references and editing, and Gladys Morris who did the multiple typings and organization of the book, as well as many of the references.

Authors

William J. Rea, MD, FACS, FAAEM, is a thoracic, cardiovascular, and general surgeon with an added interest in the environmental aspects of health and disease. Founder of the Environmental Health Center—Dallas (EHC-Dallas) in 1974, Dr. Rea is currently the director of this highly specialized Dallas-based medical facility.

Dr. Rea was awarded the Jonathan Forman Gold Medal Award in 1987 for outstanding research in environmental medicine, The Herbert J. Rinkle Award in 1993 for outstanding teaching, and the 1998 Service Award, all by the American Academy of Environmental Medicine. He was named Outstanding Alumnus by Otterbein College in 1991. Other awards include the Mountain Valley Water Hall of Fame in 1987 for research in water and health, the Special Achievement Award by Otterbein College in 1991, the Distinguished Pioneers in Alternative Medicine Award by the Foundation for the Advancement of Innovative Medicine Education Fund in 1994, the Gold Star Award by the International Biographical Center in 1997, Five Hundred Leaders of Influence Award in 1997, Who's Who in the South and Southwest in 1997, The Twentieth Century Award for Achievement in 1997, the Dor W. Brown, Jr., M.D. Lectureship Award by the Pan American Allergy Society, and the O. Spurgeon English Humanitarian Award by Temple University in 2002. He is the author of 10 medical textbooks, and Vol II The Effects of Environmental Pollutants on the Organ System *Chemical Sensitivity (V. 1–4)*, *Reversibility of Chronic Degenerative Disease and Hypersensitivity, V. 1: Regulating Mechanisms of Chemical Sensitivity*, and the coauthor of *Your Home, Your Health and Well-Being*. He also published the popular book on how to build less polluted homes, *Optimum Environments for Optimum Health and Creativity*. Dr. Rea has published more than 150 peer-reviewed research papers related to the topic of thoracic and cardiovascular surgery as well as that of environmental medicine.

Dr. Rea currently serves on the board and is the president of the American Environmental Health Foundation. He is vice president of the American Board of Environmental Medicine and previously served on the board of the American Academy of Environmental Medicine. He previously held the position of chief of surgery at Brookhaven Medical Center and chief of cardiovascular surgery at Dallas Veteran's Hospital, and he is a former president of the American Academy of Environmental Medicine and the Pan American Allergy Society. He has also served on the Science Advisory Board for the U.S. Environmental Protection Agency, on the Research Committee for the American Academy of Otolaryngic Allergy and on the Committee on Aspects of Cardiovascular, Endocrine and Autoimmune Diseases of the American College of Allergists, Committee on Immunotoxicology for the Office of Technology Assessment, and on the panel on Chemical Sensitivity of the National Academy of Sciences. He was previously adjunct professor with the University of Oklahoma Health Science Center, College of Public Health. Dr. Rea is a fellow of the American College of Surgeons, the American Academy of Environmental Medicine, the American College of Allergists, the American College of Preventive Medicine, the American College of Nutrition, and the Royal Society of Medicine.

Born in Jefferson, Ohio and raised in Woodville, Ohio, Dr. Rea graduated from Otterbein College in Westerville, Ohio, and Ohio State University College of Medicine in Columbus, Ohio. He then completed a rotating internship at Parkland Memorial Hospital in Dallas, Texas. He held a general surgery residency from 1963 to 1967 and a cardiovascular surgery fellowship and residency from 1967 to 1969 with The University of Texas Southwestern Medical School system, which includes Parkland Memorial Hospital, Baylor Medical Center, Veteran's Hospital and Children's Medical Center. He was also part of the team that treated Governor Connelly when President Kennedy was assassinated.

From 1969 to 1972, Dr. Rea was an assistant professor of cardiovascular surgery at the University of Texas S.W. Medical School; from 1984 to 1985, Dr. Rea held the position of adjunct professor of environmental sciences and mathematics at the University of Texas; while from 1972 to 1982, he acted as a clinical associate professor of thoracic surgery at The University of Texas Southwestern Medical School. Dr. Rea held the First World Professorial Chair of Environmental Medicine at the

University of Surrey, Guildford, England from 1988 to 1998. He also served as adjunct professor of psychology and guest lecturer at North Texas State University.

Kalpana D. Patel, MD, FAAP, FAAEM, is a pediatrician with an added interest in the environmental aspects of health and disease. Dr. Patel is a founder of the Environmental Health Center-Buffalo (EHC-Buffalo) in 1985, a specialized Buffalo-based medical facility. Dr. Patel was awarded the Jonathan Forman Gold Medal Award in 2006 for outstanding research in environmental medicine and the Herbert J. Rinkle Award in 2008 for outstanding teaching by the American Academy of Environmental Medicine. She was a recipient of the prestigious Hind Ratna award by the NRI organization in India. She is a coauthor of the medical textbooks *Reversibility of Chronic Degenerative Disease and Hypersensitivity, V. 1: Regulating Mechanisms of Chemical Sensitivity*. Dr. Patel has published many peer-reviewed research papers related to the topic of environmental medicine. Dr. Patel currently serves on the board and is the president of the Environmental Health Foundation of New York. She was a president of the American Board of Environmental Medicine and previously served on the board of the American Academy of Environmental Medicine. She previously held the position of Director of Child Health at Department of Health, Erie County and chief of Pediatrics at Deaconess Hospital Buffalo, New York. Dr. Patel is a fellow of the American Academy of Environmental Medicine.,

Dr. Patel was born in Pune, India and was raised in Ahmedabad, India. She graduated from St Xavier's College with honors in the state of Gujarat, India, and also with honors from B. J. Medical College, Gujarat University in Ahmedabad, India. She then completed a rotating internship at Bexar County Hospital in San Antonio, Texas. She held a pediatric residency from 1969 to 1972. Dr. Patel is an assistant professor of pediatrics at the State University of New York at Buffalo since 1973.

1 Molds

MOLD AND DAMPNESS OUTDOORS AND IN THE BUILDING

MOLD AND HEALTH

The term "mold" is a colloquial term for a group of filamentous fungi that are common on food or wet materials in outdoor or indoor environments. Outdoor, molds live in the soil, on plants, and on dead or decaying matter. Most molds consist of fungi imperfecti (Deuteromycetes) such as *Cladosporium*, *Penicillium*, and *Aspergillus*; ascospores such as *Eurotium*, *Chaetomium*; powdery mildew and Zygospores such as *Mucor* and *Rhizopus*; and the rain molds such as *Leptosphaeria* and *Phaeosphaeria*. Most of these are Ascomycetes such as *Chaetomium*, *Ascobulus deltra*, *Leptosphaeria*, powdery mildew that produce a lot of log spores. Other common forms of molds include the yeasts and the basidospores (including mushrooms, smuts, and rusts).

About 100,000 fungi species have been described, while an estimated 1.5–5.1 million species of fungi exist on Earth.[1] Different mold species are adapted to different moisture conditions, ranging from just damp to very wet.[2] Live spores act like seeds, forming new mold growths (colonies) under the right conditions.[3] Table 1.1 and Figure 1.1 show the molds by daily count in Dallas, Texas for 1 year. Although there is communality, these will be different for each area of the country and the world. The figures show the fluctuation at different times of the year. These counts are significant for the patients living in this area. They may have problems, both inside and outdoors, due to the excess environmental load.

As part of the total environmental pollutant load, the indoor and outdoor mold count have to be correlated with the total outdoor air and indoor pollutant load to assess the total body pollutant load for diagnostic and treatment tables (Figure 1.2).

HEALTH HAZARDS OF MOLDS

Molds are potential health hazards by one or more of the three major mechanisms: allergy, toxic, or infectious.[4] A brief overview of these three mechanisms is given below.

Several hundred species of molds such as *Cladosporium, Mucor, Rhizopus, Fusarium, Alternaria, Penicillium,* and *Aspergillus* commonly grow in indoor environments.[2] Samson (2010) has provided detailed descriptions, photos, and identification keys of common indoor fungi.[2]

MOLD ALLERGENS AND ALLERGIES

Allergens are the most common mold problems. Over 70 allergens from fungi have been well-characterized.[5] Some of these fungal allergens (*Alternaria* and *Aspergillus fumigatus*) have been measured in indoor and outdoor environments, and exposure to these allergens have been associated with asthma, vasculitis,[7] cardiac disease, neurological phenomena, implants, and other allergic conditions[6]. A review of 17 studies revealed that 6%–10% of the general population and 15%–50% of atopics have immediate skin sensitivity to fungi.[8]

Many patients are hypersensitive to molds and mycotoxins.[9] The most common are *Cladosporium, Alternaria*, and *Aspergillus*. These patients are indicative to the general population and those doctors who treat them to be forewarned of the etiology that may result from very long exposures to molds. As stated earlier, once a diagnosis of mold hypersensitivity is made, the clinician should be aware of these, even if they are under control. Several years later there could be a relapse leading to a fatal disease. Some of these include fatal or chronic vasculitis, arthritis, cancer, and arteriosclerosis.

TABLE 1.1

Fungal Taxa Retained and Observed from Rotorod Samples, Denoting % Frequency of Occurrence by Sampling Month and Cumulative Sampling Year 2013 EHC-Dallas

	Feb	Mar	Apr	May	Jun	Jul	Aug	Sep	Oct	Nov	Dec	Jan	Year
Class Deuteromycetes													
Hyphomycetes													
Cladosporium	82.4	80.6	93.3	96.8	93.3	96.8	90.3	80.0	93.5	90.3	77.4	64.5	87.1
Alternaria	34.4	58.1	90	93.5	76.7	74.2	83.9	83.3	6.7	60.0	51.6	67.7	70.4
Aspergillus[a]	0	0	0	0	0	0	0	0	0	0	0	0	0
Epicoccum	31.0	71.0	83.3	96.8	80.0	77.4	74.2	66.7	54.8	46.7	22.6	38.7	62.2
Drechslera	20.7	30.8	76.7	90.3	56.6	77.4	87.1	73.3	58.1	43.3	32.2	45.1	58.6
Fusarium	13.7	25.8	43.3	83.9	56.7	71.0	71.0	80.0	48.4	30.0	29.0	25.8	48.5
Nigrospora	0.0	0.0	3.3	25.8	40.0	54.8	83.9	66.7	67.7	56.7	25.8	22.5	37.5
Curvularia	6.9	3.2	0.0	35.4	40.0	67.7	87.1	73.3	51.6	33.3	22.6	0.0	35.3
Pithomyces	0.0	3.2	23.3	12.9	40.0	51.6	71.0	56.7	51.6	20.0	22.5	9.7	30.4
Stemphylium	3.4	0.0	3.3	35.5	3.3	0.0	16.1	40.0	38.7	16.7	9.7	12.9	15.1
Stachybotrys	0.0	0.0	0.0	16.1	20.0	0.0	0.0	3.3	0.0	0.0	0.0	6.5	11.5
Torula	0.0	0.0	0.0	0.0	0.0	0.0	22.6	33.3	38.7	20.0	6.5	12.9	11.2
Spegazzinia	0.0	0.0	0.0	0.0	0.0	12.9	19.4	26.7	41.9	16.7	9.7	3.2	10.7
Cercospora	0.0	0.0	0.0	9.7	13.3	3.2	38.7	10.0	0.0	0.0	0.0	0.0	6.3
Tetraplos	0.0	0.0	0.0	0.0	6.7	6.5	12.9	16.7	3.2	0.0	0.0	0.0	3.8
Corynespora	0.0	0.0	0.0	0.0	3.3	0.0	16.1	3.3	0.0	0.0	0.0	0.0	1.9
Aperisporium	0.0	0.0	0.0	0.0	0.0	0.0	6.5	0.0	6.5	0.0	0.0	0.0	1.1
Helicomyces	0.0	0.0	0.0	0.0	3.3	6.5	0.0	0.0	0.0	0.0	0.0	0.0	1.1
Dictyodesmium	0.0	0.0	0.0	0.0	0.0	0.0	3.2	0.0	3.2	0.0	0.0	0.0	0.6
Sporidylocladiella	0.0	0.0	0.0	0.0	0.0	0.0	3.2	0.0	0.0	0.0	0.0	0.0	0.3
Class Ascomycetes													
Leptosphaeria	3.4	6.5	16.7	29.0	33.3	48.4	71.0	60.0	31.4	23.3	19.4	48.4	33.2
Pharesophema													
Chaetomium	0.0	0.0	6.7	12.9	10.0	22.6	19.3	20.0	9.7	13.3	0.0	9.7	10.7
Venturia	0.0	0.0	0.0	0.0	23.3	45.2	6.5	23.3	16.1	3.3	3.2	3.2	10.7
Leptosphaerulina	0.0	0.0	6.7	3.2	10.0	12.9	19.4	6.6	3.2	0.0	0.0	0.0	5.2
Xylariaceae	0.0	0.0	0.0	0.0	0.0	3.2	6.5	26.7	12.9	3.3	0.0	0.0	4.4
Sporomiella	0.0	0.0	0.0	0.0	6.6	9.7	3.2	3.3	6.5	3.3	3.2	16.1	4.4
Pleospora	0.0	0.0	0.0	0.0	0.0	3.2	12.9	10.0	9.7	3.3	3.2	6.5	4.1
Massarina	0.0	0.0	0.0	0.0	3.3	6.5	6.5	20.0	6.5	6.7	0.0	3.2	3.8
Powdery mildew	0.0	0.0	0.0	16.1	16.7	3.2	3.2	6.6	0.0	0.0	0.0	0.0	3.8
Diatrypeceae	0.0	0.0	0.0	0.0	3.3	3.2	6.5	0.0	3.2	0.0	0.0	0.0	1.4
Ascobolus	0.0	0.0	0.0	0.0	3.3	3.2	0.0	3.3	0.0	0.0	0.0	0.0	0.8
Gliomastix	0.0	0.0	0.0	0.0	0.0	3.2	3.2	0.0	0.0	0.0	0.0	0.0	0.6
Delitschia	0.0	0.0	0.0	0.0	0.0	0.0	3.2	0.0	3.2	0.0	0.0	0.0	0.6
Lembosia	0.0	0.0	0.0	0.0	3.3	0.0	0.0	0.0	0.0	0.0	0.0	0.0	0.3
Unidentified Ascomycetes	6.9	3.2	13.3	0.0	0.0	3.2	6.5	0.0	3.2	10.0	3.2	0.0	4.1
Class Basidiomycetes													
Coprinus	0.0	0.0	0.0	0.0	33.3	64.5	58.1	70.0	35.5	6.7	3.2	16.1	24.1
Pucciniaceae rust	0.0	0.0	3.3	54.8	30.0	35.5	35.5	23.3	54.8	36.7	0.0	6.5	23.6
Ganoderma	0.0	0.0	0.0	0.0	3.3	0.0	3.2	3.2	3.2	0.0	0.0	0.0	0.8
Agrocybe	0.0	0.0	0.0	0.0	0.0	0.0	3.2	3.2	3.2	0.0	0.0	0.0	0.8
Agaricus	0.0	0.0	0.0	0.0	0.0	0.0	0.0	0.0	0.0	3.3	0.0	0.0	0.3

(*Continued*)

TABLE 1.1 (*Continued*)
Fungal Taxa Retained and Observed from Rotorod Samples, Denoting % Frequency of Occurrence by Sampling Month and Cumulative Sampling Year 2013 EHC-Dallas

	Feb	Mar	Apr	May	Jun	Jul	Aug	Sep	Oct	Nov	Dec	Jan	Year
					Unidentifiable								
Sphaerial Phaeosporae	0.0	0.0	3.3	61.3	83.3	83.9	87.1	80.0	64.5	60	54.8	58.1	54.4
Other		100.0	100.0	100.0	100.0	100.0	100.0	100.0	100.0	100.0	100.0	100.0	100.0

Note: EHC-Dallas airborne mycofloral components.
[a] Aspergilli are the third most common mold, but it cannot be sampled with rotorods.

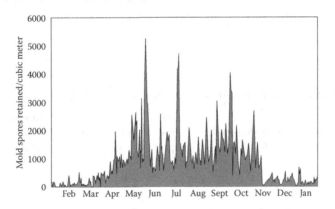

FIGURE 1.1 Variation in total spore counts for the sampling year. Counts represent an average daily 24-hour mean of total fungal spores retained and observed by rotorods.

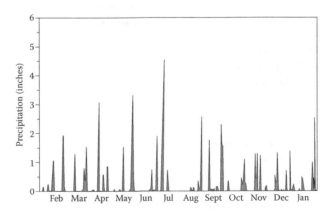

FIGURE 1.2 Total daily precipitation in inches recorded throughout the sampling year. Graph data reflect precipitation observed and recorded in both Dallas and Tarrant counties.

Some of the other molds that have been found to be very sensitive in humans are the *Rhizopus, Sporobolomyces, Trichoderma, Stachybotrys, Monilia situ, Drechslera, Curvularia, Hormodendrum, Fusarium, Streptomyces*, including the rain molds such as *Leptosphaeria*.

Phaeosphaeria: These molds in Table 1.2 represent the most common molds that have been diagnosed and used successfully for treatment at the EHC-Dallas and Buffalo.

The mold mixes as desensitizing vaccines are composite used as vaccines which the patients can take every 4–7 days. Mold Mix 1 consists of *Alternaria, Aspergillus*, and *Hormodendrum. Mold Mix* 2 consists of *Epicoccum, Fusarium*, and *Pullularia*. Mold Mix 3 consists of *Mucor, Phoma, Fomes*, and *Rhodotorula;* and Mold Mix 4 consists of *Cephalosporium, Helminthosporium, Stemphylium*, and *Geotrichum*. These molds can be very sensitive in humans and some chemically sensitive patients as proved by intradermal and inhaled provocation tests.[10] A total of 167 patients in EHC-Dallas and Buffalo sensitive to mold by intradermal challenges, and their immune blood tests under environmentally controlled conditions are shown in Tables 1.3 and 1.4.

Since ancient times, asthma, cancer, wasting, hemorrhage, inanition, and death have been linked to mold exposures.[11] The current wave of sickness from molds has developed since World War II, and paralleled in time when the construction of the interior walls of homes shifted to plasterboard (gypsum sandwiched between paper-cellulose layers) from less toxic wood or metal lath, plaster with a lime coat. Mold grew when inner walls became damp from inadequate venting or moisture from[12] leaky walls, roofs, or plumbing; in addition, mold grew on paper, cellulose, and gypsum.[13]

TABLE 1.2
Aerobiology Report December 05, 2014—Outdoors: EHC-Dallas

Pollution Index	Ozone 24 ppm	Carbon Monoxide 0.3 ppm	Nitric Oxide 5.2 ppm	Sulfur Dioxide 0.4 ppm	Nitrogen Dioxide 12.2 ppm	Particulates 23.7
						Pollen ragweed weed 30 pecan
Fungal genera						194.7
Class Deuteromycetes		Class Ascomycetes		Class Basidiomycetes		Grass 22 Pollen
Asperiosporium		*Ascobolus*		Agarocis		Algae genera 0
Alternaria	127	*Chaetomium*		Agrocybe		Fern spore 0
Cladosporium	193	*Delitshia*		Ganoderma		unidentified 83
Cercospora		*Diatripacaeae*		Coprinus		
Corynespora		*Gliomastix*		Rusts		
Curvularia		*Lembosia*		Smuts		
Diplococcocium		*Leptosphaeria*				
Drechslera	6	*Leptosphaerulina*				
Epicoccum		Massaria				
Fusarium		*Massarina*				
Elycomycus		*Pleospora*				
Nigrospora	17	Powdery mildew				
Pithomycess		*Sporomiella*				
Spegazzinia		*Venturia*				
Stachybotrys		*Xylariaceae*				
Stemphylium		*Paraphaeosphaeria*				
Tetraploa						
Torula						
Temperature 57–83°F		Humidity 65%			Total fungal count 426	Fungal total pollen and algae 2394

TABLE 1.3

Test Result Summary of Molds and Mycotoxins, Intradermal Skin Test in a Controlled, 20% Less Polluted Environment and Mold Environments at Patient's Homes with a Total of 167 Patients Tested in the EHC-Dallas 2014

Old Molds Abnormal	Other Molds Colonies Per Culture Plate	Mycotoxins Blood ppb	Urine ppb Mycotoxins	Environmental Molds at the Patients Home Colonies Culture Plate
Mold mix 1: 40	*Monilia* 18	Aflatoxin 25	Aflatoxin 7	*Penicillium* sp. 2
Aspergillus 29				*Aspergillus* 8
				Cladosporium 3
Mold mix 2: 40	*Drechslera* 17	Fusaric acid 20	Ochratoxin 4	
Mold mix 3: 36	*Aspergillus* 29	*Trichocethecine* 29	*Trichothecene*	
Mold mix 4: 34	*Curvularia* 18			*Mucor* 3
Rhizopus 25	*Cladherbarum* 19	TOE fungus 11		*Sporotrichum* 2
Soporobolomyces 5	*Cladfulvum* 21	*Candida* 26		*Rhizopus* 2
Trichoderma 22	*Streptomyces* 17			*Alternaria* 1
Lake algae 19	*Leptosphaeria* 16			*Chaetomium* 1
Stachybotrys 31	*Phaeosphaeria* 16			*Drechslera* 1

TABLE 1.4

Immune Test Results Summary in 167 Patients Diagnoses with Toxic Effect of Mycotoxins EHC-Dallas 2014

T and B cells	Control Cells	IgG Subclass	Control Cells	IgM/IgA/IgE	Control
T cells	1260–2850 μm/	Subclass 1	382–922 mg/dL	IgM	48–271 mgm/dL
8 Low	mL	(5 Low)		5 Low	
0 High				1 High	
Helper T cells	287–1770 μm/	Subclass 2	241–700 mgm/dL	IgA	81–463 mgm/dL
6 Low	mL	(8 Low)		3 Low	
Suppressor T cells	328–1050 μm/	Subclass 3	0 or 114/24	IgE	
11 Low	mL	(8 Low)		3 High	
1 High					
B cells	82–177 mgm/dL	Subclass 4	22–178 mg/dL		
3 Low		(3 Low)			
3 High		(3 High)			
NK cells		IgG Serum			
2 High		(7 Low)			
1 Low					
CD4–CD8 ratio					
11 High					
1 Low					
% Lymphocytes					
2 High					
1 Low					

ANAs	Control	Complement	Control	CMI	Control
5 Positive	0 Negative	C3	31–60 μm/mL	13 Positive	4 positive
18 Negative		(2 Low)		5 Negative	
		C4			
		(2 Low)			
		CH50			
		(8 High)			
		(2 Low)			

Antidotes that are a lower dilution for the mold sensitivities as well as higher doses for provocation injection treatment of the intradermal neutralizing dose q-4 days

Mold Mix 1	Mold Mix 2	Mold Mix 3	Mold Mix 4
Alternaria	*Epicocum*	*Mucor*	*Cephalosporium*
Aspergillus	*Fusarium*	*Phome*	*Helmenthosporium*
Hormodendrum	*Pullaria*	*Rhodotorula*	*Stemphlyium*
			Geotrichum

Drying after being wet appears to stress molds to produce spores and toxins such as trichothecenes and satratoxins that escape into living and working spaces. Recently, these toxins have been measured in serum from people exposed in moldy homes. Plaster is strongly alkaline and discourages the growth of toxigenic molds.

Randolph[14] was one of the first modern physicians to evaluate and treat people for indoor air pollution. His observations taught us to look for mold in the indoor environment as well as toxic chemicals in the sick building syndrome. Mycotoxins found in buildings are very devastating to the mycotoxin and mold-sensitive patients because they can suppress the immune system (T and B cells complement gamma globulin) as well as the enzyme detoxification systems such as superoxide dismutase, glutathione peroxidase, etc.

Modest wetting and drying in buildings and in ventilation systems are normal and generally poses little risk for occupant health. Similarly, very brief episodes of wetting are not usually a problem provided that steps are taken to rapidly dry all materials.[15] "Chronic dampness" is the presence of unwanted and excessive moisture in buildings.[16] This can lead to the growth of mold, fungi, environmental bacteria, and, in homes, house dust mites.

Some patients had to have only the four mold mixes, while others had to have not only the mixes but also the non-grouped molds such as *Monilia, Drechslera, Phaesopheria, Curvelure,* and *Streptomycetes.* Some patients had taylorized molds that were not among the standard commercial molds. These were trapped in elevators, drainage ditches, isolated basement rooms, and places only where the individual patient lived or worked. These were necessary for survival and optimum function. The most common clinical problems are followed by small vessel vasculitis, rhinosinusitis, and hypersensitivity pneumonitis. Hypersensitivity pneumonitis is an interstitial lung disease caused by repeated inhalation of certain fungal, bacteria, animal protein, and reactive chemical particles. In some people, the body's immune reaction to these particles causes inflammation of the lungs. Also, allergic bronchopulmonary aspergillus can occur. Leptosphaeria and *Phaeosphaeria* are rain molds which occur after a rain. These bother some patients who have to be desensitized in order to feel well. Record rains occurred in Dallas in 2015, and molds of the *Phaesophaeria* and *Leptosphaeria* classes were a real problem.

MYCOTOXINS

Molds produce a wide range of chemicals known as the mycotoxins. Mycotoxins include a wide range of different chemicals, including many molecules of several hundred Daltons in size (which are generally solids at room temperatures), as well as volatile liquids or gases that give molds their distinctive must odor.[1,17]

Common mycotoxins produced by indoor molds include: (1) The Trichothecenes: A group of mycotoxins that have strong neurotoxic and immunotoxic properties.[18] Trichothecenes inhibit protein synthesis and can cause hemorrhage and vomiting. Trichothecenes are produced mostly by *Fusarium, Stachybotrys,* and *Memnoniella.* Also, they can damage the immune system, eventually suppressing T-cell and B-cell function, depressing complements and, at times, gamma globulin subsets. They can cause rhinosinutitis, asthma, neurological dysfunction, and vasculitis;

(2) Aflatoxin is an immune modulatory agent, which will stimulate T2 that acts primarily on cell-mediated immunity and phagocytic cell function. Aflatoxins are highly carcinogenic mycotoxins produced by some species of *Aspergillus*; (3) Ochratoxins: carcinogens and kidney toxins produced by some Aspergillus and *Penicillium* species; (4) Fuminosins are produced by *Fusarium* species and are carcinogenic, hepatotoxic and may have estrogenic properties; (5) Sterigmatocystin is a liver toxin and immunosuppressant produced by some *Aspergillus* species; (6) Hemolysin is produced by *Stachybotrys* and causes blood hemorrhage; (7) Gliotoxin, which has several immunosuppressive properties, is genotoxic and an inducer of apoptotic cell death, can promote demyelination, and promotes increased virulence of fungal infections. Gliotoxins are produced by a number of genera of common fungi including *Aspergillus, Penicillium,* and *Candida*; (8) Patulin, which has diverse toxic effects including mutagenicity, genotoxicity, and inducer of oxidative stress. Patulin is produced by a number of species of *Aspergillus* and *Penicillium*.[17,19–21] Unfortunately, only half of the trichothecene, ochratoxin, aflatoxin, and gliotoxin, can be measured practically for patients through urine.

While most mycotoxin research has dealt with foodborne exposures, mycotoxins can also be absorbed via inhalation in mycotoxin-contaminated environments. Various studies have linked indoor exposures to trichothecenes,[22] aflatoxins, hemolysin,[23] and ochratoxins[24] to significantly elevate levels of mycotoxins in blood or urine[25] coming from mold-contaminated building. Some mycotoxins can now be readily detected in urine and other body fluids of humans exposed to indoor mold. Hooper et al.[25] tested mycotoxins (trichothecene, aflatoxin, and ochratoxins) in human tissue and body fluids from patients exposed to mold and mycotoxins in the environment. Croft[22] has developed assays for two toxins. Level of detection for the various mycotoxins varies, which is 0.2 ppb for trichothecene, 1.0 ppb for aflotoxins, and 2.0 ppb for ochratoxins (Table 1.5).

Patients exposed to environmental mycotoxins included 178 urine samples, 47 nasal secretions, 28 tissue samples, and 7 samples from other body fluids. Trichothecene levels varied in urine, sputum, and tissue biopsies (lung, liver, and brain) from undetectable (<0.2) to levels up to 18 ppb. *Aflatoxin* level from the same types of tissues varies from 1.0 to 5.0 ppb. Ochratoxins isolated in the same type of tissue varied from 2.0 to >10.0 ppb. Negative control patients had no detectable mycotoxins in their tissue or fluids, which included 58 urine samples, 27 nasal secretions, and 15 tissue samples. These data show that mycotoxins can be detected in body fluids and tissue from patients exposed to mycotoxin producing mold in the environment.[25]

There are no known antidotes for mold toxins.[11] However, methoxymethane (dimethylether) removes aflatoxins from peanuts,[26] but no evidence has been found that it applies to the removal of satratoxins or trichothecenes or to other agents. Agents developed to lessen mold exposure must not be toxic. Cholestyrmine, an oral cholesterol lowering agent has been administered to lower trichothecene burdens in the gut.[27] Certainly, intradermal neutralization has helped attenuate the mycotoxins in the chemically sensitive patient. Vitamin C 5–25 g daily; Glutathione 80 and 1000 mgm daily; and multi-B and multi-minerals administration over a period of 1–6 months, along with avoidance of molds and mycotoxins, have been found to have counteracted mycotoxins; additionally, sauna has been found to be effective to counteract mycotoxins.

TABLE 1.5
Mycotoxins: EHC-Dallas 178 Patients in 2009

Mycotoxins	Range–Abnormal	Neg. Control	Normal
Urine 178	Trichocethene 0.2–18 ppb	58	<0.2 ppb
Nasal 47	Aflatoxin 1–5 ppb	27	<1 ppb
Tissue 28	Ochratoxin 2 to >10 ppb	15	<2 ppb
Other Body Fluids (lung, liver, and brain) 7			

MOLD INFECTIONS

Fungi such as *Candida, Histoplasmosis, Cryptococcus,* and *Coccidiosis* can infect immune incompetent people.[28] In recent decades, there have been significant increases in rates of life-threatening invasive infections by *Candida, Aspergillus,* and other fungi, such as *Mucor* and *Fusarium,* can occur.[29–31] These invasive fungal infections most commonly infect immuno compromised patients such as bone and organ transplant patients, HIV+ patients, or patients with certain cancers such as lymphoma and leukemia.[29,31] However, they can also infect immune competent individuals.[29,31] *Aspergillus* is a common cause of life-threatening infection in immune compromised patients. Invasive *Aspergillus* infections occur in 5%–24% of acute leukemia cases with about 34%–40% mortality, occur in 3%–15% of bone marrow transplant cases with a mortality between 50% and 90%, and occur in 11%–14% of solid organ transplant cases with a mortality of about 60%.[29,30,32]

The recent outbreak of *Exserohilum rostratum* meningitis has been linked to epidural injections of methylprednisolone by McCarthy et al.[33] These are uncommon and often devasting and are difficult to treat. The common pathogens for the central nervous system (CNS) affecting molds are *Aspergillus, Fusarium, Seedosperium, Mucarales,* and *Dermatiacoas* molds. Infection caused by these pathogens group have distinctive profiles and therapeutic implication, all of which clinicians must understand.[33]

Hemi dissemination to the CNS: Direct inoculation of CNS or paraspinal tissue as a result of surgery, trauma, intravenous drug use, or contaminated medical supplies may also occur in immunocompetent persons, including those with *Exophiala dermatitidis* (formerly known as *Wangiella dermatitidis*) and *E. rostratum*.[34] Organisms may also spread to the CNS from adjacent structures, including the sinuses, mastoid, and orbit. Infection of the ethmoid sinuses may lead to cavernous sinus thrombosis as a result of invasion of the emissary veins that drain the sinuses. Hyphae can invade from the ethmoid sinuses through the lamina papyracea and into the periorbital space, thus, threatening the eye, extraocular muscles, and posterior apical structures, including the optic nerve.

Angioinvasion is common in immunocompromised patients and accounts for the hematogenous dissemination from the lungs that causes focal neurologic deficits. Histopathological examination of involved brain tissue reveals hyphal angioinvasion with thrombosis in small and large vessels, hemorrhagic infarction, and coagulative necrosis, as well as vasculitis and granuloma formation. Susceptibility to angioinvasion also confers a predisposition to the formation of mycotic aneurysms. Without effective management, mold infections of the CNS carry poor prognosis, particularly in immunocompromised patients; such patients may present with isolated brain abscesses that stimulate tumors of the CNS.

There are four cornerstones of the management of mold infections of the CNS: early diagnosis, administration of antifungal chemotherapy, neurosurgical assessment and intervention, and management of immunologic impairment.

Two distinct patterns characterize mold infections of the CNS. In some patients, the disease arises by direct extension from the paranasal sinuses, eye, or middle ear, causing a single abscess or a few abscesses.[35,36] These lesions usually occur in the frontal or temporal lobe. Other patients have hematogenous infection, which may lead to solitary or multiple small abscesses that are often seen at the junction of cerebral gray and white matter and in the putamen-striatal aterial distribution. Mycotic aneurysms may form and rupture, which creates the potential for hemorrhagic strokes, subarachnoid hemorrhage, and empyema formation.

EARLY DIAGNOSIS

Detection of galactomannan antigen and 1,3-β-D-glucan in cerebrospinal fluid (CSF) may be helpful in establishing the diagnosis of CNS asperfillosis or other mold infections, such as fusariosis.[37,38] However, because galactomannan antigen and 1,3-β-D-glucan can also be expressed by *Fusarium* species, its presence in CSF does not constitute a definitive diagnosis of CNS aspergillosis;[39]

1,3-β-D-glucan may also be expressed by *Scedosporium* species and *E. rostratum*. A polymerase chain reaction assay that is specific for *Aspergillus* also may prove useful, but standardized platforms are lacking.[40]

Aspergillus Species

The risk factors for CNS aspergillosis include neutropenia, systemic glucocorticoid treatment, mastoidectomy, spinal anesthesia, and paraspinal glucocorticoid injections.[41] *A. fumigates* was isolated from the index patient in the 2012 outbreak of fungal meningitis.[42]

Focal neurologic deficits and seizures caused by stroke or mass effect are the most common clinical manifestations of CNS aspergillosis.[43] Meningeal signs are uncommon, and their presence is indicative of a subarachnoid hemorrhage.[44] CNS aspergillosis should be high on the list of disorders in the differential diagnosis for patients with immunosuppression and focal brain lesions, especially those with characteristic pulmonary infiltrates in whom focal neurologic deficits or focal seizures develop. Recovery of *Aspergillus* from pulmonary lesions with the use of bronchoalveolar lavage or fine-needle aspiration should be pursued when possible. An enzyme immunoassay for detection of galactomannan in serum or bronchoalveolar lavage fluid should be performed when feasible.[45] As described above, galactomannan and 1,3-β-D-glucan may be found in the serum or CSF of patients with CNS aspergillosis.[37,38]

Mucorales

Cerebral mucormycosis, which is perhaps the most aggressive mold infection of the CNS, constitutes a medical emergency. Early cases were uniformly fatal. However, recent studies have shown improved survival, possibly as a result of earlier diagnosis and better control of underlying diseases.[46] Diabetes mellitus and iron-overload conditions are distinctive risk factors for the development of mucormycosis.[47] In patients with neutropenia or patients receiving glucocorticoid therapy, mold infections occur through hematogenous dissemination of pulmonary mucormycosis.[48] In contrast, patients with diabetes mellitus usually present with sino-orbital mucormycosis and seldom present with pulmonary or disseminated infection.[47,49] Among intravenous drug users, CNS mucoromycosis is a relatively common cause of intracerebral fungal abscesses.[49]

Fusarium Species

CNS fusariosis develops predominantly in patients with prolonged neutropenia. These organisms are highly angioinvasive and cause hemorrhagic infarction with stroke-like events.[50] Portals of entry include the lungs, sinuses, vascular catheters, and distinctively, periungual lesions (paronychia in patients with neutropenia).[51] Fusarium species are also most frequently associated with fungemia, multiple erythematous nodular cutaneous lesions, and septic arthritis. A positive blood culture growing a hyaline (i.e., colorless or lightly pigmented) mold in a patient with persistent neutropenia is most likely to indicate the presence of *Fusarium*. A definitive mycologic diagnosis can be rapidly established by biopsy and culture of these cutaneous lesions. As compared with other mold infections of the CNS, disseminated fusariosis is more commonly associated with bilateral endophthalmitis, which may lead to blindness. Hematogenously disseminated fusarium infections cause chorioretinitis at a rate that is disproportionally higher than that seen with other organisms causing mold infections of the CNS.[52] Because disseminated fusariosis commonly causes fungemia and cutaneous lesions, early diagnosis and therapy may prevent progression to encephalitis and endophthalmitis.

Dematiaceous Molds

Dematiaceous fungi are a group of molds characterized by the presence of melanin-like pigment within the cell wall that is pale brown to black.[53] These organisms can be pathogens to plants or livestock and may cause chromoblastomycosis and black-grain mycetoma. Dematiaceous molds may also cause deeply invasive infections (phaeohyphomycosis), including infections of the CNS.

Most of the agents causing phaeohyphomycosis grow very slowly, so classic mycologic identification can take 3 weeks or longer. In comparison with *Aspergillus, Mucorales,* and *Fusarium,* dematiaceous molds commonly cause infections of the CNS in immunocompetent hosts. Some dematiaceous molds within a narrow geographic range cause cerebral phaeohyphomycosis.[54]

Until October 2012, most known cases of CNS phaeohyphomycosis were caused by *Cladophialophora bantiana* (also called *Xylohypha bantiana*), *Rhinocladiella mackenzei,* and *Ochroconis gallopava* (also called *Dactylaria gallopava*).[53] *E. rostratum* has since emerged as a cause of meningitis in a nationwide outbreak associated with tainted epidural glucocorticoid injections.[55,56] Prolonged receipt of antifungal chemotherapy, surgical resection of abscesses, and reversal of immunosuppression are mainstays of the treatment of CNS phaeohyphomycosis. Persistence or recurrence of disease is common.

Mold infections of the CNS caused by *C. bantiana* are manifested as a slowly expanding space occupying lesion causing headache, seizure, and localizing neurologic signs that stimulate a brain tumor.[53] Among immunocompetent patients, CNS infection may occur in the absence of pulmonary lesions. Patients who have survived had easily resectable, encapsulated masses on CT or MRI scans, whereas those who have died had a solitary lesion that was not entirely resected, poorly demarcated abscess borders, or multiple satellite lesions.[57] There is no clearly effective antifungal therapy.[58] Surgical resection remains the most definitive treatment.

Sedosporium Species

Sedosporium apiospermum is readily isolated from soil, polluted water, and sewage. Mold infections of the CNS caused by *S. apiospermum* are strongly associated with drowning events in immunocompetent hosts, when the organism invades through the cribriform plate or disseminates from pneumonic foci.[59,60] Among immunocompromised patients, the features of CNS sedosporiosis resemble those of aspergillosis, including hematogenous dissemination from pulmonary lesions or by extension from the sinuses. Although *Sedosporium* species form branching septate hyphae that are similar to those of aspergillus, in rare cases, terminal *C. annelloconidia* is seen in tissue. Nonetheless, culture is required for a definitive diagnosis. Voriconazole is licensed as second-line therapy for *S. apiospermum* infections.

O. gallopava is a neurotropic dematiaceous mold that causes pulmonary and CNS infection in domestic poultry and in immunocompromised humans.[61] Exposure to infested aerosolized warm water may be a risk factor. In one study involving transplant recipients, the CNS was involved in 50% of patients (6 of 12) with *O. gallopava* infection and a poor outcome.[62] The most effective antifungal regimen for treatment of this infection is not known. Interpretive breakpoints for *in vitro* antifungal susceptibility tests have not been established for this organism. Combination antifungal therapy with voriconazole and a lipid formulation of amphotericin B, pending the availability of *in vitro* susceptibility data, is recommended in conjunction with surgery and reversal of immunosuppression.

E. rostratum is an opportunistic mold that until recently was an uncommon cause of disease in immunocompromised and immunocompetent human hosts.[63] On September 18, 2012, health officials began to react to a large multistate outbreak of fungal meningitis traceable to three lots of preservative-free methylpredinisolone from one compounding pharmacy in Massachusetts. This outbreak resulted in 751 cases of CNS infection and 64 deaths across the United States. Three molecular assays and assays for 1,3-β-D-glucan in serum and CSF have been developed and may serve as adjunctive diagnostic tools.[64–67] Most of the infected patients in the outbreak presented with signs and symptoms that were consistent with fungal meningitis; however, cases of spinal osteomyelitis or epidural abscess and septic arthritis or osteomyelitis were also reported.[68] *In vitro* susceptibility data indicate that voriconazole and amphotericin B have activity against *E. rostratum*; this has led to recommendations that voriconazole, liposomal amphotericin B, or both be used for initial management in conjunction with neurosurgical consultation, when appropriate.[55,56] A more detailed review of the management of *E. rostratum* meningitis is reported elsewhere.[55,69]

REVIEW OF LITERATURE OF MOLD AND WATER DAMAGE

MOLD/WATER DAMAGE EXPOSURE AND ASTHMA/RHINITIS AND OTHERS

Well-conducted epidemiology studies in several countries have consistently shown that exposures from building/house dampness and mold have been associated with increased risks for respiratory symptoms, asthma, hypersensitivity pneumonitis, rhinosinusitis, bronchitis, respiratory infections,[70,71] cardiovascular disease, and neurological degenerative disease.

Many papers have documented that exposure to molds or water damaged indoor environments are associated with significantly higher rates of wheezing, asthma, and rhinitis.[72,73] Meta-analysis of 16 published cohort and incident studies reported that significantly higher rates of asthma were associated with indoor dampness (EE 1.33%, 95% CI of 1.04–1.60, p = 0.001) and visible mold growth (EE 1.29%, 95% CI of 1.04–1.60, p = 0.001).[71] A study of 31,742 children in eight European nations reported that exposure to visible mold or dampness in the first 2 years after birth was associated with significantly higher risk of asthma symptoms early in life (OR or odds ratio 1.39%, 95% CI of 1.05–1.84) and rhinitis by 6–8 years (OR 1.12, 95% CI of 1.02–1.23).[72]

In studies conducted in the nonindustrial workplace, individuals with asthma or hypersensitivity pneumonitis were found to be at risk for progression to more severe disease if the relationship between illness and exposure to the damp building was not recognized and exposures continued.[73]

Recent, high quality, systematic reviews of the available evidence concluded that the implementation of interventions that combine elimination of moisture intrusion and leaks and removal of moldy items help to reduce mold exposure, respiratory symptoms, and new onset asthma.[70,71,74]

INDOOR MOLD AND SICK BUILDING SYNDROME

People's adverse health effects were attributed to indoor air after the 1973 energy crisis increased air recycling and decreased air leaks from buildings.[75–77] Mold disease emerged in the 1990s with infantile pulmonary hemosiderosis in Cleveland, Ohio.[78–80] Literally, people's descriptions of sickness related to musk odors and black mold on walls were not believed.[81–85] Mold in buildings also emphasized the new awareness of problems from storms particularly from hurricanes.

Epidemiological studies[86–91] showed flu-like symptoms, eye and respiratory tract irritation, chronic fatigue, skin irritations, joint pain, dizziness and impaired balance, and inability to co-process or to remember frequently used information. Initially, symptoms diminished during days out of the building, later they persisted[91] even after air turnovers were increased.[87–90]

MOLD EXPOSURE AND INFANT LUNG HEMORRHAGE

Life-threatening infant pulmonary hemorrhage has been associated with high indoor exposures to indoor water damage and high levels of *Aspergillus* and *Stachybotrys* molds.[79,80] Mean indoor air levels (in colony forming units per cubic meter of air or CFU/m^3) of viable *Stachybotrys* were 43 in the homes of nine homes of infants with lung hemorrhage as compared to four in 27 control homes, while mean airborne Aspergillus levels were 23,311 in the lung hemorrhage homes and 445 in the control homes.[79] *Stachybotrys* produce a number of mycotoxins including trichothecenes (including satratoxins and roridins) and a hemolyric protein hemolysin.[17,19]

Intranasal administration of satratoxin from *Stachybotrys* was found to cause marked damage to the olfactory nerve in laboratory mice[92] and eventually in humans. This damage eventually caused and produced the chemically sensitive problem. This generation of the mold and mycotoxin in the chemically sensitive patient was a viscous cycle, where their presence decreased T and B cells, complements, and, at times, gamma globulins. This decrease allowed the onset of mold and mycotoxin induced illness with more immune suppressions. One can see how these immune parameters were reduced on mold and mycotoxin sensitive patients (Tables 1.1 through 1.3).

Mold and mycotoxin can go up to the olfactory nerve and into the cerebrum, causing garbled thinking, depression, vertigo, imbalance, and short term memory loss. Mold can also go to the hypothalamus and the rest of the limbic system causing neurodegenerative disease, arteriosclerosis, cancer, and many other brain dysfunctions.

Contributors to the mold syndrome are *Stachybotyrus* species*: Aspergillus/Penicillium* species, *Cladosporium, Fusariam, Actinomycetes (Nocardia, Streptomyces,* especially *californicus)* and bacteria.[93,94] Moisture in poorly ventilated walls, attics, and crawl spaces encourages fungal and bacterial growth particularly on drywall (gypsum board) with paper (cellulose on both sides, which nourishes fungi). Water enters the walls from leaks of pipes, refrigerator icemaker tubes, inadequately sealed external walls and roofs, and from condensation in air conditioning ducts.[90,95] Indoor mold sickness was recognized co-temporally with the destruction of Caribbean coral reefs and growth of *A. showaii*[96] and the doubling or tripling of asthma prevalence in the United States[97-99] and several in Caribbean Islands suggesting an association.

INDOOR MOLD/MYCOTOXIN EXPOSURE AND NEUROTOXIC EFFECTS

Kilburn[100] performed extensive neuropsychological and respiratory tests on 105 symptomatic adult patients with home mold exposure (ME) and 100 consecutive chemically exposed (CE) patients. A battery of 26 physiological and neuropsychological tests as well as pulmonary spirometric tests were performed on both the ME and CE patients and were compared to 202 control referent subjects.[101] Neuropsychiatric tests were controlled for such factors as age, gender, education, and socioeconomic factors.

The group of 105 ME patients consisted of 69 women and 36 men, exposed to molds in California, Texas, and Arizona. All ME patients were exposed to visible mold growth observed on walls, floors, electrical switch and socket plates, and air conditioning systems. Mold spore concentrations in indoor air often exceeded outdoor air concentrations by four fold or more. Elevated levels of several molds such as *Aspergillus, Penicillium, Chaetomium, Alternaria, Fusarium,* and *Rhizopus* were often seen in the homes of the 105 ME patients. No visible mold growth was seen in the 100 CE patients or the 202 referents.[100]

Table 1.6 reports neuropsychiatric test scores for the 105 ME patients, 100 CE patients, and 202 referents. Compared to the referents, the ME patients had significantly slower, simple and choice reaction times, significantly greater balance, sway speed, and significantly longer blink latency ($p = 0.0001$ for all comparisons). Color discrimination and visual field performance were also significantly reduced in the ME patients as compared to controls (p values ranging from 0.0001 to 0.016). Performance on the Culture Fair, Digit Symbol, vocabulary, verbal recall, pegboard, and trail marking were all significantly reduced in the ME cohort (p 0.0001–0.004). Information and picture completion were also significantly reduced in the ME patients ($p = 0.0001$). In all, 22 of 26 physiological and neuropsychological tests were abnormal in the ME patients and 23 of 26 were abnormal in the CE patients.[100]

Table 1.7 reports POMS mood states in 108 ME patients, 100 EC patients, and 202 referents. Compared to the referents, both the ME and CE exposed patients had significantly greater levels of tension, depression, anger, fatigue, low vigor, and confusion ($p = 0.0001$ or 0.0003 for all comparisons).

Table 1.8 reports spirometric respiratory function in 108 ME patients, 100 CE patients, and 202 referents. Compared to the referents, the ME patients had significantly lower force vital capacity (FVC) ($p = 0.0001$) and significantly lower forced expiratory volume (FEV) in 1 second ($p = 0.008$).

Standardized testing and data handling ensured comparability. There was no way to quantify neither mold/mycotoxin exposures nor chemical exposures. Methods were not available to assay dozens of patients' homes for toxins from molds or other chemicals.[18,102] Many homes had had interventions to reduce exposure, especially to mold before the residents' impairment was verified

TABLE 1.6

Neurobehavioral Function for ME Subjects (105) and CE Subjects (100) Compared to 202 Referent Subjects as Percent of Predicted, Means, and Standard Deviations (SD), *p Values* by Analysis of Variance

	A 105 Mold Mean ± SD	B 100 Chemical Mean ± SD	C 202 Referent Mean ± SD	*p Values* A vs. C	*p Values* B vs. C
Age (years)	46.5 ± 13.3	46.5 ± 10.3	47.2 ± 20.2	0.621	0.98
Educational level (years)	14.7 ± 2.6	13.6 ± 2.8	12.9 ± 2.3	0.0001	0.014
Physiological Tests					
Simple reaction time (ms)	103.6 ± 6.0	105.8 ± 6.5	99.9 ± 3.7	0.0001	0.0001
Choice reaction time (ms)	102.2 ± 4.0	104.1 ± 4.1	100.0 ± 2.5	0.0001	0.0001
Balance Sway Speed (cm/s)					
Eyes open	141.3 ± 60.9	195.0 ± 193.5	100.2 ± 20.0	0.0001	0.0001
Eyes closed	174.2 ± 93.5	216.3 ± 184.1	103.1 ± 26.8	0.0001	0.0001
Blink Reflex Latency R-I (ms)					
Right	113.4 ± 13.0	112.3 ± 12.2	99.4 ± 14.6	0.0001	0.054
Left	111.9 ± 15.2	109.9 ± 10.2	96.4 ± 13.2	0.0001	0.0001
Hearing Losses					
Right	98.1 ± 36.5	98.3 ± 30.3	101.5 ± 24.5	0.673	0.454
Left	99.4 ± 35.2	97.4 ± 25.0	99.3 ± 21.7	0.533	0.606
Color Discrimination Errors					
Right	70.3 ± 43.3	74.6 ± 49.2	102.6 ± 51.1	0.0001	0.0001
Left	73.9 ± 46.1	62.1 ± 46.1	102.6 ± 51.1	0.0001	0.0001
Visual Field Performance					
Right	91.7 ± 23.2	86.9 ± 21.7	100.0 ± 22.7	0.0016	0.0002
Left	92.0 ± 24.5	88.8 ± 23.7	101.1 ± 21.6	0.0009	0.0007
Grip Strength					
Right	91.3 ± 18.7	87.9 ± 23.2	99.3 ± 17.5	0.0003	0.0001
Left	87.0 ± 20.8	83.8 ± 24.7	99.1 ± 17.5	0.0001	0.0001
Psychological Tests					
Culture fair	92.9 ± 22.6	89.9 ± 23.6	101.2 ± 20.0	0.0006	0.0001
Digit symbol	91.3 ± 11.4	90.8 ± 14.3	101.5 ± 9.2	0.0001	0.0001
Vocabulary	87.7 ± 31.9	81.6 ± 31.2	99.2 ± 30.8	0.002	0.0001
Verbal Recall					
Immediate	81.0 ± 24.2	76.0 ± 28.1	99.8 ± 31.1	0.0001	0.0001
Delayed	71.4 ± 36.4	63.9 ± 34.5	99.9 ± 41.3	0.0001	0.0001
Pegboard	92.9 ± 15.2	88.8 ± 16.0	101.8 ± 25.7	0.001	0.0001
Trails A	103.6 ± 8.1	106.6 ± 9.5	100.3 ± 8.3	0.0006	0.0001
Trails B	103.1 ± 9.0	104.5 ± 8.7	100.4 ± 7.5	0.004	0.0001

(Continued)

TABLE 1.6 (*Continued*)

Neurobehavioral Function for ME Subjects (105) and CE Subjects (100) Compared to 202 Referent Subjects as Percent of Predicted, Means, and Standard Deviations (SD), *p Values* by Analysis of Variance

	A 105 Mold Mean ± SD	B 100 Chemical Mean ± SD	C 202 Referent Mean ± SD	p Values A vs. C	p Values B vs. C
Finger Writing Errors					
Right	98.9 ± 7.6	102.7 ± 8.5	100.0 ± 7.4	0.233	0.020
Left	99.7 ± 9.6	103.5 ± 9.0	100.0 ± 7.8	0.825	0.004
Information	82.5 ± 34.9	81.9 ± 35.6	101.5 ± 39.4	0.0001	0.0001
Picture completion	81.2 ± 39.0	79.8 ± 35.6	99.3 ± 32.2	0.0001	0.0001
Similarities	93.1 ± 32.0	89.4 ± 41.5	98.1 ± 41.2	0.246	0.092
Total abnormalities	9.8 ± 4.9	10.2 ± 5.6	2.3 ± 2.4	0.0001	0.0001

Source: Adapted from Kilburn, K. H. 2003. *Arch Environ. Health* 58(8):538–542.

TABLE 1.7

Profile of Mood States for 108 ME and 100 CE Compared to 202 UE Subjects (POMS Score Is the Sum of Tension, Depression, Anger, Fatigue, and Confusion minus Vigor)

POMS	A 108 Mold Mean ± SD	B 100 Chemical Mean ± SD	C 202 Referent Mean ± SD	p Values A vs. C	p Values B vs. C
Score	69.2 ± 37.9	83.1 ± 43.4	22.1 ± 25.0	0.0001	0.0001
Tension	17.3 ± 8.3	19.8 ± 8.0	8.9 ± 4.6	0.0001	0.0001
Depression	16.1 ± 12.9	21.9 ± 15.2	7.9 ± 7.1	0.0001	0.0001
Anger	13.3 ± 10.1	15.5 ± 9.8	7.7 ± 6.5	0.0003	0.0003
Fatigue	16.8 ± 7.9	18.3 ± 7.0	8.3 ± 5.6	0.0001	0.0001
Vigor	10.8 ± 6.9	10.0 ± 6.5	17.0 ± 6.2	0.0001	0.0001
Confusion	13.9 ± 6.8	16.3 ± 6.3	6.4 ± 3.7	0.0001	0.0001
Symptom frequency	4.8 ± 1.2	5.2 ± 2.0	2.6 ± 1.1	0.0001	0.0001

Source: Adapted from Kilburn, K. H. 2009. *Toxicol. Ind. Health* 25(9–10):681–692.
Note: SD, standard deviation.

by testing. When assays become available, it would be more practical to measure people exposed in schools or office buildings, where many people shared exposures rather than in homes,[18] however, both are necessary.

People's ages, wellness, and hours per day of exposure vary more in a home-based group than in a workforce. Self-selection (bias) may increase reporting of symptoms but has not affected neurobehavioral measurements[103–105] nor have such patients' manipulated tests or malingered in previous studies.[106,107] Clinical judgment favored homes, schools, and offices that contain other toxic chemicals.[108,109]

TABLE 1.8

Pulmonary Function for 108 ME Subjects and 100 CE Compared to 202 Referent Subjects as Percentage of Predicted, Means, and Standard Deviations (SD), *p Values* by Analysis of Variance

POMS	A 108 Mold Mean ± SD	B 100 Chemical Mean ± SD	C 202 Referent Mean ± SD	p Values A vs. C	p Values B vs. C
FVC	91.2 ± 12.6	94.8 ± 16.1	101.6 ± 15.1	0.0001	0.0005
FEV$_1$	87.8 ± 14.0	90.4 ± 18.7	93.6 ± 15.8	0.0008	0.125
FEF25–75	94.1 ± 29.1	102.6 ± 37.4	88.1 ± 35.0	0.191	0.001
FEF75–85	90.2 ± 47.4	100.1 ± 53.8	78.1 ± 52.7	0.099	0.001
FEV$_1$/FVC	77.4 ± 7.5	76.5 ± 8.9	72.8 ± 9.5	0.0001	0.001

Source: Adapted from Kilburn, K. H. 2009. *Toxicol. Ind. Health* 25(9–10):681–692.

Note: FEV$_1$, forced expiration volume in 1 second, FVC = forced vital capacity, FEF25–75 = forced expiratory flow 25%–75%, FEF75–85 = forced expiratory flow 75%–85%.

Mold exposure impairments resembled those associated with formaldehyde and the indoor air syndrome, including lengthened blink reflex latency.[106] Prolonged blink reflex latency has been associated with exposure to chlorinated solvents,[105,107] including polychlorinated biphenyls[110] and chlorine,[111] and arsenic[103] and occurs from other chemicals.[104]

Bioassays for toxic activity on cells or enzymes as models to assay trichothecene activity have been explored to characterize air samples and particles[112–117] from a Montreal office building assayed by thin layer chromatography (TLC) using 4-(*p*-nitrobenzyl) pyridine to identify the 12,12-epoxy group of trichothecenes.[117] Methanol extracts of water-damaged building materials and gypsum board were 200 times as toxic as board extracts that were not water damaged for feline skin and lung cells. Another problem is that spores and fragments of three molds (*A. versicolor*, *Penicillium melinii*, and *Cladosporium cladosporiodes*) share antigens and immunological reactivity.[113] Inhibition of protein synthesis using firefly luciferase translation in rabbit reticulocytes has been correlated with fungal counts in indoor air[118] and attributed to trichothecenes. Also, trichothecenes were identified in ultra-small mold particles.[111]

Trichothecenes were identified as toxic agents for swine kidney cell cultures by MTT cleavage using 3-(4,5-dimethylthiazol-2yl)-2,5 diphenyltetrazolium bromide and characterized chemically by high-pressure liquid chromatography with a diode array detector (HPLC-DAD) and gas chromatography-mass spectrometry (GC-MS).[118] A chymotrypsin-like serin proteinase from *Stachybotrys chartarum* has been isolated and purified from the lung of an infant with pulmonary hemosiderosis. It cleaved lung proteinase inhibitors, bioactive peptides, and collagen, suggesting it could destroy lung tissue.[119] Recently, an enzyme linked immunosorbent assays (ELISA) assay, was specific for trichothecenes on tiny mold fragments caught in ultra-fine filters.[102,112]

The 105 patient study confirmed the abnormalities in balance, reaction time, recall, memory, and trail making in 20 previously evaluated patients exposed to *S. atra* in one building[89] and people exposed to various molds and mycotoxins in homes and schools.[90]

Another study reported elevated levels of neural auto-antibodies and elevated rates of abnormal nerve conduction velocities in a group of 119 patients with chronic health complaints and proven environmental mold exposure in their homes or workplaces.[120] These 119 mold exposed patients had a significantly higher rate of auto-antibodies to many nerve proteins compared with a group of 500 controls. Significantly elevated neural auto-antibodies were reported for the following antigens: myelin basic protein, myelin-associated glycoprotein, myelin oligodendrocyte, glycoprotein, glutamate, tubulin, chondroitan sulfate, and neurofilament antigen. Peripheral nerve studies were also made on these 119 mold exposed patients. Abnormal motor and sensory nerve conduction was reported in 55 patients (46%), abnormal motor conduct ion only in 17 patients (14%), abnormal sensory conduction only in 27 patients (23%), and normal nerve conduction in 20 patients (17%).[120]

MOLD/MYCOTOXIN EXPOSURE AND CANCER

A number of molds also produce highly carcinogenic mycotoxins such as aflatoxin and ochratoxin. Aflatoxins are produced by some *Aspergillus* species such as *A. flavus and A. parasiticus* and are especially common on poorly stored grains or peanuts.[120] Large human epidemiological studies have estimated that foodborne aflatoxin exposures are responsible for 25,200–155,000 new cases of liver cancer annually.[120] Persons with both foodborne exposure and aflatoxin hepatitis B infection are especially susceptible to liver cancer. Aflatoxin exposure may also significantly reduce immunity. Studies with HIV+ Ghanian adults have reported that higher foodborne aflatoxin exposure is associated with significant lower percentages of CD4+ and B cells and significantly higher HIV blood viral loads as compared with HIV+ adults not exposed to high foodborne aflatoxin exposure.[121,122] A number of studies have reported an association between foodborne aflatoxin exposure and growth stunting in children.[123] Ochratoxin A may cause cancer of the human kidney[124] and certainly trigger vasculitis in the chemically sensitive.[7] Other studies have reported a link between foodborne exposure to fuminisin mycotoxins (produced by many species of *Fusarium*) and higher levels of esophageal cancer.[123]

INDOOR MOLD EXPOSURE AND CHRONIC FATIGUE

Brewer et al.[125] conducted a study to determine if selected mycotoxins could be identified in human urine from patients suffering from chronic fatigue syndrome (CFS). Patients (n = 112) with prior diagnosis of CFS were evaluated for mold exposure and the presence of mycotoxins in their urine. Urine was tested for aflatoxins (AT), ochratoxin A (OTA) and macrocyclic trichothecenes (MT) using ELISA. Urine specimens from 104 of 112 patients (93%) were positive for at least one mycotoxin (one in the equivocal range). Almost 30% of the cases had more than one mycotoxin present. OTA was the most prevalent mycotoxin detected (83%) with MT as the next most common (44%). Urine samples from all 55 of the control patients were negative for all three mycotoxins. Exposure histories indicated current and/or past exposure to WDB in over 90% of cases. Environmental testing was performed in the WDB from a subset of these patients. This testing revealed the presence of potentially mycotoxin producing mold species and mycotoxins in the environment of the WDB.[125]

Heavy indoor exposure to molds have been linked to asthma, sinus problems, chronic fatigue and significantly reduced levels of hormones essential for energy production such as growth hormone and thyroid hormones.[126,127] A Georgia study reported on 79 subjects with chronic fatigue and chronic sinusitis (nose stuffiness) who were exposed to indoor environments with water damage and heavy mold growth.[127] Of these 79 subjects, 51% were deficient in growth hormone and 81% were deficient in the thyroid hormones T_4 and/or T_3. The 79 chronically fatigued subjects were then placed on an multifaceted treatment program including: (1) cleanup of subjects work or indoor environment to greatly reduce mold and water problems; (2) nasal salt sprays; (3) oral and nasal antibacterial and antifungal drugs; (4) replacement hormone treatment with growth hormone, thyroid hormone, and other hormones as needed; and (5) a broad range of nutritional supplements including vitamins, minerals herbs, CoQ_{10} and L-carnitine. Interdermal injections of mold antigen every four days, also is necessary for successful treatment. Following this multi-faceted treatment, complete or near complete resolution of both chronic fatigue and chronic sinusitis was seen in 93% of the subjects.[127]

Stachybotrys molds produce several neurotoxic mycotoxins including satratoxin-G. NASA installation of satratoxin-G has induced rhinitis and apoptosis of olfactory sensory neuron in Rhesus monkeys.[128] Another animal study reported that nasal installation caused olfactory neuron loss and neuroinflammation in mice.[92] *Stachybotrys* also produces a hemolytic protein called hemolysin which may be related to the hemorrhagic effects of exposure to *Stachybotrys*.[19]

MOLDS AND VASCULITIS

At the EHC-Dallas multiple patients exposed to molds have developed small vessel vasculitis. These patients developed spontaneous bruising, petechia, edema, blue and cold hands and feet, and at times acneform lesions. These patients though difficult to treat can be cleared by massive avoidance of molds and mycotoxins, intradermal neutralization of molds and mycotoxins, nutrients supplementation (vitamin C, glutathione, multiple vitamin B, and minerals), and at times immune modulators, such as antogenous and lympholytic factor, and, when deficient and necessary, gamma globulin (Table 1.9).

MOLD EXPOSURE AND MULTIPLE SCLEROSIS

Chronic fungal infection in CSF from some patients with multiple sclerosis (MS) (2013) has been found.

MS is the prototypical inflammatory disease of the central CNS and spinal cord, leading to axonal demyelination of neurons. Recently, Thrasher et al.[129] found a correlation between chronic fungal infection and MS in peripheral blood of patients. This work provides evidence of chronic fungal infection in the CSF of some MS patients. Thus, fungal antigens can be demonstrated in CSF, as well as antibodies reacting against several Candida species. Comparison was made between CSF and blood serum for the presence of fungal antigens (proteins) and antibodies against different *Candida* spp. Analyses of both CSF and serum are complementary and serve to better evaluate for the presence of disseminated fungal infection. In addition, PCR analyses indicate the presence of DNA from different fungal species in CSF, depending on the patient analyzed. Overall, these findings support the idea that chronic fungal infection can be demonstrated in CSF from some MS patients. This may constitute a risk factor in this disease and could also help in understanding the pathogenesis of MS. Our series of patients at the EHC-Dallas and Buffalo from inception to 2015 have been worked on for fungal sensitivity. Findings were always positive in those with the exposure.

MS is an inflammatory and demyelinating disease of the CNS in which sclerotic plaque form in the brain and the spinal cord.[130–132] This complex disease is thought to be triggered by an interaction between genetic and environmental factors.[133–138] MS is prototypical of inflammatory CNS

TABLE 1.9

Immune Modulators for T & B Cell Supressors and Gamma Globulin Suppression

			Control
Autogenous lymphocytic factors	–	–	< 0.1 cm^3
Gamma globulin subset deficiency	–	–	1. 382–922 mgm/dL
			2. 241–700 mgm/dL
			3. < 0–114 mgm/dL
			4. 22–178 mgm/dL

diseases and is associated with a variety of clinical symptoms. Motor impairment and sensory organ dysfunction are two major problems associated with MS. Current therapies are based on immunosuppressive and immune regulatory compounds that aim to reduce inflammation. However, these therapies are of little benefit in advanced stages of the disease.[132] Usually, these patients are never treated by antifungal medication, massive avoidance of the mycotoxins, nutrient therapy, and intradermal neutralization techniques. The treatment by the immune suppressive route may be the problem for less than successful treatments.

The exact cause of MS has been the object of intensive research in many laboratories, although the etiology of MS remains enigmatic. Autoimmunity has been put forward as a plausible cause of this disease.[139,140] Autoimmunity may result from the presence of viral proteins or other pathogenic antigens that mimic self-protein molecules in the CNS.[141,142] However, no association between antimyelin antibodies and progression to MS exists.[143] Moreover, a disorder of the immune system that attacks oligodendrocytes does not account for some clinical observations. For instance, the existence of distinct foci of degeneration cannot be explained by indiscriminate aggression against glial cells.[144] Furthermore, blood vessel inflammation is not easily explained by autoimmunity and destruction of nerve cells.[145] Intensive research to find an infectious agent that directly provokes or triggers MS has been carried out in many laboratories.

Fungal toxins have been suggested as a possible triggering factor for MS, especially the mycotoxin gliotoxin, which is produced by many common fungi including *Aspergillus*, *Penicillum*, and *Candida*.[21,146,147] A huge Danish study of 3259 MS cases and 32,590 controls reported that use of antibiotics was associated with a significantly higher risk of developing MS.[148] This suggests that development of MS may be related to changes in intestinal flora such as increased growth of *Candida*. Pesticide exposure has also been shown to significantly increase risk for MS.[149]

MOLD AND RETINOPATHY AND MS

According to Pisa,[150] Table 1.10, eight women and four men (aged 20–57 years) were involved in this study. All patients experienced early MS symptoms and all had a score of 1 on the Expanded Disability Status Scale (EDSS). None of the patients had been treated with immunosuppressive therapies and none of them had been treated with antifungal therapy or desensitization. The patients' serum and CSF were tested for antibodies and antigens to various *Candida* species such as *albicans, famata, glabrata, krusei*, and *parapsilosis*.[150]

The results obtained with the different tests carried out in this work are summarized in Table 1.10. The presence of fungal macromolecules such as fungal antigens (proteins) and DNA is taken as good evidence of fungal infection. Although the existence of anti-Candida antibodies does not constitute good proof of disseminated candidiasis, the presence of these antibodies may be of interest to provide an indication of the humoral immune response. Therefore, it is concluded that there are signs of chronic fungal infestation in the majority of MS patients. Only two patients were classified as negative (patients 5 and 6) and one as uncertain (patient 8). Future additional samples in these patients may reveal long-term fungal infection.

Antigen levels showed were considered high when the optical density value was 80 or higher; moderate when the value was between 50 and 80; low when the value was between 20 and 50, and uncertain when the value was between 10 and 20. "None" represents results for which the value was lower than 10. Antibody levels were scored according to the percentage of positivity of fluorescence assay as follows: ++++ or +++++, high; +++ or ++, moderate; +, low; −, negative; ND not done PCR results from CSF indicated presence of DNA from three different yeasts including *Malassizia globosa* (four of eight patients), *Erythrobasidium clade* (two patients), and *Rhodotorula mucilaginosa* (three patients).

This work suggests that chronic fungal infection can be found in the CSF of several MS patients.[150] Moreover, fungal DNA can be amplified with some of these samples, revealing the presence of several fungal species. The PCR results are of particular interest because they point to a variety of

TABLE 1.10

MS Patients—Molds—Age 20–57

Patient	Antigen Level CSF	Antigen Level Serum	Antibody Level CSF	Antibody Level Serum	PCR Result	Infection
1	Negative	Low	Negative	Low	Positive	Positive
2	Negative	Low	Moderate	Moderate	Positive	Positive
3	Negative	Low	Low	High	Positive	Positive
4	Negative	Negative	Low	High	Positive	Positive
5	Negative	Low	Negative	Low	ND	Negative
6	Negative	Low	Negative	Low	Negative	Negative
7	High	Low	Negative	Moderate	Positive	Positive
8	Negative	Moderate	High	High	ND	Uncertain
9	Uncertain	High	Negative	Moderate	Positive	Positive
10	Uncertain	High	Low	High	ND	Positive
11	Negative	High	High	High	ND	Positive
12	Low	High	Negative	High	Positive	Positive

Source: With kind permission from **Springer Science+Business Media**: *Eur. J. Clin. Microbiol. Infect. Dis.*, Fungal infection in cerebrospinal fluid from some patients with multiple sclerosis, 32, 2013, 795-801, Pisa, D. et al.

fungal species that infect MS patients. This may represent an important risk factor of the pathology and evolution of the disease in some patients. Also, the presence of fungal toxins can play a part in the cytotoxicity and/or inflammation of the CNS in MS patients.[146] It may be of interest to analyze the presence of gliotoxin, or other potential toxins in CSF.[151,152] Future work can measure the fungal antigens present in serum and CSF, as well as ascertain the origin of their production (which tissues are infected and/or colonized by the fungi.

The presence of chronic fungal infection in MS patients may be because the infection is the actual cause of the disease or may be a consequence of immune dysfunction in these patients.[150] Either way, the fungal infection or sensitivity should be treated appropriately with antifungal compounds or if it is a sensitivity, then it should be treated with antigen desensitization; if it is an immune deficit with T-cell, supplementation by autogeneous lymphocyte factor (ALF), or if it is gamma globulin deficiency, then supplementation by gamma globulin. The presence of such an infection, even if it does not cause MS, may negatively affect the clinical course of neurodegeneration. Patients with MS are usually treated with corticosteroids and other immunosuppressive agents, which may be favored in the long-term fungal infections.[153] In such cases, diagnosis of this type of infection must be taken into consideration in the management of these patients. Immune augmentation may be better for treatments than immune suppression.

The determination of the etiology of MS has remained elusive. The most widespread idea is the MS represents an autoimmune disease that reacts against myelin, leading to the destruction of glial cells and is followed by axonal damage of neurons. Many researchers have suggested that a microbial infection may be the cause of MS.[154,155] Particular attention has focused on CNS infection by the Epstein-Barr virus,[156] although other viruses and bacteria have also been suggested, either as a direct cause of MS or as triggers of the autoimmune reaction.[157,158]

EVIDENCE OF SIGNIFICANT FUNGAL EXPOSURE IN THE PATIENT

The best evidence of significant fungal exposure in the ill patient is the use of provocation techniques either inhaled, intradermal, or oral. In environmentally controlled mold-free rooms, the patient can have intradermally exposed provocation. Inhaled provocation is not used because it is too difficult to keep the chamber mold free for the next challenge. With intradermal provocation, the clinician can challenge multiple molds one at a time in sequence, and see if wheals 7 × 7 mm will grow or even better provoke signs and symptoms. This technique was conceived and perfected by Lee[159] and advanced by Miller[160] and members of the American Academy of Environmental Medicine and the Pan American Allergy Society. Otolaryngic allergy has been a significant advance in the assay of where the molds bother or are a significant factor in the evaluation of moldy environments. Oral challenge can be performed on a food that has already been tested for food sensitivity and is negative.

MELATONIN: DETOXIFICATION OF OXYGEN AND NITROGEN-BASED TOXIC REACTANTS

In the last decade, melatonin has been found to be highly protective against damage to macromolecules resulting from oxygen and nitrogen-based reactants. Considering this, numerous studies have examined the mechanisms whereby this indoleamine directly detoxifies these damaging agents. The evidence is compelling that melatonin scavenges several oxygen-derived reactive agents including the hydroxyl radical (OH), hydrogen peroxide (H_2O_2, singlet oxygen (O_2) and hypochlorous acid (HOCl). Additionally, melatonin reportedly reacts with nitric oxide (NO), the peroxynitrite anion ($ONOO^-$) and/or peroxynitrous acid (ONOOH) to detoxify them. In some cases the products that are formed as a consequence of melatonin's scavenging actions have been identified. Whereas the ability of melatonin to neutralize these toxic agents possibly accounts, in part, for the antioxidant activity of melatonin, it is not the only means by which melatonin serves to protect molecules from oxygen and nitrogen-based reactive metabolites.[161]

SPOTLIGHTS ON ADVANCES IN MYCOTOXIN RESEARCH

Many of these advances appear around negative genetics and may not have much clinical value, although some have proved beneficial.

Fungi are ingenious producers of complex natural products which show a broad range of biological activities. On the beneficial end, we find pharmacologically used drugs, such as penicillin, other antibiotics, and the lipid-lowering lovastatin.[162] However, other fungal metabolites possess potent toxic or carcinogenic properties and threaten human, animal, or plant health. Natural products play an important role for phylogenetic and taxonomical purposes.[163] Therefore, multiple disciplines and stimuli have driven research on natural products, making it a truly interdisciplinary area of scientific endeavor.

The availability of molecular biology protocols enabled research on the biosynthesis of numerous toxins. In contrast to most genes for primary metabolism, all or most of the genes required for the synthesis of most mycotoxins are clustered on one single genetic locus.[164] The backbones of numerous mycotoxins are synthesized by polyketide synthases (PKSs) or nonribosomal peptide synthetases (NRPSs), dedicated assembly line-like multi-domain enzymes. Therefore, the genes for these enzymes have served as genetic probes to identify such clusters of biosynthesis genes. The clusters also encode genes for regulators or self-resistance as well as for tailoring enzymes to modify and diversify the scaffolds built by the PKSs or NRPSs. An early milestone result was the genetic characterization of the sterigmatocystin cluster in *A. nidulans*.[165] This cluster served as a model to study the closely related biosynthesis of aflatoxin.

According to Bohnert et al.[166] multi-gene loci for the biosynthesis of zearalenone,[167–169] fumonisins,[170,171] and trichothecenes[172] were identified and opened new avenues of research. Expression of gene clusters was analyzed in real time, for example, for zearalenone to study its transcriptional activity under infectious conditions.[173] Also, natural product biosynthesis enzymes have been overexpressed and characterized to discover new biochemistry. This was shown, for the asteri quinone group indole alkaloid terrequinone A.[174,175] Given the similarity to NRPSs, TdiA is remarkable in that it forms carbon–carbon bonds instead of peptide bonds. *Basidiomycetes* rely on a similar biosynthetic strategy to assemble atromentin to form the side chains of 4-hydorxyphenyl-pyruvate, as shown for the *Tapinella panuoides* quinine synthetase AtrA.[176]

According to Bohnert et al.[166] small peptide toxins, the diketopiperazines, gliotoxin, and sirodesmin PL (Figure 1.2), and their biosynthesis loci have received particular attention. Gliotoxin is a metabolite of various fungi, with the opportunistic human pathogen *A. fumigates* being the most relevant producer. Sirodesmin PL is a phytotoxin of *Leptosphaeria maculns*, the causative agent of canola blackleg disease. Gliotoxin and sirodesmin share disulfur bridges as key structural prerequisite to generate reactive oxygen species and to conjugate with cysteine residues of proteins. Effects on prokaryotic or eukaryotic cells include, among numerous others, necrotic and apoptotic cell death, and NFkB activation.[177] The key enzymes for gliotoxin and sirodesmin synthesis are the NRPSs GliP and SirP, respectively, which assemble the diketopiperazine core structure from L-serine and an aromatic L-amino acid. Disruption of sirP led to a mutant which lost the capacity to produce sirodesmin.

Effective Stem Colonization Were Observed Compared to Wild Type

According to Bohnert et al.[166] in the medieval Europe, endemic outbreaks of the ergot fungus *Claviceps purpurea* resulted in contaminated food and upon continued ingestion, caused the "holy fire," that is, gangrene of the extremities.[178]

Steiner[179] isolated a seed-transmitted, mutualistic *clavcipitalean* fungus from *Ipomoea asarifolia* and *Turbina corymbosa*. The fungus apparently plays a role to deter pests from the plant host and to increase its drought tolerance.[180,181] While the fungus was clearly identified as producer, the alkaloids surprisingly accumulated only in the plant partner,[182] suggesting that a dedicated alkaloid translocation system exists in this mutualistic plant–fungus association.[183]

Gliotoxin, the ergoline alkaloids and numerous other metabolites had been isolated long before the corresponding genes were identified and functionally investigated. As we have entered the fungal genomic era, the situation fundamentally changed; the number of genetic loci presumably dedicated to secondary metabolism and now revealed by genome sequencing often exceeds the number of known compounds from a species by far.[184] Using PKS and NRPS genes as indicators during genome-wide analyses, filamentous fungi are unexpectedly rich in genetic material implicated in secondary metabolism. For example, the *A. nidulans* genome harbors 27 genes for NRPSs.[185,186] The *A. oryzae* has 44 predicted NRPSs and PKSs genes located in its genome, the opportunistic human pathogen *A. fumigatus* at least 27.[187] In a majority of cases, these gene clusters and pathways are unique and not conserved between species or redundant within a genome.

Scherlach and Hertweck[188] anticipated quinazoline or quinoline products in *A. nidulans*. This was based on the observation that its genome harbors multiple genes for anthranilate synthases which besides their function in L-tryptophan biosynthesis could play a role in alkaloid metabolism. Extracts originating from 40 parallel fermentations run under different conditions in fact yielded the highly cytotoxic aspoquinolones, a new class of fungal alkaloids.

Regulation of Fungal Secondary Metabolism

Particularly pertinent to fungal toxins and secondary metabolism in general was the discovery of LadA, a nuclear protein and master regulator of natural product synthesis in several *Aspergillus* species.[189,190] LaeA was first identified during complementation experiments to restore production of sterigmatocystin in *Aspergillus nidulans*, which had lost this metabolic capacity but developed normally otherwise.[191] LaeA was also required for the synthesis of other natural products, such as penicillin, hyphal pigments, lovastatin, or gliotoxin. As laeA-overexpressing strains showed increased metabolite titers, the concept of LaeA and a pathway independent and global regulator of secondary metabolism emerged. Deletion of LaeA in *A. fumigates* correlated with changes in conidial morphology, increased susceptibility to phagocytosis by host cells in a murine model, and the absence of gliotoxin in infected lung tissue.[192] The biotechnological potential of LaeA to mine genomes for new metabolites was demonstrated in a comparative study with *A. nidulans* as the transcriptome of an laeA-deletion mutant showed a selective down regulation of clusters of a natural product genes, compared to wild type, while adjacent genes were not affected. This makes LaeA a tool to identify or verify natural product genes and thus recognize loci and their boundaries potentially relevant for toxin production.[193,194] In these studies the locus for terrequinone A served as proof of concept for LaeA-guided discovery. Neither was *A. nidulans* known as a producer of this metabolite, nor was knowledge available on these biosynthesis genes. LaeA was identified as part of a heterotrimeric protein complex, together with VelB and the velvet protein VeA, their latter being the direct binding target of LaeA.[195] This complex integrates light stimuli and morphogenesis, and the identification of LaeA as a member of this complex underlines that development and secondary metabolism are interwoven.

The model to explain the LaeA mechanism of action includes an epigenetic control by chromatin remodeling through methyltransfer to histones.[196] Chromatin-modifying proteins have been recognized as regulatory element which lock or unlock natural product gene clusters. An *A. nidulans* strain deficient in the *cclA* gene, whose product is involved in methyltransfer to lysine 4 of histone h3, expressed at least two natural product loci which are transcriptionally silent in the wild type. These loci govern biosynthesis of the polyketides F9775A and F9775B, and of monodictyphenone.[197]

Very recently, the concept of regulation of mycotoxin biosynthesis through chromatin modification was further, corroborated, again with the *A. nidulans* sterigmatocystin biosynthesis genes as proof of principle. The *stc* gene cluster is silent during normal growth and occupied and elevated levels of heterochromatin protein A (HepA), while a decrease of HepA marks is associated with the onset of sterigmatocystin synthesis. A heap deletion mutant showed strongly increased transcript levels for the biosynthesis genes of sterigmatocystin, penicillin, and terrequinone A, the genes of the AflR regulator and, interestingly, LaeA.[198] ClrD is a histone methyltransferase which trimethylates the lysine residue 9 in history H3. ClrD activity is a prerequisite for efficient HepA labeling as HepA binding requires trimethylation. Consistent with the model, the same study presents a clrD mutant, which showed increased stc gene transcription and somewhat higher sterigmatocystin titers. The authors conclude that LaeA counteracts trimethylation at natural product gene loci which then leads to decreased HepA binding and, thus, prevents formation of repressive facultative heterochromatin. LaeA-mediated pleiotropic transcriptional regulation has been found outside the genus *Aspergillus* as well. Kosalková et al.[199] identified an orthologous gene in *P. chrysogenum*, the producer of penicillin and the mycotoxin roquefortin C. Homologous overexpression of LaeA under the control of the *A. awamori* glutamate dehydrogenase promoter increased penicillin yields by 25% calculated as benzylpenicillin per mg dry weight. Attenuation of laeA transcription by RNAi decreased penicillin titers by more than 50%. RNAi also impacted upon conidial pigmentation and morphological differentiation, as conidia are colorless and their overall amount reduced by 50%. Roquefortin C production remained unaffected after these genetic manipulations, indicating an LaeA-independent regulation of its biosynthesis.

According to Bohnert et al.[166] mitogen-activated protein (MAP) kinases were identified as another regulatory element for fungal natural product biosynthesis. In *Fusarium graminearum*, trichothecene accumulation in wheat plants was dramatically reduced when the MGV1 deletion mutant was used to infect the host.[200] The deletion of mpkB, the orthologous gene in *A. nidulans*, led to decreased transcript levels of sterigmatocystin biosynthetic genes and the pathway-specific regulator gene aflR.[201] Similarly, transcription of penicillin and terrequinone genes was attenuated. Notably, the mpkB deletion mutant also showed reduced laeA transcript levels, suggesting the mpkB kinase controls, at last to a degree, expression of this master regulator of secondary metabolism.

A Spotlight on Basidiomycete Toxins

Bohnert et al.[166] reviewed two *basidiomycete* toxins. *Basidiomycete* genomics and genetic tools are less advanced compared with *Aspergilli, Penicilli,* and other ascomycetes.

More than 90% of all fatal mushroom poisonings are caused by *Amanita phalloides* (death cap) and closely related species, the toxicologically most relevant producers of the amanitin family of bicyclic octapeptides. Recent work proves that these toxins are synthesized ribosomally and do not follow the NRPS paradigm of peptide natural product assembly in fungi. A gene family was identified in *Amanita* that code for proproteins composed of a variable portion (the precursor of the actual toxin) flanked by constant regions.[202] Thus, *Amanita* and other amantin producing species are able to produce numerous similar small peptides that are processed posttranslationally using a prolyl oligopeptidase (POP). Using the *Conocybe albipes* POP as a model, Luo et al.[203] showed that it releases the toxins from the proprotein by specific hydrolysis at a conserved prolin residue. In *A. bisporigera*, two genes (*AMA1* and *PHGA1*) encode the 35 and 34 amino acids a-amantin and phalloidin proproteins.

A recent study on an Asian *Basidiomycete mushroom, Russula subnigricans,* identified cycloprop-2-ene carboxylic acid as a new mushroom toxin (and natural product in general). This fungus was known to cause rhabdomyolysis, a sometimes fatal poisoning of the muscles, which could be reproduced experimentally by oral administration of the new toxin to mice.[204] However, cycloprop-2-ene carboxylic acid does not seem to attack myocytes directly, so the authors conclude that an indirect trigger must lead to the symptoms. Rhabdomyolysis has also been reported after the presumably edible mushroom *Tricholoma equeste* had been ingested, and this new toxin may represent the causative agent.

Mushroom alcohol or 1-octen-3-ol is a mycotoxin with a musty odor producd by many fungi including the Basidiomycetes (mushrooms). Parkinson's disease may be linked to exposure to 1-octen-3-ol. A recent study has linked exposure to 1-octyen-3-ol to dopamine neurodegeneration in *Drosophila melanogaster.*[205]

Rusts and Smuts

Building Exposure

Bloom and coworkers[206] analyzed 100 water damaged building materials from 57 buildings in Sweden for molds, mycotoxins, and the fungal metabolic ergosterol.[207] Samples came from a variety of water damaged materials including gypsum board (40 samples), wood,[208] linoleum flooring, wallpaper, and other materials.[209]

In the building material samples, the amounts of Gliotoxin (GLIO) were 0.43 and 1.12 pg/mg, of Sterigmatocystin (STRG) 4.9–150,000 pg/mg (mean 7100, median 490), of trichodermol (TRID) 0.9–8700 pg/mng (mean 670, median 46) and of VER 8.8–17,000 pg/mg (mean 1800, median 190). The amounts of Satratoxins G and H (SATG and SATH) were not calculated, since the crude standards available were not useful for quantification purposes. In settled dust, the amounts of VERA were 0.6 and 1.7 pg/mg, and in RCS cultures aflatoxin B (AFLAB) (32.0 and 14,500 pg/cm^2) STRG (3.6–10,900 pg/cm^2, mean 880 pg/cm^2, median 63 pg/cm^2), *Tricoderma (TRID)* (6.5–170 pg/cm^2, mean 58 pg/cm^2, median 13 pg/cm^2), VER (15–3400 pg/cm^2, mean 500 pg/cm^2, median 29 pg./cm^2), and GLIO (400 pg/cm^2) were found.

The mycoflora and the absolute amounts of ERG in the different types of samples are shown in Table 1.11. *Aspergillus spp., Stachybotrys spp.,* and *Chaetomium spp.* were the most prevalent and were found on all building material types. *Aspergillus spp.* were found most commonly on wood-based materials, and *Stachybotrys* and *Chaetomium spp.* were most common on gypsum board samples. Mycotoxin analysis results and the relative amounts of *Ergosterol (ERG)* in mycotoxin-positive versus mycotoxin-negative samples are shown in Table 1.12, whereas the amounts of ERG in samples positive for each of the individual mycotoxins and in mycotoxin-negative samples, are shown in Table 1.13.

The mycotoxin found most commonly in building material samples was TRID (53%), especially in gypsum board (75%) (Tables 1.9 and 1.11). Molds known to produce TRID were detected in the majority of these samples, that is, Stachybotrys spp. (78%), Memnoniella 20% and Trichoderma. Levels of ERG were approximately twice as large in the TRID-positive samples as in the mycotoxin-negative samples (Table 1.10)

TABLE 1.11

Fungal Taxa Found by Microscopy and Amounts of Ergosterol in the Studied Samples

Fungal Taxa[a]	No. of Building Material Samples in which the Indicated Fungal Taxa Were Detected			No. of Dust Samples in which the Indicated Fungal Taxa Were Detected			
	Gypsum Board	Wood Based	Linoleum Flooring	Wallpaper	Other[b]	Settled Dust	RCS Culture
	n = 40	n = 37	n = 7	n = 6	n = 10	n = 18	n = 37
Aspergillus	4	13	3	3	1	na	22
Stachybotrys	26	14	1	2	4	na	12
Chaetomium	9	7	2	1	1	na	5
Memnoniella	nd	1	nd	nd	1	na	nd
Penicillium	1	2	1	nd	nd	na	27
Cladosporium	2	1	nd	nd	nd	na	23
Acremonium	nd	1	nd	nd	1	na	1
Alternaria	nd	1	nd	nd	1	na	7
Eurotium	nd	1	1	nd	nd	na	nd
Scopulariopsis	nd	nd	nd	1	nd	na	nd
Trichoderma	nd	nd	nd	nd	nd	na	2
Ulocladium	1	nd	nd	nd	nd	na	1
Mycelia sterile	nd	nd	nd	nd	nd	na	24
Yeast	nd	nd	nd	nd	nd	na	21
Ergosterol[c]	17.0;6.2	10.0;1.4	11.2;2.4	49.2;0.2	19.4;0.2	44.9;12.3	170.2;89.8

Source: Bloom, E. et al. 2009. *J. Occup. Environ. Hyg.* 6(11):671–678. Reprinted by permission (Taylor & Francis Ltd. http://www.tandfonline.com).

Note: n = number of samples analyzed; na = not analyzed; nd = not detected, Mycelia sterile denotes nonsporulating mycelium.

[a] Other taxa found in one sample only included *Scopulariopsis* (wallpaper), *Philaphora* (other, namely, plastic floor material), and *Olpitrichum, Fusairum, Geomyces, Auerobasidium* and *Mumicola* (RCS cultures).

[b] Five flooring materials, four painted wall materials, and one inventory.

[c] Amounts of ergosterol (mean; median) in the studied building materials (ng/mg), settled dust samples (ng/mg), and in RCS cultures (mg/cm^2).

All building material samples positive for SATG and/or SATH (5%) were gypsum board samples that also were positive for VER and Stachybotrys spp. Levels of ERG were almost six times as high in the SATG-positive building material samples as in mycotoxin-negative samples and three times higher in RCS cultures (Table 1.12).

Unlike TRID, VER was seldom found as a single mycotoxin in a building material sample (only 3%), although in combination with other mycotoxins it was the second most commonly found toxin (32%) (Table 1.12). Just as for TRID, ERG levels were twice as high in the VER-positive than in the mycotoxin-negative building material samples (Table 1.12). Nine RCS cultures and two settled dust samples (from a nursing home for the elderly) contained VER (Tables 1.2 and 1.3). These two dust samples contained approximately 10 times less ergosterol and the RCS cultures about half of that of the mycotoxin-negative dust samples (Table 1.13).

STRG was the third most frequently found mycotoxin (22%) in building materials and the most common in RCS cultures (41%). *Aspergillus spp.* were found in nearly all STRG-positive samples; however, analogously with *Stachybotrys*, all samples positive for *Aspergillus spp.* did not contain detectable amounts of STRG. ERG levels were almost three times higher in STRG-positive than in mycotoxin-negative building materials samples. STRG- and satratoxin-positive RCS cultures were

TABLE 1.12

Mycotoxins in the Samples, Relative Amounts of Ergosterol in Mycotoxin-Positive versus Mycotoxin-Negative Samples

Mycotoxin	No. of Samples in the Indicated Building Material in which Mycotoxins were Detected					No. of Dust Samples in which Mycotoxin(s) was Detected	
	Gypsum Board	Wood Based	Linoleum Flooring	Wallpaper	Other[a]	Settled Dust	RCS Culture
	n = 40	n = 37	n = 7	n = 6	n = 10	n = 18	n = 37
TRID	12	4	nd	2	3	nd	1
VER	nd	3	nd	nd	nd	2	1
STRG	2	3	nd	2	1	nd	7
TRID, VER	8	5	nd	nd	2	nd	nd
TRID, STRG	3	1	nd	1	nd	nd	nd
VER, STRG	1	nd	nd	nd	1	nd	2
STRG, AFLAB	nd	nd	nd	nd	nd	nd	2
TRID, VER, GLIO	nd	nd	1	1	nd	nd	1
TRID, VER, STRG	2	3	nd	nd	nd	nd	2
TRID, VER, SATG, SATH	2	nd	nd	nd	nd	nd	nd
TRID, VER, SATG	1	nd	nd	nd	nd	nd	nd
TRIC, VER, STRG, SATG SATH	2	nd	nd	nd	nd	nd	1
VER, STRG, SATG, SATH	nd	nd	nd	nd	nd	nd	1
Ergosterol/ergosterol ratio[b]	0.9	5.0	0.2	*	140	0.1	2.1

Source: Bloom, E. et al. 2009. *J. Occup. Environ. Hyg.* 6(11):671–678. Reprinted by permission (Taylor & Francis Ltd. http://www.tandfonline.com).

Note: nd = not detected; n = number of samples analyzed, * = mycotoxin-negative samples not found.

[a] Five flooring materials, four painted wall materials, and one inventory.

[b] Amounts (mean values) of ergosterol in the mycotoxin-positive versus mycotoxin-negative samples studied.

the only mycotoxin-positive samples with more ergostrol (approximately 2–3-times higher) than mycotoxin-negative RCS cultures (Table 1.13).

Bloom et al.[206] found that 66% of the 100 building materials analyzed were positive for at least one of the studied mycotoxins. This is in accordance with their previous study where 73% of the analyzed materials with visible mold growth were mycotoxin positive.[210] To date, they have not detected any mycotoxins in building materials, RCS cultures, and settled dust from indoor environments without water damage (unpublished results).

The present study was designed to provide information about the prevalence of the selected mycotoxins in mold-contaminated, water-damaged buildings in a temperate climate zone. In accordance with their previous study, Tricoderma (TRID) was the most commonly found mycotoxin and the sole mycotoxin found in as many as 21% of the samples. VERA and STRG were less common in this study than in the previous study (32% and 23% vs. 46% and 40% respectively). Notably, the proportion of gypsum paper samples and wood-based building materials were 40% and 37% respectively, in this study and 63% and 13%, respectively in the previous study.[210] The different results found in their studies may be explained by the fact that different types of materials favor growth of different molds.[102]

ERG is a fungal cell membrane compound that can be used as a fungal biomass exposure marker in environmental samples.[129,207,211] The concentrations of ERG in house dust have been reported in

TABLE 1.13

Ergosterol in the Mycotoxin-Positive and Mycotoxin-Negative Samples

Amounts of Ergosterol in Building Materials and Settle Dust and in RCS Cultures

Samples	Building Materials (ug/g)	Settled Dust (ug/g)	RCS Culture mg/cm²
TRID-positive	n = 53	n = 0	n = 6
Mean	18.0	*	26.5
Median	4.20	*	11.5
VER-positive	n = 32	n = 2	n = 9
Mean	14.5	4.70	53.7
Median	2.70	4.70	10.1
SATG-positve	n = 5	n = 0	n = 1
Mean	46.5	*	310
Median	16.0	*	310
SATH-positive	n = 4	n = 0	n = 2
Mean	17.0	*	207
Median	14.5	*	207
STRG-positive	n = 22	n = 0	n = 15
Mean	22.9	*	285
Median	3.50	*	74.9
GLIO-positive	n = 2	n = 0	n = 1
Mean	2.60	*	12.5
Median	2.60	*	12.5
AFLAB-positive	n = 0	n = 0	n = 2
Mean	*	*	2.50
Median	*	*	2.50
Mycotoxin-negative	n = 35	n = 16	n = 20
Mean	7.80	50.6	110
Median	1.30	19.0	102

Source: Bloom, E. et al. 2009. *J. Occup. Environ. Hyg.* 6(11):671–678. Reprinted by permission (Taylor & Francis Ltd. http://www.tandfonline.com).

Note: * = sample negative for the indicated mycotoxin.

the range between 0.4 and 45 ug/g[212–214] (Dennis, D. P. 2010. Atlanta Center for E.N.T. and Facial Plastic Center, Atlanta, GA, USA, Personal Communication) and on mold-affected building material samples between 0.012 and 68 ug/g,[207,215] which is in accordance with their results. In this study, the total amount of ERG in each sample was calculated as the sum of determined free ERG (in the sample extracts) and esterfied ERG (in the sample residue). Some studies have found a correlation between concentrations of ERG in floor and chair dust and respiratory illness.[213] However, other studies have failed to confirm such associations.[211] ERG is a relatively unstable molecule that may degrade when stored at high humidity[216] or at $>-20°C$.

Apart from being analyzed by microscopy, about half the building material samples were also cultured on MEA. Mold species capable of producing the detected mycotoxins were identified in all the samples, with few exceptions as in previous findings.[18,210] Colony-forming units of cultures from the building material samples did not correlate with ERG concentrations (data not shown). However, except for GLIOtoxin, mycotoxin-positive building material samples contained 2–6 times more ERG than mycotoxin-negative samples. Whether GLIO-0 producing strains produce unusually little ERG or inhibit growth of (ERG-producing) mold is not known. Similarly, it is not clear why VER-positive dust samples and cultures contain less of ERG than mycotoxin-negative samples.

Bloom et al.[206] have shown that molds growing on a range of different materials indoors in water-damaged building, generally produce mycotoxins and distribute them on variety of building materials.

Avoiding brain damage from molds and mycotoxins requires primary prevention. Molds cause neurological and respiratory damage and illnesses that appear to progress and become irreversible and so avoidance of exposure is imperative. First, the building must be designed to prevent moisture within walls. This means preventing intrusion from roofs, (Rain and snow) condensation (including with air-conditioning ducts, and plumbing leaks (supply, icemakers and sewers), facilitate ventilation of walls and roofs so they breathe. Second, construction materials that do not aid the growth of Stachybotyrus and other toxic molds should be used. Strongly alkaline building materials for repair and new construction such as lime, plaster, and concrete deter mold growth.

PREVENTION AND REMEDIATION OF WATER AND MOLD DAMAGE

Based on this evidence, is that persistent dampness and mold damage in the nonindustrial workplace, including schools and residential housing, requires prevention, management and effective remediation.

Remediation should preferably take place within 24 hours after water damage such as a flood or leak has occurred since heavy growth of molds and bacteria often occur after 24–48 hours (EHCD Dallas and Buffalo. Unpublished data. 2010).[217] If visible mold is present, it should be remediated, regardless of what species are present. Such actions possibly reduce new onset asthma and other diseases, such as vasculitis, neurodegenerative disease, and cardiovascular disease, which lead to savings in health care costs and improve public and individual health.

While the design and location of a building has the greatest impact on the onset of serious mold damage, maintenance and effective management of mold and dampness requires an ongoing strategy involving occupants, building owners, and managers; ventilation experts; and occupational hygiene professionals.[15,16]

Owners and occupants should take action to detect and correct leaks, condensation problems and floods as soon as they are discovered. The potential for building structural damage, microbial growth and increased adverse health effects can, and should, be reduced by limiting the buildup of indoor moisture. A formal mold/water prevention program with clear actions and responsibilities is required for an effective response to signs of moisture.[218,219] The actions taken by all stakeholders, including designers, contractors, owners, and occupants of buildings, are critical to effective management of prolonged dampness in buildings. An effective prevention program is evidence of appropriate due diligence to protect both the health of occupants and visitors, and to preserve the building fabric. As new buildings are constructed, or older buildings are subject to major renovation, consistent effort is needed on the part of the architects and engineers involved in the design and construction of the structure, cladding, and roof and HVAC system to make the building durable.[15,220]

It has long been recognized that, based on the application of existing methods to analyze air or dust samples, there are no quantitative, health-based microbial exposure guidelines or thresholds.[221,222] Sampling data that may be developed during an investigation must be comprehensive and communicated in a form useful to physicians and allied professionals, building occupants and decision-makers.[223,224] Both building and individuals are unique and the conditions must be tailored to suit both in order to have optimal conditions.

There are a number of audiences for the reports that are provided pursuant to a mold investigation. Regardless of the nature of the client (home owner, insurance agent, large property company, government), reports must provide information that can (a) be translated into an action plan for repair and rehabilitation of the space, (b) provide a basis for protecting occupants and remediation workers health and, in certain situations (c) be useful for the personal physician and/or public health officials.

INVESTIGATIONS FOR MOLD

Investigators should provide clear and consistent field notes with sufficient detail to allow the field work and sampling data, if any, to be interpreted, verified, and repeated. The report should include, at a minimum, appropriate documentation of sample handling and reporting results. Ideal documentation should be thorough, detailed, readable, and focused. Additionally, it should present sufficient information to allow the work to be verified and repeated, and it should describe all quality assurance procedure.[225,226]

It is recommended that clients verify that the consultant has suitable training and project experience, as well as appropriate and related references.[227] Industrial hygienists also have specialized training in ventilation engineering, environmental health, toxicology and microbiology. Unless this is waived by the client, investigators should be independent of the remediation contractor and testing laboratory associated with the project.[224,227,228] They should be cognizant of the problems that the chemically sensitive has with mold contamination.

Basic competencies that should be assessed by clients include knowledge and education in exposure characterization, microbiological assessment and remediation, general knowledge of the ecology of fungi and bacteria associated with damp or flooded buildings, building science and problem areas in heating ventilation and air-conditioning systems.[227,228] If samples are collected, laboratory analytical staff should have specific training and experience in the identification of environmental mold and bacteria, and be able to demonstrate successful participation in an external proficiency testing program.[16,229] Some States have certification requirements and other regulations regarding mold-related activities or remediation. A number of Canadian municipalities have regulations that cover mold damage in residences.

Recent guidelines focus on factors that promote allergen and contaminant production ("facilitating factors," in this case moisture) and reservoirs.[223] In this context, properly conducted building inspections, which depend on the training and experience of the investigator(s), are essential to physician evaluation. Physicians reviewing such reports should find clearly-described key elements and be able to judge the quality of a report. At a minimum, Reports should include a statement of purpose and limitations, observations, results of any testing, conclusions, and recommendations. Such reports should not include any speculation or conclusions concerning medical causation.[16,224]

Since current analytical methods do not provide information on the health risks associated with mold exposures in the built environment,[221,222] health assessment is primarily based on the nature and extent of the mold and water/moisture damage and the type of reservoirs present (e.g., carpets and soft furniture). In most studies and a recent meta-analysis on the subject, semi-quantitative estimates of the extent of visible mold/dampness has been identified as being the best predictor of long and short-term health outcomes.[71,230–232]

Air and/or settled dust sampling can be used to defend hypotheses about the nature of the contamination, "hidden" sources of contamination, and whether or not the indoor air is similar to outdoor air.[215,224]

Investigation and remediation of mold and moisture damage in buildings must be based on an informed inspection augmented by the judicious use of existing sampling methods, primarily for the purpose of detecting any hidden damage.[16,230] The protection of remediation worker and occupants during renovations is essential.[16,230] In case of occupants with more serious pre-existing respiratory or other conditions, relocation may be appropriate.[233,234]

If mold is suspected, but not visibly detected after a thorough inspection, then microbial air sampling conducted in accordance with guidance documents can be useful.[16, 215, 235] This sampling may reveal evidence of indoor mold amplification or reservoirs, particularly of mold that is considered "hidden" behind walls and other building structures. If mold is being removed and there is a question about how far the colonization extends, then surface or bulk sampling, in combination with moisture measurements from affected building materials, may be useful. Sampling for airborne mold spores can indicate whether the mix of indoor molds is "typical" of the outdoor mix or, conversely, "atypical" or unusual at the time of sampling. Mold counts from cultures are often better than spore counts. These should be used when needed on the supersensitive patient.

Any mold sampling that does occur must be performed by qualified and experienced investigators familiar with current guidelines and, if applicable, local regulations. Samples should not be taken without a clear purpose (i.e., testing a hypothesis) and a sufficient number of samples must be taken to reliably assess the existing conditions.

It is not unusual for buildings to have a number of concurrent problems that affect IEQ or the perception of IEQ. Water and moisture damage can result in the release of gasses from some building materials.[221] Investigations of apparent or suspected mold-related health complaints must consider all possibilities. While mold damage comprises a large percentage of problem situations, studies of occupant complaints find that a high percentage have an outdoor air make up, standard, inappropriate and inadequate temperature and humidity levels, inadequate control of contaminants from outdoor air (including ozone, traffic pollutants, etc.), contaminants arising from equipment or activities within the building or house (including cooking activities), and poor air distribution.[231,236,237]

The process includes three of the five key elements: anticipation, recognition, and evaluation. While the industrial hygienist can reasonably anticipate that there will be mold exposures associated with water intrusion, mold may or may not be the primary cause of any health effect(s) that may be experienced by the occupants. The IH should ensure that, while investigating mold-related complaints, whether apparent or reported, active consideration of other possibilities affecting IEQ in the space is an essential part of the investigation.[238]

In addition to mold-related exposures, contaminants that are both directly and indirectly associated with water-related damages may also be affecting the occupants. These contaminants may include, but are limited to particulate and/gas/vapor contaminants associated with improper combustion ventilation or improperly operating utilities, such as carbon monoxide, nitrogen, and sulfur compounds, soot and other fine particles, fuel, and other volatile organic compounds (VOCs), etc.; VOCs from construction product degradation and/or off gassing, such as formaldehyde and other aldehydes, phenolics, and amines; organisms that proliferate under damp conditions or when maintenance is substandard, such as bacteria, amoeba, dust mites, cockroaches, and rodents; and animal and chemical-based allergens already present and/or exacerbated by the water damage.

Many potential contaminants may be present along with mold damage that can affect health or the safety of investigators, remediation workers, and occupants. For example, failure to recognize the presence of asbestos, radon, or lead-based paint could lead to their disturbance during investigative or remedial activities unnecessarily creating a new hazard.

Finally, there is a need to recognize the potential hazards associated with remedial alternative that may lead to the introduction of pesticides, ozone, chlorine dioxide, and other chemicals that could exacerbate existing health conditions or lead to new health issues.

TESTING FOR WATER DAMAGE

Problems with water and moisture are the most common trigger for indoor problems with mold and bacteria. It is critical to test for nonobvious sources and collection areas for water in building materials. Traditionally, nondestructive methods for non-destructive measurement of water in building materials have included the use of moisture meters and flexible fiberoptic devices such as WallChek.[239] Recently, the use of infrared cameras have proven very helpful in quickly detecting water in many types of building materials and providing useful photos.[240] Infrared devices are also being developed to quickly detect and identify spores in buildings.[241]

TESTING FOR MOLD SPORES

The most common means for testing for mold involves collecting air samples and then either observing them immediately under a microscope for total spores counts (living and dead spores), or growing them in a culture for several days to several weeks for viable or living spores. Most mold experts use several methods for collecting mold spores in air.

According to Curtis[4] it is important to collect mold air samples both indoors and outdoors, as an outdoor sample is often very useful for comparison. If the level of a certain mold is high in both indoor and outdoor samples, this would suggest that most of the indoor spores are from outdoor sources. Low outdoor levels of a particular mold (example *Cladosporium*) and high indoor levels of the same mold suggest there is an indoor source of mold contamination and water intrusion.

In addition to air samples, it is also important to collect samples for molds on surfaces such as walls, carpets, ceilings, furniture, wet wood, or wet drywall. These samples can be collected by using swabs or taking bulk samples of the material (such as water-damaged or mold-contaminated drywall) and then growing these samples in culture for several days on culture plates and then examining them under a microscope. Such bulk mold sampling is critical for testing Stachybotrys, a mold which is not readily airborne and found mostly indoors rather than outdoors. This mold usually puts out the trichothecenes mycotoxin, which can be devastating to the chemically sensitive patient. Mold cultures appear to be much more yielding than spore counts. We prefer cultures to mold spore counts.

TESTING FOR MYCOTOXINS

In high concentrations, mycotoxins cause the musty odor associated with mold contamination. Chemicals specific to molds such as aflatoxins, ochratoxins, and trichothecenes can be measured in dust, building materials, or in the air of buildings. To provide a sufficient amount for analysis, this testing requires a gram or more of the affected building material or at least one cubic meter of air obtained after several hours of air sampling.

Indoor areas can also be analyzed for volatile organic chemicals, which is another category of chemicals emitted by molds. Positive levels of benzene, hexane, acetone, and other organic chemicals can further document the presence of mold by air analysis for chemicals of moldy building. These samples are then sent to a commercial laboratory that can measure the mycotoxin content.

Testing for mycotoxins both before and after remediation can document the effectiveness of the remediation. If positive levels of mold toxins exist after an attempt at remediation, further remediation is necessary to bring the mycotoxin levels down to zero. Frequently after clean up, the mold count is extremely low but the mycotoxin count is still very high for the sensitive patient.[217]

Several companies can detect mold DNA (the genetic material) in dust or air samples. Dust DNA samples can be analyzed for the presence of approximately 100 types of common indoor molds. An Environmental Relative Moldiness Index (ERMI) score has been developed by comparing the concentrations of common indoor molds to the concentrations of common outdoor molds.[242] The ERMI scale has a range from −10 to +20. A level above +5 is considered high. Several scientific studies have found that homes with an ERMI score of +5 or above are associated with significantly higher levels of asthma.[243–246]

Dogs trained to sniff mold have been employed by a number of investigators.

Bacteria can grow in conditions similar to mold and can be collected on airborne viable samples or on surfaces, grown in culture, and measured in laboratories. Special testing is available for specific bacteria which cause infection such as Legionella.

Dehumidifier(s) are needed to keep the relative humidity (ambient air moisture) between 30 and 50 Rh during remediation, and sometimes after remediation.

Before effective remediation can begin, the cause of the water intrusion or damage must be repaired or corrected. Cracks or breaches in the foundation walls, leaks in the roof, leaky windows, plumbing leaks or drips, or heavy condensation from unwrapped piping. Any source of excess moisture or dampness needs to be corrected.

DECONSTRUCTION

The next critical step in effective mold remediation is the removal of all non-salvageable wet or contaminated building materials-and all means *all*. All materials must be removed, even those inside tight spaces and crevices. This includes damaged wallboards, paneling, decorative wood boards, wallpaper, and fiberboards. Insulation in ceilings, walls or floors, must also be removed. Non-salvageable carpeting, floor boards, vinyl flooring, hardwood flooring, sub-flooring, etc. must be removed too and preferably double-bagged and then discarded. No contaminated materials must remain. Any remaining mold can grow back inside the ceiling, wall, or floor cavities after reconstruction. Often padded furniture such as couches, love seats padded chairs, box springs, mattresses, etc. must also be discarded. Books and other paper items often transport mold spores and mold toxins and may need to be discarded as well. Remember, it is critical, that all work be done with negative air pressure.

CONTAINMENT

Heavy duty plastic sheeting, usually at least 6 mm thick, must be installed over entries or openings in walls or ceilings, separating work areas from non-affected areas prior to beginning work. Remember, no one should be inside the containment area except those performing the remediation, and the flaps should be kept taut at all times.

After removal of contaminated materials, the next stage is cleaning exposed framing an surfaces. First, there is the rough or initial cleaning. Second, the detailed surface cleaning and sanitizing. Rough or initial cleaning may involve media blasting, such as baking soda or dry ice blasting which removes viable mold. With smaller jobs, wire brushing or power brushing and light sanding may be used instead of media blasting.

After the initial removal of heavy visible mold, all of exposed remaining surfaces must be thoroughly wet-wiped, sanitized, and Hepa-vacuumed. That is everything must be meticulously wet-wiped (not dry-wiped) and Hepa-vacuumed: furniture, contents such as books, knick knacks, walls, ceiling, windows and floors, utilities, plumbing pipes—everything! They must be cleaned (wet-wiped) to as near dust-free as possible. Remember, cloths have to be wet or damp with a cleaning agent or biocide—a product that can kill mold.

CHEMICALS AND MORE

There is a plethora of chemical agents that can be used. Many of these products, while quite effective, can be mild to very caustic and require extensive ventilation (supplied air). Bleach is not recommended but many people use it. There are a number of non-caustic and non-allergenic products on the market, such as commercial grade hydrogen peroxide, vinegar, and enzyme-based cleaners which are effective and safer for occupants and technicians releasing little or no VOCs (volatile organic compounds).

After treating surfaces with a biocide, a good soap or cleaner is needed to remove heavy debris and staining. This can range from a household soap to a commercial low-VOC degreaser.

The efficacy of five common antifungal agents on six common molds were recently tested against six common molds.[239] The antifungal compounds used included (1) Sanimaster (containing 5%–20% quaternary ammonium chloride compounds, 1%–5% ethanol, 1%–5% non-ionic surfactants, and 1%–5% chelating agents), (2) 17% hydrogen peroxide, (3) 70% isopropyl alcohol, (4) bleach (containing 6.15% sodium hypochlorite and <1% sodium hydroxide), and (5) Sporicidin (containing total phenol 1.93% and glutaraldehyde 1.12%). The six common indoor molds tested included *Alternaria alternata*, *A. niger*, *Chaetomium globosum*, *Cladosporium herbarium*, *P. chrysogenum*, and *S. charatarum*. Each of the six antifungal agents (along with distilled water as a control) was used to individually treat each of the common six molds (36 comparisons in all).

Several different tests were run including: (1) Spore Germination Testing: Spore suspensions 10 μl were mixed with 10 μl of the antifungal agent. These spore solutions were then incubated for 12 hours at 25°C in the dark and spore germination rates were determined. (2) Sensitivity Spore Testing: The non-germinated spores from the Spore Germinating Testing Protocol (1) were washed with distilled water, incubated for another 12 hours and (2) checked for spore germination again; (3) Fungal Growth Tests: 1 mL of one of the antifungal plates was added to 90 mm petri plates containing one of the six mold species. Fungal growth in one or two weeks was then recorded; and (4) growth of fungi on treated wood blocks. One of the six fungi was inoculated on pine blocks that were previously sterilized by autoclaving. These fungi were allowed to grow for eight weeks on the blocks at 25°C and high humidity, and then treated with one of the antifungal agents. The blocks were tested for fungal growth (colony formation).

All five of the antifungal agents reduced spore germination by almost 100% for all six fungal species (experiment #1). However, after washing with water and reincubating for another 12 hours, mold germination ranged from 2% to 20% for each of the five antifungal treatments of each of the six fungi (experiment #2). This suggests that all five of the antifungal agents initially stopped mold germination and growth (fungistasis or mycostasis) but after the antifungal agents were washed off, did not completely inhibit growth in any of the six fungi. All five of the antifungal agents showed only a modest effect of inhibiting growth of each of the six fungi (experiment #3). Similarly, anti-fungal treatment of the pine blocks with any one of the five antifungal agents was found to only modestly reduce growth of any of the six fungi (experiment #4).[239] This study emphasizes that treatment with typical antifungal agents do not completely inactivate common mold sores. The effects of antifungal agents may be further reduced if mold spores are hiding in porous surfaces, such as upholstered furniture or carpets, and may not come into direct contact with the antifungal agents.[239]

Further indoor mold growth may occur from dormant spores if suitable conditions of water are present. Many types of mold are able to grow on wet building materials, stop growth and remain dormant during dry periods, and then resume both growth and mycotoxin production following reintroduction of water/moisture to the building materials. One study reported that spores of *S. charatum* and *P. chrysogenum* can survive for 2 or 3 years in drywall on dry ceiling tile stores under warm and dry conditions (25°C and under 60% relative humidity), and then resume vigorous growth and mycotoxin production following reintroduction of water.[247] In addition, the mycotoxins produced by molds can remain potent long after the molds that produced them have died.[247]

Long term water and moisture control is critical for solving indoor mold. The remediated area should be properly cleaned and dried. Even a small number of dormant fungal spores can grow vigorously when conditions become favorable for their growth. Also, the chemicals used to treat or limit fungal growth can be very harmful.

Recently, fungi (both mold and yeast) have become one of the leading causes of IAQ complaints.[248–255] Fungi become a problem within a built environment, where excessive humidity or moisture is present for an extended period of time.[86,249–262] The problem can originate from sudden water releases such as a ruptured pipe or large spill that goes untreated, or from a chronic condition such as a leaking roof or plumbing failure. Even high humidity or warm, moist air condensing on cool surfaces can cause fungal problems. Studies have shown that fungal occurrence in indoor environments was high during fall and summer seasons.[263] Environmental factors such as high temperature and relative humidity are among the factors contributing to the high occurrence of indoor fungi.

Fungi can grow almost anywhere in a building if conditions are favorable (moisture, temperature, and substrate) for their growth and activities.[264–266] If there is visible fungal growth on painted wall surfaces, it is possible that fungi may also be growing inside the wall cavity. The environment inside the walls of a structure often differs drastically from the outside and could create perfect conditions for fungal growth. If the wall remains wet for a prolonged period, fungal growth on the back side of gypsum board will possibly be worse than that on the front. A noninvasive but limited approach for observing fungal growth within the interstitial space (e.g., wall or ceiling cavity) can be performed using a borescope. Air sampling for the presence of fungal spores within the interstitial space can be performed using an inner wall sampling adapter with sampling cassette connected to an IAQ sampling pump.

Fungal contamination in the indoor environment is a complex issue and can cause health hazards for the inhabitants. All fungi are potentially harmful when they are allowed to grow in the indoor environment. Fungal spores, whether dormant, viable, or non-viable, can be harmful when inhaled. Fungal contamination of the indoor environment has been linked to health problems including headache, allergy, asthma, irritant effects, respiratory problems, mycoses (fungal diseases), and several other non-specific health problems.[267] The longer fungi are allowed to grow indoors, the greater the chances are that fungal spores may become airborne and cause adverse health effects. If indoor fungal contamination is not effectively remediated, fungal problems can spread to other non-affected areas and can cause health problems to the occupants. Inhalation of fungal spores is implicated as a contributing factor for organic dust toxic syndrome and noninfectious fungal indoor environmental syndrome.[268] In addition, concentrations of mycotoxins found in buildings have damaged cells of the CNS.[113,269,270] Plants inside will make a building prone to mold growth.

Correcting fungal contaminants requires understanding the extent of the problem and the under-lying causes. In many cases this is quite simple, for example when an obvious moisture source has affected only a small area resulting in observable visible fungal growth. However, this can be diffi-cult when the source(s) of moisture, their interaction with building conditions, or the location(s) of the growth are not readily apparent. When a complex fungal problem exists, it is wise to carefully assess the problem thoroughly and objectively before the beginning of remediation. To achieve a durable and effective solution, it is also imperative to understand the reason(s) for the moisture problem(s). Once pathways of moisture are known, then it becomes easy to locate hidden fungal growth. Knowing the source of the excess moisture is vital to correct it and prevent recurrence of the problem.

The success of remediating a large-scale fungal problem ultimately depends on how well the moisture and contamination problem is understood. If planning the remediation relies heavily on reports from past investigations, the accuracy and completeness of those efforts should be objectively assessed. It is essential to review the findings in the reports and evaluate how completely the important issues were assessed.

It is very important that fungal growth be physically removed and contained to prevent cross contamination of the living space. Attempts to kill or inactivate fungal growth and spores with products such as fungicides, heat, or fogging does not eliminate spores and usually not mycotoxins. The remediated area should be properly cleaned and dried. Even a small number of dormant fungal spores can grow vigorously when conditions become favorable for their growth and activities. Inhaling large number of dead or dormant fungal spores can be harmful and cause health hazards to building occupants. Also, the chemicals used to treat or limit fungal growth can be very harmful. If biocides are used they must be registered with the state government pesticide control board and must be in accordance with state or federal government laws by a licensed pesticide applicator or licensed remediation companies.

Their finding indicates that the commonly used fungicides in the indoor environment cannot completely kill all the fungal inocula. Most of the fungi form dormant spores when exposed with fungicides. These dormant spores can germinate and resume growth when a favorable environment is available to them. The results provide further evidence that physical removal of indoor fungal contaminated material is necessary as a proper remediation practice when dealing with indoor air quality problems. Their study strengthens the evidence that effect of fungistasis or mycostasis, a phenomenon linked to exogenous dormancy where fungal growth is inhibited without any effect on viability.

Ammonia

A final wipe should include an ammonia solution (3%–20% ammonia) to neutralize the mold trichothecenes. Although a single agent cannot neutralize all mold toxins, ammonia has been proven to be the most effective single agent against the mycotoxins produced by mold. Trichothecenes are very toxic (poisonous to humans and other animals) and difficult to destroy. So, spraying, fogging, or wet-wiping with ammonia in the middle or final cleaning stages is important to abate this very harmful chemical. Ammonia is also an effective biocide, (however, some contractors prefer to use it only at the final stages of the cleaning process because of its pungent nature)

OZONE

Oxone (O^3) is a natural occurring gas. However, there are generators that can produce ozone. Ozone is great for destroying bacteria, viruses, VOCs, MVOCs, odors, and molds. In short, it purifies the air. It is a very good idea to ozone at the very end of the remediation process. Ozonation should be performed by a contractor experienced in ozone generation to assure no one is in the home when the ozone is applied, and that ozone levels have returned to a safe level before anyone re-enters the home.

POST-REMEDIATION TESTING AND ASSESSMENT

Post-remediation air and surface sampling, along with a visual inspection, are highly recommended to insure the remediation was successful. Measurement for high humidity, mold spores, and residual mold toxins should be made. This post clean up assessment is usually performed by a hygienist or mold inspector—preferably by a different person that the one performing the remediation. We prefer mold plates because the spore counts are erratic. Any plate that grows five of mold colonies means the room is not decontaminated. Many buildings are still contaminated after mycotoxins clean up and cannot be lived in by the mold sensitive patient.

TREATMENT

1. Avoidance of molds and mycotoxins in the living and work quarters is essential for successful health.
2. Once mold and mycotoxin sensitivity has occurred, usually injection from every 4 days to weekly is necessary for 6–18 months.
3. Adequate nutrition for detoxification is necessary.
4. Sauna is often efficacious to get rid of the mycotoxins.
5. Immune modulators such as autogenous lymphocytic factor for low T cells in aberrant functions is necessary as well as gamma globulin, when gamma globulin is low, will help clear up recent infraction, fatigue, short-term memory loss, as well as loss of balance and fibromyalgia.

CONCLUSION

Do not take mold contamination lightly, and insure that the contamination is remediated appropriately. Follow the professional protocols, and you could prevent years of suffering and spending thousands of dollars on ineffective remediations.

REFERENCES

1. Blackwell, M. 2011. The fungi: 1, 2, 3 … 5.1 Million species? *Am. J. Bot.* 98(3):426–438.
2. Samson, R., J. Houbraken, J. C. Frisvad, U. Thrane, B. Andersen. 2010. Food and indoor fungi. In *CBS Laboratory Manual Series 2*, p. 390. Utrecht, The Netherlands: CBS-Fungal Biodiversity Centre.
3. American Industrial Hygiene Association (AIHA): Facts about Mold. December 2011. Accessed February 12, 2013. http://www.aiha.org/newspubs/newsroom/Documents/Facts%20About%20Mold%20December%202011.pdf

4. Curtis, L., A. Lieberman, M. Stark, W. Rea, M. Vetter. 2004. Adverse health effects of indoor molds. *J. Nutr. Environ. Med.* 14(3):1–14.
5. Kurup, V. P., H. D. Shen, H. Vijay. 2002. Immunotherapy of fungal allergens. *Int. Arch. Allergy Immunol.* 129:181–188.
6. Prester, L. 2011. Indoor exposure to mold allergens. *Arh. Hig. Rada. Toksikol.* 62:371–380.
7. Rea, W. J. 1997. Environmentally triggered small vessel vasculitis. *Ann. Allergy* 38:245–251.
8. Institute of Medicine. 2000. *Clearing the Air. Asthma and Indoor Exposures.* Washington, DC: The National Academic Press. https://doi.org/10.17226/9610
9. Rea, W. J., K. Patel. 2014. Reversibility of chronic degenerative disease and hypersensitivity, V. II. In *The Effects of Environmental Pollutants on the Organ Systems.* Boca Raton, FL: CRC Press, Taylor & Francis Group, Chapter 7, p. 542.
10. Rea, W. J. 1994. Chemical sensitivity. In *Sources of Total Body Load.* Vol. 2. Ch. 17. Boca Raton, FL: CRC Press, pp. 1031–1039.
11. Rall, T. W., L. S. Schleifer. 1985. Drugs affecting uterine motility. In *The Pharmacological Basis of Therapeutics*, A. G. Gilmann, L. S. Goodman, T. W. Rall, F. Murad, Eds., p. 938. New York: Macmillan.
12. Hintikka, E. L., M. Salkinoja-Salonen. 1997. Bacteria, molds, and toxins, in water-damaged building materials. *Appl. Environ. Microbiol.* 63:387–393.
13. Nielsen, K. F., S. Gravesen, P. A. Neilsen. 1999. Production of mycotoxins on artificially and naturally infested building materials. *Mycopathologia* 145:43–56.
14. Randolph, T. G. 1962. *Human Ecology and Susceptibility to the Chemical Environment.* Springfield, IL: C.C. Thomas.
15. American Society for Heating, Refrigeration, and Air-Conditioning Engineers (ASHRAE): Limiting Indoor Mold and Dampness in Buildings Position Document. June 27, 2012. Accessed February 12, 2013. https://www.ashrae.org/File%20Library/docLib/About%20Us/PositionDocuments/Position-Document---Limiting-Indoor-Mold-and-Dampness-in-Buildings.pdf
16. Prezant, B., D. M. Weekes, J. D. Miller. 2008. *Recognition, Evaluation and Control of Indoor Mold.* Fairfax, VA: AIHA.
17. Brase, S., A. Encinas, J. Keck, C. F. Nising. 2009. Chemistry and biology of mycotoxins and related fungal metabolites. *Chem. Rev.* 3903–3990.
18. Brasel, T. L., J. M. Martin, C. G. Carriker, S. C. Wilson, D. C. Straus. 2005. Detection of airborne *Stachybotrys chartarum* macrocyclic trichothecenes in the indoor environment. *Appl. Environ. Microbiol.* 71:7376–7388.
19. Vesper, S. J., M. J. Vesper. 2002. Stachylysin may be a cause of hemorrhaging in humans exposed to *Stachybotrys chatarum. Infect. Immun.* 70:2065–2069.
20. Mueller, A., U. Schlink, G. Wichmann, M. Bauer, C. Braebsch, S. Human. 2013. Individual and combined effects of mycotoxins from typical indoor molds. *Toxicol. In Vitro* 27:1970–1978.
21. Menard, A. et al. 1998. A gliotoxic factor and multiple sclerosis. *J. Neurol. Sci.* 154:209–221.
22. Croft, W., A. Lieberman, M. Stark, W. Rea, M. Vetter. 2002. Clinical confirmation of trichothecene mycotoxicosis in patient urine. *J. Environ. Biol.* 23:301–320.
23. Van Emon, R. A., I. Yike, S. Vesper. 2003. ELISA measurement of stachylysin in serum to quantify human exposures to the indoor mold *Stachybotrys chartarum. J. Occup. Environ. Med.* 45:582–591.
24. Iavacoli, I., C. Brera, G. Carelli, R. Caputti, A. Mainaccio, M. Miralia. 2002. External and internal dose in subjects occupationally exposed to ochratoxin A. *Int. Arch. Occup. Environ. Health* 75:381–386.
25. Hooper, D. G., V. E. Bolton, F. T. Guilford, D. C. Straus. 2009. Mycotoxin detection in human samples from patients exposed to environmental molds. *Int. J. Mole. Sci.* 10:1465–1475.
26. Aibara, K., N. Yano. 1977. *Mycotoxins in Human and Animal Health.* Park Forest South, IL: Pathotox Publishers Inc. pp. 151–161.
27. Shoemaker, R., D. House. 2005. A time-series of sick building syndrome; chronic, biotoxin-associated illness from exposure to water-damaged buildings. *Neurotoxicol. Teratol.* 27(1):29–46.
28. Tierney, G. L., T. J. Fahey, P. M. Groffman, J. P. Hardy, R. D. Fitzhugh, C. T. Driscoll, J. B. Yavitt. 2003. Environmental control of fine root dynamics in a northern hardwood forest. *Global Change Biol.* 9:670–679.
29. Galimberti, R., A. C. Torre, M. C. Baztan, F. Rodriguez-Chiappetta. 2012. Emerging systemic fungal infections. *Clin. Dermatol.* 30:633–650.
30. Maschmeyer, G., A. Haas, O. A. Cornely. 2007. Invasive aspergillosis. *Drugs* 67:1567–1601.
31. Garber, G. 2007. An overview of fungal infections. *Drugs* 61 (Suppl. 1):1–12.
32. Segal, B. H. 2009. Aspergillosis. *N. Engl. J. Med.* 360:1870–1884.
33. Mccarthy, M., A. Rosengart, A. N. Schuetz, D. P. Kontoyiannis, T. J. Walsh. 2014. Mold infections of the central nervous system. *N. Engl. J. Med.* 371(2):150–160.

34. Perfect, J. R. 2012. Iatrogenic fungal meningitis: Tragedy repeated. *Ann. Intern. Med.* 157:825–826.

35. Walsh, T. J., D. B. Hier, L. R. Caplan. 1985. Fungal infections of the central nervous system: Comparative analysis of risk factors and clinical signs in 57 patients. *Neurology* 35:1654–1657.

36. Li, D. M., G. S. de Hoog. 2009. Cerebral phaeohyphomycosis—A cure at what lengths? *Lancet Infect. Dis.* 9:376–383.

37. Soeffker, G., D. Wichmann, U. Loderstaedt, I. Sobottka, T. Deuse, S. Kluge. 2013. *Aspergillus galactomannan* antigen for diagnosis and treatment monitoring in cerebral aspergillosis. *Prog. Transplant.* 23:71–74.

38. Mikulska, M., E. Furfaro, V. Del Bono, A. M. Raiola, C. Di Grazia, A. Bacigalupo, C. Viscoli. 2013. (1-3)-β-D-glucan in cerebrospinal fluid is useful for the diagnosis of central nervous system fungal infections. *Clin. Infect. Dis.* 56:1511–1512.

39. Tortorano, A. M., M. C. Esposto, A. Prigitano, A. Grancini, C. Ossi, C. Cavanna, G. L. Cascio. 2012. Cross-reactivity of *Fusarium* spp. in the *Aspergillus galactomannan* enzyme-linked immunosorbent assay. *J. Clin. Microbiol.* 50:1051–1053.

40. Reinwald, M., D. Buchheidt, M. Hummel, M. Duerken, H. Bertz, R. Schwerdtfeger, S. Reuter, M. G. Kiehl, M. Barreto-Miranda, W. K. Hofmann, B. Spiess. 2013. Diagnostic performance of an Aspergillus-specific nested PCR assay in cerebrospinal fluid samples of immunocompromised patients for detection of central nervous system aspergillosis. *PLoS One* 8(2):e56706.

41. Antinori, S., M. Corbellino, L. Meroni, F. Resta, S. Sollima, M. Tonolini, A. M. Tortorano, L. Milazzo, L. Bello, E. Furfaro, M. Galli, C. Viscoli. 2013. *Aspergillus meningitis*: A rare clinical manifestation of central nervous system aspergillosis: Case report and review of 92 cases. *J. Infect.* 66:218–238.

42. Pettit, A. C., J. A. Kropski, J. L. Castilho, J. E. Schmitz, C. A. Rauch, B. C. Mobley, X. J. Wang, S. S. Spires, M. E. Pugh. 2012. The index case for the fungal meningitis outbreak in the United States. *N. Engl. J. Med.* 367:2119–2125.

43. Kourkoumpetis, T. K., A. Desalermos, M. Muhammed, E. Mylonakis. 2012. Central nervous system aspergillosis: A series of 14 cases from a general hospital and review of 123 cases from the literature. *Medicine (Baltimore)* 91:328–336.

44. Iihara, K., Y. Makita, S. Nabeshima, T. Tei, A. Keyaki, H. Nioka. 1990. Aspergillosis of the central nervous system causing subarachnoid hemorrhage from mycotic aneurysm of the basilar artery—Case report. *Neurol. Med. Chir. (Tokyo)* 30:618–623.

45. Herbrecht, R. et al. 2002. *Aspergillus galactomannan* detection in the diagnosis of invasive aspergillosis in cancer patients. *J. Clin. Oncol.* 20:1898–1906.

46. Hammond, S. P., L. R. Baden, F. M. Marty. 2011. Mortality in hematologic malignancy and hematopoietic stem cell transplant patients with mucormycosis 2001–2009. *Antimicrob. Agents Chemother.* 55:5018–5021.

47. Mantadakis, E., G. Samonis. 2009. Clinical presentation of zygomycosis. *Clin. Microbiol. Infect.* 15 (Suppl. 5):15–20.

48. McNulty, J. S. 1982. Rhinocerebral mucormycosis: Predisposing factors. *Laryngoscope* 92:1140–1143.

49. Hopkins, R. J., M. Rothman, A. Fiore, S. E. Goldblum. 1994. Cerebral mucormycosis associated with intravenous drug use: Three case reports and review. *Clin. Infect. Dis.* 19:1133–1137.

50. Martino, P., R. Gastaldi, R. Raccah, C. Girmenia. 1994. Clinical patterns of *Fusarium* infections in immunocompromised patients. *J. Infect.* 28(Suppl. 1):7–15.

51. Steinberg, G. K., R. H. Britt, D. R. Enzmann, J. L. Finlay, A. M. Arvin. 1983. *Fusarium* brain abscess: Case report. *J. Neurosurg.* 58:598–601.

52. Lamaris, G. A., B. Esmaeli, G. Chamilos, A. Desai, R. F. Chemaly, I. I. Raad, A. Safdar, R. E. Lewis, D. P. Kontoyiannis. 2008. Fungal endophthalmitis in a tertiary care cancer center: A review of 23 cases. *Eur. J. Clin. Microbiol. Infect. Dis.* 27:343–347.

53. Revankar, S. G., D. A. Sutton, M. G. Rinaldi. 2004. Primary central nervous system phaeohyphomycosis: A review of 101 cases. *Clin. Infect. Dis.* 38:206–216.

54. Al-Tawfiq, J. A., A. Boukhamseen. 2011. Cerebral phaeohyphomycosis due to *Rhinocladiella mackenziei* (formerly *Ramichloridium mackenziei*): Case presentation and literature review. *J. Infect. Public Health* 4:96–102.

55. Kauffman, C. A., P. G. Pappas, T. F. Patterson. 2013. Fungal infections associated with contaminated methylprednisolone injections. *N. Engl. J. Med.* 368:2495–2500.

56. Kainer, M. A. et al. 2012. Fungal infections associated with contaminated methylprednisolone in Tennessee. *N. Engl. J. Med.* 367:2194–2203.

57. Dixon, D. M., T. J. Walsh, W. G. Merz, M. R. McGinnis. 1989. Infections due to *Xylohypha bantiana* (*Cladosporium trichoides*). *Rev. Infect. Dis.* 11:515–525.

58. Lyons, M. K., J. E. Blair, K. O. Leslie. 2005. Successful treatment with voriconazole of fungal cerebral abscess due to *Cladophialophora bantiana*. *Clin. Neurol. Neurosurg.* 107:532–534.

59. Cortez, K. J. et al. 2008. Infections caused by *Scedosporium* spp. *Clin. Microbiol. Rev.* 21:157–197.

60. Montejo, M. et al. 2002. Case reports: Infection due to *Scedosporium apiospermum* in renal transplant recipients: A report of two cases and literature review of central nervous system and cutaneous infections by *Pseudallescheria boydii/Sc. apiospermum*. *Mycoses* 45:418–427.

61. Qureshi, Z. A., E. J. Kwak, M. H. Nguyen, F. P. Silveira. 2012. *Ochroconis gallopava*: A dematiaceous mold causing infections in transplant recipients. *Clin. Transplant.* 26:E17–E23.

62. Shoham, S. et al. 2008. Transplant-associated *Ochroconis gallopava* infections. *Transpl. Infect. Dis.* 10:442–448.

63. Stevens, D. A. 2013. Reflections on the approach to treatment of a mycologic disaster. *Antimicrob. Agents Chemother.* 57:1567–1572.

64. Gade, L., C. M. Scheel, C. D. Pham, M. D. Lindsley, N. Iqbal, A. A. Cleveland, A. M. Whitney, S. R. Lockhart, M. E. Brandt, A. P. Litvintseva. 2013. Detection of fungal DNA in human body fluids and tissues during a multistate outbreak of fungal meningitis and other infections. *Eukaryot. Cell* 12:677–683.

65. Zhao, Y., R. Petraitiene, T. J. Walsh, D. S. Perlin. 2013. A real-time PCR assay for rapid detection and quantification of *Exserohilum rostratum*, a causative pathogen of fungal meningitis associated with injection of contaminated methylprednisolone. *J. Clin. Microbiol.* 51:1034–1036.

66. Lyons, J. L., K. L. Roos, K. A. Marr, H. Neumann, J. B. Trivedi, D. J. Kimbrough, L. Steiner, K. T. Thakur, D. M. Harrison, S. X. Zhang. 2013. Cerebrospinal fluid (1,3)-β-D-glucan detection as an aid for diagnosis of iatrogenic fungal meningitis. *J. Clin. Microbiol.* 51:1285–1287.

67. Litvintseva, A. P. et al. 2014. Utility of (1-3)-β-D-glucan testing for diagnostics and monitoring response to treatment during the multistate outbreak of fungal meningitis and other infections. *Clin. Infect. Dis.* 58:62230.

68. Smith, R. M. et al. 2013. Fungal infections associated with contaminated methylprednisolone injections. *N. Engl. J. Med.* 369:1598–1609.

69. Kontoyiannis, D. P., D. S. Perlin, E. Roilides, T. J. Walsh. 2013. What can we learn and what do we need to know amidst the iatrogenic outbreak of *Exserohilum rostratum* meningitis? *Clin. Infect. Dis.* 57:853–859.

70. Mendell, M. J., A. G. Mirer, K. Cheung, M. Tong, J. Douwes. 2011. Respiratory and allergic health effects of dampness, mold, and dampness-related agents: A review of the epidemiologic evidence. *Environ. Health Perspect.* 119:748–756.

71. Quansah, R., M. S. Jaakkola, T. T. Hugg, S. A. Heikkinen, J. J. Jaakkola. 2012. Residential dampness and molds and the risk of developing asthma: A systematic review and meta-analysis. *PLoS One.* 7(11):e47526.

72. Tischer, C. G. et al. 2011. Meta-analysis of mould and dampness exposure on asthma and allergy in 8 European birth cohorts: An ENRIECO initiative. *Allergy* 66:1570–1579.

73. Park, J. H., J. M. Cox-Ganser. 2011. Mold exposure and respiratory health in damp indoor environments. *Front. Biosci. (Elite Ed.)* 3:757–771.

74. Krieger, J. et al. 2010. Housing interventions and control of asthma-related indoor biologic agents: A review of the evidence. *J. Public Health Manag. Prac.* 16:S11–S20.

75. Dally, K. A., A. D. Eckman, L. P. Hanrahan. 1981. A follow up study of indoor air quality in Wisconsin homes. In *Standard Handbook of Hazardous Waste Treatment and Disposal*, H. M. Freeman, Ed., Amherst MA: McGraw Hill Book Company, International Symposium on Indoor Air Pollution, Health and Energy Conservation.

76. Kreiss, K. 1990. The sick building syndrome: Where is the epidemiologic basis? *Am. J. Public Health* 80:1172–1173.

77. Small, G. W., J. F. Borus. 1983. Outbreak of illness in a school chorus. Toxic poisoning or mass hysteria? *N. Engl. J. Med.* 308:632–635. doi: 10.1056/NEJM198303173081105.

78. Centers for Disease Control and Prevention (CDC). 1994. Acute pulmonary hemorrhage/hemosiderosis among infants—Cleveland, January 1993–November 1994. *MMWR Morb. Mortal Wkly. Rep.* 43:881–883.

79. Etzel, R. A., E. Montana, W. G. Sorenson, G. J. Kullman, T. N. Allan, D. G. Dearborn. 1998. Acute pulmonary hemorrhage in infants associated with exposure to *Stachybotrys* and other funji. *Arch. Pediatr. Adolesc. Med.* 152:757–762.

80. Montana, E., R. A. Etzel, T. Allan, T. E. Horgan, D. G. Dearborn. 1997. Environmental risk factors associated with pediatric idiopathic pulmonary hemorrhage and hemosiderosis in a Cleveland community. *Pediatrics* 99(1):e5.

81. Hardin, B. D., B. J. Kelman, A. Saxon. 2003. Adverse human health effects associated with molds in the indoor environment. *J. Occup. Environ. Med.* 45(5):470–478.

82. Institute of Medicine. 2004. *Damp Indoor Spaces and Health.* Washington DC: National Academy Press.

83. Johanning, E., R. Biagini, D. Hull, P. Morey, B. Jarvis, P. Landsbergis. 1996. Health and immunology study following exposure to toxigenic fungi (*Stachybotrys chartarum*) in a water-damaged office environment. *Int. Arch. Occup. Environ. Health.* 68(4):207–218.

84. Mazur, L. J., J. Kim. 2006. The committee in the environmental health: Spectrum of noninfectious health effects from mold. *Am. Acad. Pediatrics* 11:1909–1926.

85. Storey, E., K. H. Dangman, P. Schenck, R. L. DeBernardo, C. S. Yang, A. Bracker, M. J. Hodgson. 2004. *Guidance for Clinicians on the Recognition and Management of Health Effects Related to Mold Exposure and Moisture Indoors.* Farmington, CT: U of Connecticut Health Center, Division of Occupational and Environmental Medicine, Center for Indoor Environments and Health.

86. Dales, R. E., H. Zwanenburg, R. Burnett, C. A. Franklin. 1991. Respiratory health effects of home dampness and mold among Canadian children. *Am. J. Epidemiol.* 134:196–203.

87. Burge, S., A. Hedge, S. Wilson, J. H. Bass, A. Robertson. 1987. Sick building syndrome: A Study of 4373 office workers. *Ann. Occup. Hyg.* 31:493–504.

88. Andersson, M. A., M. Nikulin, U. Kooljalg, M. C. Anderson, K. Rainey, K. Reuula, E. L. Hintikka, M. Salkinoja-Salonen. 1997. Bacteria, molds, and toxins in water-damaged building materials. *Appl. Environ. Microbiol.* 63:387–393.

89. Kilburn, K. H. 2002. Inhalation of molds and mycotoxins. *Eur. J. Oncol.* 7:197–202.

90. Kilburn, K. H. 2003. Summary of the 5th International conference on bioaerosols, fungi, bacteria, mycotoxins, and human health. *Arch Environ. Health* 58(8):538–542.

91. Menzies, R., R. Tamblyn, J. P. Farant, J. Hanley, F. Nunes. 1993. The effect of varying levels of outdoor—Air supply on the symptoms of sick building syndrome. *N. Engl. J Med.* 328:821–827.

92. Islam, Z., J. R. Harkema, J. J. Pestka. 2006. Satratoxin G from the black mold *Stachybotrys chartarum* evokes olfactory sensory neuron loss and inflammation in the murine nose and brain. *Environ. Health Perspect.* 114(7):1099–1107.

93. Mirocha, C. J., C. M. Christensen, G. H. Nelson. 1967. Estrogenic metabolite produced by *Fusarium graminearum* in stored grain. *Appl. Microbiol.* 15:497–503.

94. Bennett, J. W., M. Klich. 2003. Mycotoxins. *Am. Soc. Microbiol.* 16(3):497–512.

95. Vojdani, A., J. D. Thrasher, R. A. Madison, M. R. Gray, A. W. Campbell, G. Heuser. 2003. Antibodies to molds and satratoxin in individuals exposed in water-damaged buildings. *Arch. Environ. Health* 58:421–432.

96. Shinn, E. A., G. W. Smith, J. M. Prospero, P. Betzer, M. L. Hayes, V. Garrison, R. T. Barber. 2000. African dust and the demise of Caribbean coral reefs. *Geophys. Res. Lett.* 27:3029–3032.

97. Burge, H. A., C. A. Rogers. 2000. Outdoor allergens. *Environ. Health Perspect.* 108(Suppl. 4):653–659.

98. Burr, M. L. 1993. Epidemiology of asthma. *Monogr. Allergy* 31:80–102.

99. Howitt, M. E., T. C. Roach, R. Naidu. 1998. Prevalence of asthma and wheezing illnesses in Barbadian school children: The Barbados National Asthma and Allergy Study [Abstract]. *West Indian Med. J.* 47 (Suppl. 2):22–23.

100. Kilburn, K. H. 2009. Neurobehavioral and pulmonary impairment in 105 adults with indoor exposure to molds compared to 100 exposed to chemicals. *Toxicol. Ind. Health* 25(9–10):681–692.

101. Kilburn, K. H., J. C. Thornton, B. Hanscom. 1998. A field method for blink reflex latency R-1 (BRL R-1) and prediction equations for adults and children. *Electromyogr. Clin. Neurophysiol.* 38(1):25–31.

102. Straus, D. C. 2009. Molds, mycotoxins, and sick building syndrome. *Toxicol. Ind. Health* 25:617–635.

103. Kilburn, K. H. 1997a. Exposure to reduced sulfur gases impairs neurobehavioral function. *South. Med. J.* 90(10):997–1006.

104. Kilburn, K. H. 1997b. Chlordane as a neurotoxin in humans. *South. Med. J.* 90(3):299–304.

105. Kilburn, K. H., R. H. Warshaw. 1993. Neurobehavioral testing of subjects exposed residentially to groundwater contaminated from an aluminum die-casting plant and local referents. *J. Toxicol. Environ. Health* 39:483–496.

106. Kilburn, K. H. 2000a. Visual and neurobehavioral impairment associated with polychlorinated biphenyls. *Neurotoxicology* 21(4):489–499.

107. Kilburn, K. H. 2000b. Effects of diesel exhaust on neurobehavioral and pulmonary functions. *Arch. Environ. Health* 55(1):11–17.

108. Dally, K. A., L. P. Hanrahan, M. Ann Woodbury, M. S. Kanarek. 1981. Formaldehyde exposure in nonoccupational environments. *Arch. Environ. Health* 36(6):277–284.

109. Storey, E., K. H. Dangman, P. Schenck, R. L. DeBernardo, C. S. Yang, A. Bracker, M. J. Hodgson. 2004. Guidance for clinicians on the recognition and management of health effects related to mold exposure and moisture indoors. University of Connecticut Health Center Division of Occupational and Environmental Medicine-Center for Indoor Environments and Health.

110. Kilburn, K. H. 2000c. Chlorine-induced damage documented by neurophysiological, neuropsychological, and pulmonary testing. *Arch. Environ. Health* 55(1):31–37.

111. Kilburn, K. H., R. H. Warsaw, M. G. Shields. 1989. Neurobehavioral dysfunction in firemen exposed to polychlorinated biphenyls (PCBs): Possible improvement after detoxification. *Arch. Environ. Health* 44 (6):345–350.

112. Brasel, T. L., D. R. Douglas, S. C. Wilson, D. C. Straus. 2005. Detection of airborne *Stachybotrys chartarum* macrocyclic trichothecene mycotoxins on particulates smaller than conidia. *Appl. Environ. Microbiol.* 71(1):114–122.

113. Gorny, R. L., T. Reponen, K. Willeke, D. Schmechel, E. Robine, M. Boissier, S. A. Grinshpun. 2002. Fungal fragments as indoor air biocontaminants. *Appl. Environ. Microbiol.* 68:3522–3531.

114. Johanning, E., M. Gareis, K. F. Nielsen, R. Dietrich, E. Martbauer. 2002. Airborne mycotoxins sampling and screening anaylsis. In *Indoor Air 2002, The 9th International Conference on Indoor Air Quality and Climate*, Monterey, CA, June 30–July 5, 2002, H. Levin, G. Bendy, J. Cordell, Eds., Vol. 5, pp. 1–6. Santa Cruz: The International Academy of Indoor Air Sciences.

115. McLaughlin, C. S., M. H. Vaughan, I. M. Campbell, C. M. Wei, M. E. Stafford, B. S. Hansen. 1997. Inhibition of protein synthesis by trichothecenes. In *Mycotoxins in Human and Animal Health*, J. V. Rodricks, C. M. Hesseltime, M. A. Mehlman, Eds., pp. 263–273, *Proceedings of a Conferences on Mycotoxins in Human and Animal Health*, University of Maryland, College Park, Md., Oct. 4–8, 1976. Park Forest South, IL.: Pathotox Publishers.

116. Savilahti, R., J. Uitti, P. Laippala, T. Husman, P. Roto. 2000. Respiratory morbidity among children following renovation of a water-damaged school. *Arch. Environ. Health* 55(6):405–410.

117. Smoragiewicz, W., B. Cossette, A. Boutard, K. Krzystyniak. 1993. Trichothecene mycotoxins in the dust of ventilation systems in office buildings. *Int. Arch. Occup. Environ. Health* 65(2):113–117.

118. Yike, I., T. Allan, W. G. Sorenson, D. G. Dearborn. 1999. Highly sensitive protein translation assay for trichothecene toxicity in airborne particulates: Comparison with cytotoxicity assays. *Appl. Environ. Microbiol.* 65:88–94.

119. Kordula, T., A. Banbula, J. Macomson, J. Travis. 2002. Isolation and properties of stachyrase A, a chymotrypsin-like serine proteinase from *Stachybotrys chartarum*. *Infect. Immun.* 70(1):419–421.

120. Campbell, A. W., J. D. Thrasher, R. A. Madison, A. Vojdani, M. R. Gray, A. Johnson. 2003. Neural autoantibodies and neurophysiologic abnormalities in patients exposed to molds in water-damaged buildings. *Arch. Environ. Health* 58(8):464–474.

121. Jiang, Y., P. E. Jolly, P. Preko, J. Wang, W. O. Ellis, T. D. Phillips, J. H. Williams. 2008. Aflatoxin-related immune dysfunction in health and in human immunodeficiency virus disease. *Clin. Dev. Immunol.* 2008:1–12.

122. Jolly, P. E., S. Inusah, B. Lu, W. O. Ellis, A. Nyarko, T. D. Phillips, J. H. Williams. 2013. Association between high aflatoxin B 1 levels and high viral load in HIV-positive people. *World Mycotoxin J.* 6 (3):255–261.

123. Wu, F., J. D. Groopman, J. J. Pestka. 2014. Public health impacts of foodborne myctoxins. *Annu. Rev. Food Sci. Technol.* 5:351–372.

124. Creppy, E. E., I. Baudrimont, A. Marie. 1998. How aspartame prevents the toxicity of ochratoxin A. *J. Toxicol. Sci.* 23(Suppl. 2):165–172.

125. Brewer, J., J. Thrasher, D. Straus, R. Madison, D. Hooper. 2013. Detection of mycotoxins in patients with chronic fatigue syndrome. *Toxins* 5(4):605–617.

126. Curtis, L., W. Rea, P. Smith-Willis, E. Fenyves, Y. Pan. 2006. Adverse health effects of outdoor air pollutants. *Environ. Int.* 32(6):815–830.

127. Dennis, D., D. Robertson, L. Curtis, J. Black. 2009. Fungal exposure endocrinopathy in sinusitis with growth hormone deficiency: The Dennis-Robertson syndrome. *Toxicol. Ind. Health* 25(9–10):669–680.

128. Carey, S. A., C. G. Plopper, D. M. Hyde, Z. Islam, J. J. Petska, J. R. Harkema. 2012. Satratoxin from the black mold *Stachybotrys charatarum* induces rhinitis and apoptosis of olfactory sensory neurons in the nasal airways of Rhesus monkeys. *Toxicol. Pathology* 40:887–898.

129. Thrasher, J. D., M. R. Gray, K. H. Kilburn, D. P. Dennis, A. Yu. 2012. A water-damaged home and health of occupants: A case study. *J. Environ. Public Health.* 2012:1–10

130. Barnett, M. H., I. Sutton. 2006. The pathology of multiple sclerosis: A paradigm shift. *Curr. Opin. Neurol.* 19(3):242–247.

131. Hawker, K. 2011. Progressive multiple sclerosis: Characteristics and management. *Neurol. Clin.* 29 (2):423–434.

132. Stadelmann, C. 2011. Multiple sclerosis as a neurodegenerative disease: Pathology, mechanisms and therapeutic implications. *Curr. Opin. Neurol.* 24(3):224–229.

133. Burrell, A. M., A. E. Handel, S. V. Ramagopalan, G. C. Ebers, J. M. Morahan. 2011. Epigenetic mechanisms in multiple sclerosis and the major histocompatibility complex (MHC). *Discov. Med.* 11 (58):187–196.

134. Giovannoni, G., G. Ebers. 2007. Multiple sclerosis: The environment and causation. *Curr. Opin. Neurol.* 20(3):261–268.

135. Holmoy, T., H. Harbo, F. Vartdal, A. Spurkland. 2009. Genetic and molecular approaches to the immunopathogenesis of multiple sclerosis: An update. *Curr. Mol. Med.* 9(5):591–611.

136. Kakalacheva, K., C. Munz, J. D. Lunemann. 2011. Viral triggers of multiple sclerosis. *Biochem. Biophys. Acta.* 1812(2):132–140.

137. Marrie, R. 2011. Demographic, genetic, and environmental factors that modify disease course. *Neurol. Clin.* 29(2):323–341.

138. Van der Mei, I. A., S. Simpson Jr., J. Stankovich, B. V. Taylor. 2011. Individual and joint action of environmental factors and risk of MS. *Neurol. Clin.* 29(2):233–255.

139. Goverman, J. M. 2011. Immune tolerance in multiple sclerosis. *Immunol. Rev.* 241(1):228–240.

140. Hollifield, R. D., L. S. Harbige, D. Pham-Dinh, M. K. Sharief. 2003. Evidence for cytokine dysregulation in multiple sclerosis: Peripheral blood mononuclear cell production of pro-inflammatory and anti-inflammatory cytokines during relapse and remission. *Autoimmunity* 36(3):133–141.

141. McCoy, L., Tsunoda, I., Fujinami, R. S. 2006. Multiple sclerosis and virus induced immune responses: Autoimmunity can be primed by molecular mimicry and augmented by bystander activation. *Autoimmunity* 39(1):9–19.

142. Westall, F. C. 2006. Molecular mimicry revisited: Gut bacteria and multiple sclerosis. *J. Clin. Microbiol.* 44(6):2099–2104.

143. Kuhle, J. et al. 2007. Lack of association between antimyelin antibodies and progression to multiple sclerosis. *N. Engl. J. Med.* 356(4):371–378.

144. Kutzelnigg, A., C. F. Lucchinetti, C. Stadelmann, W. Bruck, H. Rauschka, M. Bergmann, M. Schmidbauer, J. E. Parisi, H. Lassmann. 2005. Cortical demyelination and diffuse white matter injury in multiple sclerosis. *Brain* 128(Pt. 11):2705–2712.

145. D'Haeseleer, M., M. Cambron, L. Vanopdenbosch, J. De Keyser. 2011. Vascular aspects of multiple sclerosis. *Lancet Neurol.* 10(7):657–666.

146. Purzycki, C. B., D. H. Shain. 2010. Fungal toxins and multiple sclerosis: A compelling connection. *Brain. Res. Bull.* 82(1–2):4–6.

147. Benito-León, J., D. Pisa, R. Alonso, P. Calleja, M. Díaz-Sánchez, L. Carrasco. 2010. Association between multiple sclerosis and Candida species: Evidence from a case–control study. *Eur. J. Clin. Microbiol. Infect. Dis.* 29(9):1139–1145.

148. Norgaard, M., R. B. Nielsen, J. F. Jacobsen, J. L. Gradus, E. Stenager, N. Koch-Henriksen, T. L. Lash. 2011. Use of penicillin and other antibiotics and risk of multiple sclerosis: A population-base case-control study. *Am. J. Epidemiol.* 174(8):945–948.

149. Parron, T., M. Requena, A. F. Hernandez, R. Alarcon. 2011. Association between environmental exposure to pesticides and neurodegenerative diseases. *Toxicol. Appl. Pharmacol.* 256:379–385.

150. Pisa, D., R. Alonson, F. J. Jimenez-Jimenez, L. Carrasco. 2013. Fungal infection in cerebrospinal fluid from some patients with multiple sclerosis. *Eur. J. Clin. Microbiol. Infect. Dis.* 32:795–801.

151. Malcus-Vocanson, C., P. Giraud, E. Broussolle, H. Perron, B. Mandrand, G. Chazot. 1998. A urinary marker for multiple sclerosis. *Lancet* 351(9112):1330.

152. Rieger, F., R. Amouri, N. Benjelloun, C. Cifuentes-Diaz, O. Lyon-Caen, D. Hantaz-Ambroise, T. Dobransky, H. Perron, C. Gemy. 1996. Gliotoxic factor and multiple sclerosis. *CR Acad. Sci.* 319(4):343–350.

153. Gutwinski, S., S. Erbe, C. Munch, O. Janke, U. Muller, J. Haas. 2010. Severe cutaneous Candida infection during natalizumab therapy in multiple sclerosis. *Neurology* 74(6):521–523.

154. Gilden, D. H. 2005. Infectious causes of multiple sclerosis. *Lancet Neurol.* 4(3):195–202.

155. Giovannoni, G., G. R. Cutter, J. Lunemann, R. Martin, C. Munz, S. Sriram, I. Steiner, M. R. Hammerschlag, C. A. Gaydos. 2006. Infectious causes of multiple sclerosis. *Lancet Neurol.* 5(10):887–894.

156. Wingerchuk, D. M. 2011. Environmental factors in multiple sclerosis: Epstein-Barr virus, vitamin D, and cigarette smoking. *Mt. Sinai J. Med.* 78(2):221–230.

157. Jacobson, D. M. 1996. Acute zonal occult outer retinopathy and central nervous system inflammation. *J. Neuroophthalmol.* 16(3):172–177.
158. Cermelli, C., S. Jacobson. 2000. Viruses and multiple sclerosis. *Viral Immunol.* 13(3):255–267.
159. Lee, C. 1983. Pioneer in diagnosing food allergy and treating by neutralization. *Clinical Ecology* 1 (3–4):181–184.
160. Miller, J. B. 1972. *Food Allergy: Provocative Testing and Injection Therapy.* Springfield: Thomas.
161. Reiter, R. J., D. Tan, C. Manchester, S. Lopez Burillo, M. Sainz Juan, C. Mayo. 2003. Melatonin: Detoxification of oxygen and nitrogen-based toxic reactants. In *Developments in Experimental Medicine and Biology Developments in Tryptophan and Serotonin Metabolism*, pp. 539–548. USA: Springer.
162. Keller, N. P., G. Turner, J. W. Bennett. 2005. Fungal secondary metabolism—From biochemistry to genomics. *Nat. Rev. Microbiol.* 3(12):937–947.
163. Stadler, M., N. P. Keller. 2008. Paradigm shifts in fungal secondary metabolite research. *Mycol. Res.* 112(2):127–130.
164. Hoffmeister, D., N. P. Keller. 2007. Natural products of filamentous fungi: Enzymes, genes, and their regulation. *Nat. Prod. Rep.* 24(2):393–416.
165. Brown, D. W., J. H. Yu, H. S. Kelkar, M. Fernandes, T. C. Nesbitt, N. P. Keller, T. H. Adams, T. J. Leonard. 1996. Twenty-five coregulated transcripts define a sterigmatocystin gene cluster in *Aspergillus nidulans. Proc. Natl. Acad. Sci. USA* 93:1418–1422.
166. Bohnert, M., B. Wackler, D. Hoffmeister. 2010. Spotlights on advances in mycotoxin research. *Appl. Microbiol. Biotechnol.* 87(1):1–7.
167. Kim, Y. T., Y. R. Lee, J. Jin, K. H. Han, H. Kim, J. C. Kim, T. Lee, S. H. Yun, Y. W. Lee. 2005. Two different polyketide synthase genes are required for synthesis of zearalenone in *Gibberella zeae. Mol. Microbiol.* 58:1102–1113.
168. Gaffoor, I., F. Trail. 2006. Characterization of two polyketide synthase genes involved in zearalenone biosynthesis in *Gibberella zeae. Appl. Environ. Microbiol.* 72:1793–1799.
169. Lysøe, E., S. S. Klemsdal, K. R. Bone, R. J. Frandsen, T. Johansen, U. Thrane, H. Giese. 2006. The *PKS4* gene of *Fusarium graminearum* is essential for zearalenone production. *Appl. Environ. Microbiol.* 72:3924–3932.
170. Proctor, R. H., D. W. Brown, R. D. Plattner, A. E. Desjardins. 2003. Co-expression of 15 contiguous genes delineates a fumonisin biosynthetic gene cluster in *Gibberella moniliformis. Fungal Genet. Biol.* 38:237–249.
171. Proctor, R. H., R. D. Plattner, D. W. Brown, J. A. Seo, Y. W. Lee. 2004. Discontinuous distribution of fumonisin biosynthetic genes in the *Gibberella fujikuroi* species complex. *Mycol. Res.* 108:815–822.
172. Desjardins, A. E. 2009. From yellow rain to green wheat: 25 years of trichothecene biosynthesis research. *J. Agric. Food Chem.* 57:4478–4484.
173. Lysøe, E., K. R. Bone, S. S. Klemsdal. 2009. Real-time quantitative expression studies of the zearalenone biosynthetic gene cluster in *Fusarium graminearum. Phytopathology* 99:176–184.
174. Schneider, P., M. Weber, K. Rosenberger, D. Hoffmeister. 2007. A one-pot chemoenzymatic synthesis for the universal precursor of antidiabetes and antiviral bis-indolylquinones. *Chem. Biol.* 14:635–644.
175. Balibar, C. J., A. R. Howard-Jones, C. T. Walsh. 2007. Terrequinone A biosynthesis through l-tryptophan oxidation, dimerization and bisprenylation. *Nat. Chem. Biol.* 3:584–592.
176. Schneider, P., S. Bouhired, D. Hoffmeister. 2008. Characterization of the atromentin biosynthesis genes and enzymes in the homobasidiomycete *Tapinella panuoides. Fungal Genet. Biol.* 45:1487–1496.
177. Fox, E. M., B. J. Howlett. 2008. Biosynthetic gene clusters for epipolythiodioxopiperazines in filamentous fungi. *Mycol. Res.* 112:162–169.
178. Elliott, C. E., D. M. Gardiner, G. Thomas, A. Cozijnsen, A. V. De Wouw, B. J. Howlett. 2007. Production of the toxin sirodesmin PL by *Leptosphaeria maculans* during infection of *Brassica napus. Mol. Plant. Pathol.* 8:791–802.
179. Steiner, U., S. Hellwig, E. Leistner. 2008. Specificity in the interaction between an epibiotic clavicipitalean fungus and its convolvulaceous host in a fungus/plant symbiotum. *Plant Signal. Behav.* 3 (9):704–706.
180. Kucht, S., J. Groß, Y. Hussein, T. Grothe, U. Keller, S. Basar, W. A. König, U. Steiner, E. Leistner. 2004. Elimination of ergoline alkaloids following treatment of *Ipomoea asarifolia* (Convolvulaceae) with fungicides. *Planta* 219:619–625.
181. Steiner, U. et al. 2006. Molecular characterisation of a seed transmitted clavicipitaceous fungus occurring on dicotyledoneous plants (Convolvulaceae). *Planta* 224:533–544.

182. Markert, A., N. Steffan, K. Ploss, S. Hellwig, U. Steiner, C. Drewke, S. M. Li, W. Boland, E. Leistner. 2008. Biosynthesis and accumulation of ergoline alkaloids in a mutualistic association between *Ipomoea asarifolia* (Convolvulaceae) and a clavicipitalean fungus. *Plant Physiol.* 147:296–305.

183. Lorenz, N., T. Haarmann, S. Pazoutová, M. Jung, P. Tudzynski. 2009. The ergot alkaloid gene cluster: Functional analyses and evolutionary aspects. *Phytochemistry* 70:1822–1832.

184. Chiang, Y. M., K. H. Lee, J. F. Sanchez, N. P. Keller, C. C. Wang. 2009. Unlocking fungal cryptic natural products. *Nat. Prod. Commun.* 4:1505–1510.

185. Cramer, R. A. Jr. et al. 2006a. Disruption of a nonribosomal peptide synthetase in *Aspergillus fumigatus* eliminates gliotoxin production. *Eukaryot. Cell* 5:972–980.

186. von Döhren, H. 2009. A survey of nonribosomal peptide synthetase (NRPS) genes in *Aspergillus nidulans*. *Fungal Genet. Biol.* 46 (1):S45–S52.

187. Coleman, J. J. et al. 2009. The genome of *Nectria haematococca*: Contribution of supernumerary chromosomes to gene expansion. *PLoS Genet.* 5:e1000618.

188. Scherlach, K., C. Hertweck. 2006. Discovery of aspoquinolones A–D, prenylated quinoline-2-one alkaloids from *Aspergillus nidulans*, motivated by genome mining. *Org. Biomol. Chem.* 4:3517–3520.

189. Perrin, R. M., N. D. Fedorova, J. W. Bok, R. A. Cramer, J. R. Wortman, H. S. Kim, W. C. Nierman, N. P. Keller. 2007. Transcriptional regulation of chemical diversity in *Aspergillus fumigatus* by LaeA. *PLoS Pathog.* 3:e50.

190. Kale, S. P., L. Milde, M. K. Trapp, J. C. Frisvad, N. P. Keller, J. W. Bok. 2008. Requirement of LaeA for secondary metabolism and sclerotial production in *Aspergillus flavus*. *Fungal Genet. Biol.* 45:1422–1429.

191. Bok, J. W., N. P. Keller. 2004. LaeA, a regulator of secondary metabolism in *Aspergillus* spp. *Eukaryot. Cell* 3:527–535.

192. Bok, J. W., S. A. Balajee, K. A. Marr, D. Andes, K. F. Nielsen, J. C. Frisvad, N. P. Keller. 2005. LaeA, a regulator of morphogenetic fungal virulence factors. *Eukaryot. Cell* 4:1574–1582.

193. Bok, J. W., D. Hoffmeister, L. A. Maggio-Hall, R. Murillo, J. D. Glasner, N. P. Keller. 2006a. Genomic mining for Aspergillus natural products. *Chem. Biol.* 13:31–37.

194. Bouhired, S., M. Weber, A. Kempf-Sontag, N. P. Keller, D. Hoffmeister. 2007. Accurate prediction of the *Aspergillus nidulans* terrequinone gene cluster boundaries using the transcriptional regulator LaeA. *Fungal Genet. Biol.* 44:1134–1145.

195. Bayram, Ö. et al. 2008. VelB/VeA/LaeA complex coordinates light signal with fungal development and secondary metabolism. *Science* 320:1504–1506.

196. Bok, J. W., D. Noordermeer, S. P. Kale, N. P. Keller. 2006b. Secondary metabolic gene cluster silencing in *Aspergillus nidulans*. *Mol. Microbiol.* 61:1636–1645.

197. Bok, J. W. et al. 2009. Chromatin-level regulation of biosynthetic gene clusters. *Nat. Chem. Biol.* 5:462–464.

198. Reyes-Dominguez, Y., J. W. Bok, H. Berger, E. K. Shwab, A. Basheer, A. Gallmetzer, C. Scazzocchio, N. Keller, J. Strauss. 2010. Heterochromatic marks are associated with the repression of secondary metabolism clusters in *Aspergillus nidulans*. *Mol. Microbiol.* 76(6):1376–1386.

199. Kosalková, K., C. García-Estrada, R. V. Ullán, R. P. Godio, R. Feltrer, F. Teijeira, E. Mauriz, J. F. Martín. 2009. The global regulator LaeA controls penicillin biosynthesis, pigmentation and sporulation, but not roquefortine C synthesis in *Penicillium chrysogenum*. *Biochimie* 91:214–225.

200. Hou, Z., C. Xue, Y. Peng, T. Katan, H. C. Kistler, J. R. Xu. 2002. A mitogen-activated protein kinase gene (MGV1) in *Fusarium graminearum* is required for female fertility, heterokaryon formation, and plant infection. *Mol. Plant Microbe Interact.* 15:1119–1127.

201. Atoui, A., D. Bao, N. Kaur, W. S. Grayburn, A. M. Calvo. 2008. *Aspergillus nidulans* natural product biosynthesis is regulated by MpkB, a putative pheromone response mitogen-activated protein kinase. *Appl. Environ. Microbiol.* 74:3596–3600.

202. Hallen, H. E., H. Luo, J. S. Scott-Craig, J. D. Walton. 2007. Gene family encoding the major toxins of lethal *Amanita* mushrooms. *Proc. Natl. Acad. Sci. USA* 104:19097–19101.

203. Luo, H., H. E. Hallen-Adams, J. D. Walton. 2009. Processing of the phalloidin proprotein by prolyl oligopeptidase from the mushroom *Conocybe albipes*. *J. Biol. Chem.* 284:18070–18077.

204. Matsuura, M., Y. Saikawa, K. Inui, K. Nakae, M. Igarashi, K. Hashimoto, M. Nakata. 2009. Identification of the toxic trigger in mushroom poisoning. *Nat. Chem. Biol.* 5:465–467.

205. Inamdar, A. A., M. M. Hossain, A. I. Bernstein, G. W. Miller, J. R. Richardson, J. W. Bennett. 2013. Fungal-derived semiochemical 1-octen-3-ol disrupts dopamine packaging and causes neurodegeneration. *Proc. Natl. Acad. Sci.* 110 (48):19561–19566.

206. Bloom, E., E. Nyman, A. Must, C. Pehrson, L. Larsson. 2009. Molds and mycotoxins in indoor environments—A survey in water-damaged buildings. *J. Occup. Environ. Hyg.* 6 (11):671–678.
207. Thrasher, J. D., S. Crawley. 2009. The biocontaminants and complexity of damp indoor spaces: More than meets the eyes. *Toxicol. Ind. Health* 25:583–615.
208. Ohtomo, T., S. Murkakoshi, S. Sugiyama, H. Kurata. 1975. Detection of aflatoxin B1 in silkworm larvae attached by an *Aspergillus flavus* isolate from a sericultural farm. *Appl. Microbiol.* 39:1034–1035.
209. Park, J. H., K. Kreiss, J. M. Cox-Ganser. 2012. Rhinosinusitis and mold as risk factors for asthma symptoms in occupants of a water-damaged building. *Indoor Air* 22:396–404.
210. Dennis, D. P. 2003. Chronic defective T-cells responding to superantigens, treated by reduction of fungi in the nose and air. *Arch. Environ. Health* 58:433–451.
211. Pestka, J. J., I. Yike, D. G. Dearborn, M. D. Ward, J. R. Harkema. 2008. *Stachybotrys chartarum*, trichothecenes mycotoxins, and damp building-related illness: New insights into a public health enigma. *Toxicol. Sci.* 104:4–26.
212. Ponikau, J. U., D. A. Sherris, E. B. Kern, H. A. Homeburger, E. Frigas, T. A. Gaffey, G. D. Roberts. 1999. The diagnosis and incidence of allergic fungal sinusitis. *Mayo Clin. Proc.* 74:877–884.
213. Braun, H., W. Buzina, F. Freudenschuss, A. Beham, H. Stammberger. 2003. Eosinophilic fungal rhinosinusitis: A common disorder in Europe? *Laryngoscope* 113:264–269.
214. Murr, A. H., A. N. Goldberg, S. D. Pletcher, K. Dillehay, L. J. Wymer, S. J. Vesper. 2012. Some chronic rhinosinusitis patients have elevated populations of fungi in their sinuses. *Laryngoscope* 122:1438–1445.
215. Ostry, V., F. Malir, J. Ruprich. 2013. Producers and important dietary sources of ochratoxin A and citrinin. *Toxins* 5:1574–1586.
216. El-Morsy, S. M., Y. W. Khafagy, M. M. El-Naggar, A. A. Beih. 2010. Allergic fungal rhinosinusitis: Detection of fungal DNA in sinus aspirate using polymerase chain reaction. *J. Layrngol. Otol.* 124:152–160.
217. HCRC Institute for Inspection, Cleaning and Restoration. 2003. *HCRC S520 Standard and Reference Guide for Professional Mold Remediation*. Vancouver, Washington: HCRC Press.
218. American Industrial Hygiene Association (AIHA). 2008. Mold prevention programs (Chap. 19). In *Recognition, Evaluation and Control of Indoor Mold*, B. Prezant, D. M. Weekes, J. D. Miller, Eds., pp. 223–225. Fairfax, VA: AIHA.
219. National Institute for Occupational Safety and Health (NIOSH). 2012. Appendix A: Building inspection checklist. In *Preventing Occupational Respiratory Disease from Exposures Caused by Dampness in Office Buildings, Schools, and Other Nonindustrial Buildings*. Cincinnati, OH: NIOSH Publication # 2013–2102, www.cdc.gov/niosh
220. National Academy of Science. 2004. Prevention and remediation of damp indoor environments (Chapt. 6). In *Damp Indoor Spaces and Health*. Institute of Medicine, pp. 270–310. Washington, DC: National Academy Press.
221. National Institute for Occupational Safety and Health (NIOSH). 2012. *Preventing Occupational Respiratory Disease from Exposures Caused by Dampness in Office Buildings, Schools, and Other Nonindustrial Buildings*. Cincinnati, OH: NIOSH Publication # 2013–2102, www.cdc.gov/niosh
222. Health Canada: Residential Indoor Air Quality Guidelines: Moulds. 2007. Accessed February 12, 2013. http://www.hc-sc.gc.ca/ewh-semt/alt_formats/hecssesc/pdf/pubs/air/mould-moisissures-eng.pdf
223. Ciaccio, C. E., K. Kennedy, J. M. Portnoy. 2012. A new model for environmental assessment and exposure reduction. *Curr. Allergy Asthma Rep.* 12:650–655.
224. Horner, W. E., C. Barnes, R. Codina, E. Levetin. 2008. Guide for interpreting reports from inspections/investigations of indoor mold. *J. Allergy Clin. Immunol.* 121:592–597.
225. American Industrial Hygiene Association (AIHA). 2008. Documentation (Chapt. 9). In *Recognition, Evaluation and Control of Indoor Mold*, B. Prezant, D. M. Weekes, J. D. Miller, Eds., pp. 105–125. Fairfax, VA: AIHA.
226. American Industrial Hygiene Association (AIHA). 2008. Documentation and reporting (Chapt. 13). In *Recognition, Evaluation and Control of Indoor Mold*. Prezant, B., D. M. Weekes, J. D. Miller, Eds., pp. 171–176. Fairfax, VA: AIHA.
227. American Industrial Hygiene Association (AIHA): Guidelines for Selecting an Indoor Air Quality Consultant. 2009. Accessed February 12, 2013. http://www.aiha.org/newspubs/newsroom/Documents/Guidelines%20for%20Selecting%20An%20Indoor%20Air%20Quality%20Consultant.pdf.
228. American Industrial Hygiene Association (AIHA). 2004. *Assessment, Remediation, and Post-Remediation Verification of Mold in Buildings*. Fairfax, VA: AIHA.

229. Canadian Construction Association: Mould Guidelines for the Canadian Construction Industry. CCA-82-2004. Accessed February 12, 2013. http://www.ccaacc.com/documents/cca82/cca82.pdf.

230. Health Canada: Fungal Contamination in Public Buildings: Health Effects and Investigation Methods. 2004. Accessed February 12, 2013. http://www.hc-sc.gc.ca/ewhsemt/alt_formats/hecs-sesc/pdf/pubs/air/fungal-fongique/fungal-fongique-eng.pdf

231. Dales, R., L. Liu, A. J. Wheeler, N. L. Gilbert. 2008. Quality of indoor residential air and health. *Can. Med. Assoc. J.* 179:147–152.

232. Park, J. H., P. L. Schleiff, M. D. Attfield, J. M. Cox-Ganser, K. Kreiss. 2004. Building-related respiratory symptoms can be predicted with semi-quantitative indices of exposure to dampness and mold. *Indoor Air* 14:425–433.

233. Hoppe, K. A., N. Metwali, S. S. Perry, T. Hart, P. A. Kostle, P. S. Thorne. 2012. Assessment of airborne exposures and health in flooded homes undergoing renovation. *Indoor Air* 22:446–456.

234. Iossifova, Y. Y., J. M. Cox-Ganser, J. H. Park, S. K. White, K. Kreiss. 2011. Lack of respiratory improvement following remediation of a water-damaged office building. *Am. J. Ind. Med.* 54:269–277.

235. Hung, L. L., J. D. Miller, K. H. Dillon. 2005. *Field Guide for the Determination of Biological Contaminants in Environmental Samples*, 2nd ed. Fairfax, VA: AIHA.

236. Davis, P. J. 2001. *Molds, Toxic Molds, and Indoor Air Quality.* Accessed February 12, 2013. http://www.library.ca.gov/crb/01/notes/v8n1.pdf

237. Nathanson, T., J. D. Miller. 1989. Studies of fungi in indoor air in large buildings. In *Airborne Deteriogens and Pathogens*, B. Flannigan, ed., pp. 129–138. Kew, UK: Biodeterioration Society.

238. American Industrial Hygiene Association (AIHA). 2006. *The IAQ Investigator's Guide*, 2nd ed. Fairfax, VA: AIHA.

239. Chakravarty, P., B. Kovar. 2013. Evaluation of five antifungal agents used in remediation practices against six common indoor fungal species. *J. Occup. Environ. Hyg.* 10:D11–D16.

240. Ceteras, N., S. Wood. 2006. Infrared Thermography and Water Damage Assessment. 2006. Accessed November 4, 2014. http://www.buildingsciencethermography.com/uploads/InfraMation2006_CeretasWood.pdf

241. Dixit, V., B. K. Cho, K. Obendorf, J. Twari. 2014. Identifications of household's spores using mid infrared spectroscopy. *Spectrochem. Acta. Mol. Biomol. Spectrosc.* 123:490–496.

242. Vesper, S., C. McKinstry, D. Cox, G. Dewalt. 2009. Correlation between ERMI values and other moisture and mold assessments of homes in the American Health Homes Survey. *J. Urban Health.* 86:850–860.

243. Blanc, P. D., P. J. Quinlan, P. P. Katz, J. R. Balmes, L. Trupin, M. G. Cisternas, L. Wymer, S. J. Vesper. 2013. Higher environmental relative moldiness index values measures in homes of adults with asthma, rhinitis, or both conditions. *Environ. Res.* 122:98–101.

244. Reponen, T. et al. 2011. High environmental relative moldiness index during infancy as a predictor of asthma at 7 years of age. *Ann. Allerg. Asthma Immunol.* 107:120–126.

245. Vesper, S., C. McKinstry, R. Haugland, L. Neas, E. Hudgens, B. Heidenfelder, J. Gallagher. 2008. Higher Environmental Relative Moldiness Index (ERMI) values measured in Detroit homes of severely asthmatic children. *Sci. Total Environ.* 394:192–196.

246. Vesper, S. et al. 2013. Higher environmental relative moldiness index (ERMI) values measured in homes of asthmatic children in Boston, Kansas City, and San Diego. *J. Asthma* 50:155–161.

247. Wilson, S., C. Carriker, T. Brasel. 2004. Culturability and toxicity of sick building related fungi over time. *J. Occup. Environ. Hyg.* 1:500–504.

248. Fernandez, D., R. M. Valencia, T. Molnar, A. Vega, E. Sagues. 1998. Daily and seasonal variations of *Alternaria* and *Cladosporium* airborne spores in Leon (North-West Spain). *Aerobiologia* 14:215–220.

249. Gregory, P. H. 1961. *The Microbiology of the Atmosphere.* New York: Interscience Publishers, Inc.

250. Grinn-Gofron, A., P. Rapiejko. 2009. Occurrence of *Cladosporium* spp. and *Alternaria* spp. spores in Western, Northern and Central Eastern Poland in 2004–2006 and relations to some meterological factors. *Atmospheric Res.* 93 (4):747–758.

251. Horner, W. E., A. Helbling, J. E. Salvaggio, S. B. Lehrer. 1995. Fungal allergens. *Clin. Microbiol. Rev.* 40:161–179.

252. Henriquez, V. I., G. R. Villegas, J. M. R. Nolla. 2001. Airborne fungi monitoring in Santiago, Chile. *Aerobiologia* 17:137–142.

253. Kasprzyk, I. 2008. Aeromycology—Main research fields of interest during the last 25 years. *Ann. Agri. Environ. Med.* 15:1–7.

254. Lacey, M. E., J. S. West. 2008. *The Air Spora.* Dordrecht, The Netherlands: Springer, 2006.

255. Simmon-Nobbe, B., U. Denk, V. Poll, R. Rid, M. Breitenbach. 2008. The spectrum of fungal allergy. *Int. Arch. Allergy Immunol.* 145:58–86.

256. Andrae, S., O. Axelson, Bjorksten, M. Fredriksson, N. I. Kjellman. 1988. Symptoms of bronchial hyper-reactivity and asthma in relation to environmental factors. *Arch. Dis. Child.* 63:473–478.
257. Strachan, D. P., C. H. Sanders. 1989. Damp housing and childhood asthma; respiratory effects of indoor air temperature and humidity. *J. Epidemiol. Community Health* 43:7–14.
258. Brunekreff, B. 1992. Associations between questionnaire reports of home dampness and childhood respiratory symptoms. *Sci. Total Environ.* 127:79–89.
259. Jaakkola, J. J., N. Jaakkola, R. Ruotsalainen. 1993. Home dampness and molds as determinants of respiratory symptoms and asthma in preschool children. *J. Expo. Anal. Environ. Epidemiol.* 3 (1):129–142.
260. Yang, C. Y., J. F. Chu, M. F. Cheng, M. C. Lin. 1997. Effects of indoor environmental factors on respiratory health of children in subtropical climate. *Environ. Res.* 75:49–55.
261. Pirasts, R., C. Nellu, P. Greco, U. Pelosi. 2009. Indoor exposure to environmental tobacco smoke and dampness: Respiratory symptoms in Sardinian children-DRIAS study. *Environ. Res.* 109:59–65.
262. Hwang, B. F., I. P. Liu, T. P. Huang. 2011. Molds, parental atopy and pediatric incident asthma. *Indoor Air* 2:472–478.
263. Shelton, B. G., K. H. Kirkland, W. D. Flanders, G. K. Morris. 2002. Profiles of airborne fungi in buildings and outdoor environments in the United States. *Appl. Environ. Microbiol.* 68:1743–1753.
264. Kirk, P. M., P. F. Cannon, J. C. David, J. A. Stalpers. 2001. *Ainsworth and Bisby's Dictionary of the Fungi*, 9th ed. Egham, UK: CABI Bioscience.
265. Barnet, H. L., B. B. Hunter. 1987. *Illustrated Genera of Imperfect Fungi*, 4th ed. New York: MacMillan Publishing Co.
266. Ellis, M. B. 1983. *Dematiaceous Hyphomycetes*. Slough, UK: Commonwealth Agricultural Bureau.
267. Burge, P. S. 2004. Sick building syndrome. *Occup. Environ. Med.* 61:185–190.
268. Nielsen, K. F. 2003. Mycotoxin production by indoor molds. *Fungal Gen. Biol.* 39:103–117.
269. Brasel, T. L., J. M. Martin, C. G. Wilson, D. C. Straus. 2005. Detection of airborne *Stachybotrys chartarum* macrocylic trichothecene mycotoxins in the indoor environment. *Appl. Environ. Microbiol.* 71:7376–7388.
270. Karunasena, E., M. D. Larranaga, J. S. Simoni, D. R. Douglas, D. C. Straus. 2010. Building-associated neurological damage modeled in human cells: A mechanism of neurotoxic effects by exposure to mycotoxins in the indoor environment. *Mycopathologia* 170:377–390.

2 Clinical Effects of Pollution

CLINICAL EFFECTS OF AIR POLLUTION

The clinical effects of air pollution are legion and have been elicited in Volume 2; newer information is discussed in this chapter. However, we have tried to categorize these areas in distinct anatomical physiological areas of the body. We will utilize them as follows: nasal, neurological, respiratory, cardiovascular, reproductive, immune, genitourinary (GU), and gastrointestinal (GI) systems. There is much overlap and therefore at times the lines will be hazy just as the clinician sees the individual patient. Many of the quoted studies are epidemiological and therefore the clinician will have to interpret for the individual patient. Each category will now be discussed.

OLFACTORY: NEUROLOGICAL

According to Guyton and Hall,[1] smell is the least understood of our senses but probably one of the most important senses to study because of the high potential for pollutant intake–induced hypersensitivity and hyposensitivity generation. Most have a supersensitive sense of smell that often incapacitates them even when it is masked. They can smell minute odors even those that appear to be one molecule or less. Hyperosmia is their true state. However, a few chemically sensitive patients have hyposmia and anosmia besides being chemically sensitive. These patients are usually in a masked or adaptive states resulting in their hyposmia.

Humans can accurately discern thousands of odors, yet there is considerable interindividual variation in the ability to detect different odors, with individuals exhibiting low sensitivity (hyposmia), high sensitivity (hyperosmia), chemical sensitivity (CS), or even "blindness" (anosmia) to particular odors as seen in chronic degenerative disease. Such differences are thought to stem from genetic differences in olfactory receptor (OR) genes, which include proteins that initiate olfactory signaling, while other differences appear to be environmentally induced particularly through the epigenes. OR-segregating pseudogenes, which have both functional and inactive alleles in the population, are excellent candidates for producing this olfactory phenotype diversity. Here, they provide evidence that a particular segregating OR gene is related to sensitivity to a sweaty odorant, isovaleric acid. They show that hypersensitivity toward this odorant is seen predominantly in individuals who carry at least one copy of the intact allele.[2] Furthermore, they demonstrate that this hyperosmia is a complex trait, being driven by additional factors affecting general olfactory acuity. Their results highlight a functional role of segregating pseudogenes in human olfactory variability, and constitute a step toward deciphering the genetic basis of human olfactory variability. Even though this segregation is possible, one cannot forget the significance of the complex environment in which we are exposed to daily. For this fact, it may overwhelm any type of genetics causing diseases. It is clear that the toxic environment of 80,000 chemicals can overwhelm genetics causing CS and chronic degenerative disease.

The genetic basis of odorant-specific variations in human olfactory thresholds, and in particular of enhanced odorant sensitivity (hyperosmia), remains largely unknown. In fact, the hyperosmia may be all environmentally induced if the pollutant load is in excess. OR-segregating pseudogenes, displaying both functional and nonfunctional alleles in humans, are excellent candidates to underlie these differences in olfactory sensitivity. Once the olfactory membrane is penetrated, the chemically sensitive in fact has a partially different pathway of cerebral tracts going first to the prefrontal cortex (PFC) and various areas there and later and probably less intense to the hypothalamus.[2] This is a different pathway from that of the normal individual where impulse goes from the olfactory tract directly to the hypothalamus with more intensity than to the PFC. We do not know whether this is a genetic variation or the tract is just altered by environmental overload.[3] We expect the latter to be the cause. To explore this hypothesis, Jacob et al.[3] examined the association between olfactory detection threshold phenotypes of four odorants and segregating pseudogene genotypes of 43 ORs genomewide. A strong association signal was observed between the single nucleotide polymorphism variants in OR11H87P and sensitivity to the odorant isovaleric acid. This association was largely due to the low frequency of homozygous pseudogenized genotype in individuals with specific hyperosmia to this odorant, implying a possible functional role of OR11H7P in isovaleric acid detection. This predicted receptor–ligand function relationship was further verified using the *Xenopus* oocyte expression system, whereby the intact allele of OR11H7P exhibited a response to isovaleric acid. Notably, they uncovered another mechanism affecting general olfactory acuity that manifested as a significant interodorant threshold concordance, resulting in an overrepresentation of individuals who were hyperosmic to several odorants. An involvement of polymorphisms in other downstream transduction genes is one possible explanation for this observation. Thus, human hyperosmial to isovaleric acid is a complex trait, contributed to by both receptor and other mechanisms in the olfactory signaling pathway. This sensitivity does not explain why some people get sensitive and others do not but may be one reason chemically there is some individual responses to illness. However, Hennies[4] has shown that an incitant (bacteria, virus, mold, mycotoxin, chemical, or EMF) can combine with protein kinase and phosphorylation will increase the sensitivities up to 1000% (Figures 2.1 through 2.3).

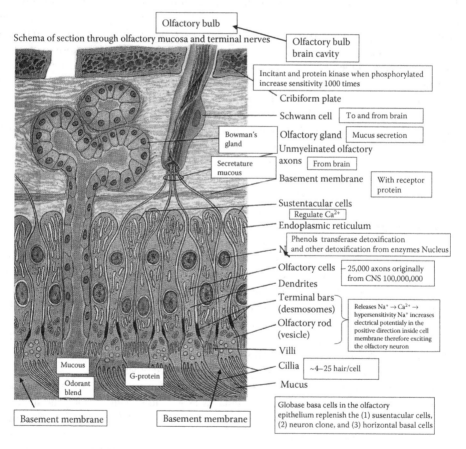

FIGURE 2.1   Areas of the odor-sensing apparatus and their potential places that may be sensitized by foods and chemicals. Schema of section through olfactory mucosa and terminal nerves. (Adapted from EHC-Dallas. 2002; Rea, W. J., K. Patel. 2015. *Reversibility of Chronic Degenerative Disease and Hypersensitivity*, Vol. 2, page 59, Figure 2.4. Copyright 2009. Reproduced by permission of Taylor and Francis Group, LLC, a division of Informa plc.)

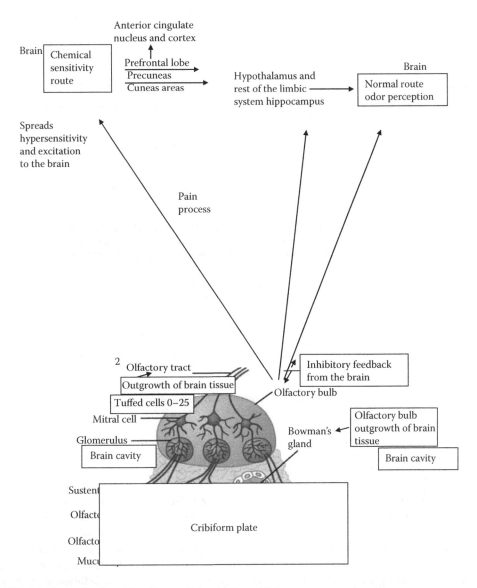

FIGURE 2.2 (See color insert.)   Route of chemical sensitivity versus normal route.

The CS will often increase constantly due to chronic stimulation. Chemically sensitive patients have a more intense impulse going to PFC in this anterior cingulate cortex than the hypothalamus, which is triggered more intensely in normal individuals. Therefore, chemically sensitive patients are different from normal individuals. These studies were performed by Azuma et al. by near-infrared (NIR) imaging.[1223]

The following case report is of a patient who had hyperosmia.

Nonaka et al.[5] reported a 42-year-old woman of nonherpetic acute limbic encephalitis (NHALE) whose CT perfusion (CTP) images revealed abnormalities of limbic system at the early stage. The patient had high fever, convulsion, and memory disturbance soon after having caught a common cold, and was admitted to a hospital where she developed progressive disturbance of consciousness. Although enhanced CT images of the brain failed to find any lesion, CTP images revealed a focal increase in the cerebral blood flow (CBF) and shortening of mean transit time in the bilateral hippocampi and amygdalae. MRI on the subsequent day showed high-signal-intensity lesions on

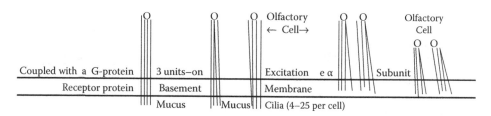

Coupled with a G-protein	3 units–on	Excitation e α	Subunit
Receptor protein	Basement	Membrane	
	Mucus	Mucus Cilia (4–25 per cell)	

Odor→

1. α subunit breaks away activating adenyl cyclase attached to the inside of the cilia membrane.

2. Adenyl cyclase converts many molecules of intracellular adenosine triphosphate into cyclic adenosine monophosphate (cAMP)

3. cAMP activates nearby membrane protein (gated Na^+ channel) that opens the gate allowing Na^+ and Ca^{2+} (large numbers) to pore through the membrane into the receptor cell cytoplasm.

4. Na^+ increases the electrical potential in a positive direction inside the cell—*exciting the olfactory neuron* transmitting action potentials to the CNS.

5. In the chemically sensitive, the Ca^{2+} combines with protein kinase A and C, and when phosphorylated, increases sensitivity up to 1000 times.

6. Number of action potential normal increases to 20–30 per second. In the chemically sensitive, it is more.

FIGURE 2.3 Receptor protein membrane inside and outside of receptors; protein threads its way through the membrane seven times folding inward and outward.

diffusion, T2-weighted and FLAIR images at the same area. Her consciousness improved by intravenous administration of high-dose methyl prednisolone together with other combination therapies. Her CTP images improved by 5 weeks after the onset, but she was left with mild memory disturbance, amenorrhea secondary to hypothalamic failure, hypersomia, and hypogeusia. In conclusion, CTP is sensitive enough to detect the lesions of the limbic system even in the early stage of NHALE. This patient was a setup for CS due to her prolonged hyperosmia to hypothalmic failure even though her health improved and she left the hospital. This condition was clearly environmentally induced by the viral infection.

Olfactory Sensitivity in Medical Laboratory Workers Occupationally Exposed to Organic Solvent Mixtures

According to Zibrowski and Roberson,[6] published epidemiological information relating to the effects of occupational exposure to organic solvents (OSs) to olfaction is limited and but in the view of the EHC-Dallas and the EHC-Buffalo, it is rapidly expanding. We have seen this type of CS patients numerous times.

The objectives of this pilot study of Zibrowski and Robertson[6] were to measure the chemosensory abilities of medical laboratory employees occupationally exposed to OS mixtures, to compare these with control workers employed within the same occupational setting and to correlate chemosensory performance with OS exposure history and with employees' hedonic (pleasantness) perceptions about workplace OS odors.

Twenty-four medical laboratory employees (OS-exposed technicians plus control workers minimally exposed to OS) completed a health-related questionnaire, a test of pyridine odor detection threshold, along with a gustatory detection threshold test involving aqueous quinine solutions. Estimates of cumulative hours of OS exposure (CSI) were calculated from self-reports.

OS-exposed laboratory technicians detected weaker concentrations of pyridine odor. Positive correlations were detected between CSI estimates to both pyridine detection and the degree that participants reported that OS odors were present in the workplace. However, no association was detected between pyridine detection and how unpleasant workplace OS odors were perceived. The OS-exposed participants were able to detect weaker concentrations of quinine. Compared to controls, OS-exposed workers complained more of experiencing several symptoms while working, including headaches, nasal irritation, and mild cognitive impairment. These are the symptoms that we see in several chemically sensitive patients.

The results of this cross-sectional pilot study indicated that, compared with controls, medical laboratory technicians exposed to low-level OS mixtures displayed evidence of elevated olfactory sensitivity (hyperosmia) to pyridine odor. The relation of this study's results to chemical intolerance warrants further investigation.[6] We have now seen thousands (18,000) of patients who fit this category. We have learned that many of these chemically sensitive patients subsequently develop vasculitis, and/or neuropathies or even malignancies or arteriosclerosis.

Olfactory Function in Migraine Both during and between Attacks

According to Marmura et al.,[7] people with migraine often report being osmophobic, both during and between acute migraine attacks. It is not clear, however, whether such reports are associated with changes in olfaction such as hyperosmia as measured by psychophysical testing. In this case–control study, they quantitatively assessed olfactory identification ability, which correlates with threshold tests of olfactory acuity, in patients with migraine at baseline (no headache), during migraine episodes, and after a treated attack and compared the test scores to those of matched control subjects.

A total of 50 episodic migraine subjects and 50 sex- and age-matched controls without headache were tested. All completed the University of Pennsylvania Smell Identification Test (UPSIT), a standardized and well-validated olfactory test.

At baseline, the UPSIT scores did not differ significantly between the migraine and the control study groups (median paired score difference: -1, $p = 0.18$). During migraine attacks, a minority of migraine subjects (8 of 42) developed microsmia (i.e., lower test scores by at least four points), suggesting that, as compared with their matched controls, olfactory acuity was somewhat impaired during migraine attacks ($p = 0.02$). This difference was less pronounced and not statistically significant after a successfully treated attack ($p = 015$).

People with episodic migraine were found to have similar olfactory function as age- and sex-matched controls, but a minority exhibit microsmia or hyposmia during acute attacks. The cause of this dysfunction is unknown, but could relate to autonomic symptoms, limbic system activation, or disorders of higher order sensory processing. We see this frequently with the chemically sensitive who then will have episodes of hypersomia but with hyposmia during the attacks because of the masking or adaptation phenomenon.

BASIC PHYSIOLOGY OF CS

Olfactory Membrane

Odors are inhaled by the nose and hit the olfactory membrane. The olfactory membrane, the histology of which is shown in Figure 2.2, lies in the superior part of each nostril. Medially, the olfactory membrane folds downward along the surface of the superior septum; laterally, it folds over the superior turbinate and even over a small portion of the upper surface of the middle turbinate. In each nostril, the olfactory membrane has a surface area of about 2.4 cm^2. This area could be sensitized in chemically sensitive patients, but most likely the nerve higher up is also damaged. Frequently due to pollen, food, or pollutant exposure, the membrane swells and will give partial or total blockages and also appears to leak dripping fluid. However, it is open enough to perceive the enhanced odor perception in the chemically sensitive, which often can give a local as well as a regional reaction in the brain.

Olfactory Cells

The receptor cells for the smell sensation are the olfactory cells (Figure 2.2), which are actually bipolar nerve cells derived originally from the central nervous system (CNS). There are about 100 million of these cells in the olfactory epithelium interspersed among sustententacular cells, as shown in Figure 2.2. The mucosal end of the olfactory cell forms a knob from which 4–25 olfactory hair (also called olfactory cilia), measuring 0.3 μm in diameter and up to 200 μm in length, project into the mucus that coats the inner surface of the nasal cavity. These projecting olfactory cilia form a dense mat in the mucus, and it is these cilia that react to odors in the air and stimulate the olfactory cells, as discussed later. Spaced among the olfactory cells in the olfactory membrane are many small Bowman's glands that secrete mucus onto the surface of the olfactory membrane. Often the chemically sensitive will drip constantly due to pollutant stimulation of these glands.

TASTE

Imagine the worst cold you have ever had in your life. Your nose is completely blocked. You struggle for air. The pressure in your sinuses sends pain streaking around your head. You cannot smell. So eating food is like chewing on cardboard; you are nauseated and you feel utterly miserable. Now imagine that the symptoms, even if they ease for a week or so, always come back. You are never free. Unfortunately, this is the very real life of patients with chronic sinusitis—a disease of the nose and other regions of the upper airway that affects about 35 million Americans. For many of these people, treatment often involves prolonged course of antibiotics and steroids. If those drugs do not work, sufferers have to undergo delicate surgery to clean out infected cavities in their skull.

This surgery seems to be happening more often these days because modern society's excessive use of antibiotics has perversely caused those medications to become less effective.

According to Lee and Cohen,[8] today one out of every five antibiotic prescriptions in the United States is for an adult with rhinosinusitis, and the illness has become part of vicious cycle, contributing to the rise of such dangerous antibiotic-resistant bacteria as methicillin-resistant *Staphylococcus aureus* (MRSA). These are the patients without proper serial dilution in neutralization intradermal techniques.

The average person breathes in more than 10,000 L of air a day, much of it through the nose, and that air contains countless bacteria, fungi, and viruses. Our nose is the front line of respiratory defense. Every time we breathe, particles of debris, viruses, bacteria, and fungal spores get trapped there. Yet, amazingly, most people walk around breathing freely without any kind of airway infection. It turns out that one previously unsuspected reason may be, literally, on our tongue. Proteins—called taste receptors—that detect bitter flavors have been found to do double duty, also defending against bacteria. Our own research has shown that these receptors, also found in the nose, trigger three bacteria-fighting responses. First, they send signals that cause the cells to flick invaders away by moving cilia—tiny, hairlike projection—on the cells' surface. Second, the receptor proteins tell cells to release nitric oxide, which kills bacteria. Third, receptors signal still other cells to send out antimicrobial proteins called defensins.

Even more astonishing, several researchers have found these receptors not just on the tongue and nose but elsewhere in the airways, as well as the in the heart, lungs, intestines, and more body organs. Along with other scientists, we now believe these receptors are a part of an innate human immune system that is different—but potentially faster—than the more familiar features of antibodies and invader-fighting cells that circulate through the body. It can take many hours or days for the immune system to produce specific antibodies against viruses or bacteria. The taste receptor response, though more of a general reaction and less tightly targeted to particular bacteria, happens in just minutes—a true early warning system.

TASTE FOR DANGER

If you think of taste receptors as sentinels that react to substances that come into the body, then their immune system role makes sense. When they reside in the cells that form taste buds on the tongue, the receptors prompt the cells to send signals to the brain that inform it about the nutritional value or potential toxicity of the foods in the mouth. According to Lee and Cohen,[8] the tongue detects five basic types of tastes: bitter, sweet, salty, sour, and savory, also known as umami. Our sense of taste acts as the gatekeeper to the digestive system, giving us information about the food we are eating so that we can decide whether or not to swallow it. Bitter taste receptors can detect the presence of poisonous plant chemicals, including a class of chemicals called alkaloids that include strychnine and nicotine. The tastes described as "bitter" are often perceived by the brain as unpleasant because receptors evolved to signal the presence of potentially harmful chemicals. Warning against harm is a key to survival, which may be why there are so many different bitter receptors. Sweet, salty, sour, and umami have only one type of receptor each, but at least 25 types of receptors detect bitter compounds. Known as taste family type 2 receptors (T2Rs), they probably evolved to recognize and protect from swallowing a wide variety of poisons. Early hints of a role elsewhere in the body emerged in 2009, when researchers at the University of Iowa discovered T2Rs on epithelial cells that line the lungs. A sticky layer of mucus on top of these cells traps microbes and irritants when inhaled. Then the tiny cilia on the cells beat 8–15 times each second, in synchrony, to push the irritants toward the throat, where you swallow them or spit them out. The Iowa team discovered that cilia in human lung cells actually beat faster when their T2Rs were stimulated by bitter compounds, suggesting that the T2Rs help the airway clear potentially dangerous inhaled substances that, in the mouth, would taste bitter. Around the same time, investigators at the University of Colorado Anschutz Medical Campus were studying bitter taste receptors found on a special type of cell in the rat nose that appears to react to irritants. They discovered that these cells, termed solitary chemosensory cells, become more active when they detect bacterial molecules called acyl-homoserine lactones (AHLs). AHLs are released by dangerous gram-negative bacteria when these microbes form biofilms.[8] Biofilms are communities of bacteria, such as *Pseudomonas aeruginosa*, that stick to one another by forming a matrix, making them up to 1000-fold more resistant to antibiotics than less organized bacteria and thus are much harder to kill. The researchers from Colorado showed the biofilm-inducing AHL molecules stimulated activity in the chemosensory cells.[8] AHLs were thus the first specific bacterial chemical shown to stimulate cells with bitter taste receptors, supporting the notion that receptors respond to outside invaders. Intrigued by these findings, they began searching for taste receptors in human nasal epithelial cells in 2011, collaborating with experts in taste at the Monell Chemical Senses Center in Philadelphia, a premier institution for smell and taste research. Their investigation started out as a small side project to determine whether they could find bitter taste receptors in nasal cells just as the Iowa researchers found them in the lung. However, it quickly became a big focus in our laboratory when they saw hints that certain taste receptors might affect people's susceptibility to rhinosinusitis.

SUPERTASTERS

According to Lee and Cohen,[8] they looked specifically for one bitter taste receptor, T2R38, the most well studied of the T2R family. The human T2R38 protein comes in several varieties, the result of slight differences, called polymorphisms, in the genes that encode them. And they did find several most common versions in the cilia lining the nose and sinuses. The discovery of this receptor menagerie led them to explore how the different T2R38 forms affect the behavior of sinus and nasal cells. Two forms in particular have dramatically different effects on taste when present in the tongue. One of these versions is very sensitive as a taste detector in the mouth, and the other one does not respond

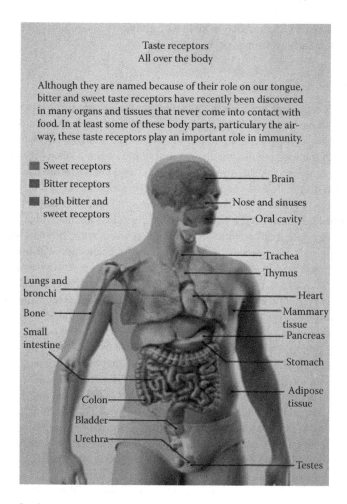

Taste receptors
All over the body

Although they are named because of their role on our tongue, bitter and sweet taste receptors have recently been discovered in many organs and tissues that never come into contact with food. In at least some of these body parts, particulary the airway, these taste receptors play an important role in immunity.

■ Sweet receptors
■ Bitter receptors
■ Both bitter and sweet receptors

Brain
Nose and sinuses
Oral cavity
Trachea
Thymus
Heart
Mammary tissue
Pancreas
Stomach
Adipose tissue
Lungs and bronchi
Bone
Small intestine
Colon
Bladder
Urethra
Testes

FIGURE 2.4 (See color insert.)   Taste receptors all over the body. (Adapted from Lee, R. J., N. A. Cohen. 2016. *Sci. Am.* 314(2):38–43; Reproduced with permission. Copyright © 2016 Scientific American, a division of Nature America, Inc. All rights reserved.)

at all. About 30% of Caucasians inherit two copies of the gene for the insensitive T2R38 variant (one from each parent), and these individuals are "nontasters" for certain bitter compounds. About 20% of Caucasians have two copies of the gene for the functional T2R38, and these individuals perceive those same compounds as intensely bitter; such people are known as "supertasters." Those with one copy of each gene variant fall somewhere in between these extremes (Figure 2.4).

Examining tissue removed during sinus and nasal surgeries, Lee and Cohen[8] compared the behaviors of nasal cells possessing one or the other of these two forms. (Lee and Cohen[8] knew which types were in the cells by sequencing their genes.) To get the receptors to react, they exposed the cells to a chemical called phenylthiocarbamide (PTC), often used for T2R38 taste testing. And they were excited to see that the cells from supertaster patients, but not those from the nontasters, produced large amounts of nitric oxide.[8] This finding gave another boost to their idea of a taste–immunity connection. Nitric oxide does two important things against bacteria in the airway. It can stimulate airway cells to increase ciliary beating. It can also directly kill bacteria. As nitric oxide molecules form a gas, they can rapidly diffuse out of the cells lining the airway into the mucus and then into bacteria. Once inside, the substance can damage membranes, enzymes, and DNA.

Ordinarily, sinuses produce large amounts of nitric oxide that travel through the airway, which helps to keep it free of infection. These twin modes of antibacterial activity made us think that different T2R38 versions might alter people's susceptibility to upper respiratory infections. And indeed, in the lab, Lee and Cohen[8] found that the nitric oxide produced by supertaster nasal cells during T2R38 activation caused faster ciliary beating and directly killed more bacteria than nontaster nasal cells. Lee and Cohen[8] next discovered that the same class of bacterial compounds that were previously shown to activate mouse nasal chemosensory cells, AHLs, directly activates human T2R38 receptors. Nasal cells from supertasters detect bacterial AHLs through T2R38 and produce nitric oxide, whereas cells from nontasters do not. These properties make cells from supertasters much better at killing AHL-producing bacteria than cells from nontasters. From these observations, we concluded that the T2R38 bitter receptor is used by airway epithelial cells to detect bacterial activity and activate defenses. Since the discovery of T2R38 in cilia of human nasal epithelial cells, the knowledge of the role of taste receptors in the nose has expanded even further.

These receptors also appear in solitary chemosensory cells in the human nose, similar to those found in mice. Solitary chemosensory cells are solitary, dispersed widely throughout the nasal cavity, making up about only 1% of the cells. The cells have both T2R bitter receptors and T1R sweet receptors. When T2Rs in these cells get stimulated, it has been found that the solitary cells release a signal to surrounding cells that prompts them to release antimicrobial proteins called defensins into the airway mucus. Defensins are capable of killing many illness-causing bacteria, including *P. aeruginosa* and MRSA. The sweet taste receptors, when stimulated, shut down the activity of the bitter ones, probably to prevent cells from releasing too many proteins at an inappropriate time. Sweet receptors had already been found in other body parts, such as the pancreas, where they sense sugars in the blood and stimulate cells to produce insulin that regulates glucose levels. The work on the nasal cells, however, showed that sweet and bitter receptors in the same cell have opposing roles. These experiments suggest to us that taste receptors constitute an early-warning alarm of the airway immune response. They seem different from the most well-studied class of early-warning proteins, which are known as toll-like receptors (TLRs). The TLRs also activate immune responses when stimulated by certain bacterial molecules, as the T2Rs appear to do. However, there is at least one important difference: some TLR responses—such as signaling genes to start creating antibodies that mark invaders for destruction—are much slower, taking several hours or even days. T2R38 and its bitter cousins, in contrast, produce responses within seconds to minutes. These taste receptors might be very important during the onset of infection by activating a kind of "locked and loaded" instant reaction. Other immune receptors may be more crucial for fighting a prolonged infection, calling up the troops when the first response is not sufficient.

VULNERABLE PEOPLE

The large number of genetic varieties in T2R bitter taste receptors makes their role in immunity even more intriguing. Most of the 25 bitter receptors have genetic variations that increase or decrease their abilities, thus making people who have them more or less sensitive to bitter-tasting substances. If a reaction to bitterness is indeed a part of the immune response to invading bacteria, these same genetic variations may also create differences in the way people combat infections. Increased bitter receptor function may confer greater protection against infection, whereas lower function may increase susceptibility. Lee and Cohen[8] have begun to test this idea in people and have hints that it is correct. The millions of patients with chronic rhinosinusitis constitute a natural test population and a group in need of help. When given quality-of-life questionnaires, rhinosinusitis patients report worse scores than patients with several heart and lung diseases. Plus, rhinosinusitis patients can develop dangerous lung infections and exacerbate lower airway diseases such as asthma.

Lee and Cohen[8] have looked at microbiology cultures from patients with the condition. Supertasters did get rhinosinusitis—they are not immune—but they had a much lower frequency of nasal infections with gram-negative bacteria than did nontasters. That makes sense because gram-negative bacteria produce AHLs, the compounds that, by triggering receptors, lead cells in these people to release microbe-killing nitric oxide. Other bacteria do not produce AHL, so they would not run afoul of these immune defenses. Further clinical research has supported the role of T2R38 in sinusitis. Two studies from the group at Pennsylvania demonstrated that people with two copies of the T2R38 supertaster gene are less likely to get severe rhinosinusitis than are patients with two nontaster copies or even patients with one copy of each. A study by otolaryngologist Martin Desrosiers of CHUM in Montreal and his colleagues verified that the T2R38 nontaster gene occurs more often in patients than in healthy people. That study found that rhinosinusitis severity is also associated with variants in two other T2R receptor types, T2R14 and T2R49. In organs beyond the nose, connections between taste receptors and immunity are starting to show up. In 2014, scientists showed that when confronted with pathogenic *Escherichia coli*, chemosensory cells in the urinary tract use T2Rs to stimulate the bladder to release urine. This could be the body trying to flush bacteria out and prevent bladder infections. Another recent study has shown that white blood cells—which include neutrophils and lymphocytes and are crucial components of the immune system—also use T2R38 to detect *Pseudomonas* AHLs. At present, we are trying to learn whether chemicals that activate T2R receptors can work as medicine for rhinosinusitis patients by stimulating stronger bacteria-killing responses. The vast array of bitter compounds in foods and drink everyday could be potential therapeutics, including humulones and lupulons from hoppy beers, isothiocyanates from green vegetables such as brussels sprouts, and bitter chemicals from citrus such as limonin. Absinthin, a bitter chemical isolated from the wormwood plant and found in the liquor absinthe, has been shown to stimulate solitary chemosensory cell T2Rs. In the lab, we are investigating several formulations that could work as drugs. Novel medications based on bitter compounds might someday be used to combat infection without using conventional antibiotics. Lee and Cohen[8] believe it is also possible that taste or genetic testing of T2Rs might eventually be used to predict susceptibility to infections. The natural variations in these taste receptors may help us answer an age-old question: Why do some people frequently get respiratory infections, whereas others never seem to get sick? Using bitter receptors to solve this puzzle would be sweet indeed.

STIMULATION OF THE OLFACTORY CELLS

Mechanism of Excitation of the Olfactory Cells

According to Guyton and Hall,[1] the portion of each olfactory cell that responds to the olfactory chemical stimuli is the olfactory cilia. The odorant substance, when come in contact with the olfactory membrane surface, first diffuses into the mucus that covers the cilia. Then it binds with receptor proteins in the membrane of each cilium (Figure 2.1). Each receptor protein is actually a long molecule that threads its way through the membrane about seven times, folding inward and outward. The odorant binds with the portion of the receptor protein that folds to the outside. The inside of the folding protein, however, is coupled to a G-protein, a combination of three subunits. On excitation of the receptor protein, an alpha subunit breaks away from the G-protein and immediately activates adenylyl cyclase, which is attached to the inside of the ciliary membrane near the receptor cell body. The activated cyclase, in turn, converts many molecules of intracellular adenosine triphosphate into cyclic adenosine monophosphate (cAMP). Finally, this cAMP activates another nearby membrane protein, a gated sodium ion channel that opens its "gate" and allows large numbers of sodium and calcium ions to pour through the membrane into the receptor cell cytoplasm. The sodium ions increase the electrical potential in the positive direction inside the cell membrane, thus exciting the olfactory neuron and transmitting action potentials into the CNS by way of the olfactory nerve. In the chemically sensitive, the mechanism of the hyperexcitation of the nerve occurs in the Ca^{2+} influx and liberation of Ca^{2+} stored within the cell that combines with protein kinases A and C and is phosphorylated, increasing sensitivity 1000 times.[4] This nerve is clearly sensitized in chemically sensitive patients, spreading its oxidation and inflammatory reaction distally to the frontal cortex and hypothalamus and the rest of the nervous system. This hypersensitivity to odors will trigger varied reactions to many incitants and thus varied symptoms in the chemically sensitive.

Therefore, even the minutest concentration of a specific odorant initiates a cascading effect that opens extremely large numbers of sodium and calcium channels. This accounts for the exquisite sensitivity of the olfactory neurons to even the slightest amount of odorant normally. Of course, this process is aggravated in the chemically sensitive, and minute odors are magnified many times. It appears as if the chemically sensitive can perceive one molecule or less clearly at times.

In addition to the basic chemical mechanism by which the olfactory cells are stimulated, several physical factors affect the degree of stimulation. First, only volatile substances that can be sniffed into the nostrils can be smelled. Second, the stimulating substance must be at least slightly water soluble so that it can pass through the mucus to reach the olfactory cilia. Third, it is helpful for the substance to be at least slightly lipid soluble, presumably because lipid constituents of the cilium itself are a weak barrier to nonlipid-soluble odorants.

MEMBRANE POTENTIALS AND ACTION POTENTIALS IN OLFACTORY CELLS

According to Guyton and Hall,[1] the membrane potential inside *unstimulated olfactory cells*, as measured by microelectrodes, averages about 55 mV. At this potential, most of the cells generate continuous action potentials at a very slow rate, varying from once every 20 seconds up to two or three per second.

Most odorants cause depolarization of the olfactory cell membrane, decreasing the negative potential in the cell from the normal level of 55–30 mV or less, that is, changing the voltage in the positive direction. Along with this, the number of action potentials increases to 20–30 per second, which is a high rate for the minute olfactory nerve fibers.

There are ~1000 ORs coded in the human genome.[9] Less than 500 receptors are functional in the nasal epithelium. Each receptor neuron is a single type of OR and is not specific to any one odorant.[10] An odorant is recognized by more than one type of receptor and thus odorants are recognized by a combination of receptors. The olfactory system relies on different excitation patterns to obtain different codes for different odorants. Buck[11] compared this system to combining different letters of the alphabet to produce different words. In this case, each word represents an odor. This coding explains why we can detect more odors than there are receptors in the nasal epithelium.[11] Certainly, this area can become hypersensitive with hyperosmia resulting as seen in the chemically sensitive. At times, it could result in the spreading phenomenon observed in the severe chemically sensitive where they develop sensitivity to a variety of and myriad of odors.

The olfactory nerve fibers leading backward from the bulb are called cranial nerve I, or the olfactory tract. However, in reality, both the tract and the bulb are an anterior outgrowth of brain tissue from the base of the brain; the bulbous enlargement at its end, the olfactory bulb, lies over the cribriform plate, separating the brain cavity from the upper reaches of the nasal cavity. The cribriform plate has multiple small perforations through which an equal number of small nerves pass upward from the olfactory membrane in the nasal cavity to enter the olfactory bulb in the cranial cavity. Figures 2.1 through 2.3 demonstrate the close relation between the olfactory cells in the olfactory membrane and the olfactory bulb, showing short axons from the olfactory cells terminating in multiple globular structures within the olfactory bulb called glomeruli. Each bulb has several thousands of such glomeruli, each of which is the terminus for about 25,000 axons from olfactory cells. Each glomerulus also is the terminus for dendrites from about 25 large mitral cells and about 60 smaller tufted cells, the cell bodies of which lie in the olfactory bulb superior to the glomeruli. These dendrites receive synapses from the olfactory cell neurons, and the mitral and tufted cells send axons through the olfactory tract to transmit olfactory signals to higher levels in the CNS. The physiology of this process is accentuated in the chemically sensitive (Figure 2.5).

Transmission of signals into the olfactory bulb

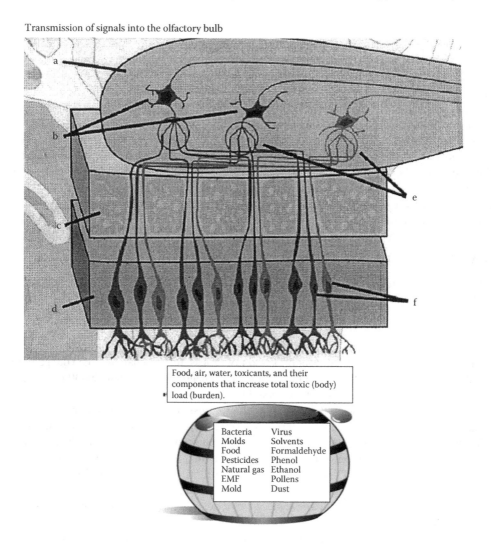

FIGURE 2.5 Human olfactory system: (a) olfactory bulb, (b) mitral cells, (c) bone, (d) nasal epithelium, (e) glomerulus (olfaction), and (f) olfactory receptor cells. (Modified from Lynch, P. J. 2007. Vulvodynia as a possible somatization disorder. More than just an opinion. *Reprod Med.* 2007 Feb;52(2):107–10.)

Some of the research has suggested that different glomeruli respond to different odors. It is possible that specific glomeruli are the real clue to the analysis of different odor signals transmitted into the CNS.

Sustentacular Cells

These cells are part of the olfactory membrane. They regulate Ca^{2+} in several ways. Also they contain phenol sulfotransferase and perhaps many other enzymes that detoxify chemicals,[12] which help an odorant perception and detoxification. Also, when combined action with chromaffin cells their action increases catacholamine output.

Globose Basal Cells

These cells are also present in the olfactory epithelium. They have infused replication-incompetent retroviral vectors into the nasal cavity of adult rats 1 day after exposure to the olfactotoxic gas methyl bromide (MeBr) to assess the lineage relationships of cells in the regenerating olfactory epithelium. The vast majority of the retrovirus-labeled clones fall into three broad categories: clones that invariably contain globose basal cells (GBCs) and/or neurons, clones that always include cells in the ducts of Bowman's glands, and clones that are composed of sustentacular cells only. Many of the GBC-related clones contain sustentacular cells and horizontal basal cells as well. Most of the duct-related clones contain gland cells, and some also include sustentacular cells. MeBr activates two distinct types of multipotent cells. The multipotent progenitor that gives rise to neurons and nonneuronal cells is a basal cell, whereas the progenitor that gives rise to duct, gland, and sustentacular cells resides within the ducts, based on the patterns of sparing after lesion and the analysis of early regeneration by using cell-type-specific markers. They conclude that the balance between the multipotency and elective neuropotency, which is characteristic of GBCs in the normal olfactory epithelium, is determined by which cell types have been depleted and need to be replenished rapidly.

They have used a replication-incompetent retrovirus to analyze the lineage of OR neurons in young rats. At 5–40 days after infection, clusters of infected cells comprised two major types: one consisted of one to two horizontal basal cells, and a second consisted of variable numbers of GBCs and immature and mature sensory neurons. Olfactory nerve lesion (which enhances neuronal turnover) increased the frequency of the globose–sensory neuron clusters as well as the number of cells in such clusters. No clusters contained both horizontal basal cells and GBCs, and none contained sustentacular cells. These data suggest, at least in young rats, that horizontal basal cells are not precursors of olfactory neurons, that there is a lineage path from globose cells to mature neurons, and that sustentacular cells may arise from a separate lineage.[13]

Not only methyl bromide can knock out the olfactory epithelium as shown in the rats but also in the human who are chemically sensitive. Multiple toxics such as natural gas, herbicides, pesticides, solvents, formaldehyde, phenols, alcohol, and mycotoxins can damage the olfactory epithelium allowing the chemically sensitive to flourish (Table 2.1).

Over a wide range, the rate of olfactory nerve impulses changes approximately in proportion to the logarithm of the stimulus strength, which demonstrates that the ORs obey principles of transduction similar to those of other sensory receptors. This area could be another generator of CS, if any of these areas swell or have enlarged pores or holes due to toxic injury or hypersensitivity seen in the chemically sensitive.

TABLE 2.1

Nose and Brain Areas Where Chemical Sensitivity Might Occur

1. Nasal basement membrane and receptor protein
2. Olfactory nerve—swelling below, above, and through cribriform plate
3. Sustentacular cells
   a. Regulates Ca^{2+}
   b. Phenol sulfate and transferase and many other detoxified enzymes
4. Olfactory bulb and cells
5. Mitrial cells
6. Tuffed cells
7. Prefrontal cortex = anterium cingulate nucleus precuneas, cuneas
8. Hypothalamus and limbic system
   a. Hippocampus
   b. Pineal gland
9. Mitochondria

Source: Adapted from Rea, W. J., K. Patel. 2014. *Reversibility of Chronic Degenerative Disease and Hypersensitivity*, Boca Raton, FL: CRC Press.

Rapid Adaptation of Olfactory Sensations

According to Guyton and Hall,[1] the ORs adapt about 50% in the first second or so after stimulation. Thereafter, they adapt very little and afterward very slowly. This is one of the reasons why the chemically sensitive has so many rapid problems when exposed to a toxic substance. This adaptation or masking can be harmful to many people because they get used to a toxic odor and it goes to the brain cavity making dysfunction. This is not true for the chemically sensitive who may take days to weeks to months to adapt; some may never adapt. Yet, we all know from our own experience that smell sensations adapt almost to extinction within a minute or so after entering a strongly odorous atmosphere. As this physiological adaptation is far greater than the degree of adaptation of the receptors themselves, it is almost certain that most of the additional adaptation occurs in the taste sensations and brain areas as well.

According to Guyton and Hall,[1] postulated neuronal mechanism for the adaptation is the following: large numbers of centrifugal nerve fibers pass from the olfactory regions of the brain backward along the olfactory tract and terminate on special inhibitory cells in the olfactory bulb, the granule cells. It has been postulated that after the onset of an olfactory stimulus, the CNS quickly develops strong feedback inhibition to suppress relay of the small signals through the olfactory bulb. This phenomenon is either damaged or eliminated in the chemically sensitive who continue to perceive the odor as long as it exists. Apparently, the area of feedback inhibition is damaged in the chemically sensitive.

It is certain that this list does not represent the true primary sensations of smell. In recent years, multiple clues, including specific studies of the genes that encode for the receptor proteins, suggest the existence of at least 100 primary sensations of smell in marked contrast to only three primary sensations of color detected by the eyes and only four or five primary sensations of taste detected by the tongue. Some studies suggest that there may be as many as 1000 different types of odorant receptors. Further support for the many primary sensations of smell is that people have been found who have odor blindness for single substances; such discrete odor blindness has been identified for more than 50 different substances. It is presumed that odor blindness for each substance represents lack of the appropriate receptor protein in olfactory cells for that particular substance. Apparently, the receptor protein in the chemically sensitive develops hypertrophy or hyperplasia resulting in the exquisite and prolonged odor sensitivity although some do have selective odor blindness.

Affective Nature of Smell

According to Guyton and Hall,[1] smell, even more than taste, has the affective quality of either pleasantness or unpleasantness. Due to this, smell is probably even more important than taste for the selection of food. Indeed, a person who has previously eaten food that disagreed with him or her is often nauseated by the smell of that same food on a second occasion or they might just be repelled. This happens routinely with the food and chemically sensitive patient. Conversely, not only food odors but perfume of the right quality can also be a powerful stimulant of human emotions but not to the chemically sensitive—it is often a downer and some people are even devastated and incapacitated by its odor. In addition, in some lower animals, odors are the primary excitant of sexual drive. This phenomenon is also true in some chemically sensitive patients who are easily aroused and often have to have sexual relief or conversely at times can shut off the sex drive completely.

Threshold for Smell

According to Guyton and Hall,[1] one of the principal characteristics of smell is the minute quantity of stimulating agent in the air that can elicit a smell sensation. This characteristic is even more severe in chemically sensitive patients; for instance, the substance methyl mercaptan can be smelled by a normal person when only one 25 trillionth of a gram is present in each milliliter of air. Due to this very low threshold, this substance methyl mercaptan is mixed with natural gas, especially methane, ethane, propane, and butane to give the gas an odor that can be detected when even small amounts of gas leak from a pipeline occurs. However, again the odor gets masked in the chemically sensitive due to the adaptation phenomena and the patient continues to take in natural gas and can get very ill. In the chemically sensitive, many of these odors give a similar effect and cause the patients dysfunction and have actual illness. The number one trigger of CS is the odor of and exposure to natural gas (which is masked) tied with pesticides and herbicides.

GRADATIONS OF SMELL INTENSITIES

Although the threshold concentrations of substances that evoke smell are extremely slight, for many (if not most) odorants, concentrations only 10–50 times above the threshold evoke maximum intensity of smell. This is in contrast to most other sensory systems of the body, in which the ranges of intensity discrimination are tremendous, for example, 500,000:1 in the case of the eyes and $1 \times 10^{12}:1$ in the case of the ears. This difference might be explained by the fact that smell is concerned more with detecting the presence or the absence of odors rather than with quantitative detection of their intensities. The chemically sensitive certainly can detect most odors whether they are harmful or nontoxic when they are unmasked with avoidances in areas like the less-polluted ECU.

TRANSMISSION OF SMELL SIGNALS INTO THE CNS

Olfactory Cortex

Signals from odor sensation are sent from the olfactory bulb through mitral and tufts cell axons via the lateral olfactory tract and synapse at the primary olfactory cortex. The primary olfactory cortex includes the anterior olfactory nucleus, the piriform cortex, the anterior cortical nucleus of the hippocampus and amygdala, the periamygdaloid complex, and the rostral entorhinal cortex.

A unique characteristic of olfaction is its independence from the thalamus. The odor signals are sent directly from the sensory receptor neuron to the primary cortex. However, communication between the primary and the secondary olfactory cortex requires connections with the thalamus.[10,11] If damaged with the result of swelling, one could see the onset of CS here. Chemically sensitive patients have a different path for odors to the brain. Many of the odors travel to the PFC in the anterior cingulate cortex including the cuneus/precuneus area and then impulses are sent to the hypothalamus secondarily. It appears that some travel through the normal route to the olfactory cortex, periform cortex, and the anterior cortical nucleus of the hippocampus and amygdala.

Odor Perception

Odor identity, quality, and familiarity are mainly deciphered by the piriform cortex. Consciousness of smell is achieved by projections from the piriform cortex to the medial dorsal nucleus of the thalamus and to the orbitofrontal cortex, which the secondary olfactory cortex is part of.[11] One sees the onset of odor supersensitivity, which may occur with pollutant, mold, or food sensitivity in this area.

According to Guyton and Hall,[1] the olfactory portions of the brain were among the first brain structures developed in primitive animals, and much of the remainder of the brain developed around these olfactory beginnings. Certainly, in the CS, the majority of function reverts around the odor perception, which frequently determines his/her behavior. Avoidance predominates in the chemically sensitive behavior and pathway through life. In fact, a part of the brain that originally subserved olfaction later evolved into the basal brain structures that control emotions and other aspects of human behavior; this is the *limbic system*. This system is clearly accentuated in chemically sensitive patients who often have difficulty controlling the temperature (low) and the endocrine system; at times, they also have trouble with behavior becoming hyperactive or depressed, for example, intake of food and chemical odors, motivational drive, vegetative function, and emotions that are triggered in the limbic system. Figure 2.6 shows a vast expansion of the olfactory system.

THREE PATHWAYS LEADING TO THE BRAIN

Very Old, the Less Old, and the Newer Olfactory Pathways into the CNS

The olfactory tract enters the brain at the anterior junction between the mesencephalon and the cerebrum; there, the tract divides into two pathways, as shown in Figure 2.7, one passing medially into the medial olfactory area of the brain stem and the other passing laterally into the lateral olfactory *area*. The medial olfactory area represents a very old olfactory system, whereas the lateral olfactory area is the input to (1) a less old olfactory system and (2) a newer system.

Very Old Olfactory System: The Medial Olfactory Area

According to Guyton and Hall,[1] the medial olfactory area consists of a group of nuclei located in the midbasal portions of the brain immediately anterior to the hypothalamus in the paraolfactory area.

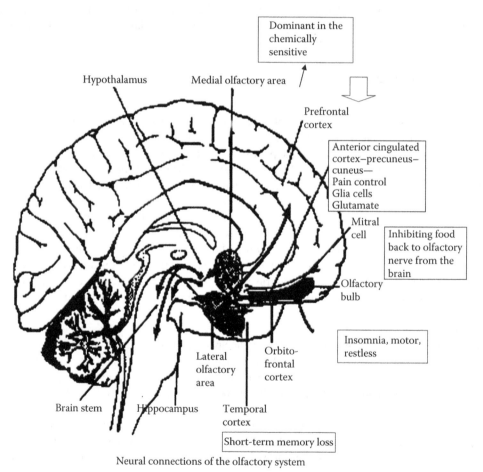

Neural connections of the olfactory system

FIGURE 2.6 Neural connections of the olfactory system in the chemically sensitive. (Modified from Guyton, A. C., J. E. Hall. 2002. In *Treaty of Medical Physiology*, 10th ed., A. C. Guyton, J. E. Hall, Eds., pp. 570–577. Rio de Janeiro: Guanabara Koogam SA; Rea, W. J., K. Patel. 2015. *Reversibility of Chronic Degenerative Disease and Hypersensitivity*, Vol. 2, page 58, Figure 2.3. Copyright 2009. Reproduced by permission of Taylor and Francis Group, LLC, a division of Informa plc.)

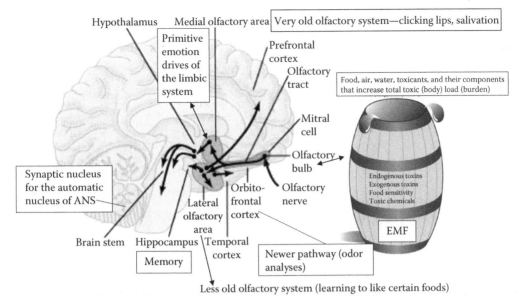

FIGURE 2.7 (See color insert.)　Neural connections of the olfactory system. (Modified from Guyton, A. C., J. E. Hall. 2002. In *Treaty of Medical Physiology*, 10th ed., A. C. Guyton, J. E. Hall, Eds., pp. 570–577. Rio de Janeiro: Guanabara Koogam SA; Rea, W. J., K. Patel. 2015. *Reversibility of Chronic Degenerative Disease and Hypersensitivity*, Vol. 2, page 58, Figure 2.3. Copyright 2009. Reproduced by permission of Taylor and Francis Group, LLC, a division of Informa plc.)

Most conspicuous are the septal nuclei, which are midline nuclei that feed into the hypothalamus and other primitive portions of the brain's limbic system. This area of the brain is mostly concerned with basic behavior (emotions).

The importance of this medial olfactory area is best understood by considering what happens in animals when the lateral olfactory areas on both sides of the brain are removed and only the medial system remains. The answer is that this hardly affects the more primitive responses to olfaction, such as licking the lips, salivation, and other feeding responses caused by the smell of food or by primitive emotional drives associated with smell. Conversely, the removal of the lateral areas abolishes the more complicated olfactory conditioned reflexes. When exposed to toxic chemicals with an increase in total body pollutant loads, the chemically sensitive cannot salivate just like in a stressful situation.

Less Old Olfactory System: The Lateral Olfactory Area

According to Guyton and Hall,[1] the lateral olfactory area is composed mainly of the prepyriform and pyriform cortex, and the cortical portion of the amygdaloid nuclei. From these areas, signal pathways pass into almost all the portions of the limbic system, especially into less primitive portions such as the hippocampus, which seem to be most important for learning to like or dislike certain foods depending on one's experiences with them. For instance, it is believed that this lateral olfactory area and its many connections with the limbic behavioral system cause a person to develop an absolute aversion to foods that have caused nausea and vomiting. This area appears to be damaged in many chemically sensitive patients.

An important feature of the lateral olfactory area is that many signal pathways from this area also feed directly into an older part of the cerebral cortex called the paleocortex in the anteromedial

TABLE 2.2
Triggering Agents

Patient	No. Foods Sensitive/Tested	No. Chemicals Sensitive/Tested	Systems
1	12/28	13/15	CV
2	34/48	5/12	Vasc.
3	78/94	5/13	GI vasc. cerebral
4	20/36	10/15	Resp. vasc.
5	41/57	6/9	Vasc. cerebral
6	50/66	3/11	Vasc.
7	25/41	7/15	Vasc. cerebral
8	10/26	1/10	Vasc.
9	42/58	2/10	Vasc. GI
10	3/19	2/10	Vasc. GI
11	0/16	0/8	Vasc.
12	1/17	0/8	CV

Source: Adapted from Environmental Health Center-Dallas, 2000. Under environmentally less (5× less polluted) conditions.

portion of the temporal lobe. This is the only area of the entire cerebral cortex where sensory signals pass directly to the cortex without passing first through the thalamus.

These signals trigger automatic but partially learned control of food intake, and aversion to toxic and unhealthy foods. When damaged by toxic chemicals, mold toxins, or certain EMF frequency, they may cause an aversion to healthy and formerly found safe foods. This malady can cause the chemically sensitive individual to be sensitive to many foods and at times all foods. When this occurs if the human loses all food he/she will rapidly lose weight and die if intravenous hypoalimentation is not used until the body is detoxified from pollutants and neutralized intradermally for foods (Table 2.2).

Newer Pathway

A newer olfactory pathway that passes through the thalamus, passing to the dorsomedial thalamic nucleus and then to the lateroposterior quadrant of the orbitofrontal cortex, has been found. On the basis of studies in monkeys, this newer system probably helps in the conscious analysis of odor.[14] This pathway is usually used in the exposed chemically sensitive but often an older reflex pathway is also involved.

Centrifugal Control of Activity in the Olfactory Bulb by the CNS

Many nerve fibers that originate in the olfactory portions of the brain pass from the brain in the outward direction into the olfactory tract to the olfactory bulb (i.e., "centrifugally" from the brain to the periphery). These terminate on a large number of small granule cells located among the mitral and tufted cells in the olfactory bulb. The granule cells send inhibitory signals to the mitral and tufted cells, which may be difficult in the chemically sensitive because of the interference of the cortex causing cloudy brain function, which is usually seen in chemically sensitive patients. According to Guyton and Hall,[14] it is believed that this inhibitory feedback might be a means for sharpening one's specific ability to distinguish one odor from another. Often the chemically sensitive can differentiate specific odors when many are combined judging which ones are toxic and the patients should try to avoid them. They also with practice can discern the benign odors so they do not always have to run. At times, the toxic odors can rapidly mask and chemically sensitive patients stay too long and will become ill for hours to days because the toxic odors are masked with weakness, fatigue, and cloudy brain becoming nonfunctional.

CNS Affects of Air Pollution

Air pollution impacts the brain through multiple pathways according to Block and Calderon-Garciduenas.[15] Through these pollutant-derived responses, the individual will not only initially malfunction but will also develop CS or chronic degenerative disease through oxidative stress followed by inflammation where odors are entirely masked but continue to cause damage.

Air pollution contains complex toxins causing diverse CNS pathology through several interrelated mechanisms that may lead to CNS disease or other degenerative diseases. These effects can be categorized into groups: (1) rhino-hypothalamic–limbic mechanism that is triggered by mold or severe toxins can trigger malbehavior, which can cause CS or chronic degenerative disease; (2) systemic oxidative stress and inflammation; (3) particulate matter (PM) (from 10–2.5 μm to <0.200 μm); and absorbed compounds; compounds such as ozone, nitrogen dioxides, carbon monoxide, sulfur dioxide, pesticides, natural gas, phenols, formaldehyde, mycotoxins, etc. can trigger the oxidative stress and inflammation.

While some CNS effects have been attributed to specific components of air pollution, a single clear pathway responsible for CNS damage has now been identified. In fact, due to the complex nature of this environmental toxin, it is very likely that CNS pathologies are due to the synergistic interaction of the multiple pathways listed in Figure 2.7, making air pollution a potent, biologically relevant environmental exposure and significant challenge for mechanistic inquiry. Many areas can be damaged by incitant entry.

Rhino-Hypothalamic–Limbic Mechanism

This mechanism (just discussed) includes the nose when pollutants go right up the olfactory nerves to the hypothalamus. This pathway and the respiratory pathway are the two largest pathways through which inhaled pollutants enter the body. The GI tract is the third largest though through a circuitous peripheral route. Skin, bladder, and vaginal absorption also can absorb, but these routes are usually slower and at times milder though the chemically sensitive can react severely at times. Recent studies by Kissel et al.[16] show that phthalates that are endocrine disruptors are absorbed through the skin. The olfactory nerve may become hypersensitive to any pollutant odor including toxic volatile organic and inorganic odors including car exhaust, pesticide, natural gas, mercury, lead, and mycotoxins, etc., all creating the chemically sensitive individual (locally in the nasal membrane and olfactory cells) or by transmitting impulses from the olfactory membrane and cells across the cribriform plate to the olfactory bulb and nerve into the prefrontal brain olfactory area and hypothalamus. This odor then can trigger a series of adverse responses in the frontal lobe like short-term memory loss, confusion, weakness, and fatigue including limbic abnormalities such as vegetative functions, endocrine functions, body temperature (low or high), emotional behavior, motivational drives, and eventually autonomic functions and dysfunctions as well as motivational misbehavior.

Conversely, the odors can be masked causing the entry of pollutants not known to the individual resulting in any of the aforementioned symptoms but especially weakness and fatigue resulting in the lack of perception of unknown reasons for the illness. Unmasking in a less-polluted, controlled area is often necessary so that the individual can recognize the true triggering agents.

Either with enhanced or masking of odors, these toxic impulses will trigger altered homeostasis and eventually brain, peripheral nerve, and vascular damage observed in CS. Especially, the small microvessels are involved resulting in spasm and lack of oxygen–CO_2 exchange and waste drainage. Pollutant withdrawal will aid in return to normal function.

In addition to their roles in behavior control, these areas control many internal conditions of the body, such as body temperature (chemically sensitive patients are almost always cold) as modality of body fluid, and the drives to eat and drink. (Many chemically sensitive are addicted to sugar, candy, chocolate, or beverages such as coffee, tea, and sweet drinks.) This hypothalamus helps control weight. These internal functions are collectively called vegetative function of the brain and their control is closely related to behavior. Much of this behavior will be addictive either consciously

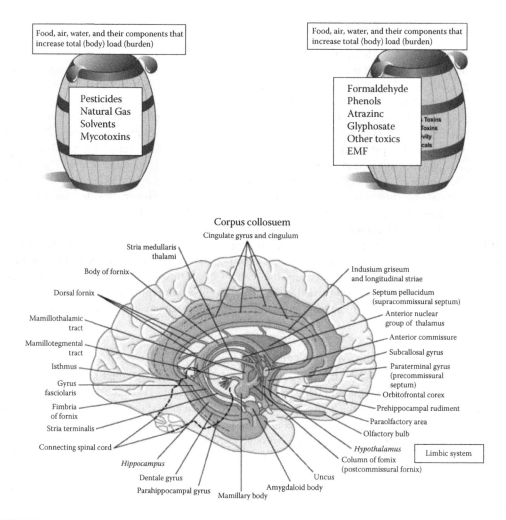

FIGURE 2.8 Anatomy of the limbic system and olfactory system in the chemically sensitive. (Redrawn from Warwick, R., Williams, P. L. 1973. *Gray's Anatomy*, 35th Br. ed. London: Longman Group Ltd; modified from Guyton, A. C., J. E. Hall. 2002. In *Treaty of Medical Physiology*, 10th ed., A. C. Guyton, J. E. Hall, Eds., pp. 570–577. Rio de Janeiro: Guanabara Koogam SA; Rea, W. J., K. Patel. 2015. *Reversibility of Chronic Degenerative Disease and Hypersensitivity*, Vol. 3, page 87, Figure 3.41. Reproduced by permission of Taylor and Francis Group, LLC, a division of Informa plc.)

or unconsciously as observed in the chemically sensitive and/or the chronic degenerative diseased patient.

The pollutant overload through the olfactory hypothalamus and limbic axis causes at times a varied physical stimulus, which at times is misinterpreted as psychological rather than the physiological phenomena which it is. Irreversible pathology can develop if the intake process goes on too long or is too severe as shown in the Mexico City dogs and humans when undergoing constant pollutant stress. Therefore, reduction in the total ambient pollutant load and thus the total body pollutant load is necessary for good health and restoration from CS. The anatomy of the limbic system is shown in Figure 2.8.

Figure 2.9 shows the anatomical structures of the limbic system, demonstrating that it is an interconnected complex of basal brain elements. Located in the middle of all these pollutants are the central elements of the limbic system, which can be disturbed in the chemically sensitive.

Surrounding the subcortical limbic areas is the limbic cortex, composed of a ring of cerebral cortex in each side of the brain (1) beginning in the orbitofrontal area on the ventral surface of the

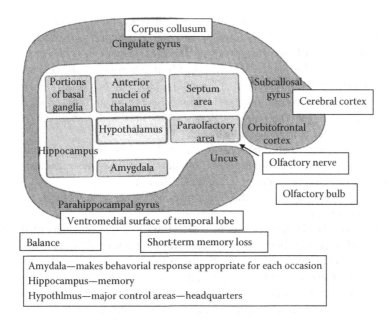

FIGURE 2.9 Limbic system showing the key position of the hypothalamus. (Modified from Guyton, A. C., J. E. Hall. 2002. In *Treaty of Medical Physiology*, 10th ed., A. C. Guyton, J. E. Hall, Eds., pp. 570–577. Rio de Janeiro: Guanabara Koogam SA; Rea, W. J., K. Patel. 2015. *Reversibility of Chronic Degenerative Disease and Hypersensitivity*, Vol. 3, page 87, Figure 3.42. Reproduced by permission of Taylor and Francis Group, LLC, a division of Informa plc.)

frontal lobes, (2) extending upward into the subcallosal gyrus, (3) then over the top of the corpus callosum onto the medial aspect of the cerebral hemisphere in the cingulate gyrus, and finally (4) passing behind the corpus callosum and downward onto the ventromedial surface of the temporal lobe to the parahippocampal gyrus and uncus.

Thus, on the medial and ventral surfaces of each cerebral hemisphere is a ring mostly of the paleocortex that surrounds a group of deep structures intimately associated with overall behavior and emotions. In turn, this ring of limbic cortex function has a two-way communication and association linkage between the neocortex and the lower limbic structures.

Many of the behavioral functions elicited from the hypothalamus and other limbic structures are also mediated throughout the reticular nuclei in the brain stem and their associated nuclei. Stimulation of the excitatory portion of this reticular formation can cause high degrees of cerebral excitability while also increasing the excitability of much of the spinal cord synapses. This condition is often seen in chemically sensitive patients when they have a reaction. We see that most of the hypothalamic signals for controlling the autonomic nervous system (ANS) are also transmitted through synaptic nuclei located in the brain stem. The ANS is one of the first systems to get deregulated in CS. When deregulated, the ANS will account for much vascular dysfunction and many symptoms.

According to Guyton and Hall,[14] an important route of communication between the limbic system and the brain stem is the medial forebrain bundle, which extends from the septal and orbitofrontal regions of the cerebral cortex downward through the middle of the hypothalamus to the brain stem reticular formation. This bundle carries fibers in both directions, forming a trunk-line communication system. A second route of communication is through short pathways among the reticular formation of the brain stem, thalamus, hypothalamus, and most other contiguous areas of the basal brain.

According to Guyton and Hall,[14] the hypothalamus is a major control headquarters for the limbic system. The hypothalamus, despite its small size of only a few cubic centimeters, has two-way communicating pathways with all levels of the limbic system. In turn, the hypothalamus and its closely allied structures send output signals in three directions: (1) backward and downward to the brain stem, mainly into the reticular areas of the mesencephalon, pons, and medulla and from these areas into the peripheral nerves of the ANS, resulting in vascular, GI, genital, urinary, and other dysfunctions observed in the chemically sensitive (2) upward toward many higher areas of the diencephalon and cerebrum, especially to the anterior thalamus and limbic portions of the cerebral cortex, which can result in mental confusion, depression, and weakness seen in the chemically sensitive, and (3) into the hypothalamic infundibulum to control or partially control most of the secretory functions of both the posterior and the anterior pituitary glands, which may be dysfunctional in the chemically sensitive. Also it can influence a change in behavior.

Thus, the hypothalamus, which represents less than 1% of the brain mass, is one of the most important control pathways of the limbic system. It controls most of the vegetative and endocrine functions of the body and many aspects of emotional behavior.

According to Guyton and Hall,[14] the vegetative and endocrine ·control functions of the hypothalamus are important.

The different hypothalamic mechanisms for controlling multiple functions of the body are so important to the malfunction in the chemically sensitive. To illustrate the organization of the hypothalamus as a functional unit, let us summarize its more important vegetative and endocrine functions.

Figure 2.10 shows enlarged sagittal and coronal views of the hypothalamus, which represents only a small area in Figure 2.11. Take a few minutes to study these diagrams, especially Figure 2.12 to see the multiple activities that are excited or inhibited when respective hypothalamic nuclei are stimulated. In addition to the centers shown in Figure 2.13, a large lateral hypothalamic area (Figure 2.10) is present on each side of the hypothalamus. The lateral areas are especially important in controlling thirst, hunger, and many of the emotional drives. The triggering of these is often seen and aberrant in the food and chemically sensitive patient.

AREAS OF DIFFERENT CONTROLS

Cardiovascular Regulation

According to Guyton and Hall,[14] cardiovascular regulation is important (Figure 2.11). In the chemically sensitive, it is paramount because of the oxygen and from which is necessary for normal function of all the cells in the body. Stimulation of different areas throughout the hypothalamus causing many neurogenic effects on the cardiovascular system, including increased and decreased arterial pressure, increased heart rate (HR), and decreased HR. In general, stimulation in the posterior and lateral hypothalamus increases the arterial pressure and HR, whereas stimulation in the preoptic area often has opposite effects, causing a decrease in both HR and arterial pressure. These effects are transmitted mainly through specific cardiovascular control centers in the reticular regions of the pons and medulla. Many chemically sensitive patients have hypertension and some have hypotension. Sinus tachycardia is common, while atrial (PACs) arrhythmia as well as atrial fibrillation (AF) can be present. Occasional episodes of PVC (nonischemic) occur. Episodes of ventricular tachycardia and fibrillation occur constituting an emergency. These areas, if triggered, in the chemically sensitive cause cardiovascular dysfunction.

The microcirculation where oxygen extraction occurs is also very regulatory with shunting and elimination of microvessels when pollutant injury occurs. Here, O_2 may be shunted from the microarterial to the venous side with lack of oxygen extraction resulting in tissue hypoxia. This leaves chemically sensitive patients weak, fatigued, and lacking stamina for carrying out normal tasks.

Body Temperature Regulation

According to Guyton and Hall,[14] the regulation of body temperature occurs in the hypothalamus. This area is apparently deregulated in the chemically sensitive and therefore they are usually cold. The anterior portion of the hypothalamus, especially the preoptic area, is concerned with regulation of body temperature. An increase in the temperature of the blood flowing through this area increases the activity of temperature-sensitive neurons, whereas a decrease in temperature decreases their

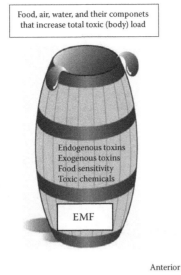

Food, air, water, and their componets
that increase total toxic (body) load

Endogenous toxins
Exogenous toxins
Food sensitivity
Toxic chemicals

EMF

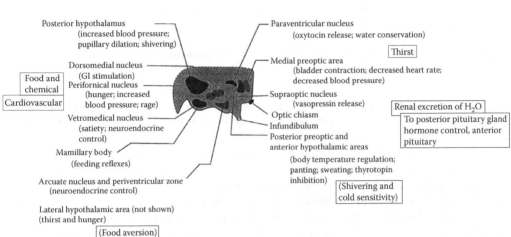

Posterior   Anterior

Posterior hypothalamus
(increased blood pressure;
pupillary dilation; shivering)

Paraventricular nucleus
(oxytocin release; water conservation)

Thirst

Dorsomedial nucleus
(GI stimulation)
Perifornical nucleus
(hunger; increased
blood pressure; rage)

Food and
chemical

Cardiovascular

Vetromedial nucleus
(satiety; neuroendocrine
control)

Mamillary body
(feeding reflexes)

Arcuate nucleus and periventricular zone
(neuroendocrine control)

Lateral hypothalamic area (not shown)
(thirst and hunger)

(Food aversion)

Medial preoptic area
(bladder contraction; decreased heart rate;
decreased blood pressure)

Supraoptic nucleus
(vasopressin release)

Optic chiasm
Infundibulum
Posterior preoptic and
anterior hypothalamic areas
(body temperature regulation;
panting; sweating; thyrotopin
inhibition)

(Shivering and
cold sensitivity)

Renal excretion of H$_2$O

To posterior pituitary gland
hormone control, anterior
pituitary

FIGURE 2.10 Control centers of the hypothalamus (sagittal view). *Note:* 15 aberrant responses are found in the chemically sensitive. (Modified from Guyton, A. C., J. E. Hall. 2002. In *Treaty of Medical Physiology*, 10th ed., A. C. Guyton, J. E. Hall, Eds., pp. 570–577. Rio de Janeiro: Guanabara Koogam SA; Rea, W. J., K. Patel. 2015. *Reversibility of Chronic Degenerative Disease and Hypersensitivity*, Vol. 3, page 89, Figure 3.43. Reproduced by permission of Taylor and Francis Group, LLC, a division of Informa plc.)

activity. In turn, these neurons control mechanisms for increasing or decreasing body temperature. Chemically sensitive patients noted for vasospasm usually are cold with temperatures running from 96°F to 97.5°F. Some other chemically sensitive patients are always hot.

Regulation of Body Water

According to Guyton and Hall,[14] the hypothalamus is involved in regulation of body water. The hypothalamus regulates body water in two ways: (1) by creating the sensation of thirst, which drives a person to drink water and (2) by controlling the excretion of water into the urine. An area called the thirst center is located in the lateral hypothalamus and can be damaged by excess pollutant exposure. When the fluid or electrolytes in either this center or closely allied areas become too concentrated, chemically sensitive patients develop an intense desire to drink water. They will search out the nearest source of water and drink enough to return the electrolyte concentration of the thirst

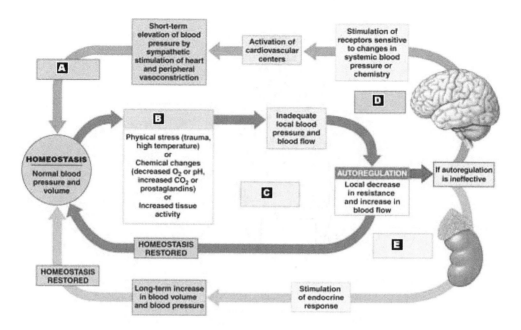

FIGURE 2.11 (See color insert.) Cardiovascular regulation of hemodynamics occurs via local autoregulation, neural control, and hormones.

to normal. We have seen CS patients, in the peak of a reaction, drink several pints of water until the reaction is over. They then develop edema and feel ill until the reaction is over and the water is released.

Control of renal excretion of water is vested mainly in the supraoptic nuclei. When the body fluids become too concentrated, the neurons of these areas become stimulated. Nerve fibers from these neurons project downward through the infundibulum of the hypothalamus into the posterior pituitary gland, where the nerve endings secrete the antidiuretic hormone—vasopressin. This hormone is then absorbed into the blood and transported to the kidneys, where it acts on the collecting ducts of the kidneys to cause increased reabsorption of water. This stimulation decreases loss of water into the urine but allows continuing excretion of electrolytes, thus decreasing the concentration of the body fluids back toward normal. Chemically sensitive patients often have problems with this apparatus causing a loss in homeostasis resulting in peripheral and periorbital edema because they have difficulty urinating or they may urinate too frequently.

Regulation of Uterine Activity

According to Guyton and Hall,[14] regulation of uterine contractility and milk ejection from the breasts is a function of the hypothalamus. Stimulation of the paraventricular nuclei causes their neuronal cells to secrete the hormone oxytocin. This hormone may be imbalanced in some chemically sensitive patients causing dysfunction.

Abnormal GI Function

GI and feeding regulation occurs and is distorted in chemically sensitive patients. Stimulation of several areas of the hypothalamus causes an animal to experience extreme hunger, a voracious appetite, and an intense desire to search for food. One area associated with hunger is the lateral hypothalamic area, which when pollutant overloaded causes a CS patient to want to eat continually even if the food is harmful to him/her; sometimes these patients gain excessive weight. Conversely, damage to this area on both sides of the hypothalamus causes the person to lose desire for food, sometimes causing lethal starvation as seen in some types of chemically sensitive patients. Some

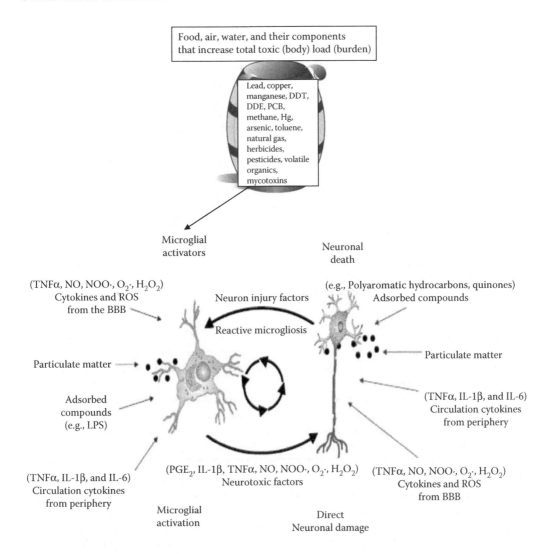

FIGURE 2.12 Microglial activation. (Adapted from Environmental Health Center-Dallas; Rea, W. J., K. Patel. 2015. *Reversibility of Chronic Degenerative Disease and Hypersensitivity*, Vol. 2. Boca Raton, FL: CRC Press.)

chemically sensitive patients develop massive weight loss when they can tolerate few foods. It is not uncommon to see weight loss of 70–90 pounds.

ENDOCRINE ACTIVITIES

According to Guyton and Hall,[14] the hypothalamic control of endocrine hormone secretion by the anterior pituitary gland occurs. Stimulation of certain areas of the hypothalamus also causes the anterior pituitary gland to secrete its endocrine hormones. Briefly, the basic mechanisms are the following.

Behavior

According to Guyton and Hall, behavioral functions of the hypothalamus and associated limbic structures are varied.[14] Effects caused by stimulation of the hypothalamus are varied. In addition to these vegetative and endocrine functions of the hypothalamus, stimulation of or lesions in the

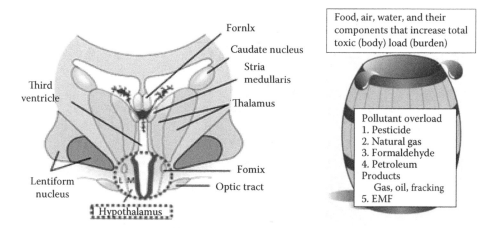

FIGURE 2.13 Connection of the olfactory tract and hypothalamus to the third ventricle, thalamus, etc. (Modified from Guyton, A. C., J. E. Hall. 2002. In *Treaty of Medical Physiology*, 10th ed., A. C. Guyton, J. E. Hall, Eds., pp. 570–577. Rio de Janeiro: Guanabara Koogam SA.)

hypothalamus often have profound effects on emotional behavior of animals and human beings. Many chemically sensitive patients go into rages, depression, agitation, fear, anxiety, increased sexual drive, and various other emotional stages during reaction to molds, food, or chemicals for which they are exposed and sensitive to.

Some of the behavioral effects of stimulation are the following: (1) Stimulation in the lateral hypothalamus not only causes thirst and eating, as discussed earlier, but also increases the general level of activity of the animal, sometimes leading to overt rage and fighting as discussed subsequently. (2) Stimulation in the ventromedial nucleus and surrounding areas mainly causes and affects opposite to those caused by lateral hypothalamic stimulation, that is, a sense of satiety, decreased eating, and tranquility. The clinician rarely sees this tranquility in chemically sensitive patients, but it does occur especially after a 3–7-day fast and little toxic exposures, when the nutrition is right and all injections are steady. (3) Stimulation of a thin zone of periventricular nuclei, located immediately adjacent to the third ventricle (or also stimulation of the central gray area of the mesencephalon that is continuous with this portion of the hypothalamus), usually leads to fear and punishment reactions. One frequently observes these tougher reactions in the chemically sensitive upon exposure to excessive molds, and mycotoxins, pesticides or natural gas, or other toxics. (4) Sexual drive can be stimulated from several areas of the hypothalamus, especially the most anterior and most posterior portions of the hypothalamus.

Effects Caused by Hypothalamic Lesions

Lesions in the hypothalamus, in general, cause effects opposite to those caused by stimulation especially in the chemically sensitive. For instance,

1. Bilateral lesions in the lateral hypothalamus will decrease drinking and eating almost to zero, often leading to lethal starvation. These lesions cause extreme passivity of the animal as well, with loss of most of its overt drives including lack of intake of calories. A subgroup of chemically sensitive patients has to have total parental nutrition until these triggers are eliminated or neutralized and the general nutrition is replaced. The following case is illustrative.

   A 50-year-old white female hardware worker developed food intolerance. She lost 40 lbs. and could not eat any food. A feeding tube was placed in her small intestine. However, she could not tolerate any foods, especially nutrients. This would be accompanied by bloating, nausea, and vomiting. Due to the intolerance of the tube feeding, a central venous catheter was placed and intravenous nutrients were supplied. At this time, she was transferred to the EHC-Dallas claiming she could only tolerate 600–700 calories. She was placed in the controlled environment and depurated. She was tested on multiple individual food, molds, and chemicals and these antigens, as well the intravenous calories she was taking. In addition, she had intravenous hyperalimentation of glucose, amino acids, and lipids. She increased her hyperalimentation calorie intake to 1700 calories/day. After taking food, mold, pollen, and chemical antigens as well as decreasing particulate and toxic solvents and pesticide intake, she gradually could tolerate foods. She got to the point of being able to tolerate 25 foods and nutrients. She had her jejunostomy food tube pulled, which was causing a frequent reaction to the rubber. She eventually could eat and did well off the total parenteral nutrition. Central intravenous hyperalimentation has now been used in several patients.

2. Bilateral lesions of the ventromedial areas of the hypothalamus cause effects that are mainly opposite to those caused by lesions of the lateral hypothalamus, which are excessive drinking and eating, as well as hyperactivity and often continuous savagery along with frequent bouts of extreme rage on the slightest provocation can occur. Frequently, at this stage, selective CS patient's symptoms are misinterpreted as psychological and proper treatment is delayed, with the patient's health is deteriorating when in fact this is a pathophysical phenomenon. Stimulation of lesions in other regions of the limbic system, especially in the amygdala, the septal area, and areas in the mesencephalon, often causes effects similar to those elicited from the hypothalamus.

According to Guyton and Hall,[14] "Reward" and "Punishment" function of the limbic system occurs with stimulation. We have observed this phenomenon in a subset of chemically sensitive patients.

From the discussion thus far, it is already clear that several limbic structures are particularly concerned with the affective nature of sensory sensations, that is, whether the sensations are pleasant or unpleasant. These affective qualities are also called reward or punishment, or satisfaction or aversion. Electrical stimulation of certain limbic areas pleases or satisfies the animal, whereas electrical stimulation of other regions causes terror, pain, fear, defense, escape reactions, and all the other elements of punishment. The degrees of stimulation of these two oppositely responding systems greatly affect the behavior of human chemically sensitive patients. Not only chemical exposures but EMF frequency derived from cell phones, Wi-Fi, smart meters, and other stray impulses also can trigger these responses.[14] These reactions are pathophysiological and not psychologically triggered reactions.

Reward Centers

Experimental studies in monkeys have used electrical stimulators to map out the reward and punishment centers of the brain. The technique that has been used is to implant electrodes in different areas of the brain so that the monkey can stimulate the area by pressing a lever that makes electrical contact with a stimulator. If stimulating the particular area gives the animal a sense of reward, then it will press the lever again and again, sometimes as much as hundreds or even thousands of times per hour. Furthermore, when offered the choice of eating some delectable food as opposed to the opportunity to stimulate the reward center, the animal often chooses the electrical stimulation.[14]

By using this procedure, the major reward centers have been found to be located along the course of the medial forebrain bundle, especially in the lateral and ventromedial nuclei of the hypothalamus. It is strange that the lateral nucleus should be included among the reward areas; indeed, it is one of the most potent of all because even stronger stimuli in this area can cause rage. However, this is true in many areas, with weaker stimuli giving a sense of reward and stronger ones a sense of punishment.[14] Less potent reward centers, which are perhaps secondary to the major ones in the hypothalamus, are found in the septum, the amygdala, certain areas of the thalamus and basal ganglia, and extending downward into the basal tegmentum of the mesencephalon. These studies illustrate the phenomenon the clinician sees in the hypersensitive patient who has mold, food, and chemical hypersensitivity, before preventive neutralization diagnosis and treatment. This procedure when performed under environmentally controlled conditions appears to step into the low-dose and high-dose stimulation by injecting specific doses of higher and lower coordination of antigens. Thus, the clinician can stimulate chemically sensitive patients or inhibit antigens with the overreaction by finding the proper dose of the antigen.

PUNISHMENT CENTERS

According to Guyton and Hall,[14] the stimulator apparatus discussed earlier can also be connected so that the stimulus to the brain continues all the time except when the lever is pressed. In this case, the animal will not press the lever to turn the stimulus off when the electrode is in one of the reward areas; but when it is in certain other areas, the animal immediately learns to turn it off. Stimulation in these areas causes the animal to show all the signs of displeasure, fear, terror, pain, punishment, and even sickness as seen in the pollutant-overloaded chemically sensitive and EMF-sensitive patients.

By means of this technique, the most potent areas for punishment and escape tendencies have been found in the central gray area surrounding the aqueduct of Sylvius in the mesencephalon and extending upward into the periventricular zones of the hypothalamus and thalamus. Less potent punishment areas are found in some locations in the amygdala and hippocampus. It is particularly interesting that stimulation in the punishment centers can frequently inhibit the reward and pleasure centers completely, demonstrating that punishment and fear can take precedence over pleasure and reward.

RAGE: ITS ASSOCIATION WITH PUNISHMENT CENTERS

According to Guyton and Hall,[14] an emotional pattern that involves the punishment centers of the hypothalamus and other limbic structures, and has also been well characterized, is the rage pattern, described as follows.

Strong stimulation of the punishment centers of the brain, especially in the periventricular zone of the hypothalamus and in the lateral hypothalamus, causes the animal to (1) develop a defense posture, (2) extend its claws, (3) lift its tail, (4) hiss, (5) spit, (6) growl, and (7) develop piloerection, wide-open eyes, and dilated pupils. Furthermore, even the slightest provocation causes an immediate savage attack. This is approximately the behavior that one would expect from an animal being severely punished, and it is a pattern of behavior that is called rage. Some chemically sensitive patients who have experienced rage have learned to prevent it and if it occurs, stop it, by eliminating the food, mold, chemical, or EMF that triggers this response. Humans also can neutralize the reaction by taking vitamin C, bicarbonates, oxygen, and taking their intradermal injections of the neutralizing dose of the specific mold, food, or chemical or by using the generalized neutralizing dose of histamine, serotonin, and capsaicin.

Fortunately, in the normal animal, the rage phenomenon is held in check mainly by inhibitory signals from the ventromedial nuclei of the hypothalamus. In addition, portions of the hippocampi and anterior limbic cortex, especially in the anterior cingulate gyri and subcallosal gyri, help suppress the rage phenomenon.

PLACIDITY AND TAMENESS

Exactly the opposite emotional behavior patterns occur when the reward centers are stimulated: placidity and tameness. At times, this phenomenon is seen in the chemically sensitive when they have eliminated the toxic substances, given the intradermal neutralizing dose of the offending food, mold or chemical, or used vitamin C or bicarbonate.

Finally, excitation of still other portions of the amygdala can cause sexual activities that include erection, copulatory movements, ejaculation, ovulation, uterine activity, and premature labor.

EFFECTS OF BILATERAL ABLATION OF THE AMYGDALA: THE KLUVER–BUCY SYNDROME

When the anterior parts of both temporal lobes are destroyed in a monkey, this removes not only portions of temporal cortex but also of the amygdalas that lie inside these parts of the temporal lobes. This causes changes in behavior, called the Kluver–Bucy syndrome, which is demonstrated by an animal that (1) is not afraid of anything, (2) has extreme curiosity about everything, (3) forgets rapidly, (4) has a tendency to place everything in its mouth and sometimes even tries to eat solid objects, and (5) often has a sex drive so strong that it attempts to copulate with immature animals, animals of the wrong sex, or even animals of a different species. Although similar lesions in human beings are rare, afflicted people respond in a manner not too different from that of the monkey or dog.

OVERALL FUNCTION OF THE AMYGDALAS

The amygdalas seem to be behavioral awareness areas that operate at a semiconscious level. They also seem to project into the limbic system one's current status in relation to both surroundings and thoughts. On the basis of this information, the amygdala is believed to make the person's behavioral response appropriate for each occasion.

FUNCTION OF THE LIMBIC CORTEX

The most poorly understood portion of the limbic system is the ring of cerebral cortex called the limbic cortex that surrounds the subcortical limbic structures. This cortex functions as a transitional zone through which signals are transmitted from the remainder of the brain cortex into the limbic system and also in the opposite direction. Therefore, the limbic cortex in effect functions as a cerebral association area for control of behavior.

According to Guyton and Hall,[14] stimulation of the different regions of the limbic cortex has failed to give a real idea of any of their functions. However, as is true of so many other portions of the limbic system essentially all behavioral patterns can be elicited by stimulation of specific portions of the limbic cortex. Likewise, ablation of some limbic cortical areas can cause persistent changes in an animal's behavior, as follows.

ABLATION OF THE ANTERIOR TEMPORAL CORTEX

When the anterior temporal cortex is ablated bilaterally, the amygdalas are almost invariably damaged as well. It was pointed out that the Kluver–Bucy syndrome occurs. The animal especially develops consummatory behaviors. It investigates any and all objects, has intense sex drives toward inappropriate animals or even inanimate objects, and loses all fear and thus develops tameness as well.

ABLATION OF THE POSTERIOR ORBITAL FRONTAL CORTEX

Bilateral removal of the posterior portion of the orbital frontal cortex often causes an animal to develop insomnia associated with intense motor restlessness, becoming unable to sit still and moving about continuously. Many chemically sensitive patients have seen problems such as insomnia. Often sleep medication and even melatonin will not allow them to sleep until the total body pollutant load is decreased or the specific chemical incitant that causes insomnia is removed. We see this in mold-infested buildings, pesticides, and solvent exposures and many other situations.

ABLATION OF THE ANTERIOR CINGULATE GYRI AND SUBCALLOSAL GYRI

The anterior cingulate gyri and the subcallosal gyri are the portions of the limbic cortex that communicate between the prefrontal cerebral cortex and the subcortical limbic structures. Destruction of these gyri bilaterally releases the rage centers of the septum and hypothalamus from prefrontal inhibitory influence. Therefore, the animal can become vicious and much more subject to fits of rage than normally.

Until further information is available, it is perhaps best to state that the cortical regions of the limbic system occupy intermediate associative positions between the functions of the specific areas of the cerebral cortex and functions of the subcortical limbic structures for control of behavioral patterns. Thus, in the anterior temporal cortex, one especially finds gustatory and olfactory behavioral associations. In the parahippocampal gyri, there is a tendency for complex auditory associations and complex thought associations derived from Wernicke's area of the posterior temporal lobe. In the middle and posterior cingulate cortex, there is reason to believe that sensorimotor behavioral associations occur. Short-term memory loss is often seen in the chemically sensitive and this improves by decreasing the total body pollutant load by eliminating and neutralizing specific triggering agents.

SYSTEMIC INFLAMMATION: PERIPHERAL IMPACT ON THE BRAIN

Systemic inflammation is implicated in CS,[17,18] vasculitis neurogenerative diseases,[19] and sickness behavior.[20,21] The peripheral immune system communicates with the CNS through oxidative stress and cytokines, where circulating cytokines impact peripheral innate immune cells, activate peripheral neuronal afferents,[22] and physically enter the brain through diffusion and active transport to impact the CNS.[21] This phenomenon is usually seen in the chemically sensitive. In addition to cellular damage and modification of the ROS/cytokine milieu in the brain, systemic inflammation has recently been shown to alter the cellular makeup of innate immune cells in the brain. Specifically, in response to peripheral tumor necrosis factor-α (TNF-α) injection, mice were shown to recruit larger amounts of circulating monocytes to the brain.[20]

It is becoming increasingly accepted that air pollution causes proinflammatory signals originating in peripheral tissues/organs such as the lung,[23] liver,[24] GI tract, GU and cardiovascular system,[25] giving rise to a systemic-induced cytokine response[26] that transfers inflammation to the brain.[23,27,28] We have observed this fact in thousands of chemically sensitive patients. For example, mercury in teeth causes local inflammation, then causes a mild inflammation in colon or vagina or bladder, which aggravates the chemically sensitive and thus triggers brain dysfunction and exacerbates the chemically sensitive.

Particulate effects (10 µg/m, 2.5 µg/m; nanoparticulates $\geq$100 nm) as well as carbon monoxide, sulfur dioxide, nitrogen dioxide, pesticides, ozone, solvents, mycotoxins, natural gas, and EMF can trigger inflammation and cause CS.

Exposure to PM has been shown to elevate plasma cytokine concentrations (IL-1β, IL-6), granulocyte-macrophage colony-stimulating factor (GMCF), which are believed to be released into circulation as a consequence of interactions between particles, alveolar macrophages, and airway epithelial cells.[29] Further, PM has been shown to mobilize bone-marrow-derived neutrophils and monocytes into the circulation in both human and animal studies.[29] Given these findings, it is not surprising that air pollution is associated with neuroinflammation particularly in the chemically sensitive who get constant pollutant exposure reactions. This fact of particulate reduction of at least five times over a normal environment in our environmental control facilities (clinic and environmentally safe housing) has cleared or reduced the hypersensitivity response in around 9000 of the chemically sensitive patients without any medication. Antigen or nutrient supplementation may be important. This reduction in pollution allows for a clearance of external pollutants resulting in an augmentation of antipollutant enzymes and detoxification systems. It then relieves symptoms and results in resuming of energy and elimination of fatigue. These are then downplayed giving relief of toxicity and hypersensitivity resulting in avoidance of permanent cerebral damages.

Circulating cytokines produced in systemic inflammation, such as TNF-α and IL-aβ, are well known to cause neuroinflammation,[30–33] neurotoxicity,[30,32,33] and cerebral vascular damage.[34] For example, chronic, low-grade inflammation associated with multiple systemic injections of low concentrations of lipopolysaccharide (LPS), a cell wall component of gram-negative bacteria that is a potent proinflammatory stimulus, in adult mice results in mild neuroinflammation, rendering animals more susceptible to further proinflammatory insult.[32] However, a single large proinflammatory insult in adult animals administered with one IP injection of a high concentraton of LPS (and TNF-α injection) results in chronic neuroinflammation that persists months after peripheral inflammation abates, resulting in delayed and progressive neuron death, beginning only after 7–10 months post-LPS treatment in mice.[30] This can occur in chemically sensitive as seen in many patients at the EHC-Dallas and the EHC-Buffalo. Animal studies have also shown that exposure to systemic inflammation early in development can both cause and potentiate neuron damage seen later, in adult animals.[33] A similar situation occurs in chemically sensitive patients who have a nidus of inflammation, that is, the GI tract, vaginal, bladder, or mouth or arteriosclerosis, etc. A chemically sensitive patient may have a nidus for bacteria, which can emanate a toxic producing the LPS. Thus, mercury-laden fillings or just an inflammation of a tooth socket will make chemically sensitive patients prone later to brain damage if this local and then systemic process is not brought under control.

In addition to neuron damage, it is also proposed that systemic inflammation caused by air, food, or water contaminant pollution may contribute to deteriorating olfactory, respiratory, and blood–brain barriers (BBB) to enhance access to the CNS and further increase neuropathology.[35] Thus, systemic inflammation caused by air pollution is very likely to give rise to both neuroinflammation and neuropathology[36] where neurotoxic effects may be cumulative. We frequently see progressive neurodamage in the history of chemically sensitive patients as they go through life with unidentified triggering agents. This is evidenced by a history of common inhaled sensitivity from rhinosinusitis to vertigo to brain fog. There is aggressive intolerance to biological inhalant (mold) to food, and chemical (benzene styrene, toluene, natural gas, herbicide, pesticides, etc.) sensitivity to chemical overload, and inflammation continues.

To define the degree of systemic inflammation, substances measured are inflammatory mediators such as C-reactive protein, prostaglandin E metabolite, and heat shock protein 60; IL-10 was the selected TH2 anti-inflammatory cytokine. Given that controlled ozone exposures are associated with upregulation of mCD14 on airway macrophages and monocytes, and that a synergistic action on the CD14 effect has been suggested between PM-LPS and ozone,[37] they selected mCD14, sCD14, and LPS-binding protein (LBP)[38,39] to characterize the LPS-recognition complex components. LPS forms a complex with an acute-phase protein called LBP responsible for the binding and transport of LPS in the circulation.[39] A major response to LPS is mediated by its interaction with CD14, a 55-kDa myeloid differentiation antigen that allows endotoxin to interact with the TLR4.[39] Finally, TLR4 specifically recognizes LPS and is part of the endotoxin signaling receptor complex that initiates proinflammatory signaling. Since missense mutations such as Asp299Gly are associated with a blunted response to inhaled LPS, it was determined the allelic frequencies of Asp299Gly TLR4 polymorphism in both cohorts and included only children fully capable of responding to LPS.[40] Certainly, the chemically sensitive can go down this pathway eventually causing permanent brain damage.

Evidence that olfactory bulb pathology is clearly associated with olfactory dysfunction is illustrated very well in both Alzheimer's and Parkinson's diseases (AD and PD)[41–43] as well as chemical and electrical sensitivity.[44]

Olfactory loss is a very early finding in both AD and PD, and this loss of pollutant perception precedes cognitive and motor symptoms, respectively, by years.[45,46] Odor identification deficits in

APOE ε 4 allele AD siblings (aged 59–88 years) are considered to be early cognitive markers of incipient AD.[47] In older adults, unexplained olfactory dysfunction in the presence of an ε 4 allele is associated with a high risk of cognitive decline (OR: 4.9).[48] APO ε 4 allele subjects have a more rapid decline in odor identification than in odor threshold or dementia rating scale scores.[49] Thus, their findings of APOE ε 4 subjects failing more items in the 10-item smell identification scale related to AD raises a key question: does residency in a highly polluted city accelerate olfactory deficits associated with increased risk for AD? In this small study, APOE 4 subjects had significantly less residency time in Mexico (p = 0.02) compared with their APOE 2 and 3 counterparts, but displayed the same deficits in UPSIT scores, along with significantly increased failure rates in the 10 UPSIT items most sensitive to AD.[50]

This suggests there may be an acceleration of their olfaction deficits. Given that functional brain abnormalities and cognitive decline are detected in young APOE 4 carriers decades before the clinical onset of dementia, it remains to be determined whether olfactory deficits precede the abnormally low rates of cerebral glucose metabolism in the posterior cingulate, parietal, temporal, and PFC and/or the lowered Mini-Mental and Verbal Learning Test scores.[51,52]

The findings of Calderón-Garcidueñas et al.[50] suggest olfactory tests may be of value along with cognitive testing in young persons with complaints of olfactory dysfunction but with no known risk factors for dementia.[47] Physicians should be aware that exposures to polluted urban environments can result in olfactory deficits. In the United States alone, 29 million people are exposed to PM_{10}, 88 million to $PM_{2.5}$, and millions more to nanopans occupationally and in the setting of disasters, including war, fires, and the aftermath of terrorist attacks such as occurred at the World Trade Center.[53] The chemically sensitive may add to the population of damaged individuals with their increased odor sensitivity leading to diminishing brain function.[44,54,55]

The long-term significance of olfactory deficits in young individuals residing in a highly polluted environment, particularly those carrying an APOE 4 allele, remains to be defined. However, Calderón-Garcidueñas et al.[50] are of the opinion that such individuals living in regions of high pollution are likely to be of high risk for later development of progressive olfactory and cognitive deficits, including neurotoxicity, AD, and PD as well as degenerative diseases such as cancer and arteriosclerosis. This possibility is based upon their findings of pollution-related (a) neuroinflammation in key brain areas, (b) altered innate immune brain responses, (c) the presence of PM in olfactory neurons, endothelial cells, and their basement membranes, and (d) the accumulation of beta amyloid 42 and alpha-synuclein in olfactory bulb, supra- and infratentorial locations.[27,56,57]

HYPERSENSITIVITY TO ODORS

It should be pointed out that none of these studies involved or discussed hypersensitivity to odor, which a large group of ENT surgeons have observed in Mexico City, Aquocalienties, Monterey, and Tlaxcala. The patients they treated had the opposite reaction to pollution in that they developed odor intolerance. This intolerance may drive these patients out of Mexico City, or they are in an earlier stage than the degeneration of smell than in Calderón-Garcidueñas's cohort. They are, in fact, a significant group of patients who may later on develop a central neuropathy as the pollution exposure progresses.

Surprisingly, little is known about the effects of big-city air pollution on olfactory function and even less about its effects on the intranasal *trigeminal system*, which elicits sensations like burning, stinging, pungent, or fresh and contributes to the overall chemosensory experience. Using the Sniffin' Sticks olfactory test battery and an established test for intranasal trigeminal perception, Guarneros et al.[58] compared the olfactory performance and trigeminal sensitivity of residents of Mexico City, in a region with high air pollution, with the performance of a control population from the Mexican state of Tlaxcala, a geographically comparable but less-polluted region. Guarneros et al.[58] compared the ability of 30 young adults from each location to detect a rose-like odor (2-phenylethanol), to discriminate between different odorants, and to identify several other common odorants. The control subjects from

Tlaxcala detected 2-phenylethanol at significantly lower concentrations than the Mexico City subjects, they could discriminate between odorants significantly better, and they performed significantly better in the test of trigeminal sensitivity. Guarneros et al.[58] concluded that Mexico City air pollution impairs olfactory function and intranasal trigeminal sensitivity, even in otherwise healthy young adults. In addition, some ENT groups had to evacuate Mexico City to survive.

Sensory mismatch induces autonomic responses associated with hippocampal theta waves in rats.[59] Aitake et al.[59] have shown that the hippocampal (HIP) theta power increases during sensory mismatch, which has been suggested. The patient with CS often exhibits this phenomenon when he or she is exposed to external pollutant overload. Pollutants induce motion sickness with autonomic abnormality. To investigate relationships between hippocampal theta rhythm and autonomic functions, theta waves in the HIP and electrocardiograms (ECGs) were recorded during sensory mismatch by backward translocation in awake rats. The rats were placed on a treadmill affixed to a motion stage that was translocated along a figure 8-shaped track. The rats were trained to run forward on the treadmill at the same speed as that of forward translocation of the motion stage (a forward condition) before the experimental (recording) sessions. In the experimental sessions, the rats were initially tested in the forward condition, and then tested in a backward (mismatch) condition, in which the motion stage was turned around by 180° before translocation. That is, the rats were moved backward by translocation of the stage although the rats ran forward on the treadmill. In this condition, the theta (6–9 Hz) power was significantly increased in the backward condition compared with the forward condition. Spectral analysis of HR variability indicated that sympathetic nervous activity increased in the backward condition. These data (theta power and sympathetic nervous activity) were positively correlated. Furthermore, electrical stimulation of the HIP at theta rhythm (8 Hz) increased HR. These results suggest that sensory mismatch information activates the HIP to induce autonomic alteration in motion sickness of the patient. The sensory mismatch is also seen in the hypersensitivity to odors group. These patients usually have a sympathetic increase or a parasympathetic decrease response or irritate variable measurements, while the advanced cases have a combination of hypoparasympathetic and hypersympathetic response.

As shown in Chapter 1 of Volume III,[60] studies have shown that the sensory nerves are initially involved in finding pollutant overload. These nerves once disturbed can alter the peripheral sensory and ANS and then the immune system, allowing for pollutant clearing or, if overloaded, disturbance of the body's local, regional, or total physiology. Brain studies have shown that the limbic system is involved.[60]

There are a myriad of effects due to this air pollution including chronic fatigue, fibromyalgia, asthma, arthritis, GI upset, GU dysfunction, and CS, and resultant cancer and cardiovascular disease.

Due to the mixture of chemicals and particulates, bacteria, molds, etc. in transportation polluted air, it cannot only be lethal but also cause chronic, debilitating illness. It can cause abnormal nerve function, CS, and chronic fatigue.

NEUROLOGICAL

Neurological dysfunction is a major part of the CS entity. The neurological dysfunction can develop as sensitized nerves and receptors as well as imbalance of the ANS. As shown throughout the series of books on CS, there are, at present, multiple studies from around the world that shows the olfactory and trigeminal nerves to be involved in pollutant injury which goes directly to the brain and causes numerous areas to be out of balance resulting in dysfunction (Volumes II and III—Reversibility of Chemical Sensitivity).[60,61] We will not repeat all these studies. However, a few new ones will be discussed to emphasize the neurological changes of CS versus normal control. For example, Alobid et al.[62] in the otolargyology smell clinic at the University of Barcelona, Spain showed that changes occur. However, an intensity fact occurs according to smell in noses.

According to Bower,[63] humans can tell apart an average of more than 1 trillion odors.

That estimate of smell's reach vastly exceeds the roughly several million colors and 340,000 sounds a typical person can distinguish.

Previous investigations found that humans have 400 genes that code for odor-sensing molecules.[63] That is a sign that smell discrimination played a significant role in human evolution. It now plays a role in human survival for the chemically sensitive.

The ability to distinguish among vast numbers of odors proves especially important that women's emotional tears contain substances that influence men's behavior via smell.

Voshall and colleagues tested the ability of 26 men and women to distinguish scents concocted from 128 odor molecules, such as banana-scented isoamyl acetate. Participants were unfamiliar with most of the resulting smells, which were randomly presented in mixtures of 10, 20, or 30 odor molecules.

In each of 264 trials, volunteers sniffed three vials. Two vials contained the same odor; the task was to pick the scent that differed. Paired odor mixtures shared varying fractions of molecules in different trials.

Participants had little difficulty telling the difference between mixtures that shared as much as 51% of their odor molecules. The number of volunteers able to tell scents apart declined steadily as pairs of odor mixes increasingly shared components. No one could discriminate between mixtures that chemically overlapped by more than 90%. This phenomenon and the ability to mask in the human can be detrimental causing a trending toward CS.

Based on individuals' accuracy rates, the number of possible odor mixtures in the order of 10^{30}, and the amount of overlap among those mixtures, the researchers calculated that the average participant could discriminate a minimum of more than 1 trillion smells containing 30 odor molecules. This is lost in the chemically sensitive, though the ones they can define are accentuated. Often the CS allows the patient to sense and react to odors others have difficulty in perceiving.

There were big differences among participants. The best performing volunteers could have distinguished many more mixtures than 1 trillion, while the least accurate sniffer could have identified almost 80 million distinct scents.

Humans undoubtedly distinguish more than 1 trillion smells. Many more odor molecules and scent mixtures exist than that were tested. This phenomenon can be detrimental to the chemically sensitive since they may perceive one molecule of a substance, which may be detrimental to their health or advantageous to their survival. At times, they have difficulty in convincing the cohorts of their perceptions. This is particularly true for chemically sensitive patients.

In contrast to the human perception, nonhuman animals often focus on a relatively narrow range of species-specific scent signals that they discern with exquisite sensitivity. Limited scent learning is possible, as in dogs trained to recognize the smell of hidden cocaine or explosives. It appears that some chemically sensitive with or without a supersense of smell do learn some odors of substances that are particularly toxic for them and they have to avoid them at all costs, when they are not made especially ill.

Many other animals may also discriminate a trillion or more odors. For instance, mice possess about 1000 genes that code for odor-sensing molecules, and flys have about 50 such genes. Studies by several investigators have shown that the olfactory system constantly makes new neurons when new exposure occurs.

STRUCTURAL AND FUNCTIONAL FEATURES OF CNS LYMPHATIC VESSELS

Louveau et al.[64] discovered functional lymphatic vessels lining the dural sinuses. These structures[65] express all of the molecular hallmarks of lymphatic endothelial cells (LECs),[66] are able to carry both fluid and immune cells from the *cerebrospinal fluid* (CSF), and are connected to the deep cervical lymph nodes (dCLN).[67] The unique location of these vessels may have impeded their discovery to date, thereby contributing to the long-held concept of the absence of lymphatic vasculature in the CNS. The discovery of the CNS lymphatic system may call for a reassessment of basic assumptions in neuroimmunology and shed new light on the etiology of neuroinflammatory and neurodegenerative diseases associated with immune system dysfunction, especially in the chemically sensitive.

Louveau et al.[64] investigated the meningeal spaces and the immune cells that occupy those spaces. First, a wholemount preparation of dissected mouse brain meninges was developed and stained by immunohistochemistry for endothelial cells, T cells, and major histocompatibility complex II (MHCII)-expressing cells. Labeling of these cells revealed a restricted partitioning of immune cells throughout the meningeal compartments, with a high concentration of cells found in close proximity to the dural sinuses.

The dural sinuses drain blood from both the internal and the external veins of the brain into the internal jugular veins. If these arterioles and venules of the microcirculation work as the rest of the body, the environmental pollutants there can result in a shunting of oxygen returning to the jugular vein. This shunting through the microcirculation can create areas of hypoxia in areas most needed resulting in brain function aberration such as cloudy thinking, weakness, and fatigue. Due to the autophagic phenomenon, the chemically sensitive cannot release toxics that are handled by the lymphatic system. The exact localization of the T lymphocytes around the sinuses was examined to rule out the possibility of artifacts caused by incomplete intracardial perfusion. Coronal sections of the dura mater were stained for CD3e (T cells) and for CD31 (endothelial cells). Indeed, the vast majority of the T lymphocytes near the sinuses were abluminal. To confirm this finding, mice were injected intravenously (IV) with DyLight 488 lectin or fluorescent anti-CD45 antibody before euthanasia and the abluminal localization was confirmed and quantified. Unexpectedly, a portion of T cells (and of MHCII-expressing cells) was aligned linearly in CD31-expressing structures along the sinuses (only few cells were evident in meningeal blood vessels of similar diameter), suggesting a unique function for these perisinusal vessels.

Lymphatic System of the Brain

In addition to the cardiovascular system, the lymphatic vessels represent a distinct and prominent vascular system in the body.[68,69] Prompted by observations that the perisinusal vessels were tested for markers associated with LECs. Wholemount meninges from adult mice were immunostained for the LEC marker, Lyve-1. Two to three Lyve-1-expressing vessels were identified running parallel to the dural sinuses. Analysis of coronal sections labeled for Lyve-1 and the endothelial cell marker, CD31, revealed that Lyve-1 vessels are located adjacent to the sinus and exhibit a distinct lumen. Intravenous injection of DyLight 488 lectin before euthanasia confirmed that these Lyve-11 vessels do not belong to the cardiovasculature.

The lymphatic character of the perisinusal vessels was further interrogated by assessing the presence of several classical LEC markers. Expression of the main LEC transcription factor, Prox1, was indeed detectable in the Lyve-1$^+$ vessels using immunostaining in wild-type mice or in transgenic mice expressing tdTomato (tdT) under the Prox1 promoter (Prox1^{tdT}). Similar to peripheral lymphatic vessels, the Lyve-1 vessels were also found to express podoplanin and the vascular endothelial growth factor receptor 3 (VEGFR3). Injection of VEGFR3-specific recombinant VEGF-c into the cisterna magna resulted in an increase in the diameter of the meningeal lymphatic vessels, when examined 7 days after the injection, suggesting a functional role of VEGFR3 on meningeal LECs. Finally, the presence of LECs in the meninges was confirmed by flow cytometry; a CD45$^-$CD31$^+$ podoplanin1 population of cells (LECs) was detected in the dura mater, and is similar to that found in the skin and diaphragm. They identified a potentially similar structure in human dura (Lyve-1podoplanin1 CD68$^-$), but further studies will be necessary to fully assess and characterize the location and organization of meningeal lymphatic vessels in the human CNS.

Two types of afferent lymphatic vessels exist: initial and collecting. They differ anatomically (i.e., the presence or the absence of surrounding smooth muscle cells [SMCs] and lymphatic valves), in their expression pattern of adhesion molecules,[68,70,71] and in their permissiveness to fluid and cell entry.[70] In contrast to the sinuses, the meningeal lymphatic vessels are devoid of SMCs.

Furthermore, meningeal lymphatic vessels were also positive for the immune-cell chemoattractant protein, CCL2. Unlike the blood vessels that exhibit a continuous pattern of Claudin-5 and vascular endothelial (VE)-cadherin, the meningeal lymphatic vessels exhibit a punctuate expression pattern of these molecules similarly to diaphragm lymphatic vessels.[70] Also, expression of integrin-a9, which is characteristic of lymphatic valves,[72] was not found on meningeal lymphatic vessels, but was readily detectable in the skin lymphatic network. Collectively, these findings indicate that the meningeal lymphatic vessels possess anatomical and molecular features characteristic of initial lymphatic vessels. Furthermore, electron microscopy of wholemount meninges revealed typical ultrastructural characteristics[73] of the lymphatic vessels, which exhibited a noncontinuous basement membrane surrounded by anchoring filaments.

While possessing many of the same attributes as peripheral lymphatic vessels, the general organization and distribution of the meningeal lymphatic vasculature displays certain unique features. The meningeal lymphatic network appears to start from both eyes and track above the olfactory bulb before aligning adjacent to the sinuses. Compared to the diaphragm, the meningeal lymphatic network covers less of the tissue and forms a less complex network composed of narrower vessels. The vessels are larger and more complex in the transverse sinuses than in the superior sagittal sinus. The differences in the vessel network could be due to the environment in which the vessels reside— the high CSF pressure in the CNS compared to the interstitial fluid pressure in peripheral tissues could affect the branching of the vessels and also limit their expansion. Because of this anatomy one can see the fragility of the network and how blows to the head could be the start of CS when these channels are disrupted as we see in many chemically sensitive patients who initially had head injuries at a younger age.

Next, the functional capability of the meningeal lymphatic vessels to carry fluid and cells from the meninges/CSF was examined. Anaesthetized adult mice were simultaneously injected with fluorescein IV and with fluorescent tracer dye (QDot655) intracerebroventricularly (ICV), and then imaged through thinned skull by multiphoton microscopy. Vessels filled with QDot655, but not with fluorescein, were seen aligned along the superior sagittal sinus, suggesting that noncardiovascular vessels drain CSF. This CSF drainage into meningeal vessels may occur in addition to the previously described CSF filtration into the dural sinuses via arachnoid granulations.[74,75] Injection of Alexa488-conjugated anti-Lyve-1 antibody ICV labeled the meningeal lymphatic vessels. Moreover, coinjection of a QDot655 and an Alexa488-conjugated anti-Lyve-1 antibody ICV demonstrated that the meningeal lymphatic vessels were indeed filled with QDot655, and thus were draining the CSF. Imaging of the QDot655-filled lymphatic vessels revealed a slower flowrate but similar direction of flow in the meningeal lymphatic vessels compared to the adjacent blood vessels, similar to what is observed outside of the CNS.[76]

Classic lymphatic vessels, in addition to draining interstitial fluids, allow cells to travel from tissues to draining lymph nodes.[77] They therefore examined whether the meningeal lymphatic vessels were capable of carrying leukocytes. Immunohistochemical analysis of wholemount meninges revealed that 24% of all sinusal T cells and 12% of all sinusal MHCII1 cells were found within these vessels. Moreover, CD11c1 cells and B2201 cells are also found in the meningeal lymphatic vessels of naive mice. Therefore, a significant number of immune cells can be distorted or blocked if the brain lymphatics are blocked by trauma or pollutant injury. When this occurs, brain toxics will clog the brain causing potentially memory loss, cloudy thinking, loss of balance, etc.

Cellular and soluble constituents of the CSF have been shown to elicit immune responses in the cervical lymph nodes.[78–81] Their proposed path is via the cribriform plate into lymphatic vessels within the nasal mucosa.[82] To determine whether meningeal lymphatic vessels communicate with dCLN directly, they injected mice with Evans blue ICV and examined peripheral lymph nodes for the presence of the dye over a 2-hour period. Thirty minutes after injection, Evans blue was detected in the meningeal lymphatic vessels and the sinus, as expected, and had also drained into the dCLN, but not into the superficial cervical lymph nodes. At later time points, Evans blue was also present in the superficial cervical lymph nodes. Virtually, no Evans blue was seen in the surrounding nonlymphatic tissue at the time points tested. Interestingly, no Evans blue was detected in the dCLN 30 minutes after direct injection into the nasal mucosa, suggesting that meningeal lymphatic vessels and not nasal mucosa lymphatic vessels represent the primary route for drainage of CSF-derived soluble and cellular constituents into the dCLN during this time frame.

Resection of the dCLN affected the T cell compartment of the meninges, resulting in an increase in the number of meningeal T cells. This presumably resulted from an inability of T cells to drain from the meningeal spaces, consistent with a direct connection between the meninges and the dCLN. To further demonstrate this connection, they ligated the lymph vessels that drain into the dCLNs, and injected the mice ICV with Evans blue. No accumulation of Evans blue was evident in the dCLN of ligated mice, as opposed to dye accumulation in the sham-operated controls. Moreover, an increase in the diameter of the meningeal lymphatic vessels was observed, similar to lymphedema observed in peripheral tissues emphasizing how polluted triggered immune reactions could cause the blocking lymphaction.[83] These results further suggest physical connection between the meningeal lymphatic vessels and the dCLN.

Drainage of the CSF into the periphery has been a subject of interest for decades and several routes have been described regarding how CSF can leave the CNS.[82,84] The newly discovered meningeal lymphatic vessels are a novel path for CSF drainage and represent a more conventional path for immune cells to egress the CNS. Their findings may represent the second step in the drainage of the interstitial fluid from the brain parenchyma into the periphery after it has been drained into the CSF through the recently discovered glymphatic system.[85,86]

The presence of a functional and classical lymphatic system in the CNS suggests that current dogmas regarding brain tolerance and the immune privilege of the brain should be revisited. Malfunction of the meningeal lymphatic vessels could be a root cause of a variety of neurological disorders in which altered immunity is a fundamental player such as multiple sclerosis, CS, AD, and some forms of primary lymphedema that are associated with neurological disorders[87–89] that are pollutant triggered.

Until now, it was believed that the brain was the only organ in the body that did not have a classical lymphatic drainage system that transports and eliminates cellular waste products. This newly discovered meningeal lymphatic system is a novel path for CSF drainage and represents a more conventional path for immune cells and degradation products of neural activity, including neuro-inflammation, to egress the CNS. This pathway strengthens the observation seen in the chemically sensitive of immune, vascular olfactory dysfunction seen in chemically sensitive patients.

Through immunohistochemical techniques, the researchers demonstrate that the meningeal lymphatic system drains into the dCLN, which then deliver the waste into the general peripheral circulation to exit the body by the urine, bile, and sweat routes. Prior to this finding, it was believed that CSF drained from the subarachnoid space into nasal lymphatics or did not drain at all.[84] These facts explain why sauna with sweating is so offacious in chemically sensitive patients, and also why chemically sensitive patients have a myriad of types of brain dysfunctions that can disable them.

The researchers discovered that the found structures were not blood vessels, but rather lymphatic vessels that carried leukocytes (T lymphocytes). Further imaging studies confirmed that the meningeal lymphatic vessels provided a drainage route from the CSF. Now, we know that lymphatic vessels exist in the brain, and that they drain immune cells and macromolecules from the CSF to the draining lymph nodes.

This step may be the second step in the drainage of interstitial fluid from the brain parenchyma. The first is the recently discovered perivascular pathway known as the glymphatic system.[90] The term glymphatic is derived from the system's reliance on glial cells and its resemblance to the lymphatic system.[91] The glymphatic system works as a "macroscopic waste clearance system that utilizes a unique system of perivascular tunnels, formed by astroglial cells, to promote efficient elimination of soluble proteins and metabolites from the CNS."[90] Besides waste elimination, the glymphatic system also enhances the distribution of several compounds in the brain, including glucose, lipids, amino acids, growth factors, and neuromodulators.[90] When the clinician gives autogenous lymphocyte factor to an immune depleted chemically sensitive patient, the patient's energy level increases and clearer brain function is observed as seen at the EHC-Dallas.

Some of the alteration of the lymphatics and the microvascular dysfunction may be due to attraction of the BBB of both the vessels and the lymphatics due to organophosphates pesticide.[92] However, it may also be triggered by head trauma that is so mild that nothing shows on brain scan.[93] Researchers at the Cleveland Clinic and Soroka Medical School and Korn et al.[93] have shown that 17 patients with neurologic symptoms revealed abnormal patterns as the generator for abnormal rhythms. SPECT scans showed local reduction of perfusion in 70%–85% of the patients. These areas were closely related to the anatomic location of the BBB lesion. These data are paired to focal cortical dysfunction in conjunction with BBB disruption. These hits can trigger the autoimmune responses; S100B protein in the blood seems to be an indicator of significant head trauma. According to Friedman et al.,[94] pyridostigmine brain penetration under stress enhances neuro net excitability and induces early immediate transcriptional responses. Pyridostigmine (PYR) obtains 20%–20% whole blood acetylcholinesterase (AGhE) inhibits, which change the treatment of poisoning by an organophosphate anticholinesterase agent. Thus, when the trauma occurs in humans, it could be a nidus for subsequent trigger of CS as we have seen in many patients at the EHC-Dallas.

RELEVANCE TO PAIN MANAGEMENT

According to Tennant,[95] the relevance to pain management of the discovery of glymphatic and lymphatic systems is big. To date, the entire discussion of brain drainage and CSF flow has been missing in pain management journals, conferences, and seminars. We have discussed this and seen problems in a subset of chemically sensitive patients at the EHC-Dallas.

Recently, we learned the pain that initially arises from a peripheral nervous system injury may become imprinted or "embedded" in the CNS, activate microglial cells (Figure 2.12), and produce neuroinflammation. This phenomenon of "central sensitization" and the resulting state is centralized pain (CP).[96–98] This pain is seen in many chemically sensitive patients and may result in blockage of areas in the brain of glia cells and lymphatic waste removal. Phantom limb pain is the classic example. Other examples include neuropathies, including complex regional pain syndrome and diabetic neuropathies. Disorders that originate in the CNS, such as trauma, stroke, infections, and arachnoiditis, also cause significant neuroinflammation (Figure 2.14).

It is now believed that these immunologic, toxic, and antigenic degradation products of painful neuroinflammation may be exiting the CNS and CSF through the newly discovered meningeal lymphatic system. This understanding gives us a scientific explanation for the peripheral, autoimmune symptoms, and syndromes we commonly see with chronic pain conditions. This explains to patients how neuroinflammatory, painful conditions in the CNS may cause chronic pain in chemically sensitive patients.

Now we know that there are glymphatic and lymphatic drainage systems in the brain; there therapeutics are opportunities. Since waste products from neuroinflammation are toxic and antigenic to peripheral tissues, the question is reasonably raised as to whether increased or more rapid lymphatic drainage from the brain is necessarily a good thing. While the answer to this question is unknown, it seems clinically prudent to simultaneously increase peripheral clearance with exercise and movement, sauna, and nutrients; at the same time, measures may be executed to increase CNS drainage. In Tennant's work,[95] he has found neuroinflammatory biomarkers in the serum to be distressingly high in CP patients. It is known why he is able to find these markers in serum. They simply drain out of the CNS through the meningeal lymphatic system, which is usually blocked in chemically sensitive patients.

A rapid drainage begets rapid healing. For example, all pain practitioners know that those patients who walk, swim, and exercise do better but often the chemically sensitive cannot do this. However, they can keep the peripheral lymphatics open to detoxify. Movement and physical activity undoubtedly accelerates lymphatic brain drainage, which would explain why Travell's rocking

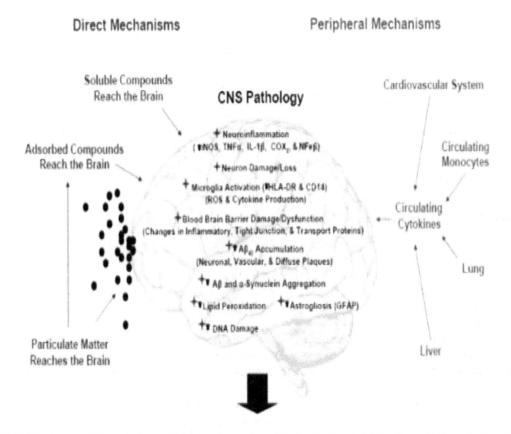

FIGURE 2.14 CNS pathology. (Adapted from Rea, W. J., K. Patel. 2015. *Reversibility of Chronic Degenerative Disease and Hypersensitivity*, Vol. 2. Boca Raton, FL: CRC Press.)

chair therapy did President John F. Kennedy some good. Rocking likely accelerates CNS lymphatic drainage. This modality tried rocking more in chemically sensitive patients who could not tolerate much exercise.

SLEEP

As clinicians, we have to ask if there is a treatment that may enhance the sweeping out of toxins through the newly discovered lymphatic drainage system. The most obvious question in chemically sensitive patients is how can we control neuroinflammation and decrease antigenic and toxic by-products, which we now know are egressing the CNS and entering the peripheral circulation to set up reactions that damage peripheral tissue.

One obscure study showed that a major function of sleep, if not its most critical function, is to clear toxic substances from the brain's interstitial spaces and CSF fluid.[85] The authors found that "natural sleep or anesthesia are associated with a 60% increase in the interstitial space, resulting in a striking increase in convective exchange of CSF with interstitial fluid. In turn, convective fluxes of interstitial fluid increased the rate of beta-amyloid clearance during sleep. Thus, the restorative function of sleep may be a consequence of the enhanced removal of potentially neurotoxic waste products that accumulate in the awake CNS."[85] This surely applies to the chemically sensitive who have difficulty in sleeping. This must be our modality that the chemically sensitive will not get well unless they get consistent good night sleep. Of course, this is not easy to obtain because of the patient's sensitivity to melatonin and many sleeping medications.

As noted above, drainage from brain tissue into the CSF occurs through a microchannel system, now called the glymphatic system. Since sleep promotes glymphatic drainage, we should be more aggressive in promoting good sleep hygiene practices and, when necessary, prescribing sleep medication for pain patients when they can tolerate them. A most interesting finding from the study was that mice given a cocktail of adrenergic receptor antagonists (prazosin [Minipress, others], atipamezole [Antisedan], and propranolol [Inderal, others]) increased drainage of cellular waste products from brain parenchyma.[85] Propranolol may prevent migraines in some patients but finding the triggering agents such as food, mold, and toxic chemicals to eliminate them is better.

Drainage of toxic waste from body tissue is as old as medicine itself. We drain abscesses, bladders, and blood. In pain management of the chemically sensitive, we now have an idea of how to "drain the brain."

Pain: AD: Neurobehavioral

The recent discovery is that pain caused by a peripheral nerve injury can imprint itself in the CNS (CP) ranks as one of the great advances in pain management.[99–101] Although there has been some debate, these brain changes appear to be the result of chronic pain and not the cause. CP is often accompanied by symptoms of hyperarousal of the sympathetic nervous system (SNS), causing responses like tachycardia and hyperarousal in the chemically sensitive, which can be used to help guide diagnosis and treatment of CP.

We do try to minimize the adrenalin response to the CNS by decreasing the total body pollutant load. By eliminating toxics in our food and water, enhance nutrition and check the hypersensitivity by intradermal serial dilution neutralization techniques occasionally the patient needs a medication like metoprolol to dampen this response.

The changing landscape of chronic pain research has yielded new ways to describe pain. IASP also offers a "simpler definition" of chronic or persistent pain: "pain that continues when it should not." "Central pain syndrome is a neurological condition caused by damage to or dysfunction of the central nervous system (CNS), which includes the brain, brain stem, and spinal cord. This syndrome can be caused by stroke, multiple sclerosis, tumors, epilepsy, brain or spinal cord trauma, CS with environmental pollutant overload or Parkinson's disease."

These well-recognized terms should not be confused with the recently used description of CP or central sensitization.[102–104] In reality, all perceived pain is centralized. Pain arises from activation of nociceptors, and the sensory receptors in skin, muscle, joints, and the viscera (exceptions being CP syndromes), which then activate second-order neurons in the CNS (spinal cord or brain stem). These, in turn, convey the "nociceptive information" to several sites in the brain, including eventually the cortex, where the conscious appreciation of the activated nociceptor is realized as pain. Therefore, most chronic pain states are driven by activation of nociceptors (or injured nerves) in peripheral tissue. The evidence in support of this derived from experiments in humans with fibromyalgia, irritable bowel syndrome, neuropathic pain, and bladder pain syndrome, in which peripheral blockage of input by local anesthetics disrupts the chronic pain for the duration of local anesthetic action.[105,106]

Magnetic resonance imaging (MRI) studies recently have shown loss of gray matter density in patients with chronic pain.[107–114] Although there has been some debate, these changes in brain volume appear to be the result of chronic pain and not the cause. In one study, researchers investigated 32 patients with osteoarthritis of the hip and found a decrease in gray matter in the anterior cingulate cortex, right insular cortex and operculum, dorsolateral PFC, amygdala, and brain stem compared with normal controls.[110] Ten patients from this study underwent total hip replacement surgery. After surgery, all 10 patients were pain free, and MRI studies showed increases in gray matter, suggesting that these brain abnormalities may be, at least partly, reversible when pain is successfully treated. We certainly have seen the reversibility in chemically sensitive patients who lost their pain and increased their memory and balance as well as their cognition.

These imaging studies and published reports are enhancing our understanding of pain mechanism, and will, hopefully, lead to improved targeted pain treatment.[101,115] It is been Tennant's[95] experience that chronic neuropathic pain (CP) causes hyperarousal of the sympathetic component of autonomic nervous system (SNS).[102,103,106,108] We have seen this augmentation in the chemically sensitive at the EHC-Dallas. According to Latremoliere and Woolf, central sensitization produces pain hypersensitivity by changing the sensory response elicited by normal inputs, including those that usually evoke innocuous sensations.[103] We see the hypersensitivity in chemically sensitive patients. At this time, the diagnosis of CP is a clinical one based on history and physical examination of ANS cases without pain. We have noticed when chemically sensitive patients lose their pain, their brain function improves, suggesting that the gray matter has improved.

Scientists have known for >40 years that the synthetic pesticide DDT is harmful to bird habitats and a threat to the environment. Recent studies have shown that exposure to DDT, banned in the United States since 1972 but still used as a pesticide in other countries, may also increase the risk and severity of AD in some people, particularly those over the age of 60. DDT has a half-life of 50 years so it will be around 150 years. We see many chemically sensitive patients with the breakdown of DDT, DDE in their blood, and many have a significant amount in their total body pollutant load.

The study published in *JAMA Neurology* discusses the findings in which levels of DDE, the chemical compound left when DDT breaks down, were higher in the blood of late-onset AD patients compared with those without the disease.[116]

DDT used in the United States for insect control in crops and livestock and to combat insect-borne diseases like malaria was introduced as a pesticide during World War II (WWII). The first to link a specific chemical compound to AD believed that research into how DDT and DDE may trigger neurodegenerative diseases like AD is crucial.

Although the levels of DDT and DDE have decreased significantly in the United States over the last three decades, the toxic pesticide is still found in 75%–80% of the blood samples collected from the Centers for Disease Control and Prevention for a National Health and Nutrition Survey. This occurs because the chemical can take decades to break down in the environment. In addition, people may be exposed to the pesticide by consuming imported fruits, vegetables, and grains where DDT is still being used and eating fish from contaminated waterways. Old houses were sprayed after WWII and this caused problems to many chemically sensitive patients.

In the Rutgers study, 74 out of the 86 AD patients involved, whose average age was 74, had DDE blood levels almost four times higher than the 79 people in the control group who did not have AD. They did no environmental measures to get it out, except in 5× less-polluted buildings, specific nutrition, sweating, and immune boosters such as autogenous lymphocytic factor and gamma globulins when indicated.

NEUROBEHAVIORAL EFFECTS OF DEVELOPMENTAL TOXICITY

Neurodevelopmental disabilities, including autism, attention-deficit hyperactivity disorder, dyslexia, and other cognitive impairments, affect millions of children worldwide, and some diagnoses seem to be increasing in frequency. Industrial chemicals that injure the developing brain are among the known causes for this rise in prevalence. In 2006, Thrasher did a systematic review and identified five industrial chemicals as developmental neurotoxicants: lead, methylmercury, polychlorinated biphenyls (PCBs), arsenic, and toluene.[117] Since 2006, epidemiological studies have documented six additional developmental neurotoxicants manganese, fluoride, chlorpyrifos, dichlorodiphenyltrichloroethane, tetrachloroethylene, and the polybrominated diphenyl ethers (PBDEs). It is postulated that even more neurotoxicants remain undiscovered. To control the pandemic of developmental neurotoxicity, there is a proposal of a global prevention strategy. Untested chemicals should not be presumed to be safe to brain development, and chemicals in existing use and all new chemicals must therefore be tested for developmental neurotoxicity. To coordinate these efforts and to accelerate translation of science into prevention, the urgent formation of a new international clearing house is proposed.

METAL EMISSIONS AND URBAN INCIDENT PD: A COMMUNITY HEALTH STUDY OF MEDICARE BENEFICIARIES BY USING GEOGRAPHIC INFORMATION SYSTEMS

According to Willis et al.,[118] PD associated with farming and exposure to agricultural chemicals has been reported in numerous studies; little is known about PD risk factors for those living in urban areas. The authors investigated the relation between copper, lead, or manganese emissions and PD incidence in the urban United States, studying 29 million Medicare beneficiaries in 2003. PD incidence was determined by using beneficiaries who had not changed residence since 1995. Over 35,000 nonmobile incident PD cases, diagnosed by a neurologist, were identified for analysis. Age-, race-, and sex-standardized PD incidence was compared between counties with high cumulative industrial release of copper, manganese, or lead (as reported to the Environmental Protection Agency [EPA]) and counties with no or low reported release of all three metals. PD incidence (per 100,000) in counties with no/low copper/lead/manganese release was 274.0 (95% confidence interval [CI]: 226.8, 353.5). Incidence was greater in counties with high manganese release: 489.4 (95% CI: 368.3, 689.5) (relative risk [RR] = 1.78, 95% CCI: 1.54, 2.07) and counties with high copper release: 304.2 (95% CI: 276.0, 336.8) (RR = 1.1, 95% CI: 0.94, 1.31). Urban PD incidence is greater in counties with high reported industrial release of copper or manganese. Environmental exposure to metals may be a risk factor for PD in urban areas.

BASIC MECHANISMS

Many pollutants such as methane, ethane, propane, butane, benzene, toluene, styrene, pesticides, herbicides, ethanol, formaldehyde, NO_2, Pb, Cd, Hg, benzene, xylene, and NO/OONO increase the N-methyl-D-aspartate (NMDA) sensitivity. This is done by membrane depolarization by moving Mg^{2+}, H^+, or redox situations by the pollutants, which liberates arachidonic acid, causing inflammation.

Ca^{2+} activates this NMDA activity and also phospholipase, protease, and NO synthetase plus protein kinases A and C and endonuclease enzymes. All of these enzymes can damage neurons, giving firing of the nerve continuously and an increase in muscle spasm; endonucleases can disrupt chromatin and DNA, and can cause other nuclear changes.

Phospholipase yields cell membrane changes with the breakdown of the membrane with an increase in arachidonic acid as well as increasing the hypersensitivity 1000 times by phosphorylating the Ca^{2+} protein kinases A and C combinations.

Membrane depolarization can be caused by Mg^{2+}, H^+, and redox pollutants. These pollutants increase arachidonic acid, giving inflammation. Brain N-arachidonoyl dopamine is a brain substance similar to capsacian, which is used to turn off certain reactions with the intradermal neutralization technique. Ethanol is another URI activator.

The N-methyl-D-aspartate receptor (also known as the NMDA receptor or NMDAR), a glutamate receptor, is the predominant molecular device for controlling synaptic plasticity and memory function[119] in chemically sensitive and chronic degenerative disease patients. These receptors are the chief excitatory receptors for neurotransmission in the brain along with glutamic acid.

The NMDA is a specific type of ionotropic glutamate receptor. NMDA is the name of a selective agonist that binds to NMDA receptors but not to other glutamate receptors. Activation of NMDA receptors results in the opening of an ion channel that is nonselective to cations with an equilibrium potential near 0 mV such as Na^+, Ca^{2+}, and K^+. A property of the NMDA receptor is its voltage-dependent activation, a result of ion channel block by extracellular Mg^{2+} and Zn^{2+} ions. This allows the flow of Na^+ and small amounts of Ca^{2+} ions into the cell and K^+ out of the cell to be voltage dependent,[120–122,1226] which when phosphorylated increases the sensitivity 1000 times. NMDA stimulates the NO/OONO receptor both short-term and long-term memory ion channels.

Calcium flux through NMDARs is thought to be critical in synaptic plasticity, a cellular mechanism for learning and memory. The NMDA receptor is distinct in two ways: first, it is both ligand-gated and voltage-dependent; second, it requires coactivation by two ligands: glutamate and either D-serine or glycine.[123]

The positively charged insert is Exon 5. The effect of this insert may be mimicked by positively charged polyamines and aminoglycosides, explaining their mode of action.

NMDA receptor function is also strongly regulated by chemical reduction and oxidation, via the "redox modulatory site."[124] Through this site, reductants dramatically enhance NMDA channel activity, whereas oxidants either reverse the effects of reductants or depress native responses. It is generally believed that NMDA receptors are modulated by endogenous redox agents such as glutathione, lipoic acid, and the essential nutrient pyroloquinoline quinine.

SRC kinase enhances NMDA receptor currents.[125] Reelin modulates NMDA function through Src family kinases and DAB1,[126] significantly enhancing LTP in the hippocampus. CDK5 regulates the amount of NR2B-containing NMDA receptors on the synaptic membrane, thus affecting synaptic plasticity.[127,128]

Proteins of the MHCI are endogenous negative regulators of NMDA-mediated currents in the adult hippocampus,[129] and modify NMDA-induced changes in AMPAR trafficking[129] and NMDAAR-dependent synaptic plasticity.[130]

RECEPTOR MODULATION

The NMDA receptor is a nonspecific cation channel that can allow the passage of Ca^{2+} and Na^+ into the cell and K^+ out of the cell. The excitatory postsynaptic potential (EPSP) produced by activation of an NMDA receptor increases the concentration of Ca^{2+} in the cell. The Ca^{2+} can in turn function as a second messenger in various signaling pathways. However, the NMDA receptor cation channel is blocked by Mg^{2+} at resting membrane potential. To unblock the channel, the postsynaptic cell must be depolarized.[131] which happens often in the pollutant plagued chemically sensitive by natural gas, pesticides, herbicides, mycotoxins, and EMF.

Therefore, the NMDA receptor functions as a "molecular coincidence detector." Its ion channel opens only when the following two conditions are met simultaneously: glutamate is bound to the receptor, and the postsynaptic cell is depolarized (which removes the Mg^{2+} blocking the channel). This property of the NMDA receptor explains many aspects of long-term potentiation (LTP) and synaptic plasticity.[132]

AGONISTS

Activation of NMDA receptors requires binding of glutamate or aspartate (aspartate does not stimulate the receptors as strongly).[133] In addition, NMDARs also require the binding of the coagonist glycine for the efficient opening of the ion channel, which is a part of this receptor.

D-serine has also been found to coagonize the NMDA receptor with even greater potency than glycine.[134] D-serine is produced by serine racemase, and is enriched in the same areas as NMDA receptors. Removal of D-serine can block NMDA-mediated excitatory neurotransmission in many areas. Recently, it has been shown that D-serine can be released both by neurons and by astrocytes to regulate NMDA receptors.

NMDAR-mediated currents are directly related to membrane depolarization. NMDA agonists therefore exhibit fast Mg^{2+} unbinding kinetics, increasing channel open probability with depolarization. This property is fundamental to the role of the NMDA receptor in memory and learning, and it has been suggested that this channel is a biochemical substrate of Hebbian learning (associative/memory learning), where it can act as a coincidence detector for membrane depolarization and synaptic transmission. However, newer data by McClelland concludes that new neurons may grow.

Glycine-site NMDA receptor agonists are now viewed with great interest for the development of new drugs with anxiolytic, antidepressant, and analgesic effects without obvious psychotomimetic activities.[135] One candidate, GLYX-13 has now completed phase 2 clinical trials for treatment-resistant clinical depression. This drug has shown an excellent safety profile and a considerably lower abuse liability than ketamine. However, withdrawing the triggering agent or interdermal neutralization (desensitization) or nutrient supplementation should be attempted first.

Known NMDA receptor agonists of the NMA receptors are (1) NMDA, (2) 3,5-dibromo-L-phenylalanine,[136] and (3) GLYX-13. The NMDA receptors are modulated by a number of endogenous and exogenous compounds and play a key role in a wide range of physiological (e.g., memory) and pathological processes (e.g., excitotoxicity).

Antagonists

Antagonists of the NMDA receptor are used as anesthetics for animals and sometimes humans, and are often used as recreational drugs due to their hallucinogenic properties, in addition to their unique effects at elevated dosages such as dissociation. When certain NMDA receptor antagonists are given to rodents in large doses, they can cause a form of brain damage called Olney's lesions. NMDA receptor antagonists that have been shown to induce Olney's lesions, include ketamine, phencyclidine, dextrophan (a metabolite of dextromethorphan), and MK-801, as well as some NDMA receptor antagonists used only in research environments. So far, the published research on Olney's lesions is inconclusive in its occurrence upon human or monkey brain tissues with respect to an increase in the presence of NMDA receptor antagonists.[137]

Clinical Significance

Memantine is approved by the U.S. FDA and the European Medicines Agency for treatment of moderate-to-severe AD,[138] and has now received a limited recommendation by the United Kingdom's National Institute for Clinical Excellence for patients who fail other treatment options.[139]

Cochlear NMDAs are the target of intense research to find pharmacological solutions to treat tinnitus. However, we doubt this will happen without many hazards. It is better to try to find triggering agents and eliminate them. Recently, NMDAs were associated with a rare autoimmune disease, anti-NMDA encephalitis, which usually occurs due to cross-reactivity of antibodies produced by the immune system against ectopic brain tissues, such as those found in teratoma. NMDA modulators are an emerging research target for mood disorders, including major depressive disorder.[140–142]

Compared to dopaminergic stimulants, the NMDA receptor antagonist PCP can produce a wider range of symptoms that resemble schizophrenia in healthy volunteers, which has led to the glutamate hypothesis of schizophrenia.[143] Experiments in which rodents are treated with NMDA receptor antagonist are today the most common model when it comes to testing of novel schizophrenia therapies or exploring the exact mechanism of drugs already approved for treatment of schizophrenia. Of course, the best treatment is curing the total body pollutant load and eliminating the specific triggering agents.

The NO/ONOO(–) cycle is primarily a local complex, biochemical, vicious cycle mechanism based on well-established processes.[144] The cycle is thought to be the possible cause of different diseases when localized in various body tissues. The most extensively documented of these is heart failure, where the impact of the cycle in the myocardium causes the vast changes that occur in heart failure.[145]

The main question being raised here is whether the impact of the NO/ONOO(–) cycle in the trabecular meshwork, and subsequently in the retinal ganglion, is the cause of open-angle glaucoma. An important idea here is that the high intraocular pressure (IOP) resulting from changes in the trabecular meshwork produces physical trauma and elevated NMDA activity; there is consequent initiation of the NO/ONOO(–) cycle in the retinal ganglion leading to retinal ganglion cell (RGC) degeneration. A second question relates to whether the high IOP in closed-angle glaucoma, and also highly variable but normal range IOP in other types of glaucoma, may both act on the retinal ganglion via physical trauma and the NO/ONOO(–) cycle to produce RGC degeneration.

According to Pall, the NO/ONOO(–) cycle has 12 different elements, which are increased by the cycle in the impacted tissue.[144] These elements include nitric oxide (NO), superoxide, peroxynitrite (OONO) oxidative stress, NF-κB, inflammatory cytokines, iNOS induction, mitochondrial dysfunction, excitotoxicity including excessive NMDA activity, intracellular calcium, elevated activity of several of the TRP receptors, and tetrahydrobiopterin depletion. All except the last two of these have been examined and shown at increased levels in the retinal ganglion in glaucoma. Most of these elements have been explored and also found at elevated levels in the trabecular meshwork in open-angle glaucoma.

Let us consider the trabecular meshwork first. According to Pall, one of the stressors that produce the trabecular remodeling found in open-angle glaucoma is H_2O_2 treatment. Li et al.[145] found that H_2O_2 treatment of the trabecular meshwork produced chronic elevation of oxidative stress, as well as that of NO, iNOS, NF-κB, inflammatory cytokines, and mitochondrial dysfunction—six elements of the NO/ONOO(–) cycle. Other studies have implicated both peroxynitrite and intracellular calcium, in addition to the aforementioned six cycle elements, in glaucoma-associated trabecular meshwork changes.

According to Pall, still other changes linked to the NO/ONOO(–) cycle in heart failure,[144] matrix metalloproteinase (MMP), calpain, and endothelin-1 elevation, are also implicated in the trabecular meshwork changes in open-angle glaucoma. The finding that the oxidant H_2O_2 treatment generates chronic changes, including oxidative stress, strongly suggests a vicious cycle in the generation of the trabecular meshwork changes. The finding of elevation of so many NO/ONOO(–) cycle elements in this trabecular meshwork process strongly suggests that the NO/ONOO(–) is the vicious cycle involved. MMP elevation and many other changes found in the tissue remodeling in heart failure can all be causally linked to NO/ONOO(–) cycle elements,[144] suggesting that remodeling of the trabecular meshwork in glaucoma may be similarly explained.

According to Pall, physical trauma has been shown to produce excessive activity of the NMDA receptors in the brain and spinal cord, subsequently leading to traumatic brain injury and spinal cord injury.[146] In various publications, the author has discussed how excessive NMDA activity may be involved in initiating cases of diseases apparently caused by the NO/ONOO(–) cycle. The role of excessive NMDA activity in causing RGC degeneration in glaucoma has been reviewed by Seki and Lipton.[147] It is reasonable, therefore, that high or highly variable IOP creates physical trauma on the RGCs in the region where the retinal ganglion leaves the eye, thereby producing excessive NMDA activity via several possible mechanisms, as discussed earlier.[147] The excessive NMDA activity may act on the RGCs to initiate the NO/ONOO(–) cycle in the retinal ganglion, causing glaucoma.

According to Pall, most of the NO/ONOO(–) cycle elements have been studied and shown to be raised in the retinal ganglion in glaucoma, namely, superoxide, nitric oxide, peroxynitrite, oxidative stress, NF-κB, inflammatory cytokines, iNOS, mitochondrial dysfunction, NMDA activity, and intracellular calcium,[148,149] with most of these having causal roles in RGC changes and apoptosis. This pattern of evidence makes it highly likely that the NO/ONOO(–) cycle has a central causal role in the retinal ganglion in glaucoma. As the NO/ONOO(–) cycle produces mitochondrial changes that can lead to apoptosis,[144] its apparent role here makes mechanistic sense.

It is Pall's view that treatments raising Nrf2 activity are likely to be promising treatments for glaucoma because of the role of Nrf2 in lowering multiple NO/ONOO(–) cycle elements. This position is also suggested by Miyamoto et al.'s recent study of quercetin acting by raising Nrf2 in glaucoma treatment.[146]

In summary, the local impact of the NO/ONOO(–) in the trabecular meshwork may lead to remodeling of that meshwork and consequent high IOP. Other mechanisms in closed angle and other types of glaucoma can also lead to high or variable normal range IOP, both of which act via physical trauma on RGC to elevate NMDA activity and initiate the NO/ONOO(–) cycle in RGC. The NO/ONOO(–) cycle in the RGC produces apoptotic cell death and other changes, including tissue remodeling. Agents that raise Nrf2 may thus be expected to be effective in glaucoma treatment; however, more studies are required.

IRON AND NEURODEGENERATION

Iron is an essential element in many physiological processes in the nervous system, including DNA synthesis, oxygen transport, mitochondrial respiration, neurotransmitter synthesis, and myelination.[150] According to Ke et al.,[151] brain iron levels increase with age, especially in those regions associated with motor function, such as the globus pallidus and substantia nigra. Age-related iron accumulation in regions associated with cognitive function, such as frontal gray matter, has also been reported.[151] Recently, abnormal brain iron accumulation was reported in a wide spectrum of neurodegenerative disorders, including AD and PD, suggesting a role for iron accumulation in neurodegeneration.[150]

BRAIN IRON TRANSPORT AND METABOLISM

The brain needs a stable environment in order to function normally. Both a deficiency and an excess of iron can cause severe damage, so it is important that iron levels in the brain are tightly regulated. The BBB forms a frontline boundary and maintains appropriate iron levels by regulating iron influx and efflux.[152] Additionally, iron exchange can take place in the blood–CSF barrier that separates circulating blood from the brain's extracellular fluid.[152] For iron inside the brain, glial cells act cooperatively to maintain appropriate iron levels to meet the need to both neurons and the brain as a whole. Astrocytes act as a bridge between neurons and BBB, and are responsible for regulating iron transport within the brain. Microglia serve as a brain iron capacitor by quickly accumulating and releasing iron, and thus contain variable iron content depending on conditions.[153,154]

IRON TOXICITY AND NEURODEGENERATION

The toxicity of iron can be explained by the fact that it is highly radioactive.[155] Under normal circumstances, most cellular iron is sequestered by proteins. However, when the level of iron exceeds the capacity of iron-binding proteins, labile iron results. Hydrogen peroxide, which is constantly generated by mitochondrial electron transport, can be converted to extremely toxic hydroxyl free radicals in the presence of labile iron via the Fenton and Haber–Weiss reactions.[155] These free radicals may elicit an array of cellular damage, including protein carboxylation and lipid peroxidation, and eventually evoke neuronal death. Since neurons normally have a high metabolic demand, they tend to be more susceptible to iron-induced oxidative damage. Moreover, iron has also been found to facilitate abnormal protein aggregation, which contributes to the pathogenesis of many neurodegenerative disorders.[156–158] However, the molecular mechanism of iron accumulation in neurodegenerative diseases such as AD and PD remains elusive.

AD AND IRON

According to Ke et al., AD is the most common form of dementia.[1227] Symptoms include impairment of memory and disturbances in reasoning, planning, and perception. This disease is characterized by the pathological hallmarks of amyloid plaques and neurofibrillary tangles (NFTs) that contain hyperphosphorylated tau aggregates, found in the hippocampus cortex, and other brain regions.

PD AND IRON

PD is the second most common neurodegenerative disorder.[159] It manifests as resting tremor, bradykinesia, rigidity, and postural instability, and is caused by the selective loss of the dopaminergic neurons in the substantia nigra pars compacta (SNpc). Abnormal accumulation of α-synclein in the form of Lewy bodies in SNpc is the major pathological hallmark.[160] There are numerous reports showing an increased level of iron in the SNpc of PD patients.[161] Studies indicate that accumulated iron in the SNpc is a critical factor in the degeneration of these neurons in PD, and that the level of iron accumulation in the SNpc is associated with the severity of PD symptoms.[161–164]

According to Ke et al.,[151] there are treatment strategies that can be used. A number of iron chelators have been suggested as possible treatments for iron-related neurodegeneration. Deferoxamine (DFO), a natural iron scavenger isolated from *Streptomyces pilosus*, was among the first-generation iron chelation drugs for treating iron overload. In one clinical trial, DFO significantly slowed PD progression,[165] but its poor BBB penetration and short half-life makes it a less than ideal therapy. Deferiprone (DFP), which can pass through BBB, has been shown to be therapeutically effective in different animal and cell culture models of neurodegeneration, including PD. Clinical trials are ongoing to assess its treatment efficacy.[166] Currently, most available iron chelators lack cellular specificity and can lead to a number of undesirable side effects. The search for better iron restriction methods is therefore ongoing.

Hepcidin is a newly discovered short peptide found to possess antimicrobial and iron-regulatory functions. It can bind to M1P1 to regulate iron levels, and inflammation and elevated iron levels can induce hepcidin expression.[167] They have shown that hepcidin is also expressed throughout the CNS and its expression increases with age. The widespread distribution of hepcidin in the brain and its presence in the peripheral organs implies that the peptide may also play a central role in brain iron homeostasis. They have also demonstrated that hepcidin may have unique functions in the brain, not only inhibiting iron release but also reducing uptake by downregulating DMT1 and TIR1 expression.[168,169] Their data also suggest reduced net iron uptake in response to hepcidin treatment, which may help relieve iron overloading.[168] It is not clear if hepcidin levels are altered in neurodegeneration characterized by brain iron accumulation. Further investigation is needed to assess the potential role of hepcidin in modifying iron-induced pathology.

Despite the indispensable role of iron in normal brain function, iron overload is known to cause oxidative damage and neurodegeneration. However, we currently lack specific and effective means of iron chelation that can slow down or reverse the progression of the resulting neurodegeneration. Understanding the molecular mechanisms of iron accumulation in the brain will hopefully lead to the identification of disease-modifying strategies that target the source of iron abnormality and the treatment of iron-related neurodegeneration.

MUSCLE DYSFUNCTION

FIBROMYALGIA

A major question in fibromyalgia is how does muscle sense exercise activity? This is by nerves and energy. The key molecular sensors of exercise include the calcium oscillations and other signaling cascades activated by neural stimulation and the profoundly altered metabolic state of contracting myofibers.

Stimulation of muscle by motor nerves generates cytosolic calcium transients that are detected by various intracellular pathways, including those regulated by the calcium/calmodulin-modulated phosphatase (calcineurin) and kinase (CaMK). Continuous low-amplitude transients, typical of endurance activity, activate calcineurin. Transgenic overexpression of calcineurin in skeletal muscle of mice promotes the formation of slow red fibers.[170] Conversely, genetic deletion of calcineurin or treatment with calcineurin inhibitors has the opposing effect, blocking exercise-induced adaptations.[171]

CaMK is likely another decoder of calcium transients.[172] CaMKII is the predominant isoform in skeletal muscle, but experiments with transgenic expression of a constitutively active CaMKIV isoform showed that CaMK can promote the formation of slow red fibers.[173] Conversely, mice with decreased CAMKII activity have lower expression of slow genes[174] by sensing of calcium exercise.[175] These observations thus suggest that mitochondria in muscle are not static objects and the mitochondrial dynamics play an important role in exercise adaptations. The specifics of that role remain poorly understood.

As shown in the cardio section, autophagy is a process by which cells selectively remove damaged organelles like mitochondria to the lysosome for subsequent degradation. This quality control process is critical for maintaining tissue integrity.[176] The process also appears important for adaptations to exercise. Exercise strongly and rapidly induces autophagy in skeletal muscle and numerous other tissues.[177–179] Moreover, genetically modified mice that lack stimulus-induced autophagy have drastically reduced treadmill-running capacity, suggesting that autophagy in muscle is thus complex. Mitochondria are not the only organelles that respond to exercise. Exercise, for example, also activates the unfolded protein response, exhibited in severe exercise intolerance.[180] In sum, burgeoning data with novel mouse models suggest that exercise helps to maintain homeostasis of multiple organelles in skeletal muscle, with likely important implications for the health of the whole organism.

Exercise also promotes neovascularization in skeletal muscle. Exercise-induced angiogenesis is a physiological process, in contrast to most post-development angiogenesis (e.g., neoplasms, retinal diseases). Exercise also remains the most efficacious intervention for peripheral artery disease. Understanding exercise-induced angiogenesis could thus inform novel approaches for the treatment of peripheral artery disease. Until recently, the prevailing paradigm had been that metabolic demands created by exercising muscle cause a supply/demand mismatch, leading to activation of ischemic sensors like AMPK and HIF-1α. Recent data with genetically modified mice, however, do not support this notion. Mice lacking AMPK activity in skeletal muscle have intact exercise-induced angiogenesis,[181] and mice lacking HIF-1α in skeletal muscle have more, rather than fewer, microvessels.[182] On the other hand, mice lacking PGC-1α in skeletal muscle lack the capacity for exercise-induced angiogenesis[183] (although, interestingly, not for exercise-induced mitochondrial biogenesis).[184,185] Conversely, mice transgenitically overexpressing PGC-1 in skeletal muscle have dramatic increases in microvascular density and are protected in a hind limb ischemia model of peripheral artery disease. B-Adrenergic and other signals induce PGC-1α in skeletal muscle, and PGC-1α directly activates the expression of VE growth factor, a canonical angiogenic factor, in an HIF-independent fashion.[186] Physiological angiogenesis in muscle is thus likely triggered more preemptively by nerve activity than reactively by ischemia.

STEPPING OUTSIDE THE MUSCLE: IS SKELETAL MUSCLE AN ENDOCRINE ORGAN?

Experiments over the last decade have made it increasingly clear that, in response to exercise, muscle sometimes secretes copious amounts of factors, now known as myokines into the circulation.[187] Muscle is the largest organ in the body and can command up to 80% of cardiac output during exercise. Muscle is thus ideally suited to disseminate blood-borne substances in response to exercise.

IL-6 was one of the earliest discovered myokines and remains one of the most studied.[188] Muscle contraction and exercise increase the expression of IL-6 in muscle and levels of IL-6 in the circulation by as much as 100-fold. IL-6 increases glucose uptake and fatty acid oxidation in muscle in an autocrine and paracrine fashion, thus facilitating fuel consumption locally.[189] At the same time, in an endocrine fashion, IL-6 stimulates lipolysis in adipose tissue and gluconeogenesis in the liver, both of which increase fuel delivery back to the muscle. Recently, IL-6 secreted by muscle has also been shown to cross-talk with the gut and pancreas to regulate insulin homeostasis.[190] IL-6 stimulates the secretion of glucagon-like peptide-1 (GLP-1) in intestinal L cells and pancreatic α cells. GLP-1, in turn, potentiates insulin secretion from pancreatic β cells. IL-6+ mice fail to induce GLP-1 during exercise and develop mature-onset obesity and glucose intolerance.[191] Conversely, exogenous IL-6 improves insulin sensitivity, but not in GLP-1+ mice.[190] This IL-6/GLP-1 axis thus likely mediates the enhanced insulin action seen in the immediate postexercise period. Interestingly, GLP-1 may also contribute to cognitive effects of exercise. GLP-1 knockout mice have learning deficits,[192] whereas GLP-1 agonists improve memory tasks in mice[193] (see below for a discussion of the cognitive effects of exercise). In sum, muscle-derived IL-6 appears to help integrate the entire organism response to the needs of exercising muscle. Other interleukins and traditional inflammatory cytokines, including IL-8 and IL-15, also likely double as exercise-induced myokines, although their functions are less clear.[188,194,195]

ABERRANT CEREBRAL BLOOD FLOW RESPONSES DURING COGNITION: IMPLICATIONS FOR THE UNDERSTANDING OF COGNITIVE DEFICITS IN FIBROMYALGIA

There is ample evidence for cognitive deficits in fibromyalgia syndrome (FMS). The present study investigated CBF responses during arithmetic processing in FMS patients and its relationship with performance. The influence of clinical factors on performance and blood flow responses was also analyzed.

A total of 45 FMS patients and 32 matched healthy controls completed a mental arithmetic task, while CBF velocities in the middle (MCAs) and anterior cerebral arteries (ACAs) were measured bilaterally using functional transcranial Doppler sonography (fTCD).

Patients' cognitive processing speeds were slower than those in healthy controls. In contrast to patients, healthy controls showed a pronounced early blood flow response (4–6 seconds after the warning signal) in all assessed arteries. MCA blood flow modulation during this period was correlated with task performance. This early blood flow response component was markedly less pronounced in FMS patients in both MCAs. Furthermore, patients displayed an aberrant pattern of lateralization, with right hemispheric dominance especially observed in the ACA. Severity of clinical pain in FMS patients was correlated with cognitive performance and CBF responses.

Cognitive impairment in FMS is associated with alterations in CBF responses during cognitive processing. These results suggest a potential physiological pathway through which psychosocial and clinical factors may affect cognition.

ACCELERATED BRAIN GRAY MATTER LOSS IN FIBROMYALGIA PATIENTS: PREMATURE AGING OF THE BRAIN?

Fibromyalgia is an intractable widespread pain disorder that is most frequently diagnosed in women. It has traditionally been classified as either a musculoskeletal disease or a psychological disorder. Accumulating evidence now suggest that fibromyalgia may be associated with CNS dysfunction, which is triggered by a variety of substances such as mycotoxins, natural gas, herbicides, pesticides, solvents, implants, and EMF. The study of Kuchinad et al.[113] investigated anatomical changes in the brain associated with fibromyalgia. Using voxel-based morphometric analysis of magnetic resonance brain images, they examined the brains of 10 female fibromyalgia patients and 10 healthy controls. Kuchinad et al.[113] found that fibromyalgia patients had significantly less total gray matter volume and showed a 3.3 times greater age-associated decrease in gray matter than healthy controls. The longer the individuals had had fibromyalgia, the greater the gray matter loss, with each year of fibromyalgia being equivalent to 9.5 times the loss in normal aging. In addition, fibromyalgia patients demonstrated significantly less gray matter density than healthy controls in several brain regions, including the cingulate, insular and medial frontal cortices, and parahippocampal gyri. The neuroanatomical changes that we see in fibromyalgia patients contribute additional evidence of CNS involvement in fibromyalgia. In particular, fibromyalgia appears to be associated with an acceleration of age-related changes in the very substance of the brain. Moreover, the regions in which we demonstrate objective changes may be functionally linked to core features of the disorder including affective disturbances and chronic widespread pain.

According to Kuchinad et al.,[113] fibromyalgia is a disorder of unknown etiology that is characterized by chronic widespread pain and often accompanied by a variety of other symptoms, including sleep impairment, chronic fatigue, affective disturbances, and altered stress responses.[196] Although the disorder has been dismissed by many physicians as purely psychological, recent neuroimaging studies show alterations in sensory processing[197] and neurochemical abnormalities,[198] indicating that fibromyalgia is associated with alterations in the brain's neural functioning.

Changes in brain morphology have been described in chronic pain conditions,[111,199,200] chronic fatigue syndrome (CFS),[201,202] and post-traumatic stress disorder.[203–205] Because fibromyalgia shares commonalities with these disorders, it is hypothesized that fibromyalgia might be associated with neuroanatomical abnormalities as well. Specifically, it was sought to determine whether fibromyalgia patients have demonstrable reductions of brain gray matter, particularly in regions involved in pain perception, pain modulation, and stress.

Interestingly, the normal age-related decrease in gray matter was accelerated in fibromyalgia patients and related to disease duration. The patients, who ranged from 27 to 61 years of age, demonstrated a yearly decrease in gray matter volume more than three times that of age-matched controls as previously shown. The age-related decrease was even greater than that observed by Resnick et al.[206] in a much older group of healthy adults (59–85 years), with the fibromyalgia patients in their study showing a decrease of 3.7 cm³/year and the older healthy subjects showing a decrease of 2.4 cm³/year. Although menopausal status can clearly have an effect on gray matter volume, the fact that more fibromyalgia patients than healthy controls in their sample were not cycling normally is not likely to account for their findings because the postmenopausal fibromyalgia patients in their study had less gray matter than the postmenopausal healthy controls. The reduced gray matter was even observed in the two patients who were on hormone replacement therapy (HRT), and Erikson et al.[207] showed increased gray matter volumes in postmenopausal women.

Accumulating evidence now indicates that a number of chronic pain and stress-related disorders, including chronic low back pain, tension-type headache, CFS, and post-traumatic stress disorder, are characterized by gray matter reductions, although the specific regions involved differ among syndromes.[111,199,201–203,205] The extensive comorbidity among these disorders suggests that mechanistic similarities may underlie brain atrophy, whereas the regional differences in gray matter decline could explain differences in symptoms.

A possible explanation for the decreased gray matter density in these disorders might be atrophy secondary to excitotoxicity and/or exposure to inflammation-related agents, such as cytokines.[111] The cytokines have been shown to be triggered by such entities as pesticides, natural gas, organic and inorganic chemicals, molds, mycotoxin, and EMF. It is noteworthy that in fibromyalgia patients, gray matter loss occurred mainly in regions related to stress (parahippocampal gyrus)[208] and pain processing (cingulate, insular, and prefrontal cortices),[209] which might reflect their long-term experience of these symptoms. As cingulate and prefrontal cortices are particularly implicated in pain modulation[209] (i.e., inhibition and facilitation of pain), structural changes in these systems could contribute to the maintenance of pain and symptom chronification in fibromyalgia. Furthermore, gray matter atrophy in areas such as parahippocampal and frontal cortices also appears consistent with cognitive deficits characteristic of fibromyalgia.[210] It is clearly seen in chemically sensitive patients. Of course, total body pollutant load will be extremely influenced in the cortices. Longitudinal studies are indicated to determine whether the observed structural changes are the cause or the consequence of the disorder. If confirmed, these findings may provide a rationale for exploring neuroprotective approaches in fibromyalgia aimed at symptom treatment or indeed at their reversal.

Odor sensitivity in chemically sensitive patients does go up through the olfactory tract to the PFC and may contribute to trigger fibromyalgia when stimulated by natural gas, herbicides, pesticides, mycotoxin, perfume, and other toxics.

MECHANISM OF AUTONOMIC DYSFUNCTION

According to Tennant,[95] the mechanism of SNS hyperarousal in CP is not well understood. A number of studies have shown that there is a loss of control of the efferent nerve pathways in CP.[211,212,1224,1225] The loss of efferent control allows excess electrical impulses to travel from the brain to the periphery via the SNS. Some like to think of this phenomenon as "uncoupling" the SNS from central brain control. For unknown reasons, however, CP does not cause much hyper-arousal of the parasympathetic system. Our findings in the chemically sensitive usually show that the parasympathetic system is depressed or neutral with an increase in sympathetic activity. There are two other responses seen in the chemically sensitive at the EHC-Dallas. One is decrease in the parasympathetic with normal sympathetic response. The other is a decrease in parasympathetic response with an increase in sympathetic response. The latter situation seems to be the most severe and prominent.

Hyperarousal of the SNS causes a wide variety of symptoms including nausea, diarrhea, urinary hesitancy, sweating or coldness from microcirculation spasm, and anxiety or nervousness (Table 2.3). The release of epinephrine and norepinephrine from the adrenal glands accounts for some complaints of nervousness, muscle spasm, and anxiety and may also cause tremors, tics, and episodes of excess body heat or coldness. Restless leg syndrome (RLS), which is associated with peripheral neuropathy, also is a frequent complaint. According to NINDS, RLS is a neurological disorder characterized by "throbbing, pulling, creeping, or other unpleasant sensations in the legs and an uncontrollable, and sometimes overwhelming, urge to move them. The sensations range in severity from uncomfortable to irritating to painful."[213]

The hallmark of intractable, chronic pain is pain that is 24/7, often is accompanied by severe insomnia, fatigue, and depression (Table 2.4). The intensity and perception of chronic pain are thought to be related to the pain-induced structural changes in the cells of the CNS.[99,102,103,109] It is believed that this implanting is the result of pain-stimulating glial cells to form excess neuroinflammation and the release of toxins such as glutamate[99–101] into the brain cells. CNS cells attempt to reform (neuroplasticity) before the pain somehow becomes imbedded in the process.[102,109] Fatigue and lack of energy, common complaints among pain patients, are probably related to chronic, constant overstimulation of the SNS with exhaustion and depletion of some neurotransmitters such as

---

TABLE 2.3

Common Symptoms Associated with Epinephrine SNS of Hyperarousal in Chronic Pain Depletion of Dopamine, Serotonin

- Anergy—decrease in T cells and/or function, occasional gamma globulin subset decrease
- Anorexia
- Anxiety
- Depression
- Diarrhea—gas
- Fatigue—chronic episode to constant
- Heat episodes—however, the chemically sensitive usually has subnormal temperatures, 98–97.5°F. Increased temperature—hands and feet are cold
- Insomnia
- Nausea
- Restless legs
- Tremors
- Urinary hesitancy
- Brain dysfunction
- Vascular spasm—cold hands and feet
- Tachycardia
- Dilated pupils
- Increased blood pressure, pulse

Source: Adapted from Rea, W. J., K. Patel. 2015. *Reversibility of Chronic Degenerative Disease and Hypersensitivity*, Vol. 2. Boca Raton, FL: CRC Press; Environmental Health Center-Dallas.
Note: SNS, sympathetic nervous system.

TABLE 2.4

Heart Rate Variability Analysis of 50 Patients with Chronic Pain

ANS Functional State	%	Physical Fitness Evaluation	%
Parasympathetic systems decreased and sympathetic system increased	80	Functioning of physiological systems reduced and adaption reserve reduced	80
Parasympathetic systems decreased and sympathetic system decreased	10	Functioning of physiological systems reduced and adaption reserve average level	10
Parasympathetic systems decreased and sympathetic system average	10	Functioning of physiological systems average level and adaption reserve increased	10
Parasympathetic systems increased and sympathetic system increased	0	Functioning of physiological systems increased and adaption reserve increased	0

Source: Adapted from EHC-Dallas. 2016.

dopamine, serotonin, and norepinephrine with vascular spasm. The presence of hyperarousal of the endocrine system requires laboratory testing.[214–216] Often the intradermal neutralizing doses of histamine, serotonin, capsacian, dopamine, and norepinephrine will sometimes control the pain when given frequently with the proper amount of dose in chemically sensitive patients.

PHYSICAL SIGNS OF SNS HYPERAROUSAL

The physical signs of SNS hyperarousal are quite specific, objective, and extremely useful in determining the presence of chronic pain (Table 2.5). As illustrated in Table 2.5, there are a number of potential sympathetic "signs." These include dilated pupil size (mydriasis), elevation of blood pressure and pulse rate, and vasoconstriction (cold hands and/or feet). Sometimes, there will be cold spots over the body, particularly over the spine or knee where there has been former tissue injury. Interestingly, if the patient has a pain flare with excess outpouring of catecholamines from the adrenals, they may report heat and an elevated body temperature, whereas the hands or feet may be cold. Other chemically sensitive patients are hypothermic with temperatures ranging from 89°F to 97°F. Hyperreflexia will be present, but it may not be uniform. Hyperhidrosis is present, and the best anatomical place to clinically spot and feel it is the skin under the eyes. On the other hand, chemically sensitive patients often with pain cannot sweat as always.

TABLE 2.5

Physical Signs of SNS Hyperarousal

- Mydriasis (dilated pupils)
- Hyperhidrosis—often chemically sensitive patients cannot sweat as the disease progresses
- Hyperreflexia
- Hypertension
- Tachycardia
- Vasoconstriction (cold hands and/or feet) muscle spasm
- Exaggerated skin sensitivity
- Chronic tremors—tics

Source: Adapted from EHC-Dallas. 2000.
Note: SNS, sympathetic nervous system.

PARTIAL FALLACY: YOU CANNOT MEASURE PAIN

Pain that has imprinted in the CNS, which now appears to affect a high proportion of the chronic pain population, will demonstrate objective, physical signs of SNS hyperarousal if the patient's pain is poorly controlled. Every pain practitioner should develop some simple clinical techniques to routinely search for SNS hyperarousal. A simple protocol at the initial examination and at each follow-up visit is highly recommended. For example, there is a checklist for the signs of SNS hyperarousal on intake forms and physical examination. Taking a patient's blood pressure and pulse rate is routine at each follow-up visit. Always shake hands with each patient during follow-up visits, in part to see if the patient has cold hands. Scanning each patient's face and pupil to look for pupillary dilation and hyperhidrosis under the eye is helpful but often they cannot sweat.

IMPACT ON TREATMENT

In addition to taking a personal history, a quick assessment of SNS hyperarousal tells if the patient has good pain control, and if dosages in the treatment regimen need to be increased or decreased.[216] Chronic overstimulation of the SNS may demand more treatment than the standard pain medications (i.e., anti-inflammatory or opioid medications; more turn off of allergy reactions; avoidance of environmental triggers; and intradermal neutralization of triggering antigens is often essential). Fatigue, insomnia, and depression are hallmarks of chronic pain and SNS hyperarousal. The addition of sleep medications, that is, melatonin, magnesium, antidepressants, antianxiety agents, and neuropathic agents, all will be necessary in various patients if triggering agents are not found, eliminated, or neutralized, which usually they can when studied and treated in a less-polluted, controlled environment. The most important treatment is avoidance of any triggering agent. This stimulates the ANS when exposed to the fumes of natural gas, pesticides, herbicides, diesel exhaust, and many more solvents.

Some of the symptoms and signs of chronic SNS hyperarousal are undoubtedly related to chronic release of epinephrine, norepinephrine, and other neurotransmitters. Consequently, there may be depletion of neurotransmitters such as histamine, serotonin, capsacian, and dopamine, which may have to be replaced by intradermal injection of the neutralization dose obtained by serial dilution (1–5) and reaction of the active ingredient. This may account for some of the tremors, tics, and other symptoms that CP patients frequently report. Interestingly, the use of stimulants, such as dextroamphetamine or methylphenidate, may have a diabolic or counterintuitive effect on blood pressure and pulse rate. They may calm or depress the SNS rather than stimulate it because these agents are adrenergic (dopamine, norepinephrine) agonists and may substitute for depleted neurotransmitters. This is probably why the intradermal neutralization helps with chronic pain patients. It can balance the ANS with minimum doses of these neurotransmitters.

Remember, SNS symptoms are a guidepost for the clinician to judge how a pain patient is doing. If a chronic pain patient does not have any SNS symptoms but complains of severe pain, the clinicians should not discount the patient's report. There is no substitute for good, old-fashioned clinical judgement.

ALZHEIMER'S DISEASE

Many studies are now linking AD to environmental contributors. Radiologists identify early brain marker of AD; high blood pressure and dementia; and blood pressure tied to dementia.

LUMBAR PUNCTURE, CHRONIC FATIGUE SYNDROME, AND IDIOPATHIC INTRACRANIAL HYPERTENSION: A CROSS-SECTIONAL STUDY

According to Higgins et al.,[217] unsuspected idiopathic intracranial hypertension (IIH) is found in a significant minority of patients attending clinics with named headache syndromes. CFS is frequently associated with headache. Moreover, there are striking similarities between the two conditions. They describe the results of a change in clinical practice aimed at capturing patients with chronic fatigue who might have IIH.

The result shows mean CSF pressure was 19 cm H_2O (range 12–41 cm H_2O). Four patients fulfilled the criteria for IIH. Thirteen others did not have pressures high enough to diagnose IIH but still reported an improvement in headache after drainage of CSF. Some patients also volunteered an improvement in other symptoms, including fatigue. No patient had any clinical signs of raised intracranial pressure.

The conclusions are an unknown but possibly substantial; minority of patients with CFS may actually have IIH.

MRI Evidence of Impaired CSDF Homeostasis in Obesity-Associated IIH

According to Alperin et al.,[218] impaired CSF homeostasis and altered venous hemodynamics are proposed mechanisms for elevated pressure in IIH. However, the lack of ventricular expansion steered the focus away from CSF homeostasis in IIH. This study aims to measure intracranial CSF volumes and cerebral venous drainage with MRI to determine whether increased CSF volume from impaired CSF homeostasis and venous hemodynamics occur in obesity-related IIH.

Two homogeneous cohorts of 11 newly diagnosed pretreatment overweight women with IIH and 11 overweight healthy women were prospectively studied. 3D volumetric MRI of the brain was used to quantify CSF and brain tissue volumes, and dynamic phase contrast was used to measure relative cerebral drainage through the internal jugular veins.

Findings confirm normal ventricular volume in IIH. However, extraventricular CSF volume is significantly increased in IIH (290 ± 52 vs. 220 ± 24 mL, p = 0.001). This is even more significant after normalization with intracranial volume (p = 0.0007). GM interstitial fluid volume is also increased in IIH (602 ± 57 vs. 557 ± 31 mL, p = 0.037). Total arterial inflow is normal, but relative venous drainage through the IIV is significantly reduced in ($65\% \pm 7\%$ vs. $81\% \pm 10\%$ p = 0.001).[218] Increased intracranial CSF volume that accumulates in the extraventricular subarachnoid space provides direct evidence for impaired CSF homeostasis in obesity-associated IIH. The finding of large GM interstitial fluid volume is consistent with increased overall resistance to cerebral venous drainage, as evident from reduced relative cerebral drainage through that IJV. The present study confirms that both impaired CSF homeostasis and venous hemodynamics coexist in obesity-associated IIH.[218]

Environmental Toxicants and Autism Spectrum Disorders: A Systematic Review

According to Rossignol et al.,[219] although the involvement of genetic abnormalities in autism spectrum disorders (ASDs) is well accepted, recent studies point toward an equal contribution by environmental factors, particularly environmental toxicants. Toxicants implicated in ASD included pesticides, phthalates, PCBs, solvents, toxic waste sites, air pollutants, and heavy metals, with the strongest evidence found for air pollutants and pesticides. Gestational exposure to methylmercury (through fish exposure) and childhood exposure to pollutants in water supplies (two studies) were not found to be associated with ASD risk. In the second category of studies investigating biomarkers of toxicants and ASD, a large number of studies were dedicated to examining heavy metals. Such studies demonstrated mixed findings, with only 19 of 40 (47%) case–control studies reporting higher concentrations of heavy metals in blood, urine, hair, brain, or teeth of children with ASD compared with controls. Other biomarker studies reported that solvent, phthalate, and pesticide levels were associated with ASD, whereas PCB studies were mixed. Seven studies reported a relationship between autism severity and heavy metal biomarkers, suggesting evidence of a dose–effect relationship. Overall, the evidence linking biomarkers of toxicants with ASD was weaker compared with the evidence associating estimated exposures to toxicants in the environment and ASD risk (the first category) because many of the biomarker studies contained small sample sizes and the relationships between biomarkers and ASD were inconsistent across studies. Regarding the third category of studies investigating potential genetic susceptibilities to studies reporting that such polymorphisms were more common in ASD individuals (or their mothers, one study) compared with controls (one study examined multiple polymorphisms). Genes implicated in these studies included paraoxonase (PON1, three of five studies), glutathione 5-transferase (GSTM1 and GSTP1, three of four studies), δ-aminolevulinic acid dehydratase (one study), SLC11A3 (one study), and the metal regulatory transcription factor 1 (one of two studies). Notably, many of the reviewed studies had significant limitations, including lack of replication, limited sample sizes, retrospective design, recall and publication biases, inadequate matching of cases and controls, and the use of nonstandard tools to diagnose ASD. The findings of this review suggest that the etiology of ASD may involve, at least in a subset of children, complex interactions between genetic factors and certain environmental toxicants that may act synergistically or in parallel during critical periods of neurodevelopment, in a manner that increases the likelihood of developing ASD. Due to the limitations of many of the reviewed studies, additional high-quality epidemiological studies concerning environmental toxicants and ASD are warranted to confirm and clarify many of these findings.

Crib Mattresses Emit High Rates of Potentially Harmful Chemicals

A team of environmental engineers from the Cockrell School of Engineering at the University of Texas, Austin, found that infants are exposed to high levels of chemical emissions from crib mattresses while they sleep.

Analyzing the foam padding in crib mattresses, the team found that the mattresses release significant amounts of volatile organic compounds (VOCs), potentially harmful chemicals also found in household items such as cleaners and scented sprays.

They studied samples of polyurethane foam and polyester foam padding from 20 new and old crib mattresses.[220]

The study found that new crib mattresses release about four times as many VOCs as old crib mattresses. Body heat increases emissions. Chemical emissions are strongest in the sleeping infant's immediate breathing zone.

They concluded that on average, mattresses emitted VOCs at a rate of 87.1 μg/m^2/hour, while older mattresses emitted VOCs at a rate of 22.1 μg/m^2/hour. Boor found crib mattresses release VOCs at rates comparable to other consumer products and indoor materials, including laminate flooring (20–35 μg/m^2/hour) and wall covering (51 μg/m^2/hour).[220] Boor became motivated to conduct the study after finding out that infants spend 50%–60% of their day sleeping.[220]

The 20 mattress samples are from 10 manufacturers.[220] Among the many chemicals considered VOCs are formaldehyde, benzene, toluene, perchlorethylene, and acetone. The crib mattresses analyzed in this study did not contain those organic compounds.

They identified more than 30 VOCs in the mattresses, including phenol, neodecanoic acid, and linalool. The most abundant chemicals identified in the crib mattress foam, such as limonene (a chemical that gives products a lemon scent), are routinely found in many cleaning and consumer products.

They found that VOC levels were significantly higher in a sleeping infant's breathing zone when compared with bulk room air, exposing infants to about twice the VOC levels as people standing in the same room. Additionally, because infants inhale significantly higher air volume per body weight than adults and sleep a longer time, they experience about 10 times as much inhalation exposure as adults when exposed to the same level of VOCs.

Texas Plant Agrees to Cut Air Pollution

Flint Hills Resources has agreed to spend $44.5 million to install new emission reduction technology to control air pollution from industrial flares and leaking equipment at its olefins plant in Port Arthur, Texas, as part of a settlement with the Department of Justice and EPA.[221]

West Virginia Tap Water Still Contaminated, River Clear

Trace amounts of 4-methylcylohexanemethanol (MCHM) have been found in water, leaving the treatment plant in Charleston, West Virginia, contaminated but not in the Elk River, which provides water to the facility.

Main study shows possible link between arsenic in drinking water and intelligence.

Research involving hundreds of Maine children might represent a breakthrough about whether exposure to arsenic in drinking water—even at very low levels—could lead to reduced intelligence, scientists who conducted the study said.[222]

Study Fuels Toxicity Debate

A review of studies carried out to assess the safety of industrial chemical substances has concluded that 11 substances including certain metals, OSs, pesticides, and flame retardants can now reliably be classified as developmental neurotoxicants. Such substances have the potential to cause permanent brain damage in developing fetuses and young children. We have observed many more chemicals that the chemically sensitive can define and perceive. Many of these cause brain damage.

In the review, Grandjean and Landrigan[117] concluded that exposure to the identified substances is contributing to a "global pandemic of developmental neurotoxicity" that mirrors smoking cigarettes, alcohol abuse, and processed foods as a public health problem. These people in our opinion are the ones who develop CS. Eventually, they can develop chronic degenerative disease especially men due to the masking phenomenon of testosterone.

The study comes at a time when Congress is looking to update laws that regulate chemical testing and risk assessment. Current regulations require that once a chemical is in the market, there must be proof that it is toxic before its use is restricted or it is removed from commerce. Toxicities of many chemicals used in industry and in consumer products have not been adequately tested, often because they were in the market prior to current regulations.

Grandjean and Landrigan[117] advocate taking a precautionary approach to risk assessment that emphasizes preventing early-life exposures to the suspected chemicals even in the absence of proof of their toxicity. In 2006, they published an initial report identifying lead, methylmercury, PCBs, arsenic, and toluene as neurotoxicants that could interfere with early-childhood brain development. The researchers have now updated their list by adding manganese, fluoride, chlorpyrifos, DDT, tetrachloroethylene, and PBDEs. This is only a partial list of the toxics that are in the current air, food, and water that we at the EHC-Dallas have shown to be toxic for human consumption. Organophosphate and pyrethrum pesticides, natural gas, formaldehyde, OSs, mycotoxins, and EMS shall be added to that list.[117]

The researchers concluded that 214 industrial chemicals could be labeled human neurotoxicants. Many of these substances have been detected in umbilical cord blood and breast milk. We would agree but might take issue that this number is too small.

Grandjean and Landrigan[117] point out that low-level exposure to these chemicals might have little or no effect on adults. However, this may not be true since the combinations are not tested in humans especially the chemically sensitive. Researchers postulated that the chemicals can cause subtle disruptions in critical brain development during pregnancy or in young children and lead to learning and behavioral disabilities. They add that these effects could hamper academic achievement and economic welfare later in life, as well as lead to criminal behavior. This speculation certainly has come true in the chemically sensitives who have shown to be affected from obtaining the maximum in their lives.

The Grandjean and Landrigan review provides a powerful summary of the mounting scientific evidence documenting the individual and societal tolls from IQ deficits to impacts on national GDP of early-life exposure to the neurodevelopmental toxicants.[117] The significance of this situation is further elevated by the real-world cumulative exposures.

It is the opinion of the physicians and scientists at the EHC-Dallas and EHC-Buffalo that they have seen the same in our patients. We have preformed thousands of challenges in the deadapted state as with the CS patient, under less-polluted, environmentally controlled conditions using ambient doses (low parts per million) of toxics that trigger symptoms and signs (Chemical Sensitivity Volumes I—IV).

"No one can really argue with identifying lead or methylmercury as developmental neurotoxicants."

Listing fluoride as a developmental neurotoxicant in the study was based primarily on research studying exposure to fluoride in areas of the world where it is at a naturally high concentration in drinking water. That is different from an acute work-related exposure or consumption of the low levels added to drinking water and toothpaste to prevent cavities. Often, chemically sensitive patients cannot tolerate these. There may be problems over time.

According to Alobid,[223] CS is characterized by a loss of tolerance to a variety of environmental chemicals. CS is frequently triggered by exposure to chemical agents, especially insecticides. The aim of the study was to measure the sense of smell and quality of life in patients with CS compared with the control group. They studied the sense of smell, both sensitive and sensorial characteristics, in female patients with CS (n = 58, mean 50.5 ± 8.5 years) and healthy female volunteers without rhinosinusal pathologies (n = 60, mean age 46 ± 10.2 years). Olfactometry (Barcelona Smell Test-24/BAST-24), sinonasal symptoms (visual analogue scale [VAS] 0–100 mm), and quality of life (Quick Environmental Exposure and Sensitivity Inventory/QEESI) were assessed. CS patients showed a significant impairment in smell identification (19% ± 12%; p > 0.05) and forced choice (62% ± 18%; p > 0.05), but not in smell detection (96% ± 4%) compared with the control group. CS patients reported more odors as being intense and irritating and less fresh and pleasant when compared with the control group. Patients scored a high level (40–100) in QEESI questionnaire (symptom severity, chemical intolerances, other intolerances, life impact). In CS patients, total symptom intensity (VAS/0–700 mm) score was 202 ± 135, while disease severity score was 80 ± 23. The most frequent symptoms were itching and posterior rhinorrhea. CS patients have an impairment in smell cognitive abilities (odor identification and forced choice, but not for detection) with increased smell hypersensitivity and poor quality of life.[223]

CHANGES IN CEREBRAL BLOOD FLOW DURING OLFACTORY SIMULATION IN PATIENTS WITH CS

According to Azuma et al.,[224] CS is characterized by somatic distress upon exposure to odors which clearly reflects our observations at the EHC-Dallas and EHC-Buffalo. Patients with CS process odors differently from controls. This odor-processing may be associated with activation in the prefrontal area connecting to the anterior cingulate cortex, which has been suggested as an area of odorant-related activation in CS patients. In this study, activation was defined as a significant increase in regional CBF (rCBF) because of odorant stimulation. Using the well-designed card-type olfactory test kit, changes in rCBF in the PFC were investigated after olfactory stimulation with several different odorants. Near-infrared spectroscopic (NIRS) imaging was performed in 12 CS patients and 11 controls. The olfactory stimulation test was continuously repeated 10 times. The study also included subjective assessment of physical and psychological status and the perception of irritating and hedonic odors. Significant changes in rCBF were observed in the PFC of CS patients on both the right and the left sides, as distinct from the center of the PFC compared with controls. CS patients adequately distinguished the nonodorant in 10 odor repetitions during the early stage of the olfactory stimulation test, but not in the late stage. In comparison with controls, autonomic perception and negative affectivity were poorer in CS patients. These results suggest that prefrontal information processing associated with odor-processing neuronal circuits and memory and cognition processes from past experiences of chemical exposure play significant roles in the pathology of this disorder.

RESPIRATORY HEALTH AIR POLLUTION

Low to moderate levels of outdoor air pollutants can greatly increase respiratory problems in the elderly, the physically compromised, and the immune and enzyme deficient like the chemically sensitive. A 1980–1995 study of Tokyo residents aged over 65 years found that increasing airborne outdoor PM_{10} concentrations were associated with significantly higher rates of asthma and bronchitis ($p < 0.001$ in both cases).[225] Higher levels of $PM_{2.5}$ were associated with significantly higher levels of hospitalizations for chronic obstructive pulmonary disease (COPD) in elderly subjects in Vancouver, Canada.[226] Higher outdoor levels of O_3, PM_{10}, SO_2, and NO_2 were associated with significantly higher rates of hospital COPD admissions in Minneapolis, Minnesota, but were not related to significantly higher COPD admissions in Birmingham, Alabama.[227] Dickey's and our studies in the significantly less-polluted ECU of chemically sensitive patients showed marked improvement in vascular and chemically sensitive patients.[55]

A cohort study in Los Angeles found a dose–response relationship between bronchitis and ambient PM_{10} levels.[228] A study of 4 million hospital emergency visits in Atlanta found that higher outdoor levels of PM_{10}, NO_2, and CO were associated with significantly higher emergency room visits for upper respiratory infections and COPD.[229] An Australian study found that higher airborne levels of PM_{10}, $PM_{2.5}$, NO_2, and SO_2 were all associated with significantly higher rates of childhood hospital admissions for pneumonia and acute bronchitis.[230] A two-winter-long study of adults with advanced COPD in Denver, Colorado found that higher ambient levels of CO, PM_{10}, and NO_2 were associated with poorer lung function and more rescue medication use in one of the two winters.[231] Significantly higher levels of chronic cough and phlegm production have been found in children exposed to higher ambient O_3 levels[232] and in adults exposed to higher ambient PM_{10} levels.[233] Higher outdoor $PM_{2.5}$ levels were associated with significantly higher childhood emergency room visits for pneumonia and respiratory illness in Santiago, Chile.[234] Large cohort studies in Austria and California found that high summer O_3 levels were associated with reduced lung function and growth in children over a follow-up period of 2–4 years.[235,236]

Most studies of the health effects of outdoor air pollution have dealt with respiratory health issues. Many of the studies have involved children and most of these studies have linked higher rates of asthma and other respiratory problems to higher outdoor air levels of priority pollutants such as particulates, ozone, sulfur and nitrogen oxides, and carbon monoxide.

Table 2.6 summarizes 10 ecologic studies in which higher levels of many common pollutants (PM_{10} or $PM_{2.5}$, O_3, CO, SO_2, NO_2, benzene) are associated with higher levels of asthma symptoms, asthma consultations, and/or hospital admissions.

Many of these air pollutants can worsen childhood asthma at relatively modest concentrations. The limits for CO and O_3 were rarely exceeded in any of these studies listed in Table 2.6.

The mean concentrations of PM_{10}, SO_2, and O_3 were well below the U.S. EPA standards in all but two of the eight studies.[238,244] This suggests that PM_{10}, CO, O_3, NO_2, and SO_2 can worsen asthma in children at levels below the U.S. EPA standards.

A Chilean study found a significant relationship between higher outdoor $PM_{2.5}$ levels and more wheezing bronchitis in infants.[246] A study conducted during the 1996 Atlanta Olympic Games found that morning traffic was reduced by 29% during this period, peak O_3 levels dropped by 28%, and asthma-related physician visits in children dropped by about 40%.[247] A French study found that increasing levels of outdoor PM_{10}, O_3, and SO_2 were associated with significantly higher rates of childhood asthma and rhinitis.[248]

GSTP1 IS A HUB GENE FOR GENE–AIR POLLUTION INTERACTIONS ON CHILDHOOD ASTHMA

According to Su,[249] there is growing evidence that multiple genes and air pollutants are associated with asthma. They conducted the Taiwan Children Health Study (TCHS) to investigate the influence of gene–air pollution interactions on childhood asthma. Their results show a

TABLE 2.6

Childhood Studies Linking Exposure to Higher Air Pollutant Levels with Significantly Worsened Asthma

Study	Outcome Measured	Particulates (PM$_{10}$ or PM$_{2.5}$)	Ozone (O$_3$)	Carbon Monoxide (CO)	Sulfur Dioxide (SO$_2$)	Nitrogen Dioxide (NO$_2$)	Benzene (C$_6$H$_6$)
Barnett et al.[230]	Respiratory hospital admissions	X				X	
Buchdahl et al.[237]	Asthma/wheezing emergency room (ER visits)		X				X
Lee et al.[238]	Asthma hospitalizations	X		X	X	X	X
Lin et al.[239]	Asthma hospitalizations	X					
Linaker et al.[240]	Worsening asthma following upper respiratory infections						X
Thompson and Patterson[241]	Asthma emergency room (ER) visits	X					X
Tolbert et al.[242]	Asthma emergency room (ER) visits	X	X				
White et al.[243]	Asthma emergency room (ER) visits		X				
Wong et al.[244]	Asthma hospitalizations		X	X			
Yu et al.[245]	Worsening asthma symptoms	X		X			

Source: Adapted from Lee, J. T. et al. 2002. *Epidemiology* 13:481–484.

Note: X in box indicates pollutant associated with significant increase (p < 0.05) in asthma.

significant two-way gene–air pollution interaction between glutathione *S*-transferase P (GSTP1) and PM$_{10}$ in the risk of childhood asthma. Interactions between GSTP1 and different types of air pollutants have a higher information gain than other gene–air pollutant combinations. Their study suggests that interaction between GSTP1 and PM$_{10}$ is the most influential gene–air pollution and combined with the GHSTP1 gene may alter the susceptibility to childhood asthma. It implies that GSTP1 is an important hub gene in the antioxidative pathway that buffers the harmful effects of air pollution. It, however, should be emphasized that although genes are involved with responses to air pollution, the overwhelming data show that environmental pollutants are the triggers of disease.

Nishimura et al.'s[250] objectives were to assess a causal relationship between air pollution and childhood asthma using data that address temporality by estimating air pollution exposures before the development of asthma and to establish the generalizability of the association by studying diverse racial/ethnic populations in different geographic regions.

This study included Latino (n = 3,343) and African-American (n = 977) participants with and without asthma from five urban regions in the mainland United States and Puerto Rico. After adjustment for confounders, a 5-ppb increase in average NO$_2$ during the first year of life was associated with an odds ratio (OR) of 1.17 for physician-diagnosed asthma (95% CI: 1.04–1.31).

Early-life NO$_2$ exposure is associated with childhood asthma in Latinos and African-Americans.

According to Zhou,[251] studies have shown diverse strength of evidence for the associations between air pollutants and childhood asthma but these associations have scarcely been documented in the early life.

Adjusted ORs were estimated to assess the relationships between exposures to air pollutants and single- and multidimensional asthma phenotypes in the first year of life in children of the EDEN mother–child cohort study (n = 1765 mother–child pairs). The generalized estimating equation (GEE) model was used to determine the associations between prenatal maternal smoking and in utero exposure to traffic-related air pollution and asthma phenotypes (data were collected when children were at birth, and at 4, 8, and 12 months of age). Adjusted Population Attributable Risk (aPAR) was estimated to measure the impacts of air pollutants on health outcomes.

In the first year of life, both single- and multidimensional asthma phenotypes were positively related to heavy parental smoking, traffic-related air pollution, and dampness, but negatively associated with contract with cats and domestic wood heating. Results persisted for prenatal maternal smoking and in utero exposure to traffic-related air pollution, although statistically significant associations were observed only with the asthma phenotype of ever bronchiolitis.

After adjusting for potential confounders, traffic-related air pollution in utero life and in the first year of life had a greater impact on the development of asthma phenotypes compared to other factors.

Review of the time series and panel studies on the short-term effects of PM_{10} on the increases of the illness in childhood was performed by Romeo, etc. Meta-analysis of panel and time series studies was performed. All studies cited in PubMed that were published between 1909 and 2003 were selected. Exposure to PM_{10} was associated with an increase in hospitalizations for asthma (ORRE = 1.017, 95% CI: 1.008; 1.025), with episodes of wheezing (ORRE = 1.063, 95% CI: 1.038; 1.087) and coughing (ORRE = 1.026, 95% CI: 1.013; 1.039), in the use of medications for asthma (ORRE = 1.033, 95% CI: 1.008; 1.059), and to a decrease in lung function (PRE = −0.269, 95% CI: −0.451; −0.087).

In conclusion, exposure to PM_{10} was associated with an increase in hospitalizations for asthma and, in asthmatic children, with the frequency of asthmatic symptoms (wheezing and cough), the use of antiasthma medications (in addition to regular therapy) and a decrease in lung functioning.

Traffic pollution, coal-fired power plants, and industrial pollution may also be important outdoor triggers to asthma and other respiratory problems. A review of 18 papers found that higher traffic exposure (as measured by traffic density, distance from roads, or vehicle-produced pollutants) was related to significantly higher levels of asthma, wheezing, or cough in 14 of these studies.[252]

An Israeli study found that childhood asthma was significantly more common in children living near a coal-fired power plant.[253] Releases of hydrogen sulfide by a pulp mill were found to cause significant breathing problems in one-third of the residents living in a nearby community.[254] A Utah study of a community near a steel mill which closed and then reopened found that childhood hospital respiratory admissions were two to three times greater during periods in which the steel mill was open.[255]

High airborne levels of mold, pollen, and algae can also worsen respiratory problems. Higher outdoor mold concentrations have been linked to higher rates of asthma mortality[256] and higher asthma incidence[257–259] in children or young adults. A study in 10 Canadian cities found that the effects of ozone and pollen had synergistic associations with increased asthma hospitalizations.[259] An Ohio study reported that airborne PM_{10} and pollen had synergistic associations with increased pediatric asthma hospital admissions.[260] The increases in asthma often seen after gusty thunderstorms are mainly due to the increased levels of airborne mold and pollens blown into the air.[261] A Mexico City study found that higher levels of outdoor pollen and/or fungi were associated with significantly higher rates of hospital asthma admissions.[262] Outdoor, rain, mold, leptosphaeria and phaesophaeria, and pollen exposure also play a major role in the development of rhinitis.[263] Epidemiological evidence and environmental chamber studies suggest that exposure to low levels of ozone, diesel exhaust, and other outdoor air pollutants react synergistically with pollen and mold spores and produce much greater drops in lung function than exposure to either the pollutants or molds/pollen our results with pollen and mold separate separately.[264–266] Ambient air exposure to brevotoxins from the saltwater algae *Karenia brevis* has been associated with significantly poorer lung function in asthmatics.[267]

Outdoor levels of some bioaerosols such as flour dust, latex, and endotoxin are generally very low, but can be present in significant concentrations in outdoor areas near the source of these bioaerosols. A study in Barcelona found that unloading soybean flour was associated with significantly higher rates of asthma attacks in subjects living within several blocks of the unloading docks.[268] Latex PM_{10} levels (from tire tread) were as high as 1 ng/m³ near a Los Angeles freeway.[269] Hospital studies have reported that PM_{10} latex levels as low as 0.6 ng/m³ can induce respiratory symptoms in latex-sensitive subjects.[270]

The burning of wood, leaves, and agricultural residue creates large amounts of PM_{10}, CO, and other pollutants that can worsen asthma and other breathing problems. Higher rates of asthma symptoms, lower lung function, and/or more respiratory hospitalizations have been reported among populations exposed to outdoor smoke from rice straw burning,[271,272] wildfire/brush fire,[273,274] leaf burning,[275] and wood burning.[276] Studies in both Seattle and San Francisco found that higher wood-burning-related PM_{10} levels were associated with significantly higher rates of asthma symptoms, medication use, and asthma-related hospitalizations.[277,278]

From July to October 1997, large Indonesian forests were deliberately burned and created dense smoke which traveled for hundreds of kilometers into Malaysia. In September 1997, all 28 Malaysian air stations recorded concentrations of PM_{10} above 150 μg/m³. At hospital in Kuala Lumpur, respirator admissions were only 912 in June 1997, but were 5000 in September 1997, during the heavy Indonesian forest-burning period.[279]

Sand particles usually contain particles of an aerodynamic diameter in excess of what is respirable.[280] However, many areas of the Persian Gulf contain many unusually small sand particles which can be easily inhaled into the lung alveoli during sandstorms. Inhaling such fine sand can cause a syndrome called Al Eskan disease, which involves a variety of respiratory and immunological problems.[280] Al Eskan disease may be a major factor in the development of Gulf War syndrome.[280] Dust can also trigger respiratory problems thousands of kilometers away from the source. A Trinidad study found that dust from African dust clouds was associated with significantly higher levels of asthma-related emergency room visits in children.[281] For years, we have immunized patients for African dust hypersensitivity.

Volcanic eruptions can emit large quantities of sulfur dioxide; particulates; fluorides; hydrogen fluoride; hydrogen chloride; and toxic metals such as mercury, arsenic, and iridium into the air. Emissions of volcanic fog (vog) can travel and produce significantly elevated levels of air pollution more than 1400 km from the volcano.[282] A New Zealand study reported personal air exposures of 75 ppm SO_2, 25 ppm HCl, and 8 ppm HF in 10 human volunteers who spent 20 minutes near volcanic vents during a quiet period of the White Island volcano.[283]

Exposure to volcanic emissions may worsen asthma. Many residents on the big island of Hawaii had reported breathing difficulties, headaches, and watery eyes after being exposed to smog from the active Kilauea volcano.[284] A study of 10,000 government workers in Anchorage, Alaska noted that asthma medical visits increased significantly following an eruption of a nearby volcano in August 1992.[285]

EXHALED METALLIC ELEMENTS AND SERUM PNEUMOPROTEINS IN ASYMPTOMATIC SMOKERS AND PATIENTS WITH COPD OR ASTHMA

EBC was obtained from 50 healthy subjects (30 healthy smokers, 30 asthmatics, and 50 patients with stable COPD) and was collected by cooling exhaled air. Trace elements and toxic metals in the samples were measured by means of inductively coupled plasma mass spectrometry and electro-thermal atomic absorption spectroscopy. The serum pneumoproteins were immunoassayed.

The EBC of COPD subjects had higher levels of such toxic elements as lead, cadmium, and aluminum, and lower levels of iron and copper than that of the nonsmoking control subjects.

There were no between-group differences in surfactant protein (SP)-A and SP-B levels. Clara cell protein and SP-D levels were negatively and positively influenced respectively by tobacco smoke. Their results show that toxic metals and transition elements are detectable in the EBC of studied subject.

Volatile organics and other "air toxics" in outdoor air may also trigger asthma, although data from outdoor air exposures are sparse. A study of 8549 West Virginia children found that asthma rates were significantly more common in areas with higher concentrations of industry-released volatile organic chemicals.[286] Decreased lung function and skin/eye/nose/throat irritation was noted in many members of a Texas community of 3000 exposed to a HF spill from a nearby oil refinery.[287] Significantly higher wheezing levels have been reported in areas in which methyl tertiary butyl ether (MTBE) has been added to gasoline,[288] while other studies report no relationship between asthma and MTBE in gasoline.[289]

A California report noted that about 165 residents had wheezing and eye/skin irritation from the drift of chloropicrin soil fumigant applied about a quarter mile away.[290] On the other hand, another study reported no community adverse respiratory or other health effects following aerial spraying of *Bacillus thuringiensis*, a biological pesticide.[291]

According to Young et al.,[292] to aid in diagnostic chest film interpretation of coal workers' pneumoconiosis (CWP), a composite profile of common radiologic patterns was developed in 98 Appalachian former coal miners who were diagnosed having CWP and who applied for black lung benefits.

Rapid Decline in Lung Function in Coal Miners: Evidence of Disease in Small Airways

According to Stansbury et al.,[293] coal mine dust exposure can cause both pneumoconiosis and chronic airflow limitation. Prevalence of abnormal spirometry results increases with increasing category of simple CWP and progressive massive fibrosis. Abnormal spirometry in coal miners is associated with CWP; these two health outcomes have similar geographic distributions.

Prevalence of CWP in China: A Systematic Analysis of 2001–2011 Studies

Nowadays, CWP is still believed to be the main occupational disease in China. The total populations from these reports were 173,646 and 10,821 for dust-exposed coal workers and patients with CWP, respectively. The pooled prevalence of CWP was 6.02% (95% CI: 3.43%–9.26%) and the pooled rate of CWP patients combined with tuberculosis (TBC) was 10.82% (95% CI: 8.26%–13.66%).

Graber et al.[294] evaluated respiratory-related mortality among underground coal miners after 37 years of follow-up. Underlying cause of death for 9033 underground coal miners from 31 U.S. mines enrolled between 1969 and 1971 was evaluated with life table analysis. Excess mortality was observed from pneumoconiosis (SMR = 79.70, 95% CI: 72.1–87.67), COPD (SMR = 1.11, 95% CI: 0.99–1.24), and lung cancer (SMR = 1.08; 95% CI: 1.00–1.18). Coal mine dust exposure increased risk for mortality from pneumoconiosis and COPD. Respirable silica was positively associated with mortality from pneumoconiosis. A significant relationship between coal mine dust exposure and lung cancer mortality (HR = 1.70; 95% CI: 1.02–2.83) but not with respirable silica (HR = 1.05; 95% CI: 0.90–1.23) occurred. In the most recent follow-up period (2000–2007), both exposures were positively associated with lung cancer mortality and coal mine dust, significantly.

According to Wang et al.,[295] this study aims to provide understanding due to exposure to silica, asbestos, and coal dusts.

ASBESTOSIS

Geometric mean (GM) concentrations were higher in cases than in the controls for chrysotile fibers 5–10 μ long in patients with asbestosis with or without lung cancer; for tremolite fibers 5–10 μ long in all patients; for crocidolite, talc, or anthrophyllite fibers 5–10 μ long in patients with mesothelioma; for chrysotile ad tremolite fibers ≥10 μ long in patients with asbestosis; and crocidolite, talc, or anthophyllite fibers ≥10 μ long in patients with mesothelioma. Average length to diameter ratios of the fibers were calculated to be larger in patients with asbestosis and lung cancer than in those without lung cancer for crocidolite fibers ≥10 μ long, for chrysotile, amosite, and tremolite fibers across the disease groups when they were calculated in each patient. Cumulative smoking index (pack-years) was higher in the group with asbestosis and lung cancer but was not statistically different from the two other disease groups.

According to Langer et al.,[296] tissues obtained at autopsy or biopsy from 81 workers and 2 household persons were chemically digested. The asbestos fibers recovered were characterized by analytical transmission electron microscopy. Among the 83 causes of death, 33 were due to mesotheliomas, 35 were due to lung cancers, 12 were due to asbestosis, and 3 were due to other cancers.

Amosite was present in all of the insulation workers' lungs studied and was found in the highest concentration in this exposure category. The highest chrysotile concentration was found among works in general trades. Although most prevalent in shipyard workers lungs, crocidolite concentration is not statistically different among the exposure groups studied. Although crocidolite was found in 20 cases, amosite accompanied it in 18 of these. Of the 20 cases, 11 were from shipyard workers. Of the eight mesothelioma cases, seven also contained amosite. Crocidolite alone only occurred in 1 of the 33 mesothelioma cases analyzed. They concluded the following: crocidolite exposure occurred among the U.S. insulators and a large percentage of other workers as well.

According to Lippmann et al.,[297] a review of the literature on chronic inhalation studies in which rats were exposed to miner fibers at known fiber number concentrations was undertaken to examine the specific roles of fiber length and composition on the incidences of both lung cancer and mesothelioma. Combining the data from various studies by fiber type, the percentage of mesotheliomas was 0.6% for Zimbabwe (Rhodesian) chrysotile, 2.5% for the various amphiboles as a group, and 4.7% for Quebec (Canadian) chrysotile.

According to Davis et al.,[298] fiber type, fiber size, deposition, dissolution, and migration are all factors of importance in miner fiber carcinogenesis. One where fiber dissemination has been suggested as being very important is that of transport from the lung tissue to the pleural cavity.

Asbestos is composed of silicon, oxygen, hydrogen, and various metal cations (positively charged metal ions).

Asbestos appealed to manufacturers and builders for a variety of reasons. It is strong yet flexible, and will not burn. It is a poor conductor of heat and electricity, and resists corrosion. Asbestos may have been so widely used because few other available substances combine the same qualities.

One study estimated that 3000 different types of commercial products contained asbestos. Many older plastics, paper products, brake linings, floor tiles, and textile products contain asbestos, as do many heavy industrial products such as sealants, cement pipe, cement sheets, and insulation. It is still legal to manufacture process and import most asbestos products.

When asbestos fibers are in the air, people may inhale them. As asbestos fibers are small and light, they can stay in the air for a long time. It is estimated that between 1940 and 1980, 27 million Americans had significant occupational exposure to asbestos. Some materials which are considered "nonfriable," such as vinyl-asbestos floor tile, can also release fibers when sanded, sawed, or otherwise aggressively disturbed. Materials such as asbestos cement pipe can release asbestos fibers if broken or crushed when buildings are demolished, renovated, or repaired.

People who touch asbestos may get a rash similar to the rash caused by fiberglass.

There is no effective treatment for asbestosis; the disease is usually disabling or fatal. Those who renovate or demolish buildings that contain asbestos may be at significant risk, depending on the nature of the exposure and precautions taken.

Lung Cancer

Lung cancer causes the highest number of deaths related to asbestos exposure. One study found that asbestos workers who smoke are about 90 times more likely to develop lung cancer than people who neither smoke nor have been exposed to asbestos.

Mesothelioma

Mesothelioma is a rare form of cancer which most often occurs in the thin membrane lining of the lungs, chest, abdomen, and (rarely) heart. About 200 cases are diagnosed each year in the United States. Virtually all cases of mesothelioma are linked with asbestos exposure. The younger people are when they inhale asbestos, the more likely they are to develop mesothelioma. Evidence suggests that cancers in the esophagus, larynx, oral cavity, stomach, colon, and kidney may be caused by ingesting asbestos.

Beryllium

Identification of Beryllium-Dependent Peptides Recognized by CD+ T Cells in Chronic Beryllium Disease

According to Falta et al.,[299] chronic beryllium disease (CBD) is a granulomatous disorder characterized by an influx of beryllium (BE)-specific CD4+ cells into the lung. The vast majority of these T cells recognize BE in an HLA-DP-restricted manner, and peptide is required for T cell recognition. However, the peptides that stimulate Be-specific T cells are unknown. Using positional scanning libraries and fibroblasts expressing HLAS-DP2, the most prevalent HLA-DP molecule linked to disease, they identified mimotopes and endogenous self-peptides that bind to MHCII and Be, forming a complex recognized by pathogenic CD4+ T cells in CBD. These peptides possess aspartic and glutamic acid residues at p4 and p7, respectively, that surround the putative Be-binding site and cooperate with HLA-DP2 in Be coordination. Endogenous plexin A peptides and proteins, which share the core motif and are expressed in lung, also stimulate these TCRs. Be-loaded HLA-DP2-mimotope and HLA-DP2 plexin A4 tetramers detected high frequencies of CD4+ T cells specific for these ligands in all HLADP2+ CBD patients tested. Thus, our findings identify the first ligand for a CD4+ T cell involved in metal-induced hypersensitivity and suggest a unique role of these peptides in metal ion coordination and the generation of a common antigen specificity in CBD.

Depending on genetic susceptibility and the nature of the exposure, CBD occurs in up to 20% of exposed workers. Genetic susceptibility has been associated with particular HLA-DP alleles, especially those possessing a negatively charged glutamic acid residue at the 69th position of the beta-chain.

Beryllium Presentation to CD4+ T Cells Is Dependent on a Single Amino Acid Residue of the MHC Class II Beta-Chain

According to Bill et al.,[300] CBD is characterized by a CD4+ T cell alveolitis and granulomatous inflammation in the lung. Thus, they hypothesized that beryllium presentation to CD4+ T cells was dependent on a glutamic acid residue at the identical position of both HLA-DP and -DR.

According to Maier et al.,[301] exposure to beryllium results in beryllium sensitization, or development of a beryllium-specific, cell-mediated immune response, in 2%–19% of exposed individuals. Sensitization usually precedes the development of the scarring lung disease, CBD. The development of granulomatous inflammation in patients with CBD is associated with the production of numerous inflammatory cytokines, including IFN-gamma, IL-2, and TNF-alpha.

Two copies of the Glu69 gene may be a disease-specific genetic risk factor. The TNF-alpha-308 A variant is associated with beryllium-stimulated TNF-alpha production, which, in turn, is associated with more severe CBD. Whether the TNF-alpha-38 A is a genetic risk factor in CBD, sensitization and CBD are multigenetic processes, and that these genes interact with exposure to determine risk of disease.

According to Schuler et al.,[302] CBD, which primarily affects the lungs, occurs in sensitized beryllium-exposed individuals.

Participation was 83%. Prevalences of sensitization and CBD were 7% (10/153) and 4% (6/153), respectively; this included employees with abnormal BeLPTs from two laboratories, four diagnosed with CBD during the survey, and one each diagnosed preceding and following the survey. CBD risk was highest in rod and wire production (p < 0.05), where air levels were highest.

According to Henneberger et al.,[303] workers at a beryllium ceramics plant were tested for beryllium sensitization and disease in 1998 to determine whether the plant-wide prevalence of sensitization and disease had declined since the last screening in 1992.

Of 167, 151 participants represented eligible workers, that is, 90%. Fifteen (9.9% of 151) had an abnormal BeLPT and were split between long-term workers (8/77 = 10.4%) and short-term workers (7/74 = 9.5%). Beryllium disease was detected in 9.1% (7/77) of long-term workers but in only 1.4% (1/74) of short-term workers (p = 0.06), for an overall prevalence of 5.3% (8/151). These prevalences were similar to those observed in the earlier survey. The prevalence of sensitization was elevated in 1992 among machinists, and was still elevated in 1998 among long-term workers (7/40 = 18%) but not among short-term workers (2/36 = 6%) with machining experience. The data suggested a positive relationship between peak beryllium exposure and sensitization for long-term workers. Long-term workers with either a high peak exposure or work experience in forming were more likely to have an abnormal BeLPT (8/51 = 16%) than the other long-term workers (0.26, p = 0.05). All seven sensitized short-term workers either had high mean beryllium exposure or had worked longest in forming or machining (7/5 = 13% vs. 0.19, p = 0.18).

A plant-wide decline in beryllium exposures between the 1992 and 1998 surveys was not matched by a decline in the prevalence of sensitization and disease.

Fifty-nine employees (9.4%) had abnormal blood tests, 47 of whom underwent bronchoscopy. Twenty-four new cases of beryllium disease were identified, resulting in a beryllium disease prevalence of 4.6%, including five known cases (29/632). Employees who had worked in ceramics had the highest prevalence of beryllium disease (9.0%).

TEXTILES

According to Fishwick et al.,[304] the objective was to document the prevalence of work-related ocular (eyeWRI) and nasal (noseWRI) irritation in workers in spinning mills of cotton and synthetic textile fibers and to relate the prevalence of symptoms to atopy, byssinotic symptoms, work history, and measured dust concentrations in the personal breathing zone and work area.

They did a cross-sectional study of 1048 cotton workers and 404 synthetic fiber workers.

A total of 3.7% of all operatives complained of symptoms of byssinosis, 253 (17.5%) complained of eye WRI and 165 (11%) of nose WRI.

Work-related ocular and nasal irritations are the most common symptoms complained of by cotton textile workers. There was no relation between these symptoms and atopy, byssinosis, or dust concentration. It is likely that they relate to as yet unidentified agents unrelated to concentration of cotton dust.

A total of 2991 workers were investigated for the presence of symptoms compatible with chronic bronchitis. Airborne endotoxin exposure was measured using a quantitative turbidometric assay. Lung function tests were performed to measure forced expiratory volume in 1 second (FEV1) and forced vital capacity (FVC). A control group of workers exposed to man-made fiber textiles was identified. Two case referent studies were also performed; cases of chronic bronchitis were separately matched with controls from the cotton and control populations to determine the effect of the symptomatic state on lung function.

After controlling for smoking (pack-years), workers in a cotton environment were significantly more likely to suffer from chronic bronchitis and this was most marked in workers over 45 years of age (OR: 2.51 (CI: 1.3–4.9); $p < 0.01$). Regression analysis of all possible influencing parameters showed that cumulative exposure to cotton dust was significantly associated with chronic bronchitis after the effects of age, sex, smoking, and ethnic group were accounted for ($p < 0.0005$). In the intra-cotton population case–control study, a diagnosis of chronic bronchitis was associated with a small decrement in lung function compared with controls: percentage predicted FEV1 in cases 81.4% (95% CI 78.3–84.6), controls 86.7% (84.9–88.5); FVC in cases 89.9% (95% CI 87.0–92.9), controls 94.6% (92.8–96.4). After controlling for cumulative past exposure and pack-years of smoking, the effect of the diagnostic state remained significant for both FEV1 ($p < 0.01$) and FVC ($p < 0.05$).

According to Fishwick et al.,[304] this survey was conducted to investigate current lung function levels in operatives working with cotton and man-made fibers.

A cross-sectional study of respiratory symptoms and lung function was made in 1057 textile spinning operatives of white Caucasian extraction. This represented 96.9% of the total available working population to be studied. Almost 713 worked currently with cotton. The remainder worked with man-made fiber.

A total of 3.5% of all operatives had byssinosis, 55 (5.3%) chronic bronchitis, 36 (3.5%) work-related persistent cough, 55 (5.3%) nonbyssinotic work-related chest tightness, and 56 (5.3%) work-related wheeze. A total of 212 static work area dust samples (range 0.04–3.23 mg/m^3) and 213 personal breathing zone samples (range 0.14–24.95 mg/m^3) were collected. Percentage of predicted FEV1 was reduced in current smokers (mean 89.5, 95% CI currently working with a man-made fiber [95.3, 93.8–96.9] in comparison with cotton [97.8, 96.6–99.0]). Regression analysis identified smoking ($p < 0.01$), increasing age ($p < 0.01$), increasing time worked in the waste room ($p < 0.01$), and male ($p < 0.05$) as being associated with a lower FEV1 and FVC.

ENDOTOXINS

According to Zhang et al.,[305] occupational exposure to endotoxin is associated with decrements in pulmonary function.

Two SNPs were found to be significant ($p < 6.29 \times 10^{-5}$), including rs 1910047 ($p = 3.07 \times 10^{-5}$, FDR = 0.0778) and rs 9469089 ($p = 6.19 \times 10^{-5}$, FDR = 0.0967), as well as other eight suggestive ($p < 5 \times 10^{-4}$) associated SNPs. Gene–gene and gene–environment interactions were also observed, such as rs 1910047 and rs 1049970 ($p = 0.0418$, FDR = 0.0895); rs 9469089 and age ($p = 0.161$, FDR = 0.0264). Genetic risk score analysis showed that the more risk loci the subjects carried, the larger the rate of FEV1 decline occurred ($p_{trend} = 3.01 \times 10^{-18}$). However, the association was different among age subgroups ($p = 7.11 \times 10^{-6}$) and endotoxin subgroups ($p = 1.08 \times 10^{-2}$). Functional network analysis illustrates potential biological connections of all interacted genes.

According to Kennedy et al.,[306] endotoxin exposure has been implicated in the etiology of lung disease in cotton workers. They investigated this potential relationship in 443 cotton workers from 2 factories in Shanghai and 439 control subjects from a nearby silk mill. Multiple area air samples were analyzed from total elutriated dust concentration (range: 0.15–2.5 mg/m^3) and endotoxin (range: 0.002–0.55 μg U.S. Reference Endotoxin/m^3). The cotton worker population was stratified by current and cumulative dust, or endotoxin exposure. Groups were compared for FEV1, FVC, FEV1/FVC%, % change in FEV1 over the shift (delta FEV1%), and prevalences of chronic bronchitis and byssinosis, and linear and logistic regression models were constructed. A dose–response trend was seen with the current endotoxin level and FEV1, delta FEV1%, and the prevalence of byssinosis and chronic bronchitis, except for the highest exposure-level group in which a reversal of the trend was seen. The regression coefficients for current endotoxin exposure were significant ($p < 0.05$) in the models for FEV1 and chronic bronchitis but not in the models for delta FEV1% (i.e., acute change in FEV1) or byssinosis prevalence. The coefficient for dust level was never significant in the models.

GRAPHENE OXIDE

Robinson et al.[307] developed nanosized, reduced grapheme oxide (nano-rGO) sheets with high NIR light absorbance and biocompatibility for potential photothermal therapy. The single-layered nano-rGO sheets were 20 nm in average lateral dimension, functionalized noncovalently by amphiphilic PEGylated polymer chains to render stability in biological solutions and exhibited sixfold higher NIR absorption than nonreduced, covalently PEGylated nano-GO. Attaching a targeting peptide bearing the Arg–Gly–Asp (RGD) motif to nano-rGO afforded selective cellular uptake in U87MG cancer cells and highly effective photoablation of cells *in vitro*. In the absence of any NIR irradiation, nano-rGO exhibited little toxicity *in vitro* at concentrations well above the doses needed for photothermal heating. This work established nano-rGO as a novel photothermal agent due to its small size, high photothermal efficiency, and low cost as compared to other NIR photothermal agents, including gold nanomaterials and carbon nanotubes.

According to Sanchez et al.,[308] graphene is a single-atom thick, two-dimensional sheet of hexagonally arranged carbon atoms isolated from its three-dimensional parent material, graphite. Related materials include few-layer-graphene (FLG), ultrathin graphite, grapheme oxide (GO), reduced grapheme oxide (rGO), and graphene nanosheets (GNSs). Several unique modes of interaction between GFNs and nucleic acids, lipid bilayers, and conjugated small molecule drugs and dyes occur. Generation of reactive oxygen species (ROS) in target cells is a potentiation mechanism for toxicity, although the extremely high hydrophobic surface area of some GFNs may also lead to significant interactions with membrane lipids leading to direct physical toxicity or adsorption of biological molecules leading to indirect toxicity. Limited *in vivo* studies demonstrate systemic biodistribution and biopersistence of GFNs following intravenous delivery. Similar to other smooth, continuous, biopersistent implants or foreign bodies, GFNs have the potential to induce foreign-body tumors. Long-term adverse health impacts must be considered in the design of GFNs for drug delivery, tissue engineering, and fluorescence-based biomolecular sensing.

TALCOSIS

According to Marchiori et al.,[309] talc is a mineral widely used in the ceramic, paper, plastics, rubber, paint, and cosmetic industries. Four distinct forms of pulmonary disease caused by talc have been defined. Three of them (talcopsilicosis, talcoasbestosis, and pure talcosis) are associated with aspiration and differ in the composition of the inhaled substance. The fourth form, a result of intravenous administration of talc, is seen in drug users who inject medications intended for oral use. Presentation of patients with talc granulomatosis can range from asymptomatic to fulminant disease. Symptomatic patients typically present with nonspecific complaints, including progressive exertional dyspnea and cough. Late complications include chronic respiratory failure, emphysema, pulmonary arterial hypertension, and cor pulmonale. History of occupational exposure or of drug addiction is the major clue to the diagnosis. The high-resolution computed tomography (HRCT) finding of small centrilobular nodules associated with heterogeneous conglomerate masses containing high-density amorphous areas, with or without panlobular emphysema in the lower lobes, is highly suggestive of pulmonary talcosis. The characteristic histopathologic feature in talc pneumoconiosis is the striking appearance of birefringent needle-shaped particles of talc seen within the giant cells and in the areas of pulmonary fibrosis with the use of polarized light. The presence of these patterns in drug abusers or in patients with an occupational history of exposure to talc is highly suggestive of pulmonary talcosis.

According to Igbal et al.,[310] pulmonary disease due to talc, a group of hydrous magnesium silicates, is almost exclusively encountered secondary to occupational exposure or intravenous drug abuse. Very often, the history of exposure is not recognized by the patient, and it is only the finding of granulomatous cellular interstitial lesions containing birefringent crystals, which indicates considerable talc exposure.

WELDER'S LUNG

Welder's Pneumoconiosis: Diagnostic Usefulness of HRCT and Ferritin Determinations in Bronchoalveolar Lavage Fluid

According to Yoshii et al.,[311] they assessed usefulness of HRCT and ferritin determinations in bronchoaleolar lavage (BAL) fluid for diagnosis of welder's pneumoconiosis.

They investigated 11 patients with welder's pneumoconiosis who were 34–67 years old and had been welding for 17–45 years. Ten patients were current smokers.

HRCT revealed small centrilobular nodules in nine cases, mild fibrotic changes in three, and emphysematous changes in three. Serum ferritin concentrations were elevated (>240 ng/mL) in 10 cases. Ferritin concentrations in BAL fluid were higher in welder's pneumoconiosis than in the occupational control group.

They obtained BAL fluid in nine cases and transbronchial lung biopsy (TBLB) specimens in seven. Ferritin concentrations in BAL fluid were compared with those in welders without pneumoconiosis and other pneumoconiosis cases.

In welder's pneumoconiosis, small centrilobular nodules are frequently seen in HRCT, and ferritin shows elevations in serum and/or BAL fluid. Such ferritin determinations are of value in diagnosis.

EFFECTS OF GENETICS AND NUTRITION ON POLLUTANT-RELATED ADVERSE HEALTH EFFECTS

Genetic factors play a role in the susceptibility to respiratory, cardiac, and cerebral effects of air pollution. A number of studies have linked alleles on chromosomes 2q, 5q, 6p 12q, and 13q as being related to differing rates of asthma.[312] Several studies have also found that genes on certain alleles can increase the respiratory health effects of ambient air pollutant exposure. A Taiwanese study found that in high-pollution areas, the risk of asthma was significantly greater in children with the Ile-105 allele of the glutathione-S-transferase gene as compared to the Val-105 alleles.[313] Risk of asthma was very similar between children with the Ile-105 allele and Val-105 alleles in areas of low air pollution.[313] Glutathione-S-transferase plays a major role in reducing cell oxidative damage and the Ile-105 subjects may be less efficient in controlling cellular oxidative damage.

NUTRITION

Adequate nutrition is also useful in reducing the respiratory effects of air pollution. A Mexico City study found that asthmatic children when given antioxidant vitamin supplements were less affected by ozone than a control group which did not receive the supplements.[314] Another study found that supplemental antioxidants (400 IU vitamin E/500 mg vitamin C) significantly reduced lung function declines in adult volunteers exposed to 45 minutes of 0.12 ppm ozone and 10 minutes of 0.10 ppm SO_2.[315] Many, but not all, studies have linked higher consumption of many nutrients to less asthma and better lung function, including fruits and vegetables (at least five servings daily); phytochemicals (such as beta-carotene, lutein, and lycopene); magnesium; vitamins B_6, B_{12}, E, and C; manganese; and copper.

LEAD AND ZINC MINERS: 1960–1988

According to Cocco et al.,[316] the mortality of 4740 male workers of two lead and zinc mines was followed up from 1960 to 1988. Exposure to respirable dust was comparable in the two mines, but the median concentration of silica in respirable dust was 10-fold higher in mine B (12.8%) than in mine A (1.2%), but the mean annual exposure to radon daughters in underground workplaces differed in the opposite direction (mine A: 0.13 working levels [WLs], mine B: 0.011 WL). Total observed deaths (1205) were similar to expected figures (1156.3) over a total of 119,390.5 person-years at risk.

Underground workers of mine B had significant increases in risk of pulmonary TBC (SMR 706, 95% CI: 473–1014) and nonmalignant respiratory diseases (SMR 518; 95%CI: 440–1606), whereas the only significant excess at mine A was for nonmalignant respiratory diseases (SMR 246; 95% CI: 191–312). Total cancer and lung cancer mortality did not exceed the expectation in the two mines combined. A 15% excess mortality of lung cancer, increased up to an SMR 204 (95% CI: 89–470) for subjects employed ≥26 years, was, however, found among underground workers in mine A who on the average experienced an exposure to radon daughters 10-fold higher than those of mine B. By contrast, despite their higher exposure to silica, mine B underground workers experienced a lower than expected lung cancer mortality. A ninefold increase in risk of peritoneal and retroperitoneal cancer combined was also found among underground workers of mine A (SMR 917; 95% CI: 250–2347; based on four deaths). A causal association with workplace exposures is unlikely, however, as the SMR showed an inverse trend by duration of employment. These findings are consistent with low-level exposure to radon daughters as a risk factor for lung cancer among metal miners. Exposure to silica at the levels estimated for the mine B underground environment did not increase the risk of lung cancer.

VOCs in Breath as Markers of Lung Cancer: A Cross-Sectional Study

According to Phillips et al.,[1228] many VOCs, principally alkanes and benzene derivatives, have been identified in breath from patients with lung cancer. They investigated whether a combination of VOCs could identify such patients. They collected breath samples from 108 patients with an abnormal chest radiograph who were scheduled for bronchoscopy. The samples were collected with a portable apparatus, and then assayed by gas chromatography and mass spectroscopy. The alveolar gradient of each breath VOC, the difference between the amount in breath and in air, was calculated. Forward stepwise discriminant analysis was used to identify VOCs that discriminated between patients with and without lung cancer. Lung cancer was confirmed histologically in 60 patients. A combination of 22 breath VOCs, predominantly alkanes, alkane derivative, and benzene derivatives, discriminated between patients with and without lung cancer, regardless of stage (all p < 0.0003). For stage 1 lung cancer, 22 VOCs had 100% sensitivity and 81.3% had specificity. Cross-validation of the combination correctly predicted the diagnosis in 71.7% patients with lung cancer and 66.7% of those without lung cancer. Interpretation in patients with an abnormal chest radiograph, a combination of 22 VOCs in breath samples distinguished between patients with and without lung cancer.

Prospective studies are needed to confirm the usefulness of breath VOCs for detecting lung cancer in the general population.

Rea and Pan analyzed 200 patients for CS by breath analysis. The top 40 showed from 348 types of chemicals at the EHC-Dallas (Table 2.7).

ENVIRONMENTAL ASPECTS OF CARDIOVASCULAR DYSFUNCTION

Pollutant Injury to the Microvessels and Myocardium Especially from PM

According to Brook et al.,[317] air pollution is a heterogeneous complex mixture of gases, liquids, and PM. Epidemiological studies have demonstrated a consistent increased risk for cardiovascular events in relation to both short- and long-term exposure to present-day concentrations of ambient PM. Several plausible mechanistic pathways have been described including enhanced coagulation/thrombosis, a propensity for arrhythmias, acute arterial vasoconstriction, systemic inflammatory responses, and the chronic promotion of atherosclerosis. The purpose of this statement is to provide clinicians and regulatory agencies with a comprehensive review of the literature on air pollution and cardiovascular disease.

TABLE 2.7

Top 40 of 200 Patients Analyzed for Chemical Sensitivity by Breath Analysis

Chemical Name	Positive (%)	Chemical Name	Positive (%)	Chemical Name	Positive (%)
Cyclopropane ethylidene-	54	Acetone	39	D-Limonene	19
Benzeneethanol, a'a''-dimethyl-	17	Heptane,5-ethyl-2,2,3-trimethyl-	11	Hexane	16
Pentane	16	Butane	15	2-Butanol	11
Butane,2,3-dimethyl-	10	Butane,2,2,3,3-tetramethyl	10	1,3-Pentadiene(E)-	10
Octane2,3,3-trimethyl-	10	Tetradecane	10	(2-Azridinyl ethyl)amine	9
Benzene,1-methyl-2-(1-methylethyl)-	9	Bicyclo(2.1.1.)hex-2-ene,2-ethenyl-	9	Bicyclo(4.2.0)octa-1,3,5-triene	9
Cyclohexene,1-methyl-5-(1-methylethenyl)-	9	Decane,2,5,6-trimethyl-	9	2,3-Epoxycarane,(E)-	9
Ethanol	9	Toluene	9	Undecane,3,7-dimethyl-	9
1,2-Butadiene,3-methyl-	8	Butane,2-methyl-	8	Cyclohexane	8
Cyclohexene,1-methyl-4-(1-methylethenyl)-,(n)-	8	Cyclopentasiloxane,decamethyl-	8	Dodecane	8
Dodecane,4,6-dimethyl-	8	Hexane,2,2-dimethyl-	8	Nonane	8
Octane,2,3,6,7-tetramethyl-	8	Pentadecane	8	Pentane,2,2,45,4-tetramethyl-	8
Pentane,2,2,4-trimethyl-	8	1-Propene,1-(methylthio)-,(E)-	8	Undecane	8
Tetrachloroethylene	7				

Source: Adapted from Rea, W., Y. Pan. Environmental Health Center-Dallas. 2016.

The association between air pollution and myocardial infarction (MI) remains controversial. Some studies illustrated an increased risk of MI, whereas other studies showed no significant effect. However, the later section puts the triggering agents into a new light. The common air pollutants are ozone (O_3), carbon monoxide (CO), nitrogen dioxide (NO_2), sulfur dioxide (SO_2), and PM within <10 μm (PM_{10}), PM within 2.5 μm ($PM_{2.5}$), and PM <200 ng. Brook et al.[317] hypothesized that air pollution is associated with an increased risk of MI.

According to Brook et al.,[317] two independent reviewers determined studies eligibility and extracted methodological and outcome data. According to Brook et al.,[317] the RRs were pooled across studies using random effects model. The I2 statistic and Egger's test were used to, respectively, assess heterogeneity and publication bias.[317]

Thirty-three studies were included, consisting of 18 time series and 15 case-crossover studies. All common air pollutants, except ozone, were significantly associated with MI; even ozone was in some studies. The pooled RRs were 1.058 (1.030–1.087), I2 = 93% for CO, 1.012 (1.006–1.017), I2 = 70% for NO_2, 1.012 (1.004–1.020), I2 = 67% for SO_2, 1.007 (1.004–1.011), I2 = 51% for PM_{10}, 1.025 (1.015–1.0361), I2 = 52% for $PM_{2.5}$ and 1.003 (0.996–1.0101), I2 = 84% for O_3 sensitivity showed a similar effect size while reducing the heterogeneity. Moreover, no statistical argument for publication bias was found. Population attributable fractions on the pollutant were between 0.7% and 5.5%.

Despite the low levels of RRs, the high frequency (HF) of exposure to air pollution corresponds to an elevated population on attributable fraction and therefore, may have considerable public health implications. However, compared with changes witnessed in rats that had breathed only clean air, vessel dilation in those that had inhaled nanoparticles was lessened and O_2 extraction was less just as the humans with CS and chronic fatigue[318] who were supersensitive to air pollution.

This diminished vessel lacking relaxation and O_2 extraction is similar to what elicits as muscle cramps, chest pain in the heart, or transient stroke in the brain.[318] In another experiment, rats inhaled or ingested particles known as multiwalled carbon nanotubes. Made from rolled-up sheets of carbon, these tubes are about 50 billionths of a meter across and are being explored for use in delivering drugs via the nose, mouth, or injections. As with the nanospheres, the nanotubes made it harder for microarterioles to dilate. The nanotubes also developed exaggerated constriction when the body commanded arterioles to reduce blood flow, which of course resulted in local hypoxia.

Effects peaked at about 24 hours after exposure to the particles, after which the microarterioles' responsiveness began to improve. However, even a week later, the vessels had not fully returned to normal.[318] This similar response is seen in the severe chemically sensitive patient with vasculitis, which often incapacitates them. This delayed continuous microvessel spasm makes the chemically sensitive very vulnerable to arrhythmia and if it involves the cerebral vessels, confusion, short-term memory loss, weakness, and fatigue result.

The finding also showed that vessel impairments did not require long exposures; in these experiments, ingested nanotubes produced the most dramatic change in arteriole reactivity with short-term hypersensitivity reactions. Microvessel reactivity is seen in coronary vessel, as well as peripheral and cerebral vessel spasms, resulting in symptoms of spastic blood supply to the appropriate microvessels of the cerebrum or extremities. Microvessel studies have now shown that the nonocculsives reaction and hypersensitivity states cause tissue changes.

Considerable evidence has accumulated to counter older concepts of a categorical definition of ischemic heart disease (IHD) and ischemic peripheral and cerebral vascular disease as simply the presence or absence of a flow-limiting stenosis. According to Petersen and Pepine,[319] revised concepts increasingly recognize nonocclusive IHD in addition at the EHC-Dallas of nonocclusive ischemic cerebral and distal extremity peripheral vascular disease. The ischemia is a continuous spectrum that is not limited to obstructive plaque seen by angiography in an epicardial coronary artery or cerebral arteries or distal extremity vessels. Included in this spectrum are vascular diseases, functional disorders of the large and smaller coronary, cerebral, gut, and distal extremity peripheral blood vessels, which result in spasm or glucose inhibition of oxygen extraction[319] causing ischemia and chest pain, cerebral, or distal extremity peripheral vascular, dysfunction, resulting in memory loss, confusion, weakness, and fatigue. These smaller vessels, collectively the coronary, cerebral, and distal extremity peripheral microcirculation, along with the gut vascular system comprise a large share of the small vessels of the microcirculation. They control the volume and distribution of blood flow to the myocardium, brain or distal peripheral extremity muscles as well as oxygenation in these organs. In our experience at the EHC-Dallas and EHC-Buffalo, microvessels can, when dysfunctional, develop oxidative stress and inflammation resulting in vascular dysfunction. This vascular spasm and functional obstruction result in the tissue (muscles, nerves) that does not extract sufficient oxygen; therefore, they also release neurotransmitters. This lack of O_2 extraction due to shunting with spasm, edema, and metabolic dysfunction is caused by many triggering agents such as natural gas (Randolph, T.G. 1985. Personal communication), pesticides,[320] formaldehyde,[321] solvents,[322] mold, mycotoxins,[323] heavy metals,[324] implants, excess glucose, and EMF, etc.[325] These vessels can develop oxidative stress and become inflamed causing more spasms or shunting with lack of oxygen extraction and delivery to the local heart, cerebrum, GI tract, or other distal extremity peripheral vessel and muscle and nerve areas supplied by the microcirculation with the resulting area of ischemia. According to Stapelton,[318] these reactions of the microvessels exposed to the toxic exposure may result in a different recovery pattern of up to a week. This slow recovery would make the microvascular tree vulnerable to subsequent exposures causing more hypersensitivity, headache, muscle pains, weakness, and fatigue. Certainly, hypersensitive reactions seen in the mold, food, chemical, and EMF challenge reactions can last from a few minutes to 1–2 hours in the severely chemically sensitive patients. PvO_2s have been observed to last in this way in some chemically sensitive patients.

Although not visualized by angiography, the coronary or other microcirculation may be indirectly assessed from the speed of radiographic contrast movement through the microvascular area as the corrected thrombolysis in MI (TIMI) frame count or the level of PvO_2 above 28 mm Hg as measured in the antecubital fossa without a tourniquet. The higher the PvO_2, the more hypoxia in the body (extremity, brain, gut, etc.) even though the PaO_2 is 95%–100%. Shunting without O_2 extraction occurs.[325,326] According to Petersen and Pepine,[319] this simple, objective, continuous index is accurate, reproducible, and highly correlated with Doppler blood flow measurements, and provides information for risk stratification in the myocardium and in our observation in the distal extremity peripheral and cerebral tissues.[327-329] The microcirculation of the heart can be directly assessed in the absence of flow-limiting stenosis, by coronary flow reserve (CFR) and also by the index of microvascular resistance. Noninvasive methods, such as positron emission tomography (PET), Doppler echocardiography, gadolinium perfusion cardiac MRI, triple-3D-camera SPECT scan, and micro-CT (cryostatic) scan are also increasingly being used to evaluate microvascular function of the myocardium or other vascular organs. Especially, the brain SPECT (Figures 2.3 and 2.4) scan appears efficacious.

Patients with symptoms and signs of ischemia, referred for invasive coronary evaluation, increasingly appear without obstructive epicardial coronary artery disease (CAD).[330,331] This same invasive angiogram is also true for cerebral, GI tract, or distal extremity peripheral vascular obstruction. This hypoxia also happens in cerebral and other peripheral vascular organs such as gut. Many other chemically sensitive patients clearly have systemic microvessel peripheral artery disease clinically presenting with not only local hypoxia but also with symptoms and signs of spontaneous bruising, peripheral edema, petechial, and at times acneiform lesions and blue and cold distal extremities of both hands and feet as well as abdominal cramps and cerebral fogginess; or in the case of brain imbalance (cannot stand on toes or walk straight line with eyes closed), confusion, and short-term memory loss. We and others identified that symptomatic patients with nonobstructive CAD may have an elevated risk of adverse outcomes compared with cohorts without symptoms or signs of IHD. This is also true for cerebral dysfunction (episodic confusion with short-term memory loss), peripheral microvascular dysfunction (distal muscle fatigue, bloating, GI upset), and cold extremities and weakness (Figure 10.3).[331] Unfortunately, because of lack of evidence-based results, the treatment and management of these symptomatic patients is often frustrating for the patients and their physicians. Studies and treatment in less-polluted, controlled environments appear to be a solution for this problem. If they do not have a less-polluted, controlled environment, which decreases overall pollution five times over a regular hospital or clinic to work in, to diagnose and treat their patients, they will fall short in their results of diagnosis and treatment.[60] However, chemically sensitive patients with nonobstructive vasculitis have to be considered. Since there is a long history at the EHC-Dallas and other environmental centers of diagnosing and treating these patients in a controlled environment, they manifest lack of oxygen exchange in the local tissue, which results in vascular spasm and mediator release.[60] As a result, these CAD, gut, cerebral, and distal extremity peripheral small-vessel disease individuals consume medical resources rivaling those for patients with obstructive cardiac (CAD)[332] carotid and peripheral artery disease. Peripheral effectiveness of the microvascular circulation can also be measured by the PvO_2 taken from the antecubital fossa without a tourniquet. A PvO_2 above 28 mm Hg indicates a lack of oxygen extraction in the microcirculation presumably therefore due to vascular spasm of the microcirculation and/or shunting past the oxygen extraction areas of the end tissue (Table 2.10).

Approximately 45%–60% of coronary microvascular disease (CMD) patients have coronary vascular deregulation (endothelial- or nonendothelial-dependent macrovascular or microvascular dysfunction) capable of causing ischemia due to lack of oxygen extraction.[330,342] Numerous reports linked coronary vascular deregulation, usually referred to as CMD with adverse clinical outcomes,[343–345] but these data have mostly been derived from cohorts of women. Indeed, the finding from the National Heart, Lung, and Blood Institute–sponsored Women's Ischemic Syndrome Evaluation (WISE) show that CMD predicted adverse outcomes.[344] This finding has resulted in multiple attempts to link CMD with female reproductive hormones and other female-specific issues, with variable results. It has been shown that men now have CMD in large numbers though female hormones do have a place in regulatory CMD in certain females.[319] We have treated many female patients with microvascular disease successfully using female hormone intradermal neutralization as well as with mini doses of estrogen, progesterone, and luteinizing hormone supplementation. Molds, mycotoxins, pesticides, natural gas, and many organic and inorganic chemicals trigger the microvascular disease in others resulting in environmentally triggered vasculopathy and vasculitis seen at the EHC-Dallas. It has been shown that men have an equal amount of nonocclusive CMD; etiologic agent must be found, eliminated, or neutralized. (Our series have 50 patients with microvascular-dysfunction-triggering agents [Table 2.8] and immune deficiency.)

Patients with chemical and electrical sensitivity as triggering agents fall into this category for a large proportion of both female and male sensitive patients with coronary chest pain and normal large coronary arteries as well as large vessels and cerebral or peripheral microcirculation. CMD patients have a clean vascular tree on coronary angiograms but still have chest pain that at times is incapacitating. Most of these patients with CS have peripheral small-vessel vasculitis as well as along with their CS. This means that a whole host of environmental triggering agents cannot only trigger the microvascular hypersensitivity but can also trigger the vascular response of spasm and/ or shunting past the oxygen extraction area. Many a times, the triggering agents can be eliminated or neutralized by the intradermal neutralization (desensitization) (Lee and Miller method) and by nutrient supplementation and also with withdrawal of the prime offending incitants.[346] Their T and B lymphocytes, complements, and gamma globulin can be replaced or improved for successful treatment if needed.

According to Petersen and Pepine,[319] the strengths of their work included a large sample size of both men (n = 405) and women (n = 813) with CMD. Of course, nonocclusive cerebrovascular disease or distal extremity peripheral vascular disease was not noted in their series. Using a CFR < 2.0 to define CMD, they found that, in both sexes, CMD was highly prevalent (>50%) and significantly associated with adverse outcomes. Even in the presence of subclinical CAD (e.g., coronary calcification), CFR remained significantly associated with adverse outcomes. The adjusted hazard decreased 20% for every 10% increase in CFR. These new data confirm and extend previous findings about

TABLE 2.8

Characteristics of the Study Sample of Avoidance of Pollutants in Air, Food, and Water Long Term in a Chemically Sensitive Group Compared with the Nonstudy Subjects

	Study Sample (n = 3896)	Nonstudy Sample (n = 2918)
Age (years)	61.4 ± 10.1	63.2 ± 10.4
Female (%)	52.6	53.2
Race (%)		
White	39.9	36.6
Chinese	12.5	10.8
African-American	25.6	30.6
Hispanic	22.0	22.0
Height (cm)	166.4 ± 9.9	166.3 ± 10.2
Weight (kg)	77.4 ± 16.2	80.3 ± 18.6
Body mass index (kg/m²)	27.8 ± 5.0	29.0 ± 6.0
Educational attainment (%)		
No high school degree	15.8	21.1
High school degree	18.1	18.3
Some college	16.1	16.7
Bachelor's degree	18.5	15.5
Higher than bachelor's degree	19.1	16.5
Cigarette smoking status (%)		
Never	52.6	47.3
Former	35.1	38.7
Current	12.4	14.0
Pack-years of smoking	10.8 ± 22.8	12.3 ± 21.4
Hypertension (%)	42.5	48.4
Systolic blood pressure (mm Hg)	125.3 ± 20.9	128.3 ± 22.1
Diabetes mellitus (%)	12.3	15.3
Fasting plasma glucose (mg/dL)	95.9 ± 28.2	99.3 ± 32.8
Study site (%)		
St. Paul	16.0	15.2
Los Angeles	18.2	20.9
Baltimore	17.7	13.6
Chicago	14.1	21.1
New York City	20.3	10.7
Winston-Salem	13.8	18.5
Stable residential neighborhood (%)		
>5 years	79.8	76.0
>10 years	63.8	61.8
NO_2 (ppb)	22.6 ± 10.3	22.2 ± 9.2[a]
NO_x (ppb)	50.5 ± 26.9	50.4 ± 26.7[a]

Note: NO_2, nitrogen dioxide; cm, centimeters; kg, kilograms; m², meter square; mm Hg, millimeters of mercury; ppb, parts per billion.

[a] 1055 participants with NO_2 and NO_x estimates not included in the study sample because of missing MRI or covariates.

TABLE 2.9

Multivariable Linear Regression Estimating the Associations between NO$_2$ Exposure and Right Ventricular Structure and Function

Model	Per Interquartile Increase in NO$_2$		
	Difference	95% CI	p-Value
RV mass, g (limited model[a])	0.4	0.2, 0.7	<0.001
RV mass, g (limited model[a] + city)	0.9	0.3, 1.4	0.002
RV mass, g (full model[b])	1.0	0.4, 1.5	0.001
RV mass, g (full model[b] + LV mass)	0.9	0.3, 1.4	0.001
RVEDV, mL (limited model[a])	2.9	1.4, 4.7	<0.001
RVEDV, mL (limited model[a] + city)	2.7	−0.9, 6.2	0.14
RVEDV, mL (full model[b])	4.1	0.5, 7.7	0.03
RVEDV, mL (full model[b] + LVEDV)	2.7	0.0, 5.4	0.05
RVEF, % (limited model[a])	−0.1	−0.5, 0.5	0.80
RVEF, % (limited model[a] + city)	−0.2	−1.2, 0.8	0.69
RVEF, % (full model[b])	−0.2	−1.2, 0.8	0.72
RVEF, % (full model[b] + LVEF)	0.0	1.0, 0.9	0.92

Source: Reprinted with permission of the American Thoracic Society. Copyright 2017 American Thoracic Society. Leary, P. J. et al. 2014. Traffic-related Air Pollution and the Right Ventricle. *The American Journal of Respiratory and Critical Care Medicine.* 189(7):1093–1100.

Note: NO$_2$, nitrogen dioxide; CI, confidence interval; RV, right ventricular; LV, left ventricular; RVEDV, right ventricular end-diastolic volume; LVEDV, left ventricular end-diastolic volume; RVEF, right ventricular ejection fraction; LVEF, left ventricular ejection fraction.

[a] Adjusted for age, sex, race ethnicity, height, and weight.

[b] Adjusted for age, sex, race/ethnicity, height, weight, city, education, income, smoking, pack-years, hypertension, diabetes, cholesterol, and impaired glucose tolerance.

the high prevalence of CMD and predictions of adverse outcomes in women and men. The findings are highly relevant for clinical trials evaluating therapeutic agent's especially massive avoidance and intradermal neutralization (desensitization) of offending particulates and chemicals. Otherwise, this field lacks evidence-based data to inform patient management. Future study is also necessary to determine whether CMD, nonocclusive ischemic cerebral vascular or peripheral microvascular disease significantly strengthens the prediction of adverse outcomes beyond that provided by traditional risk models.[319] In our experience, these patients with microvascular dysfunction often improve with specific intradermal antigens of the dose that triggers neutralization of symptoms and signs, avoidance of specific pollutants when they are sensitive to mold, food, and toxic chemicals, and specific nutrient supplementation. Only long-term studies initially performed under less-polluted, environmentally controlled conditions and then followed by avoidance of pollutants and particulates at home and work will signify the efficacy of treatment.[319]

Tables 2.8 and 2.9 show that we at the EHC-Dallas clearly have followed MVD nonocclusive, microvascular cerebral and distal extremity peripheral vascular diseased patients and those with GI upset for 30 years with excellent results for those who can comply with less-polluted living quarters neutralizing (optimum dose desensitization) injections therapy, nutrients, and rotary diets at home.

The prevalence and associated adverse prognosis of CMD in those patients with a normal perfusion scan included in Petersen and Pepine's cohort are impressive. The true prevalence of CMD is likely to be even higher when the chemically sensitive vasculitis diagnosis is included.[319]

Patients with stenotic perfusion defects were excluded from the Petersen and Pepine's[319] current study because their perfusion defect was presumed to be caused by obstructive CAD. However, others have shown that 70% of the patients with an abnormal myocardial perfusion study but angiographically "normal" epicardial coronaries had CMD.[347] Therefore, some of the patients excluded from Murthy et al.'s study[348] likely also had CMD. In those with CMD, it is probable that the triggering agents can be found and eliminated or neutralized stopping the progression of the disease by the avoidance of triggering agents by methods developed at the EHC-Dallas. We have performed the definition and avoidance of pollutants and elimination and intradermal neutralization (desensitization) of triggering agents in over 2000 patients with microvascular disease by using a less-polluted, environmentally controlled diagnostic and treatment environment (EHC-Dallas). The primary triggering agents under environmentally controlled conditions by individual intradermal and inhaled challenge were of natural gas, formaldehyde, phenol, ethanol, particulates (<200 µg), molds/mycotoxins, and herbicides/ pesticides with ambient doses in the low parts per million or high parts per billion. These are triggering agents and ambient doses of what is found in daily living at home and at work and are able to be defined under strict and precise less-polluted, environmentally controlled conditions.

According to Petersen and Pepine,[319] the high prevalence of CMD is noteworthy because CMD likely contributes not only to chest discomfort but also to ischemia-related left ventricular dysfunction. Diastolic dysfunction is the earliest functional abnormality documented in patients with ischemia secondary to vascular smooth muscle dysfunction (which is commonly thought to be spontaneously occurring coronary spasm).[349] In the studies from the WISE (Randolph, T.G. 1985. Personal communication), which included a high prevalence of CMD among women with normal left ventricular systolic function at baseline, a heart failure hospitalization was the most prevalent adverse outcome during follow-up.[319] Patients with endothelial dysfunction related to microvascular oxidative stress, inflammation/deregulation, have a high incidence of left ventricular diastolic dysfunction, and this likely contributes to the symptoms of patients with heart failure with preserved ejection fraction.[350] Similarly, in the study by Murthy et al.,[348] patients with a CFR < 2.0 were two times more likely to have a heart failure hospitalization versus those with a CFR > 2.0. Thus, CMD is a potentially important therapeutic target for the growing population of patients with heart failure with preserved ejection fraction. The antecubital PvO_2 discussed above can be the indicator of lack of oxygen extraction in these peripheral, cerebral, gut, and cardiac microvessels. This finding gives us an opportunity to recognize that environmental triggering agents occur, causing coronary artery spasms and thus eliminate them. These patients improved as the PvO_2 and thus oxygen extraction became normal when levels reached 28 mm Hg or less.

Due to its high prevalence and associated adverse prognosis, it is important to consider testing for CMD in patients with chest discomfort or left ventricular dysfunction of unclear cause. The investigators used a well-validated method to determine absolute myocardial blood flow reserve with PET.[351,352] Their study design exemplified the importance of considering absolute or regional measures of flow compared with relative distribution of flow. Although a large proportion of patients had documented impairment in CFR, all patients included in the current study by Peterson and Pepine[319] had "normal" relative perfusion by PET perfusion imaging. Therefore, when considering a more diffuse process, such as CMD, it is important to use a test that can evaluate absolute myocardial blood flow. The same is true to evaluate distal extremity peripheral or cerebral vascular flow. In the WISE, they performed coronary reactivity testing using a Doppler guide wire in a proximal left coronary artery branch. Change in blood flow velocity in response to intracoronary adenosine is used to determine CFR, and change in coronary flow and coronary cross-sectional area in response to intracoronary acetylcholine are used to define endothelial-dependent vascular function.[353] However, because most of these patients also have endothelial dysfunction, there is very limited flow-mediated dilation in response to adenosine, so coronary velocity provides a very good estimate of the absolute change in blood flow.[342] Many of our chemically sensitive patients respond both adversely and positively to different dilutions of acetylcholine at the EHC-Dallas. Intradermal neutralization with acetylcholine will help some patients temporarily improve with CMD. Prostigmine blocking acetylcholine and naltrexone blocking the opioid reaction have been shown to temporarily reduce vascular spasm in the microcirculation.

In addition to the PET techniques described by these investigators, there are other noninvasive methods available for the evaluation of coronary blood flow and CFR to assess CMD. Transthoracic Doppler echocardiography provides assessment of coronary blood flow velocity in the left anterior descending coronary that can be used to determine CFR after hypoxia.[354] Doppler echo-derived measures of CFR were shown to correlate significantly with invasive measures of CFR.[355] In contrast to PET, Doppler echo does not require radiation exposure and is available at most centers. A limitation of transthoracic Doppler echo–determined CFR is the feasibility of detecting left anterior descending flow in all of the patients. Studies reported that as few as 34% and as many as 96% of the patients included in various cohorts had successful evaluation of left anterior descending flow.[354] Echo-contrast agents can enhance the Doppler signal and led to improvement in measuring left anterior descending flow responses.[355]

In conclusion, the present studies highlight the importance of considering CMD as an explanation for chest discomfort or heart failure among both women and men without flow-limiting epicardial stenosis. Our studies also show that cerebral and distal extremity peripheral small-vessel disease exists and can be diagnosed and treated. Also, it opens the diagnosis and treatment for areas of nonocclusive coronary, cerebrovascular GI, and distal extremities peripheral vascular changes causing multiple symptoms. In this setting, the link between cerebral and peripheral small-vessel disease to CMD and adverse outcomes appears firmly established. Fortunately, many invasive and noninvasive techniques are available to evaluate CMD and possibly the cerebral or peripheral vascular dysfunction. The possibility of CMD occurring in the presence of flow-limiting stenosis is also highly likely and warrants additional study relative to its contribution to symptoms and adverse outcomes. Identification of CMD will not only assist in counseling patients on prognosis but also has the potential to serve as a novel therapeutic target for avoidance of pollutants, intradermal neutralization (desensitization), and specific nutrition if environmental measures are used. Apart from the techniques of avoiding pollutants in and out of a less-polluted, controlled environment and other toxics as well as clinicians learning and practicing intradermal neutralization (desensitization) and specific nontriggering rotational diets, clinicians might have a different view of the prevention and treatment of microvascular coronary, cerebral, GI, and peripheral nonocclusive vascular disease. Although microvascular spasm and/or lack of oxygen extraction is gaining support as a potential possibility,[329] the specific mechanism(s) responsible for CMD, GI, cerebral, and peripheral microvascular dysfunction remains elusive to only the uninformed who do not work with less-polluted environmental techniques. Using this physiology warrants continued study. However, the patients do respond to treatment for immune regulation of the T and B cell depression, complement, and abnormalities resulting in gamma globulin subset deficiency. Also, the findings and definition of the triggering agents due to pollution whether they are molds, mycotoxins, pesticides, natural gas, toxic organic or inorganic chemicals, or ultrafine particulates (UFP) can now be defined under less-polluted, environmentally controlled conditions. These can be countered not only by avoidance and intradermal neutralization (desensitization) of pollutants but also by using autogenous lymphocytic factor for enhancing T cells and their function and supplementation replacement of gamma globulin when gamma globulin deficiency occurs or giving oxygen therapy via the von Ardenne techniques[326] when tissue hypoxia is found.

Vasa Vasorum in Normal and Diseased Arteries

According to Mulligan-Kehoe and Simons,[356] Murthy et al.,[348] and Petersen and Pepine,[319] the incidence of nonobstructive CMD can cause chest pain, myocardial dysfunction, heart failure; and according to the EHC-Dallas, a multitude of problems in cerebral, gut, and distal peripheral arteries. These dysfunctions can be significant or not in the chemically sensitive because some of their small-vessel disease concentrates are in the brain, skin, or other organs such as the heart, gut, bladder, kidneys, and other peripheral blood vessels. Certainly, if the triggering agents are not identified, the disease may progress to atherosclerosis and it may also progress to end-stage neurovascular

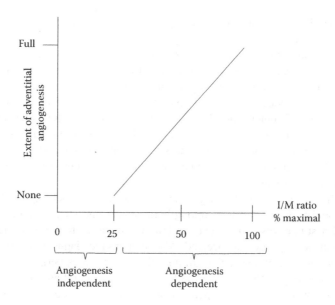

FIGURE 2.15 Angiogenesis-dependent and -independent development of neointima. Correlation between the extent of neointima formation that occurs after vessel injury in the presence and absence of adventitial angiogenesis. Note formation of some neointima even when adventitial angiogenesis is fully suppressed and a linear relationship between the growth of neointima and the extent of adventitial angiogenesis once it starts. I/M indicates intima/media. (Adapted with permission from Khurana, R. et al. 2005. *Circulation* 111:2828–2836. Authorization for this adaptation has been obtained both from the owner of the copyright in the original work and from the owner of copyright in the translation or adaptation.)

disease, which results in hypersensitivity vasculitis and/or end-stage fibrosis (Figure 2.15), biopsy with lymphocytes surrounding the blood vessels.

According to Mulligan-Kehoe and Simons,[356] the vasa vasorum are a specialized microvasculature that play a major role in normal vessel wall biology and pathology and may be of importance in chemically sensitive vasculitis. These vasa vasorum consist of small arterioles which enter the adventitia and media, then arborize to the outer media and accompanying veins (VVV) for returning blood (Figure 2.16). Under physiological conditions, the external adventitial vasa vasorum (AVV) and internal medial vasa vasorum (AVV) take up molecules carrying oxygen and nutrients that are transmitted from the blood to the media and adventitia by mass transport through the arterial wall or its branches. If the vascular membrane containing the blood is slightly damaged, dysfunction occurs, which one sees in CS. This dysfunction can involve transient offensive chemicals as triggering agents (natural gas, solvents, preoxidant molecules [pesticides, formaldehyde, phenol, metals], mycotoxins, or PM [nanoparticles], etc.) that can lead to vascular dysfunction and eventually pathology.[325] Normally, the AVV also absorbs nutrients for the detoxification and healthy maintenance and repair process of the vessels as well as keeping immune cells such as T and B cells healthy. The adventitia of the vasa vasorum is the primary early site for vessel wall response to arterial injury that occurs on the luminal side whether it is traumatic or environmentally disruptive by toxics, hypoxia, or infection. The vasa vasorum expand in response to the injury, which alters vessel homeostasis (vessel injury component triggering agent for small vessels).[356] Vasa vasorum interna originate directly from the lumen.

Part of the cardiovascular system, the vasa vasorum are a network of small blood vessels, that help supply larger vessels with blood. The vasa vasorum provide blood and oxygen to large arteries and veins, and returns that supply blood depleted of oxygen through the VVV eventually going to the lungs. Toxins are also delivered to the largest blood vessels in the body. The aorta depends on this support network of vasa vascular to maintain healthy function. All vessels with a wall less than

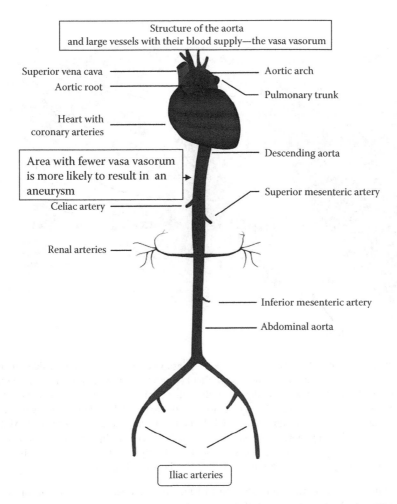

FIGURE 2.16 Vasa vasorum are small vessels which enter the large vessels and arborize. These vasa vaso-rum supply the large vessels with walls more than 500 mm (or 29 cell layers thick). Vessels whose walls <500 μm thick (or 29 cell layer normally do not have vasorum). (Adapted from Leary, P. J. et al. 2014. *Am. J. Respir. Crit. Care Med.* 189(9):1093–1100.)

500 μm thick (or 29 cell layers) do not have vasa vasorum.[357] Vasa vasorum are found in vessels 0.5 mm in diameter or greater and an arterial wall media more than 29 lamellar thick.[358,359] The vasa vasorum are needed to supply large arteries and veins because of their large size. In order to effectively receive oxygen from the bloodstream, cells must be very close to a small blood vessel or capillary so that oxygen can pass into each individual cell. Most blood vessels and veins absorb oxygen from the blood flowing inside them. However, because the large pressure big arteries are by necessity so thick, their outer and middle cell layers cannot be adequately be nourished without this additional network of blood vessels to support them by providing oxygenated blood and nutri-ents and carrying away deoxygenated blood and toxic waste materials. This vasa vasorum network stretches from the carotid to the femoral arteries possibly beyond (Figure 2.17).

There are three major types of vasa vasorum, classified by where they originate and where they lead. The vasa vasorum internal originate from inside the main large artery or vein and pass into the vessel walls. Vasa vasorum external originate in the main artery branches, then return to the main artery or vein to nourish the cells farther away from the vessels interior. Venous vasa vaso-rum (VVV) have their origins in the main vein, and then drain into the artery concomitant vein, or

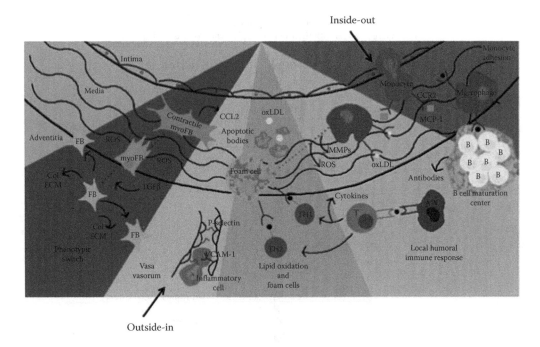

FIGURE 2.17 (See color insert.) Theories of origin of vasa vasorum. Depiction of inside-out and outside-in theories of vascular inflammation. The outside-in theory assumes that inflammatory cells enter the vessel wall from the luminal side. The outside-in theory predicts that the inflammatory cells gain entry to the vessel wall via the adventitial vasa vasorum. APC, antigen-presenting cell; CCL2, chemokine ligand 2; Col, collagen; ECM, extracellular matrix; FB, fibroblast; MCP-1, monocyte chemoattractant protein 1; MMPS, matrix metalloproteinases; myoFB, myofibroblast; oxLDL, oxidized low-density lipoprotein; ROS, reactive oxygen species; TGFβ, transforming growth factor-β; Th1 and Th2, T helper cells 1 and 2; VCAM-1, vascular cell adhesion molecule 1. (Reprinted with permission from Maiellaro and Taylor.)

partner vein. The exact structure and function of these blood vessels vary depending on which of these types it is and where it is located. The function of vasa vasorum in supporting the aorta has been the subject of many studies. In some areas, the human aorta does not have vasa vasorum, and in these areas, the aorta's walls are much thinner, making aneurysm more likely to occur in those locations. By contrast, dogs and some other mammals do have these vessels in these areas of the aorta, allowing the vessel walls to be thicker and less susceptible to aneurysm. This complex network of vessels is more commonly found in arteries than in veins, possibly because arterial walls tend to be thicker and more muscular than the walls of even the largest veins and they do need oxygen and nutrients to keep them viable and robust because of the pressure in the arteries.

Vasa Vasorum and Adventitia

According to Mulligan-Kehoe and Simons,[356] the adventitia, the outermost layer of the vessel wall, has received considerable attention in recent years. It contains a heterogeneous population of cells, including macrophages,[360,361] T cells, dendritic cells[360,361] (antigen presenting to T cells, and messenger from the innate to the adaptive immune system), progenitor cells,[362,363] and fibroblasts that can differentiate into myofibroblasts.[364] It also contains an adrenergic (autonomic) nervous system[365] (which changes and releases catechol Amicar, especially adventitia in the chemically sensitive and a lymphatic network).[366] The vasa vasorum are a specialized microvasculature that plays a major role in normal vessel wall biology and pathology. All of these tissues or cells have potential environmental triggering agents such as natural gas, pesticides, herbicides, solvents, mycotoxins, synthetic implants, EMF, etc. that often can be defined, neutralized, detoxified, and eliminated (with good environmental control technique) that render the vasa vasorum and large vessels they supply to be very clean and functioning normally. However, if the toxic environmental agents are not neutralized or eliminated, they then cause pathology such as oxidative stress, inflammation, lack of oxygen extraction, and even occlusion or rupture.

Under physiological conditions, the AVV and lymphatic vessels take up nutrients and toxic molecules that are transmitted from the blood to the adventitia by mass transport through the arterial wall.[367-369] At times, they may be nutrients, detoxifying enzymes and immune cells that keep the vessels clean. At other times, they may contain toxic environmental triggering agents (i.e., natural gas, pesticides, formaldehyde, phenol, mycotoxins, etc.) for the beginning of disturbed physiology and eventually pathology. They can also be allergens that sensitize the endothelium and affect the other immune elements that can result in endothelial dysfunction. Vascular injury at the luminal side of the vessel wall significantly impacts the adventitia by convection of soluble factors, microparticles and macroparticles, mediators such as products of oxidation, inflammation, tissue cytolysis, and proteolysis from the intima to the adventitia by hydraulic conductance.[370] The AVV can harbor toxic chemicals like natural gas, pesticides, benzene, mercury, molds, mycotoxins, food, and particle matter in CS patients. As a result, the adventitia becomes the primary in early site for the vessel wall response to arterial injury, which includes myofibroblast migration into the vessel wall,[371,372] with oxidative and inflammatory cell accumulation,[373-375] and expansion of vasa vasorum[376,377] (Figure 2.18). The latter process has the potential of affecting many aspects of the vessel homeostasis, including the development of neointima, growth of atherosclerotic plaque, and/or severe inflammation in the vessels. Often, fibrotic scar due to the inflammation develops without the atherosclerosis, which is the result of environmentally induced vasculitis.

Vasa Vasorum Structure/Function

The vasa vasorum are specialized vessels. All types of arterial vasa vasorum (AVV) are recognized. The first type is the vasa vasorum interna, which originate from the large vessel going to the[378] media[359,379] and branching out into the adjacent artery wall.[380] The second type is the vasa vasorum externa, which are found primarily in the adventitia at its border with the media. They originate from various anatomic locations like the nearby major branches (external vasa vasorum) of the large vessel. These small vessels nourish the larger vascular wall and clean them of toxic substances and debris. These vasa vasorum include the brachiocephalic and coronary arteries in the ascending aorta, the intercostal branches in the descending thoracic aorta, the lumbar and mesenteric arteries in the abdominal aorta, and bifurcation segments of epicardial vessels in coronary arteries.[381] These vessels supply nutrients and oxygen to the arterial walls and microcirculation and help detoxify substances (Figure 2.19).

In addition to its function of transporting molecules from the blood to the adventitia, the vasa vasorum externa respond to oxygen and nutrient needs of the adventitial and outer medial layers. When the supplies are not met by diffusion from the luminal surface, chemically sensitive patients will develop local tissue hypoxia. At times, this can result in vascular spasm and even local fibrosis.[359] This need for oxygen is found clinically in elevated PvO_2 in the antecubital vein (drawn without a tourniquet) above 28 mm Hg can be detrimental, the higher it goes indicates shunting or lack of tissue oxygen extraction.[326] The more diffuse the lack of O_2 extraction, the more symptoms occur such as weakness, fatigue, memory loss, cerebral confusion, and cardiac and leg pain. The blood is shunted through the microcirculation without oxygen extraction causing tissue oxidative stress and inflammation. This phenomenon can also occur with the nonextraction of nutrients causing vessel and tissue deficiency for detoxification function and lack of energy for normal function. Nutrients are needed for a process such as healing wounds and replacement of normal function of tissues and detoxification and neutralization of toxics.

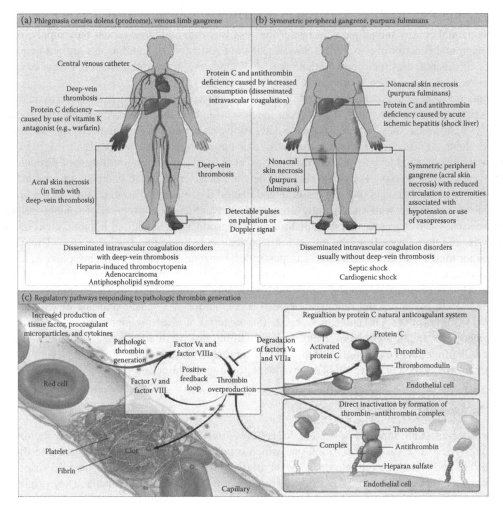

FIGURE 2.18 Clinical profile of venous limb gangrene and symmetric peripheral gangrene. Both venous limb gangrene (a) and symmetric peripheral gangrene (b) feature ischemic limb gangrene with pulses, underlying microvascular thrombosis, and a high frequency of disseminated intravascular coagulation with the failure of one or both natural anticoagulant systems (protein C and antithrombin) (c). Venous limb gangrene is characterized by acral necrosis in a distal limb with deep vein thrombosis. A reversible prodrome of this condition is phlegmasia cerulea dolens. Underlying disorders include heparin-induced thrombocytopenia, cancer (especially metastatic adenocarcinoma), and the antiphospholipid syndrome (especially the catastrophic antiphospholipid syndrome). Upper-limb venous thrombosis and limb ischemic necrosis may be associated with the use of a central venous catheter. Symmetric peripheral gangrene typically occurs in critically ill patients with cardiogenic or septic shock who have hypotension and are receiving vasopressor therapy, with acral limb necrosis that usually occurs in the absence of deep vein thrombosis. If there is additional or predominant nonacral skin necrosis, the condition is called purpura fulminans. Pathologic thrombin generation, which can be triggered or exacerbated by tissue factor, procoagulant microparticles, and proinflammatory or prothrombotic cytokines (among other factors), requires regulatory control (c). This control occurs through two major systems. In the protein C natural anticoagulant system, thrombin that is bound to endothelial thrombomodulin converts protein C to activated protein C, which degrades activated factors V and VIII (Va and VIIIa, respectively), thereby downregulating thrombin generation. In the antithrombin system, thrombin is inactivated by the formation of covalently linked thrombin–antithrombin complexes, a process that is catalyzed by endothelial heparan sulfate (a proteoglycan that binds to a variety of protein ligands and regulates a wide variety of biologic activities) or circulating pharmacologic heparin. (From *The New England Journal of Medicine*, Warkentin, T. E. Ischemic limb gangrene with pulses, 373(7). Copyright 2015. Massachusetts Medical Society. Reprinted with permission from Massachusetts Medical Society.)

Vasa vasorum occur when the vessel wall exceeds a certain thickness resulting in deficiency of oxygen or nutrients, which in mammals is 0.5 mm, or 29 lamellar units.[382–384] Under these circumstances, the vasa vasorum externa become angiogenic and expand deeper into the media in search of oxygen and nutrients. However, vasa vasorum neovascularization may be induced by stimuli other than vessel wall thickness. These include oxidative stress and inflammation, especially from environmental causes such as exposures to natural gas, pesticides, solvents, metals, EMF, nanoparticles, and atherosclerosis that results in extensive vascularization of mouse arteries even though the

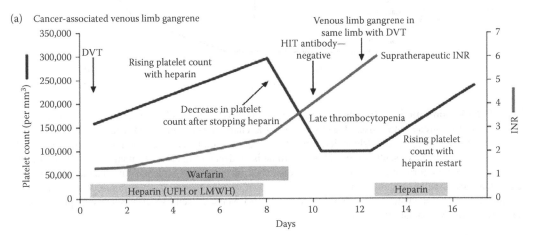

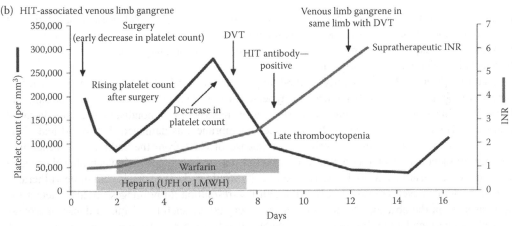

FIGURE 2.19 Changes in platelet count and INR in three clinical scenarios associated with ischemic limb gangrene with pulses. Panel (a) shows the characteristic clinical picture and associated changes in platelet counts and international normalized ratios (INRs) in patients with cancer (which is diagnosed in at least 50% of patients with venous gangrene) and disseminated intravascular coagulation. Venous limb gangrene develops in the limb affected by deep vein thrombosis (DVT) soon after the completion of the heparin phase of heparin–warfarin overlap following a rising platelet count during the initial phase of heparin treatment (with either unfractionated heparin [UFH] or low-molecular-weight heparin [LMWH]) and a rapid decrease in the platelet count after heparin is stopped. Progression to ischemic limb necrosis occurs in association with an abrupt increase in the INR to supratherapeutic levels. Patients with this syndrome test negative for heparin-dependent, platelet-activating antibodies. Panel (b) shows a scenario for patients with heparin-induced thrombocytopenia (HIT) who receive heparin during cardiac surgery with routine heparin–warfarin overlap (e.g., mechanical valve replacement). Patients with HIT test positive for platelet-activating antibodies. An alternative scenario would be later initiation of warfarin at the time that DVT occurs or during argatroban–warfarin overlap for the treatment of heparin-induced thrombocytopenia.   *(Continued)*

(c) Symmetric peripheral gangrene and purpura fulminans

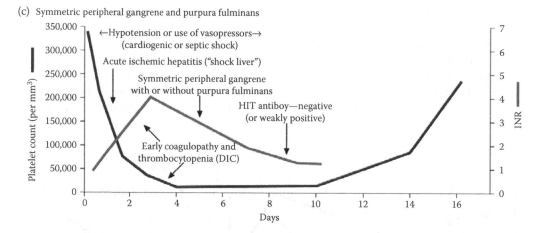

FIGURE 2.19 (Continued)   Changes in platelet count and INR in three clinical scenarios associated with ischemic limb gangrene with pulses. Panel (c) shows the characteristic interval of a few days between the onset of acute ischemic hepatitis (shock liver) and the development of ischemic limb injury in a critically ill patient with cardiogenic or septic shock. This syndrome is evidence of the role of impaired hepatic synthesis of protein C and antithrombin in exacerbating a disturbed procoagulant–anticoagulant balance during disseminated intravascular coagulation (DIC). (From *The New England Journal of Medicine*, Warkentin, T. E. Ischemic limb gangrene with pulses, 373(7). Copyright 2015. Massachusetts Medical Society. Reprinted with permission from Massachusetts Medical Society.)

murine arterial wall does not exceed the 0.5-mm diffusion limit.[385–388] Atherosclerosis studies in pigs demonstrated that growth of the vasa vasorum in coronary arteries occurs before vessel wall thickening and plaque development.[376,377] Thus, toxic environmental triggering most likely supplies the agents in which pathology originates.

According to Rea et al.,[325] as early as 1984, apparently in search of O_2 and nutrients deficiency, there were changes creating differences in hypersensitivity than in the normal microcirculation. These differences possibly were due to the vasa vasorum structure in nondiseased versus diseased arteries.[1229] Henniens[4] noted that if the blood cell membrane was damaged, K^+ would leak, Na^+ and Ca^{2+} would enter the cell triggering more release of Ca^{2+} from the endoplasmic reticulum, and then ambient Ca^{2+} would combine with protein kinases A and C, which when phosphorylated would increase sensitivity 1000 times. This sensitivity would make the vessels wall more vulnerable to toxic pollutants even at lower levels. Although low-resolution x-ray images failed to detect the vasa vasorum in the absence of human coronary artery atherosclerotic plaque, a dense microvascular plexus was evident in diseased vessels. Subsequently, high-resolution microscopic computed tomography images of coronary arteries in hypercholesterolemic pigs showed that the longitudinal vasa vasorum externa (first-order vasa vasorum) originate from the coronary artery (Figure 2.19) and branch to form a circumferential plexus (second-order vasa vasorum). Normal hearts have significantly greater first-order than second-order vasa vasorum density (ratio 3:2). However, in hypercholesterolemic pigs, the second-order vessel density is twofold greater than the first.[377,378] Furthermore, whereas vasa vasorum branching patterns in nondiseased porcine vasculature show a dichotomous tree structure with a hierarchical branching pattern similar to the vasculature of systemic circulation structure, vasa vasorum in diseased arteries present a much more disorderly image.[380] This is not surprising because the varied triggering agents will give varied responses.

The triggering agents are legion including pesticides and herbicides, solvents, molds, mycotoxins, natural gas, bacteria, virus, and PM (<200 nm as shown in small vessel/vasculitis at the EHC-Dallas). They will have different biochemical patterns and give different responses. This phenomenon occurs not only in these animals but also in humans due to contaminated feed, water, and air.

According to Mulligan-Kehoe and Simon,[356] high-resolution confocal microscopy demonstrated the presence of AVV structural hierarchy in hypercholesterolemic low-density lipoprotein (LDL) receptor-deficient/apolipoprotein B100-only mice (LDLR$^{-/-}$ApoB$^{100/100}$).[389] The vasa vasorum tree consists of a large main vessel from which smaller vessels branch; these in turn branch to form a plexus that occupies the space between two larger vessels. The vessels within the plexus collapse in response to an angiogenesis inhibitor, or even wall pressure, whereas the larger vessels of the tree remain intact. The vasa vasorum are also detectable in chow-fed mice but do not exhibit a branching pattern.[389] The cumulative data from studies using various animal models and imaging modalities clearly indicate that under disease conditions, AVV expand, frequently in a disorderly fashion. Again, this is probably in search of oxygen and nutrients to supply the normal vessel wall and function. They find nutrients to help the needed repair and for proper detoxification of the entering pollutants and for healthy wall maintenance. This plexus and disorderly growth fashion can be the result of hypersensitivity of the vascular tree due to the Ca^{2+} protein kinase phosphorylation process that will make pollutant entry and function to be very sensitive and make oxidative stress and inflammation much easier. It will magnify the pollutants response to cause hyperresponses that will earlier bring on symptoms like weakness and fatigue eventually resulting in fibrosis on arteriosclerosis.

VENOUS VASA VASORUM

According to Mulligan-Kehoe and Simons,[356] the VVV drain the arterial wall into companion veins[390] that are parallel to the AVV feeder or into the largest branches of the main vein, where they penetrate every 5–15 mm.[391] There are distinct qualitative differences between the AVV and the VVV.[392,393] The AVV are many fewer in number, with diameters ranging from 11.6 to 36.6 µm compared with the VVV diameter range of 11.1–200.3 µm. Vascular corrosion casts coupled with scanning electron microscopy show that the VVV change course at acute angles and form kinks, constrictions, and outpouchings. This spatial distribution enables the VVV to withstand vessel wall distension with increased blood pressure or vessel stretching without a dramatic effect on the VVV function.[393]

Many chemically sensitive patients have chest pain, which is apparently caused by this AVV expansion and plexus formation with resultant change to the micronerves and vessels wall or the VVV alteration in anatomy change from this anatomy and physiological mechanisms. This is in turn due to local hypoxia or change in neurotransmitters, which can alter the ANS function of these in the vascular wall. This change in ANS function usually is guided by a sympathetic nerve effect, which will result in vascular spasm.

The ANS is also thought to control blood flow in the human saphenous vein vasa vasorum.[391,393] Use of the saphenous vein for coronary artery bypass graft surgery is associated with spasm of vascular SMCs of the saphenous vein that can develop into vein-graft disease.[394,395] The conventional surgical technique for saphenous vein harvest involves stripping the connective tissue from the vein, which injures the adventitial autonomic nerves and vasa vasorum[393,394] and may trigger VVV venospasm[396] or AVV spasm. Moreover, studies suggest that the VVV play a role in vein vasorelaxation; any VVV damage during saphenous vein harvesting may impair flow-induced vasodilation in the graft.[395,397,398] These anatomy and physiology phenomena have a very practical angle.

ADVENTITIAL ANGIOGENIC GROWTH FACTORS

Studies performed in hypercholesterolemic LDLR$^{-/-}$ApoB$^{100/100}$ mice suggest that fibroblast growth factor-2 (FGF2) is the primary angiogenic growth factor expressed in the CMD AVV. Quantitative polymerase chain reaction measured an eightfold increase in FGF2 mRNA copy number in the hypercholesterolemic mice compared with age- and sex-matched chow-fed mice, whereas VE growth factor mRNA was at control levels.[385] Furthermore, fluorescein isothiocyanate–labeled lectin infusions in hypercholesterolemic mice have shown that FGF2 is associated with a well-developed vasa vasorum plexus. On the other hand, the vasa vasorum in nondiseased mice do not form a plexus, and diffuse FGF2 staining is observed in the matrix.[389] A FGF2/perlecan complex appears critical for specifying FGF2 spatial distribution.[389] It remains to be determined whether FGF2 provides a pattern for the vasa vasorum to form a plexus-like network or whether the vasa vasorum form a plexus and then produce and release FGF2 into the matrix. In one study, FGF2 delivered to the adventitia of apolipoprotein E-deficient (ApoE$^{-/-}$) mice results in vasa vasorum expansion and accelerated plaque progression.[399] Certainly, there may be a change in vascular tissue with resultant other mediator releases causing oxidative stress leading to inflammation and eventually scar formation.

Another potentially important player is a placental growth factor (PlGF), a member of the VE growth factor family of proteins. Delivery of PlGF into the carotid artery periadventitial space in hypercholesterolemic rabbits significantly increased adventitial neovascularization and macrophage accumulation,[400] whereas the absence of PlGF significantly reduced plaque size and macrophage number in ApoE$^{-/-}$PlGF$^{-/-}$ mice.[401]

AVV and the Stem/Progenitor Cells Niche

According to Mulligan-Kehoe and Simons,[356] recent studies have suggested the existence of a stem/progenitor cell (SMC) niche in the adventitia of the arterial wall. Such a niche is thought to contain mural cell progenitors, which may be positioned to respond to injury in the vessel wall[402] to promote either repair or disease.[403]

Accumulation of SMCs in the neointima of atherosclerotic plaque has been thought to be triggered by their transformation from a quiescent, contractile state to a proliferating, synthetic phenotype, which enables them to migrate from the media to the intima. Recent studies have demonstrated that a DNA demethylation protein, Ten-Eleven Translocation-2 (TET2) enzymes, plays a significant role in reversible SMC differentiation in human SMCs, human arterial tissue, and mouse models of atherosclerosis and injury-induced intimal hyperplasia.[403] Mechanistic studies show that TET2 regulates SMC phenotype by converting 5-methylcytosine to unmethylated cytosine, which results in DNA demethylation and activation of key SMC differentiation genes; knockdown of TET2 increases expression of synthetic SMC phenotype markers. Furthermore, knockdown studies indicate that TET2 differentially regulates the chromatin accessibility of contractile and dedifferentiation genes. The collective data suggest that TET2 is a master epigenetic regulator of SMC differentiation.[1230]

An alternative theory suggests that adult SMCs in the plaque originate from a variety of sources that include adventitial vessel wall progenitor cells[404] and can migrate from the adventitia into the media and intima after arterial injury.[362,405] The labeling of adventitial cells in rat common carotid arteries with β-galactosidase before a balloon catheter injury demonstrated their appearance in the media then the intima 7 and 14 days later.[406] Analysis of cellular content of the adventitia in aortic roots of ApoE$^{-/-}$ mice demonstrates the presence of cells with a number of stem cell markers, including Sca-1. The latter are thought to have the ability to differentiate into SMCs when stimulated with platelet-derived growth factor-BB[362] and to contribute to progression of atherosclerotic lesions in ApoE$^{-/-}$ mice.[362] AVV may be a conduit for mobilized progenitor cells into the intima, where they differentiate into SMCs.[407]

Regulators of Vasa Vasorum Expansion

According to Mulligan-Kehoe and Simons,[356] vasa vasorum are thought to proliferate and grow to meet the nutritional needs of the larger artery's outer medial layer when metabolic needs exceed the amount of oxygen that can diffuse from the luminal blood.[359,379] The hypoxia-inducible transcription factors HIF-1 and HIF-2 induce transcription of hypoxia-responsive genes[408] such as proangiogenic VE growth factor,[409] which promotes vessel growth. Hypoxia also stimulates increased expression of key enzymes required for heparan sulfate chain synthesis in microvascular endothelial cells. This leads to creation of new binding sites for FGF2,[410] a potent mediator of endothelial cell growth and vasa vasorum stability.[389]

Experimental evidence in hypercholesterolemic pigs[376,377] suggests that the vasa vasorum begin to sprout before aortic wall thickening and that the sprouting is in turn preceded by infiltration of inflammatory cells into the adventitia. One likely possibility is that infiltrating adventitial inflammatory cells secrete a number of angiogenic growth factors, including VE growth factor. Periadventitial fat may also contribute to this process via stimulation of inflammation[411,412] or release of angiogenic growth factors.[413,414]

The impact of cardiovascular risks on vasa vasorum dynamics and adventitial remodeling differs in various experimental models.[415–418] Hypercholesterolemia is associated with an increase in vasa vasorum density, whereas hypertension is marked more by an increase in adventitial matrix,[417] and diabetes mellitus may in fact impair vasa vasorum growth.[419] Furthermore, the absence of increased neovascularization in diabetic animal models contrasts with findings in patients with diabetes mellitus, whose plaques demonstrate elevated microvessel density, inflammatory cell content, and intraplaque hemorrhage.[420,421] The latter is thought to be the major driver for atherosclerosis progression because of an increase in a hemoglobin–haptoglobin complex, which impairs hemoglobin clearance and amplifies oxidative stress and endothelial cell dysfunction.[422]

Vasa Vasorum and Vascular Inflammation

According to Mulligan-Kehoe and Simons,[356] there is an "outside-in" theory whereby vascular inflammation begins in the adventitia and advances to the media and intima[423] (Figure 2.15). This theory opposes the long-held "inside-out" concept that monocytes infiltrate the vessel wall from the luminal side. Among the arguments favoring the outside-in theory are the presence of resident immune cells in the adventitia and the homing of macrophages to that site.[360] Additionally, balloon angioplasty experiments in pig coronary arteries demonstrate that the adventitia is the primary site for acute inflammation after mechanical vascular injury.[375] These results are consistent with reports from human studies that show inflammatory cell infiltration from the adventitia to plaque and formation of adventitial lymph follicles that contain plasma cells.[424,425] P-selectin and vascular cell adhesion molecule 1 are upregulated in vasa vasorum endothelial cells very soon after balloon angioplasty injury, which provides a means for inflammatory cells trafficking in and out of the adventitia.[375]

The outside-in concept is further demonstrated in a model of aortic transplantation between histocompatible rat strains.[426] Thirty days after transplantation, the vasa vasorum in the adventitia of aortic allografts mount a robust angiogenic response, which is found in graft rejection. Electron microscopy was used to detect leukocytes infiltrating the AVV of the rejected graft, thus indicating that the vasa vasorum serve as a conduit for inflammatory cell entry into the graft during the rejection process.

Data in humans also support this scenario. A study of coronary artery segments from 99 patients with and without atherosclerotic plaque demonstrated expression of the leukocyte adhesion molecules: vascular cell adhesion molecule 1, intercellular adhesion molecule 1, and E-selectin, predominantly on the intimal vasa vasorum rather than on the arterial luminal endothelium.[427] The presence of T cells, B cells, macrophages, and dendritic cells in the adventitia has also been documented in humans.[361,425,428] In the chemically sensitive with small-vessel vasculitis, one sees a depletion of T cells, complement, and at times g-globulin (variable) subsets (EHC-Dallas data). These may be found in the vasa vasorum or adventitial of the microcirculation. Intradermal provocation shows sensitivity to food, chemical, mold (mycotoxin), EMF, and pesticides at lower levels (EHC-Dallas data). These are of the microcirculation and of the adventitial. This adventitial area may be where they hide in mouse models vascular inflammation and of atherosclerosis.[360,374,429] For often with sauna and macronutrient supplementation, these chemicals come out and the immune cells return to normal (EHC-Dallas and EHC-Buffalo).

Pigs after coronary artery angioplasty do show changes in these areas.[375] Aortas of children who have not developed atherosclerosis have leukocytes surrounding the AVV [430] suggesting an early form of vasculitis. Studies in mice show that adventitial immune cells are present in noninflamed wild-type mice, and their numbers increase in hypercholesterolemic ApoE$^{-/-}$ mice, with T cells being the most predominant over the course of plaque development,[360,374] whereas at the same time, such accumulation is not reflected in the intima. The adventitial T cell dominance in mice is consistent with human studies.[425] Clustered immune cells in the mouse adventitia structurally organize into aortic tertiary lymphoid structures,[360,361,374,431] found predominantly at sites that border on the elastic lamina adjacent to atherosclerotic plaque.[431] Although the function of aortic tertiary lymphoid structures has not been identified clearly, there is some evidence that the aggregates are sites for selection of specific subsets of B cells.[361] They also can be the storage sites for toxics like pesticides, OSs, natural gas, heavy metals, mycotoxins, etc. that can cause additive stress and inflammation as seen in the vascular adventitial.

The inside-out theory has stimulated numerous investigations into the role of resident adventitial immune cells and the growth of the vasa vasorum in relation to atherosclerosis. The studies indicate that they play an important role in disease progression and require ongoing investigations to determine their relevance in human atherosclerosis and/or nonatherschlerotic microcirculation disease.

VASA VASORUM AND NEOINTIMA FORMATION

According to Mulligan-Kehoe and Simons,[356] neointima formation after mechanical vascular injury such as balloon angioplasty or in the setting of vessel wall disease such as atherosclerosis or environmentally triggered incitants of inflammation (vasculitis) is the key event responsible for much of the morbidity and mortality. Neointima in these settings is composed of proliferating SMCs and extracellular matrix (ECM). The key event has long been held to be the proliferation of medial SMCs.[432] Recent studies suggest additional possibilities for the origin of neointimal SMCs and the factors that control it.

Although expansion of vasa vasorum has been linked to neointima formation, the detailed molecular link between these events has been elusive.[433] Studies in normal rabbit and rat carotid arteries showed that the addition of angiogenic growth factors to the vessel adventitia resulted in expansion of adventitial vasculature and neointima formation even in the absence of any endovascular trauma. Conversely, inhibition of growth factor signaling reduced it.[433–435] Microcomputed tomography imaging further demonstrates a direct correlation between the computed tomography–determined extent of adventitial angiogenesis and the extent of neointima.[377,436] Thus, there is a strong correlation between the extent of the adventitial vasculature and the extent of neointima formation. Overall, the entire process appears to be composed of two parts: angiogenesis-independent growth, likely driven by SMC proliferation in the media, and angiogenesis-dependent growth (Figure 2.17).

The latter, characterized by the appearance of extensive adventitial vasculature (and, by extension, vasa vasorum) correlates with the influx of blood mononuclear cells and local inflammation. One of the consequences of inflammation is the development of *endothelial-to-mesenchymal transition* (EndMT). During EndMT, normal endothelial cells acquire mesenchymal characteristics that include changes in cell shape and polarity; expression of mesenchymal markers such as α-smooth muscle actin, calponin, and vimentin; and decline or outright loss of endothelial marker expression. As a result, endothelial cells transform into cells of mesenchymal lineages, including SMCs and fibroblasts, and begin producing large amounts of ECM, including collagen.[437,438] These sequences result in fibrosis, which can occlude the microcirculation. When this occurrs it is nonfunctional disrupting normal physiology like oxygen extraction, nutrition, and detoxification.

This sequence of events occurs during normal embryonic development, in which EndMT plays a crucial role in formation of cardiac valves.[439–441] However, it also occurs in a number of pathological settings in adult tissues, including MI,[438,442] fibrosis,[443–445] portal hypertension,[446] vascular malformations,[447] and transplant rejection.[437] We see this lack of oxygen extraction in the chemical sensitive and CDD patients. The final common event leading to EndMT is activation of TGF-β signaling, which plays a central role in driving endothelial cells to mesenchymal fate.[443,448] Subsequent intracellular events are less clear but probably involve both canonical (SMAD2)[437,446] and noncanonical TGF signaling pathways, changes in microRNA (miRNA) expression,[449,450] and activation of expression of the Snail gene.[451] Events leading to endothelial TGF-β signaling activation are less clear. A number of processes have been implicated, including shear stress,[452–454] stimulation with endothelin-1,[445] Notch,[455] and caveolin deficiency,[456] among others.

One of the recently identified mechanisms regulating TGF-β signaling in the endothelium involves FGF-mediated suppression of TGF receptor expression. Baseline FGF signaling is responsible for the maintenance of let-7 miRNA expression in normal endothelial cells. Let-7 miRNAs target expression of a number of TGF family members, including TGFR1; in the absence of FGF input, let-7 levels decline and TGFR1 levels increase, thus enabling activation of TGF-β signaling.[437] The importance of this FGF/TGF signaling link lies in the fact that the continuous FGF signaling input needed to suppress TGF-β signaling activation depends on expression of the key endothelial FGF receptor, FGFR1.[437] Interestingly, certain inflammatory conditions associated with production of TNF-α, interleukin 1β, or interferon-γ result in a profound decline of FGFR1, activation of TGF-β signaling, and the onset of EndMT (Figure 2.18). Thus, this mechanism likely explains the previously reported link between inflammation and EndMT.[438,457–459] Atherosclerosis, a chronic inflammatory disease potentiated by TNF-α[460] and interferon-γ,[461] is associated with infiltration of T cells and macrophages into diseased blood vessel wall; thus, EndMT may well be an important contributor to altered cellular and ECM composition in the vessel wall that promotes atherosclerotic disease progression of low T cells. It is also maybe the key contributor to peripheral, cerebral, and coronary vasculitis, which can result in simple fibrosis resulting in scar tissue.

With these considerations in mind, it is reasonable to suggest that expansion of adventitial vasculature, including vasa vasorum, in inflammatory settings provides the endothelial substrate and the milieu needed for EndMT. Functionally, induction of EndMT contributes to accumulation of SMCs, which leads to formation of neointima, extensive deposition of collagen, and other ECM proteins that lead to fibrosis and a potential for greater accumulation of white blood cells and platelets because of increased expression of various adhesion molecules (Figure 2.21). It is clear that in CS vasculitis, the T cells, complements, and at times gamma globulins decrease in the blood indicating immune deregulation as well as microcirculation dysfunctions such as augmented PvO_2 indicating lack of microcirculation and extraction of oxygen.

MICROBLEEDS

New technological advances offer an opportunity to clarify details of human pathology and pathophysiology. The advent of T2*-weighted gradient-recalled echo (GRE) MRI imaging allowed recognition of a relatively new finding, brain microbleeds. These lesions are very small (most often 2–5 mm in diameter), round, hypointense foci that were not evident on other standard MRI sequences. Susceptibility-weighted images are probably even more reliable than T2*-weighted GRE images for showing these microbleeds.[462] Hemosiderin within these small foci are mostly responsible for producing the alteration in magnetic resonance that allows recognition of microbleeds.

Histopathological studies of microbleeds show that they represent microscopic bleeding.[463,464] Many lesions contain hemosiderin-laden macrophages, often perivascular in location. Lipohyalinosis, a pathology intrinsic to small arteries and arterioles, is highly prevalent within and adjacent to these microbleeds. Microaneurysms may also be present. The two most frequently known causes are hypertension and cerebral amyloid angiopathy. Both of these conditions are known to predispose to brain hemorrhages. In these conditions, microbleeds represent very small hemorrhages and tiny infarcts with associated diapedesis of red blood cells. Microbleeds in patients with cerebral amyloid angiopathy are located in the cerebral lobes, whereas hypertension is associated with deep and lobar microbleeds.[465]

MRI studies of patients with known cerebrovascular diseases show that microbleeds represent one or two basic pathologies: (1) chronic, intrinsic, small vessel disease, including lipohyalinosis, microaneurysms, and cerebral amyloid angiopathy, and (2) small, old hemorrhages in patients with diverse causes such as head trauma, endocarditis, bleeding diathesis, AF, and disseminated intravascular coagulation (DIC) and seen after thrombolysis and carotid artery stenting. This second group represents microscopic bleeding related to bleeding diatheses, and present or past acute vascular injuries often localized vascular processes, including reperfusion. Bleeding diathesis should be recognizable by bleeding into other sites and the presence of systemic symptoms and findings.

According to Caplan,[466] microbleeds, especially when multiple, are a recognized risk factor for the development of new strokes in patients with known cerebrovascular diseases. They have also been found in patients with AD and are recognized to be a risk factor for cardiovascular and cerebrovascular disease in these patients.[467,468] Many microbleeds in patients with AD are caused by cerebral amyloid angiopathy because patients with amyloid within cerebral blood vessels have associated amyloid deposition within the brain and clinical AD dementia.

AIR POLLUTION AND HEART ATTACKS

The cardiovascular effects of air pollution are growing in numbers. It appears that they are equal to or exceeds those of the respiratory, reproduction, and genital urinary effects.

Outdoor air pollutants such as PM_{10} or $PM_{2.5}$, nano particles <0.200 μm, O_3, and NO_2 have been associated with significantly higher rates of cardiac mortality and morbidity. Table 2.10 reports on seven epidemiological studies, which have examined the associations between increasing levels of common outdoor pollutants with rates of heart-related health conditions.

TABLE 2.10
Studies Linking Exposure of Higher Levels of Air Pollutants with Adverse Heart Disease Events

Study	Outcome Measured	Particulates (PM_{10} or $PM_{2.5}$)	Ozone (O_3)	Carbon Monoxide (CO)	Nitrogen Dioxide (NO_2)	Oxygenated Volatile Organic Compounds
D'Ippoliti et al.[333]	Myocardial infarction (MI)	X		X	X	
Peters et al.[334]	Myocardial infarction (MI)	X		X	X	
Ruidavets et al.[335]	Acute MI (subjects with no previous MI)		X			
Chen et al.[336]	Fatal myocardial infarction	X (women only—little effect in men)				
Metzger et al.[337]	MI hospital admissions	X		X	X	X
Zanobetti and Schwartz[338]	MI hospital admissions	X				
Pantazopolou et al.[339]	MI and respiratory hospital admissions	X		X	X	
Yang et al.[340]	MI and respiratory hospital admissions	X		X	X	
Morris et al.[341]	Congestive heart failure hospital admissions			X		

Source: Adapted from Sheffield, A. K. 1994–1998.

Note: X in box indicates pollutant associated with significantly ($p < 0.05$) greater rates of adverse heart events.

As with respiratory effects, air pollutants can increase the risk of heart and vascular problems at levels below standards set by such agencies as the U.S. EPA or WHO. For example, Peters et al.[334] found that higher PM_{10} levels were associated with significantly more cardiac admissions even though median and 95% PM_{10} levels were only 19.4 and 37.0 $\mu g/m^3$, respectively.

Exposure to short-term traffic pollution can also trigger heart attacks. A German study of 691 patients who experienced nonfatal heart attacks found that the risk of MI was 2.9 times higher ($p < 0.0001$) within 1 hour after exposure to traffic as compared with periods that were >6 hours after the last traffic exposure.[469]

The effects of air pollutants on cardiovascular disease may be especially strong in certain populations such as women, diabetics, and the elderly, although they can occur at all ages. A 22-year prospective study of 3239 California adults found that higher outdoor levels of PM_{10} and $PM_{2.5}$ were associated with significantly higher rates of fatal coronary heart disease (CHD) in postmenopausal females but little association was found between PM_{10} or $PM_{2.5}$ and fatal heart disease in males.[336] A study in four U.S. cities found that increasing PM_{10} concentrations had a significantly stronger effect in increasing hospital cardiovascular admissions in diabetic versus nondiabetic subjects under 76 years of age.[470] Oddly, in subjects over 75 years old, the cardiovascular effect of PM_{10} in eight U.S. counties was associated with higher levels of cardiovascular hospital admissions, but not younger patients.[471]

At the EHC-Dallas, we described a 5-year-old girl who lost her toes due to a pesticide or herbicide exposure. This was the first known description of small-vessel vasculitis due to an environmental incitant. We have reported in over 500 cases of small-vessel vasculitis that we were able to prevent gangrene since then. All those had multiple environmental triggers such as natural gas, pesticides, herbicides, solvents, mycotoxins, and EMF. Warkentin[472] has reported in several cases and a nice review of the problem but he has the misconception of what having a controlled environment is. He could not define the triggering agents.

There are two distinct syndromes of microthrombosis-associated ischemic limb injury (Table 2.11).

Venous limb gangrene can complicate thrombocytopenic disorders that are strongly associated with deep vein thrombosis (e.g., cancer-associated DIC[473] and heparin-induced thrombocytopenia [HIT]).[474] In these conditions, microthrombosis occurs in the same limb with acute large vein thrombosis, resulting in acral (distal extremity) ischemic necrosis. Usually, only one limb is affected. The potentially reversible, prodromal state of limb-threatening ischemia is phlegmasia cerulea dolens, indicating the respective features of a swollen, blue (ischemic), and painful limb.

In contrast, two and sometimes all four limbs are affected in symmetric peripheral gangrene, also featuring acral limb ischemic necrosis but usually without deep vein thrombosis.[475,476] The limb necrosis is often strikingly symmetric; lower limbs are most often affected, with additional involvement of fingers or hands in approximately one-third of patients. When there is additional or predominant nonacral tissue necrosis, the term purpura fulminans is applicable. Patients are usually critically ill with cardiogenic or septic shock. In 1904, Barraud[477] discussed limb gangrene as a complication of acute infection, a complication that continues to occur today. The two syndromes have common pathophysiological features of microthrombosis associated with a disturbed procoagulant–anticoagulant balance.

DISSEMINATED INTRAVASCULAR COAGULATION AND NATURAL ANTICOAGULANT FAILURE

Disseminated intravascular coagulation is characterized by systemic activation of hemostasis (pathologic thrombin generation), impaired fibrinolysis, and intravascular formation and deposition of fibrin, with a potential for thrombotic occlusion of the microvasculature.[478] Depending on the inciting disorder, mediators include tissue factor expressed on endothelium and monocytes, enhanced leukocyte–endothelial interactions, proinflammatory cytokines (e.g., TNF-α), interleukin-1β, and interleukin-[478,479] and cytokine-mediated endothelial downregulation of thrombomodulin.[480]

TABLE 2.11

Two Syndrome of Ischemic Limb Gangrene with Pulses

Variable	Venous Limb Gangrene[a]	Symmetric Peripheral Gangrene[b]
Underlying disseminated intravascular coagulation	Heparin-induced thrombocytopenia, metastatic adenocarcinoma, antiphospholipid syndrome	Septic shock (e.g., meningococcemia), cardiogenic shock
Deep-vein thrombosis in ischemic limb[c]	Yes	Usually not
Number of limbs affected	Usually 1 limb with deep-vein thrombosis	Usually 2 or a limbs (symmetric)
Warfarin implicated	Often	Usually not
Congenital hypercoagulability state	Usually not	Usually not
Thrombocytopenia	Yes	Yes
Peak international normalized ratio	Typically >4.0, especially if associated with coumarin[d]	Typically >2.0
Fibrin-specific marker (fibrin D-dimer, fibrin monomer)	Greatly elevated	Greatly elevated
Thrombin-antithrombin complexes	Greatly elevated	Greatly elevated
Protein C <10%	Yes, especially if associated with coumarin	Yes
Acute liver dysfunction or failure	Usually not	May be common

Source: Adapted from Warkentin, T. E. et al. 1997. *Ann. Intern. Med.* 127:804–812.

[a] The prodromal state of venous limb gangrene is called phlegmasia cerula dolens, indicating the features of a swollen, blue, and painful limb.

[b] Symmetric peripheral gangrene can present with or without purpura fulminans (nonacral skin necrosis).

[c] Iliofemoral deep-vein thrombosis (i.e., thrombosis of the iliac vein or common femoral vein) can also be associated with phlegmasia cerulea dolens in the absence of disseminated intravascular coagulation. Risk factors include hypercoagulable disorders (e.g., cancer), a postoperative or post-traumatic state, pregnancy or postpartum state, vena cave filter insertion, and the May-Thurner syndrome (an anatomical variant in which the right common iliac artery overlies the left common iliac vein and compresses it against the lumbar spine).

[d] Coumarin derivatives include oral vitamin K antagonists, such as warfarin, acenocoumarol, and phenprocoumon.

Triggering or potentiating factors include the presence of bacterial endotoxin, shock, acidemia, tissue injury, and platelet- or tumor-derived procoagulant microparticles.[481,482]

Venous limb gangrene and symmetric peripheral gangrene (with or without purpura fulminans) are cutaneous manifestations of DIC that are modified and aggravated by interacting clinical factors such as warfarin therapy, deep vein thrombosis, hypotension, and vasopressor therapy.[473–476] Associated failure of the natural anticoagulant systems, both the protein C system (crucial for down-regulating thrombin generation in the microvasculature)[483] and the antithrombin system (catalyzed by circulating pharmacologic heparin and endogenous endothelial-bound heparan sulfate), helps to explain why risk factors for microthrombosis include the use of warfarin (a vitamin K antagonist) and hepatic dysfunction or failure, since the liver synthesizes protein C (a vitamin K–dependent anticoagulant) and antithrombin.

Venous Limb Gangrene

Venous limb gangrene indicates acral ischemic necrosis in a limb with deep vein thrombosis. Early investigators described virtually complete occlusion of the proximal venous limb vasculature, including collateral vessels, often in patients in the postpartum or postoperative period or in those with cancer. Limb ischemic necrosis was explained by sufficiently increased venous and interstitial pressures that collapsed small arteries or arterioles when closing pressure was exceeded.[484,485] However, in recent years, patients with venous gangrene have often been reported with underlying acquired hypercoagulability states, such as cancer-associated consumptive coagulopathy,[473,486] HIT,[474,487] and the antiphospholipid syndrome,[488,489] with associated macrovascular and microvascular thrombosis that is frequently exacerbated by protein C depletion associated with the administration of warfarin or other coumarin derivatives.[473,474,486–488] The characteristic laboratory picture includes thrombocytopenia and an international normalized ratio (INR) that typically exceeds 4.0; a supratherapeutic INR is a proxy for a severely reduced protein C level.[473,474,486]

Cancer-Associated Venous Limb Gangrene

At least 50% of patients with venous gangrene have underlying cancer,[485] together with DIC. In a recent series,[473] a characteristic clinical picture was described in which patients with apparent idiopathic deep vein thrombosis were found to have phlegmasia or venous limb gangrene soon after completing the heparin phase of heparin–warfarin overlap. The patients had a rising platelet count during the initial phase of heparin treatment (with either unfractionated or low-molecular-weight formulations), consistent with heparin control of cancer-associated hypercoagulability,[490] with a rapid decrease in the platelet count after heparin was stopped. Progression to ischemic limb necrosis occurred in association with an abrupt increase in the INR to supratherapeutic levels (usually, >4.0). Unlike patients with HIT, patients with this syndrome test negative for heparin-dependent, platelet-activating antibodies, and the platelet count increases if heparin is restarted.[473] Metastatic cancer, usually adenocarcinoma, is characteristic.

Laboratory studies support a model of profoundly disturbed procoagulant–anticoagulant balance in patients with cancer in whom venous gangrene develops during warfarin anticoagulation. Uncontrolled thrombin generation is shown by greatly elevated thrombin–antithrombin complexes (a marker of *in vivo* thrombin generation) together with greatly reduced levels of protein C activity—in other words, the ratio of thrombin–antithrombin complex to protein C is elevated as compared with that in controls.[473,486] In essence, warfarin does not inhibit cancer-associated hypercoagulability while at the same time, it predisposes the patient to microthrombosis by depleting protein C activity (often to <10% of normal levels).

Unfortunately, the idiopathic syndrome was not studied in a less-polluted, controlled environment. In our experience at the EHC-Dallas, most idiopathic vascular syndromes have triggering agents such as the fumes of natural gas, pesticides, herbicides, solvents, foods, mold, and mycotoxins, when often neutralized by injections or eliminated can reverse the vasculitis syndrome and prevent the thrombosis.

Venous Limb Gangrene and Heparin-Induced Thrombocytopenia

In patients with HIT, the decrease in the platelet count usually begins 5–10 days after the immunizing exposure to heparin, often caused by the intraoperative use of heparin (e.g., in cardiac or vascular surgery) or during the early postoperative period (for thromboprophylaxis).[491] Sometimes, thrombocytopenia begins while the patient is still receiving heparin (called typical onset), although often the decrease in the platelet count begins—or worsens—after heparin is discontinued (called delayed onset).[492] Ischemic limb injury develops in up to 5% of patients with HIT,[493] either because of arterial occlusion by a platelet-rich thrombus (a so-called white clot) or because of venous limb gangrene.

Since this syndrome occurs 5–10 days after the heparin-induced thrombocytopenia, it can usually be prevented by fasting the patient in the less-polluted, controlled environment for 5–7 days. This procedure allows the microvascular to clean out the debris that leads to the clotting phenomena before the gangrene occurs.

Warfarin therapy is implicated in the majority of patients with HIT in whom venous limb gangrene develops. Again, a characteristic feature is a supratherapeutic INR.[474,487] In such patients, a markedly elevated ratio of thrombin–antithrombin complex to protein C[2] supports a model of profoundly disturbed procoagulant–anticoagulant balance. In the minority of patients with HIT in whom venous gangrene develops in the absence of warfarin administration, unusually severe thrombocytopenia (platelet count, <20,000/mm³) and laboratory evidence of decompensated DIC (e.g., elevated INR, hypofibrinogenemia, and circulating nucleated red cells) are found.[494]

SUPRATHERAPEUTIC INR

Analysis of the vitamin K–dependent coagulation factors that influence the INR—factors II (pro-thrombin), VII, and X—explains the basis for the supratherapeutic INR that is characteristic of warfarin-associated venous limb gangrene. The elevated INR correlates closely with reduced factor VII levels, with factor VII showing a strong colinear relationship with protein C. In essence, the supratherapeutic INR is a surrogate marker for severely reduced protein C (<10% activity levels) caused by a parallel severe reduction in the factor VII level. This close correlation between pro-coagulant factor VII and anticoagulant protein C is interesting, given that both factors have short half-lives (5 and 9 hours, respectively) and low (nanomolar) plasma concentrations (10 and 65 nM, respectively), values much lower than those of the major procoagulant factor, prothrombin (60 hours and 1400 nM, respectively).[495] These characteristics help to explain the unique susceptibility to depletion of factor VII and protein C in consumptive coagulopathic states with compromised factor synthesis associated with the use of warfarin. Ironically, despite the high INR, thrombin generation persists and microthrombosis occurs.[473,474,486]

VENOUS LIMB GANGRENE VERSUS WARFARIN-INDUCED SKIN NECROSIS

Warfarin-associated venous limb gangrene differs from classic warfarin-induced skin necrosis in that for the latter disorder, necrosis is usually localized to skin or subdermal tissues, predominantly in nonacral locations (e.g., breast, abdomen, thigh, and calf),[496,497] whereas venous gangrene affects acral skin and underlying tissues (e.g., bone).[473,474,486,487] In two disorders, the onset of tissue necrosis begins approximately 2–6 days after the initiation of warfarin therapy.[496,497] This characteristic delay probably reflects the time needed for a critical reduction in protein C levels. Congenital abnormalities in the protein C anticoagulant system (e.g., protein C deficiency and factor V Leiden) are often implicated in patients with classic warfarin-induced necrosis but are usually not found in patients with venous limb gangrene. These observations suggest that the profound consumptive coagulopathy associated with HIT or cancer, combined with deep vein thrombosis, are sufficient to cause the conditions for warfarin-induced microthrombosis that is manifested as venous gangrene without the additional need for an underlying heritable defect.

Again in the noncancer patients, nonheritable defects may lower the pollutant load during fasting. This appears to reverse the inflammatory process and stop the clotting sequence from the docin wall irritability and then calms down.

Prevention and Treatment of Venous Limb Gangrene

Venous limb gangrene can be prevented if warfarin therapy is avoided (or reversed in a timely manner with vitamin K) in a patient with acute deep vein thrombosis in whom the presence of associated thrombocytopenia or coagulopathy indicates a potential diagnosis of cancer-associated coagulopathy or HIT.[474,475] Consensus conference guidelines recommend the avoidance of warfarin during the acute (thrombocytopenic) phase of HIT.[494,498] Furthermore, low-molecular-weight heparin (LMWH) is superior to warfarin in patients with cancer-associated deep vein thrombosis.[499] Also, the use of inferior vena cava filters should be avoided in patients with hypercoagulable states, such as cancer or HIT, since their use can predispose the patient to venous gangrene.[500]

These filters are synthetic and can add another trigger agent to the clotting and inflammatory mechanism.

In a patient who is recognized to have phlegmasia or venous limb gangrene, treatment is based on two principles. The first—for a patient with a prolonged INR that is caused by treatment with a vitamin K antagonist—is the administration of vitamin K (at least 10 mg by slow intravenous infusion, with 5–10 mg repeated 12–24 hours later if the prolongation in the INR persists or recurs). The second is therapeutic-dose anticoagulation. These measures can be limb saving in a patient with phlegmasia.[474,500]

However, the use of anticoagulation in a patient with an underlying coagulopathy is inherently problematic if an agent that is monitored by the activated partial thromboplastin time (APTT) is used. This is because the systematic administration of an inappropriately reduced dose of anticoagulant therapy, called APTT confounding, can result when a standard APTT-adjusted treatment nomogram is applied to a patient whose baseline (pretreatment) APTT is already elevated.[501] Such an effect can occur if unfractionated heparin is used to treat cancer-associated hypercoagulability or if argatroban is given for thrombosis complicating severe HIT with associated DIC.[501,502] Warfarin also prolongs the APTT, further contributing to less effective administration of heparin or argatroban.[501,503] This problem can be avoided by the use of LMWH or monitoring of unfractionated heparin by measuring levels of antifactor Xa (for treating cancer-associated hypercoagulability) or the use of an anticoagulant that does not require APTT monitoring (e.g., danaparoid or fondaparinux for treating HIT).

Adjunctive surgical considerations include fasciotomies (to reduce compartment pressures, if elevated)[504] and thrombectomy,[505] but prolonged wound healing, risk of infection, and a delay in or interruption of anticoagulation are drawbacks. Local pharmacomechanical thrombolysis is another option,[506] but the choice of the most effective agent, dose, and adjunctive anticoagulation is uncertain, and risks in patients with thrombocytopenia are increased. Finally, fasting with only water and bicarbonate should be tried because it has been found in vasculitis patients that this will stop the vascular wall irritation preventing clotting.

SYMMETRIC PERIPHERAL GANGRENE AND PURPURA FULMINANS

Symmetric peripheral gangrene and purpura fulminans are two syndromes typically associated with thrombocytopenia and coagulopathy in patients who are critically ill. Symmetric peripheral gangrene indicates predominantly acral necrosis, which affects the distal limbs (with more frequent and extensive involvement of the feet than the fingers or hands [Figure 2.20]) but sometimes also the nose, lips, ears, scalp, and genitalia.[475,476] The term *purpura fulminans* is used when there is extensive, multicentric, nonacral skin necrosis, although patients usually have acral limb necrosis as well. Septicemia and cardiac failure are the most common underlying disorders, and patients usually have metabolic (lactic) acidosis.[494,507] Although underlying infection may suggest septic embolization, the presence of pulses and findings on histopathological analyses show the role of microthrombosis associated with DIC. Most patients with symmetric peripheral gangrene have shock, but this complication can occasionally also occur in a normotensive patient with a severe systemic inflammatory state and in the absence of overt DIC.

Septic shock that is caused by meningococcemia is a well-recognized underlying disorder with considerable evidence for failure of the protein C natural anticoagulant pathway. More recently, acute ischemic hepatitis ("shock liver") has been identified as a potential risk factor for symmetric peripheral gangrene or purpura fulminans.[494,501]

Clinical Picture

Patients with septicemia-associated DIC that is complicated by dermal manifestations usually present with fever, hypotension, and a petechial rash that evolve to more extensive confluent nonacral and acral purpuric areas of evolving ischemic necrosis. Early signs of ischemic limb injury include marked coldness, pallor, and distal limb pain. Bullae (often hemorrhagic) indicate tissue necrosis, as does nonblanching acral cyanosis. The dermal abnormalities are often sharply demarcated and strikingly symmetric, with initial gray, blue, or purple discoloration that progresses to black as the

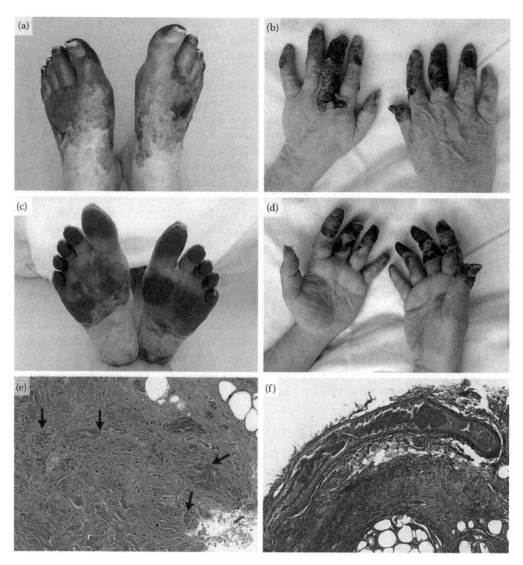

FIGURE 2.20 Symmetric peripheral gangrene. In a 62-year-old man with severe, uncontrolled ulcerative colitis that was resistant to infliximab therapy, an acute onset of swollen, discolored, and painful feet was followed 2 days later by pain and cyanosis in the fingers, with progression to ischemic necrosis of both forefeet (a and c) and hands (b and d) over the next several days. No evidence of bacterial endocarditis or macrovascular aortic disease was found. Laboratory evidence of inflammation included elevated C-reactive protein levels, along with hyperfibrinogenemia, hyperferritinemia, thrombocytosis, and anemia of inflammation. Testing for autoimmune markers and antiphospholipid antibodies was negative. Laboratory studies performed at the time of admission did not strongly support a diagnosis of decompensated disseminated intravascular coagulation, with the following values: platelet count, 472,000/mm³; international normalized ratio (INR), 1.1; activated partial thromboplastin time, 39 seconds; fibrinogen, 650 mg/dL (reference range, 160–420); and fibrin D-dimer, 1390 µg/mL of fibrinogen equivalent units (reference value, <500). Skin biopsy of the left hallux showed multiple fibrin thrombi within small vessels, as seen on hematoxylin and eosin staining (e, with arrows indicating the vessel–lumen interface) and Martius scarlet blue staining, in which fibrin is dark colored (f). The patient's proinflammatory process improved after treatment with high-dose glucocorticoids and unfractionated heparin. (Courtesy of Dr. Ahmed Barefah, Department of Medicine [a through d], and Dr. Linda Kocovski, Department of Pathology [e and f], both at McMaster University.) (From *The New England Journal of Medicine*, Warkentin, T. E. Ischemic limb gangrene with pulses, 373(7). Copyright 2015. Massachusetts Medical Society. Reprinted with permission from Massachusetts Medical Society.)

skin tissues die. Autoamputation of digital tips can occur, although more extensive necrosis usu-ally requires surgical debridement, with or without amputation. Limb ischemic necrosis typically involves lower limbs before upper limbs; approximately one-quarter of patients require four limb amputations.[508] Mortality exceeds 50%. When the bullae cold petechrol stage occurs, often the sequence of total vascular shutdown can be prevented by the administration of O_2 8 L/min and fast-ing using bicarbonate both orally and intravenously. These will often overcome the vasculitis and allow the arteries and vessels to dilate. This procedure has to be performed in a <20% less-polluted environment to reduce the totally toxic pollutant load.

Pathological Features

The histopathological features of symmetric peripheral gangrene and purpura fulminans are dermal microthrombosis involving venules and capillaries.[509] Edematous endothelial cells, capillary dilata-tion, and red cell extravasation contribute to the petechial appearance of early lesions, which over time can coalesce into confluent areas of ischemic necrosis with associated hemorrhagic bullae. Although nonacral necrosis is typically localized to dermal and subdermal tissues, when extensive acral necrosis develops, underlying tissues, including bone, can become involved; bone scans can be used to judge the extent of tissue injury.[510]

Concomitant multiple organ failure (e.g., respiratory, renal, and hepatic) is common. Postmortem studies can show microthrombi in kidneys (cortical necrosis), lungs, liver, spleen, adrenal glands, heart, brain, pancreas, and GI tract.[511,512] When bilateral adrenal hemorrhage occurs in children (most often, associated with meningococcemia), the term Waterhouse–Friderichsen syndrome applies, with evidence of fibrin microthrombi within adrenal sinusoids.[513]

Implicated Microorganisms

Purpura fulminans in young children and adolescents is usually associated with meningococcemia (caused by *Neisseria meningitidis*), whereas in adults, *Streptococcus pneumoniae* (pneumococcus) is most often implicated.[475,476,508,514] Encapsulated bacteria (meningococcus, *Haemophilus influen-zae*, or pneumococcus) are usually found when purpura fulminans occurs in a patient who has undergone splenectomy or who has functional asplenia.[515] Numerous other bacteria, both gram-positive (e.g., *Streptococcus pyogenes* and *Staphylococcus* species) and gram-negative (e.g., *E. coli*), have been implicated, as well as rickettsia,[516] malaria,[517] disseminated TBC,[518] and viral infections (e.g., rubeola[519] and varicella[475]). Infection with *Capnocytophaga* species associated with a dog bite or human saliva has a high risk of purpura fulminans.[520] Of course, these patients are usually not screened for immune parameters such as T and B lymphocytes complement or gamma globulin subsets. The T and B might be treated with autogenous lymphocytic factor and the gamma globulin, which might dampen or stop the infection.

Meningococcemia

Meningococcemia represents the quintessential disease in which bacterial endotoxin (LPS), in a dose-dependent fashion, activates the hemostatic cascades (both procoagulant and anticoagulant), fibrinolysis, and complement, kinin, and cytokine networks.[521] Tissue factor–bearing microparticles contribute to the pathogenesis of DIC.[522] Severely reduced protein C activity is associated with an increased extent of skin lesions and rate of death in children with meningococcemia.[523] A case–con-trol study showed that patients with meningococcemia who also had factor V Leiden—a mutation that impairs factor V proteolysis by activated protein C—had a rate of death that was similar to that of controls but had a tripling (from 7% to 21%) in the risk of tissue necrosis associated with purpura fulminans.[524]

Differential Diagnosis

Sometimes, symmetric peripheral gangrene can occur in the absence of definite DIC.[525,526] Representative disorders include frostbite, ergotism,[527] vasospasm (idiopathic or scleroderma-associated

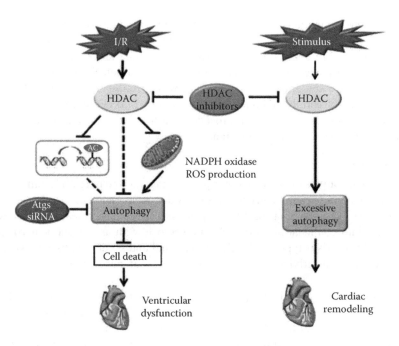

FIGURE 2.21   Role of autophagy in histone deacetylase (HDAC) inhibition–elicited protection against cardiac pathologies. The possible role of autophagy regulation in the cardioprotective effect of HDAC inhibitors in ischemia/reperfusion (I/R) heart injury is depicted. Stimulus (load and agonist)-induced cardiac hypertrophy is also displayed for comparison. HDAC inhibitors (e.g., suberoylanilide hydroxamic acid) restore autophagy homeostasis in ischemic hearts possibly through reactivation of autophagy flux deemed beneficial to infarct boarder zone. In cardiac hypertrophy, HDAC inhibitors may suppress excessive autophagy flux to maintain cardiac autophagy homeostasis. Dashed lines represent likely, although unproven, cell signaling mechanisms. AC, acetylation; ROS, reactive oxygen species. (Adapted from Zhang, Y., J. Ren. 2014. *Circulation* 129:1088–1091. http://circ.ahajournals.org/content/early/2014/01/06/CIRCULATIONAHA.113.008115.Permission by Wolters Kluwer Health, Inc.)

Raynaud's phenomenon),[526] calciphylaxis,[528] postoperative thrombotic thrombocytopenic purpura,[529] myeloproliferative or lymphoproliferative disorders (including monoclonal gammopathies), vasculitis,[530] certain rheumatologic or immunologic disorders (e.g., adult-onset Still's disease[531] and the antiphospholipid syndrome[532]), and uncontrolled proinflammatory disorders such as ulcerative colitis (UC) (Figure 2.21).[533]

Treatment

Venous limb gangrene and symmetric peripheral gangrene are observed in a small minority (<1%) of patients with DIC, so treatment considerations are based primarily on theoretical considerations and case-based observations, rather than on results of clinical trials. Theoretical considerations include pharmacologic interruption of thrombin generation (e.g., heparin anticoagulation), coagulation-factor replacement aimed at correcting depletion of natural anticoagulants such as protein C and antithrombin (given either as frozen plasma or specific factor concentrates), and efforts to minimize risk factors for decreased limb perfusion (e.g., correction of hypotension and reduction or avoidance of vasopressors). However, since ischemic limb injury that is associated with profoundly disturbed procoagulant–anticoagulant balance can occur quickly when the "perfect storm" conditions are met, initiating anticoagulation even at the first signs of ischemic limb injury may already be too late. Some experts advise early protein C replacement therapy in patients with severe meningococcemia.[534,535] However, in order to become activated, protein C requires the presence of thrombomodulin on the surface of endothelial cells. Since injured endothelial cells downregulate and shed thrombomodulin, current experimental approaches include the infusion of recombinant human soluble thrombomodulin.[536]

In choosing an anticoagulant, many practitioners favor heparin,[501,537] since its anticoagulant effect can be monitored directly (by measuring antifactor Xa levels), thus avoiding the potential for systematic underadministration in a patient with an elevated APTT at baseline. Also, heparin clearance remains normal even with liver and renal failure, and heparin has anti-inflammatory properties independent of its role as an anticoagulant.[538] Moreover, drug regimens that involve prophylactic and therapeutic doses are available, depending on the clinical situation. However, heparin requires its cofactor, antithrombin, and antithrombin levels can be reduced in patients with consumptive coagulopathies, particularly with concomitant liver dysfunction.

A recent meta-analysis suggested that the use of heparin (as compared with placebo or usual care) in patients with sepsis, septic shock, and infection-associated DIC may be associated with a relative decrease of 12% in the rate of death.[537] Whether there is any potential benefit for the use of heparin in the prevention of microthrombosis and ischemic limb injury is unknown. Recombinant-activated protein C, although theoretically attractive, was withdrawn from the market after a large, randomized trial did not show improved survival in septic shock.[539] High-dose antithrombin concentrates did not improve mortality in a trial involving patients with severe sepsis,[540] although the rate of death appeared to be lower in the antithrombin-treated subgroup with DIC who did not receive heparin.[541]

Surgical Considerations

Some surgeons advocate the use of fasciotomy in patients in whom compartment syndromes related to tissue edema can compromise flow into a limb.[508,515] However, fasciotomy disrupts the skin barrier and usually results in the interruption or postponement of anticoagulant therapy and so is not without risk. Early amputation should be avoided, whenever possible, since it can be difficult to distinguish viable tissue from nonviable tissue. Indeed, patience to the point of autoamputation in some cases can minimize ultimate tissue losses. A multidisciplinary team that involves plastic surgery or wound care, medicine or infectious diseases, and podiatry, with management in a burn unit, can be helpful.

Neonatal Purpura Fulminans

Although purpura fulminans is most commonly associated with bacterial infection, in neonates, it can be caused by a congenital deficiency in protein C or protein S. Such disorders may require lifelong treatment with frozen plasma or protein C concentrates or possibly liver transplantation.[542]

Idiopathic and Postviral Purpura Fulminans

Idiopathic purpura fulminans is a rare disorder characterized by onset without any known trigger or that occurs a few weeks after an otherwise unremarkable varicella infection. In the latter disorder, transient autoantibodies that inhibit protein S have been implicated.[543]

Conclusions

The concept that venous limb gangrene and symmetric peripheral gangrene are usually associated with microvascular thrombosis with underlying DIC provides a framework for a rational approach to diagnosing and treating these diverse and potentially devastating disorders. Prevention and treatment of venous gangrene requires correction of abnormalities associated with the use of vitamin K antagonists and aggressive anticoagulation, whereas treatment of symmetric peripheral gangrene (with or without purpura fulminans) theoretically involves heparin-based anticoagulation and the substitution of natural anticoagulants.

Roadway Proximity and Risk of Sudden Cardiac Death in Women

Though end-stage disease is emphasized in medicine, as it should be, we can learn a lot about environmental pollution to help the chronic disease patient such as the chemically sensitive who may develop end-stage disease.

According to Hart et al.,[544] sudden cardiac death (SCD) accounts for 180,000–400, 000 deaths in the United States each year.[545] SCD is responsible for more than half of the cardiovascular deaths and 15%–20% of total deaths each year and is the first manifestation of heart disease for a large proportion of victims,[546] especially women.[547] Therefore, there is a need to identify risk factors that can be modified on a population level to broadly affect SCD risk.

Unfortunately, the medical profession is not taught about avoidance of pollutants and less-polluted, controlled environments in order to avoid or minimize triggering agents.

Long-term exposures associated with traffic such as air pollution and noise have been associated with increased mortality from CHD,[548–551] and associations with fatal CHD have typically been stronger than those with nonfatal events.[552,553] Short-term exposure to air pollution or traffic has also been associated with ventricular arrhythmias in patients with implantable cardioverter defibrillators[554] and with elevations in the risk of out-of-hospital cardiac arrest in most but not all studies.[555–563] Therefore, long-term exposure to traffic may be associated with SCD, both through the development of underlying atherosclerosis and by influencing myocardial vulnerability to lethal ventricular arrhythmias[564] due to the increase in pollution causing sensitivity.

Previous studies, including our own, have observed modest elevations in incident CHD (combined nonfatal and fatal) among individuals who live closer to major roadways,[565–568] but the impact of this exposure on SCD risk is unknown. Certainly, we have observed that CS pollutants who live near freeways and busy roads are much sicker and have their vasculitis triggered much easier. The maintenance of their hypersensitivity is longer.

According to Hart et al.,[544] during the 26 years of follow-up, a total of 523 cases (328 definite, 195 probable) of SCD were observed. The associations of roadway proximity with SCD are presented in Table 2.8. In basic models adjusted for age, race, and calendar time, women living within 50 m of a roadway had a higher risk of SCD (HR, 1.56; 95% CI = 1.18–2.05) compared with women living farther away ($\geq$500 m). The dose–response relationship between roadway proximity and SCD risk was linear as determined by cubic lines, and each 100 m closer to roadways was associated with an 8% increased risk for SCD (95% CI = 3–14). In multivariable models controlling for potential confounders, HRs were attenuated but remained statistically significant in both the categorical (HR, 1.40; 95% CI = 1.06–1.85 for <50 vs. 500 m) and continuous (HR, 1.06; 95% CI = 1.01–1.12 per 100 m) analyses. Additional adjustment for incident comorbidities, including incident CHD, potentially on the causal pathway had little effect on the HRs (4.3% mediation). In sensitivity analyses, excluding probable SCDs or nonwhites, the magnitude of the associations was similar (multivariable HR, 1.33, 95% CI = 0.94–1.89; and multivariable HR, 1.32, 95% CI = 0.99–1.76 for <50 vs. 500 m). These associations also did not significantly differ by region of residence, race, or smoking status; however, the HR associated with living <50 versus 500 m from a roadway was higher among ever smokers (HR, 1.56; 95% CI = 1.08–2.23) compared with nonsmokers (HR, 1.22; 95% CI = 0.80–1.97).

Roadway Proximity and Nonfatal MI and Fatal CHD

According to Hart et al.,[544] during 24 years of follow-up, 2731 cases (1813 definite, 918 probable) of nonfatal MI and 1159 cases (794 definite, 365 probable) of fatal CHD were identified. The associations with roadway proximity and each outcome are shown in Table 2.12. In multivariable models, the risk of fatal CHD (HR, 1.24; 95% CI = 1.03–1.49) was statistically significantly higher among women living within 50 m of an A1–A3 road compared with women living $\geq$500 m away, and the HR for each additional 100 m closer in proximity was 1.04 (95% CI = 1.00–1.07). This association

TABLE 2.12

HRs (95% CIs) for the Association of Risk of SCD (1986–2012) with Residential Proximity to A1–A3 Roads among Participants (n = 107,130)

Distance, m	Cases, n	Person-Years	Basic[a]	Multivariable[b]	Multivariable[c]
0–49	103	354,901	1.56 (1.18–2.05)	1.40 (1.06–1.85)	1.38 (1.04–1.82)
50–199	150	661,072	1.27 (0.98–1.63)	1.19 (0.92–1.53)	1.17 (0.91–1.51)
200–499	169	770,257	1.26 (0.98–1.61)	1.20 (0.94–1.54)	1.20 (0.93–1.53)
≥500	101	594,129	Reference	Reference	Reference
Linear (per 100 m closer)[d]	523	2,380,358	1.08 (1.03–1.14)	1.06 (1.01–1.12)	1.06 (1.01–1.11)

Source: Hart, J. E. et al. 2014. *Circulation* 130(17):1474–1482. http://circ.ahajournals.org/content/130/17/1474.

Note: n, person-years, and number of cases apply for all models. CI, confidence interval; HR, hazard ratio; NHS, Nurses' Health Study; SCD, sudden cardiac death.

[a] Models adjusted for age, race, and calendar time.

[b] Models additionally adjusted for smoking status; secondhand smoke exposure during childhood, at home, and at work; body mass index; menopausal status and postmenopausal hormone use; the Alternative Healthy Eating Index; alcohol consumption; physical activity; family history of myocardial infarction; aspirin, multivitamin, and vitamin E use; region of residence; census tract median home value and median income; and incidence of diabetes mellitus or cancer.

[c] Models additionally adjusted for comorbidities: incidence of high cholesterol, high blood pressure, stroke, or coronary heart disease.

[d] Linear models for distances of 0–499 m compared with addresses ≥500 m away.

was slightly attenuated when fatal CHD events also considered SCDs (n = 152) were excluded from the end point (multivariable HR, 1.21, 95% CI = 0.99–1.48 for <50 vs. 500 m; and multivariable HR, 1.03, 95% CI = 0.99–1.07 per 100 m). Risks of nonfatal MI were more modest in magnitude and were not statistically significant in multivariable models. Similar to Hart's results for SCD, results for fatal CHD and nonfatal MI were essentially unchanged when additionally adjusted for incidence of other comorbidities that might be in the causal pathway (0.1% and 0.2% mediation for nonfatal MI and fatal CHD, respectively), when other categorical cut points were considered, and in models excluding probable events or nonwhites (data not shown). There was also no evidence of effect modification by race or region of residence (data not shown) or smoking status.

Population-Attributable Risks

According to Hart et al.,[544] over the course of the study, 75% of the total person-years observed were spent at residences within 499 m of an A1–A3 roadway. The multivariable adjusted HRs for the categorical variable (0–49, 50–199, and 200–499 vs. ≥500 m) translate into population-attributable risks of 17.9% (95% CI = 0.1–34.7), 11.6% (95% CI = −1.1–23.9), and 6.8% (95% CI = −1.4–14.9) for SCD, fatal CHD, and nonfatal MI, respectively, in this sample of women (Table 2.13).

Among this sample of middle-aged and older women, roadway proximity was associated with an elevation in the risk of SCD. Even after adjustment for potential confounders and mediators, women who lived within 50 m of a major roadway had a 38% higher hazard (95% CI = 1.04–1.82) of experiencing SCD compared with women living ≥500 m away. The association was linear, and each 100 m closer to a major roadway was associated with a 6% elevation in the HR (95% CI = 1–11). Proximity to a major roadway was also statistically significantly associated with fatal CHD but to a lesser magnitude. These results suggest that traffic exposure, as measured by roadway proximity,

TABLE 2.13

HRs (95% CIs) for Associations of the Risk of Nonfatal MI and Fatal CHD (1986–2010) with Residential Proximity to A1–A3 Roads among NHS Participants (n = 107,130)

Outcome	Distance, m	Cases, n	Person-Years	Basic[a]	Multivariable[b]	Multivariable[c]
Nonfatal MI	0–49	445	326,705	1.14 (1.00–1.29)	1.08 (0.96–1.23)	1.08 (0.96–1.23)
	50–199	819	611,508	1.13 (1.02–1.26)	1.09 (0.98–1.22)	1.09 (0.98–1.21)
	200–499	861	711,732	1.05 (0.95–1.17)	1.03 (0.92–1.14)	1.03 (0.92–1.14)
	≥500	606	541,065	Reference	Reference	Reference
	Linear (per 100 m)[d]	2731	2,191,010	1.03 (1.01–1.05)	1.02 (1.00–1.04)	1.02 (1.00–1.04)
Fatal CHD	0–49	228	331,321	1.41 (1.17–1.70)	1.24 (1.03–1.49)	1.24 (1.03–1.50)
	50–199	341	619,706	1.18 (1.00–1.40)	1.07 (0.90–1.27)	1.07 (0.90–1.27)
	200–499	362	720,015	1.12 (0.95–1.33)	1.06 (0.90–1.25)	1.07 (0.90–1.26)
	≥500	228	547,634	Reference	Reference	Reference
	Linear (per 100 m)[d]	1159	2,218,407	1.07 (1.03–1.10)	1.04 (1.00–1.07)	1.04 (1.00–1.07)

Source: Hart, J. E. et al. 2014. *Circulation* 130(17):1474–1482. http://circ.ahajournals.org/content/130/17/1474.

Note: n, person-years, and number of cases apply for all models. CHD, coronary heart disease; CI, confidence interval; HR, hazard ratio; MI, myocardial infarction; NHS, Nurses' Health Study.

[a] Models adjusted for age, race, and calendar time.

[b] Models additionally adjusted for smoking status; secondhand smoke exposure during childhood, at home, and at work; body mass index; menopausal status and postmenopausal hormone use; the Alternative Healthy Eating Index; alcohol consumption; physical activity; family history of myocardial infarction; aspirin, multivitamin, and vitamin E use; region of residence; census tract median home value and median income; and incidence of diabetes mellitus or cancer.

[c] Models additionally adjusted for comorbidities: incidence of high cholesterol, high blood pressure, or stroke.

[d] Linear models for distances 0–499 m compared with addresses ≥500 m away.

may increase the risk of death resulting from CHD and may increase the propensity for fatal ventricular arrhythmias. If the observed relationships are causal, these results suggest that roadway exposures may underlie 17.9%, 11.6%, and 6.8% of SCDs, fatal CHDs, and nonfatal MIs, respectively, in this population. For the end point of SCD, these population-attributable risks are comparable to or greater than the contributions made by smoking, diet, and obesity in this population.[568] This study is highly significant for the chemically sensitive. They are pollutant sensitive; their vascular area will be prone to pollutant injury just as Hart's implants even though they may not have SCD, they will be kept chronically ill by the pollutant exposure.

To the best of our knowledge, this is the first study to examine the impact of residential roadway proximity on the risk of SCD. However, a few case-crossover studies have examined the impact of short-term traffic-related air pollution exposures (most often fine $PM_{2.5}$, carbon monoxide, or oxides of nitrogen), and risk of out-of-hospital cardiac arrests. As summarized in a recent review,[569] the majority have used administrative databases to identify cases and local air pollution monitoring networks to assign pollution measures for a variety of pollutants on the day of the event and a varying number of previous days. In studies based in Rome, Italy,[557] Melbourne, Australia,[555] Helsinki, Finland,[560] Stockholm, Sweden,[570] Indianapolis, IN,[559] New York, NY,[561] and Houston, TX,[556] elevated risks were observed with increased levels of PM or other pollutants on the day of or up to 3 days preceding the cardiac arrest. However, in studies from Washington State[558,562] and Copenhagen, Denmark,[563] consistent associations were not found between levels of PM measured in the days before out-of-hospital cardiac arrest compared with control days from the same month. Although it is not possible to directly compare these studies with Hart's, the preponderance of evidence suggests that short-term exposures to traffic-related pollutants are associated with acute increases in risk of out-of-hospital cardiac arrests.

In terms of mechanisms underlying these associations, there is a growing body of literature supporting an association between short-term (hourly, daily) exposures to air pollution, especially those from traffic sources, and ventricular arrhythmias.[554] The majority of these studies have been conducted in selected high-risk populations of patients with implanted cardiac defibrillators in whom the events can be identified with fine temporal resolution. In the first such study, based in the Boston, MA, area, recent exposures to NO_2 were associated with an increased risk of arrhythmias, and multiple events were associated with a number of other traffic-related exposures.[571] A second study in the same geographic area observed a positive linear association between $PM_{2.5}$ and the risk of arrhythmias.[572] Similar findings with different measures of air pollution have been observed in studies from St. Louis, MO, Gothenburg, Germany, and Stockholm, Sweden, but not in studies of patients in Vancouver, BC, Canada, and Atlanta, GA.[554] Since fatal ventricular arrhythmias underlie a large proportion of SCD and thus contribute to fatal CHD deaths, these data provide a potential biological mechanism underlying at least part of the observed association between traffic-related exposures and SCD and fatal CHD.

Hart's data suggest that there may also be a more general association between roadway proximity and fatal CHD events that may not be entirely explained by effects on SCD. Short-term exposure to traffic has been associated with transiently increased risks of nonfatal MI,[469] and long-term exposure to traffic or roadways has been associated with higher risks of fatal and nonfatal CHD events.[565–567] In the Atherosclerosis Risk in Communities (ARIC) study, living within 300 m of a major road was associated with a 12% increased risk of CHD in a population of ≈13,000 middle-aged men and women, with stronger risks for those living near roads with higher traffic density.[565] In a case–control study in Massachusetts, each interquartile-range increase in traffic density was associated with a 4% (95% CI = 2–7) increased risk of acute MI.[567] Hart's previous analyses in the NHS found that women living at residences consistently close to traffic over follow-up were at a higher risk for incident total CHD (HR = 1.11; 95% CI = 1.01–1.21) than women who live consistently at addresses farther away.[566] Although these studies did not specifically compare associations for fatal and nonfatal events, other studies from Stockholm and Rome examining long-term exposures to traffic-related air pollution have demonstrated stronger associations with fatal MI end points and out-of-hospital deaths compared with nonfatal events,[573,574] consistent with Hart's results.

It is important to note that although there was minimal overlap between SCD and fatal CHD events, some degree of undetected overlap between SCD and fatal CHD events undoubtedly exists and is unavoidable in this epidemiological study. In prior studies,[575–577] CHD is detected at autopsy or on extensive clinical evaluation in slightly fewer than half of women who suffer a sudden cardiac arrest/SCD.[575–578] In their study, only 30% of SCDs were found to have evidence for CHD before or at the time of death; thus, it is probable that undetected CHD underlies a proportion of the remaining SCDs. Therefore, despite controlling for known CHD in their models, residual confounding by undetected CHD could account for part of the association with SCD. Conversely, the strict but standard[579] definition of SCD used in their study relies on the patient having been observed within the 24 hours before death, and it is probable that some of the fatal CHD events that occurred suddenly may not have been characterized as SCD, either because the deaths were unwitnessed for >24 hours or because details on the circumstances of the death were not available. Therefore, undetected SCDs may underlie some of the residual association between roadway proximity and fatal CHD.

A number of potential biological mechanisms are associated with residential proximity to roadways that could predispose patients to both SCD and fatal CHD apart from acute triggering of ventricular arrhythmias.[580] The primary comorbidities they examined as mediators (high cholesterol and high blood pressure) had little effect on their observed associations, as determined by the percent mediation, suggesting that the effects of roadway proximity on SCD and fatal CHD may be working through other mechanisms. Traffic-related air pollution has also been associated with elevations in systemic inflammation, oxidative stress, heart failure, and alterations in autonomic function and heart rate variability (HRV)[580]—such as seen in the chemically sensitive. Residential proximity to major roadways has been directly associated with higher left ventricular mass index[581] and severity of atherosclerosis as measured by coronary calcification.[582] Additionally, traffic noise has been linked to a number of these underlying mechanisms, including HR, cardiac output, and oxidative stress, suggesting that traffic exposures may act on cardiovascular disease through a number of underlying biological mechanisms.[583] However, the Ca^{2+} kinase phosphorylation phenomena causing 1000 times increase in sensitivity may have come into rhythms lowering the threshold for easier triggering of the arrhythmia.

This study has several limitations; however, the Ca^{2+} protein kinase phosphorylation phenomena causing 1000 times increase in sensitivity may have come into play, thus, lowering the threshold for easier triggering of the arrhythmia. The measure of exposure, roadway proximity, is a poor proxy for true traffic exposures such as noise or pollution levels, and it does not provide us with information on temporal changes in exposures that may be associated with triggering of events. These limitations are expected to lead to nondifferential misclassifications of exposure, which would bias results toward the null. It does have the advantage, however, of allowing us to assess the combined impact of all aspects of near-roadway exposure simultaneously. Additionally, only 15% of the person-time in the cohort was spent at addresses within 50 m of an A1–A3 roadway, limiting the ability to detect statistically significant effects at the highest exposure levels. The assumption of similar exposures from all roadways within a given roadway classification is another limitation of the study because time-varying information on traffic volume during the follow-up period is not widely available for the entire contiguous United States for the study period. We also lack information on the temporal and seasonal trends in traffic. This inability to differentiate roads and time periods with higher exposure levels likely leads to nondifferential exposure errors, which would lessen our ability to detect statistically significant effects. Similarly, they do not have information on the amount of time each participant spends at his/her home or on characteristics of each home such as age, ventilation rate, soundproofing, and orientation relative to prevailing winds and to the roadways. All of these factors would also lead to exposure misclassification and likely partially explain the wide CIs. However, the study applies to pollutant exposure and injury that is seen in chemically sensitive patients who do worse in the city; near major roadways, they have sluggish response, do not recover from pollutant exposure easily, and are always fatigued.

As with any observational study, exposures and comorbidities may be incompletely or imperfectly measured, resulting in residual confounding or an inability to adequately detect effect mediation by comorbidities. However, validation studies have suggested that the nurses accurately report many of the CHD risk factors and comorbidity risk factors examined in this study.[1231] We also do not have information on medication use just before death (such as QT-prolonging agents), which may mediate our observed associations with SCD.

This large prospective study also has major strengths. Information on residential address and roadway proximity over a 26-year period was available, allowing Hart et al.,[544] to look at the long-term effects of roadway proximity on the risk of SCD over a long timescale, as opposed to the daily or weekly exposures commonly examined. Additionally, the large number of well-validated cases of SCD, nonfatal MI, and fatal CHD allowed them to look at relatively fine-scale changes in exposure with tight control for a number of time-varying risk factors. This wealth of outcome data also provided them opportunity to compare the impacts of traffic exposure for a number of outcomes. Finally, the availability of a host of time-varying data on other potential risk factors for our outcomes allowed them to examine the impacts of roadway proximity independently of diet, personal characteristics, socioeconomic status, and other comorbidities.

In conclusion, living near a major roadway was associated with a significant increase in SCD risk in this sample of U.S. middle-aged women. Although the risk elevations are modest, given the ubiquitous nature of the exposure, the population-attributable risk is significant and comparable to that observed for other major SCD risk factors.[584] In the United States, the U.S. EPA estimated that 35 million people lived within 300 feet of a major road in 2009,[585] and a growing number of individuals live in close proximity to major roads worldwide. Therefore, exposures related to traffic such as air pollution and noise are widely prevalent and potentially modifiable population-level risk factors for SCD. Since the majority of SCDs occur in individuals considered to be at low risk within the general population, modification of population-level exposures that elevate SCD risk represents an important component of a comprehensive strategy to reduce the burden of SCD in the population. These data also support the fact that chemically sensitive patients are the canaries of the general population. They know that pollutant exposure from being close to major roadways makes them sick and therefore they avoid this source of pollution because it flares their vasculitis symptoms.

Outdoor Air Pollution and Out-of-Hospital Cardiac Arrest in Okayama, Japan

A number of studies have shown associations between short-term exposure to air pollution and cardiovascular disease.[580] Specific cardiovascular events considered to be associated with air pollution include IHD, heart failure, cerebrovascular disease, peripheral arterial and venous disease, and cardiac arrhythmia/arrest.[580] Indeed, a recent study from Japan using hourly air pollution monitoring data demonstrated that outdoor air pollution had adverse impacts on emergency hospital visits owing to cardiovascular and cerebrovascular events[586] not thought to be related to CS.

Although there is growing evidence to support an association between outdoor air pollution and cardiovascular disease, the number of studies focusing on cardiac arrest remains small and their findings are inconsistent. Cardiac arrest is defined as an "abrupt cessation of cardiac pump function which may be reversible by a prompt intervention but will lead to death in its absence," and is estimated to cause between 200,000 and 450,000 deaths annually in the United States owing to SCD.[587] Given that cardiac arrest leads directly to SCD, and that its consequences result in a significant burden for both individuals and society, prevention of cardiac arrest is a major public health priority. Although cigarette smoking, diabetes, and hypertension are well-known risk factors for SCD, the influence of air pollution on cardiac arrest has recently gained greater attention.[588] It is clear that the air pollution damages the large and small blood vessels in the chemically sensitive and vasculitis when studied in controlled environments.[589]

To date, a total of 10 studies evaluating the impacts of outdoor air pollution on cardiac arrest have been conducted in the United States,[556,558,559,561,562] Europe,[560,563,570] and Australia.[555,590] All of these studies examined the effect of exposure to PM, with seven suggesting a positive association with the onset of cardiac arrest.[555,556,559–561,563,588–590] In addition, five of these studies examined the effect of ozone,[555,556,560,561,570] with three of them demonstrating adverse effects.[556,560,570] Only two of these studies[563,590] provided evidence on other pollutants; however, the results of these previous studies, which were conducted in the United States, Europe, or Australia, may not be generalizable to an Asian context for a number of reasons, including differences in residents' health characteristics and the constituents of local air pollution.[591] This study evaluated the associations between short-term exposure to outdoor air pollution and the risk of out-of-hospital cardiac arrest among residents of Okayama, Japan, who had visited hospital emergency departments between January 2006 and December 2010. We often see the chemically sensitive patients who get ill due to pollution required to have alkalization and O_2 due to symptoms they gathered from outdoor traffic when coming from one environmentally controlled living quarters to our clinic. Usually, a period of just a half hour of these therapies will clear their symptoms. Most of these patients have small-vessel vasculitis, which triggers and makes them prone to future exposure symptoms.

Anonymized data on all ambulance calls made during the study period were provided by the Ambulance Division of the Fire Bureau in Okayama City, a city located in the western part of Japan with a population of 709,584 and an area of 790 km^2 (in 2010).[586] Data were available from calls made either by the patients themselves or by others to request an ambulance. Using the data, 110,110 residents were selected who had been brought to an emergency department in Okayama City by ambulance between January 2006 and December 2010.

Yorifuji et al.[592] initially restricted the study to 2181 patients who had been administered an ECG by ambulance personnel and who presented signs of cardiac arrest (i.e., ventricular fibrillation, asystole, and pulseless electrical activity).[587] To identify cardiac arrest owing to cardiac etiology, they used diagnoses made by physicians at the hospitals to which patients were admitted. Since the diagnoses were coded in accordance with the 10th International Classification of Disease (ICD-10), they restricted their analysis only to those subjects who were diagnosed with cardiac disease by medical doctors on arrival at a hospital (ICD-10: I20–I52). Data from a total of 558 individuals (i.e., cardiac arrest cases owing to cardiac etiology) were included in our final analysis.

AIR POLLUTION MONITORING AND METEOROLOGICAL DATA

They obtained data from the Okayama Prefectural Government on hourly concentrations of suspended PM (SPM), ozone, nitrogen dioxide (NO_2), sulfur dioxide (SO_2), and carbon monoxide (CO) during the study period as measured at monitoring stations in Okayama City. In Japan, measures of PM are typically expressed in terms of SPM and account for PM with an aerodynamic diameter of less than 7 μm (PM_7). During the period studied, 11 stations were used for SPM measurements, 8 for ozone, 11 for NO_2, 7 for SO_2, and 2 for CO. The entire area of Okayama City was covered within a 30-km radius of each monitoring station. They then calculated city-representative hourly average concentrations of each air pollutant from hourly concentrations recorded at each monitoring station. Although there were no missing data for city-representative hourly average concentrations of SPM, NO_2, and SO_2 during the entire study period, SO_2 hourly mean concentration readings for ozone (1.15% of eligible hours) and 26 hours for CO (0.06% of eligible hours) were unavailable.

Finally, Yorifuji et al.[592] obtained hourly data on temperature and relative humidity for the entire study period from one weather station managed by the Japan Metrological Agency located in Okayama City. There were no missing data for either temperature or relative humidity.

The characteristics of the study subjects are shown in Table 2.14. While 78.0% of the subjects were more than 65 years of age, 58.9% were male and 58.6% had experienced cardiac arrest during the cold season. About 10% of the subjects had a medical history of CHD or hypertension.

During the period studied, the IQRs of air pollutants were 20.6 μg/m³ for SPM, 25.8 ppb for ozone, 11.1 ppb for NO_2, 2.3 ppb for SO_2, and 0.3 ppm for CO. The mean values and Pearson correlation coefficients for hourly air pollutant concentrations and temperatures in both the warm and the cold seasons are shown in Table 2.15. As expected, the recorded mean concentration of ozone was higher in the warm season. Although the concentration of SPM was also higher in the warm season, the mean concentration of NO_2 was higher in the cold season. In both seasons, SPM was moderately correlated with all other pollutants except ozone. By contrast, concentrations of ozone showed a weak positive correlation with SO_2 in the warm season and a negative correlation with NO_2 and CO in the cold season. Their results also showed that NO_2 was correlated with SO_2 and CO in both seasons.

When they examined the effect of each pollutant at different lags, exposure to SPM, ozone, NO_2, and SO_2 was associated with an increased risk of cardiac arrest (Table 2.16). The ORs representing the increase in the risk of cardiac arrest in response to an IQR increase in exposure were 1.17 (95% CI = 1.02–1.33) for SPM (48–72-hour lag), 1.40 (95% CI = 1.02–1.92) for ozone (72–96-hour lag), 1.24 (95% CI = 1.01–1.53) for NO_2 (24–48-hour lag), and 1.16 (95% CI = 1.00–1.34) for SO_2 (48–72-hour lag). CO exposure was not associated with the increased risk of cardiac arrest.

When they stratified their analyses by patients' characteristics (Table 2.17), those in the younger age group had a higher effect estimate for SPM exposure compared with the older age group (p = 0.15) whereas the older group had a higher effect estimate for ozone compared with the younger age group (p = 0.04). Furthermore, the OR for cardiac arrest among male subjects in response to an IQR increase in SPM was higher than that for female subjects (p = 0.03). Although the effect estimate for SPM was higher in the warm season and the effect estimate for NO_2 exposure

TABLE 2.14

Patients' Characteristics and Timing of Emergency Hospital Visits Because of Cardiac Arrest among Residents of Okayama City, Japan, 2006–2010 (n = 558)

Variable	n (%)
Age, yrs	
≥65	435 (78.0)
<65	123 (22.0)
Sex	
Male	329 (58.9)
Female	229 (41.0)
Medical history	
Hypertension	58 (10.4)
Coronary heart disease	54 (9.7)
Cerebrovascular disease	47 (8.4)
Diabetes mellitus	35 (6.3)
Respiratory disease	21 (3.8)
Other diseases	192 (34.4)
None	85 (15.2)
Unknown	66 (11.8)
Time of onset	
Daytime (8 a.m. to 7 p.m.)	307 (55.0)
Nighttime (8 p.m. to 7 a.m.)	251 (45.0)
Season of onset	
Warm (April to September)	231 (41.4)
Cold (October to March)	327 (58.6)

Source: Permission by Wolters KLuwer Health, Inc. Copyright 2014. Yorifuji, T., E. Suzuki, S. Kashima. 2014. Outdoor air pollution and out-of-hospital cardiac arrest in Okayama, Japan. *J. Occup. Environ. Med.* 56(10):1019–1023. http://journals.lww.com/joem/Fulltext/2014/10000/Outdoor_Air_Pollution_and_Out_of_Hospital_Cardiac.2.aspx.

was higher in the cold season, no significant seasonal differences were detected for any of the pollutants analyzed.

In the study, Torifuji et al.[592] evaluated the associations between short-term exposure to outdoor air pollution and out-of-hospital cardiac arrest owing to cardiac etiology in Okayama, Japan. They found that exposures to SPM (48–72-hour lag), ozone (72–96-hour lag), NO_2 (24–48-hour lag), and SO_2 (48–72-hour lag) were all associated with a higher risk of cardiac arrest. They also observed different susceptibilities to SPM and ozone exposures by sex and age group. These data apply to chemically sensitive patients with cardiac arrest who have traffic-related exposure. They usually do not have cardiac arrest; they become quite ill after traffic exposure. CS takes several days of incapitation to recover.

The observed effect of SPM (which corresponds to PM_7) on the risk of cardiac arrest is consistent with findings obtained from seven previous studies conducted in the United States, Europe, and Australia.[555,556,559–561,563,590] In addition, the adverse effect of ozone exposure is also consistent with the findings from three studies conducted in the United States and Europe.[556,560,570] Although the evidence for effects of exposure to ozone on cardiovascular disease risk remains inconsistent, a recent large-scale study of 11,677 cases of cardiac arrest in Houston, Texas, demonstrated adverse

TABLE 2.15

Mean Values and Estimated Pearson Correlation Coefficients for Hourly Air Pollutant Concentrations and Temperature

	Mean (SD)			Pearson Condition Coefficients[a]					
	All	Warm Season	Cold Season	SPM	Ozone	NO$_2$	SO$_2$	CO	Temperature
SPM, µg/m^3	26.8 (183)	293 (18.2)	243 (18.1)	1	0.16	0.40	0.48	0.31	0.13
Ozone, ppb	25.9 (17.9)	31.4 (19.5)	20.5 (14.2)	−0.16	1	−0.16	0.32	−0.08	0.15
NO$_2$, ppb	17.1 (8.1)	15.5 (6.9)	18.8 (8.9)	0.49	−0.61	1	0.46	0.54	−0.24
SO$_2$, ppb	3.0 (2.5)	3.3 (2.7)	2.8 (2.3)	0.50	0.11	0.43	1	0.19	0.31
CO, ppm	0.6 (0.3)	0.5 (0.2)	0.6 (0.4)	0.45	−0.48	0.66	0.24	1	−0.16
Temperature, °C	16.7 (9.0)	23.2 (6.2)	10.2 (6.1)	0.26	0.32	−0.11	0.12	0.01	1

Source: Permission by Wolters KLuwer Health, Inc. Copyright 2014. Yorifuji, T., E. Suzuki, S. Kashima. 2014. Outdoor air pollution and out-of-hospital cardiac arrest in Okayama, Japan. *J. Occup. Environ. Med.* 56(10):1019–1023. http://journals.lww.com/joem/Fulltext/2014/10000/Outdoor_Air_Pollution_and_Out_of_Hospital_Cardiac.2.aspx

Note: CO, carbon monoxide; NO$_2$, nitrogen dioxide; SD, standard deviation; SO$_2$, sulfur dioxide; SPM, suspended particulate matter.

[a] Upper diagonal shows coefficients during the warm season and lower diagonal shows coefficients during the cold season.

effects of ozone both on the day of the event and in 1–3 hours before onset.[556] These findings, as well as those of this study, support the hypothesis that exposure to both PM and ozone increases the risk of cardiac arrest.

Different susceptibilities to SPM and ozone exposures by age category and different lags between SPM and ozone merit consideration. Cardiac arrest has a variety of causes, including CHD, arrhythmia, and cardiomyopathy.[587] In a recent study, Rosenthal et al.[560] examined the effect of exposure to PM$_{2.5}$ (with an aerodynamic diameter <2.5 µm) and ozone on the risk of cardiac arrest as a result of MI or other cardiac causes. Their results showed that the same-day PM$_{2.5}$ exposure was associated with cardiac arrest caused by MI and that lagged exposure to ozone was associated with cardiac arrest caused by other cardiac etiologies. This suggests that air pollution may induce cardiac arrest

TABLE 2.16

Adjusted Odds Ratios and 95% Confidence Intervals for Emergency Calls per Interquartile-Range Increase[a] in Exposure to Each Pollutant at Different Lags

Lag	SPM	Ozone	NO$_2$	SO$_2$	CO
0–24 hrs (0 d)	0.99 (0.87–1.13)	1.19 (0.83–1.69)	1.13 (0.90–1.42)	1.14 (0.98–1.33)	1.01 (0.83–1.22)
24–48 hrs (1 d)	1.07 (0.93–1.22)	0.83 (0.60–1.14)	1.24 (1.01–1.53)	1.07 (0.93–1.24)	1.15 (0.96–1.37)
48–72 hrs (2 d)	1.17 (1.02–133)	1.26 (0.92–1.73)	1.16 (0.94–1.42)	1.16 (1.00–1.34)	1.06 (0.89–1.26)
72–96 hrs (3 d)	0.95 (0.83–1.08)	1.40 (1.02–1.92)	0.90 (0.73–1.10)	1.01 (0.88–1.16)	0.87 (0.73–1.03)

Source: Permission by Wolters KLuwer Health, Inc. Copyright 2014. Yorifuji, T., E. Suzuki, S. Kashima. 2014. Outdoor air pollution and out-of-hospital cardiac arrest in Okayama, Japan. *J. Occup. Environ. Med.* 56(10):1019–1023. http://journals.lww.com/joem/Fulltext/2014/10000/Outdoor_Air_Pollution_and_Out_of_Hospital_Cardiac.2.aspx

Note: CO, carbon monoxide; NO$_2$, nitrogen dioxide; SO$_2$, sulfur dioxide; SPM, suspended particulate matter.

[a] Adjusted for ambient temperature (df = 6) and relative humidity (df = 3). Interquartile ranges are 20.6 µg/m^3 for SPM, 25.8 ppb for ozone, 11.1 ppb for NO$_2$, 2.3 ppb for SO$_2$, and 0.3 ppm for CO.

TABLE 2.17

Estimated Impact of an Interquartile-Range Increase in Atmospheric Concentrations of SPM (48–72-Hour Lag), Ozone (72–96-Hour Lag), and NO₂ (24–48-Hour Lag) on the Odds of Making an Emergency Call for Cardiac Arrest in Each Subgroup of Patients

	SPM (48–72 hrs)		Ozone (72–96 hrs)		NO₂ (24–48 hrs)		SO₂ (48–72 hrs)	
	OR (95% CI)[a]	P	OR (95% CI)[a]	P	OR (95% CI)[a]	P	OR (95% Or)	P
Age, yrs								
≥65	1.10 (0.93–1.29)	0.15	1.67 (1.17–2.39)	0.04	1.27 (1.01–1.60)	0.63	1.13 (0.96–1.34)	0.59
<65	1.36 (1.06–1.76)		0.74 (0.38–1.46)		1.12 (0.72–1.76)		125 (0.92–1.68)	
Sex								
Male	1.31 (1.10–1.56)	0.03	1.55 (1.03–2.33)	0.44	1.32 (1.01–1.72)	0.44	110 (0.99–1.46)	0.58
Female	0.96 (0.77–1.21)		1.20 (0.73–1.97)		1.13 (0.82–135)		1.11 (0.89–1.38)	
Time of onset								
Daytime (8 a.m. to 8 p.m.)	1.09 (0.91–1.31)	0.27	1.46 (0.95–2.23)	0.77	1.04 (0.79–138)	0.07	1.16 (0.95–1.42)	1.00
Nighttime (8 p.m. to 8 a.m.)	1.27 (1.04–1.55)		1.33 (0.83–2.12)		1.51 (1.12–2.03)		1.16 (0.94–1.43)	
Season of onset								
Warm (April to September)	1.31 (1.07–1.61)	0.13	1.43 (0.93–2.21)	0.86	0.99 (0.69–1.42)	0.14	1.10 (0.88–1.36)	0.49
Cold (October to March)	1.06 (0.88–1.28)		1.36 (0.86–2.15)		1.39 (1.07–1.80)		1.22 (1.00–1.48)	

Source: Permission by Wolters KLuwer Health, Inc. Copyright 2014. Yorifuji, T., E. Suzuki, S. Kashima. 2014. Outdoor air pollution and out-of-hospital cardiac arrest in Okayama, Japan. *J. Occup. Environ. Med.* 56(10):1019–1023. http://journals.lww.com/joem/Fulltext/2014/10000/Outdoor_Air_Pollution_and_Out_of_Hospital_Cardiac.2.aspx

Note: CI, confidence interval; NO₂, nitrogen dioxide; OR, odds ratio; SO₂, sulfur dioxide; SPM, suspended particulate matter.

[a] Adjusted for ambient temperature (df = 6) and relative humidity (df = 3). Interquartile ranges are 20.6 μg/m³ SPM, 25.8 ppb for ozone, 11.1 ppb for NO₂, and 2.3 ppb for SO₂.

via two distinct pathways: one in which exposure to PM results in MI and another in which ozone exacerbates other cardiac conditions such as arrhythmia to increase the risk of cardiac arrest.[560] These results may also provide an explanation for their findings that susceptibilities to SPM and ozone exposures differed by age category and that the effects of exposure to SPM and ozone had different lags.

Yorifuji et al.[592] also observed that NO_2 and SO_2 were associated with the risk of cardiac arrest. This result may reflect the different toxicological effects of each pollutant. Nevertheless, because SO_2 has been shown to have more spatial variability compared with other pollutants (e.g., NO_2)[593] and that concentrations of SO_2 were correlated with those of NO_2 and CO in this study, the effects of SO_2 should be interpreted with care. SO_2 might work as a maker of NO_2, which reflects local traffic-related air pollution.[594] A previous work by Wichmann et al.[563] has also shown a positive association between nitrogen oxides and cardiac arrest in Copenhagen, Denmark.

Their observation that exposure to SPM had a stronger effect in male than in female subjects is consistent with the results of previous studies conducted in Houston, Texas,[556] and Melbourne, Australia.[555] Although the cause is unclear, one explanation may be that men spend more time outdoors, or that they are more likely to have comorbidities and partake in unhealthy behaviors such as smoking when compared with women. Indeed, among the 54 subjects with a medical history of CHD (Table 2.15), 41 (76%) were men in this study. Another possibility is that testosterone masks the pollutant injury making it more prone to fatal episodes.

A further limitation was their assumption that all residents were exposed to the same concentrations of pollutants without considering their spatial distribution. This exposure measurement error may widen CIs but may lead to little or no bias (i.e., Berkson error[595]).

Finally, there may be a possibility of residual confounding because of other clinical factors, which can change during a month within each subject.

This study provides further evidence to support the hypothesis that short-term exposure to outdoor air pollution exposure increases the risk of cardiac arrest in a Japanese context. Furthermore, our results suggest that SPM and ozone may impact upon hospitalization owing to cardiac arrest via different mechanisms.

INCREASED PARTICULATE AIR POLLUTION AND THE TRIGGERING OF MYOCARDIAL INFARCTION

According to Peters et al.,[334] elevated concentrations of ambient particulate air pollution have been associated with increased hospital admissions for cardiovascular disease. Whether high concentrations of ambient particles can trigger the onset of acute MI, however, remains unknown.[334] However, it is clear that chemically sensitive patients with vasculitis who are studied in a less-polluted, controlled environment have the inflamed blood vessel exacerbated by the ambient exposure of small PM.[589]

Peters interviewed 772 patients with MI in the greater Boston area between January 1995 and May 1996 as part of the Determinants of Myocardial Infarction Onset Study. The hourly concentrations of particle mass <2.5 μm ($PM_{2.5}$), carbon black, and gaseous air pollutants were measured. A case-crossover approach was used to analyze the data for evidence of triggering. The risk of MI onset increased in association with elevated concentrations of fine particles in the previous 2-hour period. In addition, a delayed response associated with 24-hour average exposure 1 day before the onset of symptoms was observed. Multivariate analyses considering both time windows jointly revealed an estimated OR of 1.48 associated with an increase of 24 μg/m^3 $PM_{2.5}$ during a 2-hour period before the onset and an OR of 1.69 for an increase of 20 μg/m^3 $PM_{2.5}$ in the 24-hour period 1 day before the onset (95% CIs: 1.09, 2.02 and 1.13, 2.34, respectively).

The present study suggests that elevated concentrations of fine particles in the air may transiently elevate the risk of MIs within a few hours and 1 day after exposure. Further studies in other locations are needed to clarify the importance of this potentially preventable trigger of MI.

Actual challenge at the EHC-Dallas has shown an adverse response (not along enough to trigger a MI) in the chemically sensitive with small-vessel vasculitis.[589]

A Massachusetts study of 100 patients who underwent cardiac defibrillation found that cardiac arrhythmias were significantly associated with higher levels of airborne NO_2, CO, and particulates.[571] Another Massachusetts study reported that higher 3-day levels of $PM_{2.5}$, CO, and SO_2 were associated with significantly higher rates of ventricular tachyarrhythmias in 203 heart patients with implanted cardioverter defibrillators.[596] Several studies have noted significantly lower HRV in humans exposed to particulate air pollution, with this effect being particularly strong in patients with diabetes, hypertension, and IHD.[597,598]

Increases in outdoor airborne carbon monoxide concentrations were found to significantly increase systolic and diastolic blood pressure in 48 healthy traffic controllers in Sao Paulo.[599] A study of 56 German males with IHD found that exposure to $PM_{2.5}$ was associated with significant decreases in T-wave amplitude on EKGs and significant increases in T-wave complexity.[600] Exposure to organic carbon was associated with significant increases in QT wave duration.[601] A Massachusetts study found that exposure to higher levels of black carbon was associated with significantly greater postexercise ST-depression in 24 elderly subjects.[602] Such ST depression is often related to ischemia of myocardial tissue.

Exposure to ambient air pollutants may also have adverse effects on the blood and blood vessels. Rabbits exposed to PM_{10} levels similar to those found in cities experienced significantly larger atherosclerotic lesions and higher levels of polymorphonuclear leukocytes as compared to control rabbits.[603] A study of 798 human adults over age 40 years in Los Angeles found that exposure to higher levels of $PM_{2.5}$ is associated with significantly greater carotid intima-media thickness (a measure of atherosclerosis).[604] Human exposure to air pollution has been linked to arterial vasoconstriction,[605] increased plasma viscosity,[606] and increased C-reactive protein.[607] This observation has been borne out at the EHC-Dallas in chemically sensitive patients who usually have vasculitis. These patients are frequently in need of O_2 and other modalities to relieve their vascular constriction.

Exposure to nanosized particles have now been shown to damage the microcirculation.[608] This exposure from diesel particles has resulted in closure of the one cell-wide microcirculation entry due to edema.[608] The microarterioles do not dilate or extract O_2 properly when exposed to pollution. Some even disappear from the tissue. This condition can result in local hypoxia to a small area in the CV system. It can cause lack of O_2 extraction with shrinking of the microvessels in the local area. If the pollutant load becomes greater, more edema occurs at many areas of the microcirculation until one sees higher levels of PvO_2 (low levels of oxygen extraction) with 20%–80% less oxygen extraction. This phenomenon results in tissue hypoxia and oxidative stress. Exposure to nanosized particles can impair the responsiveness of the very tiny blood vessels. We see elevated PvO_2 in the chemically sensitive population significantly from 35 to 80 mm Hg, the latter which becomes up to only 10% O_2 extraction. This extraction defect is one of the major changes in their physiology resulting in weakness, fatigue, and brain dysfunction with an inability to carry out routine daily tasks. An example of high PvO_2 and CS was shown in a 60-year-old white male who had severe fatigue, fibromyalgia, tachycardia, and severe atrial arrhythmia. He was totally incapacitated and could barely walk. His PvO_2 was 80 mm Hg, which is about only 10% oxygen to extract. He also had pollutant exposure resulting in smaller vessel vasculitis. He underwent O_2 therapy daily of 8 L of O_2/day for 2 constant hours. After 6 weeks, his O_2 had not decreased appreciably. He was also given 0.5 hour daily of 15 L/O_2 mm and 8 L of O_2 for 1.5 hours. After 2 hours at 8 L/mm, his PvO_2 eventually decreased and it was found to be 26 mm. His energy was dramatically elevated and also was his brain function. His vasculitis subsided as did his CS and he returned to wellness with a decrease in tachycardia and arrhythmia. Table 6.27 in Chapter 6 shows our small series of vasculitis resulting in a high PvO_2 and how these chemically sensitive patients responded well to O_2 therapy.

CHRONIC FATIGUE SYNDROME: ASSESSMENT OF INCREASED OXIDATIVE STRESS AND ALTERED MUSCLE EXCITABILITY IN RESPONSE TO INCREMENTAL EXERCISE

According to Jammes et al.,[609] the muscle response to incremental exercise is not well documented in patients suffering from CFS. They combined electrophysiological (compound-evoked muscle action potential, M-wave) and biochemical (lactic acid [LA] production, oxidative stress) measurements to assess any muscle dysfunction in response to a routine cycling exercise.

This case–control study compared 15 CFS patients to a gender-, age-, and weight-matched control group (n = 11) of healthy subjects. All subjects performed an incremental cycling exercise continued until exhaustion.

They measured the oxygen uptake (VO_2), HR, systemic blood pressure, percutaneous O_2 saturation (SpO_2), M-wave recording from vastus lateralis, and venous blood sampling allowing measurements of pH (pHv), PO_2 (PvOs), LA, and three markers of the oxidative stress (thiobarbituric acid reactive substances [TBARS], reduced glutathione [GSH], and reduced ascorbic acid [RAA]).

Compared with control in CFS patients, (1) the slope of VO_2 versus work load relationship did not differ from control subjects and there was a tendency for an accentuated PvO_2 fall at the same exercise intensity, indicating an increased oxygen uptake by the exercising muscles; (2) the HR and blood pressure responses to exercise did not vary; (3) the anaerobic pathways were not accentuated; (4) the exercise-induced oxidative stress was enhanced with early changes in TBARS and RAA and enhanced maximal RAA consumption; and (5) the M-wave duration markedly increased during the recovery period.

The response of CFS patients to incremental exercise associates a lengthened and accentuated oxidative stress together with marked alterations of the muscle membrane excitability. These two objective signs of muscle dysfunction are sufficient to explain muscle pain and postexertional malaise reported by patients.

AIR POLLUTION AND CARDIOVASCULAR DISEASE BASIC MECHANISM

Ischemia–Reperfusion Phenomena

There is mounting evidence that environmental pollutants can trigger cardiovascular dysfunction. We have known this for 30+ years but now the basic science is in the thinking of some clinicians. They are beginning to see the adverse effects of pollutants on the cardiovascular system.

IHD is a leading cause of morbidity and mortality in the United States and other parts of the world. Despite therapeutic breakthroughs over the past decades such as coronary bypass, percutaneous coronary intervention, antiplatelet and antithrombotic therapies, and angioplasty, the prevalence of IHDs remains extremely high and constitutes a devastating factor for heart failure.[610,611] This devastating prevalence is usually due to microvascular dysfunction. Among various therapeutic strategies of IHD, enormous efforts have been made to limit ischemia/reperfusion (I/R) injury, which occurs when the ischemic myocardium is reperfused with oxygen and substrate-rich blood, which paradoxically worsens heart function.[611] This is often due to relief in vasospasm reinstitution of O_2 extraction. Ischemic myocardium, with nutrient and oxygen deprivation and buildup of ROS, uses glycolysis as the primary source of metabolic energy. As a consequence, metabolic acidosis, hyperkalemia, and Ca^{2+} overload develop in cardiomyocytes after coronary artery occlusion or glucose mandated lack of O_2 extraction, leading not only to cardiomyocyte apoptosis during the acute phase but also to delayed adverse myocardial remodeling, which further compromises cardiac function.[611] Therefore, limiting I/R-induced myocardial ROS accumulations and apoptosis benefits both short- and long-term survival and quality of life. Although the mechanism responsible for I/R-induced cardiac abnormalities has been focused largely on necrosis and type I (apoptotic) programmed cell death,[611] an intriguing and provocative paradigm has emerged recently that highlights a unique role for deregulated macroautophagy (hereafter referred to as autophagy) in the heart that may render cardiomyocytes more prone to I/R injury and long-term postinfarction cardiac remodeling.[610,612]

It has been perceived that autophagy induced by ischemic preconditioning is essential for cardio-protection. To this end, new and innovative strategies to maintain or restore myocardial autophagy homeostasis and its attendant cardiomyocyte survival have been the subject of intensive investigation. This condition occurs to a milder degree in the periphery resulting in painful weakness and fatigue, which chemically sensitive patients frequently develop after a pollutant exposure. This pollutant-induced vascular spasm or small blood vessel leak usually results in the symptoms induced in the chemically sensitive.

According to Zhang,[613] autophagy is a tightly regulated, lysosome-dependent catabolic process responsible for turnover of long-lived proteins and intracellular structures that are damaged or malfunctioning.[614,615] The evolutionarily conserved bulk degradation process is turned on when cells experience stress, including nutrient and energy deprivation, which often occurs in chemically sensitive patients. The autophagic pathway consists of four distinct but consecutive steps: (1) initiation, (2) formation of autophagosomes (i.e., the double-membrane structures that encircle cargo and debris of damaged cytosolic constituents), (3) generation of autophagolysosomes via docking and fusion with lysosomes, and finally (4) degradation of sequestered cargo. The sequestration of cytoplasmic cargo such as long-lived proteins, damaged organelles, and protein aggregates into the double-membrane vesicle autophagosomes occurs before fusion with lysosomes for degradation of its contents by acidic hydrolases. Although physiological levels of autophagy are essential for mitochondrial function, cell survival, cell function, and excessive activation of autophagy can be detrimental, leading ultimately to autophagic cell death. Recent findings identified an important role for autophagy in the pathogenesis of human diseases, in particular heart diseases, implicating the therapeutic potential of autophagy regulation against heart anomalies.[614,615] In light of the indispensable role of autophagy for cardiac as well as peripheral homeostasis, recent attention has focused on understanding the role of autophagy regulation in I/R injury.

It has been demonstrated that autophagy seems to play a paradoxical role in I/R injury. In ischemia, induction of autophagy via AMP kinase is protective, whereas reperfusion stimulates autophagy with Beclin-1 upregulation to compromise cardiac cell survival and function.[612,616] This is in line with the observation that preischemic autophagy induction (e.g., by chloramphenicol succinate) limits MI in swine hearts. In addition, cardioprotection of delayed preconditioning by sevoflurane, a general anesthetic, is mediated by upregulation of autophagy. On the other hand, autophagy inhibition has been demonstrated to be responsible for the protective properties of mitochondrial aldehyde dehydrogenase 2 and chemokine CXCL16 against reperfusion injury.[612] Many chemically sensitives are sensitive to formaldehyde and may have problems generating enough mitochondrial aldehyde dehydrogenase to combat the formaldehyde generated with the peripheral ischemic from the microcirculation spasm and lack of O_2 extraction. This dual regulatory paradigm of autophagy in the ischemia and reperfusion phases may underscore the homeostatic and drug intervention machinery for I/R heart injury. Further evidence indicates that I/R injury impairs autophagosome clearance (autophagy flux) mediated in part through an ROS-induced decline in lysosome-associated membrane protein-2 and upregulation of the autophagy initiation protein Beclin-1, leading to the ultimate cardiomyocyte death.[617] Recently, a number of pharmaceutical therapies targeting I/R injury have been designed to orchestrate multiple protein complexes and signaling pathways in autophagy. For instance, sevoflurane has been shown to offer cardio-protection through ROS-mediated upregulation of autophagy in I/R.[618] On the contrary, in vitro evidence suggested that α-lipoic acid protects H9C2 myoblasts against hypoxia/reoxygenation injury through suppression of autophagy.[619] This substance often helps the chemically sensitive possibly through this mechanism. Lipoic acid 100–200 mg often gives chemically sensitive patients clearer thinking and more energy.

The precise role of autophagy regulation contributing to cell survival and death in ischemic hearts remains controversial. Xie and colleagues[620] report that suberoylanilide hydroxamic acid (SAHA; vorinostat), a histone deacetylase (HDAC) inhibitor approved by the Food and Drug Administration for cancer treatment, attenuated myocardial reperfusion injury in rabbits. These results revealed that

SAHA reduced infarct size and partially rescued systolic function when administered either before surgery or at the time of reperfusion. SAHA was found to facilitate autophagic flux in the infarct border zone in rabbit myocardium and in mice harboring a red fluorescent protein–free fluorescent protein–LC3 transgene. In cultured myocytes subjected to I/R, SAHA overtly alleviated cell death, the effect of which was correlated with increased autophagy. The permissive role of autophagy in SAHA-related beneficial effects was consolidated by the mitigation of SAHA efficacy through RNAi knockdown of autophagy genes Atg7 and Atg5. These findings have great clinical relevance because the plasma SAHA levels were similar to those achieved in cancer patients.[620] This work has unveiled a new paradigm for the clinical utility of HDAC inhibitors and autophagy regulators in IHDs. A plethora of studies have demonstrated proven cardioprotective benefits of HDAC inhibitors in models of myocardial stress, including cardiac hypertrophy I/R and heart failure.[621–623] In particular, trichostatin A, a class I and II HDAC inhibitor structurally homologous to SAHA, reduced myocardial infarct size up to 50%.[624] HDAC inhibition caused a dramatic increase in phosphorylation of p38 and p38 activity in the heart.[624] Of note, HDAC inhibitors can be delivered as late as 1 hour after an ischemic insult and can achieve a similar degree of infarct size reduction using pretreatment, indicating the suitability of HDAC inhibitors to treat MI at the time of percutaneous coronary intervention. Although discrepancies exist in disease mechanisms in animal models relative to the human case, these data clearly show that facilitated autophagy is required for HDAC inhibition–induced protection against I/R injury.[620] Given the recent therapeutic promises using HDAC inhibitors in ischemic and hypertrophic heart diseases,[621,622,625,626] the finding that SAHA rescues I/R heart injury through modulating autophagy flux is of great clinical importance. Interestingly, a number of cardioprotective agents such as the angiotensin II receptor blocker *valsartan* may also elicit protection against I/R injury through autophagy induction. Valsartan preconditioning is believed to facilitate autophagy induction via an Akt/mammalian target of rapmycin/S6K-mediated mechanism, although the underlying molecular mechanism behind SAHA-induced autophagy flux remains unclear at this time.

NEW HORIZON OF HDAC INHIBITORS IN HEART DISEASES

Histone acetylation participates in the regulation of transcription by promoting a more relaxed chromatin structure necessary for transcriptional activation. Many proteins are regulated by reversible acetylation of ε-amino groups of lysine residues. Reversible protein acetylation is controlled by enzymes that either attach (histone acetyltransferases) or remove (HDACs) acetyl groups.[623] With the removal of acetyl groups from an ε-N-acetyl lysine amino acid on a histone to restore the positive charge to lysine residues, HDAC proteins may also be referred to as lysine deacetylases to more precisely recapitulate their function rather than targets.[626–628] Small-molecule HDAC inhibitors, acting specifically or broadly on one or more of the 4 HDACs and on nonhistone targets, are currently being tested for oncological indications.[626–628]

Gene deletion and overexpression studies have unveiled important functions of HDACs in a number of nononcological settings such as respiratory stress, inflammation, cardiac remodeling, apoptosis, necrosis, metabolism, contractility, and fibrosis.[621,625–628] HDACs have received attention as a potential new target for the treatment of heart diseases. Small-molecule HDAC inhibitors have demonstrated efficacy in animal models of heart failure.[623] For instance, MPTOEP14, a novel HDAC inhibitor, displayed remarkable HDAC 1,2 and isoenzyme suppressive properties, improved cardiac contractility, and retarded cardiac remodeling in isoproterenol-induced dilated cardiomyopathy.[629] Several explanations for MPTOEO14-induced beneficial effects have been suggested, including inhibition of migration and proliferation of cardiac fibroblasts, as well as cardiac fibrosis, decreased levels of atrial natriuretic peptide, angiotensin II type I receptor, TGF-β, and Ca^{2+}/calmodulin-dependent protein kinase IIδ.[629] Along the same lines, HDAC inhibition may retard cardiac remodeling and improve ventricular dysfunction caused by pressure overload.[623,630] Cao and colleagues[625] recently reported that the prototypical HDAC inhibitor trichostatin A attenuated both load- and agonist-induced hypertrophic myocardial growth through the inhibition of autophagy rather than facilitating autophagy as reported for SAHA.[620] Although these findings appear to be contradictory, it is imperative that the HDAC inhibitors strive to restore autophagy homeostasis through inhibition of excessive autophagy flux under pressure overload[625] or reactivation of autophagy flux beneficial to infarct boarder zone.[620] Although Xie and colleagues did not examine ROS production in ischemic hearts treated with or without SAHA, it is possible that oxidative stress may mediate SAHA-related beneficial stimulation of autophagy flux. NADPH oxidase–mediated oxidative stress is well known to stimulate autophagic flux during myocardial I/R. HDAC inhibition has been shown to promote the accumulation of ROS. However, how ROS regulate autophagy is not fully understood.

Considering the current controversy on the role of adaptive or maladaptive autophagy in cardiac pathology,[615] it is pertinent to better understand conditions in which autophagy should be inhibited or activated not only to best preserve cardiac homeostasis, but also to optimize therapy (such as the drug efficacy and resistance for HDAC inhibitors). Furthermore, it is noteworthy that the overall efficacy of HDAC inhibition is determined by the pleiotropic salutary actions in various cell types and pathophysiological processes, many of which (e.g., anti-inflammation and NADPH oxidase) may be autophagy independent.

HDACs are pivotal epigenetic regulatory enzymes with the ability to deacetylate nucleosome histones and nonhistone proteins and to elicit significant pathological effects in tumor growth and cardiovascular diseases. It is clear that lipoic acid will help the milder autophagy phenomena seen in chemically sensitive patients if it is present in the periphery. However, it may be buffered with food or bicarbonate in order not to have acidic damage. Autophagy must be recognized in the periphery to combat reprofusion when the microcirculation opens after O_2 treatment.

CLASSIFICATION: VASCULITIS

Vasculitis can be classified by the cause, the location, the type of vessel, or the size of vessel (Figure 2.22).

1. Large blood vessels: Temporal arteritis, Takayasu vasculitis, CS (Figure 2.23)
2. Medium blood vessels: Polyarteritis nodosa, Kawasaki's disease, Buerger's disease, CS
3. Small blood vessels: ANCA associated: Wegener's granulomatosis (WG), Churg–Strauss, microscopic polyangiitis, drug induced, chemical induced; non-ANCA associated: immune complex defects, Henoch–Schonlein purpura (HSP), CTD, cryoglobulinemic vasculitis, hypersensitive vasculitis, paraneoplastic vasculitis, inflammatory bowel disease

In chemically sensitive patients, all types and sizes of vascular inflammation can occur. However, the triggering agents are not the same. These responses can be predominantly a variety of different cell types. They can be eosinophilic, neutrophilic, or lymphocytic. Many vasculitis syndromes have names but the small-vessel lymphocytic vasculitis seems to be predominant in the chemically sensitive.

WEGENER'S GRANULOMATOSIS

WG commonly has the classic triad of involvement of the upper respiratory tract, lungs, and kidneys. Upper respiratory tract signs and symptoms include sinusitis, nasal ulcers, otitis media, or hearing loss. Upper respiratory tract signs and symptoms are seen in 70% of patients and pulmonary infiltrates. Serum antiprotease 3-ANCA (cANCA) is positive in 75%–90%, although 20% may have positive pANCA. Open lung biopsy is the most definitive diagnostic test. Sinus biopsy is diagnostic in only 30% of cases because inflammatory findings are often nonspecific and renal biopsy is also relatively nonspecific (Figure 2.24).

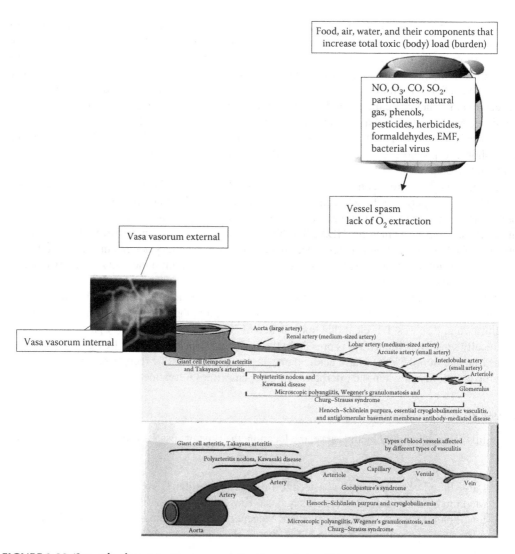

FIGURE 2.22 (See color insert.) Environmentally triggered vasculitis.

Takayasu
vasculitis diagnosis test

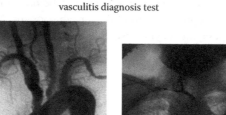

Angiography showing Takayasu's arteritis

FIGURE 2.23 Environmentally triggered vasculitis.

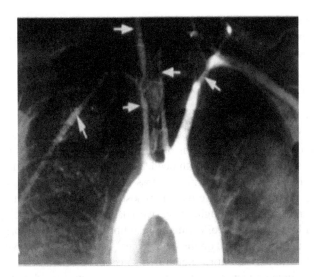

FIGURE 2.24 Wegener's granulomatosis.

MICROSCOPIC POLYANGIITIS

Microscopic polyangiitis is the most common ANCA-associated small-vessel vasculitis, and is characterized by the presence of ANCA and few or no immune deposits in the involved vessels. The kidneys are the most commonly affected organs in 90% of patients who have this type of vasculitis. Patients present with variable combinations of renal manifestations, palpable purpura, abdominal pain, cough, and hemoptysis. Most patients have positive MPO-ANCA (pANCA), although PR3-ANCA (cANCA) may also be present in 40% of patients. The most common age of onset is 40–60 years and more common in men.

ENVIRONMENTAL FACTORS ARE IMPORTANT IN PRIMARY SYSTEMIC VASCULITIS

Lane et al.[631] investigated the association between primary systemic vasculitis (PSV) and environmental risk factors.

A total of 75 PSV cases and 273 controls (220 nonvasculitis, 19 secondary vasculitis, and 34 asthma controls) were interviewed using a structured questionnaire. Factors investigated were social class, occupational and residential history, smoking, pets, allergies, vaccinations, medications, hepatitis, TBC, and farm exposure in the year before symptom onset (index year). The Standard Occupational Classification 2000 and job-exposure matrices were used to assess occupational silica, solvent, and metal exposure. Stepwise multiple logistic regression was used to calculate the OR and 95% CI adjusted for potential confounders. Total PSV, subgroups (47 WG, 12 microscopic polyangiitis, 16 Churg–Strauss syndrome [CSS]), and antineutrophil cytoplasmic antibody (ANCA)-positive cases were compared with control groups.

Farming in the index year was significantly associated with PSV (OR 2.3 [95% CI: 1.2–4.6]), WG (2.7 [1.2–5.8]), MPA (6.3 [1.9–21.6]), and perinuclear ANCA (pANCA) (4.3 [1.5–12.7]). Farming during working lifetime was associated with PSV (2.2 [1.2–3.8]) and with WB (2.7 [1.3–5.7]). Significant associations were found for high occupational silica exposure in the index year (with PSV 3.0 [1–8.4], with CSS 5.6 [1.3–23.5], and with ANCA 4.9 [1.3–18.6]), high occupational solvent exposure in the index year (with PSV 3.4 [0.9–12.5], with WB 4.8 [1.2–19.8], and with classic ANCA [cANCA] 3.9 [1.6–9.5]), high occupational solvent exposure during working lifetime (with PSV 2.7 [1.1–6.6], with WG 3.4 [1.3–8.9], and with cANCA 3.3 [1.0–10.8]), drug allergy (with PSV 3.6 [1.8–7.0], with WG 4.0 [1.8–8.7], and with cANCA 4.7 [1.9–11.7]), and allergy overall (with PSV 2.2 [1.2–3.9], with WG 2.7 [1.4–5.7]). No other significant associations were found.

A significant association between farming and PSV has been identified for the first time. This is probably due to the repeated exposure to pesticides and herbicides as well as solvents. Results also support previously reported associations with silica, solvents, and allergy.

EXPOSURE TO ORGANIC SOLVENTS: VASCULITIS

Exposure to Organic Solvents: Report of Two Cases

Braufbar et al.,[632] in the article, present case studies of two patients with systemic vasculitis and prior occupational exposure to OSs. A 44-year-old male electrician, employed as a building control panels operator for 23 months, presented with headaches and blurred vision, fatigue, night sweats, tingling sensations in legs and arms, intermittent loss of balance, and joint pain and sores on his legs, severely limiting his ambulation. He had an exposure history of inhalation and skin contact with chemical fumes and vapors throughout the workday. The patient developed diplopia, with headaches and partial loss of vision. Following a presumptive diagnosis of large-vessel vasculitis, most probably Takayasu arteritis, based on the involvement of the aorta and large vessels, the patient was started on steroids with partial improvement in his vision.

Another 51-year-old male painter, a construction worker, was presented with purpuric skin rash, intermittent abdominal pain, anorexia and weight loss, and progressive weakness of his left hand and both legs. Following a diagnosis of systemic vasculitis, the patient was treated with prednisone and cyclophosphamide. He had rapid improvement of abdominal pain, skin rash, all laboratory measures of inflammation, hematuria, and proteinuria. At the EHC-Dallas, the patients would have been treated with nutrition to aid the detoxification mechanisms, injection of the neutralizing doses of the toxics and oxygen therapy. This has always helped in clearing the inflammation and healed the blood vessels.

Case of MPO-ANCA-Related Vasculitis after Asbestos Exposure with Progression of a Renal Lesion after Improvement of Interstitial Pneumonia

Inoue et al.[633] reported on a 72-year-old woman who was admitted complaining of productive cough. She had worked for an asbestos factory for 20 years. She was positive for MPO-ANCA. The chest HRCT showed interstitial pneumonia without any UIP pattern. A specimen obtained by video-assisted thoracoscopic lung biopsy revealed chronic interstitial pneumonia associated with an asbestos body. Although the interstitial pneumonia improved after the administration of a corticosteroid and an immunosuppressive agent, hematuria and renal dysfunction developed about 9 months later. The serum MPO-ANCA titer was elevated and the renal biopsy specimen revealed the presence of vasculitis. As the interstitial pneumonia improved after this treatment, the correct diagnosis may have been, not asbestosis, but MPO-ANCA-related interstitial.

Silicon Exposure and Vasculitis

According to Tervaert et al.,[634] a combination of risk factors is involved in susceptibility to a primary or secondary form of vasculitis. Many forms of vasculitis are probably genetically based but environmentally triggered. This review discusses currently available evidence for a pathophysiologic role of one possible environmental trigger, silica. Since 1960, several patients with pulmonary silicosis have been described, which developed pauci-immune necrotizing crescentic glomerulonephritis (Figure 2.25), that is, with either completely negative immunofluorescence findings or nonspecific granular IgM or C3 deposits along the capillary wall. Recently, it was reported that these patients have ANCAs that are in most cases directed to myeloperoxidase. Further, patients with pulmonary silicosis may develop microscopic polyangiitis, the syndrome of lung hemorrhage and nephritis, or WG. To further substantiate the relation between silicon exposure and renal failure or vasculitis, several case–control studies have been reported. Exposure to silicon-containing compounds was found to be related to chronic renal failure (CRF) (OR, 1.7:2.5) or vasculitis (OR, 6.5:14.0). The mechanisms by which silica may induce ANCA-associated

Necrotizing glomerulonephritis   Normal glomerulus

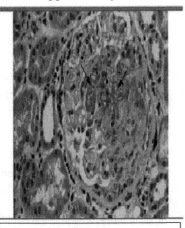   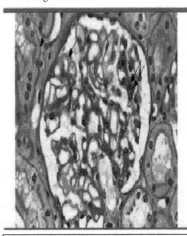

Light micrograph showing fresh segnencalro necrotizing lesions with bright red fibrin ceposizon (arrows). A necrotizing glomerulonephrtis can be seen in a rarity of inflammation disorders including vasculitis and lupus nephritis. The latter is prominent immune complex deposition, which is generally absent in vasculitis.

Light micrograph of a normal glomerulus. There are only 1 or 2 cells per capillary tuft, the capillary lumens are open, the thickness of the glomerular capillary wall (long arrows) is similar to that of the nodular basement membranes (short arrows), and the mesangial cells and mesangial matrix are located in the central or stalk regions of the tuft (arrows).

FIGURE 2.25   Necrotizing glomerulonephritis and normal glomerulus. (Courtesy of Helmut Rencke, MD.)

glomerulonephritis or vasculitis are not well known. Silicon-containing compounds have a pronounced adjuvant effect on immune responses, and silica particles are potent stimulators of lymphocytes and monocytes of macrophages. Further, silica may induce apoptosis of monocytes of macrophages and possible neutrophils. In conclusion, at present there is ample evidence that occupational exposure to silicon-containing compounds is related to the development of ANCA-associated glomerulonephritis and vasculitis, and silica is one of the first well-documented environmental triggers in these diseases.

ROLE OF METALS IN AUTOIMMUNE VASCULITIS: EPIDEMIOLOGICAL AND PATHOGENIC STUDY

According to Stratta et al.,[635] a possible relationship between silica (Si) exposure and ANCA-associated vasculitis has been reported. Furthermore, TBC has been frequently described in patients with silicosis, and TBC infection shares with ANCA-associated vasculitis the formation of granulomas. Therefore, an intriguing network including silica vasculitis, TBC, and ANCA might be hypothesized. The aim of this work was to further investigate these correlations using both epidemiological and pathogenic approaches.

Study I: Epidemiological Study

A case–control study to compare the occupational histories of 31 cases of biopsy-proven vasculitis (18 pauci-immune crescentic glomerulonephritis, 9 microscopic polyangitis, 4 WG) with those of 58 age-, sex-, and residence-matched controls (affected by other kidney diseases) was performed. Occupational health physicians designed an appropriate questionnaire in order to evaluate a widespread of exposures and calculate their entity by the product of intensity × frequency × duration.

Study II: Tuberculosis Association

A case–control study to evaluate the frequency of a previous history of TBC in 45 patients with vasculitis and 45 controls was performed.

Study III: ANCA Positivity

A case–control study to evaluate the presence of ANCA was performed by testing blood samples of 64 people with previous professional exposure and 65 sex/age-matched patients hospitalized in a General Medicine Unit. Furthermore, the same evaluation was made in a pilot study in 16 patients with ongoing or previous TBC.

Study IV: Experimental Study

The oxygen free radicals (OFRs) and IL-12 production (both involved in the pathogenesis of vasculitis) from human phagocytic cells stimulated with an amorphous (diatomaceous earth) and a crystalline (quartz form of Si) at the doses of 10 and 100 μg/mL were evaluated.

Study 1: A positive history of exposure to Si was significantly more present in cases ($14/31 = 45\%$) than in controls ($14/58 = 24\%$, $p = 0.04$, OR = 2.4) and no other significant exposure association was found (including asbestos, mineral oil, formaldehyde, diesel and welding fumes, grain and wood dust, leather, solvents, fungicides, bitumen, lead, and paint).

Study 2: Pat TBC infection was significantly more present in patients with vasculitis ($12/45 = 26\%$) than in controls ($4/45 = 8\%$, $p < 0.05$).

Study 3: ANCA was present in 2/64 exposed people (vs. 0.65 controls, $p =$ NS) and 0.16 patients with TBC.

Study 4: Both amorphous and crystalline Si forms represented a stimulus for OFR and IL-12 production, but quartz resulted as a greater inductor.

They conclude that Si exposure might be a risk factor for ANCA-associated vasculitis, possibly enhancing endothelial damage by phagocyte generation of OFRs and Th1 differentiation by an excessive IL-12 phagocyte production. Frequency of TBC was significantly higher in vasculitis patients. ANCA was not frequent in the preliminary examination of people with previous profession exposure or patients with TBC, but the number of samples evaluated is too small to allow conclusions.

Henoch–Schonlein Purpura Following Thiram Exposure

According to Duell and Morton,[636] HSP is an uncommon, nonthrombocytopenic hypersensitivity vasculitis that is often idiopathic, but may be induced by infectious agents, drugs, foods, environmental chemicals, or insect bites. To our knowledge, they report the first recognized case of HSP following exposure to the widely used industrial and agricultural agent, tetramethylthiuram disulfide. Few reports of HSP or other vasculitis resulting from exposure to structurally similar compounds are available. Despite the widespread use of tetramethylthiuram disulfide, many cases of exposure may remain unrecognized, resulting in a subsequent failure to properly identify sequelae.

Role of Nitric Oxide in Mercury Chloride–Induced Vasculitis in the Brown Norway Rat

According to Nakamura,[637] nitric oxide (NO) is an important factor in tissue trauma, but its detailed role in the pathogenesis remains unknown. In autoimmune vasculitis, it is possible that NO is one of the factors underlying tissue trauma and induction of autoimmune antibodies. To study its role on an animal model using mercury chloride ($HgCl_2$), brown Norway rats (BN rats) were given five injections of $HgCl_2$, each 1 mg/kg, over 10 days. Vasculitis and production of some autoimmune antibodies developed after $HgCl_2$ injections. Urine nitrate/nitrite, metabolic production of NO, was produced in advance of the production of other autoimmune antibodies. To elucidate the role of NO, NG-nitro-L-arginine methyl ester (L-NAME), which is a nitric oxide synthase (NOS) inhibitor, was given in addition to $HgCl_2$, at their daily dose of 30 mg/kg. There was no difference in production

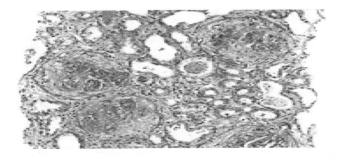

FIGURE 2.26 Biopsy of kidney.

of autoimmune antibodies between this group and the control group, but urine protein excretion was suppressed in the $HgCl_2$ + L-NAME group (p < 0.001). By immunohistochemical study, inducible NOS was positive in small vessels and mesangial cells in rat kidney. They conclude that in this animal model, overproduction of NO leads to the production of autoimmune antibodies and inhibition of NOS production ameliorates proteinuria. These results suggest that NO plays an important role in the induction of renal injury in the rat model of autoimmune vasculitis.

GOODPASTURE SYNDROME

GPS, also known as Goodpasture's disease (antiglomerular basement antibody disease, or anti-GBM disease), is a rare autoimmune disease in which antibodies attack the lungs and kidneys, leading to bleeding from the lungs and to kidney failure; exposure to OSs (e.g., chloroform) or hydrocarbons as well as metal dust inhalation can also cause this syndrome (Figure 2.26).

CHURG–STRAUSS SYNDROME

It has three phases: allergic rhinitis and asthma, eosinophilic infiltrative disease resembling pneumonia, and systemic small-vessel vasculitis with granulomatous inflammation. The vasculitic phase usually develops within 3 years of the onset of asthma. Almost all patients have more than 10% eosinophils in the blood. Coronary arteritis and myocarditis are the principal causes of morbidity and mortality (Figure 2.27).

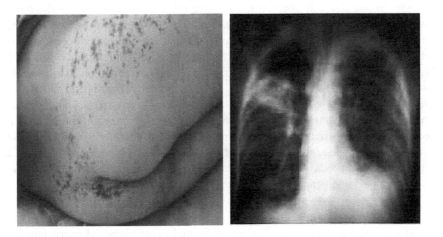

FIGURE 2.27 Churg–Strauss syndrome. (Adapted from EHC-Dallas.)

ENVIRONMENTALLY TRIGGERED LARGE-VESSEL VASCULITIS

Nonarteriosclerotic inflammatory disease of large-caliber arteries results in acute or chronic spasm and eventually, occlusion in some patients. Depending on collateral circulation, severe complications can follow, with a spectrum of symptoms ranging from organ necrosis to transient signs of ischemia.

Occlusion, when it occurs, is preceded by recurrent vasospasm with resultant transient ischemia. Although a few specific named clinical entities such as Takayasu disease and a giant cell arteritis have been delineated, there appears to be another category of inflammation. This is with usually monocytic infiltration, which results in occlusion in some patients but produces only severe vasospasm in most patients. The large-vessel involvement appears to be a part of a spectrum of environmentally triggered vascular disease characterized by acneiform lesions, spontaneous bruising and/or purpura, petechia, and peripheral and periorbital edema in addition to the vascular spasm. This inflammatory syndrome usually occurs within the first 40 years of life but can occur any time. Earlier publications by senior author Rea[589] have shown a direct cause–effect relationship between a similar inflammation of the veins and small arteries and incitants in the patient's environment. Unfortunately, in this series, because of the size of blood vessels involved, biopsies could only be done at the time of amputation or on the cutaneous manifestations, which accompany some patients with this syndrome. Therefore, the complete pathology remains unclear.

The first section of this work will present specific cases of large-vessel involvement which aroused the author's suspicions of environmental triggering. The second section reports on a prospective, controlled study designed to determine whether environmental factors contribute to large-vessel vasculitis as they do to small-vessel vasculitis.

Case Reports

Case 1

A 26-year-old paperhanger developed a cyanotic, pulseless right lower extremity rapidly progressing to no pulses in either leg. An arteriogram showed normal-sized vessels with a rise of severe spasm. Intra-arterial papaverine opened the vessels to normal caliber for 5 minutes but then spasm returned. Oral and intravenous vasodilators did not relieve the spasms nor did intravenous heparin. Hospitalization in a controlled environment (EHC-Dallas) alleviated the cyanosis, with femoral, popliteal, dorsalis pedis, and posterior tibial pulses returning to normal. Challenge with food caused no problems nor did ingested chemicals; however, inhalation challenge with pesticide used in the wallpaper paste that he used daily reproduced the symptoms and resulted in the patient's changing jobs.

Case 2

A 43-year-old white female underwent sudden onset of arterial occlusion of her left leg. Eventually, amputation was performed after an attempted bypass was unsuccessful. Microscopic sections of the leg showed that a nonarteriosclerotic fibrosis surrounded by severe inflammation had occluded all arteries. Significant past history included two pulmonary emboli, recurrent phlebitis, sinusitis, recurrent gastrointestinal upset, and sensitivity to odors. Six months later, her peripheral pulses disappeared and her remaining leg became cyanotic. An arteriogram showed severe spasm and the patient developed rest pain refractory to antispasmodics. Limb loss appeared imminent. Institutionalization in a relatively particle- and fume-free controlled environment (EHC-Dallas) for 5 days resulted in restitution of 4+ dorsalis pedis pulse, normal color, and function of the limb without problems. Challenge with numerous individual foods and chemicals entirely reproduced the abovementioned symptoms. The patient is now in environmental control 3 years after diagnosis, with symptom-free leg.

Case 3

A 45-year-old ex-chocolate factory worker was admitted complaining of excruciating leg pain that rendered him unable to walk. Eleven years prior to the current admission, the patient had experienced an episode of leg pain, chest pain, and shortness of breath, which had necessitated hospitalization. Findings indicated heart failure accompanied by pulmonary infiltration and eosinophilia. Steroids were required to bring the situation under control. Eventually, vessel biopsy revealed an inflammation, compatible with periarteritis nodosa or Wegener granuloma. The patient had to retire from his job because of his excruciating leg pain. For 11 years, he had required morphine injections (grains ¼ every 4 hours) for pain relief. He had not been able to walk extensively for 5 years and had developed paralysis of his left foot.

On admission to the Environmental Unit (EHC-Dallas), he exhibited an inability to walk more than a few steps. His left foot was pulseless, the three smaller toes were paralyzed, and the patient could not dorsiflex his feet. Light touch elicited extreme hyperesthesia with excruciating pain. During the first 5 days of environmental control (after removal of all medications), severe withdrawal symptoms occurred. However, on the sixth day, peripheral pulses were noted, the toe paralysis disappeared, the color returned, and he was able to walk without problems. No morphine was required after the fourth day. Random challenge of single, less chemically contaminated foods demonstrated the following sequential reactions:

1. 0 minute—Immediate repulsion to odor with nausea
2. 5 minutes—Itching in throat
3. 35 minutes
   a. General malaise
   b. Arms and legs aching
   c. Blueness of hands
   d. Stomach bloating
4. 45 minutes
   a. Vomiting
   b. Blueness of hands and feet
5. 50 minutes—Pulse decrease in left foot, unable to walk, toe paralyzed, hyperesthesia

Five foods gave similar reproducible sequential reactions. Chocolate was the worst offender. Challenge with 20 other foods resulted in no reactions. Inhaled odor of cigarette smoke produced symptoms similar to those of the reactive ingested foods.

Case 4

A 41-year-old vocational nurse reported a 20-year history of vague complaints associated with fatigue and mild muscle aches. A 2-year history of near-incapacitating, lower extremity arterial spasm resulted in absent dorsalis pedis and posterior tibial pulses. Incapacitating left gastrocnemius spasms, lasting several days, developed and required constant administration of Demerol and an antispasmodic to relieve the unrelenting spasm. The patient had a history of sensitivity to several chemical fumes, such as chlorine, perfume, pesticide, and cigar smoke, and to various drugs. This history and clinical course suggested environmentally triggered disease. The patient was placed in the Environmental Control Unit (EHC-Dallas) and, after 6 days without food or medication, all signs and symptoms cleared. When safe water was found, the patient had challenge in ingestions of single, less chemically contaminated foods. A typical example of the sequence of events during reactions was as follows: two bites of squash produced immediate vomiting, then generalized aching and malaise, and within 5 minutes, aching of legs with spasm and loss of the dorsalis pedis and posterior bibial pulses occurred. In the next 5 minutes, severe left pedal and gastrocnemius muscle spasm occurred with excruciating pain that required intravenous sodium bicarbonate and Demerol for relief. By the next 12 hours, noncontact cutaneous bruising would occur. The muscle and vessel spasm lasted for a total of 24–144 hours. Twelve different foods reproduced this sequential symptomatology.

Twenty other foods tested were safe and could be eaten without problems. One meal of chemically contaminated food, previously tested safe in less contaminated form, reproduced the above-listed reactions. When inhaled separately, the odors of 12 chemicals to which the patient was exposed daily during her work resulted in a similar reaction sequence.

Injections of 0.05 cc of the increments of 1:5 dilutions of the aqueous extract of No. 7 dilution of cotton linters, No. 7 dilution of pine terpene, and No. 3 dilution of histamine were each given intracutaneously on separate occasions, and reproduced the vascular and gastrocnemius spasm.

PROSPECTIVE STUDY MATERIAL AND METHODS

Twelve consecutive highly selected patients—aged 22–45, from the senior author's cardiovascular surgery practice—with large-vessel vasculitis (nonarteriosclerotic) of unknown etiology were studied. These were characterized by loss of peripheral pulses, cyanosis, or symptoms of the extremity from arterial spasm and mild periorbital and digital edema, usually having a few acneiform lesions, spontaneous bruising, and/or petechia.

Lifelong ecological histories were taken of all patients by Randolph's method[638] to determine the presence or absence of other symptoms of the environmental maladaptation syndrome. Specific symptom complexes or diseases (of unknown etiology) involving the smooth muscle or immune system were searched for and recorded.

All patients were admitted to the Environmental Unit for a minimum of 16 days during the course of testing and treatment. All patients were required to remove all hair sprays, cosmetics, perfumes, and polyester clothing before entering the room and to wear less chemically treated 100% cotton. All medications, including anticoagulants, were discontinued as soon as the patients were admitted. No medications were given during the stay in the unit, with the exception of oral or intravenous bicarbonate of soda and inhaled oxygen.

The Environmental Unit (EHC-Dallas) was constructed by the method of Randolph,[638] as described by the senior author in previous papers. This resulted in extraordinary control of particulate and odor/outgasing of the air. Once the patients reached the symptom-free basic state, they acted as their own controls. Arteriograms were performed on patients before their period of detoxification.

Pulses, blood pressure, temperature, color of extremities, and tenderness were monitored every 4 hours. Also, signs and symptoms related to the area of the body perfused by the involved artery(ies) were noted. After the patient stabilized in a basal state, free of signs and symptoms (including return of pulses, a HR below 80 beats per minute, ability to sleep all night and loss of hunger), challenge tests with single, less chemically contaminated source foods were begun. The food was selected individually and randomly for each patient. Only one food was tested at each meal and not more than four food sources were tested per day during the period in environmental control. Pulse rates were recorded 5 minutes before and at 20-, 40-, and 60-minute intervals after meals. ECGs were taken with the onset of any arrhythmia. All signs and symptoms were recorded. Testing of the next food was not begun until all reactions had subsided. Positive foods were rechallenged two more times to confirm sensitivity. In some patients, double-blind challenge through a nasogastric tube was done. After totally tolerated foods were found, the patients were retested with these same nonreactive foods, but this time obtained from the commercial market. The commercial forms of these foods had been contaminated by synthetic sprays, herbicides, preservatives, artificial colorings and sweeteners, gas, and plastic wrappings or other additives included during their production and processing. These items were then cooked on natural gas stoves in synthetic cookware. Individual and accumulative reactions after one to six such consecutive meals were observed and recorded.

Testing of chemical odors was done in the following manner: Each patient was given a timed exposure, from 1 to 60 minutes, to the flames of natural gas. Double-blind exposures to the ambient dose fumes of formaldehyde, cigarette smoke, perfume, pine-scented floor cleaner, pesticides, and ethyl alcohol were performed. Articles that were commonly found in the patient's home or work environment, such as home carpet, foam pillows, and polyester clothes, were also tested. Each exposure was at ambient concentrations, at a distance of 20 inches, with a constant flow of the vapor from a bottle.

The following laboratory tests were performed: complete blood count by the Coulter Model S method; sodium, potassium, chloride, carbon dioxide, blood urea nitrogen, serum protein, calcium, glucose, uric acid, alkaline phosphate, serum glutamic oxaloacetic transaminase, lactic dehydrogenase, and serum calcium by the SMA method; protein electrophoresis by the Helena cellulose acetate method; quantitative immunoglobulins (IgE, IgG, IgA, IgM), complement components 3 and 4, alpha$_1$-antitrypsin, and C-reactive protein by the Behring radial immunodiffusion method; total hemolytic serum complements (CH_{100}) and serum complement components by the hemolysis sheep cells method (CH_{50}); prothrombin time, partial thromboplastin time, platelets and Lee-White clotting time by the Dade Reagents method; phosphorus by the Hycel method; fibrinogen and fibrinolysins clot lysis by the Biuret quantitative method; fibrin split products by the Burroughs Wellcome method; C1-esterase inhibitor by the Behrin IEP method; and B and T lymphocytes by the sheep cell resetting method. All tests were performed upon the patient's entrance into the room and at the beginning and end of testing. C3 and C4 were done daily during the period of fasting. Serial IgG, THSC, m C3, and eosinophils were done before and 5 minutes after the onset of reaction, at one-half hour, 2 hours, and at the termination of the reaction.

RESULTS

All patients had many complaints related to smooth-muscle systems other than the symptoms from the involvement of the large blood vessels. Two had respiratory tree involvement, three had gastrointestinal involvement, and one had GU system involvement in addition to the vascular involvement.

Once under environmental control, 10 of the 12 patients cleared their symptoms. This included the subsiding of the inflammation and returning of pulses. All of these patients had their symptoms reproduced, including the reduction of pulses and tenderness over the involved area (from specific challenge tests). These reactions followed challenge exposures to one or more commonly eaten foods and/or chemicals (Table 2.2). Tables 2.18 and 2.19 show findings of the initial laboratory tests. Changes were seen in IgG, eosinophils, WBC, C-reactive protein, total complement and functions, and T lymphocytes. Two patients who did not clear test had no adverse reaction. Their symptoms were apparently due to some other problem.

TABLE 2.18
Immunoglobulin Levels

Patient	Age/Sex	IgG (800–1800)	IgE (1–110)	IgA (90–450)	IgM (F70-20 + 17) (60–250 + 16)
1	41F	960	25	180	294
2	23F	880	350	75	100
3	59F	900	91	200	370
4	55F	890	75	189	260
5	30F	1250	75	203	291
6	58F	1090	155	306	158
7	37F	600	21	175	90
8	50M	1420	115	273	266
9	44F	1000	70	296	159
10	37M	1240	170	195	296
11	32F	1910	100	246	348
12	50M	1140	35	304	108

Source: Adapted from Environmental Health Center-Dallas, 2000. Rea, W., Y Pan.

TABLE 2.19
Laboratory Test Results

Patient	WBC	Total Eosinophil (50–200 mm²)	CRP	THSC (CH$_{100}$) (90%–98%)	C$_3$ (80–120 mg/dL)	C$_3$ (20–40 mg/dL)	Absolute Lymphocyte (2000–4000)	T Lymph %
1	5100	50	+	85	72	36	627	91
2	3900		+	94	60	36	545	51
3	8900	156	Neg.	94	88	52		
4	5600	111	Neg.	96	64	59	786	48
5	4900	211	Neg.	80	64	34	–	–
6	7700	67	Neg.	94	74	39	–	–
7	4900	89	Neg.	60	79	52	422	32
8	4400	211	Neg.	96	80	40	–	–
9	6700	154	+	60	82	42	–	–
10	4500	67	+	90	80	40	–	–
11	7700	150	–	90	90	35	1224	53
12	7000	100	+	90	90	30	1491	71

DISCUSSION

Environmentally triggered large-vessel vasculitis can be an isolated vascular entity or, more often, it is accompanied by additional symptoms related to sensitization of the other smooth-muscle systems such as the respiratory gastrointestinal and GU tracts. Frequently, other parts of the vascular system, ranging from the heart to the precapillary arterioles and the veins, are involved. This was true in this series since two patients showed arrhythmias, while two other showed spontaneous bruises during the testing. One patient had two episodes of phlebitis. The pattern of triggering and response in these patients with associated phlebitis, small-vessel involvement, and arrhythmias appeared similar in most aspects to previously reported series by the senior author. These data certainly add much weight to the idea of a spectrum of environmentally triggered vascular disease. From this and previous studies, evidence suggests that any one individual can have one or all parts of the vascular tree involved. It also further substantiates the broader aspects of environmental maladaptation with its widely varied smooth-muscle sensitization and symptoms.

From a strictly allergic point of view, food allergy (i.e., atopy) has often been tested and disproved as an etiologic factor in many disease processes. In the true sense of the word, this conclusion is probably valid. IgE levels were not usually elevated in these vasculitis patients. However, it was evident that these patients had allergic-type responses that usually were apparent with one or more foods or chemicals prior to the diagnostic unmasking process. It should be pointed out that probably the Ca^{2+} protein kinases A and C when phosphorylated can increase sensitivity up to 1000 times; mechanism came into action with increase in membrane permeability in these patients. After unmasking was accomplished by 3–8 days of fasting and environmental control, multiple intolerances to previously unsuspected items were emphatically evident upon challenge. It was clear why these intolerances had been overlooked before the environmental control was implemented. Many reactions began with initially subtle, often fleeting symptoms such as running nose, hoarseness, or fatigue. These early symptoms were subtle; but the reaction, if allowed to proceed to termination, would crescendo into more marked symptoms over a period of several hours. The time course of the crescendo reaction, along with the failure to understand masking, could partially explain why no cause–effect relationships had previously been noted.

The bipolarity of the reaction symptom pattern was also quite striking. Most patients would experience an initial stimulatory phase in which they felt abnormally well or even euphoric.

This euphoria appeared similar to a "high" that is experienced by many individuals addicted to narcotics or alcohol. The stimulatory phase would last anywhere from minutes to hours and its pleasant sensations would mislead the patient and observers as to the significance of the response for the patient's chronic illness. This initial euphoric phase would also help explain in part why cause–effect relationships were usually overlooked in the environment outside of the Environmental Control Unit. As the stimulatory phase subsided, the withdrawal phase, with increasing physical malfunctioning, would become prominent. This would last for hours to days. The withdrawal symptoms were generally far more unpleasant and therefore more noticed than were those in the stimulatory phase. For instance, the longest observed reaction to an incitant lasted for 6 days, with the patient continuously in extreme pain from peripheral arterial and gastrocnemius muscle spasm. No triggering agents had previously been defined in this patient who had been experiencing these severe spasms for 2.5 years prior to introduction of environmental control. This was certainly partially because of the bipolarity as well as the length of the reaction and masking phenomenon.

Although the degree of sensitivity to the incitants was often extreme, the frequency of the exposures to many triggering agents hindered recognition of the problem. The incitants were commonly in the patient's daily environment and considered to be so safe that they were completely ignored as possible initiators or propagators of the disease process. A graphic example was the chocolate factory worker who was exposed daily to the fumes of chocolate. When he was forced to retire, he still went to the factory daily and continued to eat chocolate. Under Environmental Control, after temporary food and pollutant withdrawal, the patient immediately developed symptoms on re-exposure to the odor of chocolate. The essential diagnostic step therefore was temporary interruption of the chronic exposure, followed by acute challenge.

Inhalant chemical triggering gave an added effect of a generalized nonspecific depression in the body's homeostatic mechanism. When the chemical load was high enough, it would trigger symptoms such as malaise, sluggishness, jitteriness, and depression, and at the extreme, it would actually render apparently formerly safe foods unsafe. This chemical-load effect was particularly strong on days of high atmospheric ozone, high general ambient air pollution, or exposure to a severely chemically contaminated building.

Water sensitivity also frequently contributed to the total environmental load on these patients. Contamination with synthetic chemicals was apparently the chief factor in the water that caused problems. This facet of the chemical problem had to be resolved before the other food and chemical triggering incitants could be validly tested.

Emphasis on diagnostic techniques cannot be adequately stressed in this type of patient. One must begin with a lifelong environmental history as described by Randolph.[638] Usually, there are two outstanding features in these histories. The first is an extremely acute sense of smell. On admission or sometime in the past, each patient had noted that he could smell the fumes of natural gas when his peers could not. Usually, odors of substances such as fresh paint, aerosol sprays, cigarette smoke, pesticides- and perfume-produced nausea, headache, tight chest, or some other symptomatology related to smooth-muscle systems. Second, these widely varied and seemingly unrelated disease processes and symptoms, such as sinusitis colitis and cystitis, were in fact related by the common denominator of their all being inflammation of smooth-muscle systems. Many have associated laboratory findings of depressed white blood count, total hemolytic complements, C3, T-lymphocytes, and occasionally, IgG.

The pathophysiology in this entity is unclear, but the inflammation appeared to be a monocytic infiltrate surrounding the vessel wall, which proceeded to nonarteriorsclerotic fibrotic occlusion in several of these patients. If the immunoglobulins are involved in antigenic stimulation, it is those other than IgE. Possibly "reaginic" IgG is involved since IgG change occurred in some patients after incitant challenge. These reactions could be similar to Parish's findings[639] of deposits of IgG in the vessel wall of animals with vasculitis. Many chemically sensitive patients have decreased IgG subsets. However, the Ca^{2+} protein kinases A and C phosphorylation appears to be more efficacious as the mechanism. The vessel size seems to be the only difference in comparing this type of patients to Theorell's patients,[640] who showed similar deposition after food challenges.

It is presumed that the abnormal uptake of synthetic chemicals such as phenol, which has an extreme affinity for the vessel wall, triggers either the complement or other mediator systems. Complement activation would, in turn, lead to swelling, inflammation, and finally fibrosis. Certainly, complement changes after chemical challenge occurred in some patients with this entity. C-reactive protein also could be a factor in triggering the patients. T lymphocyte abnormality may also be important in this type patient. T lymphocyte changes occurred with ambient-dose incitant challenge in some patients. Abnormality could lead to lymphokine triggering with resultant blood vessel inflammation. All T-lymphocytes measured in these patients were depressed, suggesting a suppressor deficiency or helper-function depression causing overuse of this system. However, too few patients were studied for valid statistical analysis.

Eosinophils monitored during incitant challenge apparently shifted out of the blood to the site of reaction, while the return to normal levels in the blood appeared to signal the end of the reaction.

SUMMARY

Twelve carefully selected patients with large-vessel vasculitis resulting in symptoms from vessel spasm to severe organ necrosis were studied in a highly controlled, relatively fume- and particle-free, rigidly controlled environment. Of the 12 patients, 10 had their spasm and related symptoms relieved. The spasm could be reproduced in 10 patients with challenge of individual foods and chemicals to which they were susceptible. IgG, eosinophil, and complement changes accompanied these changes. T lymphocytes were altered in the affected patients measured.

SMALL-VESSEL INVOLVEMENT

Small-vessel vasculitis has long been an ill-defined clinical entity until recently, studies are sparse and most dissertations on the subject are vague. It has become apparent that there is a whole spectrum of vasculitis stretching from very minor vessel involvement to devastating organ necrosis. Triggering agents are generally unknown except for a few bacterial infections and drug included inflammation. Various other clinical entities such as some arthritis, nephritis, lupus, erythematosus, and periarteritis are known to have vasculitis as part of their individual syndromes but their triggering agents are also unknown. Other types of vasculitis are apparently nonspecific but also have no known etiology. A randomly selected group of patients with nonspecific vasculitis of unknown etiology was chosen for this prospective study to see whether triggering agents could be more specifically found and the clinical course more clearly defined when studied under rigid environmentally controlled conditions less polluted.

Ten consecutive patients with nonspecific vasculitis (petechiae, spontaneous bruising, vascular spasm, and recurrent edema) from this author's cardiovascular practice were selected as they presented. This section deals with the patients with small blood vessel involvement in contrast to a series where the large vessels are involved.

Detailed lifelong ecological histories were taken by Randolph's[638] method, searching for other parts of the environmental maladaptation syndrome. Specific symptom complexes and recurrent inflammations such as sinusitis, laryngitis, hoarseness, bronchitis, cystitis, spastic colon, enteritis, colitis, migraine or vascular headaches, myalgia, arthritis, arthralgia, depression, cardiac arrhythmia, or phlebitis of unknown etiology were recorded.

An attempt was made to create less-polluted (5× and in particularly organic chemicals) environment that was as free as possible from inhaled and ingested contaminations and where triggering agents could be clearly defined. Thus, cause and effect could be established.

All patients, during the course of diagnosis and treatment, were kept in the less-polluted rooms for at least a 16-day period. Patients were required to remove all hair sprays, cosmetics, perfumes, and polyester clothing before entering the room and to wear less chemically treated 100% cotton. Upon entering the room, all medications including anticoagulants and steroids were stopped. Once the patients reached the symptom-free basal state, they could act as their own controls. No medications were given during the stay in the unit with the exception of oral or intravenous bicarbonate of soda and oxygen. Pulses, blood pressure, temperature, bruising, petechiae, and color changes were monitored every 4 hours. After the patient was in a basal state free of signs and symptoms, including absence of petechiae and bruises, with normal pulses and a HR below 80, able to sleep all night and had lost hunger, challenge with single, less chemically contaminated source food was begun. The food was selected individually and randomly. In order not to miss delayed reactions, no more than four source foods were tested in one 24-hour period. As many as 60 individual source foods were tested sequentially during the period in environmental control. Pulses were recorded 5 minutes before and at 5-, 20-, 40-, and 60-minute intervals after meals. Electrocardiograms were taken with the onset of any arrhythmia. The time of onset after the challenge was noted. All signs and symptoms were recorded. Testing of the next food was not begun until all previous reactions had subsided.

After totally tolerated foods were found, the patients were retested with these same nonreactive foods but this time obtained from the commercial market. The commercial foods were naturally contaminated by synthetic sprays, herbicides, preservatives, artificial colorings and sweeteners, wax and plastic wrappings, or other additives occurring during their production and processing. These were cooked on gas stoves in synthetic cookware. Individual and cumulative reactions from one to six consecutive meals were observed and recorded.

Testing of odors was done in the following manner. Each patient was given a time exposure of 1–60 minutes to the flames of natural gas, cigarette smoke, chlorine, perfume, pine scented floor wash, ethyl alcohol, formaldehyde, phenol, and pesticides. In addition, challenge to the fumes of common odor-producing material such as home carpet, foam pillows, polyester clothes, which the individual breathed daily in the home, and work environment was done. Each exposure was at a distance of 20 inches with a constant flow of the vapor. All odors tested were of a double-blind nature in that neither the examiner nor the patient knew the content of container until after the test. Saline was used as a control.

The following laboratory tests were performed. Complete blood count, sodium, potassium, chloride, carbon dioxide, blood urea nitrogen, serum protein, protein electrophoresis, immunoglobulins (IgE, IgG, IgA, IgM), total hemolytic and serum complements (C_3 and C_4), prothrombin time, partial thromboplastin time, platelets, Lee and White clotting time, calcium, phosphorus, fibrinogen, fibrinolysins, fibrin split products, glucose, uric acid, alkaline phosphatase (ALP), serum glutamic oxaloacetic transaminase, lactic dehydrogenase, alpha-1 antitrypsin, and C_1 esterase inhibitor were obtained upon entrance into room at the beginning and at the end of testing; C_3 and C_4 were done daily during the period of fasting. Biopsies were taken of the spontaneous bruises and petechial hemorrhages.

Results

As shown in Table 2.20, there was an impressive number of associated signs and symptoms related to the environmental maladaptation syndrome occurring during the patient's lifetime. Each patient averaged more than 10 distinct recurrent signs and symptoms. Few episodes of vasculitis required hospitalization but usually rendered the patient incapacitated for the duration, which was usually 4–5 days. The average time of onset of the disease to the time of diagnosis was about 20 years. Four patients had lifelong problems with recurring symptomatology related to the respiratory, gastrointestinal, and GU systems. Prior to development of the vasculitis, all patients gave histories of being supersensitive to odors of things like car exhausts, perfumes, fabric stores, natural gas, etc. They usually also reacted adversely to medications. The difficulty in making the diagnosis was manifested by the fact that each patient had seen at least 10 physicians prior to being admitted to the Environmental Control Unit.

Once under environmental control, all 10 patients cleared their active symptoms, including their ongoing vasculitis, in 3–7 days. Frequently, symptoms were accentuated in the first 2–3 days. Most patients underwent withdrawals. Each patient initially had hunger followed by complaints of

TABLE 2.20

Associated Signs and Symptoms

Recurrent spontaneous bruising and/or petechiae	10
Recurrent edema	10
Recurrent nasal stuffiness	10
Extremity vascular spasm	10
Cold susceptibility	10
Tonsillectomy	9
Increased sense of smell	9
Adult acne	8
Recurrent myalgia	7
Recurrent sinusitis	6
Recurrent headaches	6
Spastic colon and/or nonspecific colitis	5
Recurrent nonspecific chest pain	5
Recurrent bronchitis or bronchopneumonia	5
Recurrent overwhelming fatigue	5
Recurrent sore throats	5
Asthma	4
Recurrent arrhythmias	4
Recurrent cystitis	4
Recurrent depression	2

Source: Adapted from Rea, W., Patel, K.

"nervousness," "jitters," and headaches. There were observable signs of agitation, trembling, and depression. Insomnia or disturbed sleep was the rule the first night, which was followed by assorted symptoms such as nausea, diarrhea, wheezing, and/or headaches. Finally, backaches, sometimes excruciating, usually signaled the terminations of the symptoms. At this time, all tenderness, bruises, petechiae, extremity discoloration, and other associated signs and symptoms were gone. The patients were asymptomatic and all stated that they had not been that well in years. This feeling of well-being was confirmed by observable signs of animation, walking, or even riding a stationary bicycle. None had previously been able to do this because of uncontrollable fatigue.

After testing started, it became quite obvious that reactions fell into three categories. The first consisted of unmistakable signs, such as rhinorrhea, nasal stuffiness, hoarseness, cough, wheezes, peripheral blanching, cyanosis, swelling or loss of pulses, bruising, polyuria, fever, increased pulse rate, blood pressure decreased or elevated, arrhythmia, petechiae, bruising, and phlebitis. The second category consisted of equivocal signs and the third category of no observed reactions. The latter two were lumped together for statistical purposes and considered as having no observed reactions.

All 10 patients clearly had their vasculitis reproduced on at least three separate occasions. Usually, there was a sequential progression of symptoms of color change of the hands, feet, nose, and skin followed by pulse alteration, periorbitol and peripheral edema, and petechial and/or spontaneous bruising. It is evident by the data shown in Table 2.18 that many different susceptibilities existed in each patient. Also, it was observed that some individual incitants would produce only portions, while others would produce all the patient's original signs and symptoms. These reactions were further substantiated by the benign asymptomatic course after ingestion or inhalation of nonreactive foods and food odors plus the reproducibility of signs by retesting of reacting foods. Ninety-five percent of the reactions that occurred within the first 4 hours started within the first 5 minutes after ingestion, leaving no doubt in the minds of observing personnel and patients that there was a cause–effect relationship. The severe reactions lasted up to 48 hours with lesser effects lasting up to 5 days. The moderate reactions lasted 4–8 hours while the mild ones were terminated within a 4-hour period. One hundred percent of the associated signs and symptoms were reproduced (Table 2.21).

Testing for ingested chemicals resulted in symptoms and signs after the initial meal in two patients, while eight patients took two to six meals to produce signs although symptoms were often produced at least one meal earlier.

All reactions to inhalant chemicals were within the first 1.5 hours and their after effects lasted up to 48 hours although most were terminated within a 4-hour period. Ten patients reacted to the fumes of the flame of the gas pilot, reproducing assorted signs and symptoms in all patients and reproducing the vascular signs in six. The most striking examples were those of 33-year-old and 34-year-old females who had a 15-second exposure to the natural gas pilot. Patient A developed immediate dizziness, staggering, and then premature ventricular contractions followed by severe leg pain and bruises over both extremities. Recovery took 36 hours. Patient B developed immediate abdominal cramps, irritability, chills, and vascular spasm of hands and feet vessels followed by spontaneous bruising and depression. Recovery took 48 hours under oxygen with the patients writhing in pain and complaining of abdominal cramps most of this time.

Double-blind exposures to the various inhaled chemicals are seen in Table 2.22. One can see the widespread involvement of susceptibilities to these chemicals. Not shown is the fact that the transient

TABLE 2.21
Associated Signs and Symptoms

Offending Agents	Associated Signs and Symptoms Reproduced	Vasculitis Reproduced
1. Beef, chicken, cig. smoke, shrimp, pork gas heat, ingested chemicals	Diarrhea, pulse increase 30 b/m, nasal stuffiness, bigeminy, multifocal PVCs	Pork, inhaled chemicals, wheat
2. Wheat, rice, inhaled chemicals	Vomiting, pulse increase 40 b/m, catatonia	Wheat, rice, inhaled chemicals
3. Corn, cane sugar, eggs, inhaled chemicals, milk	Wheezing, rhinorrhea, red nose, nasal stuffiness, tender muscles, cystitis	Corn, inhaled chemicals, milk
4. Beef, potatoes, ingested chemicals, wheat, corn	Peripheral pulse from 4 to 1+, tachypnea, shortness of breath, cyanosis, belching	Beef, wheat, corn, inhaled chemicals
5. Pork, pork fumes, ingested chemicals, inhaled chemicals	Edema—generalized, tender muscles, colitis, dizzy, headaches	Pork, shrimp, inhaled chemicals
6. Legumes, seafood, cane sugar, wheat, chicken, cig. smoke, ingested chemicals, inhaled chemicals	Syncope, wheezing, muscle tenderness, hives, paroxysmal atrial tachycardia, headaches	Cigarette smoke, ingested chemicals, inhaled chemicals, seafood, corn
7. Beef, chicken, lettuce, petrochemicals inhaled, corn, milk	GI bloat, belching diarrhea, PVC's vent. tach.	Wheat, corn, milk, ingested chemicals
8. Turkey, chicken, peas, cig. smoke, beef, inhaled chemicals	Decrease in pulse left arm only, left neck and arm tenderness, tender over arm veins	Chicken, beef, inhaled chemicals
9. Coffee, peanut butter, cane sugar, ingested chemicals, wheat, rice, turkey	Dyspnea, wheezing, eyes watering, hoarse, pulse increase to 50 b/m	Apples, rice, turkey, inhaled chemicals
10. Corn, wheat, beef, eggs, inhaled chemicals, chicken, peanut butter	Cystitis, diarrhea, skin rash, itching, dyspnea, pulse increase	Chicken, wheat, peanut butter, inhaled chemicals

Source: Adapted from Rea, W. Patel, K. 2004.

TABLE 2.22

Reaction to Double-Blind Exposure to the Fumes of Chemicals (1–15-Minute Exposures—ppb or Less)

Patient	Saline Control	Petroleum Alcohol	Phenol	Chlorine	(Mixture) Pesticides	Pine Scented Floor Wash	Formaldehyde
1	−	+	+	+	+	+	+
2	−	+	−	+	+	+	+
3	−	+	+	−	+	−	+
4	−	+	−	−	+	+	+
5	−	+	+	+	−	−	+
6	−	−	+	+	+	+	+
7	−	−	−	+	+	+	+
8	−	+	+	+	+	+	+
9	−	+	+	+	+	−	−
10	−	+	+	+	+	+	+

exposures produced spontaneous bruising in all patients at least on two different occasions. Vascular spasm with cyanosis was seen in all patients frequently, as were petechiae and periorbital edema.

Skin biopsies of the bruises and petechiae on occurrence showed the following:

1. Spontaneous bruises: precapillary arteriole involvement with monocellular infiltrate and either rupture or leak of red blood cells outside the vessel.
2. Petechiae showed intradermal hemorrhage of a capillary.

Table 2.23 shows a tendency for the white blood count to be depressed. Immunoglobulins generally were within normal limits. Alterations in total serum hemolytic complements were seen in only one patient and presumably this was due to abnormality in one of the unmeasured components. All C_3s were abnormally lower, but mildly so, in all cases. C_4s were altered in only two patients, both being slightly elevated in one. Bleeding studies were all normal.

TABLE 2.23

Control 10 Patients

Control 10 Patients	5–10,000 WBC	10–200 IgE	800–1800 IgG	90–450 IgA	60–280 IgM	90%–100% THC	80–120 C-3	20–40 C-4	50–200 Total Eosinophil
1	6000	15	920	231	84	90	67	25	67
2	3500	30	1560	474	116	93	62	30	150
3	4500	60	1540	201	460	91	68	28	300
4	4700	40	1420	273	266	95	70	40	75
5	5000	120	1127	210	100	80	65	47	90
6	3800	80	1290	220	124	93	58	45	140
7	4200	20	1060	290	160	91	59	36	200
8	4100	25	1580	158	160	99	60	39	66
9	5500	38	1140	104	143	96	63	29	190
10	2800	40	1040	254	240	90	61	40	88

We at the EHC-Dallas have treated over 2000 patients and proven CV disease of the small-vessel type. We have been able to clear the signs and symptoms reproduced by them with challenge and keep them well long-term with medication.

Discussion

Environmentally triggered vasculitis has been alluded in reports from many observers, starting the early 1900s. Hare[641] first observed peripheral vasoactive phenomena when he withdrew and rechallenged certain foods. Later, Harkavy[642] in the 1930s was able to link some arterial disease to sensitivity to cigarette smoke as well as induce cardiac arrhythmias with isolated food challenges in susceptible individuals. In 1970, Taylor and Hern[643] reported a fatal arrhythmia due to inhalation of aerosolized fluorocarbon. Randolph[638] performed the first studies under environmentally controlled conditions, showing that the whole spectrum of arrhythmias could be triggered by inhaled and ingested chemicals. Recently, Yevick[644] reported further evidence of chemically triggered vasculitis when he demonstrated inflammation and fibrosis of the cardiovascular system in sea life exposed to oil spills. Nour-Elden[645] further substantiated this phenomenon by showing that arteries have 15 times more affinity for phenol than any other tissue in the body. The sensitivity to phenol was borne out on our inhaled challenges. In 1976, Stewart and Hake[646] reported a case of fatal triggering of an MI by furniture refinishing solution. Last, a series of environmentally triggered phlebitis was described by the senior author of this book.

This series of patients fits the general pattern described by these aforementioned observers although distinguished by their wide variety of symptoms involving many of the major organ systems. Also, in addition to frequent peripheral vasospasms, all had the spontaneous cutaneous bruising and/or pete-chiae, plus facial and/or peripheral edema, indicating inflamed blood vessels. These vascular responses apparently act as mirrors to the pathology occurring internally, thus explaining the occurrence of unusual and even bizarre symptoms. Since these symptoms were reproducible with repeated, known, blind, and double-blind challenges, vascular involvement of that specific area of the body would be the logical explanation of underlying pathophysiological response. Frequently, they did, indeed, cor-respond with the visible bruising, purpura, petechiae, and edema. Usually, if the pathologic responses could not be explained or correspond with the vascular involvement, other components of the smooth muscle systems such as the respiratory, gastrointestinal, or GU systems were involved.

In viewing the lifelong histories, it is difficult to say when the vasculitis started. However, several facts were evident. Most patients had symptoms due to abnormal responses to environmental stimuli in early childhood. These increased insidiously over many years before exhibiting the full vasculi-tis syndrome. Many could clearly relate accentuation of their allergic manifestations with apparent spreading of intolerances to commonly used foods and outgasing objects such as newsprint, perfume, plastics, etc. very early in life. Frequently, precipitating overexposure episodes such as having the house fumigated would trigger the cascade of spreading intolerances to both foods and chemicals. This spreading phenomenon seemed to occur in patients with a background of susceptibility though two patients on careful scrutiny were totally asymptomatic at the time of the precipitating exposure. A careful review of the clinical course in these patients revealed three or four of the smooth muscle systems to be involved, indicating widespread disease. This multisystem involvement clearly dis-tinguishes the patient with environmentally triggered disease from the average atopic patient. Even though the patients presented with multisystem complaints due to apparent spreading of intolerances, many isolated clues were present years before the onset of the vasculitis. Ninety-plus percent had ton-sillectomies, indicating involvement of the respiratory and immune systems in early childhood and even infancy, thereby pointing out the importance of obtaining this information early in life. Family histories were also very important; in that, 60% had ancestors who suffered and eventually died from a nonarteriosclerotic cardiovascular entity. Finally, most patients had isolated chemical intolerances with years of complaints of a hypersensitive sense of smell to these. Usually, odors of various chemi-cals such as chlorine, newsprint, fabric stores, pesticides, etc. would cause them to be nauseated or ill. All gave histories of being able to smell natural gas, when others could not.

Water quality apparently plays a significant role in the development and treatment of vasculitis. Eighty percent of the patients in this series were tried on at least four different nonchlorinated spring and filtered waters before their symptoms cleared. One hundred percent of the patients reacted strongly to a blind challenge of chlorinated water. It repeatedly became apparent that use of well water was hazardous due to widespread permeation of the water table with pesticides. As pointed out by Randolph,[638] the patient's water intolerances must be solved or symptoms will not clear and other testing results will be suspect.

Food as a trigger to pathological responses has been mentioned by past generations of food allergists. Its importance in the pathogenesis of disease has been overlooked until recently. Responses to food testing have frequently been confusing for numerous reasons, including alteration of reactions by extraneous environmental insults and the so-called delayed food reactions. Apparently, food reactions in susceptible individuals are influenced by many factors, including the quantity and frequency of ingestions, temperatures of the foods, multiplicity of ingested synthetic elements in the food, the ambient inhaled air quality including temperature, humidity, barometric pressure, amount of ionization, the number and type of pollutants, the quality of ingested water, cyclical hormone influences, and the state of nutritional balance of the individual. This complexity explains why few triggering agents have previously been found with certainty. The controlled environment decreases the complexity and adds to the clear definition of foods as one facet of the triggering agent for vasculitis and possibly many other diseases of unknown etiology.

In a controlled environment, it becomes clear that most food reactions are immediate rather than delayed. However, many reactions are insidious and start with relatively minor symptoms such as transient nasal stuffiness, malaise, hoarseness, depression, or belching. Later, they frequently crescendo into devastating symptomatology. Once the physician and the patient observe this sequential phenomena under controlled conditions, they are able to dissect out other influential environmental triggering agents.

One factor is dominant in testing food and, that is, the food must be as uncontaminated as possible. With the environment steadily deteriorating, the difficulty of acquiring pure food is at times almost overwhelming. Food is contaminated from the point of growing by artificial fertilizers, pesticides, and herbicides. Further, contamination continues during processing by the different washes, additives, preservatives, stabilizers, polyvinyl chloride wrappings, etc. Cooking with gas in synthetic cookware adds more contamination. Due to this chemical adulteration of food, it was necessary to develop a network of food growers who farmed without the use of synthetics. Then, one must be sure that the food was not contaminated during transportation or preparation. Once this detail was managed, testing results were reproducible in the 95% range. Food monitoring by treated chemically susceptible individuals appears to be the best mode of monitoring at present and is a necessity.

The increase in the ambient air pollution further adds to the difficulty of defining triggering agents. There appears to be two types of effects from inhaled pollution. One is an overall depressant effect which is very subtle. This appears to be volume load effect and may account for the fact that certain reactions are accentuated in days when there is more air pollution with all other facets remaining constant. These observations were first observed by Randolph[638] and later supported by analytical studies of ambient air by Whitby et al.,[647] who measured air in various areas of the world. They found that sea air had the fewest fumes and particles (excluding salt). Comparable standards for clean continental air showed a 10-fold increase in pollution while air blowing from cities, but still on continental areas, increased pollution at least 35 times. The city on a good day had 150-fold more pollution while on bad days it increased, 1000–4000 times. The abnormal responses of patients to food in this series were more frequent and accentuated when they were taken out of the Environmental Control Unit to areas of higher nonspecific air pollution. This was further evidenced when the same patients went to areas of the country with less air pollution and found reactions to certain foods to be much less or even absent in a few instances. With less ambient air pollution, they also found ingested chemicals, formerly intolerable, to be less harmful. Due to this effect, it became clear that patients had to have 10–12 hours in a less-polluted environment to keep their vasculitis under control out of the hospital. This necessitated cleaning up the home by removing the high out-gasing plastics (polyvinyls, polyethylene, polyurethane, foam rubber, etc.) and other synthetics (oil base paints, natural gas, etc.) as well as eliminating particle producing materials. Most of all, none got well until their natural gas appliances, including heating, were removed.

While developing instrumentation for the orbital space laboratory, Poehlmann et al.[648] observed that the fine tuning of instruments was initially distorted, giving disastrous results. They measured outgasing potentials of all materials and found glass, steel, metal, and stone to be inert while the soft-plastics, such as polyvinyl chloride, polyethylene, polyurethane, and silicone, to be constantly fum-ing. Some of the hardest synthetics like masonite, polycarbonate, and formica had initial fuming but little thereafter. Knowledge of these phenomena is crucial in diagnosing and treating a chemically susceptible vasculitis patient. This nonspecific pollution effect usually explains why patients are not clearing all symptoms periodically and also explains sudden susceptibility to formerly safe foods.

The second type of response to air pollution followed the more classic allergic reactions with a sudden precipitating onset followed by the usual sequence of symptoms. This was also present to the same incitants and was easily reproducible. In addition to occasional pollen, dust and mold trig-gering incitants were mainly due to halogenated petrochemicals such as pesticides, floor cleaning compounds, and/or metals like copper, aluminum, cadmium, and nickel. This effect was always most evident if the patient's ambient overall pollution level was low.

Environmentally triggered small-vessel vascular disease is probably part of a spectrum of inflammatory diseases of all sizes of arteries since smooth muscle appears to be the sensitized system involved. This particular group of patients had blood vessel involvement at the precapillary arteriole level and/or small arteries of the intraoral type. At times, there were large-vessel responses but minimal in this group of patients.

The pathologic vascular damage seen in this series fell into the mild to moderate categories and would be considered to be stage I and II responses. As seen in all pathologic sections, this resulted in mild vessel damage resulting in localized or mild generalized edema. This appeared to be reversible even when the vasculitis had been long-standing. Also, rupture of the capillaries was present, manifested by bruising and petechiae. Frequently, noninflammatory purpura was seen and it seemingly reflected a more severe, but still reversible, clinical course. The pathologic involvement fell short of organ necrosis apparently because of the size of vessels involved and the scarcity of involvement in any one area and the lack of intravascular coagulation. This probably accounted for the diversity of symptoms and multiple complaints of the patients.

Laboratory data were unremarkable other than the change in the serum complements. Immunoglobulins were not elevated and did not change much although gamma globulin subsets were often low. The fact that patients had immediate type I reactions (Gell and Coombs) with some challenges makes one suspect that there was alteration of IgE at the local level. However, as shown recently in allergic lung diseases, this response may be more a reflection of IgG alteration.[649] Direct triggering of the kinin and complement systems bypassing the a-a reaction also apparently occurs. The complement mechanism is involved in producing the inflammation since all patients had mild depression of the C_3 and some elevation of the C_4. It would have been interesting to measure kinin levels but these were unavailable in our laboratory at the time of these studies. Many of the clinical characteristics in this series are similar to those of Garner and Diamond,[650] who found kinin eleva-tion associated with bruising but thought the triggering was due to autoerythrocyte sensitization, and by Leibe,[651] who actually introduced bruising by kinin injection in a single patient. T and B cells are involved as small vasculitis but were not available in the early series. They were abnormal in the 1500 small-vessel vasculitis studied since then.

The intrinsic mechanism of the environmentally triggered arteritis is unclear but probably encompasses a variety of mechanisms. Some incitants probably trigger the deposition of antigen–antibody complexes in the vessel walls. Another possible mechanism which occurs in other vascu-litis would be the alteration of a native component of the vessel wall so that it becomes antigenic and induces hormonal or cellular immunity. Deposition of an antigenic foreign substance within the vessel should also be considered in some patients. Finally, alteration of a vessel wall component so that it directly induces an inflammatory response surely occurs in other patients. Regardless of these different pathways for the final production of vasculitis, it is now possible to define a multiplicity of incitants in any given patient, thus allowing us the opportunity to remove the triggering agent.

Summary

1. Ten randomly selected patients with recurrent, nonspecific small-vessel vasculitis of unknown etiology were placed in a therapeutic diagnositic Environmental Control Unit.
2. All patients had multiple recurrent symptoms in addition to their vasculitis, including such complexes as sinusitis, colitis, bronchitis, asthma, myalgia, arrhythmias, depression, and otitis.
3. All patients were cleared of their symptoms, including their vasculitis, without medications while in the unit.
4. With each patient acting as his own control, the whole spectrum of associated symptoms could be reproduced by direct challenge with individual foods and chemicals immediately and repeatedly.
5. Ten patients had a direct cause–effect relationship demonstrated by challenge with individual foods and chemicals causing reproduction of their vasculitis. Multiple individual incitants were found to trigger the vasculitis in each of 10 patients.

Subsequently, 2000 more vasculitis patients were seen and followed demonstrating the same observations and clinical course.

STROKE

Evidence for an Association between Air Pollution and Daily Stroke Admissions in Kaohsiung, Taiwan Occurred

According to Tsai,[652] many studies have reported increases in daily cardiovascular mortality and hospital admissions associated with increases in levels of air pollutants. This study was undertaken to determine whether there is an association between air pollution and hospital admissions for stroke in Kaohsiung, Taiwan.

Data on a total of 23,179 stroke admissions were obtained for the period 1997–2000. The RR of hospital admissions was estimated with a case-crossover approach.

In the single-pollutant models, on warm days ($\geq 20°C$), significant positive associations were found between levels of PM_{10}, NO_2, SO_2, and O_3 and both primary intracerebral hemorrhage and ischemic stroke admissions. On cool days ($< 20°C$), only CO levels and ischemic stroke admissions were significantly associated with admissions for both types of stroke on warm days. They observed estimated RRs of 1.54 (95% CI: 1.31–1.81) and 1.56 (95% CI: 1.32–1.84) for primary intracerebral hemorrhage for each interquartile range increase in PM_{10} and NO_2. The values for ischemic stroke were 1.46 (95% CI: 1.32–1.61) and 1.55 (95% CI: 1.40–1.71), respectively. The effects of CO, SO_2, and O_3 were mostly nonsignificant when either NO_2 or PM_{10} was controlled for.

This study provides an association between exposure to air pollution and hospital admissions for stroke.[652]

Air Pollution and Hospital Admissions for Ischemic and Hemorrhagic Stroke among Medicare Beneficiaries

According to Wellenius et al.,[653] the association between short-term elevations in ambient air particles and increased cardiovascular morbidity and mortality is well documented.

Ambient Particles May Similarly Increase the Risk of Stroke

They evaluated the association between daily levels of respirable PM (aerodynamic diameter $\leq 10 \mu m$ PM_{10}) and hospital admission for ischemic and hemorrhagic stroke among Medicare recipients (age ≥ 65 years) in nine U.S. cities using a s-stage hierarchical model.

Ischemic (n = 155,503) and hemorrhagic (19,314) stroke admissions were examined separately. For ischemic stroke, an interquartile range increase in PM_{10} was associated with a 1.03% (95% CI: 0.04%–2.04%) increase in admissions on the same day only. Similar results were observed with CO, NO_2, and SO_2. For hemorrhagic stroke, no association was observed with any pollutant 0–2 days before admission.

These results suggest that elevations in ambient particles may transiently increase the risk of ischemic, but not hemorrhagic stroke.

Ambient Air Pollution and the Risk of Acute Ischemic Stroke

According to Wellenius et al.,[654] the link between daily changes in level of ambient fine PM air pollution (PM <2.5 μm in diameter [$PM_{2.5}$]) and cardiovascular morbidity and mortality is well established. Whether $PM_{2.5}$ levels below current U.S. National Ambient Air Quality Standards also increase the risk of ischemic stroke remains uncertain.

They reviewed the medical records of 1705 Boston area patients hospitalized with neurologist-confirmed ischemic stroke.

These results suggest that exposure to $PM_{2.5}$ levels considered generally safe by the U.S. EPA increases the risk of ischemic stroke onset within hours of exposure.

Daily changes in levels of ambient fine PM air pollution (PM <2.5 μm in diameter [$PM_{2.5}$]) have been associated with higher risk of acute cardiovascular events, excess hospitalizations, and deaths.[580] These cardiovascular effects of $PM_{2.5}$ appear to be mediated through a combination of autonomic, hemostatic, inflammatory, and vascular endothelial disturbances with consequent changes in cardiac and vascular function.[607,655–659] Relying on the current evidence, the U.S. EPA regulates mean daily and annual $PM_{2.5}$ levels. Whether the current regulatory standards are sufficient to protect public health remains controversial[660] but in our opinion are clearly too high for proper function.

Hong et al.[661] conducted a time-series study to examine the evidence of an association between air pollutants and stroke over 4 years (January 1995–December 1998) in Seoul, Korea. When they examined the associations among PM_{10} levels stratified by the level of gaseous pollutants and vice versa, they found that these pollutants are interactive with respect to their effects on the risk of stroke mortality. They also observed that the effects of PM_{10} on stroke mortality differ significantly in subgroups by age and sex. They concluded that PM_{10} and gaseous pollutants are significant risk factors for acute stroke death and that the elderly and women are more susceptible to the effect of particulate pollutants.

Associations of Fine and Ultrafine Particulate Air Pollution with Stroke Mortality in an Area of Low Air Pollution Levels Found by Kettunen et al.[662]

According to Kettunen et al.,[662] daily variation in outdoor concentrations of inhaled particles (PM_{10} <10 μm in diameter) has been associated with fatal and nonfatal stroke. Toxicological and epidemiological studies suggest that smaller, combustion-related particles are especially harmful. They therefore evaluated the effects of several particle measures including ultrafine particles (<0.1 μm) on stroke.

Levels of particulate and gaseous air pollution were measured from 1998 to 2004 at central outdoor monitoring sites in Helsinki. Associations between daily levels of air pollutants and deaths caused by stroke among persons aged 5 years or older were evaluated in warm and cold seasons using Poisson regression.

There were a total of 1304 and 1961 deaths from stroke in warm and cold seasons, respectively. During the warm season, there were positive associations of stroke mortality with current and previous day levels of fine particles (<2.5 μm, $PM_{2.5}$) (6.9%, 95% CI: 0.8%–13.8%; and 7.4%, 95% CI: 1.3%–13.8% for an interquartile increase in $PM_{2.5}$) and previous day levels of ultrafine particles (8.5, 95% CI: 1.2%–19.1%) and carbon monoxide (8.3; 95% CI: 0.6%–16.6%). Associations for fine particles were mostly independent of other pollutants. There were no associations in the cold season.

These results suggest that especially $PM_{2.5}$, but also ultrafine particles and carbon monoxide, are associated with increased risk of fatal stroke, but only during the warm season. The effect of season might be attributable to seasonal differences in exposure or air pollution mixture.

AUTONOMIC NERVOUS SYSTEM AND VASCULAR DEREGULATION

Over the last 10 years, epidemiologic studies have increasingly found higher daily morbidity and mortality associated with acute changes in ambient PM exposures.[663,664] These changes have been reported at concentrations at or near current ambient levels especially nanoparticles <0.200 mm and have raised concerns about the adequacy of the National Air Quality Standards for Particulate Matter in protecting human populations with an adequate margin of safety. Recent toxicologic and human clinical studies have suggested a variety of PM-mediated mechanisms, including ANS responses, particularly among patients with preexisting cardiovascular diseases.[665,666]

HRV (Volumes II and III of this series in the Cardiovascular chapter), which is under the control of the ANS, has been demonstrated to vary with air pollution.[655,667] Reduced HRV has been associated with increased risk of MI in population studies[668] and considered a predictor of increased risk of mortality in patients with heart failure. Although these studies did not assess the impact of acute changes in HRV, a recent study reported that ischemic events are preceded by decreases in HF HRV in the hour before the event,[669] and a decrease in HRV also has been reported to precede paroxysmal AF.[670] Hence, short-term changes in HRV also may be risk factors for more serious consequences.

Local and regional traffic has been proposed as an important source of PM pollution that may increase cardiovascular risk, perhaps through triggering short-term autonomic changes. A recent German study demonstrated that exposure to local traffic within the previous hour was a trigger of MI, but the mechanism through which this occurred was not determined.[469] Traffic can be a source not only of PM pollution but also of stress, a known risk factor for adverse cardiac outcomes, and psychologic stress has been known to influence HRV and autonomic function.[671] In a study of traffic patrol troopers, traffic pollution inside the vehicle was demonstrated to increase HRV, systemic inflammation, and cardiac arrhythmias.[672] Most other studies have found reduction in HRV with pollution,[317] but the directionality and clinical implications of the pollution-related cardiac autonomic changes likely vary with patient vulnerability.

Zanobetti et al.[673] suggest that short-term traffic exposure and ambient exposure to air pollution are associated with significant reductions in HRV in free-living patients with underlying heart disease, and that recent traffic exposure can cause reductions in HRV as great as 39% in patients 2–6 weeks after hospitalization for CAD. As in previous studies,[655,674,675] Zanobetti et al.[673] found stronger autonomic dysfunction for HRV measures that represent vagal tone (r-MSSD and HF) than for HRV measures representing overall autonomic responses or sympathetic tone (SDNN and TP). Zanobetti et al.[673] found associations for both at shorter (2 hour) and at longer averaging times (up to 5 days). They observed the greatest effects of PM and BC for longer cumulative averages.

Zanobetti et al.[673] may not have found an influence of indoor air pollution on HRV because the indoor levels were lower with few indoor sources of indoor pollution. However, studies at the EHC-Dallas have shown that many indoor toxics such as the fumes of natural gas, pesticides, formaldehyde, and volatile organics and mycotoxins change the HRV similar to the outdoor air pollutants. However, in this same cohort, Zanobetti et al.[673] found an effect of both outdoor and indoor BC with an increase in T-wave alternans (TWA)[676] (an electrophysiologic measure of alternating repolarization waveform indicative of instabilities in cardiac membrane voltage and disruptions in intracellular calcium cycling dynamics). In Zanobetti et al.'s cohort,[676] the TWA was more influenced by short-term cumulative averages of pollution and may be linked to pollution exposure through pathways different from those of HRV. Pollution may influence HRV through direct stimulation of pulmonary reflexes, leading to cardiac or systemic autonomic dysfunction, or through pulmonary systemic inflammation or oxidative stress, which may lead to autonomic dysfunction.[36,598,665,677,678]

The associations of ambient (central site measured) BC with their outcomes were uniformly stronger than the associations of BC outside the home. It is possible that ambient central site measures of BC had stronger and larger associations with reduced HRV than did outdoor measures because the measures of Zanobetti et al.[673] provided a better measure of regional average exposure during the times when the participants were away from home. The association of reduced HRV in single pollutant models with only NO_2, which can be considered another marker of traffic in addition to BC, provides further support for the effects of pollution of traffic origins. The data also suggest that mixtures of pollutants may influence autonomic cardiac tone, in both PM pollution and O_3, which had independent associations with reduced HRV in two pollutant models.

The results of Zanobetti et al.[673] are consistent with those of the previous literature on potentially high-risk patients (defined as elderly subjects with or without documented CHD).[655,656,679–681] Others who have studied pollution responses in patients with stable CHD,[682,683] in studying their subjects 2–6 weeks after hospitalization for MI, have found unstable angina pectoris or worsening stable CAD. Autonomic dysfunction can precede more serious cardiac electrophysiologic disturbances in vulnerable patients.[684–686] HRV is a predictor of long-term cardiac mortality,[687] although the debate continues as to whether it is a marker or cause of increased cardiac risk. Previously, Zanobeti et al.[676] described pollution-associated ST segment depression[688] and increases in T-wave alternates in the subjects participating in their study; the finding of traffic- and pollution-associated autonomic dysfunction adds to the evidence that pollution is increasing cardiac risk in this vulnerable population.

Within this population that was vulnerable on the basis of CAD, people with diabetes were even more vulnerable due to their microvascular involvement. This adds to cumulative evidence that type 2 diabetes, which is accompanied by a chronic autonomic dysfunction, is a source of vulnerability to population.[470,689–692]

Although it is possible that being in traffic represents a combination of exposures, Zanobetti et al.[673] found that the effects of traffic are not a result of chance or the specific vulnerability of a few subjects. Being in traffic for either part or all of 2 hours before and including HRV measurement was associated with reduced HRV. Although there are only 27 observations for six subjects who were in traffic for a full 2 hours, 40 subjects contributed 315 observations when they were in traffic for a part of the previous 2 hours (at least one-half hour). It is, however, possible that being in traffic is a measure of combination of factors with adverse effects. Studies have suggested that stress can trigger adverse cardiac events, including MI or arrhythmias.[693] A limitation of their study is that they did not measure stress while in traffic and therefore cannot disentangle the combination of pollution and stress exposures that "being in traffic" represents. Nevertheless, in the models including "being in traffic" and in the models stratified by being indoors and not in traffic, the independent associations of measured pollution with reduced HRV are not likely to be confounded by the stress of being in traffic. They did not have details on pollution levels in the cars of their study participants. Ventilation in vehicles can vary widely. It would be useful for future studies to evaluate whether reduction of in-vehicle pollution improves HRV and other indicators of cardiac risk in vulnerable populations.

This study provides further evidence that exposure to ambient pollution to both $PM_{2.5}$ and BC alters autonomic function, particularly among subjects with a history of previous myocardial injury. Traffic exposure, which likely represents a complex combination of local pollution exposure and stress, independently adds to risk incurred by the background of regional pollution. Mixtures with gases such as ozone may add to the risk of PM pollution exposure. Susceptible populations such as individuals with CAD should be considered when setting national policies and regulations to control levels of particle matter air pollution and traffic.

TEMPERATURE—AIR AND BODY

Air temperature has also been found to trigger myocardial reaction. Working in a less-polluted, controlled environment, Rea et al.[694] found reductions of pollutants to lower CS and cold was also a factor. Numerous studies have shown that elevated ambient air pollutants and changes in air temperature are associated with increases in hospital admissions and mortality due to cardiovascular events.[694–696] The effects of air pollution on HR and HRV have been studied more extensively since the initial publications by Rea et al.,[694] Pope et al.,[597] Peters et al.,[697] and Gold et al.[655] For example, researchers reported a reduced HRV in susceptible participants such as senior adults[698] and patients with CADCAD.[683] Increased levels of air pollution have been shown to enhance the risk for ST-segment depression[699] and arrhythmia.[700] It is hypothesized that the observed associations between HR and HRV and air pollutants are a consequence of the activation of the ANS or a direct affliction of the electric system of the heart.[696] Little is known about the influence of temperature on HR and HRV. Drops in temperature may activate the SNS via stimulation of cold receptors in the skin (TRPV8), which may result in increased catecholamine levels. The consequences are vasoconstriction and increased blood pressure.[701,702] The chemically sensitive usually has subnormal temperatures ranging from 96°F to 97°F and this drop in temperature will trigger their vasculitis and thus at times cardiac dysfunction.

Potential mechanisms of the influence of air pollutants and temperature on repolarization have received less attention. Some researchers have hypothesized that a prolonged QT interval and T-wave abnormalities might trigger the onset of arrhythmias[703] and increase the risk for coronary deaths.[704] Only a few studies have investigated the relationship between elevated levels of PM air pollution and repolarization thus far,[601,705,706] and little is known about the temperature influence on these parameters.

The main objective of Hampel et al.'s[707] study was to evaluate the influence of air pollutants and air temperature on repeated measurements of HR and repolarization parameters, such as Bazett-corrected QT interval (QT_c)[708] and T-wave amplitude (T_{amp}).

As specific single nucleotide polymorphisms (sympathetic nerves system pathways) have been reported to modulate the QT interval,[709] they examined modifications of the association between air pollution and ECG parameters by sympathetic nervous system pathways (SNPs) involved in detoxification pathways. Hampel et al.'s[707] analyses showed no main effects of air pollutants on HR overall, but they observed significant positive associations between PM_{0-23} HR before and HR among participants with BMI > 30 kg/m^2 and among those not using beta-blocker medications. They observed a prolonged QT_c interval in association with increases in PM levels 24–47 hours before ECG transmission, with stronger associations among participants with one or two minor alleles of the nFEV2l2 sympathetic nervous system pathways rs236N4725. However, patients with at least one minor allele showed shortened QT_c in association with an increase in PNC 96–119 hours before.

T_{amp} decreased in association with both cold and warm temperatures, with maximum T_{amp} around 5°C which is 41°F.

Several authors have reported inverse associations between air pollutants and HRV in the elderly.[675,698] Pollutants activate the SNS directly or indirectly, which possibly leads to an increased HR and reduced HRV. UFP might even translocate into the systemic circulation and affect the electric system of the heart directly.[696] It has been shown that patients not using beta-blocker medications exhibit a stronger reduction in HRV in association with PM exposure compared with patients using beta blockers.[710] Hampel et al.[707] observed an increased HR with exposure to air pollutants only among patients with 200 ECGs not using beta blockers. Beta blockers constrain the activation of the sympathetic tone; thus, participants using beta blockers might be less susceptible to activation of the SNS by air pollutants. Due to the small number of participants not taking beta blockers and even if patient characteristics did not differ significantly between individuals with and without beta-blocker intake, it is still possible that the observed differences in the estimated air pollution effects are related to something other than medication intake. Consistent with their findings, Chen et al.[711] reported stronger positive associations between $PM_{2.5}$ and HR in individuals with BMI >30 kg/m². CO will increase HR.

Henneberger et al.[601] detected an immediate positive association of 24-hour averages of organic carbon with QT_c. Furthermore, Liao et al.[712] reported immediate and delayed QT_c prolongations associated with elevated 30-minute averages of $PM_{2.5}$. However, Lux and Pope[713] observed no association between $PM_{2.5}$ and repolarization parameters in elderly participants. Hampel et al.'s[707] analysis found lagged associations between PM and QT_c.

Associations were more pronounced among participants with one or two minor alleles of the NFE2L2 SNP rs 2364725. The NFE2L2 gene is believed to be involved in the defense against oxidative stress.[714] Speculation that the defense is more activated in patients with common alleles, whereas patients with at least one minor allele are more susceptible to PM. In contrast, they observed inverse associations between QT_c and PNC, a proxy for UFP, in accordance with two chamber studies[706,715] that reported QT_c shortening in healthy nonsmoking subjects who were exposed to UFP.

Different effects of PM and PNC might reflect different biological pathways activated by different particle properties. T_{amp} indicates the repolarization of the ventricles, and Henneberger et al.[601] reported a 7.3% decrease in T_{amp} in association with an increase in UFP 0–23 hours before ECG measuring. A subsequent analysis of Yue et al.[716] suggested that this association was driven by traffic-related UFP specifically. Hampel et al.[707] observed a 4-day delayed decrease and an immediate elevation of T_{amp} in relation with all PM parameters, which cannot be explained by a single patient characteristic such as BMI.

It can only be speculated that a combination of medication intake and disease history may be involved in the susceptibility of air pollution. It also needs to see if the cold susceptibility holds with this premise. A study by Schneider et al.[717] also observed opposed variations in T_{amp} responses depending on the considered $PM_{2.5}$ lag. In general, changes in repolarization might be the result of changes in the ion channel function or a direct effect of the ANS on the ventricular myocardium.[601,705,706] However, the understanding of the complex biologic pathways is still very limited.

It has been shown that TWA is a reliable predictor for SCD.[718] Zanobetti et al.[676] observed an association between black carbon on TWA in CAD patients. Prolonged QT_c is a risk factor for cardiac arrhythmia[703] and cardiovascular mortality.[719] Hampel et al.'s[707] results suggest that elevated levels of air pollutants might trigger changes in T_{amp} and QT_c and therefore might predispose to additional cardiovascular problems in individuals who had already experienced an MI. Extremes in temperature may also influence these outcomes.

Yamamoto et al.[720] found increased HR and reduced HRV after exposing six healthy Japanese to a heated condition (37°C) in a chamber study. Bruce-Low et al.[721] observed similar results among participants with ECG measurements before and during exposure to heat in a sauna. In Hampel et al.'s[707] analyses, HR did not appear to be altered by temperature changes, but during the study period, 24-hour averages of temperature never exceeded 28°C, which is similar to the temperature conditions before heat exposures in the previously described studies.

Several studies reported a U- or J-shaped influence of apparent temperature on cardiorespiratory mortality; the lowest mortality was observed for temperatures between 15°C and 25°C.[722,723] However, Baccini et al.[722] conducted their study only in the summer, whereas Hampel et al.'s[707] study took almost 1 year with low temperatures during the winter. A study conducted by McMichael et al.[693] also included Asian and South American cities with high mean temperatures.

Lin et al.[724] reported an increased risk of cardiovascular events during a follow-up of 30 days among patients with T-wave flattening at the time of the emergency department visit. In their study, T_{amp} decreased with temperature increases as well as decreases. Wolf et al.[725] observed an inverse relation between temperature and MI occurrence. Therefore, temperature might act as a trigger for T-wave flattening in susceptible individuals, leading to an enhancement of already existing cardiovascular problems. In chemically sensitive patients with cardiovascular involvement, the senior author of this book has observed the U- and J-shaped curve in many situations with both low and high temperatures.

As core temperature should not be affected by small changes in ambient temperature, we can only speculate that Hamel et al.'s observed associations are probably affected by changes in the ANS or by loading effects on the heart possibly mediated by cutaneous blood flow regulation or neural input from temperature sensors in the skin.

Large-Vessel Disease and Small-Vessel Disease in Combination

Outdoor air pollution may increase the risk of strokes coupled with macrovessel and microvessel disease. A Georgia (U.S.) study found that admissions for strokes and peripheral vascular disease (thrombosis, claudication, aneurysm, vasculitis) were significantly associated with higher outdoor levels of CO, $PM_{2.5}$, and NO_2.[337] A study of 19,005 stroke deaths in a 7-year period in Seoul, South Korea, found that higher levels of particulates and sulfur dioxide were associated with significantly higher rates of stroke mortality.[726] A study in Shanghai found that higher levels of outdoor particulates and nitrogen oxides were associated with significantly higher stroke mortality rates.[727] However, a study in eight European cities found that increased levels of PM_{10} had little effect on stroke incidence.[728] A 1994–1998 study in Sheffield, United Kingdom found that stroke mortality was significantly higher at the highest quintile of exposure to NO_2 (37% higher mortality), PM_{10} (33% higher), and CO (26% higher) as compared to lowest quintile of exposures to these pollutants.[729] Presumably, many of these were not only macrovascular occlusions but also microvascular spasms and lack of O_2 extraction.

Air pollutants (both NO_2 and $PM_{2.5}$) were positively associated with stroke mortality in this study based in Japan, but the associations were stronger for hemorrhagic stroke, especially for subarachnoid hemorrhage, than for ischemic stroke mortality. Of course, pollutant injury can weaken the walls of the microcirculation and vasa vasorum causing a wall weakness with a blood leak or blow out.

The present finding that both pollutants were positively associated with ischemic stroke is consistent with the previous studies conducted in Western[653] as well as Asian contexts.[726] In addition, the finding that NO_2 was positively associated with intracerebral hemorrhage mortality was also consistent with the previous study conducted in Asia.[652] The pattern found that both air pollutants (especially $PM_{2.5}$) were more strongly associated with subarachnoid hemorrhage mortality that has not been reported previously, which may be attributable to the HF of strokes of the hemorrhagic type or stronger effects of air pollution for stroke mortality in Japan (Tables 2.24 and 2.25).[729]

Air pollution is hypothesized to raise the risk of ischemic stroke through increased plasma viscosity.[726] However, vascular loads from the hypoxia may have occurred more than just edema resulting in hemorrhage or severe vascular spasm. In contrast, the potential mechanisms linking air pollution to hemorrhagic stroke may include the following: first, direct ischemic damage to blood vessels induced by air pollution might lead to brain hemorrhage[730] due to small- or medium-sized vessel inflammation and leak or spasm; second, air pollution has been associated with acute endothelial dysfunction (atherosclerosis or vasculitis),[696] which may lead to the brain vessels' vulnerability to rupture[603] or severe spasm; third, air pollution may trigger vasoconstriction or hypertension,[696] which might also lead to hemorrhagic stroke or spasm; and fourth, coughing due to air pollution may result in raised intracranial pressure (Valsalva effect), which may rupture vulnerable aneurysms or fragile inflamed vessels that are already leaking fluid or just causing spasm. Furthermore, the finding that the associations were stronger for hemorrhagic stroke than for ischemic stroke mortality may be attributable to the existence of potential effect modifiers (environmental and genetic factors such as hypertension, pesticide or severe natural gas exposure, or heavy drinking), which might be associated with HF of hemorrhagic stroke in Japan.[731] In addition, the entry of Ca^{2+} and the release of intracellular Ca^{2+} combine with protein kinases A and C; and when the complex is phosphorylated, it effects the cell wall increasing sensitivity up to 1000 times, which will allow incitants to be able to punch more holes in the cell wall to bleed at lower levels of pressure intensity.[4]

TABLE 2.24

Air Pollutants Concentrations, Meteorological Variables, and Stroke Mortality from April 2003 to December 2008 in 23 Special Wards, Tokyo, Japan

	Mean (SD)	Minimum	Maximum
Air pollutants			
NO_2, ppb	344 (11.1)	7.0	74.0
$PM_{2.5}$, μg/m³	21.6 (10.8)	2.5	80.0
Meteorology			
Temperature, °C	16.6 (7.8)	0.9	33.1
Relative humidity, %	66.7 (14.5)	26.8	96.1
Barometric pressure, hPa	1009.4 (6.7)	986.0	1031.5
Mortality (no. of daily mortality)			
Stroke (160–161, 163, 169–169.3)	19.7 (5.1)	3	39
Subarachnoid hemorrhage (160, 169.0)	2.4 (1.5)	0	9
Intracerebral hemorrhage (161, 169.1)	5.6 (2.5)	0	20
Ischemic stroke (163, 169.3)	11.7 (3.7)	1	27

Source: Adapted from Lippincott Williams and Wilkins. 2011.

Note: NO_2, nitrogen dioxide; $PM_{2.5}$, particulate matter < 2.5 μm; SD, standard device.

MITOCHONDRIAL UCPS AND BIOGENESIS FACTORS IN mROS GENERATION

Mitochondrial uncoupling is a process involving the disassociation of mitochondrial respiration from ATP generation that is characterized by increased permeability of the inner mitochondrial membrane to protons and subsequent dissipation of mitochondrial membrane potential.

Respiratory burst is a large increase in oxygen consumption and ROS generation that accompanies the exposure of neutrophils to microorganisms and/or inflammatory mediators.

NADPH oxidase is a plasma membrane– and phagosomal membrane–bound enzyme complex that transfers electrons from NADPH to molecular oxygen, promoting the generation of the ROS superoxide.

UCP2 is a member of a family of mitochondrial uncoupling proteins that are homologous to UCP1. Although UCP2 shares 60% sequence identity with UCP1 and both proteins localize to the IM, UCP2 exhibits a broad tissue distribution and is abundantly expressed in monocytes and macrophages,[732] whereas UCP1 expression is restricted to brown adipose tissue. UCP2 has been shown to induce mild mitochondrial uncoupling, which increases the rate of respiration and is thought to reduce electron leak from oxidative phosphorylation complexes, thereby decreasing mitochondrial superoxide generation.[733]

IMMUNOMODULATION BY LEAD

According to Singhy et al.,[734] lead, a potential human carcinogen, is a ubiquitous environmental pollutant in the industrial environment that poses a serious threat to human health. This toxic lead can modulate the immune response of animals as well as humans. In some instances, the immune system appears to be exquisitely sensitive to lead as compared with other toxicological parameters. Both stimulation and suppression of immune response have been demonstrated in lead-exposed animals and humans depending on the T helper (Th) 1 versus Th2 response. Although the majority of data accumulated to date pertain to the effects of lead in small laboratory rodents, there is little reason to believe that similar quantifiable effects do not occur in domestic and food-producing animals owing to basic functional similarities of the immune system of mammals.

TABLE 2.25

Adjusted Rate Ratios[a] with a 10-Unit Increase in Pollutants and 95% Confidence Intervals for Stroke Mortality

	RR (95% CI)				
	Lag 0	Lag 1	Lag 2	Lag 0–1	Lag 0–2
NO2 (per 10 ppb increase)					
Stroke	1.015 (1.003–1.027)	0.997 (0.98–1.009)	1.001 (0.990–1.012)	1.009 (0.995–1.024)	1.009 (0.993–1.026)
Subarachnoid hemorrhage	1.002 (0.969–1.036)	1.034 (1.002–1.068)	1.012 (0.982–1.044)	1.031 (0.988–1.075)	1.037 (0.989–1.088)
Intracerebral hemorrhage	1.023 (1.001–1.046)	0.996 (0.975–1.017)	0.995 (0.976–1.016)	1.015 (0.987–1.043)	1.009 (0.978–1.041)
Ischemic stroke	1.013 (0.998–1.029)	0.991 (0.977–1.005)	1.001 (0.988–1.015)	1.003 (0.984–1.022)	1.004 (0.982–1.025)
PM2.5 (per 10 μg/m3 increase)					
Stroke	1.013 (1.002–1.024)	0.999 (0.989–1.010)	0.998 (0.989–1.008)	1.009 (0.995–1.023)	1.006 (0.991–1.022)
Subarachnoid hemorrhage	1.012 (0.980–1044)	1.041 (1.011–1.072)	1.009 (0.981–1.038)	1.043 (1.004–1.084)	1.044 (1.000–1.090)
Intracerebral hemorrhage	1.012 (0.991–1033)	0.986 (0.966–1006)	0.994 (0.975–1.012)	0.997 (0.971–1.022)	0.992 (0.964–1.021)
Ischemic stroke	1.014 (0.999–1.028)	0.997 (0.984–1.011)	0.998 (0.986–1.011)	1.008 (0.990–1.025)	1.005 (0.986–1.025)

Source: Adapted from Lippincott Williams and Wilkins. 2011.

Note: CI, confidence interval; NO_2, nitrogen dioxide; $PM_{2.5}$, particulate matter < 2.5 μm; RR, rate ratio.

[a] Adjusted for same-day temperature (df = 6), same-day relative humidity (df = 3), the number of patients with influenza, seasonal variation (df = 12/year), barometric pressure, public holiday, and day of the week.

INFLAMMATION

Acute inflammation is an early response to injury/infection, usually lasting days. Classic signs and symptoms are localized swelling, redness, heat, and pain.

Cytokines are usually beneficial, leading to elimination of infection and subsequent tissue healing by innate cells and mediators.

Chronic inflammation is a late or sustained response to intracellular pathogens, toxicants, or self-antigens (autoimmunity), which is harmful, resulting in tissue destruction. These are using the adaptive and innate cells and mediators.

RIGHT HEART ABNORMALITIES

Right heart failure is a cause of morbidity and mortality in obstructive and restrictive lung disease, left ventricular dysfunction, and when pulmonary arterial hypertension occurs.[735–737] Right ventricular (RV) hypertrophy is also associated with increased risk for heart failure and cardiovascular death in community-dwelling adults without known cardiac disease at baseline.[738] Despite important epidemiologic and clinical roles of the RV, little is known about modifiable determinants of RV structure function.[739]

Traffic-related air pollution is linked to left ventricular hypertrophy, heart failure, and cardiovascular death,[552,581] as shown previously. Air pollution may affect the left ventricle through oxidative stress, inflammation, and autonomic dysfunction, and these mechanisms could also affect the RV.[659,740,741] These effects are seen in the majority of the chemically sensitive heart vascular patients treated in Dallas. There are symptoms of vasculitis and cardiovascular disease in the earlier stages. The lungs have substantial exposure to traffic-related air pollution and inhalants, which may directly increase RV afterload and lead to disproportionately greater changes in the RV compared to the left ventricle.[742,743] The impact of traffic-related air pollution on the RV, however, is not well studied. However, Leary et al.[744] have emphasized epidemiologically in situations that the EHC-Dallas has observed over the last 30 years of studying patients in the controlled environments.

Leary et al.[744] examined the relationship between nitrogen dioxide (NO_2), a surrogate for traffic-related air pollution and total environmental pollutant load, and MRI measures of RV structure and function in a multiethnic cohort of adults free of clinical cardiovascular disease. They hypothesized that increased exposure to NO_2 would be independently associated with greater RV mass and larger RV end-diastolic volume (RVEDV). Some of the results in these studies have been previously reported in the form of an abstract (Tables 2.26 through 2.29).[745]

Leary et al.[744] Multi-Ethnic Study of Atherosclerosis (MESA) is a multicenter prospective cohort study designed to investigate subclinical cardiovascular disease.[746,747] Exclusion criteria included clinical cardiovascular disease (physician diagnosed heart attack, stroke, transient ischemic attack, heart failure, angina, current AF, any cardiovascular procedure), weight >136 kg (300 lbs), pregnancy, or impediment to long-term participation.

Using weighted averages of residential addresses over the year prior to cardiac MRI, individual outdoor home exposure to NO_2 and NO_x was estimated using spatiotemporal modeling and maximized via maximum likelihood.[748,749] Estimates were fit using monitoring data from the Environmental Protection Agencies Air Quality System database and extensive cohort-specific air monitoring including home-based monitoring conducted as a part of MESA Air.[750] Geographical variables incorporated into the model included information on land use (e.g., industrial, residential), vegetative index, distance to various features (e.g., airports, coastline), road density, population density, elevation, urban topography, emissions sources, and dispersion model outputs integrating road position, traffic volume, diurnal traffic patterns, and meteorology.

According to Leary et al.,[744] methods for acquisition and interpretation of LV and RV MRI parameters have been previously reported.[751,752] Endocardial and epicardial borders of the RV were manually traced on short-axis cine images at end-systole and end-diastole. The outflow tract was

TABLE 2.26

Multivariable Linear Regression Estimating the Associations between NO$_2$ Exposure and Right Ventricular Structure and Function in the Full Model[a] with Further Adjustment for Differences in Roadway Noise, Inflammation, and Lung Disease

Model	Per Interquartile Increase in NO$_2$		
	Difference	95% CI	p-Value
RV Mass, g, full model (n = 3896)	1.0	0.4, 1.5	0.001
Full + roadway noise (n = 3890)	1.0	0.4, 1.5	0.001
Full + CRP and IL-6 (n = 3804)	1.1	0.5, 1.6	<0.001
Full + % emphysema (chest CT) and self Reported asthma or emphysema (n = 3893)	0.9	0.4, 1.5	0.001
RVEDV, mL, full model (n = 3896)	4.1	0.5, 7.7	0.03
Full + roadway noise (n = 3,890)	3.9	0.3, 7.6	0.04
Full + CRP and IL-6 (n = 3,804)	4.2	0.5, 7.8	0.03
Full + % emphysema (chest CT) and self Reported asthma or emphysema (n = 3893)	3.7	0.1, 7.3	0.04

Source: Reprinted with permission of the American Thoracic Society. Copyright 2017. Leary, P. J. 2014. Traffic-related air pollution and the right ventricle. *The American Journal of Respiratory and Critical Care Medicine.* 189(7):1093–1100.

Note: NO$_x$, nitrogen dioxide; CI, confidence interval; RV, right ventricular, CRP, C-reactive protein; IL-6, interleukin-6; CT, computed tomography; RVEDV, right ventricular end-diastolic volume.

[a] Adjusted for age, sex, race/ethnicity, height, weight, city, education, income, smoking, pack-years, hypertension, diabetes, cholesterol, and impaired glucose tolerance.

included in RV volume. Papillary muscle and trabeculae were included in RV volumes and excluded from RV mass, as is commonly done for LV mass.[753,754] RV end-systolic volume and RVEDV were calculated using Simpson's rule by summation of areas on each slice multiplied by the sum of slice thickness and image gap. RV mass was determined at end-diastole as the difference between RV free wall end-diastolic epicardial and endocardial volumes multiplied by the specific gravity of the heart (1.05 g/mL). RVEF was calculated by subtracting RV end-systolic volume from RVEDV and dividing this difference by RVEDV.

Leary et al.[744] has shown that higher estimates of long-term outdoor residential NO$_2$ exposure are associated with greater RV mass and larger RVEDV in a multiethnic, multicity cohort of adults without clinical cardiovascular disease. MESA participants had a 1.0 g (5%) increase in RV mass and 4.1 mL (3%) increase in RVEDV with an interquartile increase in NO$_2$. This difference in RV mass is quantitatively similar to that seen in LV mass in MESA participants with diabetes (2.4%) and current smokers (5.3%), supporting clinical and biologic relevance.[755,756] RV hypertrophy in MESA participants is associated with a threefold increased risk for heart failure or cardiovascular death.[738] This is the first report to suggest traffic-related air pollutants, of which NO$_2$ is a well-recognized surrogate for the pollutant mix (total environmental load), are associated with morphologic changes in the right ventricle of the heart.

Their study provides initial insight into timing of this association. Duration of exposure to traffic-related air pollutants appears to be important. Participants who lived in the same neighborhood for several years had the strongest associations between NO$_2$ and RV mass. This suggests that a dose–response may provide insight for duration of necessary exposure, and supports a causal relationship.

The finding of both increased RV mass and RVEDV may suggest that the exposure of interest increased RV afterload.[757] Previous studies have suggested that air pollution increases endothelin-1, a potent pulmonary vasoconstrictor,[758] which could lead to increased pulmonary vascular resistance,

TABLE 2.27

Residential Stability as a Proxy for the Timing of Exposure to Traffic-Related Air Pollution: A Sliding Time Window Analysis of the Full Model[a]

Number of Years Lived in the Same Neighborhood	n	Per Interquartile Increase in NO_2		
		RV mass (g)	95% CI	p-Value
0–5 years	785	1.0	(−0.2, 2.4)	0.09
1–6 years	834	1.1	(−0.2, 2.3)	0.09
2–7 years	848	1.3	(0.0, 2.5)	0.04
3–8 years	816	1.8	(0.5, 3.0)	0.005
4–9 years	743	1.6	(0.3, 2.9)	0.02
5–10 years	773	1.6	(0.3, 2.9)	0.02
6–11 years	727	1.6	(0.3, 2.9)	0.01
All years	3896	1.0	(0.4, 1.5)	0.001
	n	RVEDV (mL)	95% CI	p-Value
0–5 years	785	4.8	(−3.2, 12.8)	0.24
1–6 years	834	4.7	(−3.1, 12.5)	0.24
2–7 years	848	4.4	(−3.5, 12.3)	0.28
3–8 years	816	7.5	(−0.5, 15.5)	0.07
4–9 years	743	7.2	(−1.2, 15.6)	0.10
5–10 years	773	3.8	(−4.6, 12.2)	0.37
6–11 years	727	4.6	(−3.7, 13.0)	0.28
All years	3896	4.1	(0.5, 7.7)	0.03

Source: Reprinted with permission of the American Thoracic Society. Copyright 2017. Leary, P. J. 2014. Traffic-related air pollution and the right ventricle. *The American Journal of Respiratory and Critical Care Medicine.* 189(7):1093–1100.

Note: NO_2, nitrogen dioxide; CI, confidence interval; RV, right ventricular; RVEDV, right ventricular end-diastolic volume.

[a] Adjusted for age, sex, race/ethnicity, height, weight, city, education, income, smoking, pack-years, hypertension, diabetes, cholesterol, and impaired glucose tolerance.

increased RV afterload, and ultimately RV hypertrophy and dilation. Alternatively, air pollutants can irritate the respiratory epithelium and lead to heterogeneous ventilation with decreased regional ventilation.[759] Regional hypoxia can cause hypoxic pulmonary vasoconstriction, increased resistance, and RV enlargement.[760] Increases in afterload may compound oxidative stress and autonomic dysfunction, which have been implicated in the relationship between air pollution and LV mass and could directly contribute to RV pathology.[659,740,741,761]

Other mechanisms are possible as well. Air pollution may upregulate myocardial inflammatory genes and proteins in the RV.[762] While it is not feasible to study myocardial gene and protein profiles in such a large study of the general population, their findings remained after adjustment for C-reactive protein and interleukin-6 blood levels, which suggests that their findings were independent of systemic inflammation. Roadway noise, which accompanies traffic-related air pollution and may disrupt sleep, could mediate some aspects of the relationship between roadway proximity and heart disease.[763] Adjusting for traffic-related noise did not attenuate relationships between NO_2 and RV morphology in our analyses.

Air pollution has also been linked to obstructive lung disease severity, which could increase RV afterload leading to increased RV mass.[764,765] However, they have previously shown that increasing

TABLE 2.28

Multivariable Linear Regression Estimating the Associations between NO_x Exposure and Right Ventricular Structure and Function

Model	Per Interquartile Increase NO_x (48 ppb)		
	Difference	95% CI	p-Value
RV mass, g (limited model[a])	0.2	(0.0, 0.4)	0.04
RV mass, g (limited model[a] + city)	0.4	(0.0, 0.8)	0.04
RV mass, g (full model[b])	0.5	(0.1, 0.8)	0.03
RVEDV, mL (limited model[a])	1.3	(0.0, 2.7)	0.05
RVEDV, mL (limited model[a] + city)	0.8	(−1.7, 3.3)	0.52
RVEDV, mL (full model[b])	1.7	(−0.9, 4.2)	0.20
RVEF, % (limited model[a])	0.0	(−0.4, 0.4)	0.98
RVEF, % (limited model[a] + city)	0.1	(−0.6, 0.8)	0.78
RVEF, % (full model[b])	0.1	(−0.6, 0.9)	0.72

Source: Reprinted with permission of the American Thoracic Society. Copyright 2017. Leary, P. J. 2014. Traffic-related air pollution and the right ventricle. *The American Journal of Respiratory and Critical Care Medicine.* 189(7):1093–1100.

Note: NO_x, oxides of nitrogen; CI, confidence interval; ppb, parts per billion; RV, right ventricular; LV, left ventricular; RVEDV, right ventricular end-diastolic volume; LVEDV, left ventricular end-diastolic volume; RVEF, right ventricular ejection fraction; LVEF, left ventricular ejection fraction.

[a] Adjusted for age, sex, race/ethnicity, height, and weight.

[b] Adjusted for age, sex, race/ethnicity, height, weight, city, education, income, smoking, pack-years, hypertension, diabetes, cholesterol, and impaired glucose tolerance.

airflow obstruction is associated with decreased RVEDV in MESA.[766] In addition, adjustment for structural or self-reported lung disease did not change relationships between NO_2 and RV morphology in this analysis. Finally, LV mass may increase with traffic-related air pollution and LV hypertrophy can contribute to diastolic dysfunction and increased RV afterload, potentially explaining their results.[581,767] However, adjusting for the LV did not affect the results.

Relationships between NO_2 and RV morphology were similar, but mildly attenuated compared to those with NO_2. In addition, the relationship between NO_2 and RVEDV was sensitive to adjustment. The NO_2 analyses reinforce that the observed relationships are consistent with associations of a pollutant mix (total environmental pollutant load) not a specific pollutant and that relationships between these pollutants and RV mass are stronger than relationships with RVEDV.

It is clear that higher estimated exposure to NO_2 is associated with greater RV mass and larger RVEDV. This relationship is independent of markers of socioeconomic status, cardiovascular risk factors, left-side cardiovascular disease, and markers of inflammation and lung disease. This is the first report to implicate traffic-related air pollution with changes in RV morphology. Air pollution may therefore play a role in determining the RV response and outcomes in cardiopulmonary disease.

AGE-SPECIFIC INCIDENCE, OUTCOME, COST, AND PROJECTED FUTURE BURDEN OF ATRIAL FIBRILLATION–RELATED EMBOLI

The increase in life expectancy, partly attributable to prevention of premature vascular deaths, and the consequent increase in the elderly population have implications for the effective targeting of preventive medicine and healthcare costs. A key issue for prevention of vascular disease and for future burden is the extent to which incidence of nonfatal events is also moving to older ages.

TABLE 2.29

Multivariable Linear Regression Estimating the Associations between NO$_2$ Exposure by Calendar Year and Right Ventricular Structure and Function in the Full Model[a]

Model	Per Interquartile Increase in NO$_2$		
	Difference	95% CI	p-Value
Calendar year 2000 (NO2 IQR 17.7 ppb)			
RV mass, g	0.8	0.2, 1.3	0.005
RVEDV, mL	4.3	0.8, 7.8	0.02
RVEF, %	0.1	−0.9, 1.1	0.82
Calendar year 2001 (NO2 IQR 17.0 ppb)			
RV mass, g	0.9	0.4, 1.4	0.001
RVEDV, mL	4.4	1.0, 7.8	0.01
RVEF, %	−0.1	−1.1, 0.8	0.77
Calendar year 2002 (NO2 IQR 17.5 ppb)			
RV mass, g	0.9	0.3, 1.4	0.002
RVEDV, mL	4.1	0.6, 7.6	0.02
RVEF, %	−0.3	−1.3, 0.7	0.56

Source: Reprinted with permission of the American Thoracic Society. Copyright 2017. Leary, P. J. 2014. Traffic-related air pollution and the right ventricle. *The American Journal of Respiratory and Critical Care Medicine.* 189(7):1093–1100.

Note: NO$_2$, nitrogen dioxide; CI, confidence interval; IQR, interquartile range; RV, right ventricular; LV, left ventricular; RVEDV, right ventricular end-diastolic volume; LVEDV, left ventricular end-diastolic volume; RVEF, right ventricular ejection fraction; KVEF, left ventricular ejection fraction.

[a] Adjusted for age, sex, race/ethnicity, height, weight, city, education, income, smoking, pack-years, hypertension, diabetes, cholesterol, and impaired glucose tolerance.

Stroke

Stroke is a major cause of death and disability,[768,769] leaving 5 million people permanently disabled in Europe each year at a cost of 38 billion euros in 2006.[770] AF is one of the most common preventable causes of stroke. AF-related ischemic strokes tend to be severe and to incur high mean costs,[771] and noncerebral systemic embolism secondary to AF is also a major clinical burden.[772,773] With 2.3 million people estimated to have AF in the United States,[774] with prevalence increasing from 0.5% at 50–59 years to 10% at ≥80 years, and with age-specific prevalence possibly also increasing,[774–776] the burden and cost of AF-related stroke and systemic embolism could increase dramatically. However, anticoagulation with warfarin is highly effective in primary prevention of AF-related embolic events,[777,778] and several new oral anticoagulants may be of at least equivalent clinical benefit,[779] albeit with some disadvantages.[780,781] Yet, there is widespread underuse of warfarin for AF,[782–784] particularly in the elderly.[785–787] Although there are few published data on the safety of newer anticoagulants at age ≥80 years,[779,788] there is good evidence that warfarin is more effective than aspirin in primary prevention in high-risk elderly patients with AF.[789]

We could therefore be facing a substantial increase in potentially preventable AF-related embolic events at older ages because of the multiplicative effects of increased life expectancy, and low rates of use of anticoagulation in older people with AF with little evidence of any recent improvement.[782,787] One major barrier to action at the public health policy level is that in contrast to the numerous studies documenting low rates of anticoagulation, there are few published data on the consequences and costs of such undertreatment in terms of potentially preventable embolic events at the population level and no data on projected future burden. Gabriel et al.[790] therefore performed a prospective population-based study of all stroke and systemic embolism associated with AF in

Oxfordshire, United Kingdom, during 2002–2012 to determine age- and sex-specific incidence; rates of prior AF; premorbid treatment in relation to age, sex, risk scores, and contraindications; premorbid disability; clinical outcome; and cost. By comparison with a sister study in the same population in 1981–1986, they also determined the change in numbers of AF-related ischemic strokes, reflecting the combined impact of trends in age-specific incidence of AF, aging of the population, and the impact of anticoagulation. Finally, they projected future numbers of AF-related thromboembolic events in older people if prevention is not improved.

Although the high prevalence of AF in the elderly and the widespread underuse of anticoagulation are well described, the impact on event rates at the population level has not been determined previously. By studying the combined burden of AF-related stroke and peripheral embolic events, they have made several observations that have important implications for the future burden of disease and improving prevention. As expected in view of the aging population, the number of AF-related ischemic strokes (and presumably also other embolic events) at older ages have increased over the last 25 years. However, this increase in absolute numbers is greater than expected on the basis of demographic change alone because of a concomitant increase in incidence of AF-related ischemic stroke at age ≥80 years, despite the advent of convincing trial evidence of the effectiveness of anticoagulation. Crucially, from an overall burden of disease perspective, this increase in events at older ages has not been counterbalanced by a reduction in incidence of events at younger ages (i.e., there has been no right shift in age-specific incidence). Even assuming, as we have, that age-specific incidence of AF-related stroke at older ages does not continue to increase, without improved prevention the absolute number of AF-related ischemic strokes and systemic emboli will treble again by 2050 on the basis of demographic change alone (Figure 2.28).

They also documented in detail the consequences and costs of potentially preventable AF-related ischemic events at the population level. Only 9% of patients aged ≥80 years with ischemic stroke or systemic emboli related to known prior AF were on premorbid anticoagulants (despite the vast majority having a high CHADS2 score and low bleeding risk and despite the low rate of documented contraindications). Consequently, there was a 50-fold imbalance in this age group between numbers of AF-related embolic events (n = 208) and numbers of anticoagulant-associated intracerebral hemorrhages (n = 4). Importantly, more than half of patients aged ≥80 years and not anticoagulated were previously independent (mRS score ≤2), and nearly 90% were independently mobile (mRS score ≤2), but nearly three quarters were dead or more disabled 6 months after the event. Consequently, half of all disabling or fatal incident ischemic strokes at age ≥80 years in the OXVASC population were AF related. This underuse of anticoagulation was in stark contrast to the high rates of use of antihypertensive drugs and statins in these patients. Given our projection that by 2050 >80% of AF-related embolic events will occur at age ≥80 years and >90% at age ≥90 years, this underuse of anticoagulants in relatively fit older individuals is a major problem for public health.

Rates of anticoagulation for AF at age ≥80 years in the United Kingdom range from 21% to 46%, despite the Birmingham Atrial Fibrillation Treatment of the Aged (BAFTA) Study [789] having shown safety and effectiveness in the elderly. We found relatively high rates of premorbid antiplatelet drug use in older patients with known prior AF, consistent with evidence that physicians overestimate the bleeding risks of warfarin and underestimate its benefits and overestimate the benefits of antiplatelet drugs for stroke prevention in AF.[783] Although the benefit of anticoagulants over antiplatelet drugs in high-risk patients with AF is maintained at older ages,[789,791] there is a particular reticence to prescribe warfarin in healthy elderly patients with AF.[792] The availability of new oral agents, which postdated our study period, might change this, but there is little evidence thus far of any impact on rates of anticoagulation in older age groups.[793,794]

They found no evidence of any reduction in AF-related ischemic events during 2002–2012, despite the introduction in 2006 of AF registers in primary care as part of a remuneration scheme in the United Kingdom and publication of the BAFTA trial results in 2007.[789] AF registers are clearly potentially useful tools, but only 118 (26%) of 454 patients with incident AF-related ischemic

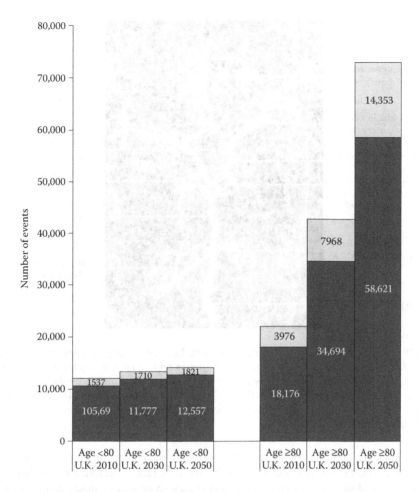

FIGURE 2.28 Projected number of atrial fibrillation–related incident ischemic strokes (dark gray bar) and incident systemic emboli (light gray bar) extrapolated from the Oxford Vascular Study to the U.K. population in 2010, 2030, and 2050 stratified by age and based on the current incidence rate in the Oxford Vascular Study. (Permission by Wolters Kluwer Health, Inc. Gabriel, S. C. Yin et al., Age-specific incidence, outcome, cost, and project future burden of atrial fibrillation-related embolic vascular events clinical perspective. *Circulation*. 130(15)1236–1244. https://www.ncbi.nlm.nih.gov/pubmed/25208551.)

strokes or systemic emboli in OXVASC did not have documented prior AF and were not aware of the diagnosis, and in some of these apparently undocumented cases, the AF would have been either very recent or potentially induced by the ischemic event itself. Overall, therefore, their findings show that most of the clinical burden of potentially preventable embolic events is attributable to undertreatment and not underdetection.

In conclusion, without improved prevention, the United Kingdom faces a substantial increase in potentially preventable AF-related embolic events because of the multiplicative effects of increased life expectancy and prevalence rates at older ages, without any evidence of a counterbalancing reduction in age-specific incidence at younger ages. AF projection studies in the United States[774,775] suggest that the findings will be generalizable to North America. Ongoing monitoring and improved prevention of embolic events in people with AF should be a major public health priority throughout the developed world and will become increasingly important in the developing world as populations age.

On the basis of the literature review described above, they have developed the following working model: intracranial arteries and especially the small circle of Willis arteries have a specific

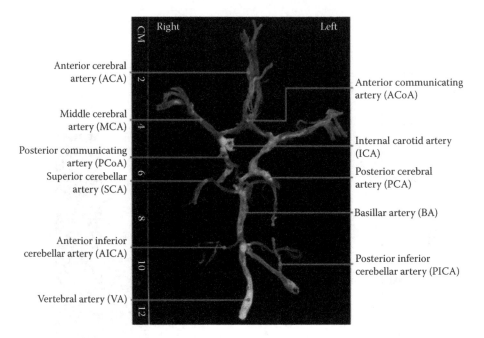

FIGURE 2.29   Circle of Willis of a 90-year-old subject. Macroscopically, atherosclerotic lesions can be identified by the white vessels, whereas nondiseased arteries appear largely transparent. This case shows prominent atherosclerosis mainly in the internal carotid artery, vertebral artery, basilar artery, left middle cerebral artery, and posterior cerebral artery. (Permission by Wolters Kluwer Health, Inc. Ritz, K. et al. Cause and mechanisms of intracranialo atherosclerosis. *Circulation* 130(16)1407–1414. http://circ.ahajournals.org/content/130/16/1407.full.)

constitution. They are muscular-type arteries that contain only a few medial elastic fibers, a thick and dense internal elastic lamina, and a few AVV, and they lack an external elastic lamina. A low endothelial permeability, a special glycocalyx, and enhanced protective mechanisms against oxidative stress suggest the presence of a barrier function. Early in life, the compliance of the aorta and carotid arteries maintains a low pulse pressure in the intracranial arteries, retarding the development of intracranial atherosclerosis. With increasing age and accelerated by hypertension, diabetes mellitus, and an enhanced stiffness of aorta and carotid arteries, the protective effect of a low pulse pressure is lost, and the enhanced pulsed-wave propagation may become a major driver of intracranial atherosclerosis later in life and explain the steep increase in incidence. The atherogenic effect of an increased pulse pressure can be modified by variations in the anatomy of the circle of Willis (Figure 2.29). Intracranial atherosclerotic lesions show special features such as fibrosis, small lipid pools, and a low grade of inflammation (macrophages and T-cells). This so-called stable plaque morphology may also explain the relatively low numbers of complicated (ruptured or eroded) plaques in intracranial arteries. The underlying mechanisms remain largely unknown but may be related to the abovementioned special constitution and characteristics of the intracranial arteries such as the scarceness of vasa vasorum, a high antioxidant capacity, low inflammasome activation and response, and protective effects of the CSF.

Cause and Mechanisms of Intracranial Atherosclerosis

Chemically sensitive patients may give us insight into the nonhypersensitive vascular pollutant because pollutant injury appears to be the same etiology to both types of vascular disease.

Intracranial atherosclerosis, one of the leading causes of ischemic stroke, is associated with an increased risk for recurrent stroke and dementia.[795,796] Individuals of Asian, Hispanic, and

African-American ancestry are especially affected. Recent European studies revealed a much higher prevalence of intracranial lesions than commonly presumed, suggesting that intracranial atherosclerotic disease is potentially the most common cause of ischemic stroke worldwide.[795,797] Ischemic strokes are clinically categorized into five subtypes based on their underlying cause: (1) large-artery atherosclerotic stenosis, (2) small-artery disease (lacunes), (3) cryptogenic, (4) major-risk-source cardiogenic embolism, and (5) unusual (e.g., dissections, arteritis). Most nonlacunar ischemic strokes are thought to be thromboembolic, which presumably also accounts for most cryptogenic strokes. Embolic sources include minor-risk or covert cardiac sources, veins via paradoxical embolism, and nonocclusive atherosclerotic plaques in the aortic arch or cervical or cerebral arteries.[798] Besides embolic strokes, two other mechanisms have been associated with intracranial atherosclerosis-related strokes, namely, hypoperfusion through a stenotic artery causing watershed or border-zone stroke and plaque overgrowth of perforator artery ostia, which is associated with penetrating artery disease and lacunar infarcts and has been related to cryptogenic strokes.[799–801] Even mild stenosis of intracranial atherosclerotic arteries (<50%) may therefore be clinically relevant, and high-resolution MRI studies are needed to identify and determine the degree and location of stenosis in this patient group.[799,802] The possibly causal role of nonstenotic plaques in ischemic stroke highlights the need for more insight into the mechanisms and occurrence of intracranial atherosclerosis.

In the 1960s and 1970s, large, descriptive autopsy studies were conducted, providing classic morphological features of intracranial arteries. Despite the importance of intracranial atherosclerosis to stroke and dementia, there is a lack of more recent mechanistic studies. Therefore, Ritz et al.[803] intends to draw attention to this neglected research field by providing an overview of available literature and a working model for intracranial atherosclerosis.

In 45%–62% of patients with ischemic stroke, intracranial plaques or stenosis were identified, which were causal in ≈10%–20% of cases (reviewed elsewhere[804]). The estimated prevalence of symptomatic intracranial stenosis in literature ranges from 20% to 53%, depending on the study population, race, and method of choice. Most studies revealed a higher incidence of intracranial atherosclerosis in Asians and African-Americans compared with white Americans. The few studies on white Europeans that are available suggest a high prevalence of intracranial plaques or stenosis. One French autopsy study detected intracranial plaques and stenosis in 62% and 43% of stroke cases, respectively, and in a Dutch study, 82% of asymptomatic patients showed calcification of the intracranial internal carotid artery (ICA) by computed tomography.[797,802] Notably, magnetic resonance angiography, computed tomography angiography, and transcranial Doppler, which measure luminal changes, may underestimate the number of intracranial plaques, partly explaining the large differences in the literature.[802]

In the 1960s and 1970s, several large-scale autopsy studies performed in asymptomatic cohorts from fetuses to patients in their 10th decade of life revealed intracranial atherosclerotic changes from the first to second decade, progressing with age.[805,806] Advanced atherosclerotic lesions are almost nonexistent up to the fourth decade.[807] Overall, intracranial atherosclerosis develops ≈20 years later in life compared with atherosclerosis in extracranial arterial beds.[808] Progression of atherosclerosis was not parallel in different vascular beds. Although aortic atherogenesis progressed linearly, intracranial atherosclerosis increased more slowly initially and paralleled aortic lesions thereafter.[807] The steepest gradient for the incidence of intracranial atherosclerosis was reported in the sixth and seventh decades,[805] with a steady increase beyond the eighth and ninth decades,[806] whereas coronary atherosclerosis progressed more rapidly initially and attenuated between the fifth and eighth decades.[807] A total of 3%–4% of individuals >80 years of age exhibited only mild intracranial atherosclerotic changes.[805,807] Intracranial atherosclerotic stenosis were described as dynamic lesions showing progression and regression, but they were less dynamic than coronary stenosis. Repeated magnetic resonance angiography over a 7-year period in patients with IHD showed a 1.1% annual progression of the average intracranial stenosis. Differences among the intracranial vessels were evident with stable atherosclerosis in the intracranial ICA and dynamic lesions in the ACA, MCA, and posterior cerebral arteries (PCAs), with 2.6% annual progression of average stenosis. Regression was noted in 14% of intracranial ICAs and 28% of ACAs, MCAs, and PCAs.[809] A 5-year longitudinal study of 41 Japanese patients with IHD reported the progression of cervical carotid artery stenosis in five patients (12%) and in only one patient with intracranial stenosis.[810] During a 2–3-year follow-up of 40 stroke patients, 33% of MCA stenosis progressed and 8% regressed.[811] Intracranial lesions were identified predominantly in the anterior circulation.[812] Overall, American and European studies showed a similar pattern: the ICA was most commonly affected, followed by the MCA, basilar artery (BA), intracranial vertebral artery (VA), PCA, and ACA (Figure 2.29).[805,813] The MCA appeared to be most commonly involved in Asians, followed by the ICA, BA, VA, PCA, and ACA.[812] In all cohorts, cerebellar and communicating arteries were barely affected. Atherosclerosis in the intracranial ICA was observed mainly in the cavernous and also in the supraclinoid segment.[813,814] The BA was commonly affected in the upper and lower parts and less affected in the middle part.[815] MCA lesions were mainly found in the M2 segment.[813]

One major characteristic that distinguishes healthy intracranial from extracranial arteries is that extracranial arteries such as the aorta and carotid arteries are elastic arteries rich in elastin filaments in the tunica media. In contrast, intracranial arteries are muscular arteries with few elastic fibers.[816] The transition from elastic to muscular artery is at the level of the carotid bifurcation[817] and embryological junctions between segments of the VA and ICA, which has been attributed to different embryological sites of origin of their primordial mesodermal cells.[818] Compared with extracranial arteries of a similar size, a thinner media, less abundant adventitia, and only a few elastic fibers have been reported for intracranial vessels[818] with a denser internal elastic lamina and without an external elastic lamina.[808,816] The external elastic lamina is still present in the petrous portion of the ICA but disappears within the cavernous portion, which forms a hotspot of stenosis.[819] A distinct vessel wall metabolism was suggested for intracranial arteries. Intima-media preparations of unaffected intracranial arteries showed lower contents of hexosamine, uronic acid, and sulfur, a lower proportion of hyaluronic acid and chondroitin sulfates in the total glycosaminoglycans (GAGs), and a lower ratio of ester to total cholesterol, whereas the percentage of heparin sulfate was higher compared with normal aorta and coronary arteries.[820] In addition, unaffected intracranial arteries of all ages revealed elevated antioxidant enzyme activity (manganese superoxide dismutase, copper-zinc superoxide dismutase, catalase) compared with extracranial arteries. Animal studies in rats and rabbits reported that the BA had less vesicles and caveolae and exhibited tight junctions between endothelial cells, leading to a reduced intimal permeability compared with the aorta and suggesting the presence of a barrier function.[821,822] In monkeys and rabbits, a distinct composition of the glycocalyx on luminal endothelial cells was suggested in cerebral arteries; the carbohydrate-binding protein concanavalin A reacted with aorta, coronary, and carotid arteries but not with cerebral arteries. It has been speculated that a specific glycocalyx composition inhibits trapping of chylomicrons and very-low-density lipoprotein, resulting in a reduced deposition of apolipoproteins in the intima of intracranial vessels.[823] In cats, histamine stimulation showed a threefold-stronger contraction of extracranial compared with intracranial arteries.[824] SMCs of rabbit intracranial arteries were relatively insensitive to sympathomimetic stimulation compared with systemic vessels.

PLAQUE CHARACTERISTICS AND AGE-RELATED CHANGES

In intracranial arteries, aging was associated with a gradual loss of elastic fibers and muscular elements in the media and an increase in collagen tissue replacing medial muscle fibers.[825] From the second to third decade, reduplication and splitting of the thick internal elastic lamina were observed frequently in combination with intimal thickening, which was most prominent from the fifth to sixth decade. In the same age group, fibrosis and hyalinization of media and adventitia prevailed.[815] In the aorta and coronary arteries, fragmentation and reduplication of the internal elastic lamina were common in fetuses, infants, and young juveniles. In contrast to the aorta, lipids were rarely observed in intracranial arteries in patients <15 years of age.[825]

Intracranial lesions not only developed later in life compared with extracranial vessels but also developed mainly as fibrous plaques with fewer fatty streaks and complicated lesions. Complicated lesions, which contain calcifications or a plaque rupture, appeared after the fifth decade with a degree of involvement and lipid content similar to that observed in coronary arteries and were limited mainly to proximal segments of the ICA, VA, and BA.[807,808] Hoff[826,827] reported no major differences in chemical and enzymatic plaque characteristics in intracranial compared with extracranial arteries and no qualitative differences in apolipoproteins (apolipoprotein A1 from high-density lipoprotein, apolipoprotein B from LDL, apolipoprotein CIII from very-low-density lipoprotein).

Intracranial arteries of human fetuses from hypercholesterolemic mothers showed fewer intimal macrophages and less intimal LDL, and oxidized LDL compared with extracranial arteries, which is suggestive of divergent atherogenic responses.[828,829] Evidence for intracranial protective mechanisms comes from animal studies in rabbits. Hypercholesterolemia alone evoked a reduced intimal permeability and foam cell accumulation in the aorta but not in the BA, whereas the combination of hypercholesterolemia and hypertension also affected the permeability of intracranial arteries.[822]

Review of the literature made clear that histological data in a recent cohort are lacking. Therefore, they screened 283 circle of Willis segments from 18 asymptomatic patients (mean age, 70.2 ± 10.9 years; range, 51–90 years; male, 9; causes of death: cardiovascular disease, 8; malignancy, 3; subarachnoid hemorrhage, 2; AD, 2; sickle cell disease, 1; acute stroke, 1; HIV/hepatitis, 1) for basic structural features (Methods in the online-only Data Supplement) (Table 2.30). In accordance with previous literature, we identified mainly early lesions (63%) and a few advanced atherosclerotic lesions (15%). Calcifications were rare (6%). Two patients presented with complicated lesions (chronic total occlusion and intraplaque hemorrhage). Intracranial arteries, especially the smaller arteries (ACA, PCA, and cerebellar and communicating arteries), show a distinct structure such as the lack of vasa vasorum and an external elastic lamina and only a few medial elastic fibers compared with extracranial arteries. The larger intracranial arteries such as the ICA, MCA, VA, and BA, however, show an intermediate phenotype sharing structural features of both the larger extracranial and the smaller intracranial arteries, which may explain the conflicting results in literature. Macrophage load was low in their series, which is in line which previous observations[829] (0.9% ± 0.7% CD68 positivity per plaque area compared with 1.8% ± 2.4% in

---

TABLE 2.30

Data from This Review on the Basic Characteristics of the Large Intracranial Arteries of 18 Asymptomatic Patients

	ICA	VA	MCA	BA
Type of lesion, % (n/N)				
Early	57 (17/30)	54 (15/28)	68 (19/28)	75 (24/32)
Advanced	33 (10/30)	25 (7/28)	25 (7/28)	16 (5/32)
High content of elastin fibers, % (n/N)	37 (11/30)	43 (12/28)	29 (8/28)	13 (4/32)
Continuous EEL, % (n/N)	17 (5/30)	79 (22/28)	21 (6/28)	9 (3/32)
Calcification, % (n/N)	20 (6/30)	18 (5/28)	14 (4/28)	9 (3/32)
Vasa vasorum, % (n/N)	53 (16/30)	43 (12/28)	11 (3/28)	16 (5/32)
Macrophages (mean ± SD), %	0.9 ± 0.7	0.4 ± 0.5	0.8 ± 0.7	0.9 ± 0.9

Source: See methods in the online-only Data Supplement for more information. Adapted from Ritz, K. et al. 2014. *Circulation* 130(16):1407–1414. http://circ.ahajournals.org/content/130/16/1407.

Note: BA, basilar artery; EEL, external elastic lamina; ICA, intracranial internal carotid artery; MCA, middle cerebral artery; and VA, intracranial vertebral artery.

coronaries).[830] In general, intracranial arteries exhibited fewer and more stable lesions, and the few advanced atherosclerotic lesions were identified predominantly in the large intracranial arteries such as the ICA, MCA, and VA.

Age is one of the most important independent risk factors for both intracranial and extracranial atherosclerosis. Several autopsy and imaging studies showed that aging is associated with increasing prevalence and severity of intracranial atherosclerosis among all investigated races with, as mentioned above, a distinct disease progression compared with extracranial arteries.[797,805,814,831]

African-Americans show a comparable or more severe degree of atherosclerosis compared with white Americans.[832] In Asians, intracranial atherosclerosis developed earlier and more extensively compared with white Americans and Europeans.[833] In symptomatic patients with transient ischemic attack or ischemic stroke, studies consistently reported the highest incidence and severity of intracranial atherosclerosis in Asians and Hispanics, followed by African-Americans and whites. The reverse order was found for extracranial lesions.[834,835] Differences in incidence and location of atherosclerosis were also observed within countries. Intracranial lesions in symptomatic patients were more common in North than in South China, which has been attributed to a more Westernized lifestyle in North China.[836] Within African populations, Nigerians had lower atherosclerotic scores compared with Senegalese, Ugandans, and African-Americans, with highest scores in the last group.[837,838] Therefore, observed differences among races cannot be attributed to genetic factors only but are highly influenced by lifestyle and other risk factors. In addition, most studies do not take into account differences in the prevalence of vascular risk factors being higher in Hispanic and African-American populations and maybe resulting in an overrepresentation of specific races in intracranial atherosclerosis.[839]

The incidence of extracranial atherosclerosis is higher in men; this correlation is less evident in patients with intracranial lesions.[814,831,840] This discrepancy may be attributed to the different disease course in men and women. Men showed a high increase in intracranial lesions in the fourth and fifth decades, which steadily progressed with age, whereas women exhibited relatively mild atherosclerotic lesions until the sixth decade, with rapidly increasing lesion formation thereafter. In the eighth and ninth decades, the degree of intracranial atherosclerosis was comparable between sexes, whereas women showed higher atherosclerotic scores in the 9th and 10th decades.[805,836] It has been speculated that the observed sex differences can be explained by a distinct risk factor profile resulting from the influence of sex hormones such as the known hypocholesterolemic effect of estrogens.[841]

It has been suggested recently that the circle of Willis and its communicating arteries protect the cerebral artery and BBB from hemodynamic stress.[842] In line with this hypothesis, variations in the circle of Willis were shown to influence the volume flow rates of the bilateral ICA and BA in healthy individuals and the development of atherosclerosis.[843,844] Racial differences in atherogenesis that have been discussed before could not be linked to anatomic variations of the circle of Willis.[845] No clear genetic risk factors such as 9p21 for CHD have been identified for intracranial atherosclerosis. Notably, most studies have been conducted in Asian cohorts; data for other countries, especially European countries, are lacking.

One of the most important risk factors for atherosclerosis, especially intracranial lesions, is hypertension. Hypertension has been correlated to the degree of atherosclerosis in intracranial arteries in different ethnic cohorts.[812,814,846] Some studies reported a higher incidence of hypertension in populations of African and Asian ancestry, which may explain their higher prevalence of intracranial atherosclerosis.[834,837,847]

Diabetes mellitus is a specific risk factor for intracranial lesions regardless of race in symptomatic and asymptomatic cohorts.[797,802,814,831,835] In Koreans, diabetes mellitus was an independent risk factor for intracranial lesions only after 50 years of age[841] and only in posterior, not anterior, circulation diseases in a prospective study.[812] As for hypertension, the aforementioned higher incidence of intracranial lesions in patients of African and Asian ancestry may be partly attributed to an increased prevalence of diabetes mellitus.[847]

Recent magnetic resonance angiography studies showed an independent association of the metabolic syndrome with intracranial atherosclerosis.[812,835] In a prospective Korean study, the metabolic syndrome was related more to intracranial than to extracranial lesions and to posterior and not anterior circulation strokes.[812]

Dyslipidemia is a known risk factor for coronary atherosclerosis and MI, but its role in intracranial atherosclerosis is less clear.[839,848] High LDL cholesterol was associated mainly with extracranial lesions, whereas a high ratio of apolipoprotein B to apolipoprotein I and low levels of apolipoprotein AI, the major protein component of high-density lipoprotein, correlated with intracranial lesions.[840,849] In China, low level of high-density lipoprotein cholesterol is one of the most common types of dyslipidemia and was associated with the development of intracranial artery stenosis in a cohort of acute ischemic stroke.[850] Sex-specific differences were reported in two Asian studies. Hypercholesterolemia was an independent risk factor for intracranial atherosclerosis only in asymptomatic men, whereas elderly symptomatic women >63 years of age had significantly more intracranial atherosclerotic lesions and hyperlipidemia than men.[836,841] Race and environmental factors may influence the effect of dyslipidemia on atherogenesis. Generally, individuals of Asian and African ancestry exhibited lower serum lipid levels than whites, which may be one factor explaining the lower incidence of extracranial and coronary atherosclerosis in both populations.[806,834]

Extracranial atherosclerosis was suggested as a risk factor for intracranial lesions. Extensive coronary atherosclerotic disease correlated with intracranial lesions,[802,806,851] and patients with concurrent lesions had a higher risk of suffering further (fatal) vascular events.[852] In a cohort of symptomatic intracranial atherosclerosis, 52% of cases were diagnosed with silent myocardial ischemia caused by CAD.[853] The American Heart Association Stroke Council recommends testing for asymptomatic CAD in patients who have had ischemic events associated with intracranial atherosclerosis.[804,854] In contrast, other studies reported correlations between coronary and carotid but not intracranial lesions[855] or failed to show a correlation.[810,813] A few studies suggested that smoking, especially duration of smoking, is a risk factor for intracranial lesions.[797,840] However, large-scale studies of the effects of smoking on intracranial atherosclerosis are scarce. As for extracranial lesions, moderate hyperhomocysteinemia was a predictor for severity of intracranial atherosclerosis in Asian patients with cerebral infarction.[856] A few reports associated AD, sickle cell disease, systemic lupus erythematosus, radiotherapy, bacterial meningitis, and herpes zoster infection with intracranial atherosclerosis, but their contribution needs further research.[857–862]

In conclusion, age, hypertension, diabetes mellitus, and probably the metabolic syndrome are the most consistent risk factors for intracranial atherosclerosis. Race may represent a predisposing factor, which is unfavorable in combination with other risk factors and especially lifestyle. Sex appears to influence intracranial atherosclerosis, and its effects are age dependent. Genetics may predispose to intracranial atherosclerosis, but large-scale association studies in different ethnic groups are lacking.

Two major characteristics that distinguish intracranial and extracranial atherosclerosis are the later onset and the more stable plaque phenotype in intracranial arteries, which may be explained by the distinct characteristics of the intracranial arteries. These characteristics may also be linked to the role of intracranial arteries in regulating the cerebrovascular resistance. The control mechanisms of CBF encompass cerebrovascular responsiveness to O_2 and CO_2, cerebral autoregulation and neurogenic control of the cerebral vasculature, endothelium-mediated signaling, and neurovascular coupling meeting local cerebral metabolic demand.[863] Cerebral artery endothelial cells and pericytes produce nitric oxide in direct proportion to the arterial CO_2 partial pressure[864] and contribute to the resting tone of cerebral arteries and arterioles.[865] Impairment of cerebral autoregulation results in pressure-passive CBF, that is, CBF increases and decreases together with cerebral perfusion pressure, whereas reduced CO_2 responsiveness affects the vasodilatory reserve of the brain.

EVALUATION OF THE ENDOCRINE SYSTEM

Evaluation of the endocrine system is discussed in detail in Rea, Chemical Sensitivity, Volume III, Chapter 24[60] and Reversibility of Chemical Sensitivity, Volumes II and III.[60,61]

Endocrine malfunction is often associated with CS. Imbalance in the affected endocrine organ may be hyper- or hypofunction, though the majority of patients experience hypofunction. There are a lot of hormone mimics, endocrine stimulants, and endocrine suppression avenues in the chemical contamination of the air, food, and water. Therefore, the endocrine system must be evaluated.

ADRENAL

The urine catecholamine profile and blood platelet–bound catecholamine are tests that provide a differential determination of the individual adrenal catecholamines, epinephrine, norepinephrine, dopamine, metanephrine, normetanephrine, MHPG, VMS, and serotonin. These may or may not be elevated in the chemically sensitive individual,[866] with data revealed in Table 2.31.

However, when these are elevated, the patient is usually hyperactive, and when they are depressed, the patient exhibits depression.

Assessment of Adrenocortical Function

Testing is indicated when blood or urine ratios of sodium/potassium are significantly abnormal or when Addison's disease or Cushing's syndrome is suspected. The most thorough tests are basal urine steroid profiles followed by ACTH challenge. Weakness in many chemically sensitive patients may suggest mild adrenal insufficiency, but usually weakness is due to mitochondrial damage.

Blood adrenal function tests are occasionally found to be abnormal in environmentally sensitive patients. However, gross changes are not found. Therefore, stress challenge tests must be done in order to make a complete evaluation of the adrenal pituitary axis. This assessment involves measuring urinary levels of androsterone (An) and etiocholanoline (Et), their ratio Et/An, and sums An + Et, dehydroepiandrosterone (DHEA), 11-ketoandrosterone, and 11-ketoetiocholanolone, 11-hydroxyanderosterone, 11-hyroxyetioallochalan-olone, pregnanediol, pregnanetrial, 11-deoxy tetrahydrocortisone, and tetrahydrocortisone. Then, the patient is stimulated with 0.25 mg ACTH (Cortrosyn), and the results are remeasured. At this point, a comparison of the two levels may be made. Various patterns will emerge; these include hypostimulation of the adrenal from lack of pituitary output and total adrenal response. Examples of each are shown in Table 2.32.[866]

These tests also measure DHEA, pregnanalol, pregnanetriol, androsterone, tetrahydrocortisones, 11-ketosteroid, and ACTH. Less comprehensive are measurements of plasma ACTH, plasma cortisol, urine 17-keto, and hydroxy steroids used to define diurnal variation.

Although uncommon, some patients with CS have abnormal cortical function tests.

Pineal Gland

A notable feature of sulfate is that it is difficult to transport.[867] Seneff's[868] extensive work on sulfur deficiency has led her to consider the important but perhaps underestimated role of the pineal gland in the transport process.

Seneff [868] suggests that one of the critical purposes of melatonin, in turn, is to deliver sulfate to the neurons at night during sleep. Seneff[868] outlined this intricate and elegant delivery system as follows:

1. With sunlight exposure serving as a catalyst, the pineal gland builds up supplies of sulfate by day, storing it in heparin sulfate molecules.
2. The pineal gland produces melatonin in the evening, transporting it as melatonin sulfate to various parts of the brain, including the third ventricle, where the melatonin releases the sulfate into the CSF.

TABLE 2.31

Adrenal Medullary Depression Profile Catecholamine Analysis of Platelets

Tests	Patient 9-6-87	Patient 12-20-89	Control ng/10 platelets		
Norepinephrine	0.07	3.0	3.3	–	10.6
Epinephrine	0.20	4.5	3.4	–	28.6
Normetanephrine	0.39	0.1	4.1	–	36.8
Metanephrine	0.89	1.5	4.0	–	37.2
Dopamine	0.23	11.6	1.4	–	10.3
Serotonin (SHT)	10.2	4.5	19.2	–	286.8
Tyramine				<5	
Cortisol/plasma	10.3	14.0	AM–7.25 µg%		
			PM–2.9 µg%		

Compound	Level	Urine
Norepinephrine	73.1	8.7–45.6 µg/24 hour
Epinephrine	7200	31.5–136.8 µg/24 hour
Normetanephrine	34	14.0–106.4 mg/24 hour
Metanephrine	3.9	99.0–419.3 µg/24 hour
Dopamine	<1.0	19.0–59.9 µg/24 hour
Serotonin	158.1	19.2–68.9 µg/24 hour
5-Hydroxyl inalacetic acid	–	0–10 mg/24 hour
3-Methoxy-4 pygroxyphenol glycol	158.3	128–1980 µg/24 hour
Vanilylmandelic acid	4.1	8–9.6 mg/24 hour
Homovanillic acid	–	0–15 µg/24 hour
Cortisol	115.7	20–90 µg/24 hour
Tyramine, free	–	0.68–3.3 mg/24 hour
Tyramine, total	–	1.0–7.3 mg/24 hour

		Blood
Monoamine	3.3	10.7–23.6 nmol/10 platelets/hour
Adrenal cortical antibody	+	
Testosterone antibody	–	

Source: Adapted from EHC-Dallas. 1990.

The association of autism with heparin sulfate depletion in the lateral and third venticles[869,870] now gets more interesting, because the tip of the third ventricle is encased in the pineal gland. The pineal recess is in fact the "main site of penetration of melatonin into the CSF."[871] In other words, under normal circumstances the pineal gland delivers melatonin sulfate to the third ventricle, which then diffuses the sulfate throughout the CSF. In addition, melatonin not only transports sulfate but also is an outstanding antioxidant and binds toxic metals to help dispose them off. It may come as no surprise, then, that melatonin impairment has not only been implicated in autism but also in CS.

Melatonin also plays an important role in inducing REM sleep, which may be the most important stage of sleep. Interestingly, AD is associated with reduced REM sleep and a calcified pineal gland. Sleep disorders are also linked to autism as well as other neurological diseases, including depression, schizophrenia, ALS, PD, and others.

TABLE 2.32
Adrenal Steroid Profile

Steroid	Random (mg/24 hour)			Reference Range (mg/24 hour)	
	Pre-ACTH (mg/24 hour)	Post-ATCH (mg/24 hour)	% Change	Post-pubertal Male	Post pubertal Pre-menopausal Female
Androsterone (AN)	Low 0.19	Low 0.37	+95	2.0–5.0	0.5–3.2
Etiocholanolone (Et)	Low 0.38	1.01	+166	1.4–5.0	0.5–5.0
Et/An	High 2.00	High 2.73	+37	0.31–0.89	0.21–1.83
An + Et	Low 0.57	1.38	+142	3.4–10.0	1.0–8.2
Dehydroepiandrosterone	Low 0.04	Low 0.09	+125	0.2–2.0	0.2–2.0
11-Keto-anderosterone and 11-Keto-epietiocholanolone	Low 0.06	Low 0.27	+350	0.4–2.1	0.4–2.6
11-Hydroxyandrosterone	0.19	0.46	+142	0.3–2.8	0.1–1.5
11-Hydroxyetiocholanolone	Low trace	Low 0.09	–	0.1–1.5	0.1–1.5
Pregnanediol	Low 0.06	0.37	+517	0.2–1.2	Fol. Phase: 0.2–2.4
					Lut Phase: 2.0–6.0
Pregnanetroil	Low 0.16	0.78	+388	0.5–2.0	0.8–2.0
11-Deoxy tetra hydrocortisone	0.05	0.27	+440	Trace–1.0	Trace–1.0
Tetrahydrocortisone	Low 0.96	4.01	+318	1.6–9.8	1.2–6.0
Aldosterone					

Source: Adapted from EHC-Dallas. 1991.

Heavy metals play a part in the modern-day epidemic of neurological diseases and part of the explanation for the sleep disorders encountered in various neurological diseases, which may be that both aluminum and mercury (thimerosal) disrupt the pineal gland and its ability to make sulfate. When the pineal gland's ability to make sulfate is impaired, this, in turn, reduces production of melatonin, all important for adequate and healthy sleep. The pineal gland is particularly susceptible to aluminum and other heavy metals because it is not protected by the BBB and has a very high blood perfusion rate.

According to Seneff,[868] melatonin makes an important link between autism and sulfation, concluding that children with abnormal sulfation chemistry (among other factors) may be particularly susceptible to the toxic effects of the thimerosal in flu and other childhood vaccines.[872]

Role of Sunlight

Seneff[868] underscored the important and neglected fact that sunlight is absolutely essential for human health because of its role in catalyzing sulfate production. Sulfate-deficiency occurs if the individual does not get enough sunlight. The pineal gland plays an important role in this process. Specifically, endothelial and neuronal NOS both of which are present in the pineal gland produce sulfate from reduced sulfur sources catalyzed by sunlight. When this process is impaired through lack of sunlight exposure, the result is sulfate deficiency and when a serum sulfate deficiency is present, an individual will also have an impaired ability to dispose of aluminum.[873] Aluminum accumulation in the pineal gland over time will disrupt sulfate supplies to the brain by interfering with the pineal gland's ability to make sulfate. A 2012 study found that nanoalumina destroyed mitochondria (thus severely depleting ATP, induced autophagy and programmed cell death in brain endothelial cells, and decreased expression of tight-junction proteins), thereby contributing to elevated BBB permeability.[874] The nanoparticle effects were persistent and damaging. Thus, contrary to popular opinion, use of sunscreen is neither beneficial nor safe.

Sunlight May Be Protective against Autism

Seneff[868] further assessed the importance of sunlight by compiling data from demographic studies in 50 states (Table 2.33).

Public schools in the United States keep track of the number of students enrolled in each grade, and they also keep track of the number of students enrolled in programs specifically targeting autism. Using a ratio of these numbers, Seneff[868] and coinvestigators calculated a measure for autism in each state (using grades one to six for the 2007–2008 school year). They also obtained data for weather-related factors, using these as proxies for sun exposure (e.g., number of clear days and a combination variable capturing latitude and rainfall) and looked at states' vaccination rates as a proxy measure for aluminum and thimerosal exposure.

They calculated Pearson's correlation coefficients as a way of understanding the strength of the relationship (or correlation) between sunlight exposure and autism. (Correlation coefficients range from −1 to 1, and a coefficient that is close to zero signals a weak relationship.) Bearing in mind that correlation does not necessarily mean causation, their analysis nonetheless produced correlations suggesting that sunlight is protective against autism, although other factors also clearly explain some of the variability.

Glyphosate: The Elephant in the Room

Both glyphosate and autism are associated with low melatonin, impaired sulfur metabolism (and low serum sulfate), low vitamin D, sleep disorders, disrupted gut bacteria, etc. Glyphosate, already a very dangerous chemical on its own, causes aluminum to be much more toxic. Glyphosate and aluminum can be viewed as "partners in crime," working synergistically. This partnership plays out in several ways:

1. First, glyphosate preferentially kills beneficial bacteria in the gut, which allows pathogens such as *C. difficile* to overgrow. Not only does this lead to leaky gut syndrome, but *C. difficile* produces *p*-cresol, a phenolic compound that is toxic to other microbes via its ability to interfere with metabolism. (*C. difficile* is one of only a few bacteria able to ferment tyrosine into *p*-cresol.) As it happens, *p*-cresol also promotes aluminum uptake by cells. *p*-Cresol is a known biomarker for autism and also an important factor in kidney failure, which leads to aluminum retention in tissues and eventually to dementia.

2. *Glyphosate* also serves to increase aluminum toxicity by "caging" aluminum to promote its entry into the body. Glyphosate promotes calcium uptake by voltage-activated channels, which allow aluminum to gain entry as calcium mimetic. Aluminum then promotes calcium loss from bones, contributing to pineal gland calcification. Ca^{2+} triggers more release of Ca^{2+} and when combined with protein kinases A and C, it is phosphorylated increasing sensitivity to environmental agents 1000 times.

TABLE 2.33
Correlation of Sunlight Exposure and Autism in Public School Students in 50 States (Grades 1–6, 2007–2008)

Demographic	Coefficient	Category
Number of clear days	−0.40	Sunlight exposure
Rainfall and latitude	+0.34	Sunlight exposure
Vaccination rate	+0.38	Aluminum, mercury

Source: Adapted from Seneff S. et al. 2015. *Agric. Sci.* 6:42–70.

3. Bringing melatonin back into the discussion, glyphosate interferes with what is known as the shikimate pathway. Although humans do not have the shikimate pathway, the gut flora depends on bacteria and green vegetables to supply essential amino acids and many other things. Disruption of the shikimate pathway in the gut results in depletion of tryptophan, which is the sole precursor to melatonin. Besides needing melatonin to transport sulfate into the brain, also needed is melatonin to reduce heavy metal toxicity since it is an anti-oxidant eight times over other ones. Where supplies of melatonin are adequate, melatonin will bind to aluminum, cadmium, copper, iron, and lead, and reduce their toxicity. Where melatonin is low, a lot of damage can result.

Levels of prolactin range from 0 to 18 ng/mL by the RAI method. Abnormalities of prolactin levels can be excessive and an indicator of pituitary dysfunction. See Rea, Chemical Sensitivity, Volume II, Chapter 12.[875]

Thyroid

Thyroid functions are measured with the standard thyroid profile TSH, T_3, and T_4. In addition, thyroid and antimicrosomal antibodies are used to evaluate the degree of thyroid that is involved. Above one degree, it is considered abnormal.

Thyroid Profiles

In the following profiles, 2% of the TSH, none of the T_7, 5% of the T_3, and 2% of the T_4 were low; none of the T_4 profiles were high in a group of 200 chemically sensitive patients. A thyroid profile, however, does not always reveal borderline thyroid dysfunction in chemically sensitive patients. Often, clinicians must use auxiliary temperatures and other signs and symptoms that are abnormal to determine the necessity of supplementation.

Anti-TSH Antibodies

Five percent of anti-TSH antibodies measured in 200 consecutive chemically sensitive patients tested positive. Most chemically sensitive patients with specific hypothyroidism or neck pain with sore throat have antibodies in the 50s–100s.

An example of chemical minimal disturbing thyroid functions is as follows:

A new study published in *American Journal of Epidemiology* (PDF) shows pesticide exposure of farmers' spouses increased their chances of developing thyroid diseases.[876] Part of the government-conducted multiyear Agricultural Health Study focused on the health of the thyroid gland in farmers' spouses. Researchers studied more than 16,500 women living in Iowa and North Carolina who were married to men who sought certification to use restricted pesticides in those states during the 1990s. The study found that wives of farmers in the two states who had been exposed to certain pesticides had a 12.5% incidence rate of thyroid diseases, while the incidence of thyroid disease in the general population ranges from 1% to 8%. When they looked at 44 different pesticides, they found that women married to men who had ever used organochlorine insecticides such as aldrin, DDT, and lindane were 1.2 times more likely to have hypothyroidism. The risk of hypothyroidism for women exposed to fungicides was 1.4-fold greater. Fungicides benomyl and maneb/mancozeb were associated with tripled and doubled risk, respectively, and the herbicide paraquat nearly doubled the likelihood of hypothyroidism. Maneb/mancozeb was the only chemical studied that upped the risk of both hypothyroidism and hyperthyroidism.

Antimicrosomal Antibodies

Five percent of antimicrosomal antibodies was measured in 200 consecutive patients; however, mitochondrial dysfunction is seen in many more chemically sensitive patients.

TABLE 2.34

Estrogen and Progesterone Levels—Controls

	Estrogen (ng/dL)	Progesterone (ng/dL)
Early follicular	G–20	2.1–15
Late follicular	40–1000	
Midluteal	20–60	3.8–28
Postmenopausal	<5	
Postpubertal fenide	<3	0–0.7
Adult male	4–16	

Parathyroid

Parathormone levels may be directly assessed and compared with serum and urine magnesium, calcium, and phosphorous levels. The levels range from 10 to 65 pg/mL. They will be abnormal in a small subgroup of chemically sensitive patients.

Ovarian Dysfunction

Standard estrogen, progesterone, and luteinizing hormones may be measured in chemically sensitive patients; 15% will be abnormal. Deregulation of ovarian function is usually shown by intradermal skin tests and occurs in the other 85% of those chemically sensitive patients with ovarian dysfunction. Antiovarian antibodies are clearly elevated in a portion of chemically sensitive patients (Table 2.34).

Testicles

Testicular dysfunction occurs in a larger subset of chemically sensitive individuals than the antibodies show. Many patients who have low testosterone can function well without lack of energy, weakness, and fatigue.

The clinician must be aware that there are many endocrine disruptors from both molds and toxic chemicals. The top 12 are used here, but there are undoubtedly many more.

There is no end to the tricks that endocrine disruptors can play: increasing production of certain hormones, decreasing production of others, imitating hormones, turning one hormone into another, interfering with hormone signaling, telling cells to die prematurely, competing with essential nutrients, binding to essential hormones, and accumulating in organs that produce hormones.

Here are 13 of the worst hormone disrupters, with some tips on how to avoid them (Table 2.35).

1. **BPA (bisphenol-A):** Plastics imitate the sex hormone, estrogen. This synthetic hormone can trick the body into thinking it is the real thing. BPA has been linked to everything from breast and other cancers to reproductive dysfunction, obesity, early puberty, and heart

TABLE 2.35

Worst Hormone Disrupters

1. Bisphenol A	8. Arsenic
2. Dioxin	9. Mercury
3. Atrazine	10. Polyfluorinated chemicals
4. Phthalate	11. Organophosphate and organophosphate insecticides
5. Perchlorate	12. Glycol ethers
6. Fire retardants—polybrominated diphenyl ethers (PBDE)	13. Glyphosate
7. Lead	

disease.[877] According to government tests, 93% of Americans have BPA in their bodies.[877] Many food cans are lined with BPA. Thermal paper is often coated with BPA. Avoid plastics marked with a "PC," for polycarbonate, or recycling label #7. Not all of these plastics contain BPA, but many do. For more tips, check out: www.ewg.org/bpa/

2. **Dioxin:** Dioxins are formed by many industrial processes when chlorine or bromine is burned in the presence of carbon and oxygen. Dioxins can disrupt the delicate ways that both male and female sex hormone signaling occurs in the body. Exposure to low levels of dioxin in the womb and early in life can both permanently affect sperm quality and lower the sperm count in men during their prime reproductive years. Dioxins are very long-lived, build up both in the body and in the food chain, are powerful carcinogens, and can also affect the immune and reproductive systems. There is an ongoing industrial release of dioxin, which has meant that the American food supply is widely contaminated. The products including meat, fish, milk, eggs, and butter are most likely to be contaminated, but you can cut down on exposure by eating fewer animal products.

3. **Atrazine:** Feminization of male frogs occurs. Exposure to even low levels of the herbicide atrazine can turn male frogs into females that produce completely viable eggs. Atrazine is widely used on the majority of corn crops in the United States, and consequently, it is a pervasive drinking water contaminant. Atrazine has been linked to breast tumors, delayed puberty, and prostate inflammation in animals, and some research has linked it to prostate cancer in people. Buy organic produce and get a drinking water filter certified to remove atrazine. For help in finding a suitable filter, check out EHC-Dallas.

4. **Phthalates:** It is totally normal and healthy for 50 billion cells in the body to die every day. But studies have shown that chemicals like phthalates can trigger what is known as "death-inducing signaling" in testicular cells, making them die earlier than they should. Studies have linked phthalates to hormone changes, lower sperm count, less mobile sperm, birth defects in the male reproductive system, obesity, diabetes, and thyroid irregularities.[877] Avoid plastic food containers, children's toys (some phthalates are already banned in kid's products), and plastic wrap made from PVC, which has the recycling label #3. Some personal care products also contain phthalates. Avoid products that simply list added "fragrance," since this catch-all term sometimes means hidden phthalates.

5. **Perchlorate:** Perchlorate, a component in rocket fuel, contaminates much of produce and milk, according to EWG and government test data.[878] When perchlorate gets into the body, it competes with the nutrient iodine which the thyroid gland needs to make thyroid hormones. Basically, this means that if ingested too much of these, it ends up in alteration of thyroid hormone balance, dysregulating metabolism in adults. It is critical for proper brain and organ development in infants and young children. Reduce perchlorate in drinking water by installing a reverse osmosis filter. As for food, it is pretty much impossible to avoid perchlorate, but you can reduce its potential effects by making sure there is enough iodine in your diet. Eating iodized salt and organic food is one good way.

6. **Fire retardants—polybrominated diphenyl ethers:** In 1999, Swedish scientists studying women's breast milk discovered something totally unexpected: the milk contained an endocrine-disrupting chemical found in fire retardants, and the levels had been doubling every 5 years since 1972. These incredibly persistent chemicals, known as PBDEs, have since been found to contaminate the bodies of people and wildlife around the globe—even polar bears. These chemicals can imitate thyroid hormones in the body and disrupt their activity that can lead to lower IQ, among other significant health effects. While several kinds of PBDEs have now been phased out, this does not mean that toxic fire retardants have gone away. PBDEs are incredibly persistent, so they are going to be contaminating people and wildlife for decades to come.

7. **Lead:** Lead (Pb) is one heavy metal; lead is toxic, especially to children. Lead harms almost every organ system in the body and has been linked to a staggering array of health

effects, including permanent brain damage, lowered IQ, hearing loss, miscarriage, premature birth, increased blood pressure, kidney damage, and nervous system problems. But few people realize that one other way that lead may affect the body is by disrupting hormones. In animals, lead has been found to lower sex hormone levels. Also, it is shown that lead can disrupt the hormone signaling that regulates the body's major stress system (called the HPA axis)—especially when this stress system is implicated in high blood pressure, diabetes, anxiety, and depression.

8. **Arsenic:** This toxin is lurking in food and drinking water. In smaller amounts, arsenic (As) can cause skin, bladder, and lung cancer. Basically, arsenic interferes with normal hormone functioning in the glucocorticoid system that regulates how bodies process sugars and carbohydrates. Disruption of the glucocorticoid system has been linked to weight gain/loss, protein wasting, immunosuppression, insulin resistance (which can lead to diabetes), osteoporosis, growth retardation, and high blood pressure.

   Reduce exposure by using a water filter that lowers arsenic levels. Do not eat commercial chicken. It is used as a growth promoter.

9. **Mercury:** Mercury (Hg), a naturally occurring but toxic metal, gets into the air and the oceans primarily through burning coal. Eventually, it can end up on the plate in the form of mercury-contaminated seafood. It rains 200 tons of Hg per year from melting of the polar ice caps due to which all seafood is contaminated. Pregnant women are mostly at risk from the toxic effects of mercury, since the metal is known to concentrate in the fetal brain and can interfere with brain development. Mercury is also known to bind directly to one particular hormone that regulates women's menstrual cycle and ovulation, interfering with normal signaling pathways. Hormones do not work so well when they have got mercury attached to them. The metal may also play a role in diabetes, since mercury has been shown to damage cells in the pancreas that produce insulin. Mercury dental amalgams are also another source of mercury.

   For people who still want to eat (sustainable) seafood with lots of healthy fats but without the presence of toxic mercury, wild salmon and farmed trout are good choices, but it still can have Hg in them.

10. **Perfluorinated chemicals:** The perfluorinated chemicals (PFCs) used to make non-stick cookware can accumulate in the patient. Perfluorochemicals are so widespread and extraordinarily persistent that 99% of Americans have these chemicals in their bodies. One particularly notorious compound PFOA has been shown to be "completely resistant to biodegradation." That means that even though the chemical was banned after decades of use, it will be showing up in people's bodies for countless generations to come. PFOA exposure has been linked to decreased sperm quality, low birth weight, kidney disease, thyroid disease, and high cholesterol, among other health issues. Animal studies have found that it can affect thyroid and sex hormone levels.[877]

    Skip nonstick pans as well as stain- and water-resistant coatings on clothing, furniture, and carpets.

11. **Organophosphate and OP pesticides:** Some chemicals are OP but not pesticides or herbicides like tricreasyl phosphate in jet fuel, which are extremely toxic, contaminating the cabin air system.

    Neurotoxic organophosphate compounds that the Nazis produced in huge quantities for chemical warfare during WWII were luckily never used. American scientists used the same chemistry to develop a long line of pesticides that target the nervous systems of insects. Despite many studies linking organophosphate exposure to effects on brain development, behavior, and fertility, they are still among the more common pesticides in use today. A few of the many ways that organophosphates can affect the human body include interfering with the way testosterone communicates with cells, lowering testosterone, and altering thyroid hormone levels.

12. **Glycol ethers:** Shrunken testicles: This is one thing that can happen to rats exposed to chemicals such as glycol ethers, which are common solvents in paints, cleaning products,

brake fluid, and cosmetics. The European Union says that some of these chemicals "may damage fertility or the unborn child."[877] Studies of painters have linked exposure to certain glycol ethers to blood abnormalities and lower sperm counts. Children who were exposed to glycol ethers from paint in their bedrooms had substantially more asthma and allergies.

13. **Glyphosate—a special herbicide—Roundup Ready:** Glyphosate is a toxic herbicide used on corn, wheat, soy, and other plants. It is detrimental to the GI tract and brain as well as other body areas.[877] It is a genetically engineered substance with all the problems these substances have (see Genetic Engineered Substances).

REPRODUCTIVE AND DEVELOPMENTAL EFFECTS

Some outdoor air pollutants have been linked to reproductive and developmental problems. A study of births in Vancouver from 1985 to 1998 found that increasing levels of outdoor carbon monoxide and sulfur oxides significantly increased risk of preterm birth.[878] Air pollution levels are fairly low in Vancouver, with values well below the U.S. EPA limits.[878] Other studies have linked increased rates of preterm births to exposure to ambient formaldehyde levels and living near an oil refinery,[879] while another study found no relationship between preterm birth and maternal residence near an oil refinery.[880]

Studies in Mexico and the Czech Republic have reported a relationship between ambient particulate levels and excess infant deaths.[881,882] A study of 4 million U.S. infants born from 1989 to 1991 has found that higher PM_{10} levels were associated with significantly higher death rates from sudden infant death syndrome (SIDS).[883] A California case–control study found that higher levels of outdoor NO_2 were associated with significantly higher SIDS deaths, while higher CO levels were not associated with higher SIDS deaths.[884] In a study of 221,406 live births in New Jersey in 1990, it was found that low birth weight, premature birth, and fetal death were significantly more common in mothers living in areas with high levels of airborne PAHs.[885] A Pennsylvania study found that higher outdoor air levels of PM_{10} and SO_2 were associated with significantly higher rates of preterm birth.[886] A Texas study found that higher levels of CO were associated with significantly higher levels of Tetralogy of Fallot, higher PM_{10} levels were associated with significantly higher levels of atrial septal defects, and higher SO_2 levels were associated with significantly higher rates of ventral septal defects.[887]

A Belarus study noted significantly increased rates of several congenital abnormalities following the 1986 Chernobyl accident.[888] Higher outdoor levels of CO in Los Angeles[889] and industrial pollution in Moravia[890] have been associated with significantly higher rates of congenital cardiac defects such as ventricular septal defects. A French retrospective cohort study found a significant relationship between traffic exposure and cardiac birth defects, a borderline relationship to urinary tract defects, and no relationship to oral cleft defects.[891]

REPRODUCTIVE SYSTEM

A brief review of the literature on the effects of three trace metals, copper, manganese, and molybdenum, that are required for human health, yet may also cause adverse reproductive effects, is as follows.

HAZARDS OF HEAVY METAL CONTAMINATION

According to Jarup et al.,[892] the main threats to human health from heavy metals are associated with exposure to lead, cadmium, mercury, and arsenic.

ENVIRONMENTAL POLLUTION AND HYPERSENSITIVITY IMMUNOLOGICAL MECHANISMS

According to Pie et al.,[893] airborne pollutants, both particulate and gaseous, represent a major environmental factor promoting hyper- and hyposensitization and disease expression. These adverse effects of PM are highly dependent upon the nature and size of the particles, their content of chemicals and metals, and the subject's genetic makeup. Diesel exhaust and gases, in particular ozone, has been shown to exacerbate cellular inflammation and to act as mucosal adjuvant to skew the immune response to inhaled antigens toward a Th_2-like phenotype. Growing evidence suggests that mechanisms of pollutant-inducted amplification of the hypersensitive reaction depend on oxidative stress that is under the control of susceptibility genes, as well as epigenetic mechanisms but mostly environmental pollutant and the triggers.

Not only can environmental pollutants trigger classic IgE mechanism but also they can trigger the IgG and subsystems to give a hypersensitive and hyposensitive response. These pollutants can also create nonimmune hypersensitivity by triggering the cell membrane and Ca^{2+} through the membrane and release those Ca^{2+} that are stored in the cell, which then combine with protein kinases A and C and are phosphorylated causing an increase in sensitivity up to 1000 times. The nonimmune process may be the most hypersensitive reaction in T and B cells in the body from pollutant injury.[4] Complement and enzyme deficiencies may also trigger the nonimmune and immune hypersensitive responses. The immune system is divided into two parts: the innate immune system and the adaptive long-term immune system. The innate immune system is the acute response system emphasized and driven by the mitochondria. The adaptive long-term immune systems are the T and B cells, the complements, and the gamma globulin system.

The dendritic cells initiate the immune response; initiate and orchestrate so that they communicate the acute response immune system with the adaptive immune system. They also present antigens to T cells.

MITOCHONDRIA AND THE INNATE IMMUNE SYSTEM

According to West et al.,[894] the innate immune system has a key role in the mammalian immune response. Recent research has demonstrated that mitochondria participate in a broad range of innate immune pathways, functioning as signaling platforms and contributing to effector responses. In addition to regulating antiviral signaling, mounting evidence suggests that mitochondria facilitate antibacterial immunity by generating ROS and contribute to innate immune activation following cellular damage and stress. Therefore, in addition to their well-appreciated roles in cellular metabolism, with energy production and programmed cell death, mitochondria appear to function as centrally positioned hubs in the innate immune system. We often see this change in the chemically sensitive damaged innate immune responses that result in recovering bacterial and viral infections. This system is commonly damaged by pesticides, herbicides, natural gas, inorganic chemicals, solvents, formaldehyde, phenols, molds/mycotoxins, EMF, etc. (EHC-Dallas).

Following infection, microorganisms are initially sensed by pattern-recognition receptors (PRRs) of the innate immune system, which bind to conserved molecular patterns that are shared by different classes of microorganisms. These pathogen-associated molecular patterns (PAMPs) include microbial structural components, nucleic acids, and proteins. The list of PRRs known to sense PAMPs is extensive and composed most notably of four families: (1) TLRs, (2) nucleotide oligomerization domain (NOD)-like receptors (NLRs), (3) C-type lectin receptors (CLRs), and (4) retinoic acid (RA)-inducible gene I (RIG-I)-like receptors (RLRs).[894–896]

PRR ligation triggers multiple signaling pathways that culminate in the activation of nuclear factor-κB (NF-κB), mitogen-activated protein kinases (MAPKs), and interferon regulatory factors (IRFs), which control the expression of proinflammatory cytokines and chemokines, type I interferons (IFNs), and costimulatory molecules.[894,895,897] The resulting proinflammatory state is necessary for the generation of a robust antimicrobial environment and proper activation of the adaptive immune response.

Mitochondria are dynamic double-membrane-bound organelles that are involved in a wide range of cellular processes, including ATP generation, programmed cell death, and calcium homeostasis as well as the biosynthesis of amino acids, lipids, nucleotides, and hemoglobin. Although mitochondria possess their own genome (mitochondrial DNA [mtDNA]) that encodes 13 proteins of the oxidative phosphorylation machinery, two ribosomal RNAs, and 22 transfer RNAs essential for translation in the mitochondria, ~1500 proteins comprising the mitochondrial proteome are nuclear encoded.[898] Most of these proteins not only function in oxidative phosphorylation or other metabolic pathways, but also include those needed for replication and expression of mtDNA (i.e., the mitochondrial transcription and translation machinery). Consequently, coordination between the mitochondrial and nuclear genomes is required for proper assembly and function of the mitochondrial network, and cellular signaling cascades mediate crosstalk between mitochondria and the nucleus.[899] The mitochondrial network forms a reticular branching structure that, through association with the cytoskeleton, is motile and undergoes regular fusion and division.[900] Mounting evidence suggests that mitochondrial dynamics regulate many aspects of mitochondrial biology and are influenced by a variety of metabolic and cellular signals.[900]

Mitochondrial regulation of apoptotic signaling has been appreciated for some time; however, more recent evidence suggests that mitochondria also participate in various additional signaling pathways.[900,901] For example, research over the past several years has unveiled previously unappreciated roles for mitochondria in the innate immune response and it is becoming increasingly apparent that mitochondria participate in RLR signaling antibacterial immunity and sterile inflammation. Although mitochondrial control of apoptosis during infection is an important aspect of the mammalian innate immune response, this topic has been reviewed thoroughly by others[902,903] and therefore is not discussed further. Instead, West et al.[894] reviewed and discussed the involvement of mitochondria in innate immune signaling pathways and the mechanisms by which these organelles facilitate effector responses of the innate immune system.

MITOCHONDRIA AND ANTIVIRAL IMMUNITY

The RLR family includes three members: RIG-I, melanoma differentiation-associated gene 5 (MDA5), and laboratory of genetics and physiology 2 (LGP2; also known as DHX58).[904,905] RLRs are expressed in the cytosol, present in both immune and nonimmune cells, and required for type I IFN and proinflammatory cytokine production in response to viral infection. RIG-I and MDA5 each possess two amino-terminal caspase recruitment domains (CARDs) that are required for signaling a DExD/H box RNA helicase domain that detects viral double-stranded RNA in the cytoplasm and a carboxy-terminal repressor domain. Although LGP2 was initially suggested to function as a negative regulator of RIG-I and MDA5 signaling, a more recent study indicates that LGP2 positively regulates RIG-I- and MDA5-dependent antiviral responses.[904,906]

Oxidative Phosphorylation

This metabolic pathway occurs at the inner mitochondrial membrane and uses an electrochemical gradient created by the oxidation of electron carriers to generate ATP.

Mitochondrial dynamics refer to the movement of mitochondria along the cytoskeleton and the regulation of mitochondrial morphology and distribution mediated by tethering and fusion and fission events.

Sterile inflammation results from trauma, ischemia-reperfusion injury, or chemically induced injury that typically occurs in the absence of any microorganisms. This is what occurs and often predominant in CS.

According to West et al.,[894] the adaptor TNFR1-associated death domain protein (TRADED) also interacts with MAVS and recruits TRAF3 and TRAF family member-associated NF-κB activator (TANK), which then activates IκB kinase-ε (IKKε) and/or TANK-binding kinase 1 (TBK1), resulting in IRF3 and IRF7 activation.[907] In addition, MAVS–TRADD signaling leads to the recruitment of FAS-associated death domain protein (FADD) and receptor-interacting protein 1 (RIP1; also known as RIPK1), which induces canonical NF-κB signaling.[907,908] Furthermore, IKKα, IKKβ, and IKKε, which are kinases responsible for NF-κB and IRF activation, respectively, have also been identified as MAVS signaling partners, and IKKε collocalizes with mitochondria following viral infection.[909,910] Finally, WD repeat containing protein 5 (WDR5) was recently shown to regulate MAVS signaling during viral infection by facilitating the assembly of active MAVS signaling complexes on the mitochondrial surface.[911] The signaling probably occurs when the intradermal neutralization of an influenza virus infection occurs, thus stopping the flu progression immediately in hundreds of patients treated at the EHC-Dallas and Buffalo.

A typical pathway of NF-κB activation that involves phosphorylation and degradation of the prototypical NF-κB inhibitor is IκBα.

The translocase of the outer membrane (TOM) is a complex of proteins localized to the outer mitochondrial membrane that recognizes and imports nuclear-encoded mitochondrial proteins into the intermembrane space.

HSP: A member of a class of functionally related proteins that function as molecular chaperones and have crucial roles in protein folding and intracellular trafficking is the heat shock protein (HSP).

MAMs: Regions of the endoplasmic reticulum that are closely juxtaposed to mitochondria and support communication between the organelles via calcium and phospholipid exchange are on the mitochondrial membrane.

Despite the identification of many cytosolic signaling molecules linking MAVS to the NF-κB, IRF3, and IRF7 pathways, the regulation of mitochondria antiviral signaling (MAVS) during viral infection is not well understood. Furthermore, how cytosolic signaling molecules are recruited to mitochondrial membrane–bound MAVS complexes during viral infection remains undocumented. As the OMM contains numerous proteins that regulate many aspects of mitochondrial biology including protein import, nutrient and ion exchange, organelle dynamics, and apoptosis regulation, it is likely that mitochondrial proteins directly influence MAVS signaling. Recently, several bona fide mitochondrial proteins have been identified as MAVS binding partners, yielding new insight into the regulation of MAVS signaling at the mitochondrion.

Mitochondrial Cofactors for MAVS Signaling

Nuclear DNA-encoded mitochondrial proteins are imported across the OMM via the TOM machinery. The multiprotein TOM complex forms the translocation pore that recognizes and localizes preproteins for import into the intermembrane space of the mitochondrion. TOM20 and TOM70 serve as the primary preprotein receptors and are anchored to the OMM via N-terminal transmembrane segments, whereas the hydrophilic domains of these proteins face the cytosol and bind mitochondrial targeting sequences (MTSs).[912] TOM20 mainly binds preproteins containing a classical N-terminal MTS, whereas TOM70 interacts with proteins that possess internal hydrophobic targeting sequences, as well as chaperones such as heat shock protein 90 (HSP90) that are required for the proper localization of some preproteins to the TOM complex.[912]

Mitochondrial Dynamics Govern Antiviral Signaling

The mitochondrial network in eukaryotic cells is highly dynamic, with both fusion and fission events occurring regularly to regulate morphology and activity. Mitochondrial dynamics determine the integrity of the mitochondrial network and maintain respiratory capacity, but also participate in several other processes, including mammalian development, neurodegeneration, and apoptosis.[913,914]

Mitofusin (MFN), an outer mitochondrial membrane protein, regulates mitochondrial fusion and ER-mitochondrial interactions by tethering adjacent organelles.

MFN proteins are the best characterized fusion regulators, whereas mitochondrial fission protein 1 (FIS1) and dynamin-related protein 1 (DRP1) control fission.[913] MFN1 and MFN2 are dynamin-related GTPases expressed on the OMM that tether mitochondria together during fusion, although MFNB2 is also expressed on MAMs and regulates mitochondrial-ER tethering.[915]

MITOCHONDRIAL ROS AND ANTIVIRAL SIGNALING

A consequence of electron transport through mitochondrial oxidative phosphorylation complexes is the generation of ROS. Although ROS can damage cellular proteins, lipids, and nucleic acids via oxidation, they are also crucial second messengers in various redox-sensitive signaling pathways. As mitochondria are a significant source of ROS in many eukaryotic cells, mitochondrial ROS (mROS) have been suggested to modulate several signaling pathways.[901] Interestingly, ROS have been implicated as both positive and negative modulators of RLR signaling.[916–918]

Mitophagy is a term referring to the selective removal of mitochondria by macroautophage under conditions of nutrient starvation or mitochondrial stress.

Autophage-related gene 5 (ATG5) and ATG12, which are crucial regulators of autophagy and mitophagy (the specific removal of damaged mitochondria), can inhibit RLR signaling, and Tal et al. demonstrated that Atg5[-1-] cells accumulate dysfunctional mitochondria and exhibit increased mROS levels and type I IFN production in response to polyI:C stimulation.[918,919] Treatment of Atg5[-1-] fibroblasts and primary macrophages with antioxidants reduces the production of type I IFNs to wild-type levels, suggesting that aberrant ROS generation potentiates RLR signaling in these cells (Figure 2.30).

Furthermore, augmentation of mROS via exposure of cells to the oxidative phosphorylation complex I inhibitor rotenone (which induces the production of mROS) increases polyI:C-induced IFNβ generation in both wild-type and Atg5[-1-] cells.[918] Therefore, increased RLR signaling and subsequent antiviral responses in the absence of ATG5 are possibly the result of heightened mROS generation from accumulated abnormal or damaged mitochondria in these cells. Furthermore, mROS induction also potentiates RLR signaling I wild-type cells, thus implicating mROS more broadly as important second messengers in RLR–MAVS signaling.[918]

MITOCHONDRIAL ROS AND ANTIBACTERIAL RESPONSES

The phagocytic response of the innate immune system is crucial for the effective clearance of microbial pathogens and indispensable for host defense. This response is initiated following microbial pathogens and indispensable for host defense. This response is initiated following microbial contact with host phagocytes (mainly macrophages and neutrophils) and results in the engulfment and killing of microorganisms within phagosomes. Phagocytosis is associated with the production of ROS via the respiratory burst, a necessary effector response for the destruction of intracellular microorganisms.[920,921] Although ROS are primarily produced by the NADPH oxidase system I phagocytes, mitochondrial oxidative metabolism is also a major source of cellular ROS. The production of mROS has traditionally been considered a deleterious consequence of electron transport, but mounting evidence indicates that mROS also facilitate antibacterial innate immune signaling and phagocyte bactericidal activity. Leukocytes and lymphocytes often are suppressed in the chemically sensitive with WBC running between 2000 and 5000, which tells that phagocytosis is impaired. These patients are not only prone to recurrent infections but also prone to all kinds of pollutant generated nonbiological inflammations.

IMMUNITY

Many new facts and ideas about the immune system have evolved. However, some old ideas have been modified or evolved into new ideas that will help chemically sensitive patients. One of the autogenous lymphocytic factors has evolved from the ideas of transfer factor from animals or other humans. The other is the replacement of gamma globulin when one or more gamma globulin subsets are abnormal in the chemically sensitive.

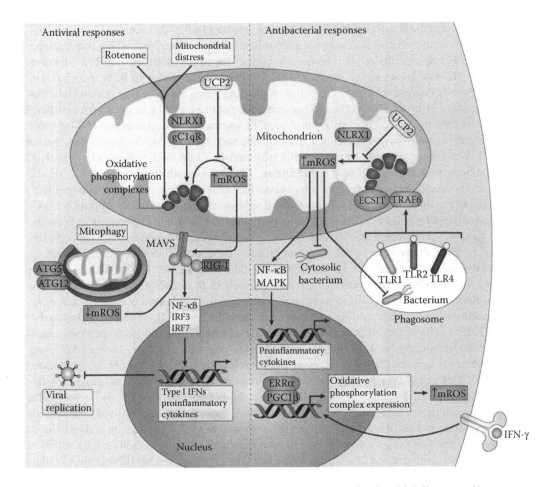

FIGURE 2.30 Mitochondrial ROS and innate immune responses. Mitochondrial distress and/or rotenone treatment augment mitochondrial reactive oxygen species (mROS) generation from oxidative phosphorylation complexes, and this potentiates RIG-I-like receptor (RLR)–mitochondrial antiviral signaling protein (MAVS) signaling to nuclear factor-κB (NF-κB) and interferon regulatory factor 3 (IRF3) and IRF7. This increases the production of type I interferons (IFNs) and proinflammatory cytokines, which limit viral replication. NLR family member X1 (NLRX1) and receptor for globular head domain of complement component 1q (gC1qR) interact with oxidative phosphorylation complexes and may increase mROS generation, whereas uncoupling protein 2 (UCP2) decreases mROS production. Mitophagy mediated by autophagy-related gene 5 (ATG5) and ATG12 also decreases mROS production and subsequent RLR–MAVS signaling by removing dysfunctional, mROS-generating mitochondria. https://www.ncbi.nlm.nih.gov/pmc/articles/PMC4281487/figure/F3/.

Lyme Disease

CD4+ T cells were responsible for the observed immune-mediated pathology. These data demonstrate directly the deleterious effect of T cells in Lyme disease.

The dominance of CD4+ Th1 cells in mouse strains susceptible to *Borrelia burgdorferi*–induced disease and in humans with Lyme arthritis has led to the notion that Th1 cell effector functions impair host control of the pathogen and promote disease.[922,923] Our present study evaluated the role of T cells in resolution of Lyme carditis and provides evidence that CD4+ Th1 cells may have a beneficial effect on this disease manifestation. In this setting, IFN-γ secreting CD4+ T cells did not exacerbate disease but instead promoted the complete resolution of carditis. These results provide the first example of a beneficial role for Th1 cells on the course of Lyme borreliosis.

They who showed the *B. burgdorferi*–vaccinated interferon gamma–deficient (IFN-γ° mice challenged with the Lyme spirochete) developed a prominent chronic severe destructive osteorthropathy. The immune response underlying the development of the severe destructive arthritis involves interleukin-17 (IL-17). Treatment of vaccinated IFN-γ° mice challenged with *B. burgdorferi* with anti-IL-17 antibody delayed the onset of swelling of the hind paws, but more importantly, inhibited the development of arthritis. Histopathologic examination confirmed that treatment with anti-IL-17 antibody prevented the destructive arthopathy seen in vaccinated and challenged IFN-γ° mice. Similar preventive results were obtained when vaccinated and challenged IFN-γ° mice were treated with anti-IL-17 receptor antibody or sequentially with anti-IL-17 antibody followed by anti-IL-17 receptor antibody. In contrast, treatment of vaccinated IFN-γ° mice with recombinant IL-17 (rIL-17) did not alter the development and progression of arthritis found in vaccinated and challenged IFN-γ° mice without treatment with rIL-17. Therapeutic intervention may be a realistic approach to prevent arthritis especially if IL-17 is involved in the perpetuation of chronic or intermittent arthritis.

CD4+ CD25+ T cells are a population for active suppression of autoimmunity. Specifically, CD4+ CD25+ T cells have been shown to prevent insulin-dependent diabetes mellitus, inflammatory bowel disease, and pancreatitis. Here, we present evidence that CD4+ CD25+ T cells also play a major role in controlling the severity of arthritis detected in *B. burgdorferi*–vaccinated gamma interferon–deficient (IFN-γ°) C57BL/6 mice challenged with the Lyme spirochete. When *B. burgdorferi*–vaccinated and –challenged IFN-γ° mice were treated with anti-IL-17 antibody, the number of CD4+ CD25+T cells increased in the local lymph nodes. Furthermore, this histopathologic examination showed the mice to be free of destructive arthritis. When these anti-IL-17-treated *B. burgdorferi*–vaccinated and –challenged mice were also administered anti-4 25 antibody, the number of CD4+ CD25+ T cells in the local lymph nodes decreased. More importantly, severe destructive arthopathy was induced. In addition, delayed administration of anti-CD25 antibody decreased the severity of the arthritis. These results suggest that CD4+ CD25+ T cells are involved in regulation of a severe destructive arthritis induced with an experimental model of vaccination and challenged with *B. burgdorferi*. Collectively, these results suggest that other immune mediators, but not IFN-γ, are responsible for the induction of arthritis. There is evidence, however, that IFN-γ can potentiate the proinflammatory effects of IL-17.

The development of Lyme arthritis has traditionally been attributed to Th1 cytokines, such as IFN-γ. However, recent studies demonstrate that IFN-γ is not absolutely required for the induction of Lyme arthritis. This suggests that the established model of Lyme arthritis as solely a Th1-mediated response has to be modified to include other inflammatory cytokines or mediators. One possible candidate for updating this paradigm is the Th176 cell subset, a recently discovered helper T cell subset distinct from Th1 and Th2 cells. The prototypical Th17 cytokine. IL-17 has been shown to play a major role in the development of arthritis in *Borrelia*-vaccinated and -challenged mice.

Many mirror the delicate balance between eradication and immune-mediated host tissue injury, that is, Th1 inflammation not only eradicates borrelia, but also causes symptoms of disease. In conclusion, asymptomatic *Borrelia*-seropositive individuals may have an enhanced innate immune activation, demonstrated as strong TNF-α and IL-12 responses to live spirochetes. Their findings support the view that proinflammatory and Th1 inducing responses in the early disease course result in an optimal resolution of LB. The results should, however, be confirmed in a larger study.

Conclusion: Patients with persisting symptoms following an EM show a decreased Th1-type inflammatory response in infected skin early during the infection, which might reflect a dysregulation of the early immune response. This finding supports the importance of an early, local Th1-type response for optimal resolution of LB.

Patients with persisting symptoms 6 months after antibiotic-treated EM showed reduced expression of Th1-like cytokines in the EM lesions prior to antibiotic treatment. This finding indicates an impact of the initial local immune response on the long-term outcome of LB and supports the hypothesis that an early and strong Th1 type response is important for optimal resolution of LB. Additional studies are, however, needed to further substantiate their findings.

Their results support the notion that a Th1-type immune response dominates in the CNS in early NG, and is then followed by a Th2-type immune response. They also show that IL-17 levels are increased in CSF in a substantial proportion of NB cases, suggesting a role for Th17 in NB. However, the precise role of Th17 in NB pathogenesis and clinical course remains to be evaluated.

Clinical applications of transfer factor are defects in cell-mediated immunity: children, elderly, immunosuppressed, and people with infections such as viral, fungi, parasites, and mycobacteria.

Cancer as well as Autoimmune Disease/Allergy

We at the EHC-Dallas have developed a transfer factor out of the patients' own blood. This takes away the complication of animal or other human transfer factor.

Our experience with ALF like the importance of mucosal immunity wherever it may be, nasal, sinus, olfactory, bronchial pulmonary, bladder, cardiovascular, as well as the GI, is extremely important in aiding chemically sensitive patients to reduce its susceptibility and allowing the restoration to health.

GASTROENTEROLOGY

The GI tract is extremely prone to pollutant injury because of the gross contamination of the food and water and the size. Even inhaled chemicals can affect the GI tract when people are exposed to pollutant overload like excess exposure to car exhaust, factory emission, gas fracking, mycotoxin inhalation exposure, etc.

There is a growing intolerance worldwide to gluten, which causes a spreading phenomena to sensitivity to other foods not only in the wheat family but also to unrelated individual foods. This spreading phenomena result in brain fog, confusion, headache, cardiovascular, and respiratory upset as well as GI gas, bloating, distention, constipation, diarrhea, etc. Thus, fatigue and weakness often prevail. Increased sensitivity to foods, molds, and other toxic chemicals is due to the extreme use of pesticides and herbicides and other toxic agents applied to the food when growing it. It is one of the main reasons for CS. Pesticides and herbicides are tied as the number one triggering agent in CS. The following data are shown on these triggering agents of natural gas and herbicide such as glyphosate.

GI Immunity

IMPORTANCE OF THE GI SYSTEM TO HUMAN HEALTH IS ENTIRELY GERMAIN

GI Immunity

Physiologic features such as the development of innate and adaptive immunity, relative susceptibilities to infections, immune tolerance, bioavailability of nutrients, and intestinal barrier function are diseased with pollutant expression.

The role of tight junctions in the mucosal cells is of upmost importance. This is because it prevents many toxic environmental substances like bacteria, virus, parasites, toxic chemicals, and molds/mycotoxins to enter the body. It can also prevent the hypersensitivity reproduction of the Ca^{2+} protein kinases A and C from becoming phosphorylated, thus increasing the hypersensitivity response 1000 times (Figure 2.31).

The surface area of the human intestinal tract is approximately equal to that of a regular singles tennis court. It must be protected with great care as it is easily disturbed in this modern area of increased chemical and EMF exposure. The food and water is grossly contaminated, and this overload can easily disturb GI balance.

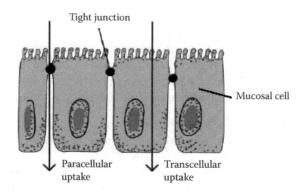

FIGURE 2.31 Many toxics disrupt the tight membranes causing the Ca^{2+} to enter the sebaceous cells and cells on the other side of the blood or gut. The tight junctions prevent infections of any type from taking hold and thus keep the human well.

Importance of Mucosal Immunity Paramount in Optimum Function

The dominating part of the immune defenses, even if flora is excluded, is localized in the gut—no less than 75% of the immune cells of the body are suggested to be found in the GI tract. Therefore, the GI system cannot be ignored in the overall optimum function of the body (Figure 2.32).

Dendritic cells are specialized APCs that orchestrate innate and adaptive immune responses. The intestinal mucosa contains numerous DCs, which induce either protective immunity to infectious agents or tolerance to innocuous antigens, including food and commensal bacteria. Several subsets of mucosal DCs have been described that display unique functions dictated in part by the local microenvironment (Figure 2.33).

Natural killer cells play a role in the innate immune system. Cytotoxic, granular lymphocytes release proteins perforin and granzyne that cause target cell to die by apoptosis. They play a major

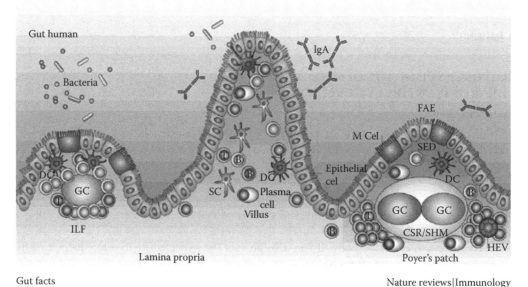

FIGURE 2.32 Bacteria–virus, parasites, pesticides, solvents, mold/mycotoxin, EMF. (Reprinted by permission from Macmillian Publishers Ltd: Nature Publishing Group. Sidonia, F., T. Honjo. 2003. Intestinal IgA synthesis: Regulation of front-line body defences. *Nat. Rev. Immunol.*)

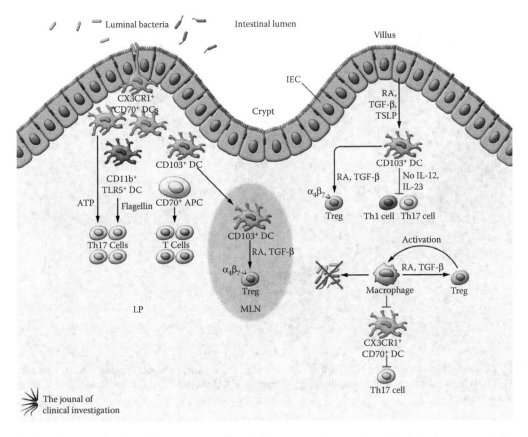

FIGURE 2.33 Dendritic cells engulf foreign substances presenting them to the phagocytes and T cell for destruction. (Permission granted by American Society for Clinical Investigation. Maria, R., A. Di Sabatino. 2009. *J. Clin. Invest.*)

role in killing viruses, tumor cells, bacteria, and protozoa. However, they cannot attack biological cells that cause inflammation.

Macrophages are derived from monocytes, which act as phagocytes in the innate immune system and antigen-presenting cells in the adaptive immune system The key to normal immune system function depends upon balanced immune system responses between cellular response, T and B cells, and humoral responses, that is, antibodies.

Cytokines are small peptides secreted by a variety of cells such as macrophages leaking to lymphocytes, which regulate both initiation and maintenance of the immune response through a complex network.

Cytokines can be divided into various categories, recognizing that many cytokines have multiple cellular sources with multiple targets and overlapping range of activities. Th1 (adaptive/memory, cell mediated): IL-2, IFN-γ; Th2 (adaptive/memory, antibodies): IL-4, IL-5, IL-13, IL-10, TGF-β; innate: TNBF-α, IL-1, IL-6, IL-12; proinflammatory: TGF-β, IL-10; regulatory: IL-10, IL-12, TGF-β (Figure 2.34).

A brief history of Th17, the first major revision in the Th1/Th2 hypothesis of T cell-mediated tissue damage, is as follows.

For over 35 years, immunologists have divided Th cells into functional subsets. Th1 cells—long thought to mediate tissue damage—might be involved in the initiation of damage, but they do not sustain or play a decisive role in many commonly studied models of autoimmunity, allergy, and microbial immunity. A major role for the cytokine IL-17 has now been described in various

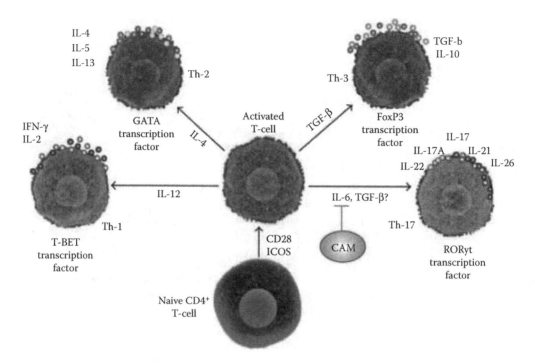

FIGURE 2.34 General scheme of T helper-cell differentiation. (Adapted from Vojdani, A., J. Lambert. 2011. The role of Th17 in neuroimmune disorders: Target for CAM therapy. Part I. *Evid. Based Complement. Alternat. Med.* 1–8.)

models of immune-mediated tissue injury, including organ-specific autoimmunity in the brain, heart, synovium and intestines, allergic disorders of the lung and skin, and microbial infections of the intestines and the nervous system.

Breath Alkanes Determination in Ulcerative Colitis and Crohn's Disease

By considering the pathophysiologic basis of inflammatory bowel diseases (IBD), a role for excessive lipid peroxidation caused by oxygen free radical compounds has been proposed repeatedly. However, to date only a few studies are available on this topic in human beings. This study was designed to assess breath alkanes in a group of patients with active inflammatory bowel disease by a technique that clearly distinguishes pentane from isoprene to prevent overestimation of values as in previous studies.

Twenty patients with a diagnosis of active inflammatory bowel disease (10 with Crohn's disease [CD] and 10 with UC) were studied. Extension of the disease was similar between patient groups, and all were treated with equivalent doses of steroids and salicylates.

Breath alkanes determination was performed by a standard procedure involving a gas chromatography column, which was able to separate pentane from isoprene.

Overall, significant differences between patients with IBD and controls were found for ethane, propane, and pentane but not for butane and isoprene. Isoprene (1,3-butadiene-2-methyl) was clearly distinguished from pentane, demonstrating that the significant elevation of pentane levels in patients with IBD is a real phenomenon and not an artifact caused by collocation with isoprene.

An excess of lipid peroxidation is probably an important pathogenetic factor in *IBD* and this may be assessed through a noninvasive method. As this method has also been shown previously to be able to evaluate disease activity, it could be a useful tool for studying patients with IBD.

Although progress has been made in understanding the pathophysiologic basis of UC and CD, the cause of these entities still remains unknown unless the clinician studies toxic and hypersensitive exposures. Among other factors, several mediators of inflammation and tissue injury have been proposed, such as the OFRs,[924–926] final common mediators of inflammation, and tissue injury in general.[1232] Clearly, pesticides, natural gas components, molds/mycotoxins, parasites, other chemicals, etc., have been found as triggering agents in some.

The production of OFRs in IBD may be caused by several processes, including xanthine oxidation, oxygen reduction by reduced neutrophilic nicotinamide adenine dinucleotide phosphate, and arachidonic acid oxidation.[927,928] These pathways led to the production of superoxide anion, which can form hydroxyl radicals.[929] Generation of the latter compounds can stimulate lipid peroxidation,[930] resulting in the production of several alkanes[931] and lipid radicals. Lipid radicals then perpetuate this reaction, attracting other lipid molecules and leading to destruction of lipidic cell membranes and eventually to cell damage.

Of the several techniques available to assess by-products of OFRs on lipids, the one currently accepted for *in vivo* measurements of lipid peroxidation is the determination of the alkanes, ethane, and pentane in exhaled air.[929] Pentane formation is observed exclusively with peroxidation of ω-6 polyunsaturated fatty acid (PUFA) whereas ethane formation is observed with ω-3 PUFA. However, it must be pointed out that small quantities of ethane, together with propane and butane, may be formed as a result of oxygen free radical attack on the branched-chain amino acids leucine and isoleucine.[932] In addition, patients exposed to natural gas (methane) for heating and cooking may become sensitive to these. They include methane, ethane, propane, and butane, which can be found in the breath of the chemically sensitive. These may occur whether the GI tract is involved or not involved. Natural gas is tied with pesticides and herbicides as the number one triggering agents of CS. Since natural gas is discussed in other sections as hypersensitivity and disturbing the immune system, it will not be further discussed in this section. Instead, the following discussions of the herbicide glyphosate will be discussed as a prime candidate for the contamination of the food supply and a representative of many chemicals that can cause CS.

Although measurement of exhaled hydrocarbons has raised interest in its use as a noninvasive method to determine the presence of inflammation in any organ and consequent lipid peroxidation,[933–936] this technique has only recently been applied to the study of patients with irritable bowel disease (IBD). In particular, only two studies in such patients are available, one showing increased breath pentane in a heterogeneous group of patients with CD[937] and the other showing elevated breath ethane (but not pentane) content in patients with active left-sided UC.[938]

Glyphosate, Pathways to Modern Diseases: Celiac Sprue and Gluten Intolerance, Nongluten Wheat Sensitivity and Other Food and Chemical Sensitivity

According to Samsel and Seneff, [939] gluten intolerance is a growing epidemic in the Unites States and, increasingly, worldwide, so is other inflammatory disease and just plain GI upset, that is, gas, bloating constipation, diarrhea, and spastic bowels, accompanied with food and chemical sensitivity. Celiac sprue is a more specific disorder, characterized by gluten intolerance along with autoantibodies to the protein, and transglutaminase, which builds crosslinks in undigested fragment of gliadin, a major constituent of gluten.[940] The autoantibodies are produced as an immune response to undergraded fragments of proteins in gluten. Other nonceliac food and chemical sensitivity results in irritable bowel and all its symptoms including bloating, sleepiness after eating, gas, diarrhea, and constipation; it is not accompanied by autoantibodies but is found with low T and B lymphocytes, total complements, and occasionally low gamma globulin and subsets. A remarkable set of symptoms develop over time in association with celiac disease, including weight loss, diarrhea, chronic fatigue, neurological disorders, anemia, nausea, skin rashes, depression, and nutrient deficiencies. This also happens with chemical and food sensitivity. Usually, but not always, a strict gluten-free diet can alleviate many of the symptoms. However, many patients have to have intradermal neutralization to specific foods, molds, and chemicals to overcome wheat sensitivity. A key associated pathology is an inflammatory response in the upper small intestine, leading to villous atrophy, which impairs their ability to function in their important role in absorbing nutrients. Also, a spreading phenomenon with specific individual food sensitivity occurs resulting in an increase in overall sensitivity and malnutrition including avoidance which is successful for treatment of both celiac disease and nonceliac food and chemical sensitivity. Also, this pollutant overload in the GI tract for chemicals in food like glyphosate can trigger remote areas such as the neurological, cardiovascular, GU dermal, and skeletal muscular systems to alter their normal efficient response to mild and severe dehydration.

Some have suggested that the recent surge in celiac disease and food and chemical sensitivity is simply due to better diagnostic tools. However, a recent study tested frozen sera obtained between 1948 and 1954 for antibodies to gluten, and compared the results with sera obtained from a matched sample from people living today.[941] They identified a fourfold increase in the incidence of celiac disease in the newer cohort compared to the old one. They also determined that undiagnosed celiac disease is associated with a fourfold increased risk of death, mostly due to increased cancer risk. They concluded that the prevalence of undiagnosed celiac disease has increased dramatically in the United States during the past 50 years. Individual food and chemical sensitivity has been observed for 50+ years. This observation has spurred the study, origination, and propagation of three giant medical societies to diagnose and treat these entities because of the food and chemical sensitivity found in their patients. Wheat sensitivity has long been found and usually is accompanied by an herbicide glyphosphate, which can cause other food sensitivity with and without the autoantibodies. The mechanism of the nonceliac wheat sensitivity autoantibodies or other immune aberrations appear to be in the phenomena of an injury, that is, glyphosate occurs to the GI cells causing to send out K^+ and to ingress Na^+ and Ca^{2+} into the cells. Ca^{2+} combines with protein kinases A and C and is phosphorylated increasing sensitivity 1000 times. This increase in sensitivity sensitizes not only wheat but also many other foods.[4]

Transglutaminases play many important roles in the body, as they form covalent crosslinks in complex proteins in connection with blood coagulation, skin barrier formation, ECM assembly, and fertilization, endowing the substrate with protection from degradation by proteases.[942] They also form crosslinks in undigested fragments of gliadin derived from wheat, and sensitivity to certain of these fragments leads to the development of autoantibodies to tissue transglutaminase[943] that inhibit its activity. Many times there is wheat sensitivity without autoantibodies, which occurs due to gut membrane leakage, blood, gut, and brain barrier, and intracellular leakage doing Ca^{2+} intake in the cell creating wheat and other sensitivity of foods.

Glyphosate is the active ingredient in the herbicide Roundup. It is a broad-spectrum herbicide considered to be nearly nontoxic to humans[944] which is entirely false as are the other toxic chemicals in food sources. Other opinions to the contrary by other physicians have deemed this nontoxicity of glyphosate and other chemicals as nonsense since many of their patients got well with a switch to organic foods. Overall, these toxic chemicals contribute to the total body pollutant load. A recent paper by Samsel and Seneff[939] and studies from the EHC-Dallas and Buffalo argued that glyphosate may be a key contributor to the obesity epidemic, CS, and the autism epidemic in the United States, as well as to several other diseases and conditions, such as AD, PD, infertility, depression, and cancer. We would agree with the fact that this idea is in concert with the clinicians of the AAEM who have found similar findings of chemically induced food sensitivity for 40 years in clinical studies. Glyphosate suppresses 5-enolpyruvylshikimic acid-3-phosphate synthase (EPSP synthase), the rate-limiting step in the synthesis of the aromatic amino acids, tryptophan, tyrosine, and phenylalanine in the shikimate pathway of bacteria, archaea, and plants.[945] In plants, aromatic amino acids collectively represent up to 35% of the plant dry mass.[946] This mode of action is unique to glyphosate among all emergent herbicides. Humans do not possess this pathway, and therefore we depend upon ingested food and out of gut microbes to provide these essential nutrients. Chemically sensitive patients have a limited number of microbes in stool analyses and are prone to a defect to digest foods, properly. Glyphosate, patented as an antimicrobial,[947] has been shown to disrupt gut bacteria in animals, preferentially killing beneficial forms and causing an overgrowth of pathogens. Two other properties of glyphosate also negatively impact human health—chelation of minerals such as iron and cobalt, and interference with cytochrome P450 (CYP) enzymes, which play many important roles in the body. Interference with iron and cobalt metabolisms and the cytochrome P450 systems has long been observed in the chemically sensitive and food sensitive patient by clinicians treating those patients.[939] Usually, mineral analyses are disturbed in the chemically sensitive and when corrected, restore not only good GI function but also eventually eliminating the weakness and fatigue seen in the chemically sensitive.

According to Samsel and Seneff,[939] a recent study on glyphosate exposure in carnivorous fish revealed remarkable adverse effects throughout the digestive system.[948] The activities of protease, lipase, and amylase were all decreased in the esophagus, stomach, and intestine of these fish following exposure to glyphosate. The authors also observed "disruption of mucosal folds and disarray of microvilli structure" in the intestinal wall, along with an exaggerated secretion of mucin throughout the alimentary tract. These features are highly reminiscent of not only celiac disease but also food and chemical sensitivity and GI tracts. Gluten peptides in wheat are hydrophobic and therefore resistant to degradation by gastric, pancreatic, and intestinal proteases.[949] Thus, the evidence from this effect on fish suggests that glyphosate may interfere with the breakdown of complex proteins in the human stomach, leaving larger fragments of wheat and other foods in the human gut that will then trigger an immune enzyme autoimmune or nonautoimmune immune response. This leads to the defects in the lining of the small intestine that are characteristic of these fish exposed to glyphosate of not only wheat sensitive but also some other patients who do not have autoantibodies like the celiac patients. This finding results in leaky gut syndrome and multiple food sensitivities. The usage of glyphosate on wheat in the United States has risen sharply in the last decade, in step with the sharp rise in the incidence of celiac disease and nonautoantibody wheat and food sensitivity.

Samsel and Seneff[939] show that glyphosate's known suppression of CYP enzyme activity in plants and animals plausibly explains this effect in humans. There is the role of excess RA in celiac disease. They link this to the known effects of glyphosate on RA, mediated by its suppression of CYP enzymes. Cobalamin deficiency occurs which is a known pathology associated with celiac disease that leads to macrocytic anemia. They argue that this follows as a direct consequence of glyphosate's ability to chelate cobalt. Section "Gut Bacteria" discusses in more depth the role of anemia in celiac disease, a consequence of both cobalamin and iron deficiency. Section "Molybdenum Deficiency" discusses molybdenum deficiency and its link to microcephaly, which is associated with celiac disease. Section "Selenium and Thyroid Disorders" discusses the link between selenium deficiency and autoimmune thyroid disease. Section "Indole and Kidney Disease" discusses kidney disease in connection with celiac disease and glyphosate. Section "Nutritional Deficiencies" discusses various nutritional deficiencies associated with celiac disease, and shows how these can be directly explained by glyphosate. Section "Cancer" discusses the link between celiac disease and certain rare cancers that have also been linked to glyphosate. Section "Proposed Transglutaminase–Glyphosate Interactions" goes into an in-depth discussion of how glyphosate might promote autoantibodies to transglutaminase, following a section which presents compelling evidence that glyphosate residues in wheat, sugar, and other crops are likely increasing in recent decades, and a section discussing the increased risk to kidney failure in agricultural workers exposed to excess glyphosate occupationally.

Gut Bacteria

In this section, the role of pathogens in inducing the breakdown of tight junctions in enterocytes lining the small intestinal wall is discussed. They show that glyphosate is associated with an overgrowth of pathogens along with an inflammatory bowel disease in animal models. A parallel exists with celiac disease and food and chemical sensitivity where the bacteria that are positively and negatively affected by glyphosate and other toxic chemicals are overgrown or underrepresented, respectively, in association with celiac disease and nonautoimmune wheat sensitivities in humans. This imbalance also occurs in the chemically sensitive with food sensitivity. The beneficial bacteria that are negatively impacted by glyphosate and other toxics can not only protect from celiac or even irritable bowel disease but also applies to chemical and food sensitivity through their enzymatic activities on gluten and other foods and point to several articles recommending treatment plans based on probiotics.[939] Probiotics are one of the mainstays for prescription of the nonceliac wheat sensitive patient with food and chemical sensitivities. Success also depends on intradermal neutralization (desensitization) of wheat and other foods which decreases immune response to multiple foods, and chemicals in those patients afflicted with GI upset.

Pathogens, through their activation of a potent signaling molecule called zonulin, induce a breakdown of the tight junctions in cells lining the gut, leading to "leaky gut" syndrome.[950] The leaky gut syndrome causes the K^+ to leave cells with an ingress of Na^+ and Ca^{2+}. Also, the Ca^{2+} stored in the cells is activated. When the Ca^{2+} is released or floods the cell, it combines with protein kinases A and C which when phosphorylated increases the hypersensitivity response up to 1000 times. Also, the Ca^{2+} triggers releases of endolymph protease, nitric oxide, snythetase, endonuclease, and protein kinase. These enzymes result in cell signals of transduction, regulatory energy output, cell metabolism, and phenotypical expansion of cell characteristics. They can change GI function radically and alter brain function. This increase in sensitivity results in individual and at times universal food sensitivity, which if unrecognized and untreated results in a viscous cycle of GI upset, augmenting the aforementioned GI upset cascade.[939] This process also leads to systemic symptoms especially neurological, one of headache, confusion, weakness, and fatigue. Concentrations of zonulin were sharply elevated ($p < 0.000001$) in subjects with celiac disease during the acute fast.[951] As many as 30% of celiac patients continue to experience GI symptoms after adopting a gluten-free diet, despite optimal adherence, a condition that was attributed to bacterial overgrowth in the small intestine.[952] This is caused by the result of other food sensitivity unrelated to gluten. There is a correlation between glyphosate application to corn and soy and the incidence of intestinal infections and hypersensitivity to these and many other foods and chemicals.

Evidence of disruption of gut bacteria by glyphosate and other toxics is available for poultry,[953] cattle,[954] and swine.[955] Glyphosate disrupts the balance of gut bacteria in poultry,[953] increasing the ratio of pathogenic bacteria to other commensal microbes. *Salmonella* and *Clostridium* are highly resistant to glyphosate, where *Enterococcus*, *Bifidobacteria*, and *Lactobacillus* are especially susceptible. Food and chemically sensitive patients often respond to *Lactobicillus*; however, they also often become sensitive to these bacteria and cannot tolerate them when needed. Thus, we have a dual problem fostered by the glyphosphate of bacterial deficiency and hypersensitivity to them causing more GI upset. Glyphosate was proposed as a possible factor in the increased risk to *C. botulinum* infection in cattle in Germany over the past 10–15 years.[956] Pigs fed GMO corn and soy developed widespread intestinal inflammation that may have been due in part to glyphosate exposure.[955]

Celiac disease and food and chemical sensitivity are associated with reduced levels of *Enterococcus, Bifidobacteria*, and *Lactobacillus* in the gut and an overgrowth of pathogenic gramnegative bacteria. We have seen these levels to be reduced or absent in the food and chemically sensitive patient. Stool analyses of chemically sensitive patients seen also can be made into stool vaccines.[957–959] In Di Cagno et al.'s study,[959] *Lactobacillus, Enterococcus*, and *Bifidobacteria* were found to be significantly lower in fecal samples of children with celiac disease compared to controls, while levels of the pathogens, *Bacteroides, Staphylococcus, Salmonella*, and *Shigella* were elevated. We have observed the same in nonceliac wheat, chemically sensitive patients. According to Collado et al.,[959] another study comparing the fecal material of celiac infants to healthy controls, *Bacteroides, Clostridium*, and *Staphylococcus* were all found to be significantly higher ($p < 0.05$). Often patients are sensitive to these remaining bacteria and stool vaccines made at the EHC-Dallas have improved the gut problem (see treatment section). Sulfate-reducing bacterial counts were also elevated ($p < 0.05$).[959,960] A significant reduction in *Bifidobacteria* was also found in celiacs.[960] An increased excretion of the bacterial metabolites *p*-cresol and phenol has also been recognized in association with celiac disease.[961] *p*-Cresol is produced via anaerobic metabolism of tyrosine by pathogenic bacteria such as *C. difficile*.[962] It is a highly toxic carcinogen, which also causes adverse effects on the CNS, the cardiovascular system, lungs, kidney, and liver.[963] Chemically sensitive patients have been exceptionally intolerant of phenol and cresol not only by ingestion but also by inhalation and intradermal challenge. All these avenues of administration have been found to trigger GI symptoms in selective patients. Tricreosol phosphate emanates from jet airplane engines and is used for cabin heat on commercial airlines. The pilots and cabin crew breathe this substance and develop after a period of time (months to years) neurodegenerative disease. Some also develop GI disease.

Probiotic treatments are recommended to aid in digestive healing in celiac disease and nonimmune wheat sensitivity. This is true for many chemically sensitive patients with chronic diseases. The proteolytic activity of *Lactobacilli* aids the breakdown of wheat into less allergenic forms. Ongoing research aims to produce gluten-containing sourdough breads fermented by *Lactobacilli* that can then serve as probiotics to help ameliorate the symptoms of celiac disease and allow celiac patients to consume wheat.[964] However, it has been our experience that most of the chemically sensitive and food sensitive patients are sensitive to wheat in any form and cannot eat wheat without the intradermal neutralization (desensitization) of wheat, then only occasionally and in small amounts. Probiotic *Lactobacilli* produces the enzyme phytase which breaks down phytates that would otherwise deplete important minerals and other cations through chelation.[965] Their activities would therefore improve absorption of these micronutrients, a known problem in celiac patients.[966] Glyphosate itself also chelates rare minerals.

Probiotic treatment with *Bifidobacteria* has been shown to alleviate symptoms associated with celiac disease.[967,968] However, if the food to which people are sensitive to is not removed and neutralized yet then absorbed, irritable bowel occurs in both the celiac, and in the food sensitive individual, gastrointestinal upset occurs. *Bifidobacteria* suppress the proinflammatory milieu triggered by the microbiota of celiac patients.[969] Live culture of *B. lactis* would promote healing of the gut if offered as treatment in conjunction with the gluten-free diet, or might even allow the celiac and nonceliac food sensitive patient to consume modest amounts of gluten without damaging effects.[970] In this *in vitro* study, it was demonstrated that *B. lactis* reduce epithelial permeability and improved the integrity of the tight junctions in human colon cells. *Bifidobacteria* and *Lactobacilli* are both capable of modifying gluten in such a way as to make it less allergenic, an idea that is being exploited in recent efforts to develop gluten-containing foods that may be safe for consumption by celiac and irritable bowel patients. Probiotics containing live forms of these bacteria are also being actively marketed today.

CYP ENZYME IMPAIRMENT AND SULFATE DEPLETION

As mentioned previously, glyphosate has been shown to suppress cytochrome P450 (CYP) enzymes in plants[971] and animals.[972] A study on rats demonstrated that glyphosate decreased the levels of CYP enzymes and monooxygenase activities in the liver and the intestinal activity of aryl hydrocarbon hydroxylase.[972] The enzyme was also seen to be depressed in chemically sensitive patients. These patients particularly not only had food sensitivity and irritable bowel and food intolerance but also they could not tolerate inhaled hydrocarbons both of the alkanes and nonmethane hydrocarbons like toluene, xylene, benzene, ethylbenzene, and 2- and 3-methylpentane.

CP enzymes are essential for detoxification of many compounds in the liver[973] which have to do with the onset or aggravation of CS. In fact when these toxic hydrocarbons are inhaled as a part of heavy traffic or other sources, they exacerbate the CS and at times may even cause the CS. Intraperitoneal exposure of rats to Roundup in acute doses over a short time interval induced irreversible damage to hepatocytes and elevated urinary markers of kidney disease. This was associated with lipid peroxidation and elevated levels of the inflammatory cytokine TNF-α.[974] CYP3A is constitutively expressed in human intestinal villi and plays an important role in drug metabolism.[975] This may be why chemically sensitive patients are so intolerant of most medications used for any prescription. Celiac disease is associated with a decrease in the intestinal CYP3A.[976] This defect is restored by a gluten-free diet. This decrease in CYP found in the chemically sensitive also results in a failure of detoxification of many chemicals.

Impaired gallbladder bile acid production[977] and biliary cirrhosis, an inflammatory liver disease characterized by obstruction of the bile duct,[978] have been shown to co-occur with celiac disease. CYP enzymes are crucial in the production of bile acids.[979] An obligatory CYP enzyme in bile acid synthesis, CYP27A, has been identified as being identical to the mitochondrial vitamin D_3 activating enzyme.[980] In Kemppainen et al.,[981] 64% of men and 71% of women with celiac disease were found to be vitamin D_3 deficient, manifested as low spinal bone mineral density. Celiac disease is associated with impaired gall bladder function and decreased pancreatic secretions[982,983] along with recurrent pancreatitis.[984] Abnormalities in bile acid secretion have been found in children suffering from celiac disease.[985] Celiac patients exhibit abnormally low synthesis of cholecystokinin,[986] but it has also become apparent that the gall bladder is less responsive to stimulation of contraction by cholecystokinin.[982] A reversible defect of gallbladder emptying and cholecystokinin release has been identified in association with celiac disease.[987] These pathologies may be related to impaired CYP enzyme activity induced by glyphosphate.

While it is clear that CYP enzymes play an important role in bile acid synthesis and in cholesterol homeostasis, the details have not yet been worked out.[979] However, some mouse knockout experiments produce embryonically lethal effects, pointing to the importance of these enzymes to biological systems. Disruption of CYP7A1, involved in bile acid synthesis in mice, induces elevated serum cholesterol and early death. Frequently, the food and chemically sensitive patient has increased cholesterol probably through this mechanism.

A link has been established between celiac disease and nonalcoholic fatty liver, which is likely due to the liver's inability to export cholesterol sulfate through the bile acids due to impaired CYP enzymes.[979] This requires a private store of fats to house the excess cholesterol that cannot be exported in bile. This would also likely lead to insufficient sulfate supplies to the small intestine and could result in impaired heparin sulfate synthesis in the GAGs and subsequent pathologies. Heparan sulfate populating the GAGs surrounding enterocytes is essential for the proper function of the small intestines. Leakage of both albumin and water in both the vasculature and tissues results when the negative charge is reduced due to insufficient sulfation of the polysaccharide units.[988] Vascular leakage may be a consequence of degradation of sulfated GAGs due to inflammatory agents.[989] A similar problem may occur in the kidneys leading to albumin loss into urine during nephrosis.[990] Intestinal protein loss in inflammatory enteropathy associated with celiac disease, CS, irritable bowel, and food sensitivity may also be due to a deficiency in the sulfated GAGs.[991,992] A case study of three infants with congenital absence of enterocyte heparin sulfate demonstrated profound enteric protein loss with secretory diarrhea and absorption failure, even though their intestines were not inflamed.[993] Some chemically sensitive patients are food sensitive with the sulfated GAGs resulting in gas, bloating, and diarrhea. Others have blood clots especially thrombophlebitis is seen in a subset of chemically sensitive patients previously presented in vascular section.

Samsel and Seneff[939] developed a hypothesis that glyphosate disrupts the transport of sulfate from the gut to the liver and pancreas due to its competition as a similarly kosmotropic solute that also increases blood viscosity. (Kosmotropes are ions that induce "structure ordering" and "salting out" of suspended particles in colloids.) Insufficient sulfate supply to the liver is a simple explanation for reduced bile acid production. The problem is compounded by impaired CYP enzymatic action and impaired cycling of bile acids through defective enterocytes in the upper small intestine. The catastrophic effect of loss of bile acids to the feces due to impaired reuptake compels the liver to adopt a conservative approach of significantly reduced bile acid synthesis, which, in turn, leads to gall bladder disease.

The protein, NF-κ-light chain-enhancer of activated B cells (NF-κB) controls DNA transcription of hundreds of genes and is a key regulator of the immune response to infection.[994] Light chains are polypeptide subunits of immunoglobulins. NF-κB responds to stimulation from bacterial and viral antigens, inflammatory cytokines like TNF-α, free radicals, oxidized LDL, DNA damage, and UV light. The incidence of acute pancreatitis has been increasing in recent years[995] and it often follows biliary disease. A local inflammatory reaction at the site of injury coincides with an increase in the synthesis of hydrogen sulfide (H_2S) gas. H_2S regulates the inflammatory response by exciting the extracellular signal-regulated (ERK) pathway, leading to production of NF-κB.[995] Samsel and Seneff[939] hypothesize that H_2S, while toxic, is a source of both energy and sulfate for the pancreas, derived from sulfur-containing amino acids such as cysteine and homocysteine. DHEA sulfate, but not DHEA, inhibits NF-κB synthesis, suggesting that sulfate deficiency is a driver of inflammation.[996] Many chemically sensitive patients have an intolerance to sulfur containing element like glutathione, cysteines, etc. This hampers their detoxification of many toxic substances and can augment chemically sensitive patients' odor sensitivity.

While H_2S is well known as a toxic gas through its inhibition of aerobic respiration, a recent paradigm shift in the research surrounding H_2S has been inspired by the realization that it is an important signaling gas in the vasculature on a par with nitric oxide.[997] H_2S can serve as an inorganic source of energy to mammalian cells.[998] 3-Mercaptopyruvate sulfurtransferase (3MST) is expressed in the vascular endothelium, and it produces H_2S derived from 3-mercaptopyruvate which stimulates additional mitochondrial H_2S production, which then is oxidized to thiosulfate via at least three different pathways[999–1001] and produces ATP. The inflammatory agent superoxide can act as substrate for the oxidation of H_2S to sulfite and subsequently sulfate and the activated form PAPS[1002] but will likely induce oxidative damage in the pancreas, particularly, as we will see in Section "Molybdenum Deficiency", if molybdenum deficiency impairs sulfite-to-sulfate synthesis. The superoxide and H_2S can constrict the microcirculation resulting in tissue hypoxia and metabolic acidosis.

According to Samsel and Seneff,[939] pancreatic beta cells express extraordinarily high levels of heparin sulfate, which is essential for their survival[1003] since it protects them from ROS-induced cell death. As sulfate transport via the hepatic portal vein is likely disrupted by glyphosate, H_2S, whether derived from sulfur-containing amino acids or supplied via diffusion following its production by sulfur-reducing bacteria in the gut, can become an important source of sulfur for subsequent sulfate production locally in the pancreatic cells. Pancreatic elastase is a serine protease that is needed to assist in protein degradation but an overabundance can lead to autolysis of tissues.[1004] Cholesterol sulfate inhibits pancreatic elastase[1004] so a deficiency in cholesterol sulfate supply due to impaired sulfate supply to the liver and impaired CYP function should increase the risk of tissue digestion by pancreatic enzymes, contributing to the loss of villi in the upper small intestine observed in celiac disease and other irritable bowel disease and nonceliac wheat and other food CS.

In the early 1990s, a newly recognized disease began to appear, characterized by eosinophil infiltration into the esophagus, which manifested as dysphagia in adults and refractory reflux symptoms in children.[1005] This disease termed eosinophilic esophagitis (EOE) is associated with a Th2 immune profile and synthesis of the cytokine IL-13, which has direct cytotoxic effects on epithelial cells. A dose-dependent induction of eosinophilia by intratracheal delivery of IL-13 confirms its association with EOE.[1006] An association has been found between EOE and celiac disease.[1007] Patients with refractory celiac disease that is not corrected by dietary gluten restriction show an increased production of IL-13 in the gut.[1008] The incidence of EOE has increased at alarming rates in Western countries in the last three decades.[1009,1010,1233] Most of these specific triggering agents are individual foods by the IGE pathway. However, many other pathways triggered by foods and chemicals can trigger the non-IGE pathway also in chemically sensitive patients.

Glyphosate is highly corrosive to the esophageal epidermal lining, with upper GI tract injury observed in 94% of patients following glyphosate ingestion.[1011] In Zouaoui et al.'s findings,[1012] the most common symptoms in an acute response from glyphosate poisoning were oropharyngeal ulceration or irritation, nausea, and vomiting. Samsel and Seneff[939] hypothesize that glyphosate induces EOE via a systemic response as well as through direct contact. The pathogenesis of EOE is related to food sensitivities, but airborne exposure to chemicals in the lungs can also induce it, so it does not require physical contact to the allergen.[1013] It is conceivable that glyphosate is responsible for the emergence of EOE. In our experience at the EHC-Dallas and Buffalo, often successful treatment can be obtained by eating organic food and using intradermal neutralization of the triggering food as well as increase in antioxidant nutrition.

The cytochrome P450 reductase (CPR) and cytochrome P450 (CP) enzyme system is essential for inducing nitric oxide release from organic nitrates.[1014] The nitrate moiety is reduced while simultaneously oxidizing NADPH to $NADP^+$. This system is invoked in organic nitrate drug treatment for cardiovascular therapy. The reaction depends on anaerobic, acidic conditions, a feature of venous rather than arterial blood. Failure to extract O_2 in the microcirculation due to microvessel abnormal physiology results in cellular hypoxia and acidosis. The elevated PvO_2 above 28 mm Hg drawn from the antecubital fossa without using a tourniquet is usually seen in chemically sensitive patients with GI symptoms and food sensitivity. We have seen 2000 patients with these clinical problems. Since L-arginine is a substrate for NO synthesis by endothelial NOS (eNOS) under oxidative conditions,[1015] it is likely that CPR and CP play an important role mainly in stimulating venous smooth muscle relation. Impaired venous relaxation would likely contribute to venous thrombosis, which is a well-established complication of celiac disease[1016–1019] as well as food and chemical sensitivity. The CRP and COP are abnormal in these chemically sensitive patients.

In summary, celiac disease and food and chemical sensitivity are associated with multiple pathologies in the digestive system, including impaired gall bladder function, fatty liver, pancreatitis, and EOE. Samsel and Seneff[939] have argued here that many of these problems can be traced to impaired CYP function in the liver due to glyphosate exposure, leading to insufficient flow of bile acids through the circular pathway between the liver and the gut. These result in a system-wide depletion in sulfate, which induces inflammation in multiple organs to produce sulfate locally. A potential sulfur source for sulfate synthesis could be hydrogen sulfide gas, provided in part by the local breakdown of sulfur-containing amino acids like cysteine and homocysteine and in part by diffusion of the gas produced from inorganic dietary sources by sulfur-reducing bacteria in the large intestine. Impaired CYP enzyme function may also contribute to venous thrombosis, for which celiac disease and food and chemical sensitivity are an established risk factor.

Retinoic Acid, Celiac Disease, and Reproductive Issues

In this section, Samsel and Seneff[939] first establish that excess RA is a risk factor for celiac disease. They then show that excess RA leads to complications in pregnancy and teratogenic effects in offspring. Glyphosate has been shown to exhibit teratogenic effects in line with known consequences of excess RA exposure to the embryo and propose that the mechanism for this effect may be glyphosates known disruption of CYP enzymes that are involved in RA catabolism. This then links glyphosate to increased risk to celiac disease via its direct effects on RA. It identifies a possibly important factor in the association of celiac disease with reproductive issues. They also discuss other adverse effects of excess RA and a possible relationship to impaired sulfate supply to the gut.

In celiac disease, T cells develop antibody responses against dietary gluten, a protein present in wheat.[1020] RA, a metabolite of vitamin A, has been shown to play a critical role in the induction of intestinal-regulatory responses.[1021–1023] The peptide in gluten, A-gliadin P31-43, induces interleukin 15 (*IL-15), a key cytokine promoting T cell activation.[949] RA synergizes with high levels of IL-15 to promote JNK phosphorylation,[1024,1025] which potentiates cellular apoptosis.[1026] IL-15 is a causative factor driving the differentiation of precursor cells into antigluten $CD4^+$ and $CD8^+$ Th1 cells in the intestinal mucosa. Furthermore, in DePaolo et al.'s study,[1025] it was discovered that RA exhibits an unanticipated co-adjuvant property to induce Th1 immunity to antigens during infection of the intestinal mucosa with pathogens. RA has also been shown to directly suppress transglutaminase activity, another way in which it would negatively impact celiac disease[1027] or even nonceliac food and chemical sensitivity. Thus, it is becoming clear that excess exposure to RA would increase risk to celiac disease, and warnings have been issued regarding potential adverse effects of RA supplements on celiac disease.

It is well established that high RA levels lead to teratogenic effects both in human and in experimental models. Brain abnormalities such as microcephaly, impairment of hindbrain development, mandibular and midfacial under development, and cleft palate are all implicated.[1028,1029] Women with celiac disease are known to have higher rates of infertility, miscarriages, and birth defects in their offspring.[1030–1033] Excess RA could be a significant factor in these complications.

A possible mechanism by which glyphosate might induce excess RA is via its interference with the CYP enzymes that metabolize RA. There are at least three known CYPs (CYP26A1, CYP26B1, and CYP26CC1) that catabolize RA, and they are active in both the embryo and the adult.[1034] A 1/5000 dilution of glyphosate was sufficient to induce reproducible malformations, characteristic of RA exposure, in frog embryos.[1035] Pathologies included shortening of the trunk, reduction in the size of the head, abnormally small eyes or the presence of only one eye (cyclopia), and other craniofacial malformations in the tadpole. Glyphosate's toxicity to tadpoles has been well demonstrated, as it killed nearly 100% of larval amphibians exposed in experimental outdoor pond mesocosms.[1036]

According to official records, there has been a recent fourfold increase in developmental malformations in the province of Chaco, Argentina, where glyphosate is used massively on GMO monocrops of soybeans.[1037] In Paraguay, 52 cases of malformations were reported in the offspring of women exposed during pregnancy to agrochemicals, including anencephaly, microcephaly, facial defects, cleft palate, ear malformations, polydactily, and syndactyly.[1038] In *in vitro* studies on human cell lines, DNA strand breaks, plasma membrane damage, and apoptosis were observed following exposure to glyphosate-based herbicides.[1039] Another factor in teratogenic effects of glyphosate may be the suppression of the activity of androgen–estrogen conversion by aromatase, a CYP enzyme.[1039]

Ingested vitamin A, a fat-soluble vitamin, is delivered to the blood via the lymph system in chylomicrons, and excess vitamin A is taken up by the liver as RA for catabolism by CYP enzymes.[1040] Remaining RA that is not catabolized is exported inside LDL particles, and it lingers much longer as retinyl esters in the vasculature in this form.[1041] Excess RA is more readily stored in this way in LDL particles in the elderly. Vitamin A toxicity can lead to fatty liver and liver fibrosis[1040] as well as hypertriglyceridemia.[1042] Vitamin A has a negative effect on cholesterol sulfate synthesis,[1043] which might negatively impact the livers ability to maintain adequate supplies of cholesterol sulfate for the bile acids, and therefore also interfere with the supply of cholesterol sulfate to the gastrointestinal tract.

In summary, glyphosate's disruption of the CYP enzymes responsible for RA catabolism could lead to an excess bioavailability of RA that could contribute adversely to celiac disease, and plain food and chemical sensitivity as well as damaging the liver and leading to teratogenic effects in offspring of exposed individuals.

In addition to higher risk of birth defects, individuals with celiac disease have increased risk to infertility.[1044,1045] Increased incidence of hypogonadism, infertility, and impotence was observed in a study of 28 males with celiac disease.[1045] Marked abnormalities of sperm morphology and motility were noted, and endocrine dysfunction was suggested as a probable cause. In studies conducted on Sertoli cells in prepubertal rat testis, exposure to Roundup (glyphosate) induced oxidative stress leading to cell death.[1046] Roundup induced the opening of L-type voltage-dependent calcium channels as well as ryanodine receptors, initiating ER stress and leading to calcium overload and subsequent necrosis, including hypersensitivity. Glutathione was depleted due to upregulation of several glutathione-metabolizing enzymes. This suggests that Roundup would interfere with spermatogenesis, which would impair male fertility.

COBALAMIN DEFICIENCY

Untreated celiac disease and food and chemical sensitivity patients often have elevated levels of homocysteine, associated with folate and/or cobalamin deficiency.[1047,1048] Species of *Lactobacillus* and *Bifidobacterium* have the capability to biosynthesize folate[1049] so their disruption by glyphosate could contribute to folate deficiency. Malabsorption in the proximal small intestine could also lead to iron and folate deficiencies. Cobalamin was originally thought to be relatively spared in celiac disease because its absorption is mostly through the terminal ileum which is unaffected by celiac disease. However, a recent study found that cobalamin deficiency is prevalent in celiac patients. A total of 41% of the patients studied were found to be deficient in cobalamin (<220 ng/L), and 31% of these cobalamin-deficient patients also had folate deficiency.[1050] Either cobalamin or folate deficiency leads directly to impaired methionine synthesis from homocysteine because these two vitamins are both required for the reaction to take place. This induces hyperhomocysteinemia[1051] and established risk factor in association with celiac disease.[1052] Long-term cobalamin deficiency also leads to neurodegenerative diseases,[1053] seen as a result of long-term food and chemical sensitivity.

Since a deficiency in cobalamin can generate a large pool of methyltetrahydrofolate that is unable to undergo reactions, cobalamin deficiency will often mimic folate deficiency. Cobalamin requires cobalt, centered within its corrin ring, to function. We depend upon our gut bacteria to produce cobalamin, and impaired cobalt supply would obviously lead to reduced synthesis of this critical molecule. Glyphosate is known to chelate +2 cations such as cobalt. Glyphosate complexes with cobalt as a dimer (Co[glyphosate]2)3 in 15 different stereoisomeric configurations, and it is facile at switching among the different stereoisomers, an unusual kinetic property compared to most Co(III) systems.[1054]

Chemically sensitive patients often have cobalamin sensitivity and deficiency as well as folic need. The GI upset and the CS can often be helped by supplementation with both.

In fact, studies have revealed that glyphosate inhibits other cytosolic enzymes besides EPSP synthase in plants and microbes that also activate steps in the shikimate pathway.[1055,1056] Glyphosate potently inhibits three enzymes in the shikimate pathway in yeast.[1056] It has been confirmed that these other enzymes depend upon cobalt as a catalyst, and glyphosate inhibition works through competitive cobalt binding and interference with cobalt supply.[1055] It has also been proposed that chelation by glyphosate of both cobalt and magnesium contributes to impaired synthesis of aromatic amino acids in *E. coli* bacteria.[1057] Thus, it is plausible that glyphosate similarly impairs cobalamin function in humans by chelating cobalt. The aromatic amino acids are often difficult to detoxify in the chemically sensitive causing deficiencies.

ANEMIA AND IRON

Anemia is one of the most common manifestations of celiac disease outside of the intestinal malabsorption issues[1019,1058] and present in up to half of diagnosed celiac patients. Celiac patients often have both cobalamin and folate deficiency, which can cause anemia, but iron deficiency may be the most important factor.[949] Celiac patients often do not respond well to iron treatment. This may be because the glyphosphate has triggered sensitivity to Fe. This frequently can be desensitized by Fe intradermal neutralization.

Glyphosate's chelating action can have profound effects on iron in plants.[1059,1060] Glyphosate interferes with iron assimilation in both glyphosate-resistant and glyphosate-sensitive soybean crops.[1060] It is therefore conceivable that glyphosate's chelation of iron is responsible for the refractory iron deficiency present in celiac disease and nonceliac GI food sensitivity.

Erythropoietin (EPO) (hematopoietin) is a cytokine produced by interstitial fibroblasts in the kidney that regulates red blood cell production. Low EPO levels, leading to a low turnover rate of red blood cells, is a feature of celiac disease.[949,1061] This can lead to megaloblastic anemia, where red blood cells are large (macrocytic) and reduced in number due to impaired DNA synthesis. A recent hematological study on mice exposed to Roundup at subacute levels for just 15 days revealed an anemic syndrome in both male and female mice with a significant reduction in the number of erythrocytes and in hemoglobin, reduced hematocrit and increased mean corpuscular volume, indicative of macrocytic anemia.[1062]

MOLYBDENUM DEFICIENCY

Molybdenum deficiency occurs as it is only needed in trace amounts. Molybdenum is essential for at least two very important enzymes: sulfite oxidase and xanthine oxidase (XO). Sulfite oxides convert sulfite, a highly reactive anion, to sulfate, which is much more stable. Sulfite is often present in foods such as wine and dried fruits as a preservative. Usually, the food and chemically sensitive patient cannot tolerate either if the sulfite is included. Sulfate plays an essential role in the sulfated proteoglycans that populate the intracellular matrices of nearly all cell types.[991,992,1063] So, impaired sulfite oxidase activity leads to both oxidative damage and impaired sulfate supplies to the tissues, such as the enterocytes in the small intestine. Many chemically sensitive patients have this GI upset when there is impaired sulfate. The excess presence of sulfur-reducing bacteria such as *Desulfovibrio* in the intestine in association with celiac disease[959,960] could be protective because these bacteria can reduce dietary sulfite to hydrogen sulfide, a highly diffusible gas that can migrate through tissues to provide a source of sulfur for sulfate regeneration at a distant site. These distal sites could reoxidize the H_2S through an alternative pathway that does not require molybdenum for sulfur oxidation.[999] This impaired sulfate supply and its tissue instability may be one of the reasons observed where instability of tissue is seen in the severe chemically sensitive patient who cannot hold intradermal endpoints for treatment. These endpoints are always changing in their precise patient doses of antigen, which are always changing off and the patient has a hard time stabilizing their physiology.

XO produces uric acid from xanthine and hypoxanthine, which are derived from purines. It is activated by iron which is often intractably deficient in association with celiac disease as well as food and chemical sensitivity. Impaired XO activity would be expected to drive purines toward other degradation pathways. Adenosine deaminase (ADA), a cytoplasmic enzyme that is involved in the catabolism of purine bases, is elevated in celiac disease, and is therefore a useful diagnostic marker.[1063] In fact, elevation of ADA is correlated with an increase in several inflammatory conditions including Ca^{2+}, irritable bowel, etc. Impaired purine synthesis is expected in the context of cobalamin deficiency as well because methylmalonic (CoA mutase) depends on catalytic action by cobalamin.[1064] Decreased purine synthesis results in impaired DNA synthesis, which then leads to megaloblastic anemia[1065] due to slowed renewal of RBCs from multipotent progenitors, a problem that is compounded by suppressed EPO activity,[1061] a feature of celiac disease.

According to Samsel and Seneff, [939] a remarkable recent case of a 3-month-old infant suffering from molybdenum deficiency links several aspects of glyphosate toxicity together, although glyphosate exposure was not considered as a possible cause in this case.[1066] This child presented with microcephaly, developmental delay, severe irritability, and lactic acidosis. Lactic acidosis is a striking feature of intentional glyphospate poisoning induced by drinking Roundup,[1012,1067] and it suggests impaired oxidative respiration, as is seen in *E. coli* exposed to glyphosate.[1068] *In vitro* studies of glyphosate in the formulation of Roundup have demonstrated an ability to disrupt oxidative respiration by inducing mitochondrial swelling and inhibiting mitochondria complexes II and III.[1069] This would explain a massive buildup of LA following ingestion of Roundup due to a switch to anaerobic metabolism. This phenomenon explains why chemically sensitive patients who are exposed to the glyphosate needs alkalization frequently to stay well. Glyphosate has also been shown to uncouple mitochondrial phosphorylation in plants.[1070,1071] The disruption of oxidative respiration by mitochondrial swelling without a reduction of ATP explains the weakness and fatigue observed in many chemically sensitive patients after ingestion of commercially grown glyphosate contaminating foods.

According to Samsel and Seneff, [939] as stated previously, microcephaly is a feature of excess RA, which could be induced by glyphosate due to its inhibitory action on CYP enzymes. In the case study on molybdenum deficiency,[1066] urinary sulfite levels were high, indicative of defective sulfite oxidase activity. Serum hypouricemia was also present, indicative of impaired XO activity. So, the induction of excess RA, depletion of molybdenum, and lactic acidosis by glyphosate prove a plausible environmental factor in this case.

One final aspect of molybdenum deficiency involves nitrate metabolism. As a source of nitric oxide, inorganic nitrite regulates tissue responses to ischemia. While nitrate reductase activity has been known to be a capability of microbes for many years, it has only recently been realized that mammals also possess a functioning nitrate reductase capability, utilizing a molybdenum-dependent enzyme to produce nitrate from nitrite.[1072] Molybdenum deficiency would impair this capability, likely contributing to the higher risk to venous thrombosis observed in celiac disease.[1016–1018] This could also explain the excess nitrates in the urine observed in association with celiac disease.[1073] For more information, see section on metals—molybdenum. Glyphosphate can also directly irritate the venous wall causing thrombophlebitis and microvasculation. This substance when ingested along with food can cause the food sensitivity as seen in our series of thrombophlebitis cases at the EHC-Dallas of environmentally triggered thrombophelbitis.[1234]

SELENIUM AND THYROID DISORDERS

Autoimmune thyroid disease is associated with celiac disease[1074] as well as with noncoeliac wheat and other food and chemical sensitivity. In Valentino et al.'s study,[1075] up to 43% of patients with Hashimoto's thyroiditis showed signs of mucosal T cell activation typical of celiac disease and/or plain food and chemical sensitivity. Selenium whose deficiency is associated with celiac disease[1076] plays a significant role in thyroid hormone synthesis, secretion, and metabolism, and selenium deficiency is therefore a significant factor in thyroid diseases.[1077–1079]

Selenium is required for the biosynthesis of the "twenty-first amino acid," selenocysteine. Twenty-five specific selenoproteins are derived from this amino acid. Selenium deficiency can lead to impairment in immune function and spermatogenesis in addition to thyroid function.[1080] One very important selenoprotein is glutathione peroxidase, which protects cell membranes and cellular components against oxidative damage by both hydrogen peroxide and peroxynitrite ($ONOO^-$).[1081]

Wheat can be a good source of selenoproteins. However, the content of selenium in wheat can range from sufficient to very low depending upon soil's physical conditions. Soil compaction, which results from modern practices of "no till" agriculture,[1082] can lead to both reduced selenium content and a significant increase in arsenic content in the wheat.[1083] Many GI patients have a high level of arsenic on intracellular mineral analyses. Since glyphosate has been shown to deplete sulfur in plants,[1084] and selenium is in the same column of the periodic table as sulfur, it is likely that glyphosate also disrupts selenium uptake in plants. A gluten-free diet will guarantee, however, that no selenium is available from wheat, inducing further depletion of selenoproteins, and therefore increasing the risk to immune system, thyroid, and infertility problems in treated celiac patients. Supplementation with selenium and even intradermal neutralization for sensitivity is often necessary in those hypersensitive patients who cannot tolerate specific foods like wheat.

The gut bacterium *Lactobacillus*, which is negatively impacted by glyphosate[953] and depleted in association with celiac disease,[958] is able to fix inorganic selenium into more bioavailable organic forms like selenocysteine and selenomethionine.[1085] Selenocysteine is present in the catalytic center of enzymes that protect the thyroid from free radical damage.[1235] Free radical damage would lead to apoptosis and an autoimmune response.[1087] Glyphosate's disruption of these bacteria would lead to depletion in the supply of selenomethionine and selenocysteine. Methionine depletion by glyphosate[1088] would further compound this problem. Of course, methane is needed for the methylation pathway for detoxification of many chemicals stored in the food in chemically sensitive patient.

According to Samsel and Seneff,[939] thus, there are a variety of ways in which glyphosate would be expected to interfere with the supply of selenoproteins to the body, including its effects on *Lactobacillus*, depletion of methionine, the no-till farming methods that are possible because weeds are killed chemically, and the likely interference with plant uptake of inorganic selenium. This aligns well with the observed higher risk of thyroid problems in association with celiac disease and non-cecliac food and chemical sensitivity, in addition to infertility problems and immune issues, which are discussed elsewhere in this volume. Further support for an association between glyphosate and thyroid disease comes from plots over time of the usage of glyphosate in the United States on corn and soy time-aligned with plots of the incidence rate of thyroid cancer in the Unites States as shown in Figure 2.3. Chemical sensitivity is fraught with thyroid problems requiring supplementation of the thyroid as well as the selenomethionine.

INDOLE AND KIDNEY DISEASE

According to Samsel and Seneff,[939] the prevalence of kidney disease and resulting dialysis is increasing worldwide, and kidney disease is often associated with increased levels of celiac disease autoantibodies. Kidney disease and thyroid dysfunction are intimately connected.[1086] A population-based study in Sweden involving nearly 30,000 people with diagnosed celiac disease determined that there was nearly a threefold increased risk for kidney failure in this population group.[1089]

Inflammation plays a crucial role in kidney disease progression.[1090–1092] Chronic kidney disease develops as a consequence of assaults on the kidney from inflammatory agents, brought on by the induction of proinflammatory cytokines and chemokines in the kidney. The toxic phenol p-cresol sulfate, found in jet engine cabin air (see OP pesticides section) jet fuel syndrome, and indoxyl sulfate, a molecule that is chemically similar to p-cresol, have been shown to induce activation of many of these cytokines and chemokines.[1093] p-Cresol and indoxyl sulfate both decrease endothelial proliferation and interfere with wound repair.[1094] p-Cresol is produced by the pathogenic bacterium *C. difficile*, and indoxyl sulfate, derived from indole through sulfation in the liver,[1095] which accumulates at high levels in association with chronic kidney disease.[1096]

The aromatic amino acid tryptophan contains an indole ring, and therefore disruption of tryptophan synthesis might be expected to generate indole as a by-product. Indeed, glyphosate has been shown to induce a significant increase in the production of indole-3-acetic acid in yellow nutsedge plants.[1097] Indole is produced by coliform microorganisms such as *E. coli* under anaerobic conditions. Glyphosate induces a switch in *E. coli* from aerobic to anaerobic metabolism due to impaired mitochondrial ATP synthesis,[1068,1098] which would likely result in excess production of indole. Besides *E. coli*, many other pathogenic bacteria can produce indole, including *Bacillus, Shigella, Enterococcus*, and *V. cholera*.[1099] At least 85 different species of both gram-positive and gram-negative bacteria produce indole, and its breakdown by certain bacterial species depends on CYP enzymes.[1099] Feeding indole to rats deprived of sulfur metabolites leads to macrocytic anemia.[1100] Indole is an important biological signaling molecule among microbes.[1099] Indole acetic acid inhibits the growth of cobalamin-dependent microorganisms, which then causes macrocytic (pernicious) anemia in the host due to cobalamin deficiency.[1101]

Experiments on exposure of mouse fetuses to indole-3-acetic acid have shown that it dramatically induces microcephaly in developing fetuses exposed at critical times in development.[1102] A case study found celiac disease associated with microcephaly and developmental delay in a 15-month-old girl.[1103,1104] A gluten-free diet restored head growth. The authors suggested that poor head growth might precede other manifestations of celiac disease or nonceliac food and chemical sensitivity in infants. A study on plants demonstrated a concentration gradient of indole-3-acetic acid in the plant embryo, similar to the gradient in RA that controls fetal development in mammals.[1105] This alternative may be another way in which glyphosate would promote microcephaly.

Thus, solely through its effect on indole production and indole catabolism in gut bacteria, chronic glyphosate exposure would be expected to lead to cobalamin deficiency, pernicious anemia, microcephaly in a fetus during pregnancy, and kidney failure. p-Cresol supply by overgrown pathogens like *C. difficile* would likely contribute in a similar way as indole, due to its similar biochemical and biophysical properties.

NUTRITIONAL DEFICIENCIES

The damaged villi associated with celiac disease, food sensitivity and CS, irritable bowel, etc. are impaired in their ability to absorb a number of important nutrients, including vitamins B_6, B_{12}

(cobalamin), and folate, as well as iron, calcium, and vitamins D and K.[1106] Thus, long-term celiac disease, CS, and irritable bowel lead to major deficiencies in these micronutrients. Cobalamin deficiency has been well addressed previously. Samsel and Seneff[939] have also already mentioned the chelation of trace minerals by phytates and glyphosate. However, other factors may be at play as well, as discussed here.

Glyphosate disrupts the synthesis of tryptophan and tyrosine in plants and gut bacteria, due to its interference with the shikimate pathway,[945,1068] which is its main source of toxicity to plants. Glyphosate also depletes methionine in plants and microbes. A study on serum tryptophan levels in children with celiac disease revealed that untreated children had significantly lower ratios of tryptophan to large neutral amino acids in the blood, and treated children also had lower levels, but the imbalance was less severe.[1107] The authors suggested a metabolic disturbance in tryptophan synthesis rather than impaired absorption, as other similar amino acids were not deficient in the serum. It was proposed that this could leak to decreased synthesis of the monoamine neurotransmitter, serotonin, in the brain associated with behavior disorders in children with celiac disease, CS, and food sensitivity such as depression.[1108] Deficiencies in tyrosine and methionine were also noted.[1108] "Functional dyspepsia" is an increasing and mainly intractable problem in the Western world, which is estimated to affect 15% of the U.S. population.[1109] Dyspepsia, a clinical symptom of celiac disease, is likely mediated by excess serotonin synthesis following ingested tryptophan-containing foods.[1110] This fact explains not only why vitamins and capasacian intradermal neutralization of serotonin help chemically sensitive patients without dyspepsia but also why seratonin neutralization is so efficacious in others.

Serotonin (5-hydroxytryptamine of 5-HT) is produced by enterochromaffin (EC) cells in the gut and an important signaling molecule for the enteric mucosa.[1111] EC cells are the most numerous neuroendocrine cell types in the intestinal lumen, and they regulate gut secretion, motility, pain, and nausea by activating primary afferent pathways in the nervous system.[1112] Serotonin plays an important role in activating the immune response and inflammation in the gut and also induces nausea and diarrhea when it is overexpressed. Anaerobic bacteria in the colon convert sugars into short-chain fatty acids which can stimulate 5-HT release from EC cells.[1113,1114] This is likely an important source of fats to the body in the case of a low-fat diet induced by impaired fatty acid metabolism due to insufficient bile acids.

The number of 5-HT expressing EC cells in the small intestine is increased in association with celiac disease, along with crypt hyperplasia,[1115,1116] and as a consequence, serotonin uptake from dietary sources of tryptophan is greatly increased in celiac patients.[1117] Postprandial dyspepsia is associated in celiac disease, nonceliac, CS, and food sensitivity with increased release of 5-HT, and this may account for the digestive symptoms experienced by celiac patients, nonceliac, chemically sensitive and food sensitive patients.[1118] An explanation for these observations is that a chronic tryptophan insufficiency due to the impaired ability of gut bacteria to produce tryptophan induces aggressive uptake whenever dietary tryptophan is available. Seratonin intradermal neutralization often turns off the GI symptoms as well as the cerebral symptoms. When the precise intradermal neutralization dose is found and given repeatedly as needed, it is one of the main stays in calming the gut and brain when it is disrupted by pesticides and herbicides in the food and chemically sensitive patient.

Glyphosate forms strong complex with transition metals, through its carboxylic, phosphonic, and amino moieties, each of which can coordinate to metal ions, and it can also therefore form complexes involving two or three atoms of the targeted transition metal.[1119–1121] This means that it is a metal chelator par excellence. One can expect therefore deficiencies in multiple transition (trace) metals such as iron, copper, cobalt, molybdenum, zinc, and magnesium in the presence of glyphosate. Glyphosate has been shown to reduce levels of iron, magnesium, manganese, and calcium in non-GMO soybean plants.[1122]

As well as in food and chemicals, zinc deficiency seems to be a factor in celiac disease, as a recent study of 30 children with celiac disease demonstrated a significantly reduced serum level of zinc (0.64 vs. 0.94 μg/mL in controls).[1123] Copper deficiency is a feature of celiac disease,[1124] and copper is one of the transition metals that glyphosate binds to and chelates.[1119,1121] Confirmed magnesium deficiency in celiac disease has been shown to be due to significant loss through the feces.[1125] This would be expected through binding to phytates and/or glyphosate. A study of 23 patients with gluten-sensitive enteropathy to assess magnesium status revealed that only one had serum magnesium levels below the normal range, whereas magnesium levels in erythrocytes and lymphocytes were markedly below normal, and this was associated with evidence of osteoporosis due to malabsorption.[1126] Daily treatment with $MgCl_2$ or Mg lactate led to a significant increase in bone mineral density, and was correlated with a rise in RBC Mg^{2+}.

A recent study investigated the status of 25(OH) vitamin D_3 in adults and children with celiac disease.[1127] It was determined that vitamin D_3 deficiency was much more prevalent in the adults than in the children, suggesting a deterioration in vitamin D_3 serum levels with age. This could be explained by a chronic accumulation of glyphosate, leading to increasingly impaired vitamin D_3 activation in the liver. The liver converts 1,25(OH) vitamin D_3 to the active form, 25(OH) vitamin D_3, using CYP27A[1128,1129] which might be disrupted by glyphosate exposure, given its known interference with CYP function in mice.[972] On a broader level, this might also explain the recent epidemic in the United States in vitamin D_3 deficiency.[1130]

Another issue to consider is whether the food being consumed by celiac and nonceliac wheat and food sensitive patients is itself depleted in nutrients. This is likely the case for the transgenic Roundup Ready crops that increasingly supply the processed food industry. Celiac as well as food and chemical sensitive patients and those with irritable bowel are usually not only depleted of nutrients but also often have brain and cardiovascular dysfunction. A recent study on the effects of glyphosate on Roundup Ready soy revealed a significant effect on growth, as well as an interference with the uptake of both macro- and micronutrients.[1084] Transgenic soybeans exposed to glyphosate are often affected by a "yellow flashing" or yellowing of the upper leaves, and an increased sensitivity to water stress. An inverse linear relationship was observed between glyphosate dosage and levels of the macronutrients, sodium, calcium, sulfur, phosphorous, potassium, magnesium, and nitrogen, as well as the micronutrients, iron, zinc, manganese, copper, cobalt, molybdenum, and boron. Glyphosate's ability to form insoluble metal complexes likely mediates these depletions.[1131] Glyphosate also interferes with photosynthesis, as reflected in several measures of photosynthesis rate[1084] and reductions in chlorophyll.[1070,1236] This could be due to depletion of zinc and manganese since chloroplasts require these micronutrients to function well.[1132,1133]

CANCER

According to Samsel and Seneff,[939] chronic inflammation, such as occurs in celiac disease, is a major source of oxidative stress, and is estimated to account for one-third of all cancer cases worldwide.[1134,1135] Oxidative stress leads to DNA damage and increased risk to genetic mutation. Several population-based studies have confirmed that patients with celiac disease suffer from increased mortality, mainly due to malignancy.[1136-1141] These include increased risk to non-Hodgkin's lymphoma, adenocarcinoma of the small intestine, and squamous cell carcinomas of the esophagus, mouth, and pharynx, as well as melanoma. The non-Hodgkins's lymphoma was not restricted to gastrointestinal sites, and the increased risk remained following a gluten-free diet.[1141]

Celiac disease is associated with lifelong risk of any malignancy between 8.1% and 13.3% with the risk for non-Hodgkin's lymphoma alone being 4.3%–9%.[1142,1143] This risk is 19-fold higher than the risk in the general population. Selenium deficiency in association with celiac disease may be a significant factor in the increased cancer risk. Selenium deficiency is associated with increased risk to several cancers, and selenium supplements are beneficial in reducing the incidence of liver cancer and decreasing mortality in colorectal, lung, and prostate cancer.[1144,1145]

Children with celiac disease, whether or not they are on a gluten-free diet, and exhibit elevated urinary biomarkers of DNA damage.[1146] Human colon carcinoma cells exposed to peptides extracted from wheat responded with a sharp increase in the GSSG/GSH ratio (ratio of oxidized to reduced glutathione), a well-established indicator of oxidative stress.[1147] The authors did not provide information as to whether the wheat plants were exposed to glyphosate, but they did suggest that this effect could explain the increased risk to intestinal cancer associated with celiac. Intriguingly, studies on pea plants have shown that glyphosate induces a sharp increase in the GSSG/GSH ratio in plant,[1148] which suggests that glyphosate contamination could explain the results observed in them.[1147]

Interestingly, it was noted in 1996 that the incidence of both non-Hodgkin's lymphoma and melanoma had been rising sharply worldwide in recent decades, and so it was decided to investigate whether there might be a link between the two cancers associated with sunlight exposure. Surprisingly, the authors found an inverse relationship between non-Hodgkin's lymphoma and UV exposure. More recently, such UV protection has been reaffirmed in a review of epidemiologic studies on the subject.[1149] This suggests that vitamin D_3 *is protective*, so vitamin D_3 deficiency due to impaired CYP function in the liver could be contributory to increased risk in celiac disease.

The incidence of non-Hodgkins lymphoma has increased rapidly in most Western countries over the last few decades. Statistics from the American Cancer Society show an 80% increase since the early 1970s when glyphosate was first introduced on the market.

While there have been only a few studies of lymphoma and glyphosate, nearly all have indicated a potential relationship.[1150–1154] A dose–response relationship for non-Hodgkin's lymphoma was demonstrated in a cross-Canada study of occupational exposure to glyphosate in men,[1153] and a larger study in the United States noted a similar result.[1153] A population-based study in Sweden showed an increased risk to non-Hodgkins lymphoma upon prior exposure to herbicides and fungicides but not insecticides.[1152] Glyphosate exposure resulted in an OR of 2.3, although the number of samples was small, and the authors suggested that further study is necessary. A study on mice showed increases in carcinoma, leukemia, and lymphoma,[1151] and an *in vitro* mutagenic test on human lymphocytes revealed increased sister-chromatid exchanges[1150] upon exposure to glyphosate.

Proposed Transglutaminase–Glyphosate Interactions

Establishing the mechanism by which glyphosate might promote autoantibodies to transglutaminase is a challenging task, not because this possibility seems unlikely but rather because multiple disruptions are plausible. In this section, Samsel and Seneff[939] present evidence from the research literature that supports various hypotheses for the interaction of glyphosate with the transglutaminase enzymatic pathways. The definitive studies that clarify which of these hypotheses are correct have yet to be conducted.

Celiac disease is thought to be primarily caused by ingestion of wheat gluten protein, particularly gliadin, due to a high concentration of proline- and glutamine-rich sequences which imparts resistance to degradation by proteases. Transglutaminase autoimmunity arises with specific epitopes of wheat gliadin activating sensitized T cells which then stimulate B-cell synthesis of IgA or IgM autoantibodies to transglutaminase.

Transglutaminase Bound to Gliadin Can Induce False Recognition by a T Cell

Transglutaminase acts on gluten in wheat to form crosslinks between glutamine residues and lysine residues, producing ammonia as a by-product. Ammonia is known to induce greater sensitivity to glyphosate in plants, and it is common practice to apply ammonium sulfate simultaneously with glyphosate for this reason.[1155] This enhanced effect is due to ammonium binding to glyphosate at three sites, one on the carbonyl group and two on the phosphonyl group, which displaces cations such as calcium and endows glyphosate with enhanced reactivity.

Transglutaminase sometimes achieves only half of its intended reaction product, by converting a glutamine residue to glutamate, and leaving lysine intact, thus not producing the desired crosslink. It has been established that gluten fragments containing "deamidated glutamine" residues instead of the crosslinks are much more highly allergenic than those that contain the crosslinks.[1156,1157] These have been referred to as "celiac disease T-cell epitopes." T cells of celiac patients preferentially recognize epitopes that are augmented with negatively charged deamidated glutamine residues, the product of the reaction when the lysine linkage does not occur. Thus, if there is a mechanism by which glyphosate interferes with crosslink formation, this would explain its ability to enhance gluten sensitivity. Low T cells are found in food and chemical sensitivity patients which can be treated with glyphosphate removal from the gut. Often, the elimination of glyphosate is not enough and autogenous lymphocytic factor is needed in chemically sensitive patients with food sensitivity (Treatment Volume V).

A clue can be found from the research literature on glyphosate sensitivity in plants, where it has been determined that the substitution of a lysine residue in a critical locale in EPSP synthase greatly increases sensitivity to glyphosate.[1158] Lysine's NH_{3+} group is highly reactive with negatively charged ions, and this makes it a common constituent of DNA binding proteins due to its ability to bind to phosphates in the DNA backbone. Glyphosate contains a phosphonyl group that binds easily to ammonia and behaves as a phosphate mimetic. It also contains a carboxyl group that substitutes well for the carboxyl group of glutamate, the intended reaction partner.

According to Samsel and Seneff,[939] it seems possible that the glyphosate would be drawn to the ammonia released when the glutamine residue is deamidated by transglutaminase, and then the ammonium glyphosate would react with the lysine residue, releasing the ammonia and resulting in the binding of glyphosate to the lysine residue. This would yield a gluten *fragment bound* to glyphosate that is likely highly allergenic. An analogous EPSP synthase–EPSP–glyphosate ternary complex has been identified in numerous studies on the physiology of glyphosate in plants.[1159] We see herbicide and pesticide overloaded in the nonceliac food and chemically sensitive patient who becomes very sensitive to the odor of ammonia. These patients can develop a spreading phenomenon becoming more sensitive to multiple food and a variety of chemicals.

Research in the food industry has concerned producing breads that, while not gluten free, may contain forms of gluten to which celiac patients are less sensitive. Such research has revealed that enzymatic modification to promote methionine binding to glutamine reduces IgA immunoreactivity.[1160] Whether methionine binding to glutamine residues in wheat takes place *in vivo* is not known, but it is established that glyphosate depletes methionine by 50%–65% in plants as well as the aromatic amino acids.[1070,1088] As we have already discussed, glyphosate interferes with cobalt bioavailability for cobalamin synthesis, and cobalamin is an essential catalyst for the conversion of cysteine to methionine.

Transglutaminase also cross-links proteins in the extracellular matrix, and therefore is important for wound healing, tissue remodeling, and stabilization of the extracellular matrix. Thus, autoimmunity to transglutaminase leads to destabilization of the microvilli lining the small intestines. Transglutaminase has 18 free cysteine residues which are targets for S-nitrosylation. A cysteine residue is also involved in the catalytic active site. A unique Ca^{2+}-dependent mechanism regulates nitrosylation by NO, mediated by CysNO (*S*-nitrosocysteine). It was shown experimentally that up to 15 cysteines of transglutaminase were nitrosylated by CysNO in the presence of Ca^{2+}, and this inhibited its enzymatic activity.[1161]

Thus, another plausible mechanism by which glyphosate might enhance the development of autoantibodies to transglutaminase is by nitrosylating its cysteines, acting similarly to CysNO. A precedent for this idea is set with research proposing nitrosylation as the means by which glyphosate interferes with the heme active site in CYP enzymes.[971] It is conceivable that cysteine nitrosylation by glyphosate at the active site inactivates the molecule, in which case glyphosate is itself acting as an "antibody."

EVIDENCE OF GLYPHOSATE EXPOSURE IN HUMANS AND ANIMALS

The U.S. EPA has accepted Monsanto's claim that glyphosate is essentially harmless to humans. Due to this position, there have been virtually no studies undertaken in the United States to assess glyphosate levels in human blood or urine. However, a recent study involving multiple countries in Europe provides disturbing confirmation that glyphosate residues are prevalent in the Western diet.[1162] This study involved exclusively city dwellers, who are unlikely to be exposed to glyphosate except through food sources. Despite Europe's more aggressive campaign against GMO foods than that of the Americas, 44% of the urine samples contained quantifiable amounts of glyphosate. Diet seems to be the main source of exposure. One can predict that, if a study were undertaken in the United States, the percentage of the affected population would be much larger.

A recent study conducted on dairy cows in Denmark shows conclusively that the cows' health is being adversely affected by glyphosate.[954] All of the cows had detectable levels of glyphosate in their urine, and it was estimated that from 0.1 to 0.3 mg of glyphosate was excreted daily from each cow. More importantly, all of the cows had serum levels of cobalt and manganese that were far below the minimum reference level for nutrient sufficiency. Half of the cows had high serum urea, and there was a positive linear relationship between serum urea and glyphosate excretion. High serum urea is indicative of nephrotoxicity. Blood serum levels of enzymes indicative or cytotoxicity such as creatine kinase (CK) and ALP were also elevated. CK is indicative of rhabdomyolysis or kidney failure. High levels of ALP indicate liver damage, and it is often used to detect blocked bile ducts.[1163]

Thus, the low cobalt levels and the indicators of liver, kidney, and gall bladder stress are all consistent with our previous discussion. The results of this study were also consistent with results of a study on rats exposed experimentally to glyphosate[1164] in which Roundup was shown to be even more toxic than its active ingredient, glyphosate.

Glyphosate-metal complexes serve to reduce glyphosate's toxicity in the soil to plants, but they also protect glyphosate from attack by microorganisms that could decompose it.[1054] The degree of reactivity of the complex depends on which metals glyphosate binds to, which in turn depends upon the particular soil conditions.[1165] Glyphosate usually degrades relatively quickly;[1166] however, a half-life of up to 22 years has also been reported in conditions where pH is low and organic matter contents are high.[1165] Therefore, glyphosate may survive much longer in certain soils than has been claimed by the industry, and could be taken up by crops planted subsequent to glyphosate application to kill weeds.

A disturbing trend of crop desiccation by glyphosate preharvest[1167–1171] may be a key factor in the increased incidence of celiac disease. According to Monsanto, glyphosate was used on some 13% of the wheat area preharvest in the United Kingdom in 2004. However, by 2006 and 2007, some 94% of the U.K. growers used glyphosate on at least 40% of cereal and 80% of oilseed crops for weed control or harvest management.[947] According to Samsel and Seneff,[939] an increasing number of farmers now consider the benefits of desiccating their wheat and sugarcane crops with glyphosate shortly before the harvest.[947] The advantage is improved harvesting efficiency because the quantity of materials other than grain or cane is reduced by 17%, due to a shutdown of growth following glyphosate treatment. Treated sugarcane crops produce drier stalks which can be bailed more easily. There is a shorter delay before the next season's crop can be planted, because the herbicide was applied preharvest rather than postharvest. Several pests can be controlled due to the fact that glyphosate is a broad-spectrum herbicide. These include Black grass, Brome grasses, and Rye grasses, and the suggestion is that this would minimize the risk of these weeds developing resistance to other herbicides.

A complete list of the latest EPA residue levels for glyphosate as of September 18, 2013 are shown in Table 2.36. Tolerances are established on all crops for both human and animal consumption resulting from the application of glyphosate.

As glyphosate usage continues unabated, glyphosate resistance among weeds is becoming a growing problem,[1172] necessitating a strategy that either involves an increase in the amount of glyphosate that is applied or a supplementation with other herbicides such as glufosinate, dicampa, 2,4-D, or atrazine. Agrochemical companies are now actively developing crops with resistance to multiple herbicides,[1173] a disturbing trend, especially since glyphosate's disruption

TABLE 2.36

Complete List of Glyphosate Tolerances for Residues in Food Crops in the United States as of September 18, 2013, as reported in EPA: Title 40: Protection of Environment

Commodity	ppm	Commodity	ppm	Commodity	ppm
Acerola	0.2	Galangal, roots	0.2	Quinoa, grain	5
Alfalfa, seed	0.2	Ginger, white, flower	0.2	Rambutan	0.2
Almond, hulls	25	Gourd, buffalo seed	0.1	Rice, grain	0.1
Aloe vera	0.5	Governor's plum	0.2	Rice, wild, grain	0.1
Ambrella	0.2	Gow kee, leaves	0.2	Rose apple	0.2
Animal feed, nongrass, group 18	400	Grain, cereal, forage, and straw, group 16, except field corn, forage and field corn, stover	100	S apod illia	0.2
Artichoke, globe	0.2	Grain, cereal, group15 except field corn, popcorn, rice sweet corn, and wild rice	30	Sapote, black	0.2
Asparagus	0.5	Grass, forage, fodder and hay, group 17	300	Sapote, mamey	0.2
Atemoya	0.2	Guava	0.2	Sapote, white	0.2
Avocado	0.2	Herbs subgroup 19A	0.2	Shellfish	3
Bamboo shoots	0.2	Hop, dried cones	7	Soursop	0.2
Banana	0.2	Ilama	0.2	Spanish lime	0.2
Barley, bran	30	Lambe	0.2	Spearmint tops	0.2
Beet, sugar, dried pulp	25	Imbu	0.2	Spice subgroup 198	200
Beet, sugar, roots	10	Jaboticaba	0.2	Star apple	7
Beet, sugar, tops	10	Jackfruit	0.2	Starfruit	0.2
Berry and small fruit, group 13-07	0.2	Kava, roots	0.2	Stevia, dried leaves	0.2
Betelnut	1	Kenaf, forage	0.2	Sugar apple	1
Birba	0.2	Leucaena, forage	200	Sugarcane, cane	0.2
Blimbe	0.2	Longan	0.2	Sugarcasne, molasses	200
Breadfruit	0.2	Lychee	0.2	Surham cherry	30
Cacao bean, bean	0.2	Mamey apple	0.2	Sweet potato	0.2
Cactus, fruit	0.2	Mango	0.2	Tamarind	3
Cactus, pads	0.5	Mangosteen	0.2	Tea, dried	0.2
Canistgel	0.2	Marmalade box	0.2	Tea, instant	1
					7

(Continued)

TABLE 2.36 (Continued)

Complete List of Glyphosate Tolerances for Residues in Food Crops in the United States as of September 18, 2013, as reported in EPA: Title 40: Protection of Environment

Commodity	ppm	Commodity	ppm	Commodity	ppm
Canola, seed	20	Mioga, flower	0.2	Teff, forage	100
Carrot	5	Noni	0.2	Teff, grain	5
Chaya	1	Nut, pine	1	Teff, hay	100
Cherimoya	0.2	Nut, tree group 14	1	Ti, leaves	0.2
Citrus, dried pulp	1	Oilseeds, group 20, except canola	40	Ti, roots	0.2
Coconut	0.1	Okra	0.5	Ugli fruit	0.5
Coffee bean, green	1	Papaya	0.2	Vegetable, bulb, group 3.07	0.2
Corn, pop, grain	0.1	Papaya, mountain	0.2	Vegetable, cucurbit, group 9	0.5
Corn, sweet, kernel plus cob with husk removed	3.5	Passionfruit	0.2	Vegetable, foliage of legume subgroup 7A, except soybean	0.2
Cotton, gin byproducts	210	Pawpaw	0.2	Vegetable, fruiting, group 8-10 (except okra)	0.1
Custard apple	0.2	Pea, dry	8	Vegetable, leafy, brassica group 5	0.2
Dried fruit	0.2	Peanut	0.1	Vegetable, leafy, except brassica, group 4	0.2
Dokudami	2	Peanut, hay	0.5	Vegetable, leaves of root and tuber, group 2, except sugar beet tops	0.2
Durian	0.2	Pepper leaf, fresh leaves	0.2	Vegetable, legume, group 6 except soybean & dry pea	5
Epazote	1.3	Peppermint, tops	200	Vegetables, root & tuber group 1 except carrot, sweet potato, and sugar beet	0.2
Feijoa	0.2	Perilla, tops	1.8	Wasabi	0.2
Fig	0.2	Persimmon	0.2	Water spinach, tops	0.2
Fish	0.25	Pineapple	0.1	Watercress, upland	0.2
Fruit, citrus, group 10-10	0.5	Pistachio	1	Wax jambu	0.2
Fruit, pome group 11-10	0.2	Pomegrante	0.2		
Fruit, stone, group 12	0.2	Pulasan	0.2		

Source: Adapted from Samsel, A., S. Seneff. 2013. *Interdiscip. Toxicol.* 6(4):159–184.

of CYP enzymes leads to an impaired ability to break down many other environmental chemicals in the liver.

KIDNEY DISEASES IN AGRICULTURAL WORKERS

According to Samsel and Seneff,[939] chronic kidney disease is a globally increasing problem,[1174] and glyphosate may be playing a role in this epidemic. A plot showing recent trends in hospitalization for acute kidney injury aligned with glyphosate usage rates on corn and soy shows strong correlation, as illustrated in Figure 2.35.

Recently, it has been noted that young men in Central America are succumbing in increasing numbers to chronic kidney disease.[1175–1179] The problem appears to be especially acute among agricultural workers, mainly in sugarcane fields.[1176–1178] Since we have shown how glyphosate can produce toxic effects on the kidneys through its disruption of gut bacteria, it is fruitful to consider whether glyphosate could be playing a role in the fate of Central American workers in the sugarcane fields (Figure 2.36).

In attempting to explain this phenomenon, physicians and pharmacists have proposed that it may be due to dehydration caused by over-exertion in high temperature conditions, combined with an acute reaction to commonly administered nonsteroidal anti-inflammatory drugs (NSAIDs) to treat pain and/or antibiotics to treat infection.[1174] NSAIDs require CYP enzymes in the liver for detoxification.[1180] so impaired CYP function by glyphosate would lead to a far more toxic effect of excessive NSAID administration. Kidney disease among agricultural workers ends to be associated with chronic glomerulonephritis and interstitial nephritis, which was proposed in Soderland et al.[1237] to be due to environmental toxins such as heavy metals or toxic chemicals. Glomerulonephritis is also found in association with celiac disease.[1181,1182] A Swedish study showed a fivefold increase in nephritis risk in celiac patients.[1182]

A strong hint comes from epidemiological studies conducted in Costa Rica.[1176] The demographic features of those with CRF revealed a remarkably specific pattern of young men, between 20 and 40 years old, with chronic interstitial nephritis. All of them were sugarcane workers.

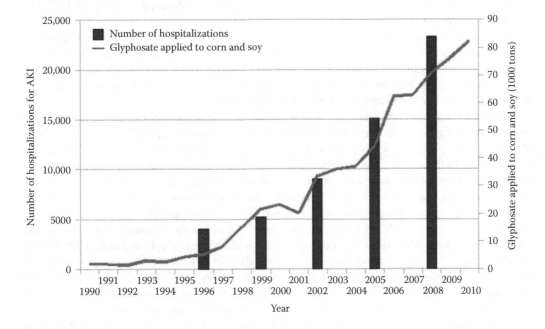

FIGURE 2.35 Number of hospitalizations, glyphosate applied to corn and soy. (Courtesy of Nancy Swanson.)

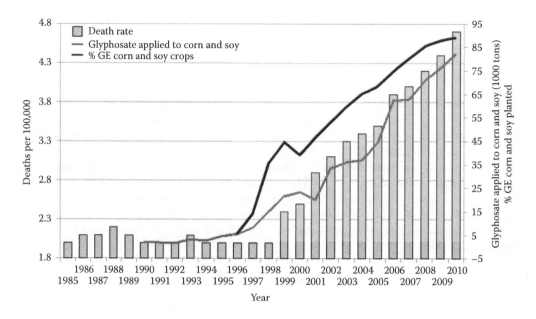

FIGURE 2.36 Death rate, glyphosate applied to corn and soy, GE corn and soy crops. (Courtesy of Nancy Swanson.)

Agriculture is an important part of the economy of the state of Louisiana in the United States, and sugarcane is a significant agricultural product. Chemical methods to ripen sugarcane are commonly used, because they can substantially increase the sucrose content of the harvest.[1183] Glyphosate, in particular, has been the primary ripener used in Louisiana since 1980.[1184] As of 2001, Louisiana had the highest rate of kidney failure in the United States (State-Specific Trends in Chronic Kidney Failure—United States, 1990–2001).[1185] Louisiana's death rate per 100,000 from nephritis/kidney disease is 26.34 as compared to a U.S. rate of 14.55 (Network Coordinating Council, 2013).[1186] The number of patients on dialysis has risen sharply in the last few years.

By 2005, it is estimated that 62% of the total harvested hectares of sugarcane in Louisiana were ripened with glyphosate.[1187] A paper published in 1990 showed that glyphosate applied as a ripener on three different sugarcane varieties grown in Costa Rica, produce up to a 15% increase in the sucrose content of the harvested sugarcane.[1188] Glyphosate applied before the harvest is the only sugarcane ripener currently registered for use in the United States.

A disturbing recent trend is the repeated application of glyphosate over the course of the season with the hope of further increasing yields.[1183] Responses to the standard application rate (0.188 lb/acre) of glyphosate have been inconsistent, and so farmers are increasing both the amount and the frequency of application. In Richard and Dalley's[1183] research, they have concluded that growers are encouraged not to apply glyphosate beyond mid-October, as results are counterproductive, and not to use higher rates in an attempt to improve yield. But it is doubtful that these recommendations are being followed. It is likely, although we have not been able to confirm this, which glyphosate usage has expanded in scope on the sugar cane fields in Central America since 2000, when the expiration of Monsanto's patent drove prices down, and that the practices of multiple applications of glyphosate in the United States are also being followed in Central America. Several other ripening agents exist, such as ethephon, trinexapacethyl, and sulfometuron-methyl, but glyphosate is likely growing in popularity recently due to its more favorable pricing and perceived nontoxicity. Larger amounts are needed for effective ripening in regions that are hot and rainy, which matches the climate of Costa Rica and Nicaragua.

In this Volume V, Samsel and Seneff[939] have developed an argument that the alarming rise in the incidence of celiac disease in the United States and elsewhere in recent years is due to an increased burden of herbicides, particularly glyphosate exposure in the diet. They suggest that a principal factor is the use of glyphosate to desiccate wheat and other crops prior to the harvest, resulting in crop residue and increased exposure. Strong evidence for a link between glyphosate and celiac disease and noncoeliac food and chemical sensitivity comes from a study on predatory fish, which showed remarkable effects in the gut that parallel the features of celiac disease.[949]

More generally, inflammatory bowel disease of many kinds has been linked to several environmental factors including a higher socioeconomic status, urban as opposed to rural dwelling, and a "Westernized" cultural context.[1189] Disease incidence is highest in North America and Europe, and is higher in northern latitudes than in southern latitudes within these regions, suggesting a beneficial role for sunlight. According to the most recent statistics from the U.S. EPA,[1190] the United States currently represents 25% of the total world market on herbicide usage. Glyphosate has been the most popular herbicide in the United States since 2001, whereas it was the 17th most popular herbicide in 1987.[1191] Since 2001, glyphosate usage has grown considerably, due to increased dosing of glyphosate resistant weeds and in conjunction with the widespread adoption of "Roundup-Ready" genetically modified crops. Glyphosate is probably now the most popular herbicide in Europe as well.[1192] Glyphosate has become the number one herbicide worldwide, due to its perceived lack of toxicity and its lower price after having become generic in 2000.[1193]

A recent estimate suggests that 1 in 20 people in North America and Western Europe suffer from celiac disease.[1194,1195] Another 5%–20% suffer CS, food sensitivity, and irritable bowel syndrome. Outdoor occupational status is protective.[1196] First generation immigrants into Europe or North America are generally less susceptible, although second generation non-Caucasian immigrants statistically become even more susceptible than native Caucasians.[1189] This may in part stem from the increased need for sunlight exposure given darker skin pigmentation.

Table 2.37 summarizes Samsel and Seneff's[939] findings relating glyphosate to celiac disease. All of the known biological effects of glyphosate cytochrome P450 inhibition, disruption of synthesis of aromatic amino acids, chelation of transition metals, and antibacterial action contribute to the pathology of not only celiac disease but also food-derived CS.

Celiac disease is associated with deficiencies in several essential micronutrients such as vitamin D_3, cobalamin, iron, molybdenum, selenium, and the amino acids, methionine and tryptophan, all of which can be explained by glyphosate. Glyphosate depletes multiple minerals in both genetically modified soybeans[1084] and conventional soybeans,[1122] which would translate into nutritional deficiencies in foods derived from these crops. This, together with further chelation in the gut by any direct glyphosate exposure, could explain deficiencies in cobalt, molybdenum, and iron. Glyphosate's effect on CYP enzymes should lead to inadequate vitamin D_3 activation in the liver.[972] Cobalamin depends on cobalt-dependent enzymes in plants, and microbes have been shown to be inhibited by glyphosate.[1055,1056] Glyphosate has been shown to severely impair methionine and tryptophan synthesis in plants,[1088] which would reduce the bioavailability of these nutrients in derived foods.

There are multiple intriguing connections between celiac disease and microcephaly, all of which can be linked to glyphosate. Celiac disease is found in association with microcephaly in infants,[1103,1104] and teratogenic effects are also observed in children born to celiac mothers.[1031,1032] Microcephaly in an infant where confirmed molybdenum deficiency was present[1066] suggests that molybdenum deficiency could be causal. However, elevated RA also induces microcephaly, as does indole-3-acetic acid, which has been dramatically linked to microcephaly in mice.[1102] Elevated RA is predicted as a response to glyphosate due to its expected inhibition of CYP enzymes which catabolize RA in the liver.[971,972] Molybdenum deficiency is expected due to glyphosate's ability to chelate cationic minerals. Glyphosate has been shown to induce indole-3-acetic acid synthesis in plants,[1097] and it induces a shift to anaerobic metabolism in E. coli,[1068] which is associated with indole synthesis.

Celiac disease and noncoeliac food sensitivity are associated with impaired serotonin metabolism and signaling in the gut, and this feature leads us to propose a novel role for serotonin in

TABLE 2.37

Illustration of the Myriad Ways in Which Glyphosate Can Be Linked to Celiac Disease or Its Associated Pathologies

Disruption of Gut Bacteria		
Glyphosate Effect	**Dysfunction**	**Consequences**
Reduced *Bifidobacteria*	Impaired gluten breakdown	Transglutaminase antibodies
Reduced *Lactobacillus*	Impaired phytase breakdown	Metal chelation
	Reduced selenoproteins	Autoimmune thyroid disease
Anaerobic *E. coli*	Indole toxicity	Kidney failure
C. difficile overgrowth	*p*-Cresol toxicity	Kidney failure
Desulfovibrio overgrowth	Hydrogen sulfide gas	Inflammation

Transition Metal Chelation		
Glyphosate Effect	**Dysfunction**	**Consequences**
Cobalt deficiency	Cobalamin deficiency	Neurodegenerative diseases
	Reduced methionine	Impaired protein synthesis
	Elevated homocysteine	Heart disease
Molybdenum deficiency	Inhibited sulfite oxidase	Impaired sulfate supply
	Inhibited xanthine oxidase	DNA damage/center
		Teratogenesis
		Megaloblastic anemia
Iron deficiency		Anemia

CYP Enzyme Inhibition		
Glyphosate Impairment	**Dysfunction**	**Consequences**
Vitamin D_3 inactivation	Impaired calcium	Osteoporosis; cancer risk
Retinoic acid catabolism	Metabolism suppressed transglutaminase	Teratogenesis
Bile acid synthesis	Impaired fat metabolism	Gall bladder disease
	Impaired sulfate supply	Pancreatitis
Xenobiotic detoxification	Increased toxin sensitivity	Liver disease
	Impaired indole breakdown	Macrocytic anemia
		Kidney failure
Nitrate reductase	Venous constriction	Venous thrombosis

Shikimate Pathway Suppression		
Glyphosate Effect	**Dysfunction**	**Consequences**
Tryptophan deficiency	Impaired serotonin supply	Depression
	Hypersensitive receptors	Nausea, diarrhea

Source: Adapted from Samsel, A., S. Seneff. 2013. *Interdiscip. Toxicol.* 6(4):159–184.

transporting sulfate to the tissues. It is a curious and little known fact that glucose and galactose, but not fructose or mannose, stimulate 5-HT synthesis by EC cells in the intestinal lumen,[1111] suggesting a role for EC cells as "glucose sensors." Glucose and galactose are the two sugars that make up the heparin sulfate chains of the syndecans and glypicans that attach to the membrane-bound proteins in most cells, serving as the innermost constituent of the ECM.[1197] In Seneff et al.'s study,[1002] it was proposed that part of the postprandial glucose that is taken up by the tissues is temporarily stored in the ECM as heparin sulfate, and that a deficiency in sulfate supply impairs this process, which impedes glucose uptake in cells. These heparin sulfate units have a high turnover rate, as they are typically broken down within three houses of their initial placement.[1198] This provides the cells with a convenient temporary buffer for glucose and galactose that can allow them to be efficiently removed from the serum. Insufficient sulfate supplies would impair this process and lead to insulin resistance, which is seen in many diabetics with a sensitivity problem.

As is the case for other monoamine neurotransmitters as well as most sterols, 5-HT is normally transported in the serum in a sulfated form. The sulfate moiety must be removed for the molecule to activate it. Therefore, 5-HT, as well as these other monoamine neurotransmitters and sterols, can be viewed as a sulfate "escort" in the plasma. In Samsel and Seneff's article,[1098] it was argued that such carbon-ring-containing molecules are necessary for safe sulfate transport, especially in the face of copresent kosmotropes like glyphosate, in order to protect the blood from excess viscosity during transport. Support for the concept that glyphosate gels the blood comes from the observation that disseminated coagulation is a characteristic feature of glyphosate poisoning.[1012] Since glyphosate disrupts sterol sulfaction and it disrupts monoamine neurotransmitter synthesis, in addition to its physical kosmotropic feature, it can be anticipated that a chronic exposure to even a small amount of glyphosate over the course of time will lead to a system wide deficiency in the supply of sulfate to the tissues. We believe that this is the most important consequence of glyphosate's insidious slow erosion of health. We see many nonceliac food and chemically sensitive patients who have severe problems with sulfur containing nutrients and cannot sulfinate these compounds at the EHC-Dallas and Buffalo. It proposes a severe problem for these patients who are unstable having fluctuating endpoints and are very fragile upon exposure to toxics.

An interesting consideration regarding a known link between celiac disease and hypothyroidism[1199] emerges when one considers that iodide is one of the few chaotyropic (structure breaking) anions available to biological systems; another important one being nitrate, which is elevated in the urine in association with celiac disease.[1200] It is intriguing that the conversion of T4 to T3 (the active form of thyroid hormone) involves selenium as an essential cofactor. Furthermore, iodide is released in the process, thus providing chaotopic buffering in the blood serum. Therefore, impaired conversion due to deficient selenium results in an inability to buffer this significant chaotrope in the blood, despite the fact that chaotropic buffering is desperately needed in the context of the kosmotropic effects of glyphosate. While speculative, it is possible that the autoimmune thyroid disease that develops in association with celiac disease is a direct consequence of the inability to activate thyroid hormone due to insufficient selenium. Indeed, celiac patients with concurrent hypothyroidism require an elevated dose of levothyroxine (T4) compared to nonceliac hypothyroid patients,[1199] which could be due to impaired activation to T3.

The link between autoimmune (type 1) diabetes and autoimmune thyroiditis is likely tied to deficiencies in selenoproteins leading to apoptosis. Diabetic rats produce significantly less glomerular heparin sulfate in the kidneys than controls, and this is associated with increased albuminurea.[1201] However, children with type 1 diabetes and celiac disease excrete lower levels of albumin than type 1 diabetic children without celiac disease, suggesting protective role for celiac disease.[1202] Wheat is a good source of tryptophan, so it is likely that tryptophan-derived serotonin induces the symptoms of diarrhea and nausea associated with wheat ingestion, but, at the same time, transports available sulfate through the vasculature, to help maintain adequate supplies of heparin sulfate to the glomerulus. Thus, increased metabolism of dietary tryptophan to serotonin observed in association with celiac disease may help ameliorate the sulfate deficiency problem. Glyphosate's interference with CYP enzymes links to impaired bile-acid production in the liver, which in turn impairs sterol-based transport, placing a higher burden on serotonin for this task.

Samsel and Seneff[939] have argued here that kidney failure, a known risk factor in celiac disease as well as nonceliac food and chemical sensitivity, is a consequence of depleted sulfate supplies to the kidneys.

While they have covered a broad range of pathologies related to celiac disease and have shown how they can be explained by glyphosate exposure, there are likely still other aspects of the disease and the connection to glyphosate that have been omitted. For example, in a remarkable case study,[1203] a 54-year-old man who accidentally sprayed himself with glyphosate developed skin lesions 6 hours later. More significantly, 1 month later he exhibited symptoms of PD. Movement disorders such as Parkinsonism are associated with gluten intolerance.[1204] Figure 2.6 shows plots of glyphosate application to corn and soy alongside plots of deaths due to PD. These and other connections will be further explored in future research.

Celiac disease as well as nonceliac food and chemical sensitivity is a complex and multifactorial condition associated with at times gluten intolerance and a higher risk to thyroid disease, cancer, and kidney disease, and there is also an increased risk to infertility and birth defects in children born to celiac mothers. While the principal diagnostic is autoantibodies to tissue transglutaminase, celiac disease as well as nonceliac food and chemical sensitivities associated with a spectrum of other pathologies such as deficiencies in iron, vitamin D_3, molybdenum, selenium, and cobalamin, an overgrowth of pathogens in the gut at the expense of beneficial biota, impaired serotonin signaling, and increased synthesis of toxic metabolites like p-cresol and indole-3-acetic acid. Samsel and Seneff[939] have systematically shown how all of these features of celiac disease can be explained by glyphosate's known properties. These include (1) disrupting the shikimate pathway, (2) altering the balance between pathogens and beneficial biota in the gut, (3) chelating transition metals, as well as sulfur and selenium, and (4) inhibiting cytochrome P450 enzymes. Samsel and Seneff[939] argue that a key system-wide pathology in celiac disease is impaired sulfate supply to the tissues, and that this is also a key component of glyphosate's toxicity to humans.

The monitoring of glyphosate levels in food and in human urine and blood has been inadequate. The common practice of desiccation and/or ripening with glyphosate right before the harvest ensures that glyphosate residues are present in our food supply. It is plausible that the recent sharp increase of kidney failure in agricultural workers is tied to glyphosate exposure. We urge governments globally to reexamine their policy towards glyphosate and to introduce new legislation that would restrict its usage.

GENITOURINARY SYSTEM

Pollutants are known to affect the GU system. Particularly, the kidneys are involved and many chemicals have been found to overload the kidneys causing renal failure.

Also, lots of cases of bladder spasm have been attributed to pollutant overload. These include the metals, volatile organics, pesticides, and mycotoxins. Generally, there is a decrease in the parasympathetic nervous system and an increase in the SNS, in chemically sensitive patients who have bladder spasms.

RENAL FUNCTION AND HYPERFILTRATION CAPACITY IN LEAD SMELTER WORKERS WITH HIGH BONE LEAD

According to Roels et al.,[1205] the study was undertaken to assess whether the changes in urinary excretion of eicosanoids (a decrease of 6-keto-PGF 1 alpha and PGF2) and an increase of thromboxane previously found in lead (Pb)-exposed workers may decrease the renal hemodynamic response to an acute oral protein load.

The renal hemodynamic response was estimated by determining the capacity of the kidney to increase the glomerular filtration rate (GFR) (in terms of creatinine clearance) after an acute consumption of cooked red meat (400 g). A cross-sectional study was carried out in 76 male Pb workers (age range 30–60 years) and 68 controls matched for age, sex, socioeconomic state, general environment (residence), and workshift characteristics.

The Pb workers had been exposed to lead on average for 18 (range 6–36) years and showed a threefold higher body burden of Pb than the controls as estimated by *in vivo* measurements of tibial Pb concentration (Pb-T) (GM 66 vs. 21 µg Pb/g bone mineral). The GM concentrations of Pb in blood (Pb-B) and Pb in urine (Pb-U) were also significantly higher in the Pb group (Pb-B: 430 vs. 141 µg Pb/l; Pb-U: 40 vs. 7.5 µg Pb/g creatinine). These conditions of chronic exposure to Pb did not entail any significant changes in the concentration of blood borne and urinary markers of nephrotoxicity, such as urinary low and high molecular weight plasma derived proteins (beta-2 microglobulin, retinal binding protein, albumin, transferrin), urinary activities of N-acetyl-beta-D-glucosamindase and kallikrein, and serum concentrations of creatinine, beta-2 microglobulin, urea, and uric acid. All participants also had normal baseline creatinine clearances ($>$80 mL/min/1.73 m^2) amounting on average to 115.5 in the controls versus 122,31.3 mL/min/1.73 m^2 in the Pb group. Both control and Pb-exposed workers showed a significant increment in creatinine clearance (on average 15%) after oral protein load, suggesting that the previously found changes in secretion of urinary eicosanoids apparently has no deleterious effect on *renal* hemodynamics in the examined Pb workers.

The finding that both baseline and stimulated creatinine clearance rates were not only significantly higher in the Pb workers but also positively correlated with Pb-T suggests that moderate exposure to Pb may be associated with a slight hyperfiltration state, which has been found to attenuate the age-related decline in baseline creatinine clearance by a factor of two. Although the relevance of this effect for the worker's health is unknown, it can be concluded that adverse renal changes are unlikely to occur in most adult male Pb workers when their blood Pb concentration is regularly kept below 700 pg Pb/L. One should, however, be cautious in extrapolating this conclusion to the general population because of preemployment screening of the Pb workers for the absence of renal risk factors.

Usefulness of Biomarkers of Exposure to Inorganic Mercury, Lead, or Cadmium in Controlling Occupational and Environmental Risks of Nephrotoxicity

According to Roels et al.,[1205] a successful prevention of renal diseases induced by occupational or environmental exposure to toxic metals such as mercury (Hg), lead (Pb), or cadmium (Cd) largely relies on the capability to detect nephrotoxic effects at a stage when they are still reversible or at least not yet compromising renal function. The knowledge of dose–effect/response relations has been useful to control nephrotoxic effects of these *metals* through a "biological monitoring of exposure approach." Chronic occupational exposure to inorganic mercury (mainly mercury vapor) may result in renal alterations affecting both tubules and glomeruli. Most of the structural or functional renal changes become significant when urinary mercury (HgU) exceeds 50 µg Hg/g creatinine. However, a marked reduction of the urinary excretion of prostaglandin E2 was found at an HgU of 35 µg Hg/g creatinine. As renal changes evidenced in moderately exposed workers were not related to the duration of Hg exposure, it is believed that those changes are reversible and mainly the consequence of recently absorbed mercury. Thus, monitoring HgU is useful for controlling the nephrotoxic risk of overexposure to inorganic mercury: HgU should not exceed 50 µg Hg/g creatinine in order to prevent cytotoxic and functional renal effects.

Several studies on Pb workers with blood lead concentrations (PbB) usually below 70 µg Pb/dL have disclosed either no renal effects or subclinical changes of marginal or unknown health significance. Changes in urinary excretion of eicosanoids were not associated with deleterious consequences on either the GFR—estimated from the creatinine clearance (C_{CR})—or renal hemodynamics if the workers' PbB is yet unknown. In terms of Pb body burden, a mean tibia Pb concentration of about 60 µg Pb/g bone mineral (that is 5–10 times the average "normal" concentration corresponding to a cumulative PbB index of 900 µg Pb/dL $\times$ year) did not affect the GFR in male workers. This conclusion may not necessarily be extrapolated to the general population, as recent studies have disclosed inverse associations between PbB and GFR at low-level environmental Pb exposure. A 10-fold increase in PbB (e.g., from 4 to 40 µg Pb/dL) was associated with a reduction of 10–13 mL/min in the C_{CR} and the OR of having impaired renal function (viz., C_{CR} $<$5th percentile (52 and 43 mL/min in men and women, respectively) was 3.8 (CI $=$ 1.4–10.4; p $=$ 0.01). However, the causal implication of Pb in this association remains to be clarified.

The Cd concentration in urine (CdU) has been proposed as an indirect biological indicator for Cd accumulation in the kidney. Several biomarkers for detecting nephrotoxic effects of Cd at different renal sites were studies in relation to CdU. In occupationally exposed males, the CdU thresholds for significant alterations of renal markers ranged, according to the marker, from 2.4 to 11.5 µg Cd/g creatinine. A threshold of 10 µg Cd/g creatinine (corresponding to 200 µg Cd/g renal cortex: the critical Cd concentration in the kidney) is confirmed for the occurrence of low-molecular-mass proteinuria (functional effect) and subsequence loss of renal filtration reserve capacity. In workers, microproteinuria was found reversible when reduction or cessation of exposure occurred timely when tubular damage was still mild (beta-2-microblobulinuria <1500 µg/g creatinine) and CdU had never exceeded 20 µg Cd/g creatinine. As the predictive significance of other renal changes (biochemical or cytotoxic) is still unknown, it seems prudent to recommend that occupational exposure to Cd should not allow that CdU exceeds 5 µg Cd/g creatinine.

HEALTH EFFECTS OF CADMIUM EXPOSURE: A REVIEW OF THE LITERATURE AND A RISK ESTIMATE

According to Jarup et al.,[1206] this study provides a review of the cadmium exposure situation in Sweden and updates the information on health risk assessment according to recent studies on the health effects of cadmium. The study focuses on the health effects of low cadmium doses and the identification of high-risk groups. The diet is the main source of cadmium exposure in the Swedish nonsmoking general population. The average daily dietary intake is about 15 µg/day, but there are great individual variations due to differences in energy intake and dietary habits. It has been shown that a high-fiber diet and a diet rich in shellfish increase the dietary cadmium intake substantially. Cadmium concentrations in agricultural soil and wheat have increased continuously during the last century. At present, soil cadmium concentrations increase by about 0.2% per year. Cadmium accumulates in the kidneys. Human kidney concentrations of cadmium have increased several folds during the last century. Cadmium in pig kidney has been shown to have increased by about 2% per year from 1984 to 1992. There is no tendency towards decreasing cadmium in the lungs 10%–50% while the absorption in the gastrointestinal tract is only a few percent.

Smokers have about 4–5 times higher blood cadmium concentrations (about 1.5 µg/L), and twice as high kidney cortex cadmium concentrations (about 20–30 µg/wet weight) as nonsmokers. Similarly, the blood cadmium concentrations are substantially elevated in persons with low body and iron stores, indicating increased gastrointestinal absorption. About 10%–40% of Swedish women of childbearing age are reported to have empty iron stores (S-ferritin, 12 µg/L). In general, women have higher concentrations of cadmium in blood, urine, and kidney than men.

The population groups at highest risk are probably smokers, women with low body iron stores, and people habitually eating a diet rich in cadmium. According to current knowledge, renal tubular damage is probably the critical health effect of cadmium exposure, both in the general population and in occupationally exposed workers. Tubular damage may develop at much lower levels than previously estimated, as shown in this report. Data from several recent reports from different countries indicate that an average urinary cadmium excretion of 2.5 µg/g creatinine is related to an excess prevalence of renal tubular damage of 4%. An average urinary excretion of 2.5 µg/g creatinine corresponds to an average concentration of cadmium in renal cortex of 50 µg/g, which would be the result of long-term (decades) intake of 50 µg/day. When the critical concentrations for adverse effects due to cadmium accumulation are being evaluated, it is crucial to consider both the individual variation in kidney cadmium concentrations and the variations in sensitivity within the general population. Even if the population average kidney concentration is relatively low for the general population, a certain proportion will have values exceeding the concentration where renal tubular damage can occur. It can be estimated that, at the present average daily intake of cadmium in Sweden, about 1% of women with low body iron stores and smokers may experience adverse renal effects related to cadmium. If the average daily intake of cadmium would increase to 30 µg/day, about 1% of the entire population would have cadmium-induced tubular damage. In risk groups, for example, women with low iron stores, the percentage would be higher, up to 5%. Both human and animal studies indicate that skeletal damage (osteoporosis) may be a critical effect of cadmium exposure. They conclude, however, that the present evidence is not sufficient to permit such a conclusion for humans. They would like to stress, however, that osteoporosis is a very important public health problem worldwide, but especially in the Scandinavia.

COEXPOSURE TO LEAD INCREASES THE RENAL RESPONSE TO LOW LEVELS OF CADMIUM IN METALLURGY WORKERS

According to Hambach et al.,[1207] research on the effect of co-exposure *to* Cd and Pb *on the kidney is scarce*. The objective of the present study was to assess the effect of co-exposure to these metals on biomarkers of early renal effect.

Cd in blood (CdB), Cd in urine (CdU), Pb-B and urinary renal biomarkers, that is, microalbumin (μ-Alb), beta-2 microglobulin (β_2–MG), retinol binding protein (RBP), *N*-acetyl-β-*d*-glucosaminidase (NAG), intestinal alkaline phosphatase (IAP) were measured in 122 metallurgic refinery workers examined in a cross-sectional survey.

The median CdB, CdU, and PbB were 0.8 μg/L (IQR = 0.5, 1.2), 0.5 μg/g creatinine (IQR = 0.3, 0.8), and 158.5 μg/L (IQR = 111.0, 219.3), respectively. The impact of CdB on the urinary excretion of NAG and IAP was only evident among workers with PbB concentrations $\geq$ 75th percentile. No statistically significant interaction terms were observed from the associations between CdB or CdU and the other renal markers under study (i.e., μ-Alb and β2-MG). Their findings indicate that Pb increases the impact of Cd exposure on early renal biomarkers.

PHYSIOCHEMICAL AND BIOCHEMICAL SIGNS OF NEPHROLITHIASIS

According to Tomakh,[1208] urolithiasis diagnosis by uroliths presence reflects insufficient knowledge of the disease pathogenesis. A total of 42 patients with oxalocalcium nephrolithiasis and 20 health patients were examined for differences in the urine and plasma composition. The authors studied factors involved in regulation of mineral metabolism and urinary elimination of crystal-forming substances. The patients with urinary stones compared to the control are characterized by low total crystal-inhibiting activity, hypersomnia, hypodipsia, decreased surface free energy, high quantities of ionized calcium, low ionized magnesium in the urine, and oligo- and uricosuria. Shifts in hormonal regulation in nephrolithiasis result from slight elevation of urinary cyclic adenosine monophosphate, a relative rise in the levels of aldosterone and parathyroid hormone, low blood calcitonin, all the changes being statistically significant.

Mechanism of Kidney Participation in Maintaining Osmotic and Ion Homeostasis in CFR

According to Bogolepova et al.,[1209] in examination of patients with CRF at GFR below 30 mL/min and blood serum ion concentration within limits of normal values, hyperosmia has been found. Under the natural regimen, essential differences have been revealed neither in variation limits of renal excretion of ions nor osmotically active substances in CRF patients as compared with healthy controls. Diuresis correlated with renal excretion of osmotically active substances. It is shown that a decrease in reabsorption of osmotically active substances depends on secretion and excretion of prostaglandin E2. A suggestion is made about the role of prostaglandins in regulation of renal changes.

Metal Ions Affecting the Pulmonary and Cardiovascular Systems Yielding Hypersensitive and Hyposensitive Responses

According to Corradi et al.,[1210] some metals, such as copper and manganese, are essential to life and play irreplaceable roles in, for example, the functioning of important enzyme systems; however, excess manganese can cause pathology. Other metals are xenobiotics, that is, they have no useful role in human physiology and, even worse, as in the case of lead, cadmium, mercury erseine, etc., may be toxic even at trace levels of exposure. Even those metals that are essential, however, have the potential to turn harmful at very high levels of exposure or at lower exposure if the tissue becomes hypersensitive. A reflection of a very basic tenet of toxicology is "the dose makes the poison." However, it must be emphasized that low doses can be triggered if the tissue is sensitized or the total pollutant load is high. Toxic metal exposure may lead to serious risks to human health. As a result of the extensive use of toxic metals and their compounds in industry and consumer products, these agents have been widely disseminated in the environment. Since metals are not biodegradable, they can persist in the environment and produce a variety of adverse effects for years. Exposure to metals can lead to damage in a variety of organ systems and, in some cases, metals also have the potential to be carcinogenic and atherogenic. Even though the importance of metals as environmental health hazards is now widely appreciated, the specific mechanisms by which metals produce their adverse effects have yet to be fully elucidated. The unifying factor in determining toxicity, hypersensitivity, and carcinogenicity for most metals is the generation of reactive oxygen and nitrogen species. Metal-mediated formation of free radicals causes various modifications to nucleic acids, enhanced lipid peroxidation, and altered calcium and sulfhydryl homeostasis. While copper, chromium, and cobalt undergo redox-cycling reactions, for metals such as cadmium and nickel the primary route for their toxicity is depletion of glutathione, and bonding to sulfhydryl groups of proteins. They can also cause sensitization. This chapter attempts to show that the toxic and hypersensitive aspects effects of different metallic compounds may be manifested in the pulmonary, neurological, urological, and cardiovascular systems. The knowledge of health effects due to metal exposure is necessary for practicing physicians, and should be assessed by inquiring about present and past occupational history and environmental exposure.

IMMUNOTOXCICITY OF HEAVY METALS

According to Bernier et al.,[1211] heavy metals including mercury, lead, and cadmium are present throughout the ecosystem and are detectable in small amounts in the Great Lakes water and fish. The main route of exposure of humans to these metals is via the ingestion of contaminated food, especially fish. Extensive experimental investigations indicated that heavy metals alter a number of parameters of the host's immune system and lead to increased susceptibility to infections, autoimmune diseases, and hypersensitive manifestations. The existing limited epidemiologic data and data derived from *in vitro* systems in which human peripheral blood leukocytes were used suggested that the human immune system may also be at increased risk following exposure to these *metals*. The magnitude of the risk that the presence of such metals in the Great Lakes may pose to the human immune system, and consequently to their health, is not known.

IMPACT OF EFFECTS OF ACID PRECIPATION ON TOXICITY OF METALS

According to Nordberg et al.,[1212] acid precipitation may increase human exposure to several potentially toxic metals by increasing metal concentrations in major pathways to man, particularly food and water, and in some instances by enhancing the conversion of metal species to more toxic forms. Human exposures to methylmercury are almost entirely by way of consumption of fish and seafood as well as dental amalgams. In some countries, intakes by this route may approach the levels that can give rise to adverse health effects for population groups with a high consumption of these food items. A possible increase in methylmercury concentrations in fish from lakes affected by acid precipitation may thus be of concern to selected population groups.

Human exposures to lead reach levels that are near those associated with adverse health effects in certain sensitive segments of the general population in several countries. The possibility exists that increased exposures to lead may be caused by acid precipitation through a mobilization of lead from soils into crops. A route of exposure to lead that may possibly be influenced by acid precipitation is an increased deterioration of surface materials containing lead and a subsequent ingestion by small children.

A similar situation with regard to uptake from food exists for cadmium (at least in some countries). Human metal exposures via drinking water may be increased by acid precipitation. Decreasing pH increases corrosiveness of water enhancing the mobilization of metal salts from soil; metallic compounds may be mobilized from minerals, which may eventually reach drinking water. Also, the dissolution of metals (Pb, Cd, Cu) from piping systems for drinking water by soft acidic waters of high corrositivity may increase metal concentrations in drinking water. Exposures have occasionally reached concentrations that are in the range where adverse health effects may be expected in otherwise healthy persons. Dissolution from piping systems can be prevented by neutralizing the water before distribution.

Increased aluminum concentrations in water as a result mainly of the occurrence of Al in acidified natural waters and the use of Al chemicals in drinking water purification. If such water is used for dialysis in patients with CRF, it may give rise to cases of dialysis dementia and other disorders. A possible influence on health of persons with normal renal function (e.g., causing AD) is uncertain and requires further investigation.

PRESENT STATUS OF BIOLOGICAL EFFECTS OF TOXIC METALS IN THE ENVIRONMENT: LEAD, CADMIUM, AND MANGANESE

According to Shukla,[1213] the number of reports concerning the chemical toxicology of metals, which are released in the environment by natural as well as anthropogenic sources, has been increasing constantly. Lead, cadmium, and manganese have found a variety of uses in industry, craft, and agriculture owing to their physical and chemical properties. The environmental burden of heavy metals has been rising substantially by smelter emission in air and waste sewage in water. Further, organic compounds of lead and manganese used as antiknock substances in gasoline are emitted into the atmosphere by automobile exhaustion. Such environmental contamination of air, water, soil, and food is a serious threat to all living kinds. Although these metals are known to produce their toxic effects on a variety of body systems, much emphasis has been placed on their effects on the nervous system owing to apparent association of relatively low or "subclinical" levels of metallic exposure with behavioral and psychological disorders. As previously stated in this chapter, clinical and animal data on environmental exposure show that while lead and manganese are most toxic to the nervous system, cadmium exerts profound adverse effects on kidney and the male reproductive system. It appears that the consequences of exposure to lead in adults are less severe than the types of exposure associated with hyperactivity in neonates. Except for a few reports, hyperactivity has indeed been observed in animals exposed to either of these three metals. Experimental work has also shown that these metals produce behavioral changes by altering the metabolism of brain neurotransmitters, especially catecholamines. Recently, it is hypothesized that these metals exert their toxic effect by damaging biological defences which exist in the body to serve as protective mechanisms against exogenous toxins. A voluminous publication list with diverse opinions on the biological effects of metals is available and there is an urgent need to compile assessment of the existing literature to identify the future theme of research work. The problem of metal toxicity becomes even more complex owing to simultaneous or successive exposure of the general population to different physical, chemical, biological, and psychological factors in the environment. The net toxic manifestations produced by multiple exposures should, therefore, be different from those produced by a single factor as the result of their additive, synergistic, or antagonistic action. Even though a metal may not exist in sufficient amounts to cause any disability, the toxicity could result when a second factor is also present.

PLATINUM COMPLEX THAT BINDS NONCOVALENTLY TO DNA AND INDUCES CELL DEATH VIA A DIFFERENT MECHANISAM THAN CISPLATIN

According to Suntharalingam et al.,[1214] cisplatinum and some of its derivatives have been shown to be very successful anticancer agents. Their main mode of action has been proposed to be via covalent binding to DNA. However, one of the limitations of these drugs is their poor activity against some tumors due to intrinsic or acquired resistance. Therefore, there is interest in developing complexes with different binding modes and mode of action. Herein, they present a novel platinum(ii)-terpyridine complex (1) which interacts noncovalently with DNA and induces cell death via a different mechanism than cisplatin. The interaction of this complex with DNA was studied by UV/Vis spectroscopic titrations, fluorescent indicator displacement (FID) assays, and circular dichroism (CD) titrations. In addition, computational docking studies were carried out with the aim of establishing the complex's binding mode. These experimental and computational studies showed the complex to have an affinity constant for DNA of $\sim10^4$ (4) M^{-1}, a theoretical free energy of binding of -10.83 kcal mol^{-1} and selectivity for the minor groove of DNA. Long-term studies indicated that one does not covalently bind (or nick) DNA. The cancer cell antiproliferative properties of this platinum(ii) complex were probed *in vitro* against human and murine cell lines. Encouragingly, the platinum(ii) complex displayed selective toxicity for the cancerous (U2OS and SH-SY5Y) and proliferating NIH 3T3 cell lines. Further cell-based studies were carried out to establish the mode of action. Cellular uptake studies demonstrated that the complex is able to penetrate the cell membrane and localize to the nucleus, implying that genomic DNA could be a cellular target. Detailed immunoblotting studies in combination with DNA-flow cytometry showed that the platinum(ii) complex induced cell death in a manner consistent with necrosis.

When an incitant reaction occurs in the body that area becomes acidotic, therefore the use of Na, K, and low Ca carbonate helps overcome the reaction. Often, patients' own physiology can then overcome the reaction. We have treated thousands of episodes with the administration of bicarbonates.

LINK BETWEEN COPPER AND WILSON'S DISEASE

According to Purchase et al.,[1215] Wilson's disease (hepatolenticular degeneration) is a rare inherited autosomal recessive disorder of copper metabolism leading to copper accumulation in the liver and extrahepatic organs such as the brain and cornea. Patients may present with combination of hepatic, neurological, and psychiatric symptoms. Copper is the therapeutic target for the treatment of Wilson's disease. But how did copper come to be linked with Wilson's disease? The answer encompasses a study of enzootic neonatal ataxiain lambs in the 1930s, the copper-chelating properties of British Anti-Lewisite, and the chemical analysis for copper of the organs of deceased Wilson's disease patients in the mid-to-late 1940s. Wilson's disease is one of a number of copper-related disorders where loss of copper homeostasis as a result of genetic, nutritional, or environmental factors affects human health.

INFLUENCE OF RATIO SIZE ON COPPER HOMEOSTASIS DURING SUBLETHAL DIETARY COPPER EXPOSURE IN JUVENILE RAINBOW TROUT, *ONCORHYNCHUS MYKISS*

According to Kamunde et al.,[1216] the influence of ratio size on homeostasis and sublethal toxicity of copper (Cu) was assessed in rainbow trout (*Oncorhynchus mykiss*) during dietary Cu exposure in synthetic soft water. A constant dietary dose of 0.24 μm Cu per gram fish per day as $CuSO_4 \cdot 5H_2O$ was delivered via diets containing 15.75, 7.87, and 5.24 μm Cu g^{-1} fed at 1.5%, 3.0%, and 4.5% wet body weight daily ration, respectively. Juvenile rainbow trout showed clear effects of ratio but not Cu on growth, suggesting that growth is hardly a sensitive endpoint for detection of sublethal dietary Cu exposure. All Cu-exposed fish accumulated the same total metal load when expressed on a per fish basis. This suggests that differences in tissue and whole-body Cu concentrations among the treatments reflected the differences in the fish size rather than total Cu accumulation, and demonstrate that absorption and accumulation of Cu from the gut during dietary exposure are independent of the food quantity in which the Cu is delivered. Fish fed a high ratio exhibited greater mass-specific unidirectional uptake of waterborne Cu than fish fed a low ratio indicating an increased need for Cu for growth processes in rapidly growing fish. Stimulated excretion of Cu was indicated by greater Cu accumulation in the bile of the Cu-exposed fish. Branchial NA^+, K^+-ATPase was not affected by dietary Cu exposure or ratio but gut Na^+, K^+-ATPase activities showed stimulatory effects of increasing ratio but not of Cu exposure. The 96-hour LC_{50} for waterborne Cu (range 0.17–0.21 μmL^{-1}, 10.52–13.20 $\mu g\ L^{-1}$) was same in all treatment groups indicating that ratio size was unimportant and that dietary Cu did not induce an increase in tolerance to waterborne Cu. Taken together, these results suggest that the nutritional status, fish size, and growth rates should be considered when comparing whole-body and -tissue Cu concentration data for biomonitoring and risk assessment. Moreover, expressing the exposure as total metal dose rather than metal concentration in the diet is more appropriate.

BIOAVAILIABILITY AND TOXICITY OF DIETBORNE COPPER AND ZINC TO FISH

According to Clearwater et al.,[1217] till date, most researchers have used dietborne metal concentrations rather than daily doses to define metal exposure and this has resulted in contradictory data within and between fish species. It has also resulted in the impression that high concentrations of dietborne Cu and Zn (e.g., >900 mg kg^{-1} dry diet) are relatively nontoxic to fish. They reanalyzed existing data using ratios and dietborne metal concentrations, and used daily dose, species, and life stage to define the toxicity of dietborne Cu and Zn to fish. Partly because of insufficient information they were unable to find consistent relationships between metal toxicity in laboratory-prepared diets and any other factor including supplemented metal compound (e.g., $CuSO_4$ or CuC_2), duration of metal exposure, diet type (i.e., practical, purified, or live diets), or water quality (flow rates, temperature, hardness, pH, alkalinity). For laboratory-prepared diets, dietborne Cu toxicity occurred at daily doses of >1 mg kg^{-1} body weight d^{-1} for channel catfish (*Ictalurus punctatus*), 1–15 mg kg^{-1} body weight d^{-1} (depending on life stage) for Atlantic salmon (*Salmo salar*), and 35–45 mg kg^{-1} body weight d^{-1} for rainbow trout (*Oncorhynchus mykiss*).

They found that dietborne Zn toxicity has not yet been demonstrated in rainbow trout or turbot (*Scophtalmus maximus*) probably because these species have been exposed to relatively low doses of metal (<90 mg kg^{-1} body weight d^{-1}) and effects on growth and reproduction have not been analyzed. However, daily doses of 9–12 mg Zn kg^{-1} body weight d^{-1} in laboratory-prepared diets were toxic to three other species: carp, *Cyprinus carpio*; Nile tilapia, *Oreochromis niloticus*; and guppy, *Poecilia reticulate*. Limited research indicates that biological incorporation of Cu or Zn into a natural diet can either increase or decrease metal bioavailability, and the relationship between bioavailability and toxicity remains unclear. They have resolved the contradictory data surrounding the effect of organic chelation on metal bioavailability. Increased bioavailability of dietborne Cu and Zn is detectable when the metal is both organically chelated and provided in very low daily doses. They have summarized the information available on the effect of phosphates, phytate, and calcium on dietborne Zn bioavailability. They also explored a rationale to understand the relative importance of exposure to waterborne or dietborne Cu and Zn with a view to finding an approach useful to regulatory agencies. Contrary to popular belief, the relative efficiency of Cu uptake from water and diet is very similar when daily doses are compared rather than Cu concentrations in each media. The ratio of dietborne dose:waterborne dose is a good discriminator of the relative importance of exposure to dietborne or waterborne Zn.

CHEMICAL-SPECIFIC HEALTH CONSULTATION FOR CHROMATE COPPER ARSENATE CHEMICAL MIXUTRE: PORT OF DJIBOUTI

According to Chou et al.,[1218] the Agency for Toxic Substances and Disease Registry (ATSDR) prepared this health consultation to provide support for assessing the public health implications of hazardous chemical exposure, primarily through drinking water, related to releases of chromate copper arsenate (CCA) in the port of Djibouti. CCA from a shipment, apparently intended for treating electric poles, is leaking into the soil in the port area. CCA is a pesticide used to protect wood against decay causing organisms. This mixture commonly contains chromium(VI) (hexavalent chromium) as chromic acid, arsenic(V) (pentavalent arsenic) as arsenic pentoxide, and copper(II) (divalent copper) as cupric oxide, often in an aqueous solution or concentrate. Experimental studies of the fate of CCA in soil and monitoring studies of wood-preserving sites where CCA was spilled on the soil indicate that the chromium(VI), arsenic, and copper components of CCA can leach from soil into groundwater and surface water. In addition at CCA wood-preserving sites, substantial concentrations of chromium(VI), arsenic, and copper remained in the soil and were leachable into water 4 years after the use of CCA was discontinued, suggesting prolonged persistence in soil, with continued potential for leaching. The degree of leaching depended on soil composition and the extent of soil contamination with CCA. In general, leaching was highest for chromium(VI), intermediate for arsenic and lowest for copper. Thus, the potential for contamination of sources of drinking water exists. Although arsenic that is leached from CCA-contaminated soil into surface water may accumulate in the tissues of fish and shellfish, most of the arsenic in these animals will be in a form (often called fish arsenic) that is less harmful. Copper, which leaches less readily than the other components, can accumulate in tissues of mussels and oysters. Chromium is not likely to accumulate in the tissues of fish and shellfish. Limited studies of air concentrations during cleanup of CCA-contaminated soil at wood-preserving sites showed that air levels of chromium(VI), arsenic, and copper were below the occupational standards. Workers directly involved in the repackaging, containment, or cleanup of leaking containers of CCA or of soil saturated with CCA, however, may be exposed to high levels of CCA through direct dermal contact, inhalation of aerosols or particulates, and inadvertent ingestion. Few studies have been conducted on the health effects of CCA. CCA as a concentrated solution is corrosive to the skin, eyes, and digestive tract.

Studies of workers exposed to CCA in wood-preserving plants have not found adverse health effects in these workers, but the studies involved small numbers of workers and therefore are not definitive. People exposed to very high levels of CCA, from sawing wood that still had liquid CCA in it or from living in a home contaminated with ash containing high levels of chromium(VI), arsenic, and copper, experienced serious health effects including nosebleeds, digestive system pain and bleeding, itching skin, darkened urine, nervous system effects such as tingling or numbness of the hands and feet and confusion, and rashes or thickening and peeling of the skin.

These health effects of the mixture are at least qualitatively reflective of the health effects of the individual components of CCA (arsenic, chromium(VI), and copper). For a given mixture, the critical effects of the individual components are of particular concern, as are any effects in common that may become significant due to additivity or interactions among the components. Effects of concern for CCA, based on the known effects of the individual components, include cancer (arsenic by the oral route, arsenic and chromium(VI) by the inhalation route), irritant or corrosive effects (all three mixture components), the unique dermal effects of arsenic, neurologic effects (arsenic and chromium(VI)), and hematologic, hepatic, and renal effects (all three components). Since arsenic, chromium(VI), and copper components affect some of the same target organs, they may have additive toxicity toward those organs.

Few studies have investigated the potential toxic interactions among the components (arsenic, chromium(VI), and copper) of CCA. The available interaction studies and also possible mechanisms of interaction were evaluated using a weight-of-evidence approach. The conclusion is that there is no strong evidence that interactions among the components of CCA will result in a marked increase in toxicity. This conclusion reflects a lack of well-designed interaction studies as well as uncertainties regarding potential mechanisms of interaction. Confidence in the conclusion is low.

Workers exposed to high levels of CCA during cleanup of leaking containers of CCA or soil heavily contaminated with CCA should wear protective clothing and respirators if air concentrations of arsenic are about 10 $\mu g/m^3$. In addition, they should not eat, drink, or use tobacco products during exposure to CCA, and should thoroughly wash after skin contact with CCA and before eating, drinking, using tobacco products, or using restrooms.

When protective clothing becomes contaminated with CCA, it should be changed, and the contaminated clothing should be disposed of in a manner approved for pesticide disposal. Workers should leave all protective clothing, including work shoes and boots, at the workplace so that CCA will not be carried into their cars and homes, which would endanger other people. People not involved in the cleanup of the CCA and who are not wearing protective clothing should be prevented from entering contaminated areas. Leaking containers of CCA must be repackaged and contained to prevent direct exposure of on-site personnel; and contaminated soil needs to be removed to prevent the CCA from leaching into surface water and groundwater thereby contaminating sources of drinking water.

EFFECTS OF DIETARY COPPER ON THE GROWTH PERFORMANCE, NONSPECIFIC IMMUNITY AND RESISTANCE TO AEROMONAS HYDROPHILA OF JUVENILE CHINESE MITTEN CRAB, *ERIOCHEIR SINENSIS*

According to Sun et al.,[1219] an 8-week feeding trial was conducted to determine the dietary copper (Cu) on growth performance and immune responses of juvenile Chinese mitten crab *Eriocheir sinensis*. Six semipurified diets with six copper levels (1.88, 11.85, 20.78, 40.34, 79.56, and 381.2 mg kg^{-1} diet) of $CuSO_4 \cdot 5H_2O$ were fed to *E. sinensis* (0.45 $\pm$ 0.01 g). Each diet was fed to the crab in five replicates. The crab fed diets with 20.78 and 40.34 mg Cu kg^{-1} diet had significantly greater weight gain and hemolymph oxyhemocyanin content than those fed diets with 1.88 and 381.2 mg Cu kg^{-1} diet. Survival rates of crab were not significantly different between all treatment groups. The activities of copper-zinc superoxide dismutase (Cu-Zn SOD), phenoloxidase (PO), and total hemocyte count (THC) significantly increased when the supplementation of dietary copper reached 20.78–40.34 mg Cu kg^{-1} diets. In the bacteria challenge experiment with *Aeromonas hydrophila*, survival rates significantly increased and reached a plateau when the dietary copper increased from 1.88 to 40.34 mg kg^{-1}, whereas significantly decreased when the dietary copper increased from 40.34 to 381.2 mg kg^{-1}. This study indicates that the level of dietary copper is important in regulating growth and immune response in crab.

IMPACT OF ALUMINUM EXPOSURE ON THE IMMUNE SYSTEM

According to Zhu et al.,[1220] aluminum (Al) is widely used in daily life and will lead to environmental release and exposure. The toxicity of Al had been documented, and which attracted a growing concern on human and animal health. The immune system appears to be sensitive to Al exposure. But few studies focused on the potential immunological responses induced by Al. It is imperative to study the effects of Al on the immune function and this review discusses the effects of Al on autoimmunity, oral tolerance, expression of the immune cells, hypersensitivity, and erythrocyte immune function. It will provide evidence to the association between Al and immune function.

OXIDATIVE STRESS DUE TO ALUMINUM EXPOSURE INDUCES ERYPTOSIS WHICH IS PREVENTED BY ERYTHROPOIETIN

According to Vota et al.,[1221] the widespread use of aluminum (Al) provides easy exposure of humans to the metal and its accumulation remains a potential problem. *In vivo* and *in vitro* assays have associated Al overload with anemia. To better understand the mechanisms by which Al affects human erythrocytes, morphological and biochemical changes were analyzed after long-term treatment using an *in vitro* model. The appearance of erythrocytes with abnormal shapes suggested metal interaction with cell surface, supported by the fact that high amounts of Al attached to cell membrane. Long-term incubation of human erythrocytes with A-induced signs of premature erythrocyte death (eryptosis), such as phosphatidylserine (PS) externalization, increased intracellular calcium, and band 3 degradation. Signs of oxidative stress, such as significant increase in reactive oxygen *s*pecies in parallel with decrease in the amount of "reduced glutathione," were also observed. These oxidative effects were completely prevented by the antioxidant *N*-acetylcysteine. Interestingly, erythrocytes were also protected from the prooxidative action of Al by the presence of EPO. In conclusion, results provide evidence that chronic Al exposure may lead to biochemical and morphological alterations similar to those shown in eryptosis induced by oxidant compounds in human erythrocytes. The antieryptotic effect of EPO may contribute to enhance the knowledge of its physiological role on erythroid cells. Irrespective of the antioxidant mechanism, this property of EPO, shown in this model of Al exposure, lets us suggest potential benefits by EPO treatment of patients with anemia associated to altered redox environment.

Stimulation of Eryptosis by Aluminum Ions

According to Niemoeller et al.,[1222] aluminum salts are utilized to impede intestinal phosphate absorption in CRF. Toxic side effects include anemia, which could result from impaired formation or accelerated clearance of circulating erythrocytes. Erythrocytes may be cleared secondary to suicidal erythrocyte death or eryptosis, which is characterized by cell shrinkage and exposure of PS at the erythrocyte surface. As macrophages are equipped with PS receptors, they bind, engulf, and degrade PS-exposing cells. The present experiments have been performed to explore whether Al^{3+} ions trigger erptosis. The PS exposure was estimated from annexin binding and cell volume from forward scatter in FACS analysis. Exposure to Al^{3+} ions (> or 10 μM Al^{3+} for 24 hours) indeed significantly increased annexin binding, an effect paralled by decrease or forward scatter at higher concentrations (> or 30 μM Al^{3+} for 24 hours). According to Fluo-3 fluorescence, Al^{3+} ions (> or 30 μM for 3 hours) increased cytosolic Ca^{2+} activity. Al^{3+} ions (> or 10 μM for 24 hours) further decreased cytosolic ATP concentrations. Energy depletion by removal of glucose similarly triggered annexin binding, an effect not further enhanced by Al^{3+} ions. The eryptosis was paralleled by release of hemoglobin, pointing to loss of cell membrane integrity. In conclusion, Al^{3+} ions decrease cytosolic ATP leading to activation of Ca^{2+}-permeable cation channels, Ca^{2+} entry, simulation of cell membrane scrambling, and cell shrinkage. Moreover, Al^{3+} ions lead to loss of cellular hemoglobin, a feature of hemolysis. Both effects are expected to decrease the life span of circulating erythrocytes and presumably contribute to the development of anemia during Al^{3+} intoxication.

REFERENCES

1. Guyton, A. C., J. E. Hall. 2002. The chemical senses: Tasting and smelling-CaO. In *Treaty of Medical Physiology*, 10th ed., A. C. Guyton, J. E. Hall, Eds., pp. 570–577. Rio de Janeiro: Guanabara Koogam SA.
2. Menashe, I., T. Abaffy, Y. Hasin, S. Goshen, V. Yahalom, C. W. Luetje, D. Lancet. 2007. Genetic elucidation of human hyperosmia to isovaleric acid. *PLoS Biol.* 5(11):e284.
3. Jacob, S., M. K. Mcclintock, B. Zelano, C. Ober. 2002. Paternally inherited HLA alleles are associated with women's choice of male odor. *Nat. Genet.* 30(2):175–179.
4. Hennies, K., H.-P. Neitzke, H. Voigt. 2000. *Mobile Telecommunications and Health*. ECOLOG-Insititut.
5. Nonaka, M., N. Ariyoshi, T. Shonai, M. Kashiwagi, T. Imai, S. Chiba, H. Matsumoto. 2004. CT perfusion abnormalities in a case of non-herpetic acute limbic encephalitis. *Rinsho Shinkeigaku* 44(8):537–540.
6. Zibrowski, E. M. 2006. Olfactory sensitivity in medical laboratory workers occupationally exposed to organic solvent mixtures. *Occup. Med.* 51(6):51–54.
7. Marmura, M. J., T. S. Monteith, W. Anjum, R. L. Doty, S. E. Hegarty, S. W. Keith. 2014. Olfactory function in migraine both during and between attacks. *Cephalalgia* 34(12):977–985.

8. Lee, R. J., N. A. Cohen. 2016. Bitter taste bodyguards. *Sci. Am.* 314(2):38–43, doi:10.1038/scientificamerican0216-38.

9. Hummel, T., B. Landis, K. B. Huttenbrink. 2011. Smell and taste disorders. *GMS Curr. Top. Otorhinolaryngol. Head Neck Surg.* 10:1865–1011.

10. Doty, R. 2009. The olfactory system and its disorders. *Semin. Neurol.* 29(1):74–81.

11. Buck, L., R. Axel. 1991. A novel multigene family may encode odorant receptors: A molecular basis for odor recognition. *Cell* 65:175–187.

12. Miyawaki, A., J. Llopis, R. Heim, J. M. McCaffery, J. A. Adams, M. Ikura, R. Y. Tsien. 1997. Fluorescent indicators for Ca^{++} based on green fluorescent proteins and calmodulin. *Nature* 388(6645):882–887.

13. Caggiano, M., J. Kauer, D. Hunter. 1994. Globose basal cells are neuronal progenitors in the olfactory epithelium: A lineage analysis using a replication-incompetent retrovirus. *Neuron* 13(2):339–352.

14. Hall, J., A. Guyton. 2016. *Guyton and Hall Textbook of Medical Physiology.* Philadelphia: Elsevier.

15. Block, M. L., L. Calderon-Garciduenas. 2009. Air pollution: Mechanisms of neuroinflammation and CNS disease. *Trends Neurosci.* 32(9):506–516.

16. Kissel, J., G. Dotson, A. Bunge, C. P. Chen, J. Cherrie, G. Kasting, H. Frasch, J. Sahmel, S. Semple, S. Wilkinson. 2013. Analysis of finite dose dermal absorption data: Implications for dermal exposure assessment. *J. Expo. Sci. Environ. Epidemiol.* 24(1):65–73.

17. McColl, B. W., S. M. Allan, N. J. Rothwell. 2009. Systemic infection, inflammation and acute ischemic stroke. *Neuroscience* 158:1049–1061.

18. Castillo, J., J. Alvarez-Sabín, E. Martínez-Vila, J. Montaner, J. Sobrino, J. Vivancos; MITICO Study Investigators. 2009. Inflammation markers and prediction of post-stroke vascular disease recurrence: The MITICO study. *J. Neurol.* 256:217–224.

19. Cunningham, C., S. Campion, K. Lunnon, C. L. Murray, J. F. Woods, R. M. Deacon, J. N. Rawlins, V. H. Perry. 2009. Systemic inflammation induces acute behavioral and cognitive changes and accelerates neurodegenerative disease. *Biol. Psychiatry* 65:304–312.

20. D'Mello, C., T. Le, M. G. Swain. 2009. Cerebral microglia recruit monocytes into the brain in response to tumor necrosis factoralpha signaling during peripheral organ inflammation. *J. Neurosci.* 29:2089–2102.

21. Dantzer, R., J. C. O'Connor, G. G. Freund, R. W. Johnson, K. W. Kelley. 2008. From inflammation to sickness and depression: When the immune system subjugates the brain. *Nat. Rev. Neurosci.* 9:46–56.

22. Tracey, K. J. 2009. Reflex control of immunity. *Nat. Rev. Immunol.* 9:418–428.

23. Tamagawa, E., S. F. van Eeden. 2006. Impaired lung function and risk for stroke: Role of the systemic inflammation response? *Chest* 130:1631–1633.

24. Folkmann, J. K., L. Risom, C. S. Hansen, S. Loft, P. Møller. 2007. Oxidatively damaged DNA and inflammation in the liver of dyslipidemic ApoE-/- mice exposed to diesel exhaust particles. *Toxicology* 237:134–144.

25. Swiston, J. R., W. Davidson, S. Attridge, G. T. Li, M. Brauer, S. F. van Eeden. 2008. Wood smoke exposure induces a pulmonary and systemic inflammatory response in firefighters. *Eur. Respir. J.* 32:129–138.

26. Ruckerl, R. et al.; AIRGENE Study Group. 2007. Air pollution and inflammation (interleukin-6, C-reactive protein, fibrinogen) in myocardial infarction survivors. *Environ. Health Perspect.* 115:1072–1080.

27. Calderón-Garcidueñas, L. et al. 2008. Air pollution, cognitive deficits and brain abnormalities: A pilot study with children and dogs. *Brain Cogn.* 68:117–127.

28. Calderon-Garciduenas, L. et al. 2008. Systemic inflammation, endothelial dysfunction, and activation in clinically healthy children exposed to air pollutants. *Inhal. Toxicol.* 20:499–506.

29. Mills, N. L., K. Donaldson, P. W. Hadoke, N. A. Boon, W. MacNee, F. R. Cassee, T. Sandström, A. Blomberg, D. E. Newby. 2009. Adverse cardiovascular effects of air pollution. *Nat. Clin. Pract. Cardiovasc. Med.* 6:36–44.

30. Qin, L., X. Wu, M. L. Block, Y. Liu, G. R. Breese, J. S. Hong, D. J. Knapp, F. T. Crews. 2007. Systemic LPS causes chronic neuroinflammation and progressive neurodegeneration. *Glia* 55:453–462.

31. Rivest, S., S. Lacroix, L. Vallières, S. Nadeau, J. Zhang, N. Laflamme. 2000. How the blood talks to the brain parenchyma and the paraventricular nucleus of the hypothalamus during systemic inflammatory and infectious stimuli. *Proc. Soc. Exp. Biol. Med.* 223:22–38.

32. Perry, V. H., C. Cunningham, C. Holmes. 2007. Systemic infections and inflammation affect chronic neurodegeneration. *Nat. Rev. Immunol.* 7:161–167.

33. Ling, Z., Y. Zhu, C. W. Tong, J. A. Snyder, J. W. Lipton, P. M. Carvey. 2006. Progressive dopamine neuron loss following supra-nigral lipopolysaccharide (LPS) infusion into rats exposed to LPS prenatally. *Exp. Neurol.* 199(2):499–512.

34. Manousakis, G., M. B. Jensen, M. R. Chacon, J. A. Sattin, R. L. Levine. 2009. The interface between stroke and infectious disease: Infectious diseases leading to stroke and infections complicating stroke. *Curr. Neurol. Neurosci. Rep.* 9:28–34.
35. Calderon-Garciduenas, L., B. Azzarelli, H. Acuna, R. Garcia, T. M. Gambling, N. Osnaya, S. Monroy, M. R. DEL Tizapantzi, J. L. Carson, A. Villarreal-Calderon. 2002. Air pollution and brain damage. *Toxicol. Pathol.* 30:373–389.
36. Peters, A., B. Veronesi, L. Calderon-Garciduenas, P. Gehr, L. C. Chen, M. Geiser, W. Reed, B. Rothen-Rutishauser, S. Schurch, H. Schulz. 2006. Translocation and potential neurological effects of fine and ultrafine particles a critical update. *Part Fibre Toxicol.* 3:13.
37. Alexis, N. E., S. Becker, P. A. Bromberg, R. Devlin, D. B. Peden. 2004. Circulating CD11b expression correlates with the neutrophil response and airway mCD14 expression is enhanced following ozone exposure in humans. *Clin. Immunol.* 111:126–131.
38. Bonner, J. C., A. B. Rice, P. M. Lindroos, P. O. O'Brien, K. L. Dreher, I. Rosas, E. Alfaro-Moreno, A. R. Osornio-Vargas. 1998. Induction of the lung myofibroblast PDGF receptor system by urban ambient particles from Mexico City. *Am. J. Respir. Cell Mol. Biol.* 19:672–680.
39. Fenton, M. J., D. T. Golenbock. 1998. LPS-binding proteins and receptors. *J. Leukoc. Biol.* 64:25–32.
40. Garantziotis, S., J. W. Hollingsworth, A. K. Zaas, D. A. Schwartz. 2008. The effect of toll-like receptors and toll-like receptor genetics in human disease. *Ann. Rev. Med.* 59:343–359.
41. Ansari, K. A., A. Johnson. 1975. Olfactory dysfunction in patients with Parkinson's disease. *J. Chronic Dis.* 28:493–497.
42. Doty, R. L. 2003. Odor perception in neurodegenerative diseases and schizophrenia. In *Handbook of Olfaction and Gustation*, 2nd ed., R. L. Doty, Ed., pp. 479–502. New York: Marcel Dekker.
43. Kovács, T. 2004. Mechanisms of olfactory dysfunction in aging and neurodegenerative disorders. *Ageing Res. Rev.* 3:215–232.
44. Rea, W. J., J. R. Butler, J. L. Laseter, I. R. DeLeon. 1984. Pesticides and brain function changes in a controlled environment. *Clin. Ecol.* 2(3):145–150.
45. Hawkes, C. 2003. Olfaction in neurodegenerative disorders. *Mov. Disord.* 18:364–372.
46. Kranick, S. M., J. E. Duda. 2008. Olfactory dysfunction in Parkinson's disease. *Neurosignals* 16:35–40.
47. Handley, O. J., C. M. Morrison, C. Miles, A. J. Bayer. 2006. ApoE gene and familial risk of Alzheimer's disease as predictors of odour identification in older adults. *Neurobiol. Aging* 27:1425–1430.
48. Graves, A. B., J. D. Bowen, L. Rajaram, W. C. McCormick, S. M. McCurry, G. D. Schellenberg, E. B. Larson. 1999. Impaired olfaction as a marker for cognitive decline: Interaction with apolipoprotein E epsilon4 status. *Neurology* 53:1480–1487.
49. Calhoun-Haney, R., C. Murphy. 2005. Apolipoprotein epsilon4 is associated with more rapid decline in odor identification than in odor threshold or Dementia Rating Scale scores. *Brain Cogn.* 58:178–182.
50. Calderón-Garcidueñas, L. et al. 2010. Urban air pollution: Influences on olfactory function and pathology in exposed children and young adults. *Exp. Toxicol. Pathol.* 62(1):91–102.
51. Reiman, E. M., K. Chen, G. E. Alexander, R. J. Caselli, D. Bandy, D. Osborne, A. M. Saunders, J. Hardy. 2004. Functional brain abnormalities in young adults at genetic risk for late-onset alzheimer's dementia. *Proc. Natl. Acad. Sci. U. S. A.* 101:284–289.
52. Kozauer, A. N., M. M. Mielke, G. K. Chan, G. W. Rebock, C. G. Lyketsos. 2008. Apolipoprotein E genotype and lifetime cognitive decline. *Int. Psychogeriatr.* 20:109–123.
53. Desai, S. C., R. L. Doty, R. de la Hoz, J. Moline, R. Herbert, P. J. Gannon, K. W. Altman. 2009. Prevalence and severity of smell dysfunction in workers at the post-9/11 World Trade Center site. *Am. J. Rhinol.*
54. Randolph, T. G. 1978. *Human Ecology and Susceptibility to the Chemical Environment.* Springfield, Illinois: Charles C. Thomas, 1962 (sixth printing 1978).
55. Dickey, L. D. Ed. 1976. *Clinical Ecology.* Springfield, IL: Charles C. Thomas.
56. Calderón-Garcidueñas, L. et al. 2004. Brain inflammation and Alzheimer's-like pathology in individuals exposed to severe air pollution. *Toxicol. Pathol.* 32:650–658.
57. Calderón-Garcidueñas, L. et al. 2008. Long-term air pollution exposure is associated with neuroinflammation, an altered innate immune response, disruption of the blood-brain-barrier, ultrafine particle deposition, and accumulation of amyloid beta 42 and alpha synuclein in children and young adults. *Toxicol. Pathol.* 36:289–310.
58. Guarneros, M., T. Hummel, M. Martinez-Gomez, R. Hudson. 2009. Mexico City air pollution adversely affects olfactory function and intranasal trigeminal sensitivity. *Chem. Senses* 34(9):819–826.
59. Aitake, M., E. Hori, J. Matsumoto, K. Umeno, M. Fukuda, T. Ono, H. Nishijo. 2011. Sensory mismatch induces autonomic responses associated with hippocampal theta waves in rats. *Behav. Brain Res.* 220(1):244–253.

60. Rea, W. J., K. Patel. 2014. *Reversibility of Chronic Degenerative Disease and Hypersensitivity*, Vol. 1. Boca Raton, FL: CRC Press.
61. Rea, W. J., K. Patel. 2015. *Reversibility of Chronic Degenerative Disease and Hypersensitivity*, Vol. 2. Boca Raton, FL: CRC Press.
62. Alobid, I., J. M. Guilemany, A. García-Piñero, S. Cardelús, S. Centellas, J. Bartra, A. Valero, C. Picado, J. Mullol. 2009. Persistent allergic rhinitis has a moderate impact on the sense of smell, depending on both nasal congestion and inflammation. *Laryngoscope* 119(2):233–238.
63. Bower, B. Human noses can sniff 1 trillion odors: Smell may have played an underappreciated role in evolution. *Science News*. Print. BODY & BRAIN.
64. Louveau, A. et al. 2015. Structural and functional features of central nervous system lymphatic vessels. *Nature* 523(7560):337–341.
65. Ransohoff, R. M., B. Engelhardt. 2012. The anatomical and cellular basis of immune surveillance in the central nervous system. *Nat. Rev. Immunol.* 12:623–635.
66. Kipnis, J., S. Gadani, N. C. Derecki. 2012. Pro-cognitive properties of T cells. *Nat. Rev. Immunol.* 12:663–669.
67. Shechter, R., A. London, M. Schwartz. 2013. Orchestrated leukocyte recruitment to immune-privileged sites: Absolute barriers versus educational gates. *Nat. Rev. Immunol.* 13:206–218.
68. Alitalo, K. 2011. The lymphatic vasculature in disease. *Nat. Med.* 17:1371–1380.
69. Wang, Y., G. Oliver. 2010. Current views on the function of the lymphatic vasculature in health and disease. *Genes Dev.* 24:2115–2126.
70. Baluk, P. et al. 2007. Functionally specialized junctions between endothelial cells of lymphatic vessels. *J. Exp. Med.* 204:2349–2362.
71. Kerjaschki, D. 2014. The lymphatic vasculature revisited. *J. Clin. Invest.* 124:874–877.
72. Bazigou, E., S. Xie, C. Chen, A. Weston, N. Miura, L. Sorokin, R. Adams, A. F. Muro, D. Sheppard, T. Msakinen. Integrin-alpha9 is required for fibronectin matrix assembly during lymphatic valve morphogenesis. *Dev. Cell* 17:175–186.
73. Koina, M. E., L. Baxter, S. J. Adamson, F. Arfuso, P. Hu, M. C. Madigan, T. Chan-Ling. 2015. Evidence for lymphatics in the developing and adult human choroid. *Invest. Ophthalmol. Vis. Sci.* 56:1310–1327.
74. Johanson, C. E., J. A. Duncan, P. M. Klinge, T. Brinker, E. G. Stopa, G. D. Silverberg. 2008. Multiplicity of cerebrospinal fluid function: New challenges in health and disease. *Cerebrospinal Fluid Res.* 5:10.
75. Weller, R. O., E. Djuanda, H. Y. Yow, R. O. Carare. 2009. Lymphatic drainage of the brain and the pathophysiology of neurological disease. *Acta. Neuropathol.* 117:1–14.
76. Liu, N. F., Q. Lu, Z. H. Jiang, C. G. Wang, J. G. Zhou. 2009. Anatomic and functional evaluation of the lymphatics and lymph nodes in diagnosis of lymphatic circulation disorders with contrast magnetic resonance lymphangiography. *J. Vasc. Surg.* 49:980–987.
77. Girard, J. P., C. Moussion, R. Förster. 2012. HEVx, lymphatics and homeostatic immune cell trafficking in lymph nodes. *Nat. Rev. Immunol.* 12:762–773.
78. Weller, R. O., I. Galea, R. O. Carare, A. Minagar. 2010. Pathophysiology of the lymphatic drainage of the central nervous system: Implications for pathogenesis and therapy of multiple sclerosis. *Pathophysiology* 17:295–306.
79. Mathieu, E., N. Gupta, R. L. Macdonald, J. Ai, Y. H. Yücel. 2013. In vivo imaging of lymphatic drainage of cerebrospinal fluid in mouse. *Fluids Barriers CNS* 10:35.
80. Cserr, H. F., C. J. Harling-Berg, P. M. Knopf. 1992. Drainage of brain extracellular fluid into blood and dep cervical lymph and its immunological significance. *Brain Pathol.* 2:269–276.
81. Harris, M. G. et al. 2014. Immune privilege of the CNS is not the consequence of limited antigen sampling. *Sci. Rep.* 4:4422.
82. Laman, J. D., R. O. Weller. 2013. Drainage of cells and soluble antigen from the CNS to regional lymph nodes. *J. Neuroimmune Pharmacol.* 8:840–856.
83. Schneider, M., A. Ny, C. Ruiz de Almodovar, P. Carmeliet. 2006. A new mouse model to study acquired lymphedema. *PLoS Med.* 3:e264.
84. Kida, S., A. Pantazis, R. O. Weller. 1993. CSF drains directly from the subarachnoid space into nasal lymphatics in the rat: Anatomy, histology and immunological significance. *Neuropathol. Appl. Neurobiol.* 19(6):480–488.
85. Xie, L. et al. 2013. Sleep drives metabolite clearance from the adult brain. *Science* 342(6156):373–377.
86. Yang, L., B. T. Kress, H. J. Weber, M. Thiyagarajan, B. Wang, R. Deane, H. Benveniste, J. J. Iliff, M. Nedergaard. 2015. Evaluating glymphatic pathway function utilizing clinically relevant intrathecal infusion of CSF tracer. *J. Transl. Med.* 11:107.

87. Berton, M., G. Lorette, F. Baulieu, E. Lagrue, S. Blesson, F. Cambazard, L. Vaillant, A. Maruani. 2015. Generalized lymphedema associated with neurologic signs (GLANS) syndrome: A new entity? *J. Am. Acad. Dermatol.* 72, 333–339.

88. Akiyama, H. et al. 2000. Inflammation and Alzheimer's disease. *Neurobiol. Aging* 21:383–421.

89. Hohlfeld, R., H. Wekerle. 2001. Immunological update on multiple sclerosis. *Curr. Opin. Neurol.* 14:299–304.

90. Jessen, N. A., A. S. Munk, I. Lundgaard, M. Nedergaard. 2015. The glymphatic system: A beginner's guide. *Neurochem. Res.* 40(12):2583–2599.

91. Wood, H. 2015. Neuroimmunology: Uncovering the secrets of the "brain drain"—The CNS lymphatic system is finally revealed. *Nat. Rev. Neurol.* 11(7):367.

92. Song, X., C. Pope, R. Murthy, J. Shaikh, B. Lal, J. P. Bressler. 2004. Interactive effects of paraoxon and pyridostigmine on blood-brain barrier integrity and cholinergic toxicity. *Toxicol. Sci.* 78(2):241–247.

93. Korn, A., H. Golan, I. Melamed, R. Pascual-Marqui, A. Friedman. 2005. Focal cortical dysfunction and blood-brain barrier disruption in patients with postconcussion syndrome. *J. Clin. Neurophysiol.* 22(1):1–9.

94. Friedman, A., D. Kaufer, J. Shemer, I. Hendler, H. Soreq, I. Tur-Kaspa. 1996. Pyridostigmine brain penetration under stress enhances neuronal excitability and induces early immediate transcriptional response. *Nat. Med.* 2(12):1382–1385.

95. Tennant, F. 2016. Brain drain: Lymphatic drainage system discovered in the brain. *Practical Pain Management.* 5 Aug. 2015. Web. 08 Jan. 2016. http://www.practicalpainmanagement.com/resources/news-and-research/brain-drain-lymphatic-drainage-system-discovered-brain&gt.

96. Graeber, M. B., M. J. Christei. 2012. Multiple mechanisms of microglia: A gatekeeper's contribution to pain states. *Exp. Neurol.* 234(2):255–261.

97. Calvo, M., D. L. Bennett. 2012. The mechanism of micro-gliosis and pain following peripheral nerve injury. *Exp. Neurol.* 234(2):271–282.

98. Finnerup, N. B. 2008. A review of central neuropathic pain states. *Curr. Opin. Anaesthesiol.* 21(5):586–589.

99. Watkins, L. R., M. R. Hutchinson, A. Ledeboer, J. Wieseler-Frank, E. D. Milligan, S. F. Maier. 2003. Norman Cousins lecture. Glia as the "bad guys": Implications for improving clinical pain control and the clinical utility of opioids. *Brain Behav. Immun.* 21(2):131–146.

100. Watkins, L. R., S. F. Maier. 2003. When good pain turns bad. *Curr. Dir. Psychol. Sci.* 12(6):232–236.

101. Milligan, E. D., L. R. Watkins. 2009. Pathological and protective roles of glia in chronic pain. *Nat. Rev. Neurosci.* 10(1):23–36.

102. Henry, D. E., A. E. Chiodo, W. Yan. 2011. Central nervous system reorganization in a variety of chronic pain states: A review. *PM R.* 3(12):1116–1125.

103. Latremollier, A., C. J. Woolf. 2009. Central sensitization: A generator of pain hypersensitivity by central neural plasticity. *J. Pain* 10(9):895–926.

104. Woolf, C. J. 2011. Central sensitization: Implications for the diagnosis and treatment of pain. *Pain* 152(Suppl. 3):S2–S15.

105. Staud, R., S. Nagel, M. E. Robinson, D. D. Price. 2009. Enhanced central pain processing of fibromyalgia patients is maintained by muscle afferent input: A randomized, double-blind, placebo controlled study. *Pain* 145(1–2):96–104.

106. Kim, S. E., L. Chang. 2012. Overlap between functional GI disorders and other functional syndromes: What are the underlying mechanisms? *Neurogastroenterol. Motil.* 24(10):895–913.

107. Tracey, I., C. M. Bushnell. 2009. How neuroimaging studies have challenged us to rethink: Is chronic pain a disease? *J. Pain* 10(11):1113–1120.

108. May, A. 2008. Chronic pain may change the structure of the brain. *Pain* 137(1):7–15.

109. May, A. 2011. Structural brain imaging: A window into chronic pain. *Neuroscientist* 17(2):209–220.

110. Rodriguez-Raecke, R., A. Niemieier, K. Ihle, W. Ruether, A. May. 2009. Brain gray matter decrease in chronic pain is the consequence and not the cause of pain. *J. Neurosci.* 29(44):13746–13750.

111. Apkarian, A. V., Y. Sosa, S. Sonty, R. M. Levy, R. N. Harden, T. B. Parrish, D. R. Gitelman. 2004. Chronic back pain is associated with decreased prefrontal and thalamic gray matter density. *J. Neurosci.* 24(46):10410–10415.

112. Teutsch, S., W. Herken, U. Bingel, E. Schoell, A. May. 2008. Changes in brain gray matter due to repetitive painful stimulation. *Neuroimage* 42(2):845–849.

113. Kuchinad, A., P. Schweinhardt, D. A. Seminowicz, P. B. Wood, B. A. Chizh, M. C. Bushnell. 2007. Accelerated brain gray matter loss in fibromyalgia patients: Premature aging of the brain? *J. Neurosci.* 27(15):4004–4007.

114. Buckalew, N., M. W. Haut, L. Morrow, D. Weiner. 2008. Chronic pain is associated with brain volume loss in older adults: Preliminary evidence. *Pain Med.* 9(2):240–248.
115. Hutchinson, M. R., Y. Shavit, P. M. Grace, K. C. Rice, S. R. Maier, L. R. Watkins. 2011. Exploring the neuroimmunopharmacology of opioids: An integrative review of mechanisms of central immune signaling and their implications for opioid analgesia. *Pharmacol. Rev.* 63(3):772–810.
116. Alzheimer's & Dementia Weekly: DDT Pesticide Linked to Alzheimer's. 2014. Web. January 08, 2016. http://www.alzheimersweekly.com/2014/02/ddt-pesticide-linked-to-alzheimers.html
117. Grandjean, P., P. J. Landrigan. 2014. Neurobehavioural effects of developmental toxicity. *Lancet Neurology* 13(3):330–338.
118. Willis, A. W., B. A. Evanoff, M. Lian, A. Galarza, A. Wegrzyn, M. Schootman, B. A. Racette. 2010. Metal emissions and urban incident parkinson disease: A community health study of medicare beneficiaries by using geographic information systems. *Am. J. Epidemiol.* 172(12):1357–1363.
119. Li, F., J. Z. Tsien. 2009. Memory and the NMDA receptors. *N. Engl. J. Med.* 361(3):302–303.
120. Dingledine R., K. Borges, D. Bowie, S. F. Traynelis. 1999. The glutamate receptor ion channels. *Pharmacol. Rev.* 51(1):7–61.
121. Liu, Y., J. Zhang. 2000. Recent development in NMDA receptors. *Chin. Med. J.* 113(10):948–956.
122. Cull-Candy, S., S. Brickley, M. Farrant. 2001. NMDA receptor subunits: Diversity, development and disease. *Curr. Opin. Neurobiol.* 11(3):327–335.
123. Kleckner, N. W., R. Dingledine. 1988. Requirement for glycine in activation of NMDA-receptors expressed in Xenopus oocytes. *Science* 241(4867):835–837.
124. Aizenman, E., S. A. Lipton, R. H. Loring. 1989. Selective modulation of NMDA responses by reduction and oxidation. *Neuron* 2(3):1257–1263.
125. Yu, X. M., R. Askalan, G. J. Keil, M. W. Salter. 1997. NMDA channel regulation by channel-associated protein tyrosine kinase Src. *Science* 275(5300):674–678.
126. Chen, Y., U. Beffert, M. Ertunc, T. S. Tang, E. T. Kavalali, I. Bezprozvanny, J. Herz. 2005. Reelin modulates NMDA receptor activity in cortical neurons. *J. Neurosci.* 25(36):8209–8216.
127. Hawasli, A. H., D. R. Benavides, C. Nguyen, J. W. Kansy, K. Hayashi, P. Chambon, P. Greengard, C. M. Powell, D. C. Cooper, J. A. Bibb. 2007. Cyclin-dependent kinase 5 governs learning and synaptic plasticity via control of NMDAR degradation. *Nat. Neurosci.* 10(7):880–886.
128. Zhang, S., L. Edelmann, J. Liu, J. E. Crandall, M. A. Morabito. 2008. Cdk5 regulates the phosphorylation of tyrosine 1472 NR2B and the surface expression of NMDA receptors. *J. Neurosci.* 28(2):415–424.
129. Fourgeaud, L., C. M. Davenport, C. M. Tyler, T. T. Cheng, M. B. Spencer, L. M. Boulanger. 2010. MHC class I modulates NMDA receptor function and AMPA receptor trafficking. *Proc. Natl. Acad. Sci. U. S. A.* 107(51):22278–22283.
130. Huh, G. S., L. M. Boulanger, H. Du, P. A. Riquelme, T. M. Brotz, C. J. Shatz. 2000. Functional requirement for class I MHC in CNS development and plasticity. *Science* 290(5499):2155–2159.
131. Nelson, P. A., J. R. Sage, S. C. Wood, C. M. Davenport, S. G. Anagnostaras, L. M. Boulanger. 2013. MHC class I immune proteins are critical for hippocampus-dependent memory and gate NMDAR-dependent hippocampal long-term depression. *Learn. Mem.* 20(9):505–517.
132. Purves, D., G. J. Augustine, D. Fitzpatrick, W. C. Hall, A. S. LaMantia, J. O. McNamara, L. E. White. 2008. *Neuroscience*, 4th ed., pp. 137–138, Sinauer Associates, ISBN 978-0-87893-697-7.
133. Chen, P. E., M. T. Geballe, P. J. Stansfeld, A. R. Johnston, H. Yuan, A. L. Jacob, J. P. Snyder, S. F. Traynelis, D. J. Wyllie. 2005. Structural features of the glutamate binding site in recombinant NR1/NR2A N-methyl-D-aspartate receptors determined by site-directed mutagenesis and molecular modeling. *Mol. Pharmacol.* 67(5):1470–1484.
134. Wolosker, H. 2006. D-serine regulation of NMDA receptor activity. *Sci. STKE* 2006(356):pe41.
135. Moskal, J., D. Leander, R. Burch. 2010. Unlocking the Therapeutic Potential of the NMDA Receptor. Drug Discovery & Development News. Retrieved December 19, 2013.
136. Ehinger, B., O. P. Ottersen, J. Storm-Mathisen, J. E. Dowling. 1988. Bipolar cells in the turtle retina are strongly immunoreactive for glutamate. *Proc. Natl. Acad. Sci. U. S. A.* 85:8321–8325.
137. Anderson, C. 2003. The Bad News Isn't In: A Look at Dissociative-Induced Brain Damage and Cognitive Impairment. Erowid DXM Vaults: Health. Retrieved December 17, 2008.
138. Mount, C., C. Downton. 2006. Alzheimer disease: Progress or profit? *Nat. Med.* 12(7):780–784.
139. NICE Technology Appraisal January 18, 2011 Azheimer's Disease—Donepezil, Galantamine, Rivastigmine and Memantine (Review): Final Appraisal Determination.
140. Flight, M. H. 2013. Trial watch: Phase II boost for glutamate-targeted antidepressants. *Nat. Rev. Drug Discov.* 12(12):897.

141. Vécsei, L., L. Szalárdy, F. Fülöp, J. Toldi. 2012. Kynurenines in the CNS: Recent advances and new questions. *Nat. Rev. Drug Discov.* 12(1):64–82.
142. Wijesinghe, R. 2014. Emerging therapies for treatment resistant depression. *Ment. Health Clin.* 4(5):56.
143. Lisman, J. E., J. T. Coyle, R. W. Green, D. C. Javitt, F. M. Benes, S. Heckers, A. A. Grace. 2008. Circuit-based framework for understanding neurotransmitter and risk gene interactions in schizophrenia. *Trends Neurosci.* 31(5):234–242.
144. Pall, M. L. 2013. The NO/ONOO-cycle as the central cause of heart failure. *Int. J. Mol. Sci.* 14(11):22274–22330.
145. Li, G., C. Luna, P. B. Liton, I. Navarro, D. L. Epstein, P. Gonzalez. 2007. Sustained stress response after oxidative stress in trabecular meshwork cells. *Mol. Vis.* 13:2282–2288.
146. Pall, M. L. 2014. Is open-angle glaucoma caused by the NO/ONOO(-) cycle acting at two locations in the eye? *Med. Hypothesis Discov. Innov. Ophthalmol.* 3(1):1–2.
147. Seki, M., S. A. Lipton. 2008. Targeting excitotoxic/free radical signaling pathways for therapeutic intervention in glaucoma. *Prog. Brain Res.* 173:495–510.
148. Almasieh, M., A. M. Wilson, B. Morquette, J. L. Cueva Vargas, A. Di Polo. 2014. The molecular basis of retinal ganglion cell death in glaucoma. *Prog. Retin. Eye Res.* 31(2):152–181.
149. Aslan, M., A. Cort, I. Yucel. 2008. Oxidative and nitrative stress markers in glaucoma. *Free Radic. Biol. Med.* 45(4):367–376.
150. Zecca, L., M. B. Youdim, P. Riederer, J. R. Connor, R. R. Crichton. 2004. Iron, brain ageing and neurodegenerative disorders. *Nat. Rev. Neurosci.* 5(11):863–873.
151. Ke, Y., Z. M. Qian. 2007. Brain iron metabolism: Neurobiology and neurochemistry. *Prog. Neurobiol.* 83(3):149–173.
152. Rouault, T. A. 2013. Iron metabolism in the CNS: Implications for neurodegenerative diseases. *Nat. Rev. Neurosci.* 14(8):551–564.
153. Dusek, P., J. Jankovic, W. Le. 2012. Iron dysregulation in movement disorders. *Neurobiol. Dis.* 46(1):1–18.
154. Dringen, R., G. M. Bishop, M. Koeppe, T. N. Dang, S. R. Robinson. 2007. The pivotal role of astrocytes in the metabolism of iron in the brain. *Neurochem. Res.* 32(11):1884–1890.
155. Sian-Hulsmann, J., S. Mandel, M. B. Youdim, P. Riederer. 2011. The relevance of iron in the pathogenesis of Parkinson's disease. *J. Neurochem.* 118(6):949–957.
156. Matsuzaki, M., T. Hasegawa, A. Takeda, A. Kikuchi, K. Furukawa, Y. Kato, Y. Itoyama. 2004. Histochemical features of stress-induced aggregates in alpha-synuclein overexpressing cells. *Brain Res.* 1004(1–2):83–90.
157. Yamamoto, A., R. W. Shin, K. Hasegawa, H. Naiki, Hiroyoki Sato, F. Yoshimsau, T. Kitamoto. 2002. Iron (III) induces aggregation of hyperphosphorylated τ and its reduction to iron (II) reverses the aggregation: Implications in the formation of neurofibrillary tangles of Alzheimer's disease. *J. Neurochem.* 82(5):1137–1147.
158. Mantyh, P. W., J. R. Ghilardi, S. Rogers, E. DeMaster, C. J. Allen, E. R. Stimson, J. E. Maggio. 1993. Aluminum, iron, and zinc ions promote aggregation of physiological concentrations of beta-amyloid peptide. *J. Neurochem.* 61(3):1171–1174.
159. de Lau, L. M., M. M. Breteler. 2006. Epidemiology of Parkinson's disease. *Lancet Neurol.* 5(6):525–535.
160. Kazantsev, A. G., A. M. Kolchinsky. 2008. Central role of alpha-synuclein oligomers in neurodegeneration in Parkinson disease. *Arch. Neurol.* 65(12):1577–1581.
161. Rhodes, S. L., B. Ritz. 2008. Genetics of iron regulation and the possible role of iron in Parkinson's disease. *Neurobiol. Dis.* 32(2):183–195.
162. Salazar, J. et al. 2008. Divalent metal transporter 1 (DMT1) contributes to neurodegeneration in animal models of Parkinson's disease. *Proc. Natl. Acad. Sci. U.S.A.* 105(47):18578–18583.
163. Martin, W. R., M. Wieler, M. Gee. 2008. Midbrain iron content in early Parkinson disease: A potential biomarker of disease status. *Neurology* 70(16 Oart 2):1411–1417.
164. Bartzokis, G., J. L. Cummings, C. H. Markham, P. Z. Marmarelis, L. J. Treciokas, T. A. Tishler, S. R. Marder, J. Mintz. 1999. MRI evaluation of brain iron in earlier- and later-onset Parkinson's disease and normal subjects. *Magn. Reson. Imaging* 17(2):213–222.
165. Cuajungco, M. P., K. Y. Faget, X. Huang, R. E. Tanzi, A. I. Bush. 2000. Metal chelation as a potential therapy for Alzheimer's disease. *Ann. N.Y. Acad. Sci.* 920:292–304.
166. Mounsey, R. B., P. Teismann. 2012. Chelators in the treatment of iron accumulation in Parkinson's disease. *Int. J. Cell. Biol.* 2012:983245.
167. Wang, Q., F. Du, Z. M. Qian, X. H. Ge, L. Zhu, W. H. Yung, L. Yang, Y. Ke. 2008. Lipopolysaccharide induces a significant increase in expression of iron regulatory hormone hepcidin in the cortex and substantia nigra in rat brain. *Endocrinology* 149(8):3920–3925.

168. Du, F., Z. M. Qian, Q., Gong, Z. J. Zhu, L. Lu, Y. Ke. 2012. The iron regulatory hormone hepcidin inhibits expression of iron release as well as iron uptake proteins in J774 cells. *J. Nutr. Biochem.* 23(12):1694–1700.

169. Du, F., C. Qian, Z. M. Qian, X. M. Wu, H. Xie, W. H. Yung, Y. Ke. 2011. Hepcidin directly inhibits transferrin receptor 1 expression in astrocytes via a cyclic AMP-protein kinase a pathway. *Glia* 59(6):936–945.

170. Naya, F. J., B. Mercer, J. Shelton, J. A. Richardson, R. S. Williams, E. N. Olson. 2000. Stimulation of slow skeletal muscle fiber gene expression by calcineurin *in vivo. J. Biol. Chem.* 275(7):4545–4548.

171. Parsons, S. A., B. J. Wilkins, O. F. Bueno, J. D. Molkentin. 2003. Altered skeletal muscle phenotypes in calcineurin Aalpha and Abeta gene-targeted mice. *Mol. Cell Biol.* 23(12):4331–4343.

172. Bassel-Duby, R., E. N. Olson. 2006. Signaling pathways in skeletal muscle remodeling. *Annu. Rev. Biochem.* 75:19–37.

173. Wu, H., S. B. Kanatous, F. A. Thurmond, T. Gallardo, E. Isotani, R. Bassel-Duby, R. S. Williams. 2002. Regulation of mitochondrial biogenesis in skeletal muscle by CaMK. *Science* 296(5566):349–352.

174. Kramerova, I., E. Kudryashova, N. Ermolova, A. Saenz, O. Jaka, A. López de Munain, M. J. Spencer. 2012. Impaired calcium calmodulin kinase signaling and muscle adaptation response in the absence of calpain 3. *Hum. Mol. Genet.* 21(14):3193–3204.

175. Chen, H., M. Vermulst, Y. E. Wang, A. Chomyn, T. A. Prolla, J. M. McCaffery, D. C. Chan. 2010. Mitochondrial fusion is required for mtDNA stability in skeletal muscle and tolerance of mtDNA mutations. *Cell* 141(2):280–289.

176. Mizushima, N., M. Komatsu. 2011. Autophagy: Renovation of cells and tissues. *Cell* 147(4):728–741.

177. Grumati, P., L. Coletto, A. Schiavinato, S. Castagnaro, E. Bertaggia, M. Sandri, P. Bonaldo. 2011. Physical exercise stimulates autophagy in normal skeletal muscles but is detrimental for collagen VI-deficient muscles. *Autophagy* 7(12):1415–1423.

178. He, C. et al. 2012. Exercise-induced BCL2-regulated autophagy is required for muscle glucose homeostasis. *Nature* 481(7382):511–515.

179. He, C., R. Sumpter Jr., B. Levine. 2012. Exercise induces autophagy in peripheral tissues and in the brain. *Autophagy* 8:1548–1551.

180. Wu, J. et al. 2011. The unfolded protein response mediates adaptation to exercise in skeletal muscle through a PGC-1α/ATF6α complex. *Cell Metab.* 13(2):160–169.

181. Zwetsloot, K. A., L. M. Westerkamp, B. F. Holmes, T. P. Gavin. 2008. AMPK regulates basal skeletal muscle capillarization and VEGF expression, but is not necessary for the angiogenic response to exercise. *J. Physiol.* 586(24):6021–6035.

182. Mason, S. D. et al. 2004. Loss of skeletal muscle HIF-1alpha results in altered exercise endurance. *PLoS Biol.* 2(10):e288.

183. Chinsomboon, J., J. Ruas, R. K. Gupta, R. Thom, J. Shoag, G. C. Rowe, N. Sawada, S. Raghuram, Z. Arany. 2009. The transcriptional coactivator PGC-1alpha mediates exercise-induced angiogenesis in skeletal muscle. *Proc. Natl. Acad. Sci. U.S.A.* 106:21401–21406.

184. Rowe, G. C., R. El-Khoury, I. S. Patten, P. Rustin, Z. Arany. 2012. PGC-1α is dispensable for exercise-induced mitochondrial biogenesis in skeletal muscle. *PLoS One* 7:e41817.

185. Leick, L., J. F. Wojtaszewski, S. T. Johansen, K. Kiilerich, G. Comes, Y. Hellsten, J. Hidalgo, H. Pilegaard. 2008. PGC-1alpha is not mandatory for exercise- and training-induced adaptive gene responses in mouse skeletal muscle. *Am. J. Physiol. Endocrinol. Metab.* 294:E463–E474.

186. Arany, Z. et al. 2008. HIF-independent regulation of VEGF and angiogenesis by the transcriptional coactivator PGC-1alpha. *Nature* 451:1008–1012.

187. Pedersen, B. K., M. A. Febbraio. 2012. Muscles, exercise and obesity: Skeletal muscle as a secretory organ. *Nat. Rev. Endocrinol.* 8:457–465.

188. Pedersen, B. K., M. A. Febbraio. 2008. Muscle as an endocrine organ: Focus on muscle-derived interleukin-6. *Physiol. Rev.* 88:1379–1406.

189. Carey, A. L. et al. 2006. Interleukin-6 increases insulin-stimulated glucose disposal in humans and glucose uptake and fatty acid oxidation *in vitro* via AMP-activated protein kinase. *Diabetes* 55:2688–2697.

190. Ellingsgaard, H. et al. 2011. Interleukin-6 enhances insulin secretion by increasing glucagon-like peptide-1 secretion from L cells and alpha cells. *Nat. Med.* 17:1481–1489.

191. Wallenius, V., K. Wallenius, B. Ahrén, M. Rudling, H. Carlsten, S. L. Dickson, C. Ohlsson, J. O. Jansson. 2002. Interleukin-6-deficient mice develop mature-onset obesity. *Nat. Med.* 8:75–79.

192. Abbas, T., E. Faivre, C. Hölscher. 2009. Impairment of synaptic plasticity and memory formation in GLP-1 receptor KO mice: Interaction between type 2 diabetes and Alzheimer's disease. *Behav. Brain Res.* 205:265–271.

193. Isacson, R., E. Nielsen, K. Dannaeus, G. Bertilsson, C. Patrone, O. Zachrisson, L. Wikström. 2011. The glucagon-like peptide 1 receptor agonist exendin-4 improves reference memory performance and decreases immobility in the forced swim test. *Eur. J. Pharmacol.* 650:249–255.

194. Quinn, L. S., B. G. Anderson, J. D. Conner, T. Wolden-Hanson. 2013. IL-15 overexpression promotes endurance, oxidative energy metabolism, and muscle PPARδ, SIRT1, PGC-1α, and PGC-1β expression in male mice. *Endocrinology* 154(1):232–245.

195. Pistilli, E. E. et al. 2011. Loss of IL-15 receptor α alters the endurance, fatigability, and metabolic characteristics of mouse fast skeletal muscles. *J. Clin. Invest.* 121:3120–3132.

196. Wolfe, F., H. A. Smythe, M. B. Yunus, R. M. Bennett, C. Bombardier, D. L. Goldenberg, P. Tugwell, S. M. Campbell, M. Abeles, P. Clark. 1990. The American College of Rheumatology 1990 criteria for the classification of fibromyalgia. Report of the Multicenter Criteria Committee. *Arthritis Rheum.* 33:160–172.

197. Gracely, R. H., F. Petzke, J. M. Wolf, D. J. Clauw. 2002. Functional magnetic resonance imaging evidence of augmented pain processing in fibromyalgia. *Arthritis Rheum.* 46:1333–1343.

198. Wood, P. B., J. C. Patterson 2nd, J. J. Sunderland, K. H. Tainter, M. F. Glabus, D. L. Lilien. 2006. Reduced presynaptic dopamine activity in fibromyalgia syndrome demonstrated with positron emission tomography: A pilot study. *J. Pain* 8:51–58.

199. Schmidt-Wilcke, T., E. Leinisch, A. Straube, N. Kampfe, B. Draganski, H. C. Diener, U. Bogdahn, A. May. 2005. Gray matter decrease in patients with chronic tension type headache. *Neurology* 65:1483–1486.

200. Schmidt-Wilcke, T., E. Leinisch, S. Gansbauer, B. Draganski, U. Bogdahn, J. Altmeppen, A. May. 2006. Affective components and intensity of pain correlate with structural differences in gray matter in chronic back pain patients. *Pain* 125(1–2):89–97.

201. Okada, T., M. Tanaka, H. Kuratsune, Y. Watanabe, N. Sadato. 2004. Mechanisms underlying fatigue: A voxel-based morphometric study of chronic fatigue syndrome. *BMC Neurol.* 4:14.

202. de Lange, F. P., J. S. Kalkman, G. Bleijenberg, P. Hagoort, J. W. van der Meer, I. Toni. 2005. Gray matter volume reduction in the chronic fatigue syndrome. *Neuroimage* 26:777–781.

203. Villarreal, G., D. A. Hamilton, H. Petropoulos, I. Driscoll, L. M. Rowland, J. A. Griego, P. W. Kodituwakku, B. L. Hart, R. Escalona, W. M. Brooks. 2002. Reduced hippocampal volume and total white matter volume in posttraumatic stress disorder. *Biol. Psychiatry* 52:119–125.

204. Corbo, V., M. H. Clement, J. L. Armony, J. C. Pruessner, A. Brunet. 2005. Size versus shape differences: Contrasting voxel-based and volumetric analyses of the anterior cingulate cortex in individuals with acute posttraumatic stress disorder. *Biol. Psychiatry* 58:119–124.

205. Chen, S., W. Xia, L. Li, J. Liu, Z. He, Z. Zhang, L. Yan, J. Zhang, D. Hu. 2006. Gray matter density reduction in the insula in fire survivors with posttraumatic stress disorder: A voxel-based morphometric study. *Psychiatry Res.* 146:65–72.

206. Resnick, S. M., D. L. Pham, M. A. Kraut, A. B. Zonderman, C. Davatzikos. 2003. Longitudinal magnetic resonance imaging studies of older adults: A shrinking brain. *J. Neurosci.* 23:3295–3301.

207. Erickson, K. I., S. J. Colcombe, N. Raz, D. L. Korol, P. Scalf, A. Webb, N. J. Cohen, E. McAuley, A. F. Kramer. 2005. Selective sparing of brain tissue in postmenopausal women receiving hormone replacement therapy. *Neurobiol. Aging* 26(8):1205–1213.

208. Herman, J. P., M. M. Ostrander, N. K. Mueller, H. Figueiredo. 2005. Limbic system mechanisms of stress regulation: Hypothalamo-pituitaryadrenocortical axis. *Prog. Neuropsychopharmacol. Biol. Psychiatry* 29:1201–1213.

209. Apkarian, A. V., M. C. Bushnell, R. D. Treede, J. K. Zubieta. 2005. Human brain mechanisms of pain perception and regulation in health and disease. *Eur. J. Pain* 9:463–484.

210. Park, D. C., J. M. Glass, M. Minear, L. J. Crofford. 2001. Cognitive function in fibromyalgia patients. *Arthritis Rheum.* 44:2125–2133.

211. Vera-Portocarrero, L. P., E. T. Zhang, M. H. Ossipov, J. Y. Xie, T. King, J. Lai, F. Porreca. 2006. Descending facilitation from the rostral ventromedial medulla maintains nerve injury-induced central sensitization. *Neuroscience* 140(4):1311–1320.

212. King, T., C. Qu, A. Okun, R. Mercado, J. Ren, T. Brion, J. Lai, F. Porreca. 2011. Contribution of afferent pathways to nerve injury-induced spontaneous pain and evoked hypersensitivity. *Pain* 152(9): 1997–2005.

213. National Institute of Neurological Disorders and Stroke. Restless leg syndrome fact sheet. http://www.ninds.nih.gov/disorders/restless_legs/detail_restless_legs.htm. Accessed February 23, 2014.

214. Moore, R. A., P. J. Evans, R. F. Smith, J. W. Lloyd. 1983. Increased cortisol excretion in chronic pain. *Anaesthesia* 38(8):788–791.

215. Strittamatter, M., O. Bianchi, D. Ostertag, M. Grauer, C. Paulus, C. Fischer, S. Meyer. 2005. Altered function of the hypothalamic-pituitary-adrenal axis in patients with acute, chronic and episodic pain. *Schmerz* 19(2):109–116.

216. Tennant, F., L. Hermann. 2002. Normalization of serum cortisol concentration with opioid treatment of severe chronic pain. *Pain Med.* 3(2):132–134.

217. Higgins, N., J. Pickard, A. Lever. 2013. Lumbar puncture, chronic fatigue syndrome and idiopathic intracranial hypertension: A cross-sectional study. *JRSM Short Rep.* 4(12). doi: 10.1177/2042533313507920.

218. Alperin, N., S. Ranganathan, A. M. Bagci, D. J. Adams, B. Ertl-Wagner, E. Saraf-Lavi, E. M. Sklar, B. L. Lam. 2012. MRI evidence of impaired CSF homeostasis in obesity-associated idiopathic intracranial hypertension. *AJNR Am. J. Neuroradiol.* 34(1):29–34.

219. Rossignol, D. A., S. J. Genuis, R. E. Frye. 2014. Environmental toxicants and autism spectrum disorders: A systematic review. *Transl. Psychiatry* 4(2):e360.

220. Boor, B. E., H. Järnström, A. Novoselac, Y. Xu. 2014. Infant exposure to emissions of volatile organic compounds from crib mattresses. *Environ. Sci. Technol.* 48(6):3541–3549.

221. Hess, G. 2016. Texas Plant Agrees To Cut Air Pollution. CEN RSS. 2014. Web. January 11, 2016. http://cen.acs.org/articles/92/i13/Texas-Plant-Agrees-Cut-Air.html

222. Lawlor, J., S. McMillan. 2016. Maine Study Shows Possible Link between Arsenic in Drinking Water and Intelligence—Central Maine. 2014. Web. January 11, 2016. http://www.centralmaine.com/2014/04/02/maine_study_shows_possible_link_between_arsenic_in_drinking_water_and_intelligence_/

223. Alobid, I., S. Nogué, A. Izquierdo-Dominguez, S. Centellas, M. Bernal-Sprekelsen, J. Mullol. 2014. Multiple chemical sensitivity worsens quality of life and cognitive and sensorial features of sense of smell. *Eur. Arch. Otorhinolaryngol.* 271(12):3203–3208.

224. Azuma, K., I. Uchiyama, H. Takano, M. Tanigawa, M. Azuma, I. Bamba, T. Yoshikawa. 2013. Changes in cerebral blood flow during olfactory stimulation in patients with multiple chemical sensitivity: A multi-channel near-infrared spectroscopic study. *PLoS One* 8(11):e80567. doi: 10.1371/journal.pone.0080567.

225. Ye, F., W. T. Piver, M. Ando, C. J. Portier. 2001. Effects of temperature and air pollutant son cardiovascular and respiratory diseases for males and females older than 65 years of age in Toyko, July and August 1980–1995. *Environ. Health Perspect.* 109:355–359.

226. Chen, Y., Q. Yang, D. Krewski, Y. Shi, R. T. Burnett, K. Mc Frail. 2004. Influence of relatively low level particulate air pollution and hospitalization for COPD in elderly people. *Inhal. Toxicol.* 16:21–25.

227. Moolgavkar, S. H., E. G. Luebeck, E. L. Anderson. 1997. Air pollution and hospital admissions for respiratory causes in Minneapolis–St. Paul and Birmingham. *Epidemiology* 8:364–370.

228. McConnell, R., K. Berhane, F. Gillihand, J. Molitor, D. Thomas, F. Lurmann, E. Avol, W. J. Gauderman, J. M. Peters. 2003. Prospective study of air pollution and bronchitic symptoms in children with asthma. *Am. J. Respir. Crit. Care Med.* 168(7):790–797.

229. Peel, J., T. Paige, M. Klein, K. B. Metzger, W. D. Flanders, K. Todd, J. A. Mulholland, P. B. Ryan, H. Frumkin. 2005. Ambient air pollution and respiratory emergency department visits. *Epidemiology* 16:164–174.

230. Barnett, A. G., G. M. Williams, J. Schwartz, A. H. Neller, T. L. Best, A. L. Petroeschevsky, R. W. Simpson. 2005. Air pollution and child respiratory health: A case-crossover study in Australia and New Zealand. *Am. J. Respir. Crit. Care Med.* 171:1272–1278.

231. Silkoff, P. E., L. Zhang, S. Dutton, E. L. Langmack, S. Vedal, J. Murphy, B. Make. 2005. Winter air pollution and disease parameters in advanced chronic obstructive pulmonary disease panels residing in Denver, Colorado. *J. Allergy Clin. Immunol.* 115:337–344.

232. Romieu, I., F. Meneses, S. Ruiz, J. Huerta, J. J. Sienra, M. White, R. Etzel, M. Hernandez. 1997. Effects of intermittent ozone exposure on peak expiratory flow and respiratory symptoms among asthmatic children in Mexico City. *Arch. Environ. Health* 52:368–376.

233. Zemp, E. et al. 1999. Long-term ambient air pollution and respiratory symptoms in adults (SAPALDIA study). The SAPALDIA Team. *Am. J. Respir. Crit. Care Med.* 159(4 pt 1):1257–1266.

234. Ilbaca, M., I. Olaeta, E. Campos, J. Villaire, M. M. Tellez-Rojo, I. Romieu. 1999. Association between levels of fine particulates and emergency visits for pneumonia and other respiratory illnesses among children in Santiago, Chile. *J. Air Waste Manage. Assoc.* 49:154–163.

235. Frischer, T., M. Studnicka, C. Gartner, E. Tauber, F. Horak, A. Veiter, J. Spengler, J. Kühr, R. Urbanek. 1999. Lung function growth and ambient ozone: A three-year population study in school children. *Am. J. Respir. Crit. Care Med.* 160:390–396.

236. Gauderman, W. J. et al. 2002. Association between air pollution and lung function growth in southern California children: Results from a second cohort. *Am. J. Respir. Crit. Care Med.* 166(1):76–84.

237. Buchdahl, R., C. D. Willems, M. Vander, A. Babiker. 2000. Associations between ambient ozone, hydrocarbons, and childhood wheezy episodes: A prospective observational study in south east London. *Occup. Environ. Med.* 57:86–93.

238. Lee, J. T., H. Kim, H. Song, Y. C. Hong, Y. S. Cho, S. Y. Shin, Y. J. Hyun, Y. S. Kim. 2002. Air pollution and asthma among children in Seoul, Korea. *Epidemiology* 13:481–484.

239. Lin, M., Y. Chen, R. T. Burnett, P. J. Villeneuve, D. Krewski. 2002. The influence of ambient coarse particulate matter on asthma hospitalization in children: Case-crossover and time-series analysis. *Environ. Health Perspect.* 110:578–581.

240. Linaker, C. H., D. Coggon, S. T. Holgate, J. Clough, L. Josephs, A. J. Chauhan, H. M. Inskip. 2000. Personal exposure to nitrogen dioxide and risk of airflow obstruction in asthmatic children with upper respiratory infection. *Thorax* 55:930–933.

241. Thompson, A. J., M. D. Shields, C. C. Patterson. 2001. Acute asthma exacerbations and air pollutants in children living in Belfast, Northern Ireland. *Arch. Environ. Health* 56(3):234–241.

242. Tolbert, P. E. et al. 2000. Air quality and pediatric emergency room visits for asthma in Atlanta, Georgia, USA. *Am. J. Epidemiol.* 151(8):798–810.

243. White, M. C., R. A. Etzel, W. D. Wilcox, C. Lloyd. 1994. Exacerbations of childhood asthma and ozone pollution in Atlanta. *Environ. Res.* 65:56–68.

244. Wong, G. W., F. W. Ko, T. S. Lau, S. T. Li, D. Hui, S. W. Pang, R. Leung, T. F. Fok, C. K. Lai. 2001. Temporal relationship between air pollution and hospital admissions for asthmatic children in Hong Kong. *Clin. Exp. Allergy* 31:565–569.

245. Yu, O., C. Sheppard, T. Lumley, J. Q. Koenig, G. G. Shapiro. 2000. Effects of ambient air pollution on symptoms of asthma in Seattle-area children enrolled in the CAMP study. *Environ. Health Perspect.* 106:1209–1214.

246. Pino, P., T. Walter, M. Oyarzun, R. Villegas, I. Romieu. 2004. Fine particulate matter and wheezing illnesses in the first year of life. *Epidemiology* 15:702–708.

247. Freidman, M. S., K. E. Powell, L. Hutwanger, L. M. Graham, W. G. Teague. 2001. Impact of changes in transportation and commuting during the 1996 Summer Olympic Games in Atlanta on air quality and childhood asthma. *JAMA* 285(7):897–905.

248. Penard-Morand, C., D. Charpin, C. Raherison, C. Kopferschmitt, D. Callaud, F. Lavaud, I. Annesi-Maesano. 2005. Long-term exposure to background air pollution related to respiratory and allergic health in schoolchildren. *Clin. Exp. Allergy* 35:1279–1287.

249. Su, M. W., C. H. Tsai, K. Y. Tung, B. F. Hwang, P. H. Liang, B. L. Chiang, Y. H. Yang, Y. L. Lee. 2013. GSTP1 is a hub gene for gene-air pollution interactions on childhood asthma. *Allergy* 68(12):1614–1617.

250. Nishimura, K. K. et al. 2013. Early-life air pollution and asthma risk in minority children. The GALA II and SAGE II studies. *Am. J. Respir. Crit. Care Med.* 188(3):309–318.

251. Zhou, C., N. Baïz, T. Zhang, S. Banerjee, I. Annesi-Maesano. 2013. Modifiable exposures to air pollutants related to asthma phenotypes in the first year of life in children of the EDEN mother-child cohort study. *BMC Public Health* 13:506.

252. Delfino, R. J. 2002. Epidemiological evidence for asthma and exposure to air toxics: Linkages between occupational, indoor and community air pollution research. *Environ. Health Perspect.* 110(Suppl. 4):573–589.

253. Goren, A., J. R. Goldssmith, S. Hellman, S. Brenner. 1991. Follow-up of schoolchildren in the vicinity of a coal-fired power plant in Israel. *Environ. Health Perspect.* 94:101–105.

254. Haahtela, T., O. Mattila, V. Vikka, P. Jappinen, J. J. Jaakkola. 1992. The South Karelia Air Pollution Study: Acute health effects of malodorous sulfur air pollutants released by a pulp mill. *Am. J. Public Health* 82:603–605.

255. Pope, C. A. 1989. Respiratory diseases associated with community air pollution and a steel mill, Utah Valley. *Am. J. Public Health* 79:623–628.

256. Targonski, P., V. Persky, V. Ramakrishnan. 1995. Effect of environmental molds on risk of death from asthma during the pollen season. *J. Allergy Clin. Immunol.* 95:955–961.

257. Neas, L. M., D. W. Dockery, H. Burge, P. Koutrakis, F. E. Speizer. 1996. Fungus spores, air pollutants, and other determinants of peak expiratory flow rates in children. *Am. J. Epidemiol.* 143:797–807.

258. Delfino, R. J., R. S. Zeiger, J. M. Seltzer, D. H. Street, R. M. Matteucci, P. R. Anderson, P. Koutrakis. 1997. The effect of outdoor fungal spore concentrations on daily asthma severity. *Environ. Health Perspect.* 105:622–635.

259. Dales, R. E., S. Cakmak, S. Judek, T. Dann, F. Coates, J. R. Brook, R. T. Burnett. 2004. Influence of outdoor aeroallergens on hospitalization for asthma in Canada. *J. Allergy Clin. Immunol.* 113:303–306.

260. Lierl, M. B., R. W. Hornung. 2003. Relationship of outdoor air quality to pediatric asthma exacerbations. *Ann. Allergy Asthma Immun.* 90:28–33.

261. Dales, R. E., S. Cakmak, S. Judek, T. Dann, F. Coates, J. R. Brook, R. T. Burnett. 2003. The role of fungal spores in thunderstorm asthma. *Chest* 123:745–750.

262. Rosas, I., H. A. McCartney, R. W. Payne, C. Calderon, J. Lacey, R. Chapela, S. Ruiz-Velazco. 1998. Analysis of relationships between environmental factors and asthma emergency admissions to a hospital in Mexico City. *Allergy* 53:394–401.

263. Burge, H., C. A. Rogers. 2000. Outdoor allergens. *Environ. Health Perspect.* 108(Suppl. 4):653–659.

264. Janssen, N. A., B. Brunekreef, P. Van Vliet, F. Aarts, K. Meliefste, H. Hars, P. Fischer. 2003. The relationship between air pollution from heavy traffic and allergic sensitization, bronchial hyper-responsiveness, and respiratory symptoms in Dutch schoolchildren. *Environ. Health Perspect.* 111:1512–1518.

265. Wyler, C., C. Braun-Fahrlander, N. Kunzli, C. Schindler, U. Ackermann-Liebrich, A. P. Perruchoud, P. Leuenberger, B. Wüthrich. 2001. Exposure to motor vehicle traffic and allergic sensitization: The Swiss study on air pollution and lung diseases in adults (SAPALDIA) team. *Epidemiology* 11(4): 450–456.

266. Molfino, N. A., S. C. Wright, I. Katz, S. Tario, F. Silverman, P. A. McClean, J. P. Szalai, M. Raizenne, A. S. Slutsky, N. Zamel. 1991. Effect of low concentrations of ozone on inhaled allergen responses in asthmatic subjects. *Lancet* 338:199–203.

267. Fleming, L. E. et al. 2005. Initial evaluation of aerosolized Florida red tide toxins (Brevetoxins) in personals with asthma. *Environ. Health Perspect.* 113:650–657.

268. Rodrigo, M. J., M. J. Cruz, M. D. Garcia, J. M. Anto, T. Genover, F. Morell. 2004. Epidemic asthma in Barcelona: An evaluation of new strategies for control of soybean dust emission. *Int. Arch. Allergy Immunol.* 134:158–164.

269. Miguel, A. G., G. R. Cass, J. Weiss, M. M. Glovsky. 1996. Latex allergens in tire dust and airborne particles. *Environ. Health Perspect.* 104:1180–1186.

270. Baur, X., Z. Chen, V. Liebers. 1998. Exposure-response relationship of occupational inhalative allergens. *Clin. Exp. Allergy* 28:537–544.

271. Torigoe, K., S. Hasegawa, O. Numata, S. Yazaki, M. Magtsunaga, N. Boku, M. Hiura, H. Ino. 2000. Influence of emission from rice straw burning on bronchial asthma in children. *Pediatr. Int.* 42:143–150.

272. Jacobs, J., R. Kreutzer, D. Smith. 1997. Rice burning and asthma hospitalizations, Butte County, California, 1983–1992. *Environ. Health Perspect.* 105:980–985.

273. Viswanathan, S., L. Eria, N. Diunugala, S. Johnson, C. McClean. 2006. An analysis of effects of San Diego wildfire on ambient air quality. *J. Air Waste Manage. Assoc.* 56:56–67.

274. Johnston, F. H., A. M. Kavanagh, D. M. Bowman, R. K. Scott. 2002. Exposure to brushfire smoke and asthma: An ecological study. *Med. J. Aust.* 176:535–538.

275. From, L. J., L. G. Bergen, C. J. Humlie. 1992. The effects of open leaf burning on spirometric measurements in asthma. *Chest* 101:1236–1239.

276. Koenig, J. Q., T. V. Larson, Q. S. Hanley, V. Reboliedo, K. Dumler, H. Checkoway, S. Z. Wang, D. Lin, W. E. Pierson. 1993. Pulmonary function changes in children associated with exposure to particulate matter. *Environ. Res.* 63:26–38.

277. Slaughter, J. C., T. Lumley, L. Sheppard, J. Q. Koenig, G. G. Shapiro. 2003. Effects of ambient air pollution on symptom severity and medication use in children with asthma. *Ann. Allergy Asthma Immunol.* 91:346–353.

278. Lipsett, M., S. Hurley, B. Ostro. 1997. Air pollution and emergency room visits for asthma in Santa Clara County, California. *Environ. Health Perspect.* 105:216–222.

279. Awang, M. B., A. F. Rahman, W. Z. Adullah, R. Lazer, M. T. Majid. 2000. Air quality in Malaysia: Impacts, management issues and future challenges. *Respirology* 5:183–196.

280. Korenyi-Both, A. L., A. L. Korenyi-Both, D. J. Juncer. 1997. Al Eskan disease: Persian Gulf syndrome. *Mil. Med.* 162:1–13.

281. Gyan, K., W. Henry, S. Lacaille, A. Laloo, C. Lamsee-Ebanks, R. McKay, R. M. Antoine, M. A. Monteil. 2005. African dust clouds are associated with increased pediatric asthma accident and emergency admission on the Caribbean island of Trinidad. *Int. J. Biometeorol.* 49:371–376.

282. Grattan, J. P., M. Brayshay, J. P. Sadler. 1998. Modeling the impacts of past volcanic gas emissions: Evidence of Europe-wide environmental impacts from gases emitted from the Italian and Icelandic volcanoes in 1783. *Quaternaire* 9:25–35.

283. Durand, M., C. Florkowski, P. George, T. Walmsley, P. Weinstein. 2005. Effects of volcanic gas exposure on urine, blood, and serum chemistry. *N. Z. Med. J.* 118(1210):U1319.

284. Durand, M., J. Grattan. 2001. Effects of volcanic air pollution and health. *Lancet* 357:164.

285. Choudhury, A., M. E. Gordon, S. S. Morris. 1997. Associations between respiratory illness and PM10 pollution. *Arch. Environ. Health* 52:113–117.

286. Ware, J. H., J. D. Spengler, L. M. Neas, J. M. Samer, G. R. Wagner, D. Couitas, H. Ozkaynak, M. Schwab. 1993. Respiratory and irritant health effects of ambient volatile organic compounds. The Kanawha county health study. *Am. J. Epidemiol.* 137:1287–1301.

287. Wing, J. S., J. D. Brender, L. M. Sanderson, D. M. Perrota, R. Beauchamp. 1991. Acute health effects in a community after a release of hydrofluoric acid. *Arch. Environ. Health* 46:155–160.

288. Joseph, P. M., M. G. Weiner. 2002. Visits to physicians after the oxygenation of gasoline in Philadelphia. *Arch. Environ. Health* 57:137–154.

289. Gordian, M. E., M. D. Huelsman, M. L. Brecht, D. G. Fisher. 1995. Health effects of methyl tertiary butyl ether (MTBE) in gasoline of Alaska. *Alaska Med.* 37:101–103.

290. O'Malley, M. A., S. Edmiston, D. Richmond, M. Ibarra, T. Barry, M. Smith. 2004. Illness associated with drift of chloropricin soil fumigant into a residential area—Kern County, California 2003. *MMWR Mort. Morb. Wkly. Rep.* 53(32):740–742.

291. Pearce, M., B. Habbick, J. Williams, M. Eastman, M. Newman. 2002. The effects of aerial spraying with Bacillus thuringiensis Kurstaki on children with asthma. *Can. J. Public Health* 93:21–25.

292. Young, R. C., R. E. Rachal, P. G. Carr, H. C. Press. 1992. Patterns of coal workers' pneumoconiosis in Appalachian former coal miners. *J. Natl. Med. Assoc.* 84(1):41–48.

293. Stansbury, R. C., L. F. Beeckman-Wagner, M. Wang, J. P. Hogg, E. L. Petsonk. 2013. Rapid decline in lung function in coal miners: Evidence of disease in small airways. *Am. J. Ind. Med.* 56(9):1107–1112.

294. Graber, J. M., L. T. Stayner, R. A. Cohen, L. M. Conroy, M. D. Attfield. 2013. Respiratory disease mortality among us coal miners; results after 37 years of follow-up. *Occup. Environ. Med.* 71(1):30–39.

295. Wang, X., D. C. Christiani. 2000. Respiratory symptoms and functional status in workers exposed to silica, asbestos, and coal mine dusts. *J. Occup. Environ. Med.* 42(11):1076–1084.

296. Langer, A. M., R. P. Nolan. 1998. Asbestos in the lungs of persons exposed in the USA. *Monaldi. Arch. Chest Dis.* 53(2):168–180.

297. Lippmann, M. 1994. Deposition and retention of inhaled fibres: Effects on incidence of lung cancer and mesothelioma. *Occup. Environ. Med.* 51(12):793–798.

298. Davis, J. M. 1989. Mineral fibre carcinogenesis: Experimental data relating to the importance of fibre type, size, deposition, dissolution and migration. *IARC Sci. Publ.* 90:33–45.

299. Falta, M. T. et al. 2013. Identification of beryllium-dependent peptides recognized by CD4+ T cells in chronic beryllium disease. *J. Exp. Med.* 210(7):1403–1418.

300. Bill, J. R., D. G. Mack, M. T. Falta, L. A. Maier, A. K. Sullivan, F. G. Joslin, A. K. Martin, B. M. Freed, B. L. Kotzin, A. P. Fontenot. 2005. Beryllium presentation to CD4 T cells is dependent on a single amino acid residue of the MHC class II beta-chain. *J. Immunol.* 175(10):7029–7037.

301. Maier, L. A. 2002. Genetic and exposure risks for chronic beryllium disease. *Clin. Chest Med.* 23(4):827–839.

302. Schuler, C. R., M. S. Kent, D. C. Deubner, M. T. Berakis, M. Mccawley, P. K. Henneberger, M. D. Rossman, K. Kreiss. 2005. Process-related risk of beryllium sensitization and disease in a copper-beryllium alloy facility. *Am. J. Ind. Med.* 47(3):195–205.

303. Henneberger, P. K., D. Cumro, D. D. Deubner, M. S. Kent, M. Mccawley, K. Kreiss. 2001. Beryllium sensitization and disease among long-term and short-term workers in a beryllium ceramics plant. *Int. Arch. Occup. Environ. Health* 74(3):167–176.

304. Fishwick, D., A. M. Fletcher, C. A. Pickering, R. M. Niven, E. B. Faragher. 1994. Ocular and nasal irritation in operatives in Lancashire cotton and synthetic fibre mills. *Occup. Environ. Med.* 51(11):744–748.

305. Zhang, R. et al. 2013. A large scale gene-centric association study of lung function in newly-hired female cotton textile workers with endotoxin exposure. *PLoS One* 8(3):e59035.

306. Kennedy, S. M., D. C. Christiani, E. A. Eisen, D. H. Wegman, I. A. Greaves, S. A. Olenchock, T. T. Ye, P. L. Lu. 1987. Cotton dust and endotoxin exposure-response relationships in cotton textile workers. *Am. Rev. Respir. Dis.* 135(1):194–200.

307. Robinson, J. T., S. M. Tabakman, Y. Liang, H. Wang, H. S. Casalongue, D. Vinh, H. Dai. 2011. Ultrasmall reduced graphene oxide with high near-infrared absorbance for photothermal therapy. *J. Am. Chem. Soc.* 133(17):6825–6831.

308. Sanchez, V. C., A. Jachak, R. H. Hurt, A. B. Kane. 2012. Biological interactions of graphene-family nanomaterials: An interdisciplinary review. *Chem. Res. Toxicol.* 25(1):15–34.

309. Marchiori, E., S. Lourenço, T. D. Gasparetto, G. Zanetti, C. M. Mano, L. F. Nobre. 2010. Pulmonary talcosis: Imaging findings. *Lung* 188(2):165–171.

310. Igbal, A., B. Aggarwal, B. Menon, R. Kulshreshtha. 2008. Talc granulomatosis mimicking sarcoidosis. *Singapore Med. J.* 49(7):e168–e170.

311. Yoshii, C., T. Matsuyama, A. Takazawa, T. Ito, K. Yatera, T. Hayashi, T. Imanaga, M. Kido. 2002. Welder's pneumoconiosis: Diagnostic usefulness of high-resolution computed tomography and ferritin determinations in bronchoalveolar lavage fluid. *Intern. Med.* 41(12):1111–1117.

312. McCunney, R. J. 2005. Asthma, genes, and air pollution. *J. Occup. Environ. Med.* 47:1285–1291.

313. Lee, Y. L., Y. C. Lin, Y. C. Lee, J. Y. Wang, T. R. Hsiue, Y. L. Guo. 2004. Gluthatione S-transferase P1 gene polymorphism and air pollution as interactive risk factors for childhood asthma. *Clin. Exp. Allergy* 34:1707–1713.

314. Romieu, I., J. J. Sinra-Monge, M. Ramirez-Aguilar. 2002. Antioxidant supplementation and lung function among children with asthma exposed to high levels of air pollutants. *Am. J. Respir. Crit. Care Med.* 166:703–709.

315. Trenga, C. A., J. Q. Koenig, P. V. Williams. 2001. Dietary antioxidants and ozone-induced bronchial hyperresponsiveness in adults with asthma. *Arch. Environ. Health* 56:242–249.

316. Cocco, P. L., P. Carta, S. Belli, G. F. Picchiri, M. V. Flore. 1994. Mortality of Sardinian lead and zinc miners: 1960-88. *Occup. Environ. Med.* 51(10):674–682.

317. Brook, R. D. et al. 2004. Air pollution and cardiovascular disease: A statement for healthcare professionals from the expert panel on population and prevention science of the American heart association. *Circulation* 109(21):2655–2671.

318. Raloff, J. 2012. Nanopollutants harm vessel health: Tiny particles and tubes diminish arteriole response in rats. *Science News* 181(8):18.

319. Petersen, J. W., C. J. Pepine. 2014. The prevalence of microvascular dysfunction, its role among men, and links with adverse outcomes: Noninvasive imaging reveals the tip of the iceberg. *Circulation* 129(24):2497–2499.

320. Laseter, J. L., R. D. Ildefonso, W. J. Rea, J. R. Butler. 1983. Chlorinated hydrocarbon pesticides in environmentally sensitive patients. *Clin. Ecol.* 2(1):3–12.

321. Formaldehyde Found in Building Materials. Global Health and Safety Initiative. 2008. Print.

322. Pan, Y., A. R. Johnson, W. J. Rea. 1987/88. Aliphatic hydrocarbon solvents in chemically sensitive patients. *Clin. Ecol.* 5(3):126–131.

323. Curtis, L., A. Lieberman, M. Stark, W. Rea, M. Vetter. 2004. Adverse health effects of indoor molds. *J. Nutr. Environ. Med.* 14(3):261–274.

324. Heavy Metal Poisoning and Safe Detoxification. Heavy Metal Poisoning Safe Detoxification. Web. January 13, 2016. http://www.evenbetterhealth.com/heavy-metal-poisoning.asp

325. Rea, W. J. 1977. Environmentally triggered small vessel vasculitis. *Ann. Allergy* 38:245–251.

326. von Ardenne, M. 1990. *Oxygen Multistep Therapy: Physiological and Technical Foundations.* W. Kruger. 65. New York: Georg Thieme Verlag Stuttgart.

327. Gibson, C. M. et al. 1996. TIMI frame count: A quantitative method of assessing coronary artery flow. *Circulation.* 93(5):879–888.

328. Manginas, A., P. Gatzov, C. Chasikidis, V. Voudris, G. Pavlides, D. V. Cokkinos. 1999. Estimation of coronary flow reserve using the Thrombolysis in Myocardial Infarction (TIMI) frame count method. *Am. J. Cardiol.* 83:1562–1565. A1567.

329. Petersen, J. W., B. D. Johnson, K. E. Kip, R. D. Anderson, E. M. Handberg, B. L. Sharaf, P. K. Mehta, S. F. Kelsey, C. N. Bairey Merz, C. J. Pepine. 2014. TIMI frame count and adverse events in women with no obstructive coronary disease: A pilot study from the NHLBI-sponsored Women's Ischemia Syndrome Evaluation (WISE). *PLoS One* 9(5):e96630.

330. Ong, P., A. Athanasiadis, G. Borgulya, H. Mahrholdt, J. C. Kaski, U. Sechtem. 2012. High prevalence of a pathological response to acetylcholine testing in patients with stable angina pectoris and unobstructed coronary arteries. The ACOVA Study (Abnormal COronary VAsomotion in patients with stable angina and unobstructed coronary arteries). *J. Am. Coll. Cardiol.* 59:655–662.

331. Jespersen, L., A. Hvelplund, S. Z. Abildstrøm, F. Pedersen, S. Galatius, J. K. Madsen, E. Jørgensen, H. Kelbæk, E. Prescott. 2012. Stable angina pectoris with no obstructive coronary artery disease is associated with increased risks of major adverse cardiovascular events. *Eur. Heart J.* 33:734–744.

332. Shaw, L. J. et al. 2006. The economic burden of angina in women with suspected ischemic heart disease: Results from the National Institutes of Health—National Heart, Lung, and Blood Institute—sponsored Women's Ischemia Syndrome Evaluation. *Circulation* 114:894–904.

333. D'Ippoliti, D., F. Forastiere, C. Ancona, N. Agabiti, D. Fusco, P. Michelozzi, C. A. Perucci. 2003. Air pollution and myocardial infarction in Rome: A case-crossover analysis. *Epidemiology* 14(5):528–535.

334. Peters, A., D. W. Dockery, J. F. Miller, M. A. Mittelman. 2001. Increased particular matter and the triggering of myocardial infarction. *Circulation* 103(23):2810–2815.

335. Ruidavets, J. B., M. Cournot, S. Cassadou, M. Giroux, M. Meybeck, J. Ferrieres. 2005. Ozone air pollution is associated with acute myocardial infarction. *Circulation* 111:563–569.

336. Chen, L. H., S. F. Knutsen, D. Shavlik, W. L. Beeson, F. Petersen, M. Ghamsary, D. Abbey. 2005. The association between fatal coronary heart disease and ambient particulate air pollution: Are females at greater risk? *Environ. Health Perspect.* 113:1723–1729.

337. Metzger, K. B., P. E. Tolbert, M. Klein, J. L. Peel, W. D. Flanders, K. Todd, J. A. Mulholland, P. B. Ryan, H. Frumkin. 2004. Ambient air pollution and cardiovascular emergency room visits. *Epidemiology* 15(1):46–56.

338. Zanobetti, A., J. Schwartz, D. Dockery. 2000. Airborne particles are a risk factor for hospital admissions for heart and lung disease. *Environ. Health Perspect.* 108(11):1071–1077.

339. Pantazopolou, A., K. Katsouyanni, J. Kourea-Kremastinou, D. Trichopoulous. 1995. Short-term effects of air pollution on hospital emergency outpatient visits and admissions in the greater Athens, Greece area. *Environ. Res.* 69:31–36.

340. Yang, C. Y., Y. S. Chen, C. H. Yang, S. C. Ho. 2004. Relationship between ambient air pollution and hospitalization for cardiovascular diseases in Kaohsiung, Taiwan. *J. Toxicol. Environ. Health A* 67:483–493.

341. Morris, R., E. N. Naumova, R. L. Mungjinshe. 1995. Ambient air pollution and hospitalization for congestive heart failure among elderly people in 7 large US cities. *Am. J. Public Health* 85:1361–1365.

342. Reis, S. E., R. Holubkov, A. J. Conrad Smith, S. F. Kelsey, B. L. Sharaf, N. Reichek, W. J. Rogers, C. N. Merz, G. Sopko, C. G. Pepine; WISE Investigators. 2001. Coronary microvascular dysfunction is highly prevalent in women with chest pain in the absence of coronary artery disease: Results from the NHLBI WISE study. *Am. Heart J.* 141:735–741.

343. Halcox, J. P., W. H. Schenke, G. Zalos, R. Mincemoyer, A. Prasad, M. A. Waclawiw, K. R. Nour, A. A. Quyyumi. 2002. Prognostic value of coronary vascular endothelial dysfunction. *Circulation* 106:653–658.

344. Pepine, C. J., R. D. Anderson, B. L. Sharaf, S. E. Reis, K. M. Smith, E. M. Handberg, B. D. Johnson, G. Sopko, C. N. Bairey Merz. 2010. Coronary microvascular reactivity to adenosine predicts adverse outcome in women evaluated for suspected ischemia: Results from the National Heart, Lung and Blood Institute WISE (Women's Ischemia Syndrome Evaluation) study. *J. Am. Coll. Cardiol.* 55:2825–2832.

345. von Mering, G. O. et al. 2004. National Heart, Lung, and Blood Institute. Abnormal coronary vasomotion as a prognostic indicator of cardiovascular events in women: Results from the National Heart, Lung, and Blood Institute-Sponsored Women's Ischemia Syndrome Evaluation (WISE). *Circulation* 109:722–725.

346. Randolph, T. G. 1961. Human ecology and susceptibility to the chemical environment. *Ann. Allergy* 19:518–540.

347. Verna, E., L. Ceriani, L. Giovanella, G. Binaghi, S. Garancini. 2000. "False-positive" myocardial perfusion scintigraphy findings in patients with angiographically normal coronary arteries: Insights from intravascular sonography studies. *J. Nucl. Med.* 41:1935–1940.

348. Murthy, V. L. et al. 2000. Effects of sex on coronary microvascular dysfunction and cardiac outcomes. *Circulation* 129(24):2518–2527.

349. Maseri, A., R. Mimmo, S. Chierchia, C. Marchesi, A. Pesola, A. L'Abbate. 1975. Coronary artery spasm as a cause of acute myocardial ischemia in man. *Chest* 68(5):625–633.

350. Paulus, W. J., C. Tschöpe. 2013. A novel paradigm for heart failure with preserved ejection fraction: Comorbidities drive myocardial dysfunction and remodeling through coronary microvascular endothelial inflammation. *J. Am. Coll. Cardiol.* 62:263–271.

351. Yoshida, K., N. Mullani, K. L. Gould. 1996. Coronary flow and flow reserve by PET simplified for clinical applications using rubidium-82 or nitrogen-13-ammonia. *J. Nucl. Med.* 37:1701–1712.

352. Dekemp, R. A. et al. 2013. Multisoftware reproducibility study of stress and rest myocardial blood flow assessed with 3D dynamic PET/CT and a 1-tissue-compartment model of 82Rb kinetics. *J. Nucl. Med.* 54:571–577.

353. Petersen, J. W. et al. 2014. Comparison of low and high dose intracoronary adenosine and acetylcholine in women undergoing coronary reactivity testing: Results from the NHLBI-sponsored Women's Ischemia Syndrome Evaluation (WISE). *Int. J. Cardiol.* 172:e114–e115.

354. Dimitrow, P. P. 2003. Transthoracic Doppler echocardiography—Noninvasive diagnostic window for coronary flow reserve assessment. *Cardiovasc. Ultrasound* 1:4.

355. Caiati, C., C. Montaldo, N. Zedda, R. Montisci, M. Ruscazio, G. Lai, M. Cadeddu, L. Meloni, S. Iliceto. 1999. Validation of a new noninvasive method (contrast-enhanced transthoracic second harmonic echo Doppler) for the evaluation of coronary flow reserve: Comparison with intracoronary Doppler flow wire. *J. Am. Coll. Cardiol.* 34:1193–1200.

356. Mulligan-Kehoe, M. J., M. Simons. 2014. Vasa vasorum in normal and diseased arteries. *Circulation* 129(24):2557–2566.
357. Okuyama, K., G. Yagimuna, T. Takahashi, H. Sasaki, S. Mori. 1988. The development of vasa vasorum of the human aorta in various conditions. A morphometric study. *Arch. Pathol. Lab. Med.* 112:721–725.
358. Zamir, M., M. D. Silver. 1985. Vasculature in the walls of human coronary arteries. *Arch. Pathol. Lab. Med.* 109:659–662.
359. Heistad, D. D., M. L. Marcus. 1979. Role of vasa vasorum in nourishment of the aorta. *Blood Vessels* 16:225–238.
360. Galkina, E., A. Kadl, J. Sanders, D. Varughese, I. J. Sarembock, K. Ley. 2006. Lymphocyte recruitment into the aortic wall before and during development of atherosclerosis is partially L-selectin dependent. *J. Exp. Med.* 203:1273–1282.
361. Houtkamp, M. A., O. J. de Boer, C. M. van der Loos, A. C. van der Wal, A. E. Becker. 2001. Adventitial infiltrates associated with advanced atherosclerotic plaques: Structural organization suggests generation of local humoral immune responses. *J. Pathol.* 193:263–269.
362. Hu, Y., Z. Zhang, E. Torsney, A. R. Afzal, F. Davison, B. Metzler, Q. Xu. 2004. Abundant progenitor cells in the adventitia contribute to atherosclerosis of vein grafts in ApoE-deficient mice. *J. Clin. Invest.* 113:1258–1265.
363. Passman, J. N., X. R. Dong, S. P. Wu, C. T. Maguire, K. A. Hogan, V. L. Bautch, M. W. Majesky. 2008. A sonic hedgehog signaling domain in the arterial adventitia supports resident Sca1+ smooth muscle progenitor cells. *Proc. Natl. Acad. Sci. U.S.A.* 105:9349–9354.
364. Stenmark, K. R., M. E. Yeager, K. C. El Kasmi, E. Nozik-Grayck, E. V. Gerasimovskaya, M. Li, S. R. Riddle, M. G. Frid. 2013. The adventitia: Essential regulator of vascular wall structure and function. *Annu. Rev. Physiol.* 75:23–47.
365. Gingras, M., P. Farand, M. E. Safar, G. E. Plante. 2009. Adventitia: The vital wall of conduit arteries. *J. Am. Soc. Hypertens.* 3:166–183.
366. Sacchi, G., E. Weber, L. Comparini. 1990. Histological framework of lymphatic vasa vasorum of major arteries: An experimental study. *Lymphology* 23:135–139.
367. Baldwin, A. L., L. M. Wilson, I. Gradus-Pizlo, R. Wilensky, K. March. 1997. Effect of atherosclerosis on transmural convection an arterial ultrastructure: Implications for local intravascular drug delivery. *Arterioscler. Thromb. Vasc. Biol.* 17:3365–3375.
368. Gössl, M., N. M. Malyar, M. Rosol, P. E. Beighley, E. L. Ritman. 2003. Impact of coronary vasa vasorum functional structure on coronary vessel wall perfusion distribution. *Am. J. Physiol. Heart Circ. Physiol.* 285:H2019–H2026.
369. Hwang, C. W., D. Wu, E. R. Edelman. 2003. Impact of transport and drug properties on the local pharmacology of drug-eluting stents. *Int. J. Cardiovasc. Intervent.* 5:7–12.
370. Michel, J. B., O. Thaunat, X. Houard, O. Meilhac, G. Caligiuri, A. Nicoletti. 2007. Topological determinants and consequences of adventitial responses to arterial wall injury. *Arterioscler. Thromb. Vasc. Biol.* 27:1259–1268.
371. Shi, Y., J. E. O'Brien, A. Fard, J. D. Mannion, D. Wang, A. Zalewski. 1996. Adventitial myofibroblasts contribute to neointimal formation in injured porcine coronary arteries. *Circulation* 94:1655–1664.
372. Shi, Y., M. Pieniek, A. Fard, J. O'Brien, J. D. Mannion, A. Zalewski. 1996. Adventitial remodeling after coronary arterial injury. *Circulation* 93:340–348.
373. Jabs, A., E. Okamoto, J. Vinten-Johansen, G. Bauriedel, J. N. Wilcox. 2005. Sequential patterns of chemokine- and chemokine receptor-synthesis following vessel wall injury in porcine coronary arteries. *Atherosclerosis* 192:75–84.
374. Moos, M. P., N. John, R. Gräbner, S. Nossmann, B. Günther, R. Vollandt, C. D. Funk, B. Kaiser, A. J. Habenicht. 2005. The lamina adventitia is the major site of immune cell accumulation in standard chow-fed apolipoprotein E-deficient mice. *Arterioscler. Thromb. Vasc. Biol.* 25:2386–2391.
375. Okamoto, E., T. Couse, H. De Leon, J. Vinten-Johansen, R. B. Goodman, N. A. Scott, J. N. Wilcox. 2001. Perivascular inflammation after balloon angioplasty of porcine coronary arteries. *Circulation* 104:2228–2235.
376. Herrmann, J., L. O. Lerman, M. Rodriguez-Porcel, D. R. Holmes Jr., D. M. Richardson, E. L. Ritman, A. Lerman. 2001. Coronary vasa vasorum neovascularization precedes epicardial endothelial dysfunction in experimental hypercholesterolemia. *Cardiovasc. Res.* 51:762–766.
377. Kwon, H. M., G. Sangiorgi, E. L. Ritman, C. McKenna, D. R. Holmes Jr., R. S. Schwartz, A. Lerman. 1998. Enhanced coronary vasa vasorum neovascularization in experimental hypercholesterolemia. *J. Clin. Invest.* 101:1551–1556.

378. Kwon, H. M., G. Sangiorgi, E. L. Ritman, A. Lerman, C. McKenna, R. Virmani, W. D. Edwards, D. R. Holmes, R. S. Schwartz. 1998. Adventitial vasa vasorum in balloon-injured coronary arteries: Visualization and quantitation by a microscopic three-dimensional computed tomography technique. *J. Am. Coll. Cardiol.* 32:2072–2079.

379. Heistad, D. D., M. L. Marcus, G. E. Larsen, M. L. Armstrong. 1981. Role of vasa vasorum in nourishment of the aortic wall. *Am. J. Physiol.* 240:H781–H787.

380. Gössl, M., M. Rosol, N. M. Malyar, L. A. Fitzpatrick, P. E. Beighley, M. Zamir, E. L. Ritman. 2003. Functional anatomy and hemodynamic characteristics of vasa vasorum in the walls of porcine coronary arteries. *Anat. Rec. A. Discov. Mol. Cell. Evol. Biol.* 272:526–537.

381. Clarke, J. A. 1965. An x-ray microscopic study of the postnatal development of the vasa vasorum in the human aorta. *J. Anat.* 99(pt 4):877–889.

382. Moss, A. J., P. Samuelson, C. Angell, S. L. Minken. 1968. Polarographic evaluation of transmural oxygen availability in intact muscular arteries. *J. Atheroscler. Res.* 8:803–810.

383. Wilens, S. L., Malcolm, J. A., Vazquez, J. M. 1965. Experimental infarction (medial necrosis) of the dog's aorta. *Am. J. Pathol.* 47:695–711.

384. Wolinsky, H., S. Glagov. 1967. Nature of species differences in the medial distribution of aortic vasa vasorum in mammals. *Circ. Res.* 20:409–421.

385. Drinane, M., J. Mollmark, L. Zagorchev, K. Moodie, B. Sun, A. Hall, S. Shipman, P. Morganelli, M. Simons, M. J. Mulligan-Kehoe. 2009. The antiangiogenic activity of rPAI-1(23) inhibits vasa vasorum and growth of atherosclerotic plaque. *Circ. Res.* 104:337–345.

386. Mollmark, J., S. Ravi, B. Sun, S. Shipman, M. Buitendijk, M. Simons, M. J. Mulligan-Kehoe. 2011. Antiangiogenic activity of rPAI-1(23) promotes vasa vasorum regression in hypercholesterolemic mice through a plasmin-dependent mechanism. *Circ. Res.* 108:1419–1428.

387. Moulton, K. S., E. Heller, M. A. Konerding, E. Flynn, W. Palinski, J. Folkman. 1999. Angiogenesis inhibitors endostatin or TNP-470 reduce intimal neovascularization and plaque growth in apolipoprotein E-deficient mice. *Circulation* 99:1726–1732.

388. Moulton, K. S., K. Vakili, D. Zurakowski, M. Soliman, C. Butterfield, E. Sylvin, K. M. Lo, S. Gillies, K. Javaherian, J. Folkman. 2003. Inhibition of plaque neovascularization reduces macrophage accumulation and progression of advanced atherosclerosis. *Proc. Natl. Acad. Sci. U.S.A.* 100:4736–4741.

389. Mollmark, J. I., A. J. Park, J. Kim, T. Z. Wang, S. Katzenell, S. L. Shipman, L. G. Zagorchev, M. Simons, M. J. Mulligan-Kehoe. 2012. Fibroblast growth factor-2 is required for vasa vasorum plexus stability in hypercholesterolemic mice. *Arterioscler. Thromb. Vasc. Biol.* 32:2644–2651.

390. Schoenenberger, F., A. Mueller. 1960. On the vascularization of the bovine aortic wall [in German]. *Helv. Physiol. Pharmacol. Acta* 18:136–150.

391. Kachlík, D., A. Lametschwandtner, J. Rejmontová, J. Stingl, I. Vanek. 2003. Vasa vasorum of the human great saphenous vein. *Surg. Radiol. Anat.* 24:377–381.

392. Kachlik, D., V. Baca, J. Stingl, B. Sosna, A. Lametschwandtner, B. Minnich, M. Setina. 2007. Architectonic arrangement of the vasa vasorum of the human great saphenous vein. *J. Vasc. Res.* 44:157–166.

393. Lametschwandtner, A., B. Minnich, D. Kachlik, M. Setina, J. Stingl. 2004. Three-dimensional arrangement of the vasa vasorum in explanted segments of the aged human great saphenous vein: Scanning electron microscopy and three-dimensional morphometry of vascular corrosion casts. *Anat. Rec. A Discov. Mol. Cell. Evol. Biol.* 281:1372–1382.

394. Ahmed, S. R., B. L. Johansson, M. G. Karlsson, D. S. Souza, M. R. Dashwood, A. Loesch. 2004. Human saphenous vein and coronary bypass surgery: Ultrastructural aspects of conventional and "no-touch" vein graft preparations. *Histol. Histopathol.* 19:421–433.

395. Loesch, A., M. R. Dashwood. 2009. On the sympathetic innervation of the human greater saphenous vein: Relevance to clinical practice. *Curr. Vasc. Pharmacol.* 7:58–67.

396. Souza, D. 1996. A new no-touch preparation technique. Technical notes. *Scand. J. Thorac. Cardiovasc. Surg.* 30:41–44.

397. Crotty, T. P. 2007. The venous valve agger and plasma noradrenaline-mediated venodilator feedback. *Phlebology* 22:116–130.

398. Maurice, G., X. Wang, B. Lehalle, J. F. Stoltz. 1998. Modeling of elastic deformation and vascular resistance of arterial and venous vasa vasorum [in French]. *J. Mal. Vasc.* 23:282–288.

399. Tanaka, K., D. Nagata, Y. Hirata, Y. Tabata, R. Nagai, M. Sata. 2011. Augmented angiogenesis in adventitia promotes growth of atherosclerotic plaque in apolipoprotein E-deficient mice. *Atherosclerosis* 215:366–373.

400. Nagy, J. A., A. M. Dvorak, H. F. Dvorak. 2003. VEGF-A(164/165) and PlGF: Roles in angiogenesis and arteriogenesis. *Trends Cardiovasc. Med.* 13:169–175.
401. Khurana, R., L. Moons, S. Shafi, A. Luttun, D. Collen, J. F. Martin, P. Carmeliet, I. C. Zachary. 2005. Placental growth factor promotes atherosclerotic intimal thickening and macrophage accumulation. *Circulation* 111:2828–2836.
402. Majesky, M. W., X. R. Dong, V. Hoglund, W. M. Mahoney Jr., G. Daum. 2011. The adventitia: A dynamic interface containing resident progenitor cells. *Arterioscler. Thromb. Vasc. Biol.* 31:1530–1539.
403. Ergün, S., H. P. Hohn, N. Kilic, B. B. Singer, D. Tilki. 2008. Endothelial and hematopoietic progenitor cells (EPCs and HPCs): Hand in hand fate determining partners for cancer cells. *Stem Cell Rev.* 4:169–177.
404. Psaltis, P. J., A. Harbuzariu, S. Delacroix, E. W. Holroyd, R. D. Simari. 2011. Resident vascular progenitor cells—Diverse origins, phenotype, and function. *J. Cardiovasc. Transl. Res.* 4:161–176.
405. Li, G., S. J. Chen, S. Oparil, Y. F. Chen, J. A. Thompson. 2000. Direct *in vivo* evidence demonstrating neointimal migration of adventitial fibroblasts after balloon injury of rat carotid arteries. *Circulation* 101:1362–1365.
406. Mallawaarachchi, C. M., P. L. Weissberg, R. C. Siow. 2005. Smad7 gene transfer attenuates adventitial cell migration and vascular remodeling after balloon injury. *Arterioscler. Thromb. Vasc. Biol.* 25:1383–1387.
407. Hu, Y., Q. Xu. 2011. Adventitial biology: Differentiation and function. *Arterioscler. Thromb. Vasc. Biol.* 31:1523–1529.
408. Lisy, K., D. J. Peet. 2008. Turn me on: Regulating HIF transcriptional activity. *Cell Death Differ.* 15:642–649.
409. Pagès, G., J. Pouysségur. 2005. Transcriptional regulation of the vascular endothelial growth factor gene: A concert of activating factors. *Cardiovasc. Res.* 65:564–573.
410. Li, J., N. W. Shworak, M. Simons. 2002. Increased responsiveness of hypoxic endothelial cells to FGF2 is mediated by HIF-1alpha-dependent regulation of enzymes involved in synthesis of heparan sulfate FGF2-binding sites. *J. Cell Sci.* 115(pt 9):1951–1959.
411. Gurtner, G. C., S. Werner, Y. Barrandon, M. T. Longaker. 2008. Wound repair and regeneration. *Nature* 453:314–321.
412. Swift, M. E., H. K. Kleinman, L. A. DiPietro. 1999. Impaired wound repair and delayed angiogenesis in aged mice. *Lab. Invest.* 79:1479–1487.
413. Fukumura, D., R. K. Jain. 2008. Imaging angiogenesis and the microenvironment. *APMIS* 116:695–715.
414. Szpaderska, A. M., C. G. Walsh, M. J. Steinberg, L. A. DiPietro. 2005. Distinct patterns of angiogenesis in oral and skin wounds. *J. Dent. Res.* 84:309–314.
415. Alexander, R. W. 1995. Theodore cooper memorial lecture. Hypertension and the pathogenesis of atherosclerosis. Oxidative stress and the mediation of arterial inflammatory response: A new perspective. *Hypertension* 25:155–161.
416. Chobanian, A. V. 1990. 1989 Corcoran lecture: Adaptive and maladaptive responses of the arterial wall to hypertension. *Hypertension* 15(6 pt 2):666–674.
417. Herrmann, J., S. Samee, A. Chade, M. Rodriguez Porcel, L. O. Lerman, A. Lerman. 2005. Differential effect of experimental hypertension and hypercholesterolemia on adventitial remodeling. *Arterioscler. Thromb. Vasc. Biol.* 25:447–453.
418. Kai, H., F. Kuwahara, K. Tokuda, R. Shibata, K. Kusaba, H. Niiyama, N. Tahara, T. Nagata, T. Imaizumi. 2002. Coexistence of hypercholesterolemia and hypertension impairs adventitial vascularization. *Hypertension* 39(2 pt 2):455–459.
419. Veerman, K. J., D. E. Venegas-Pino, Y. Shi, M. I. Khan, H. C. Gerstein, G. H. Werstuck. 2013. Hyperglycaemia is associated with impaired vasa vasorum neovascularization and accelerated atherosclerosis in apolipoprotein-E deficient mice. *Atherosclerosis* 227:250–258.
420. Moreno, P. R., V. Fuster. 2004. New aspects in the pathogenesis of diabetic atherothrombosis. *J. Am. Coll. Cardiol.* 44(12):2293–2300.
421. Purushothaman, K. R., M. Purushothaman, P. Muntner, P. A. Lento, W. N. O'Connor, S. K. Sharma, V. Fuster, P. R. Moreno. 2011. Inflammation, neovascularization and intra-plaque hemorrhage are associated with increased reparative collagen content: Implication for plaque progression in diabetic atherosclerosis. *Vasc. Med.* 16:103–108.
422. Purushothaman, M. et al. 2012. Genotype-dependent impairment of hemoglobin clearance increases oxidative and inflammatory response in human diabetic atherosclerosis. *Arterioscler. Thromb. Vasc. Biol.* 32(11):2769–2775.

423. Maiellaro, K., W. R. Taylor. 2007. The role of the adventitia in vascular inflammation. *Cardiovasc. Res.* 75:640–648.

424. Thaunat, O. et al. 2005. Lymphoid neogenesis in chronic rejection: Evidence for a local humoral alloimmune response. *Proc. Natl. Acad. Sci. U.S.A.* 102:14723–14728.

425. Watanabe, M., A. Sangawa, Y. Sasaki, M. Yamashita, M. Tanaka-Shintani, M. Shintaku, Y. Ishikawa. 2007. Distribution of inflammatory cells in adventitia changed with advancing atherosclerosis of human coronary artery. *J. Atheroscler. Thromb.* 14:325–331.

426. Thaunat, O. et al. 2008. Antiangiogenic treatment prevents adventitial constrictive remodeling in graft arteriosclerosis. *Transplantation* 85:281–289.

427. O'Brien, K. D., T. O. McDonald, A. Chait, M. D. Allen, C. E. Alpers. 1996. Neovascular expression of E-selectin, intercellular adhesion molecule-1, and vascular cell adhesion molecule-1 in human atherosclerosis and their relation to intimal leukocyte content. *Circulation* 93:672–682.

428. Schwartz, C. J., J. R. Mitchell. 1962. Cellular infiltration of the human arterial adventitia associated with atheromatous plaques. *Circulation* 26:73–78.

429. Zhao, L. et al. 2004. The 5-lipoxygenase pathway promotes pathogenesis of hyperlipidemia-dependent aortic aneurysm. *Nat. Med.* 10:966–973.

430. Wick, G., M. Romen, A. Amberger, B. Metzler, M. Mayr, G. Falkensammer, Q. Xu. 1997. Atherosclerosis, autoimmunity, and vascular-associated lymphoid tissue. *FASEB J.* 11:1199–1207.

431. Gräbner, R. et al. 2009. Lymphotoxin beta receptor signaling promotes tertiary lymphoid organogenesis in the aorta adventitia of aged ApoE-/- mice. *J. Exp. Med.* 206:233–248.

432. Marx, S. O., H. Totary-Jain, A. R. Marks. 2011. Vascular smooth muscle cell proliferation in restenosis. *Circ. Cardiovasc. Interv.* 4:104–111.

433. Khurana, R., Z. Zhuang, S. Bhardwaj, M. Murakami, E. De Muinck, S. Yla-Herttuala, N. Ferrara, J. F. Martin, I. Zachary, M. Simons. 2004. Angiogenesis-dependent and independent phases of intimal hyperplasia. *Circulation* 110:2436–2443.

434. Koga, J., T. Matoba, K. Egashira, M. Kubo, M. Miyagawa, E. Iwata, K. Sueishi, M. Shibuya, K. Sunagawa. 2009. Soluble Flt-1 gene transfer ameliorates neointima formation after wire injury in flt-1 tyrosine kinase-deficient mice. *Arterioscler. Thromb. Vasc. Biol.* 29:458–464.

435. Ohtani, K. et al. 2004. Blockade of vascular endothelial growth factor suppresses experimental restenosis after intraluminal injury by inhibiting recruitment of monocyte lineage cells. *Circulation* 110:2444–2452.

436. Cheema, A. N. et al. 2006. Adventitial microvessel formation after coronary stenting and the effects of SU11218, a tyrosine kinase inhibitor. *J. Am. Coll. Cardiol.* 47:1067–1075.

437. Chen, P. Y. et al. 2012. FGF regulates TGF-β signaling and endothelial-to-mesenchymal transition via control of let-7 miRNA expression. *Cell Rep.* 2:1684–1696.

438. Zeisberg, E. M. et al. 2007. Endothelial-to-mesenchymal transition contributes to cardiac fibrosis. *Nat. Med.* 13:952–961.

439. Chang, A. C. et al. 2011. Notch initiates the endothelial-to-mesenchymal transition in the atrioventricular canal through autocrine activation of soluble guanylyl cyclase. *Dev. Cell.* 21:288–300.

440. Flagg, A. E., J. U. Earley, E. C. Svensson. 2007. FOG-2 attenuates endothelial-to-mesenchymal transformation in the endocardial cushions of the developing heart. *Dev. Biol.* 304:308–316.

441. Garside, V. C., A. C. Chang, A. Karsan, P. A. Hoodless. 2013. Co-ordinating Notch, BMP, and TGF-β signaling during heart valve development. *Cell Mol. Life Sci.* 70:2899–2917.

442. Aisagbonhi, O., M. Rai, S. Ryzhov, N. Atria, I. Feoktistov, A. K. Hatzopoulos. 2011. Experimental myocardial infarction triggers canonical Wnt signaling and endothelial-to-mesenchymal transition. *Dis. Model Mech.* 4:469–483.

443. Goumans, M. J., A. J. van Zonneveld, P. ten Dijke. 2008. Transforming growth factor beta-induced endothelial-to-mesenchymal transition: A switch to cardiac fibrosis? *Trends Cardiovasc. Med.* 18:293–298.

444. Piera-Velazquez, S., Z. Li, S. A. Jimenez. 2011. Role of endothelial-mesenchymal transition (EndoMT) in the pathogenesis of fibrotic disorders. *Am. J. Pathol.* 179:1074–1080.

445. Widyantoro, B. et al. 2010. Endothelial cell-derived endothelin-1 promotes cardiac fibrosis in diabetic hearts through stimulation of endothelial-to-mesenchymal transition. *Circulation* 121:2407–2418.

446. Kitao, A., Y. Sato, S. Sawada-Kitamura, K. Harada, M. Sasaki, H. Morikawa, S. Shiomi, M. Honda, O. Matsui, Y. Nakanuma. 2009. Endothelial to mesenchymal transition via transforming growth factor-beta1/Smad activation is associated with portal venous stenosis in idiopathic portal hypertension. *Am. J. Pathol.* 175:616–626.

447. Maddaluno, L. et al. 2013. EndMT contributes to the onset and progression of cerebral cavernous malformations. *Nature* 498:492–496.
448. van Meeteren, L. A., P. ten Dijke. 2012. Regulation of endothelial cell plasticity by TGF-β. *Cell Tissue Res.* 347:177–186.
449. Ghosh, A. K., V. Nagpal, J. W. Covington, M. A. Michaels, D. E. Vaughan. 2012. Molecular basis of cardiac endothelial-to-mesenchymal transition (EndMT): Differential expression of microRNAs during EndMT. *Cell Signal.* 24:1031–1036.
450. Kumarswamy, R., I. Volkmann, V. Jazbutyte, S. Dangwal, D. H. Park, T. Thum. 2012. Transforming growth factor-β-induced endothelial-to-mesenchymal transition is partly mediated by microRNA-21. *Arterioscler. Thromb. Vasc. Biol.* 32:361–369.
451. Lee, S. W. et al. 2013. Snail as a potential target molecule in cardiac fibrosis: Paracrine action of endothelial cells on fibroblasts through snail and CTGF axis. *Mol. Ther.* 21:1767–1777.
452. Egorova, A. D., P. P. Khedoe, M. J. Goumans, B. K. Yoder, S. M. Nauli, P. ten Dijke, R. E. Poelmann, B. P. Hierck. 2011. Lack of primary cilia primes shear-induced endothelial-to-mesenchymal transition. *Circ. Res.* 108:1093–1101.
453. Egorova, A. D. et al. 2011. Tgfβ/Alk5 signaling is required for shear stress induced klf2 expression in embryonic endothelial cells. *Dev. Dyn.* 240:1670–1680.
454. Ten Dijke, P., A. D. Egorova, M. J. Goumans, R. E. Poelmann, B. P. Hierck. 2012. TGF- β signaling in endothelial-to-mesenchymal transition: The role of shear stress and primary cilia. *Sci. Signal* 5:pt2.
455. Li, C., F. Dong, Y. Jia, H. Du, N. Dong, Y. Xu, S. Wang, H. Wu, Z. Liu, W. Li. 2013. Notch signal regulates corneal endothelial-to-mesenchymal transition. *Am. J. Pathol.* 183:786–795.
456. Li, Z., P. J. Wermuth, B. S. Benn, M. P. Lisanti, S. A. Jimenez. 2013. Caveolin-1 deficiency induces spontaneous endothelial-to-mesenchymal transition in murine pulmonary endothelial cells *in vitro. Am. J. Pathol.* 2013;182:325–331.
457. Mahler, G. J., E. J. Farrar, J. T. Butcher. 2013. Inflammatory cytokines promote mesenchymal transformation in embryonic and adult valve endothelial cells. *Arterioscler. Thromb. Vasc. Biol.* 33:121–130.
458. Maleszewska, M., J. R. Moonen, N. Huijkman, B. van de Sluis, G. Krenning, M. C. Harmsen. 2013. IL-1β and TGFβ2 synergistically induce endothelial to mesenchymal transition in an NFκB-dependent manner. *Immunobiology* 218:443–454.
459. Rieder, F., S. P. Kessler, G. A. West, S. Bhilocha, C. de la Motte, T. M. Sadler, B. Gopalan, E. Stylianou, C. Fiocchi. 2011. Inflammation-induced endothelialto-mesenchymal transition: A novel mechanism of intestinal fibrosis. *Am. J. Pathol.* 179:2660–2673.
460. Brånén, L., L. Hovgaard, M. Nitulescu, E. Bengtsson, J. Nilsson, S. Jovinge. 2004. Inhibition of tumor necrosis factor-alpha reduces atherosclerosis in apolipoprotein E knockout mice. *Arterioscler. Thromb. Vasc. Biol.* 24:2137–2142.
461. Gupta, S., A. M. Pablo, X. Jiang, N. Wang, A. R. Tall, C. Schindler. 1997. IFN-gamma potentiates atherosclerosis in ApoE knock-out mice. *J. Clin. Invest.* 99:2752–2761.
462. Cheng, A. L., S. Batool, C. R. McCreary, M. L. Lauzon, R. Frayne, M. Goyal, E. E. Smith. 2013. Susceptibility-weighted imaging is more reliable than T2*-weighted gradient-recalled echo MRI for detecting microbleeds. *Stroke* 44:2782–2786. doi: 10.1161/STROKEAHA.113.002267.
463. Gouw, A. A., A. Seewann, W. M. van der Flier, F. Barkhof, A. M. Rozemuller, P. Scheltens, J. J. Geurts. 2011. Heterogeneity of small vessel disease: A systematic review of MRI and histopathology correlations. *J. Neurol. Neurosurg. Psychiatry* 82:126–135. doi: 10.1136/jnnp.2009.204685.
464. Shoamanesh, A., C. S. Kwok, O. Benavente. 2011. Cerebral microbleeds: Histopathological correlation of neuroimaging. *Cerebrovasc. Dis.* 32:528–534. doi: 10.1159/000331466.
465. Viswanathan, A., S. M. Greenberg. 2011. Cerebral amyloid angiopathy in the elderly. *Ann. Neurol.* 70:871–880. doi: 10.1002/ana.22516.
466. Caplan, L. R. 2015. Microbleeds. *Circulation* 132:479–480.
467. Benedictus, M. R., N. D. Prins, J. D. Goos, P. Scheltens, F. Barkhof, W. M. van der Flier. 2015. Microbleeds, mortality, and stroke in Alzheimer disease: The MISTRAL study. *JAMA Neurol.* 72:539–545. doi: 10.1001/ jamaneurol.2015.14.
468. Kester, M. I., J. D. Goos, C. E. Teunissen, M. R. Benedictus, F. H. Bouwman, M. P. Wattjes, F. Barkhof, P. Scheltens, W. M. van der Flier. 2014. Associations between cerebral small-vessel disease and Alzheimer disease pathology as measured by cerebrospinal fluid biomarkers. *JAMA Neurol.* 71:855–862. doi: 10.1001/jamaneurol.2014.754.
469. Peters, A., S. von Klot, M. Heier, I. Trentinaglia, A. Hormann, E. H. Wichmann, H. Löwel; Cooperative Health Research in the Region of Augsburg Study Group. 2004. Exposure to traffic and the onset of myocardial infarction. *N. Engl. J. Med.* 351:1721–1730.

470. Zanobetti, A., J. Schwartz. 2002. Cardiovascular damage by airborne particles: Are diabetics more susceptible? *Epidemiology* 13(5):588–592.

471. Schwartz, J. 1999. Air pollution and hospital admissions for heart disease in eight US counties. *Epidemiology* 10:17–22.

472. Longo, D. L., T. E. Warkentin. 2005. Ischemic limb gangrene with pulses. *N. Engl. J. Med.* 373(7):642–655.

473. Warkentin, T. E., R. J. Cook, R. Sarode, D. A. Sloane, M. A. Crowther. 2015. Warfarin-induced venous limb ischemia/gangrene complicating cancer: A novel and clinically distinct syndrome. *Blood* 126:486–493.

474. Warkentin, T. E., L. J. Elavathil, C. P. Hayward, M. A. Johnston, J. I. Russett, J. G. Kelton. 1997. The pathogenesis of venous limb gangrene associated with heparin-induced thrombocytopenia. *Ann. Intern. Med.* 127(9):804–812.

475. Molos, M. A., J. C. Hall. 1985. Symmetrical peripheral gangrene and disseminated intravascular coagulation. *Arch. Dermatol.* 121:1057–1061.

476. Ghosh, S. K., D. Bandyopadhyay, A. Ghosh. 2010. Symmetrical peripheral gangrene: A prospective study of 14 consecutive cases in a tertiary-care hospital in eastern India. *J. Eur. Acad. Dermatol. Venereol.* 24:214–218.

477. Barraud, S. 1904. Über Extremitätengangrän im jugendlichen Alter nach Infektionskrankheiten. *Dtsch. Z. Chir.* 74(3–4):237–297.

478. Levi, M., H. Ten Cate. 1999. Disseminated intravascular coagulation. *N. Engl. J. Med.* 341(8):586–592.

479. Gando, S. 2010. Microvascular thrombosis and multiple organ dysfunction syndrome. *Crit. Care Med.* 38(Suppl. 2):S35–S42.

480. Levi, M., T. Van Der Poll. 2013. Thrombomodulin in sepsis. *Minerva. Anestesiol.* 79:294–298.

481. Warkentin, T. E., C. P. Hayward, L. K. Boshkov, A. V. Santos, J. A. Sheppard, A. P. Bode, J. G. Kelton. 1994. Sera from patients with heparin-induced thrombocytopenia generate platelet-derived microparticles with procoagulant activity: An explanation for the thrombotic complications of heparininduced thrombocytopenia. *Blood* 84(11):3691–3699.

482. Geddings, J. E., N. Mackman. 2013. Tumor-derived tissue factor-positive microparticles and venous thrombosis in cancer patients. *Blood* 122:1873–1880.

483. Esmon, C. T. 2003. The protein C pathway. *Chest* 124(Suppl. 3):26S–32S.

484. Haimovici, H. 1965. The ischemic forms of venous thrombosis. 1. Phlegmasia cerulea dolens. 2. Venous gangrene. *J. Cardiovasc. Surg. (Torino)* 5(Suppl.):164–173.

485. Perkins, J. M., T. R. Magee, R. B. Galland. 1996. Phlegmasia caerulea dolens and venous gangrene. *Br. J. Surg.* 83(1):19–23.

486. Warkentin, T. E. 2001. Venous limb gangrene during warfarin treatment of cancer-associated deep venous thrombosis. *Ann. Intern. Med.* 135:589–593.

487. Srinivasan, A. F., L. Rice, J. R. Bartholomew, C. Rangaswamy, L. La Perna, J. E. Thompson, S. Murphy, K. R. Baker. 2004. Warfarin-induced skin necrosis and venous limb gangrene in the setting of heparin-induced thrombocytopenia. *Arch. Intern. Med.* 164:66–70.

488. Grim Hostetler, S., J. Sopkovich, S. Dean, M. Zirwas. 2012. Warfarin-induced venous limb gangrene. *J. Clin. Aesthet. Dermatol.* 5:38–42.

489. Padjas, A., B. Brzezinska-Kolarz, A. Undas, J. Musial. 2005. Phlegmasia cerulea dolens as a complication of deep vein thrombosis in a man with primary antiphospholipid syndrome. *Blood Coagul. Fibrinolysis* 16:567–569.

490. Bell, W. R., N. F. Starksen, S. Tong, J. K. Porterfield. 1985. Trousseau's syndrome: Devastating coagulopathy in the absence of heparin. *Am. J. Med.* 79:423–430.

491. Warkentin, T. E., J. G. Kelton. 2001. Temporal aspects of heparin-induced thrombocytopenia. *N. Engl. J. Med.* 344:1286–1292.

492. Warkentin, T. E. 2010. Agents for the treatment of heparin-induced thrombocytopenia. *Hematol. Oncol. Clin. North Am.* 24:755–775.

493. Warkentin, T. E., A. Greinacher, A. Koster, A. M. Lincoff. 2008. Treatment and prevention of heparin-induced thrombocytopenia: American College of Chest Physicians evidence-based clinical practice guidelines (8th edition). *Chest* 133(Suppl. 6):340S–380S.

494. Warkentin, T. E. 2015. Heparin-induced thrombocytopenia in critically ill patients. *Semin. Thromb. Hemost.* 41:49–60.

495. Vadivel, K., A. E. Schmidt, V. J. Marder, S. Krishnaswamy, S. P. Bajaj. 2013. Structure and function of vitamin K-dependent coagulant and anticoagulant proteins. In *Hemostasis and Thrombosis: Basic Principles and Clinical Practice*, 6th ed., V. J. Marder, W. C. Aird, J. S. Bennett, S. Schulman, G. C. White, Eds., pp. 208–232. Philadelphia: Lippincott Williams & Wilkins.

496. Cole, M. S., P. K. Minifee, F. J. Wolma. 1988. Coumarin necrosis—A review of the literature. *Surgery* 103:271–277.
497. Warkentin, T. E. 2013. Coumarin-induced skin necrosis and venous limb gangrene. In *Hemostasis and Thrombosis: Basic Principles and Clinical Practice*, 6th ed., V. J. Marder, W. C. Aird, J. S. Bennett, S. Schulman, G. C. White, Eds., pp. 1308–1317. Philadelphia: Lippincott Williams & Wilkins.
498. Lee, A. Y. et al. 2003. Low-molecular-weight heparin versus a coumarin for the prevention of recurrent venous thromboembolism in patients with cancer. *N. Engl. J. Med.* 349:146–153.
499. Rice, L. 2013. A clinician's perspective on heparin-induced thrombocytopenia: Paradoxes, myths, and continuing challenges. In *Heparin-Induced Thrombocytopenia*, 5th ed., T. E. Warkentin, A. Greinacher, Eds., pp. 608–617. Boca Raton, FL: CRC Press.
500. Weaver, F. A., P. W. Meacham, R. B. Adkins, R. H. Dean. 1988. Phlegmasia cerulea dolens: Therapeutic considerations. *South Med. J.* 81:306–312.
501. Warkentin, T. E. 2014. Anticoagulant failure in coagulopathic patients: PTT confounding and other pitfalls. *Expert Opin. Drug Saf.* 13:25–43.
502. Greinacher, A. 2015. Heparin-induced thrombocytopenia. *N. Engl. J. Med.* 373:252–261.
503. Smythe, M. A., T. E. Warkentin, J. L. Stephens, D. Zakalik, J. C. Mattson. 2002. Venous limb gangrene during overlapping therapy with warfarin and a direct thrombin inhibitor for immune heparin-induced thrombocytopenia. *Am. J. Hematol.* 71:50–52.
504. Qvarfordt, P., B. Eklöf, P. Ohlin. 1983. Intramuscular pressure in the lower leg in deep vein thrombosis and phlegmasia cerulae dolens. *Ann. Surg.* 197(4):450–453.
505. Meissner, M. H. 2012. Rationale and indications for aggressive early thrombus removal. *Phlebology* 27(Suppl. 1):78–84.
506. Erdoes, L. S., J. B. Ezell, S. I. Myers, M. B. Hogan, C. J. LeSar, L. R. Sprouse 2nd. 2011. Pharmacomechanical thrombolysis for phlegmasia cerulea dolens. *Am. Surg.* 77:1606–J1612.
507. Knight, T. T. Jr., S. V. Gordon, J. Canady, D. S. Rush, W. Browder. 2000. Symmetrical peripheral gangrene: A new presentation of an old disease. *Am. Surg.* 66:196–199.
508. Warner, P. M. et al. 2003. Current management of purpura fulminans: A multicenter study. *J. Burn. Care Rehabil.* 24:119–126.
509. Robboy, S. J., M. C. Mihm, R. W. Colman, J. D. Minna. 1973. The skin in disseminated intravascular coagulation: Prospective analysis of thirty-six cases. *Br. J. Dermatol.* 88:221–229.
510. Hamdy, R. C., P. S. Babyn, J. I. Krajbich. 1993. Use of bone scan in management of patients with peripheral gangrene due to fulminant meningococcemia. *J. Pediatr. Orthop.* 13:447–451.
511. Watanabe, T., T. Imamura, K. Nakagaki, K. Tanaka. 1979. Disseminated intravascular coagulation in autopsy cases: Its incidence and clinicopathologic significance. *Pathol. Res. Pract.* 165:311–322.
512. Shimamura, K., K. Oka, M. Nakazawa, M. Kojima. 1983. Distribution patterns of microthrombi in disseminated intravascular coagulation. *Arch. Pathol. Lab. Med.* 107:543–547.
513. Fox, B. 1971. Disseminated intravascular coagulation and the Waterhouse-Friderichsen syndrome. *Arch. Dis. Child* 46:680–685.
514. Betrosian, A. P., T. Berlet, B. Agarwal. 2006. Purpura fulminans in sepsis. *Am. J. Med. Sci.* 332:339–345.
515. Childers, B. J., B. Cobanov. 2003. Acute infectious purpura fulminans: A 15-year retrospective review of 28 consecutive cases. *Am. Surg.* 69:86–90.
516. Kirkland, K. B., P. K. Marcom, D. J. Sexton, J. S. Dumler, D. H. Walker. 1993. Rocky Mountain spotted fever complicated by gangrene: Report of six cases and review. *Clin. Infect. Dis.* 16:629–634.
517. Kato, Y., K. Ohnishi, Y. Sawada, M. Suenaga. 2007. Purpura fulminans: An unusual manifestation of severe falciparum malaria. *Trans. R. Soc. Trop. Med. Hyg.* 101:1045–1047.
518. Chen, C. F., J. L. Wang, Y. F. Wei. 2012. Symmetrical peripheral gangrene, an uncommon complication of tuberculosis. *QJM* 105:279–280.
519. Wynne, J. M., G. L. Williams, B. A. Ellman. 1977. Gangrene of the extremities in measles. *S. Afr. Med. J.* 52(3):117–121.
520. Christiansen, C. B., R. M. Berg, R. R. Plovsing, K. Møller. 2012. Two cases of infectious purpura fulminans and septic shock caused by Capnocytophaga canimorsus transmitted from dogs. *Scand. J. Infect. Dis.* 44:635–639.
521. Brandtzaeg, P., P. M. Sandset, G. B. Joø, R. Ovstebø, U. Abildgaard, P. Kierulf. 1989. The quantitative association of plasma endotoxin, antithrombin, protein C, extrinsic pathway inhibitor and fibrinopeptide A in systemic meningococcal disease. *Thromb. Res.* 55:459–470.
522. Hellum, M., R. Øvstebø, B. S. Brusletto, J. P. Berg, P. Brandtzaeg, C. E. Henriksson. 2014. Microparticle-associated tissue factor activity correlates with plasma levels of bacterial lipopolysaccharides in meningococcal septic shock. *Thromb. Res.* 133:507–514.

523. Fijnvandraat, K., B. Derkx, M. Peters, R. Bijlmer, A. Sturk, M. H. Prins, S. J. van Deventer, J. W. ten Cate. 1995. Coagulation activation and tissue necrosis in meningococcal septic shock: Severely reduced protein C levels predict a high mortality. *Thromb. Haemost.* 73:15–20.

524. Kondaveeti, S., M. L. Hibberd, R. Booy, S. Nadel, M. Levin. 1999. Effect of the Factor V Leiden mutation on the severity of meningococcal disease. *Pediatr. Infect. Dis. J.* 18:893–896.

525. Sharma, B. D., S. R. Kabra, B. Gupta. 2004. Symmetrical peripheral gangrene. *Trop. Doct.* 34:2–4.

526. Hotchkiss, R., T. Marks. 2014. Management of acute and chronic vascular conditions of the hand. *Curr. Rev. Musculoskelet. Med.* 7(1):747–752.

527. Wollina, U., G. Hansel, M. Gruner, J. Schönlebe, B. Heinig, E. Köstler. 2007. Painful ANA-positive scleroderma-like disease with acral ulcerations: A case of chronic gangrenous ergotism. *Int. J. Low Extrem. Wounds* 6:148–152.

528. Hammadah, M., S. Chaturvedi, J. Jue, A. B. Buletko, M. Qintar, M. E. Madmani, P. Sharma. 2013. Acral gangrene as a presentation of non-uremic calciphylaxis. *Avicenna J. Med.* 3:109–111.

529. Chang, J. C., N. Ikhlaque. 2004. Peripheral digit ischemic syndrome can be a manifestation of postoperative thrombotic thrombocytopenic purpura. *Ther. Apher. Dial.* 8:413–418.

530. Sharif, M., S. Hameed, I. Akin, U. Natarajan. 2015. HIV diagnosis in a patient presenting with vasculitis. *Int. J. STD AIDS* 27(2):152–154.

531. Ames, P. R., E. Walker, D. Aw, D. Marshall, F. de Villiers, M. Staber. 2009. Multi-organ failure in adult onset Still's disease: A septic disguise. *Clin. Rheumatol.* 28(Suppl. 1):S3–S6.

532. Grob, J. J., J. J. Bonerandi. 1989. Thrombotic skin disease as a marker of the anticardiolipin syndrome: Livedo vasculitis and distal gangrene associated with abnormal serum antiphospholipid activity. *J. Am. Acad. Dermatol.* 20:1063–1069.

533. Bhoola, P. H., G. Shtofmakher, A. Bahri, A. A. Patel, S. R. Barlizo, M. Trepal. 2016. Pedal gangrenous changes in the digits of an adolescent with ulcerative colitis: A case report. *J. Foot Ankle Surg.* 55(2):272–275.

534. Smith, O. P., B. White. 1999. Infectious purpura fulminans: Diagnosis and treatment. *Br. J. Haematol.* 104:202–207.

535. Piccin, A., A. O'Marcaigh, C. McMahon, C. Murphy, I. Okafor, L. Marcheselli, W. Casey, L. Claffey, O. P. Smith. 2014. Non-activated plasma-derived PC improves amputation rate of children undergoing sepsis. *Thromb. Res.* 134:63–67.

536. Vincent, J. L. et al. 2013. A randomized, double-blind, placebo-controlled, phase 2b study to evaluate the safety and efficacy of recombinant human soluble thrombomodulin, ART-123, in patients with sepsis and suspected disseminated intravascular coagulation. *Crit. Care Med.* 41:2069–2079.

537. Wada, H. et al.; The scientific standardization committee on DIC of the International Society on Thrombosis Haemostasis. 2013. Guidance for diagnosis and treatment of disseminated intravascular coagulation from harmonization of the recommendations from three guidelines. *J. Thromb. Haemost.* 11:761–767.

538. Zarychanski, R. et al.; Canadian Critical Care Trials Group. 2015. The efficacy and safety of heparin in patients with sepsis: A systematic review and metaanalysis. *Crit. Care Med.* 43:511–518.

539. Ranieri, V. M. et al.; PROWESS-SHOCK Study Group. 2012. Drotrecogin alfa (activated) in adults with septic shock. *N. Engl. J. Med.* 366:2055–2064.

540. Warren, B. L. et al.; KyberSept Trial Study Group. 2001. Caring for the critically ill patient: High-dose antithrombin III in severe sepsis: A randomized controlled trial. *JAMA* 286:1869–1878.

541. Kienast, J., M. Juers, C. J. Wiedermann, J. N. Hoffmann, H. Ostermann, R. Strauss, H. O. Keinecke, B. L. Warren, S. M. Opal; KyberSept investigators. 2006. Treatment effects of high-dose antithrombin without concomitant heparin in patients with severe sepsis with or without disseminated intravascular coagulation. *J. Thromb. Haemost.* 4(1):90–97.

542. Price, V. E., D. L. Ledingham, A. Krümpel, A. K. Chan. 2011. Diagnosis and management of neonatal purpura fulminans. *Semin. Fetal Neonatal Med.* 16:318–322.

543. Josephson, C., R. Nuss, L. Jacobson, M. R. Hacker, J. Murphy, A. Weinberg, M. J. Manco-Johnson. 2001. The varicella-autoantibody syndrome. *Pediatr. Res.* 50:345–352.

544. Hart, J. E., S. E. Chiuve, F. Laden, C. M. Albert. 2014. Roadway proximity and risk of sudden cardiac death in women. *Circulation* 130(17):1474–1482.

545. Nichol, G. et al. 2008. Essential features of designating out-of-hospital cardiac arrest as a reportable event: A scientific statement from the American heart association emergency cardiovascular care committee; council on cardiopulmonary, perioperative, and critical care; council on cardiovascular nursing; council on clinical cardiology; and quality of care and outcomes research interdisciplinary working group. *Circulation* 117(17):2298–2308.

546. Kannel, W. B., D. L. McGee. 1985. Epidemiology of sudden death: Insights from the Framingham study. *Cardiovasc. Clin.* 15(3):93–105.
547. Albert, C. M., C. U. Chae, F. Grodstein, L. M. Rose, K. M. Rexrode, J. N. Ruskin, M. J. Stampfer, J. E. Manson. 2003. Prospective study of sudden cardiac death among women in the United States. *Circulation* 107:2096–2101.
548. Hoek, G., R. M. Krishnan, R. Beelen, A. Peters, B. Ostro, B. Brunekreef, J. D. Kaufman. 2013. Long-term air pollution exposure and cardio-respiratory mortality: A review. *Environ. Health* 12(1):43.
549. Beelen, R., G. Hoek, D. Houthuijs, P. A. van den Brandt, R. A. Goldbohm, P. Fischer, L. J. Schouten, B. Armstrong, B. Brunekreef. 2009. The joint association of air pollution and noise from road traffic with cardiovascular mortality in a cohort study. *Occup. Environ. Med.* 66:243–250.
550. Eriksson, C., M. E. Nilsson, S. M. Willers, L. Gidhagen, T. Bellander, G. Pershagen. 2012. Traffic noise and cardiovascular health in Sweden: The roadside study. *Noise Health* 14:140–147.
551. Ndrepepa, A., D. Twardella. 2011. Relationship between noise annoyance from road traffic noise and cardiovascular diseases: A meta-analysis. *Noise Health* 13:251–259.
552. Miller, K. A., D. S. Siscovick, L. Sheppard, K. Shepherd, J. H. Sullivan, G. L. Anderson, J. D. Kaufman. 2007. Long-term exposure to air pollution and incidence of cardiovascular events in women. *N. Engl. J. Med.* 356:447–458.
553. Puett, R. C., J. Schwartz, J. E. Hart, J. D. Yanosky, F. E. Speizer, H. Suh, C. J. Paciorek, L. M. Neas, F. Laden. 2008. Chronic particulate exposure, mortality, and coronary heart disease in the nurses' health study. *Am. J. Epidemiol.* 168:1161–1168.
554. Link, M. S., D. W. Dockery. 2010. Air pollution and the triggering of cardiac arrhythmias. *Curr. Opin. Cardiol.* 25(1):16–22.
555. Dennekamp, M., M. Akram, M. J. Abramson, A. Tonkin, M. R. Sim, M. Fridman, B. Erbas. 2010. Outdoor air pollution as a trigger for out-of-hospital cardiac arrests. *Epidemiology* 21:494–500.
556. Ensor, K. B., L. H. Raun, D. Persse. 2013. A case-crossover analysis of out-of-hospital cardiac arrest and air pollution. *Circulation* 127:1192–1199.
557. Forastiere, F. et al. 2005. A case-crossover analysis of out-of-hospital coronary deaths and air pollution in Rome, Italy. *Am. J. Respir. Crit. Care Med.* 172:1549–1555.
558. Levy, D., L. Sheppard, H. Checkoway, J. Kaufman, T. Lumley, T. Koenig, D. Siscovick. 2001. A casecrossover analysis of particulate matter air pollution and out-of-hospital primary cardiac arrest. *Epidemiology* 12(2):294–299.
559. Rosenthal, F. S., J. P. Carney, M. L. Olinger. 2008. Out-of-hospital cardiac arrest and airborne fine particulate matter: A case-crossover analysis of emergency medical services data in Indianapolis, Indiana. *Environ. Health Perspect.* 116:631–636.
560. Rosenthal, F. S., M. Kuisma, T. Lanki, T. Hussein, J. Boyd, J. I. Halonen, J. Pekkanen. 2013. Association of ozone and particulate air pollution with out-of-hospital cardiac arrest in Helsinki, Finland: Evidence for two different etiologies. *J. Expo. Sci. Environ. Epidemiol.* 23(3):281–288.
561. Silverman, R. A., K. Ito, J. Freese, B. J. Kaufman, D. De Claro, J. Braun, D. J. Prezant. 2010. Association of ambient fine particles with out-of-hospital cardiac arrests in New York City. *Am. J. Epidemiol.* 172:917–923.
562. Sullivan, J., N. Ishikawa, L. Sheppard, D. Siscovick, H. Checkoway, J. Kaufman. 2003. Exposure to ambient fine particulate matter and primary cardiac arrest among persons with and without clinically recognized heart disease. *Am. J. Epidemiol.* 157:501–509.
563. Wichmann, J., F. Folke, C. Torp-Pedersen, F. Lippert, M. Ketzel, T. Ellermann, S. Loft. 2013. Out-of-hospital cardiac arrests and outdoor air pollution exposure in Copenhagen, Denmark. *PLoS One* 8:e53684.
564. Watkins, A., M. Danilewitz, M. Kusha, S. Masse, B. Urch, K. Quadros, D. Spears, T. Farid, K. Nanthakumar. 2013. Air pollution and arrhythmic risk: The smog is yet to clear. *Can. J. Cardiol.* 29:734–741.
565. Kan, H., G. Heiss, K. M. Rose, E. A. Whitsel, F. Lurmann, S. J. London. 2008. Prospective analysis of traffic exposure as a risk factor for incident coronary heart disease: The atherosclerosis risk in communities (ARIC) study. *Environ. Health Perspect.* 116:1463–1468.
566. Hart, J. E., E. B. Rimm, K. M. Rexrode, F. Laden. 2013. Changes in traffic exposure and the risk of incident myocardial infarction and all-cause mortality. *Epidemiology* 24:734–742.
567. Tonne, C., S. Melly, M. Mittleman, B. Coull, R. Goldberg, J. Schwartz. 2007. A case-control analysis of exposure to traffic and acute myocardial infarction. *Environ. Health Perspect.* 115:53–57.
568. Beelen, R., G. Hoek, P. A. van den Brandt, R. A. Goldbohm, P. Fischer, L. J. Schouten, M. Jerrett, E. Hughes, B. Armstrong, B. Brunekreef. 2008. Long-term effects of traffic-related air pollution on mortality in a Dutch cohort (NLCS-air study). *Environ. Health Perspect.* 116:196–202.

569. Teng, T. H., T. A. Williams, A. Bremner, H. Tohira, P. Franklin, A. Tonkin, I. Jacobs, J. Finn. 2014. A systematic review of air pollution and incidence of out-of-hospital cardiac arrest. *J. Epidemiol. Community Health* 68:37–43.

570. Raza, A., T. Bellander, G. Bero-Bedada, M. Dahlquist, J. Hollenberg, M. Jonsson, T. Lind, M. Rosenqvist, L. Svensson, P. L. Ljungman. 2014. Short-term effects of air pollution on out-of-hospital cardiac arrest in stockholm. *Eur. Heart J.* 35:861–868.

571. Peters, A. et al. 2000. Air pollution and risk incidence of cardiac arrhythmia. *Epidemiology* 11:11–17.

572. Rich, D. Q., M. H. Kim, J. R. Turner, M. A. Mittleman, J. Schwartz, P. J. Catalano, D. W. Dockery. 2006. Association of ventricular arrhythmias detected by implantable cardioverter defibrillator and ambient air pollutants in the St Louis, Missouri metropolitan area. *Occup. Environ. Med.* 63:591–596.

573. Rosenlund, M., S. Picciotto, F. Forastiere, M. Stafoggia, C. A. Perucci. 2008. Traffic-related air pollution in relation to incidence and prognosis of coronary heart disease. *Epidemiology* 19(1):121–128.

574. Rosenlund, M., N. Berglind, G. Pershagen, J. Hallqvist, T. Jonson, T. Bellander. 2006. Long-term exposure to urban air pollution and myocardial infarction. *Epidemiology* 17:383–390.

575. Albert, C. M., B. A. McGovern, J. B. Newell, J. N. Ruskin. 1996. Sex differences in cardiac arrest survivors. *Circulation* 93(6):1170–1176.

576. Chugh, S. S., A. Uy-Evanado, C. Teodorescu, K. Reinier, R. Mariani, K. Gunson, J. Jui. 2009. Women have a lower prevalence of structural heart disease as a precursor to sudden cardiac arrest: The Ore-SUDS (oregon sudden unexpected death study). *J. Am. Coll. Cardiol.* 54:2006–2011.

577. Chugh, S. S., K. Chung, Z. J. Zheng, B. John, J. L. Titus. 2003. Cardiac pathologic findings reveal a high rate of sudden cardiac death of undetermined etiology in younger women. *Am. Heart J.* 146:635–639.

578. Spain, D. M., V. A. Bradess, C. Mohr. 1960. Coronary atherosclerosis as a cause of unexpected and unexplained death. An autopsy study from 1949–1959. *JAMA* 174:384–388.

579. Fishman, G. I. et al. 2010. Sudden cardiac death prediction and prevention: Report from a national heart, lung, and blood institute and heart rhythm society workshop. *Circulation* 122:2335–2348.

580. Brook, R. D. et al. 2010. Particulate matter air pollution and cardiovascular disease: An update to the scientific statement from the American heart association. *Circulation* 121:2331–2378.

581. Van Hee, V. C., S. D. Adar, A. A. Szpiro, R. G. Barr, D. A. Bluemke, A. V. Diez Roux, E. A. Gill, L. Sheppard, J. D. Kaufman. 2009. Exposure to traffic and left ventricular mass and function: The multiethnic study of atherosclerosis. *Am. J. Respir. Crit. Care Med.* 179:827–834.

582. Hoffmann, B. et al. 2007. Residential exposure to traffic is associated with coronary atherosclerosis. *Circulation* 116:489–496.

583. Babisch, W. 2014. Updated exposure-response relationship between road traffic noise and coronary heart diseases: A meta-analysis. *Noise Health* 16:1–9.

584. Chiuve, S. E., T. T. Fung, K. M. Rexrode, D. Spiegelman, J. E. Manson, M. J. Stampfer, C. M. Albert. 2011. Adherence to a low-risk, healthy lifestyle and risk of sudden cardiac death among women. *JAMA* 306:62–69.

585. US Environmental Protection Agency Office of Transportation and Air Quality (OTAQ). 2014. Near roadway air pollution and health.

586. Yorifuji, T., E. Suzuki, S. Kashima. 2014. Cardiovascular emergency hospital visits and hourly changes in air pollution. *Stroke* 45:1264–1268.

587. Myeburg, R., A. Castellanos. 2012. Cardiovascular collapse, cardiac arrest, and sudden cardiac death. In *Harrison's Principles of Internal Medicine*. A. Fauci, E. Braunwald, D. Kasper et al., Eds., pp. 1707–1713. New York, NY: McGraw-Hill.

588. Teng, T. H., T. A. Williams, A. Bremner, H. Tohira, P. Franklin, A. Tonkin, I. Jacobs, J. Finn. 2014. A systematic review of air pollution and incidence of out-of-hospital cardiac arrest. *J. Epidemiol. Community Health* 68:37–43.

589. Rea, W. J., A. R. Johnson, G. H. Ross, J. R. Butler, E. J. Fenyves, B. Griffiths, J. Laseter. 1992. Considerations for the diagnosis of chemical sensitivity. *Multiple Chemical Sensitivities*. https://www.nap.edu/catalog/1988/multiple-chemical-tivities: Addendum to Biologic Markers in Immunotoxicology.

590. Straney, L., J. Finn, M. Dennekamp, A. Bremner, A. Tonkin, I. Jacobs. 2014. Evaluating the impact of air pollution on the incidence of out-of-hospital cardiac arrest in the Perth Metropolitan Region: 2000–2010. *J. Epidemiol. Community Health* 68:6–12.

591. HEI International Scientific Oversight Committee. 2010. *Outdoor Air Pollution and Health in the Developing Countries of Asia: A Comprehensive Review.* Special Report 18. Boston, MA: The Health Effects Institute.

592. Yorifuji, T., E. Suzuki, S. Kashima. 2014. Outdoor air pollution and out-of-hospital cardiac arrest in Okayama, Japan. *J. Occup. Environ. Med.* 56(10):1019–1023.

593. Ito, K., G. D. Thurston, R. A. Silverman. 2007. Characterization of PM2.5, gaseous pollutants, and meteorological interactions in the context of time-series health effects models. *J. Expo. Sci. Environ. Epidemiol.* 17(Suppl. 2):S45–S60.

594. World Health Organization. 2006. *Air Quality Guidelines: Global Update 2005: Particulate Matter, Ozone, Nitrogen Dioxide, and Sulfur Dioxide.* Copenhagen, Denmark: World Health Organization.

595. Armstrong, B. G. 1998. Effect of measurement error on epidemiological studies of environmental and occupational exposures. *Occup. Environ. Med.* 55:651–656.

596. Dockery, D. W., H. Luttmann-Gibson, D. Q. Rich, M. L. Link, M. A. Mittleman, D. R. Gold, P. Koutrakis, J. D. Schwartz, R. L. Verrier. 2005. Association of air pollution with increased incidence of ventricular tachyarrhythmias recorded by implanted cardioverter defibrillators. *Environ. Health Perspect.* 113:670–674.

597. Pope, C. A., R. L. Verrier, E. G. Lovett, A. C. Larson, M. E. Raizenne, R. E. Kanner, J. Schwartz, G. M. Villegas, D. R. Gold, D. W. Dockery. 1999. Heart rate variability associated with particulate air pollution. *Am. Heart J.* 138:890–899.

598. Park, S. K., M. S. O'Neill, P. S. Vokonas, D. Sparrow, J. Schwartz. 2005. Effects of air pollution on heart rate variability: The VA Normative Aging Study. *Environ. Health Perspect.* 113:304–309.

599. De Paula Santos, U., A. L. Braga, D. M. Giorgi, C. J. Grupi, C. A. Li, M. A. Bussacos, D. M. Zanetta, P. H. do Nascimento Saldiva, M. T. Filho. 2005. Effects of air pollution on blood pressure and heart rate variability: A panel study of vehicular traffic controllers in the city of Sao Paulo, Brazil. *Eur. Heart J.* 26:193–200.

600. Curtis, L., W. J. Rea, P. Smith-Willis, E. Fenyves, and Y. Pan. 2006. Adverse health effects of outdoor air pollutants. *Environ. Int.* 32:815–830.

601. Henneberger, A., W. Zareba, A. Ibald-Mulli, R. Rückert, J. Cyrys, J. P. Couderc, B. Mykins, G. Woelke, H.-E. Wichmann, A. Peters. 2005. Repolarization changes induced by air pollution in ischemic heart disease patients. *Environ. Health Perspect.* 113:440–446.

602. Gold, D. R. et al. 2005. Air pollution and ST-segment depression in elderly subjects. *Environ. Health Perspect.* 113:883–887.

603. Suwa, T., J. C. Hogg, K. B. Quinlan, A. Ohgami, R. Vincent, S. F. Van Eeden. 2002. Particulate air pollution induces progression of atherosclerosis. *J. Am. Coll. Cardiol.* 39:935–942.

604. Kunzli, N., M. Jerrett, W. J. Mack, B. Beckerman, L. LaBree, F. Gilliland, D. Thomas, J. Peters, H. N. Hodis. 2005. Ambient air pollution and atherosclerosis in Los Angeles. *Environ. Health Perspect.* 113:201–206.

605. Brook, R. D., J. R. Brook, B. Urch, R. Vincent, S. Rajagopalan, F. Silverman. 2002. Inhalation of fine particulate matter and ozone causes acute arterial vasoconstriction in healthy adults. *Circulation* 105:1534–1536.

606. Peters, A., A. Doring, H. E. Wichmann, W. Koenig. 1997. Increased plasma viscosity during an air pollution episode: A link to mortality. *Lancet* 349:1582–1587.

607. Peters, A., M. Froehlich, A. Doring, T. Immervoll, H. E. Wichmann, W. L. Hutchinson, M. B. Pepys, W. Koenig. 2001. Particulate air pollution is associated with an acute phase response in men: Results from the MONICA–Augsburg Study. *Eur. Heart J.* 22(14):1198–1204.

608. Rea, W. J., K. Patel. 2010. *Reversibility of Chronic Degenerative Disease and Hypersensitivity*, Vol. 1. Boca Raton, FL: CRC Press.

609. Jammes, Y., J. G. Steinberg, O. Mambrini, F. Bregeon, S. Delliaux. 2005. Chronic fatigue syndrome: Assessment of increased oxidative stress and altered muscle excitability in response to incremental exercise. *J. Intern. Med.* 257:299–310.

610. Przyklenk, K., Y. Dong, V. V. Undyala, P. Whittaker. 2012. Autophagy as a therapeutic target for ischaemia/reperfusion injury? Concepts, controversies, and challenges. *Cardiovasc. Res.* 94:197–205.

611. Jennings, R. B. 2013. Historical perspective on the pathology of myocardial ischemia/reperfusion injury. *Circ. Res.* 113:428–438.

612. Ma, H., R. Guo, L. Yu, Y. Zhang, J. Ren. 2011. Aldehyde dehydrogenase 2 (ALDH2) rescues myocardial ischaemia/reperfusion injury: Role of autophagy paradox and toxic aldehyde. *Eur. Heart J.* 32:1025–1038.

613. Zhang, Y., J. Ren. 2014. Targeting autophagy for the therapeutic application of histone deacetylase inhibitors in ischemia/reperfusion heart injury. *Circulation* 129:1088–1091.

614. Choi, A. M., S. W. Ryter, B. Levine. 2013. Autophagy in human health and disease. *N. Engl. J. Med.* 368:651–662.

615. Lavandero, S., R. Troncoso, B. A. Rothermel, W. Martinet, J. Sadoshima, J. A. Hill. 2013. Cardiovascular autophagy: Concepts, controversies and perspectives. *Autophagy* 9:1455–1466.

616. Hariharan, N., P. Zhai, J. Sadoshima. 2011. Oxidative stress stimulates autophagic flux during ischemia/reperfusion. *Antioxid. Redox Signal* 14:2179–2190.

617. Ma, X., H. Liu, S. R. Foyil, R. J. Godar, C. J. Weinheimer, J. A. Hill, A. Diwan. 2012. Impaired autophagosome clearance contributes to cardiomyocyte death in ischemia/reperfusion injury. *Circulation* 125:3170–3181.

618. Shiomi, M., M. Miyamae, G. Takemura, K. Kaneda, Y. Inamura, A. Onishi, S. Koshinuma, Y. Momota, T. Minami, V. M. Figueredo. 2013. Sevoflurane induces cardioprotection through reactive oxygen species-mediated upregulation of autophagy in isolated guinea pig hearts. *J. Anesth.* 28:593–600. doi: 10.1007/ss00540-013-1755-9. http://link.springer.com/article/10.1007%2Fs00540-013-1755-9. Accessed December 18, 2013.

619. Cao, X., A. Chen, P. Yang, X. Song, Y. Liu, Z. Li, X. Wang, L. Wang, Y. Li. 2013. Alpha-lipoic acid protects cardiomyocytes against hypoxia/ reoxygenation injury by inhibiting autophagy. *Biochem. Biophys. Res. Commun.* 441:935–940.

620. Xie, M. et al. 2014. Histone deacetylase inhibition blunts ischemia/reperfusion injury by inducing cardiomyocyte autophagy. *Circulation* 129:1139–1151.

621. Granger, A., I. Abdullah, F. Huebner, A. Stout, T. Wang, T. Huebner, J. A. Epstein, P. J. Gruber. 2008. Histone deacetylase inhibition reduces myocardial ischemia-reperfusion injury in mice. *FASEB J.* 22:3549–3560.

622. Kong, Y., P. Tannous, G. Lu, K. Berenji, B. A. Rothermel, E. N. Olson, J. A. Hill. 2006. Suppression of class I and II histone deacetylases blunts pressure-overload cardiac hypertrophy. *Circulation* 113:2579–2588.

623. Xie, M., J. A. Hill. 2013. HDAC-dependent ventricular remodeling. *Trends Cardiovasc. Med.* 23:229–235.

624. Zhao, T. C., G. Cheng, L. X. Zhang, Y. T. Tseng, J. F. Padbury. 2007. Inhibition of histone deacetylases triggers pharmacologic preconditioning effects against myocardial ischemic injury. *Cardiovasc. Res.* 76:473–481.

625. Cao, D. J., Z. V. Wang, P. K. Battiprolu, N. Jiang, C. R. Morales, Y. Kong, B. A. Rothermel, T. G. Gillette, J. A. Hill. 2011. Histone deacetylase (HDAC) inhibitors attenuate cardiac hypertrophy by suppressing autophagy. *Proc. Natl. Acad. Sci. U.S.A.* 108:4123–4128.

626. McKinsey, T. A. 2012. Therapeutic potential for HDAC inhibitors in the heart. *Annu. Rev. Pharmacol. Toxicol.* 52:303–319.

627. Bush, E. W., T. A. McKinsey. 2010. Protein acetylation in the cardiorenal axis: The promise of histone deacetylase inhibitors. *Circ. Res.* 106:272–284.

628. McKinsey, T. A. 2011. Isoform-selective HDAC inhibitors: Closing in on translational medicine for the heart. *J. Mol. Cell Cardiol.* 51:491–496.

629. Kao, Y. H., J. P. Liou, C. C. Chung, G. S. Lien, C. C. Kuo, S. A. Chen, Y. J. Chen. 2013. Histone deacetylase inhibition improved cardiac functions with direct antifibrotic activity in heart failure. *Int. J. Cardiol.* 168:4178–4183.

630. Tao, H., K. H. Shi, J. J. Yang, C. Huang, H. Y. Zhan, J. Li. 2013. Histone deacetylases in cardiac fibrosis: Current perspectives for therapy. *Cell Signal* 26:521–527.

631. Lane, S. E., R. A. Watts, L. Bentham, N. J. Innes, D. G. I. Scott. 2003. Are environmental factors important in primary systemic vasculitis? A case-control study. *Arthritis Rheum.* 48:814–823.

632. Brautbar, N., E. D. Richter, G. Nesher. 2004. Systemic vasculitis and prior recent exposure to organic solvents: Report of two cases. *Arch. Environ. Health* 59:515–517.

633. Inoue, T. et al. 2004. A case of MPO-ANCA-related vasculitis after asbestos exposure with progression of a renal lesion after improvement of interstitial pneumonia. *Nihon Kokyuki Gakkai Zasshi* 42(6):496–501.

634. Tervaert, J. W., C. A. Stegeman, C. G. Kallenberg. 1998. Silicon exposure and vasculitis. *Curr. Opin. Rheumatol.* 10(1):12–17.

635. Stratta, P. et al. 2001. The role of metals in autoimmune vasculitis: Epidemiological and pathogenic study. *Sci. Total Environ.* 270(1–3):179–190.

636. Duell, P. B. 1987. Henoch-Schonlein Purpura following Thiram Exposure. *Arch. Intern. Med.* 147(4):778–779.

637. Nakamura, S. 1997. The role of nitric oxide in mercury chloride-induced vasculitis in the brown norway rat. *Nihon Jinzo Gakkai Shi* 39(5):447–454.

638. Randolph, T. E. 1962. *Human Ecology and Susceptibility to the Chemical Environment.* Springfield, IL: Charles C Thomas.

639. Parish, W. R. 1971. Studies on vasculitis, immunoglobulins, 1C, C-reactive proteins, and bacterial antigens in cutaneous vasculitis lesions. *Clin. Allergy* 1:97–109.

640. Theorell, H., M. Blombock, C. Kockum. 1976. Demonstration of reactivity to airborne and food allergens in cutaneous vasculitis by variations in fibrinopeptide A and others blood coagulation, fibrinolysis and complement parameters. *Thrombo. Haemost.* 36:593.

641. Hare, F. 1905. *The Food Factor in Disease.* Chapter 10. London: Longmans.

642. Harkavy, J. 1963. *Vascular Allergy and Its Systemic Manifestations.* Washington: Butterworths.

643. Taylor, G. J., W. S. Hern. 1970. Cardiac arrhythmias due to aerosol propellents. *JAMA* 214(1):81–85.

644. Yervick, P. Oil pollutants in marine life. Eighth Advanced Seminar, Society of Clinical Ecology, Instatape, Tape II.

645. Nour-Elden, R. 1970. Uptake of phenol by vascular and brain tissue. *Microvasc. Res.* 2:224–225.

646. Steward, R. D., C. L. Hake. 1976. Paint-remover hazard. *JAMA* 235:398–401.

647. Willeke, K. and Whitby, K. T. 1975. Atmospheric aerosols: Size distribution interpretation. *J. Air Poll. Control Assoc.* 25:529.

648. Poehlmann, H. C. 1969. General aspects of outgassing & contamination. In *Proceedings of the Symposium on Long Life Hardware for Space.* Huntsville, AL, Vol. 2.

649. Patterson, R., M. Roberts, R. Roberts, D. Emanul, Franks J. 1976. Antibodies of different immunoglobulins. Classes against antigens causing Farmers Lung. *Am. Rev. Resp. Dis.* 114:315.

650. Garner, F. H., L. K. Diamond. 1955. Autoerythrocyte sensitization; a form of purpura producing painful bruising following autosensitization to red blood cell in certain women. *Blood* 10:675–690.

651. Leibe, H., C. H. Almag, S. Kaufman, H. Edery. 1972. Possible role of bradykinins in a patient with recurrent ecchymosis (DNA sensitization). *Isr. J. Med Sci.* 8:67–74.

652. Tsai, S. S., W. B. Goggins, H.-F. Chiu, C. Y. Yang. 2003. Evidence for an association between air pollution and daily stroke admissions in Kaohsiung, Taiwan. *Stroke* 34(11):2612–2616.

653. Wellenius, G. A., J. Schwartz, M. A. Mittleman. 2005. Air pollution and hospital admissions for ischemic and hemorrhagic stroke among medicare beneficiaries. *Stroke* 36(12):2549–2553.

654. Wellenius, G. A., M. R. Burger, B. A. Coull, J. Schwartz, H. H. Suh, P. Koutrakis, G. Schlaug, D. R. Gold, M. A. Mittleman. 2012. Ambient air pollution and the risk of acute ischemic stroke. *Arch. Intern. Med.* 172(3):229–234.

655. Gold, D. R., A. Litonjua, J. Schwartz, E. Lovett, A. Larson, B. Nearing, G. Allen, M. Verrier, R. Cherry, R. Verrier. 2000. Ambient pollution and heart rate variability. *Circulation* 101(11):1267–1273.

656. Pope, C. A. 3rd, M. L. Hansen, R. W. Long, K. R. Nielsen, N. L. Eatough, W. E. Wilson, D. J. Eatough. 2004. Ambient particulate air pollution, heart rate variability, and blood markers of inflammation in a panel of elderly subjects. *Environ. Health Perspect.* 112(3):339–345.

657. O'Neill, M. S., A. Veves, A. Zanobetti, J. A. Sarnat, D. R. Gold, P. A. Economides, E. S. Horton, J. Schwartz. 2004. Diabetes enhances vulnerability to particulate air pollution-associated impairment in vascular reactivity and endothelial function. *Circulation* 111(22):2913–2920.

658. Ruckerl, R., A. Ibald-Mulli, W. Koenig, A. Schneider, G. Woelke, J. Cyrys, J. Heinrich, V. Marder, M. Frampto, H. E. Wichmann, A. Peters. 2006. Air pollution and markers of inflammation and coagulation in patients with coronary heart disease. *Am. J. Respir. Crit. Care Med.* 173(4):432–441.

659. Brook, R. D. et al. 2009. Insights into the mechanisms and mediators of the effects of air pollution exposure on blood pressure and vascular function in healthy humans. *Hypertension* 54(3):659–667.

660. Costa, D. 2011. Air quality in a changing climate. *Environ. Health Perspect.* 119(4):154–155.

661. Hong, Y., J. Lee, H. Kim, E. Ha, J. Schwartz, D. C. Christiani. 2002. Effects of air pollutants on acute stroke mortality. *Environ. Health Perspect.* 110(2):187–191.

662. Kettunen, J., T. Lanki, P. Tiittanen, P. P. Aalto, T. Koskentalo, M. Kulmala, V. Salomaa, J. Pekkanen. 2007. Associations of fine and ultrafine particulate air pollution with stroke mortality in an area of low air pollution levels. *Stroke* 38(3):918–922.

663. Pope, C. A. III, D. W. Dockery. 1999. Epidemiology of particle effects. In *Air Pollution and Health*, S. T. Holgate, H. S. Koren, J. M. Samet, R. L. Maynard, Eds., pp. 673–705. London: Academic Press.

664. U.S. EPA. 2004. *Air Quality Criteria for Particulate Matter.* Washington, DC: U.S. Environmental Protection Agency.

665. Chuang, K. J., C. C. Chan, T. C. Su, C. T. Lee, C. S. Tang. 2007. The effect of urban air pollution on inflammation, oxidative stress, coagulation, and autonomic dysfunction in young adults. *Am. J. Respir. Crit. Care Med.* 176:370–376.

666. Zanobetti, A., J. Schwartz. 2007. Particulate air pollution, progression, and survival after myocardial infarction. *Environ. Health Perspect.* 115:769–775.

667. Delfino, R. J., C. Sioutas, S. Malik. 2005. Potential role of ultrafine particles in associations between airborne particle mass and cardiovascular health. *Environ. Health Perspect.* 113:934–946.

668. Tsuji H., M. G. Larson, F. J. Venditti Jr., E. S. Manders, J. C. Evans, C. L. Feldman, D. Levy. 1996. Impact of reduced heart rate variability on risk for cardiac events. The Framingham Heart Study. *Circulation* 94:2850–2855.

669. Kop W.J., R. J. Verdino, J. S. Gottdiener, S. T. O'Leary, C. N. Bairey Merz, D. S. Krantz. 2001. Changes in heart rate and heart rate variability before ambulatory ischemic events. *J. Am. Coll. Cardiol.* 38:742–749.

670. Bettoni, M., M. Zimmermann. 2002. Autonomic tone variations before the onset of paroxysmal atrial fibrillation. *Circulation* 105:2753–2759.

671. Anderson, J. L. et al.; American College of Cardiology; American Heart Association Task Force on Practice Guidelines (Writing Committee to Revise the 2002 Guidelines for the Management of Patients With Unstable Angina/Non-ST-Elevation Myocardial Infarction); American College of Emergency Physicians; Society for Cardiovascular Angiography and Interventions; Society of Thoracic Surgeons; American Association of Cardiovascular and Pulmonary Rehabilitation; Society for Academic Emergency Medicine. 2007. ACC/AHA 2007 guidelines for the management of patients with unstable angina/ non ST-elevation myocardial infarction: A report of the American College of Cardiology/American Heart Association Task Force on Practice Guidelines. *Circulation* 116:e148–e304.

672. Riediker, M., R. B. Devlin, T. R. Griggs, M. C. Herbst, P. A. Bromberg, R. W. Williams, W. E Cascio. 2004. Cardiovascular effects in patrol officers are associated with fine particulate matter from brake wear and engine emissions. *Part. Fibre Toxicol.* (1):2. doi: 10.1186/1743-8977-1-2 [Online December 9, 2004].

673. Zanobetti, A., D. R. Gold, P. H. Stone, H. H. Suh, J. Schwartz, B. A. Coull, F. E. Speizer. 2009. Reduction in heart rate variability with traffic and air pollution in patients with coronary artery disease. *Environ. Health Perspect.* 118(3):324–330.

674. Adar, S. D., D. R. Gold, B. A. Coull, J. Schwartz, P. H. Stone, H. Suh. 2007. Focused exposures to airborne traffic particles and heart rate variability in the elderly. *Epidemiology* 18:95–103.

675. Schwartz, J. et al. 2005. Traffic related pollution and heart rate variability in a panel of elderly subjects. *Thorax* 60:455–461.

676. Zanobetti, A., P. H, Stone, F. E, Speizer, J. Schwartz, B. A. Coull, B. C. Nearing, H. H. Suh, M. A. Mittleman, R. L. Verrier, D. R. Gold. 2009. T-wave alternans, air pollution and traffic in high-risk subjects. *Am. J. Cardiol.* 104(5):665–670.

677. Adamkiewicz, G., S. Ebelt, M. Syring, J. Slater, F. E. Speizer, J. Schwartz, H. Suh, D. R. Gold. 2004. Association between air pollution exposure and exhaled nitric oxide in an elderly population. *Thorax* 59:204–209.

678. Adar, S. D., G. Adamkiewicz, D. R. Gold, J. Schwartz, B. A. Coull, H. Suh. 2007. Ambient and micro-environmental particles and exhaled nitric oxide before and after a group bus trip. *Environ. Health Perspect.* 115:507–512.

679. Creason, J., L. Neas, D. Walsh, R. Williams, L. Sheldon, D. Liao, C. Shy. 2001. Particulate matter and heart rate variability among elderly retirees: The Baltimore 1998 PM study. *J. Expo. Anal. Environ. Epidemiol.* 11:116–122.

680. Holguin, F., M. M. Tellez-Rojo, M. Hernandez, M. Cortez, J. C. Chow, J. G. Watson, D. Mannino, I. Romieu. 2003. Air pollution and heart rate variability among the elderly in Mexico City. *Epidemiology* 14:521–527.

681. Liao, D., Y. Duan, E. A. Whitsel, Z. J. Zheng, G. Heiss, V. M. Chinchilli, H. M. Lin. 2004. Association of higher levels of ambient criteria pollutants with impaired cardiac autonomic control: A population-based study. *Am. J. Epidemiol.* 159:768–777.

682. Lipsett, M. J., F. C. Tsai, L. Roger, M. Woo, B. D. Ostro. 2006. Coarse particles and heart rate variability among older adults with coronary artery disease in the Coachella Valley, California. *Environ. Health Perspect.* 114:1215–1220.

683. Timonen, K. L. et al. 2006. Effects of ultrafine and fine particulate and gaseous air pollution on cardiac autonomic control in subjects with coronary artery disease: The ULTRA study. *J. Expo. Sci. Environ. Epidemiol.* 16:332–341.

684. Lombardi, F., A. Porta, M. Marzegalli, S. Favale, M. Santini, A. Vincenti, A. De Rosa; Implantable Cardioverter Defibrillator-Heart Rate Variability Italian Study Group. 2000. Heart rate variability patterns before ventricular tachycardia onset in patients with an implantable cardioverter defibrillator. Participating Investigators of ICD-HRV Italian Study Group. *Am. J. Cardiol.* 86:959–963.

685. Monmeneu, J. V., F. J. Chorro, V. Bodi, J. Sanchis, A. Llacer, R. GarciaCivera, R. Ruiz, R. Sanjuán, M. Burguera, V. López-Merino. 2001. Relationships between heart rate variability, functional capacity, and left ventricular function following myocardial infarction: An evaluation after one week and six months. *Clin. Cardiol.* 24:313–320.

686. Shusterman, V., B. Aysin, R. Weiss, S. Brode, V. Gottipaty, D. Schwartzman, K. P. Anderson. 2000. Dynamics of low-frequency R-R interval oscillations preceding spontaneous ventricular tachycardia. *Am. Heart J.* 139:126–133.

687. de Bruyne, M. C., J. A. Kors, A. W. Hoes, P. Klootwijk, J. M. Dekker, A. Hofman, J. H. van Bemmel, D. E. Grobbee. 1999. Both decreased and increased heart rate variability on the standard 10-second electrocardiogram predict cardiac mortality in the elderly: The Rotterdam Study. *Am. J. Epidemiol.* 150:1282–1288.

688. Chuang, K. J., B. A. Coull, A. Zanobetti, H. Suh, J. Schwartz, P. H. Stone, A. Litonjua, F. E. Speizer, D. R. Gold. 2008. Particulate air pollution as a risk factor for ST-segment depression in patients with coronary artery disease. *Circulation* 118:1314–1320.

689. Dubowsky, S. D., H. Suh, J. Schwartz, B. A. Coull, D. R. Gold. 2006. Diabetes, obesity, and hypertension may enhance associations between air pollution and markers of systemic inflammation. *Environ. Health Perspect.* 114:992–998.

690. O'Neill, M. S., A. Veves, J. A. Sarnat, A. Zanobetti, D. R. Gold, P. A. Economides, E. S. Horton, J. Schwartz. 2007. Air pollution and inflammation in type 2 diabetes: A mechanism for susceptibility. *J. Occup. Environ. Med.* 64:373–379.

691. O'Neill, M. S., A. Veves, A. Zanobetti, J. A. Sarnat, D. R. Gold, P. A. Economides, E. S. Horton, J. Schwartz. 2005. Diabetes enhances vulnerability to particulate air pollution-associated impairment in vascular reactivity and endothelial function. *Circulation* 111:2913–2920.

692. Zanobetti, A., J. Schwartz. 2001. Are diabetics more susceptible to the health effects of airborne particles? *Am. J. Respir. Crit. Care Med.* 164:831–833.

693. Albert, C. M., L. Rosenthal, H. Calkins, J. S. Steinberg, J. N. Ruskin, P. Wang, J. E. Muller, M. A. Mittleman; TOVA Investigators. 2007. Driving and implantable cardioverterdefibrillator shocks for ventricular arrhythmias: Results from the TOVA study. *J. Am. Coll. Cardiol.* 50:2233–2240.

694. Rea, W. J., Y. Pan, A. R. Johnson, G. H. Ross, H. Suyama, E. J. Fenyves. 1996. Reduction of chemical sensitivity by means of heat depuration, physical therapy, and nutritional supplementation in a controlled environment. *J. Nutr. Environ. Med.* 6(2):141–148.

695. Analitis, A. et al. 2008. Effects of cold weather on mortality: Results from 15 European cities within the PHEWE project. *Am. J. Epidemiol.* 168:1397–1408.

696. Pope, C. A. 3rd, D. W. Dockery. 2006. Health effects of fine particulate air pollution: Lines that connect. *J. Air Waste Manag. Assoc.* 56:709–742.

697. Peters, A., S. Perz, A. Doring, J. Stieber, W. Koenig, H. E. Wichmann. 1999. Increases in heart rate during an air pollution episode. *Am. J. Epidemiol.* 150:1094–1098.

698. Luttmann-Gibson, H., H. H. Suh, B. A. Coull, D. W. Dockery, S. E. Sarnat, J. Schwartz, P. H. Stone, D. R. Gold. 2006. Short-term effects of air pollution on heart rate variability in senior adults in Steubenville, Ohio. *J. Occup. Environ. Med.* 48:780–788.

699. Pekkanen, J. et al. 2002. Particulate air pollution and risk of ST-segment depression during repeated submaximal exercise tests among subjects with coronary heart disease: The Exposure and Risk Assessment for Fine and Ultrafine Particles in Ambient Air (ULTRA) study. *Circulation* 106:933–938.

700. Berger, A., W. Zareba, A. Schneider, R. Rückerl, A. Ibald-Mulli, J. Cyrys, H. E. Wichmann, A. Peters. 2006. Runs of ventricular and supraventricular tachycardia triggered by air pollution in patients with coronary heart disease. *J. Occup. Environ. Med.* 48:1149–1158.

701. Alpérovitch, A., J. M. Lacombe, O. Hanon, J. F. Dartigues, K. Ritchie, P. Ducimetiere, C. Tzourio. 2009. Relationship between blood pressure and outdoor temperature in a large sample of elderly individuals: The three-city study. *Arch. Intern. Med.* 169:75–80.

702. Pääkkönen, T., J. Leppäluoto. 2002. Cold exposure and hormonal secretion: A review. *Int. J. Circumpolar Health* 61:265–276.

703. Roden, D. M. 2008. Keep the QT interval: It is a reliable predictor of ventricular arrhythmias. *Heart Rhythm* 5:1213–1215.

704. Greenland, P., X. Xie, K. Liu, L. Colangelo, Y. Liao, M. L. Daviglus, A. N. Agulnek, J. Stamler. 2003. Impact of minor electrocardiographic ST-segment and/or T-wave abnormalities on cardiovascular mortality during long-term follow-up. *Am. J. Cardiol.* 91:1068–1074.

705. Ghelfi, E., C. R. Rhoden, G. A. Wellenius, J. Lawrence, B. Gonzalez-Flecha. 2008. Cardiac oxidative stress and electrophysiological changes in rats exposed to concentrated ambient particles are mediated by TRP-dependent pulmonary reflexes. *Toxicol. Sci.* 102:328–336.

706. Zareba, W., J. P. Couderc, G. Oberdörster, D. Chalupa, C. Cox, L. S. Huang, A. Peters, M. J. Utell, M. W. Frampton. 2009. ECG parameters and exposure to carbon ultrafine particles in young healthy subjects. *Inhal. Toxicol.* 21:223–233.

707. Hampel, R. et al. Altered cardiac repolarization in association with air pollution and air temperature among myocardial infarction survivors. *Environ. Health Perspect.* 118(12):1755–1761.

708. Bednar, M. M., E. P. Harrigan, R. J. Anziano, A. J. Camm, J. N. Ruskin. 2001. The QT interval. *Prog. Cardiovasc. Dis.* 43:1–45.

709. Pfeufer, A. et al. 2009. Common variants at ten loci modulate the QT interval duration in the QTSCD Study. *Nat. Genet.* 41:407–414.

710. de Hartog, J. J. et al. 2009. Associations between PM2.5 and heart rate variability are modified by particle composition and beta-blocker use in patients with coronary heart disease. *Environ. Health Perspect.* 117:105–111.

711. Chen, J. C., J. M. Cavallari, P. H. Stone, D. C. Christiani. 2007. Obesity is a modifier of autonomic cardiac responses to fine metal particulates. *Environ. Health Perspect.* 115:1002–1006.

712. Liao, D., M. L. Shaffer, S. Rodriguez-Colon, F. He, X. Li, D. L. Wolbrette, J. Yanosky, W. E. Cascio. 2010. Acute adverse effects of fine particulate air pollution on ventricular repolarization. *Environ. Health Perspect.* 118:1010–1015.

713. Lux, R. L., C. A. Pope 3rd. 2009. Air pollution effects on ventricular repolarization. *Res. Rep. Health Eff. Inst.* (141):3–28.

714. Goldring, C. E. et al. 2004. Activation of hepatic Nrf2 *in vivo* by acetaminophen in CD-1 mice. *Hepatology* 39:1267–1276.

715. Samet, J. M. et al. 2009. Concentrated ambient ultrafine particle exposure induces cardiac changes in young healthy volunteers. *Am. J. Respir. Crit. Care Med.* 179:1034–1042.

716. Yue, W., A. Schneider, M. Stölzel, R. Rückerl, J. Cyrys, X. Pan, W. Zareba, W. Koenig, H. E. Wichmann, A. Peters. 2007. Ambient source-specific particles are associated with prolonged repolarization and increased levels of inflammation in male coronary artery disease patients. *Mutat. Res.* 621:50–60.

717. Schneider, A., L. M. Neas, D. W. Graff, M. C. Herbst, W. E. Cascio, M. T. Schmitt, J. B. Buse, A. Peters, R. B. Devlin. 2010. Association of cardiac and vascular changes with ambient PM$_{2.5}$ in diabetic individuals. *Part Fibre Toxicol.* 7:14. doi: 10.1186/1743-8977-7-14

718. Stein, P. K., D. Sanghavi, N. Sotoodehnia, D. S. Siscovick, J. Gottdiener. 2010. Association of Holter-based measures including T-wave alternans with risk of sudden cardiac death in the community-dwelling elderly: The Cardiovascular Health Study. *J. Electrocardiol.* 43:251–259.

719. Ziegler, D., C. P. Zentai, S. Perz, W. Rathmann, B. Haastert, A. Doring, C. Meisinger; KORA Study Group. 2008. Prediction of mortality using measures of cardiac autonomic dysfunction in the diabetic and nondiabetic population: The MONICA/KORA Augsburg Cohort Study. *Diabetes Care* 31:556–561.

720. Yamamoto, S., M. Iwamoto, M. Inoue, N. Harada. 2007. Evaluation of the effect of heat exposure on the autonomic nervous system by heart rate variability and urinary catecholamines. *J. Occup. Health* 49:199–204.

721. Bruce-Low, S. S., D. Cotterrell, G. E. Jones. 2006. Heart rate variability during high ambient heat exposure. *Aviat. Space Environ. Med.* 77:915–920.

722. Baccini, M. et al. 2008. Heat effects on mortality in 15 European cities. *Epidemiology* 19:711–719.

723. McMichael, A. J. et al. 2008. International study of temperature, heat and urban mortality: The "ISOTHURM" project. *Int. J. Epidemiol.* 37:1121–1131.

724. Lin, K. B., F. S. Shofer, C. McCusker, E. Meshberg, J. E. Hollander. 2008. Predictive value of T-wave abnormalities at the time of emergency department presentation in patients with potential acute coronary syndromes. *Acad. Emerg. Med.* 15:537–543.

725. Wolf, K., A. Schneider, S. Breitner, S. von Klot, C. Meisinger, J. Cyrys, H. Hymer, H. E. Wichmann, A. Peters; Cooperative Health Research in the Region of Augsburg Study Group. 2009. Air temperature and the occurrence of myocardial infarction in Augsburg, Germany. *Circulation* 120:735–742.

726. Hong, Y. C., J. T. Lee, H. Kim, H. J. Kwon. 2002. Air pollution: A new risk factoring ischemic stroke mortality. *Stroke* 33:2165–2169.

727. Kan, H., B. Chen. 2003. Air pollution and daily mortality in Shanghai: A time course series. *Arch. Environ. Health* 58:360–367.

728. Le Tetre, A. et al. 2002. Short-term effects of particulate air pollution on cardiovascular diseases in eight European cities. *J. Epidemiol. Community Health* 56:773–779.

729. Maheswaran, R., R. P. Haining, P. Brindley, J. Law, T. Pearson, P. R. Fryers, S. Wise, M. J. Campbell. 2005. Outdoor air pollution and stroke in Sheffield, United Kingdom. A small-area level geographic study. *Stroke* 36:239–243.

730. Dickinson, C. J. 2001. Why are strokes related to hypertension? Classic studies and hypotheses revisted. *J. Hypertens.* 19:1515–1521.
731. Kitamura, A. et al. 2006. Proportions of stroke subtypes among men and women > or = 40 years of age in an urban Japanese city in 1992, 1997, and 2002. *Stroke* 37:1374–1378.
732. Fleury C. et al. 1997. Uncoupling protein-2: A novel gene linked to obesity and hyperinsulinemia. *Nat. Genet.* 15:269–272.
733. Brand, M. D., T. C. Esteves. 2005. Physiological functions of the mitochondrial uncoupling proteins UCP2 and UCP3. *Cell Metab.* 2:85–93.
734. Singh, V. K., K. P. Mishra, R. Rani, V. S. Yadav, S. K. Awasthi, S. K. Garg. 2003. Immunomodulation by lead. *Immunol. Res.* 28(2):151–166.
735. Thabut, G. G., G. G. Dauriat, J. B. Stern, D. Logeart, A. Lévy, R. Marrash-Chahla, H. Mal. 2005. Pulmonary hemodynamics in advanced COPD candidates for lung volume reduction surgery or lung transplantation. *Chest* 127:1531–1536.
736. Ghio, S. S., A. A. Gavazzi, C. C. Campana, C. Inserra, C. Klersy, R. Sebastiani, E. Arbustini, F. Recusani, L. Tavazzi. 2001. Independent and additive prognostic value of right ventricular systolic function and pulmonary artery pressure in patients with chronic heart failure. *J. Am. Coll. Cardiol.* 37:183–188.
737. D'Alonzo, G. E. et al. 1991. Survival in patients with primary pulmonary hypertension. Results from a national prospective registry. *Ann. Intern. Med.* 115:343–349.
738. Kawut, S. M. et al. 2012. Right ventricular structure is associated with the risk of heart failure and cardiovascular death: The MESA-Right Ventricle Study. *Circulation* 126:1681–1688.
739. Voelkel, N. F. et al.; National Heart, Lung, and Blood Institute Working Group on Cellular and Molecular Mechanisms of Right Heart Failure. 2006. National Heart, Lung, and Blood Institute Working Group on Cellular and Molecular Mechanisms of Right Heart Failure. Right ventricular function and failure: Report of a National Heart, Lung, and Blood Institute working group on cellular and molecular mechanisms of right heart failure. *Circulation* 114:1883–1891.
740. HEI Panel on the Health Effects of Traffic-Related Air Pollution. 2010 *Traffic related air pollution: A critical review of the literature on emissions, exposure, and health effects.* HEI Special Report 17. Boston, MA: Health Effects Institute.
741. Park, S. K., A. H. Auchincloss, M. S. O'Neill, R. Prineas, J. C. Correa, J. Keeler, R. G. Barr, J. D. Kaufman, A. V. Diez Roux. 2010. Particulate air pollution, metabolic syndrome, and heart rate variability: The multi-ethnic study of atherosclerosis (MESA). *Environ. Health Perspect.* 118:1406–1411.
742. Mills, N. L. et al. 2006. Do inhaled carbon nanoparticles translocate directly into the circulation in humans? *Am. J. Respir. Crit. Care Med.* 173:426–431.
743. Loennechen, J. P., V. Beisvag, I. Arbo, H. L. Waldum, A. K. Sandvik, S. Knardahl, O. Ellingsen. 1999. Chronic carbon monoxide exposure *in vivo* induces myocardial endothelin-1 expression and hypertrophy in rat. *Pharmacol. Toxicol.* 85:192–197.
744. Leary, P. J., J. D. Kaufman, R. G. Barr, D. A. Bluemke, C. L. Curl, C. L. Hough, J. A. Lima, A. A. Szpiro, V. C. Van Hee, S. M. Kawut. 2014. Traffic-related air pollution and the right ventricle. The multi-ethnic study of atherosclerosis. *Am. J. Respir. Crit. Care Med.* 189(9):1093–1100.
745. Leary, P. J., R. G. Barr, J. A. Bluemke, C. L. Hough, J. D. Kaufman, A. A. Szpiro, S. M. Kawut, V. C. Van Hee. 2013. The relationship of roadway proximity and NOx with right ventricular structure and function: The MESA-Right Ventricle and MESA-Air studies. *Am. J. Respir. Crit. Care Med.* 187:A3976.
746. Bild, D. E. et al. 2002. Multi-ethnic study of atherosclerosis: Objectives and design. *Am. J. Epidemiol.* 156:871–881.
747. Kaufman, J. D. et al. 2012. Prospective study of particulate air pollution exposures, subclinical atherosclerosis, and clinical cardiovascular disease: The Multi-Ethnic Study of Atherosclerosis and Air Pollution (MESA Air). *Am. J. Epidemiol.* 176:825–837.
748. Sampson, P. D., A. A. Szpiro, L. Sheppard, J. Lindström, J. D. Kaufman. 2011. Pragmatic estimation of a spatio-temporal air quality model with irregular monitoring data. *Atmos. Environ.* 45:6593–6606.
749. Szpiro, A. A., P. D. Sampson, L. Sheppard, T. Lumley, S. D. Adar, J. D. Kaufman. 2010. Predicting intraurban variation in air pollution concentrations with complex spatiotemporal dependencies. *Environmetrics* 21:606–631.
750. Cohen, M. A. et al. 2009. Approach to estimating participant pollutant exposures in the Multi-Ethnic Study of Atherosclerosis and air pollution (MESA air). *Environ. Sci. Technol.* 43:4687–4693.
751. Chahal, H., C. Johnson, H. Tandri, A. Jain, W. G. Hundley, R. G. Barr, S. M. Kawut, J. A. Lima, D. A. Bluemke. 2010. Relation of cardiovascular risk factors to right ventricular structure and function as determined by magnetic resonance imaging (results from the multi-ethnic study of atherosclerosis). *Am. J. Cardiol.* 106:110–116.

752. Bluemke, D. A., R. A. Kronmal, J. A. Lima, K. Liu, J. Olson, G. L. Burke, A. R. Folsom. 2008. The relationship of left ventricular mass and geometry to incident cardiovascular events: The MESA (MultiEthnic Study of Atherosclerosis) study. *J. Am. Coll. Cardiol.* 2008; 52:2148–2155.
753. Vogel-Claussen, J., J. P. Finn, A. S. Gomes, G. W. Hundley, M. Jerosch-Herold, G. Pearson, S. Sinha, J. A. Lima, D. A. Bluemke. 2006. Left ventricular papillary muscle mass: Relationship to left ventricular mass and volumes by magnetic resonance imaging. *J. Comput. Assist. Tomogr.* 30:426–432.
754. Winter, M. M., F. J. Bernink, M. Groenink, B. J. Bouma, A. P. van Dijk, W. A. Helbing, J. G. Tijssen, B. J. Mulder. 2008. Evaluating the systemic right ventricle by CMR: The importance of consistent and reproducible delineation of the cavity. *J. Cardiovasc. Magn. Reson.* 10:40.
755. Heckbert, S. R., W. Post, G. D. N. Pearson, D. K. Arnett, A. S. Gomes, M. JeroschHerold, W. G. Hundley, J. A. Lima, D. A. Bluemke. 2006. Traditional cardiovascular risk factors in relation to left ventricular mass, volume, and systolic function by cardiac magnetic resonance imaging: The multiethnic study of atherosclerosis. *J. Am. Coll. Cardiol.* 48:2285–2292.
756. Sader S., M. Nian, P. Liu. 2003. Leptin: A novel link between obesity, diabetes, cardiovascular risk, and ventricular hypertrophy. *Circulation* 108:644–646.
757. Leary, P. J., C. E. Kurtz, C. L. Hough, M. P. Waiss, D. D. Ralph, F. H. Sheehan. 2012. Three-dimensional analysis of right ventricular shape and function in pulmonary hypertension. *Pulm. Circ.* 2:34–40.
758. Peretz, A., J. H. Sullivan, D. F. Leotta, C. A. Trenga, F. N. Sands, J. Allen, C. Carlsten, C. W. Wilkinson, E. A. Gill, J. D. Kaufman. 2008. Diesel exhaust inhalation elicits acute vasoconstriction *in vivo. Environ. Health Perspect.* 116:937–942.
759. Pietropaoli, A. P. et al. 2004. Pulmonary function, diffusing capacity, and inflammation in healthy and asthmatic subjects exposed to ultrafine particles. *Inhal. Toxicol.* 16(Suppl. 1):59–72.
760. Scherrer-Crosbie, M., W. Steudel, P. R. Hunziker, G. P. Foster, L. Garrido, N. Liel-Cohen, W. M. Zapol, M. H. Picard. 1998. Determination of right ventricular structure and function in normoxic and hypoxic mice: A transesophageal echocardiographic study. *Circulation* 98:1015–1021.
761. Bogaard, H. J., K. Abe, A. Vonk Noordegraaf, N. F. Voelkel. 2009. The right ventricle under pressure: Cellular and molecular mechanisms of right-heart failure in pulmonary hypertension. *Chest* 135:794–804.
762. Villarreal-Calderon, R. et al. 2012. Intra-city differences in cardiac expression of inflammatory genes and inflammasomes in young urbanites: A pilot study. *J. Toxicol. Pathol.* 25:163–173.
763. Kim, M., S. I. Chang, J. C. Seong, J. B. Holt, T. H. Park, J. H. Ko, J. B. Croft. 2012. Road traffic noise: Annoyance, sleep disturbance, and public health implications. *Am. J. Prev. Med.* 43:353–360.
764. Hansel, N. N., M. C. McCormack, A. J. Belli, E. C. Matsui, R. D. Peng, C. Aloe, L. Paulin, D. L. Williams, G. B. Diette, P. N. Breysse. 2013. In-home air pollution is linked to respiratory morbidity in former smokers with chronic obstructive pulmonary disease. *Am. J. Respir. Crit. Care. Med.* 187:1085–1090.
765. Vonk-Noordegraaf, A., J. T. Marcus, S. Holverda, B. Roseboom, P. E. Postmus. 2005. Early changes of cardiac structure and function in COPD patients with mild hypoxemia. *Chest* 127:1898–1903.
766. Grau, M. et al. 2013. Percent emphysema and right ventricular structure and function: The multi-ethnic study of atherosclerosis-lung and multi-ethnic study of atherosclerosis-right ventricle studies. *Chest* 144:136–144.
767. Zile, M. R., J. S. Gottdiener, S. J. Hetzel, J. J. McMurray, M. Komajda, R. McKelvie, C. F. Baicu, B. M. Massie, P. E. Carson; I-PRESERVE Investigators. 2011. Prevalence and significance of alterations in cardiac structure and function in patients with heart failure and a preserved ejection fraction. *Circulation.* 124:2491–2501.
768. Feigin, V. L., C. M. Lawes, D. A. Bennett, S. L. Barker-Collo, V. Parag. 2009. Worldwide stroke incidence and early case fatality reported in 56 population-based studies: A systematic review. *Lancet Neurol.* 8:355–369.
769. Rothwell, P. M. et al.; Oxford Vascular Study. 2004. Change in stroke incidence, mortality, case-fatality, severity, and risk factors in Oxfordshire, UK from 1981 to 2004 (Oxford Vascular Study). *Lancet* 363:1925–1933.
770. European Society of Cardiology. How Can We Avoid a Stroke Crisis. Working Group Report: Stroke Prevention in Patients with AF. December, 2009. Accessed February 10, 2012. http://www.escardio.org/communities/EHRA/publications/papers-interest/Documents/ehra-stroke-report-recommend-document.pdf
771. Luengo-Fernandez, R., G. S. Yiin, A. M. Gray, P. M. Rothwell. 2013. Population-based study of acute- and long-term care costs after stroke in patients with AF. *Int. J. Stroke* 8:308–314.

772. Frost, L., G. Engholm, S. Johnsen, H. Møller, E. W. Henneberg, S. Husted. 2001. Incident thromboembolism in the aorta and the renal, mesenteric, pelvic, and extremity arteries after discharge from the hospital with a diagnosis of atrial fibrillation. *Arch. Intern. Med.* 161:272–276.

773. Menke, J., L. Lüthje, A. Kastrup, J. Larsen. 2010. Thromboembolism in atrial fibrillation. *Am. J. Cardiol.* 105:502–510.

774. Miyasaka, Y., M. E. Barnes, B. J. Gersh, S. S. Cha, K. R. Bailey, W. P. Abhayaratna, J. B. Seward, T. S. Tsang. 2006. Secular trends in incidence of atrial fibrillation in Olmsted County, Minnesota, 1980 to 2000, and implications on the projections for future prevalence. *Circulation* 114:119–125.

775. Go, A. S., E. M. Hylek, K. A. Phillips, Y. Chang, L. E. Henault, J. V. Selby, D. E. Singer. 2001. Prevalence of diagnosed atrial fibrillation in adults: National implications for rhythm management and stroke prevention: The AnTicoagulation and Risk Factors in Atrial Fibrillation (ATRIA) Study. *JAMA* 285(18):2370–2375.

776. Heeringa, J., D. A. van der Kuip, A. Hofman, J. A. Kors, G. van Herpen, B. H. Stricker, T. Stijnen, G. Y. Lip, J. C. Witteman. 2006. Prevalence, incidence, and lifetime risk of atrial fibrillation: The Rotterdam study. *Eur. Heart J.* 27:949–953.

777. Hart, R. G., L. A. Pearce, M. I. Aguilar. 2007. Meta-analysis: Antithrombotic therapy to prevent stroke in patients who have nonvalvular atrial fibrillation. *Ann. Intern. Med.* 146:857–867.

778. Aguilar, M. I., R. Hart, L. A. Pearce 2007. Oral anticoagulants versus antiplatelet therapy for preventing stroke in patients with non-valvular atrial fibrillation and no history of stroke or transient ischemic attacks. *Cochrane Database Syst. Rev.* CD006186.

779. Ruff, C. T. et al. 2014. Comparison of the efficacy and safety of new oral anticoagulants with warfarin in patients with atrial fibrillation: A metaanalysis of randomised trials. *Lancet* 383:955–962.

780. Harper, P., L. Young, E. Merriman. 2012. Bleeding risk with dabigatran in the frail elderly. *N. Engl. J. Med.* 366:864–866.

781. Radecki, R. P. 2012. Dabigatran: Uncharted waters and potential harms. *Ann. Intern. Med.* 157:66–68.

782. Ogilvie, I. M., N. Newton, S. A. Welner, W. Cowell, G. Y. Lip. 2010. Underuse of oral anticoagulants in atrial fibrillation: A systematic review. *Am. J. Med.* 123:638–645.

783. Gladstone, D. J., E. Bui, J. Fang, A. Laupacis, M. P. Lindsay, J. V. Tu, F. L. Silver, M. K. Kapral. 2009. Potentially preventable strokes in high-risk patients with atrial fibrillation who are not adequately anticoagulated. *Stroke* 40:235–240.

784. Lakshminarayan, K., C. A. Solid, A. J. Collins, D. C. Anderson, C. A. Herzog. 2006. Atrial fibrillation and stroke in the general Medicare population: A 10-year perspective (1992–2002). *Stroke* 37:1969–1974.

785. Perera, V., B. V. Bajorek, S. Matthews, S. N. Hilmer. 2009. The impact of frailty on the utilisation of antithrombotic therapy in older patients with atrial fibrillation. *Age Ageing* 38:156–162.

786. Zimetbaum, P. J., A. Thosani, H. T. Yu, Y. Xiong, J. Lin, P. Kothawala, M. Emons. 2010. Are atrial fibrillation patients receiving warfarin in accordance with stroke risk? *Am. J. Med.* 123:446–453.

787. Scowcroft, A. C., S. Lee, J. Mant. 2013. Thromboprophylaxis of elderly patients with AF in the UK: An analysis using the General Practice Research Database (GPRD) 2000–2009. *Heart* 99:127–132.

788. Eikelboom, J. W. et al. 2011. Risk of bleeding with 2 doses of dabigatran compared with warfarin in older and younger patients with atrial fibrillation: An analysis of the randomized evaluation of long-term anticoagulant therapy (RE-LY) trial. *Circulation* 123:2363–2372.

789. Mant, J., F. D. Hobbs, K. Fletcher, A. Roalfe, D. Fitzmaurice, G. Y. Lip, E. Murray; BAFTA Investigators; Midland Research Practices Network (MidReC). 2007. Warfarin versus aspirin for stroke prevention in an elderly community population with atrial fibrillation (the Birmingham Atrial Fibrillation Treatment of the Aged Study, BAFTA): A randomised controlled trial. *Lancet* 370:493–503.

790. Yiin, G. S. C., D. P. J. Howard, N. L. M. Paul, L. Li, R. Luengo-Fernandez, L. M. Bull, S. J. V. Welch, S. A. Gutnikov, Z. Mehta, P. M. Rothwell. 2014. Age-specific incidence, outcome, cost, and projected future burden of atrial fibrillation-related embolic vascular events: A population-based study. *Circulation* 130(15):1236–1244.

791. van Walraven, C. et al. 2009. Effect of age on stroke prevention therapy in patients with atrial fibrillation: The atrial fibrillation investigators. *Stroke* 40:1410–1416.

792. Pugh, D., J. Pugh, G. E. Mead. 2011. Attitudes of physicians regarding anticoagulation for atrial fibrillation: A systematic review. *Age Ageing* 40:675–683.

793. Kirley, K., D. M. Qato, R. Kornfield, R. S. Stafford, G. C. Alexander. 2012. National trends in oral anticoagulant use in the United States, 2007–2011. *Circ. Cardiovasc. Qual. Outcomes* 5:615–621.

794. Holt, T. A., T. D. Hunter, C. Gunnarsson, N. Khan, P. Cload, G. Y. Lip. 2012. Risk of stroke and oral anticoagulant use in atrial fibrillation: A cross-sectional survey. *Br. J. Gen. Pract.* 62:e710–e717.

795. Gorelick, P. B., K. S. Wong, H. J. Bae, D. K. Pandey. 2008. Large artery intracranial occlusive disease: A large worldwide burden but a relatively neglected frontier. *Stroke* 39:2396–2399.
796. Yarchoan, M., S. X. Xie, M. A. Kling, J. B. Toledo, D. A. Wolk, E. B. Lee, V. Van Deerlin, V. M. Lee, J. Q. Trojanowski, S. E. Arnold. 2012. Cerebrovascular atherosclerosis correlates with Alzheimer pathology in neurodegenerative dementias. *Brain* 135(12):3749–3756.
797. Bos, D., M. J. van der Rijk, T. E. Geeraedts, A. Hofman, G. P. Krestin, J. C. Witteman, A. van der Lugt, M. A. Ikram, M. W. Vernooij. 2012. Intracranial carotid artery atherosclerosis: Prevalence and risk factors in the general population. *Stroke* 43:1878–1884.
798. Hart, R. G., H. C. Diener, S. B. Coutts, J. D. Easton, C. B. Granger, M. J. O'Donnell, R. L. Sacco, S. J. Connolly; Cryptogenic Stroke/ESUS International Working Group. 2014. Embolic strokes of undetermined source: The case for a new clinical construct. *Lancet Neurol.* 13:429–438.
799. Bodle, J. D., E. Feldmann, R. H. Swartz, Z. Rumboldt, T. Brown, T. N. Turan. 2013. High-resolution magnetic resonance imaging: An emerging tool for evaluating intracranial arterial disease. *Stroke* 44:287–292.
800. Liberman, A. L., S. Prabhakaran. 2013. Cryptogenic stroke: How to define it? How to treat it? *Curr. Cardiol. Rep.* 15:423.
801. Bang, O. Y., B. Ovbiagele, J. S. Kim. 2014. Evaluation of cryptogenic stroke with advanced diagnostic techniques. *Stroke* 45:1186–1194.
802. Mazighi, M., J. Labreuche, F. Gongora-Rivera, C. Duyckaerts, J. J. Hauw, P. Amarenco. 2008. Autopsy prevalence of intracranial atherosclerosis in patients with fatal stroke. *Stroke* 39:1142–1147.
803. Ritz, K., N. P. Denswil, O. C. G. Stam, J. J. Van Lieshout, M. J. A. P. Daemen. 2014. Cause and mechanisms of intracranial atherosclerosis. *Circulation* 130(16):1407–1414.
804. Qureshi, A. I., L. R. Caplan. 2014. Intracranial atherosclerosis. *Lancet* 383:984–998.
805. Resch, J. A., A. B. Baker. 1964. Etiology mechanisms in cerebral atherosclerosis. *Arch. Neurol.* 10:617–628.
806. Leung, S. Y., T. H. Ng, S. T. Yuen, I. J. Lauder, F. C. Ho. 1993. Pattern of cerebral atherosclerosis in Hong Kong Chinese: Severity in intracranial and extracranial vessels. *Stroke* 24:779–786.
807. Mathur, K. S., S. K. Kashyap, S. C. Mathur. 1968. Distribution and severity of atherosclerosis of aorta, coronary, and cerebral arteries in persons dying without morphologic evidence of atherosclerotic catastrophe in North India: A study of 900 autopsies. *J. Assoc. Physicians India* 16:113–122.
808. Moossy, J. 1966. Morphology, sites and epidemiology of cerebral atherosclerosis. *Res. Publ. Assoc. Res. Nerv. Ment. Dis.* 41:1–22.
809. Akins, P. T., T. K. Pilgram, D. T. Cross 3rd, C. J. Moran. 1998. Natural history of stenosis from intracranial atherosclerosis by serial angiography. *Stroke* 29:433–438.
810. Uehara, T., M. Tabuchi, E. Mori, A. Yamadori. 2003. Evolving atherosclerosis at carotid and intracranial arteries in Japanese patients with ischemic heart disease: A 5-year longitudinal study with MR angiography. *Eur. J. Neurol.* 10:507–512.
811. Arenillas, J. F., C. A. Molina, J. Montaner, S. Abilleira, M. A. González-Sánchez, J. Alvarez-Sabín. 2001. Progression and clinical recurrence of symptomatic middle cerebral artery stenosis: A long-term follow-up transcranial Doppler ultrasound study. *Stroke* 32:2898–2904.
812. Kim, J. S. et al. 2012. Risk factors and stroke mechanisms in atherosclerotic stroke: Intracranial compared with extracranial and anterior compared with posterior circulation disease. *Stroke* 43:3313–3318.
813. Alkan, O., O. Kizilkilic, T. Yildirim, H. Atalay. 2009. Intracranial cerebral artery stenosis with associated coronary artery and extracranial carotid artery stenosis in Turkish patients. *Eur. J. Radiol.* 71:450–455.
814. Bae, H. J., J. Lee, J. M. Park, O. Kwon, J. S. Koo, B. K. Kim, D. K. Pandey. 2007. Risk factors of intracranial cerebral atherosclerosis among asymptomatics. *Cerebrovasc. Dis.* 24:355–360.
815. Baker, A. B., A. Iannone. 1959. Cerebrovascular disease, I: The large arteries of the circle of Willis. *Neurology* 9:321–332.
816. Velican, C. 1970. Studies on the age-related changes occurring in human cerebral arteries. *Atherosclerosis* 11:509–529.
817. Hori, E., N. Hayashi, H. Hamada, T. Masuoka, N. Kuwayama, Y. Hirashima, H. Origasa, O. Ohtani, S. Endo. 2008. A development of atheromatous plaque is restricted by characteristic arterial wall structure at the carotid bifurcation. *Surg. Neurol.* 69:586–590.
818. Bevan, J. A. 1979. Sites of transition between functional systemic and cerebral arteries of rabbits occur at embryological junctional sites. *Science* 204:635–637.
819. Masuoka, T., N. Hayashi, E. Hori, N. Kuwayama, O. Ohtani, S. Endo. 2010. Distribution of internal elastic lamina and external elastic lamina in the internal carotid artery: Possible relationship with atherosclerosis. *Neurol. Med. Chir. (Tokyo)* 50:179–182.

820. Nakamura, M., K. Imaizumi, U. Shigemi, Y. Nakashima, Y. Kikuchi. 1976. Cerebral atherosclerosis in Japanese, part 5: Relationship between cholesterol deposition and glycosaminoglycans. *Stroke* 7:594–598.

821. Kurozumi, T. 1975. Electron microscopic study on permeability of the aorta and basilar artery of the rabbit—With special reference to the changes of permeability by hypercholesteremia. *Exp. Mol. Pathol.* 23:1–11.

822. Kurozumi, T., T. Imamura, K. Tanaka, Y. Yae, S. Koga. 1984. Permeation and deposition of fibrinogen and low-density lipoprotein in the aorta and cerebral artery of rabbits: Immuno-electron microscopic study. *Br. J. Exp. Pathol.* 65:355–364.

823. Weber, G. 1985. Delayed experimental atherosclerotic involvement of cerebral arteries in monkeys and rabbits (light, Sem and Tem observations). *Pathol. Res. Pract.* 180:353–355.

824. Edvinsson, L., C. Owman. 1975. A pharmacologic comparison of histamine receptors in isolated extracranial and intracranial arteries *in vitro*. *Neurology* 25:271–276.

825. Zugibe, F. T., K. D. Brown. 1961. Histochemical studies in atherogenesis: Human cerebral arteries. *Circ. Res.* 9:897–905.

826. Hoff, H. F. 1972. A histoenzymatic study of human intracranial atherosclerosis. *Am. J. Pathol.* 67:583–600.

827. Hoff, H. F. 1976. Apolipoprotein localization in human cranial arteries, coronary arteries, and the aorta. *Stroke* 7:390–393.

828. Napoli, C., J. L. Witztum, F. de Nigris, G. Palumbo, F. P. D'Armiento, W. Palinski. 1999. Intracranial arteries of human fetuses are more resistant to hypercholesterolemia-induced fatty streak formation than extracranial arteries. *Circulation* 99:2003–2010.

829. D'Armiento, F. P., A. Bianchi, F. de Nigris, D. M. Capuzzi, M. R. D'Armiento, G. Crimi, P. Abete, W. Palinski, M. Condorelli, C. Napoli. 2001. Age-related effects on atherogenesis and scavenger enzymes of intracranial and extracranial arteries in men without classic risk factors for atherosclerosis. *Stroke* 32:2472–2479.

830. Narula, J., M. Nakano, R. Virmani, F. D. Kolodgie, R. Petersen, R. Newcomb, S. Malik, V. Fuster, A. V. Finn. 2013. Histopathologic characteristics of atherosclerotic coronary disease and implications of the findings for the invasive and noninvasive detection of vulnerable plaques. *J. Am. Coll. Cardiol.* 61:1041–1051.

831. López-Cancio, E. et al. 2012. The Barcelona-Asymptomatic Intracranial Atherosclerosis (AsIA) study: Prevalence and risk factors. *Atherosclerosis* 221:221–225.

832. Williams, A. O., J. A. Resch, R. B. Loewenson. 1969. Cerebral atherosclerosis: A comparative autopsy study between Nigerian Negroes and American Negroes and Caucasians. *Neurology* 19:205–210.

833. Resch, J. A., N. Okabe, R. B. Loewenson, K. Kimoto, S. Katsuki, A. B. Baker. 1969. Pattern of vessel involvement in cerebral atherosclerosis: A comparative study between a Japanese and Minnesota population. *J. Atheroscler. Res.* 9:239–250.

834. Inzitari, D., V. C. Hachinski, D. W. Taylor, H. J. Barnett. 1990. Racial differences in the anterior circulation in cerebrovascular disease: How much can be explained by risk factors? *Arch. Neurol.* 47:1080–1084.

835. Rincon, F., R. L. Sacco, G. Kranwinkel, Q. Xu, M. C. Paik, B. Boden-Albala, M. S. Elkind. 2009. Incidence and risk factors of intracranial atherosclerotic stroke: The Northern Manhattan Stroke Study. *Cerebrovasc. Dis.* 28:65–71.

836. Pu, Y., L. Liu, Y. Wang, X. Zou, Y. Pan, Y. Soo, T. Leung, X. Zhao, K. S. Wong, Y. Wang; Chinese IntraCranial AtheroSclerosis (CICAS) Study Group. 2013. Geographic and sex difference in the distribution of intracranial atherosclerosis in China. *Stroke* 44:2109–2114.

837. Solberg, L. A., P. A. McGarry. 1972. Cerebral atherosclerosis in Negroes and Caucasians. *Atherosclerosis* 16:141–154.

838. Owor, R., J. A. Resch, R. B. Loewenson. 1976. Cerebral atherosclerosis in Uganda. *Stroke* 7:404–406.

839. Sacco, R. L., D. E. Kargman, Q. Gu, M. C. Zamanillo. 1995. Race-ethnicity and determinants of intracranial atherosclerotic cerebral infarction: The Northern Manhattan Stroke Study. *Stroke* 26:14–20.

840. Ingall, T. J., D. Homer, H. L. Baker Jr, B. A. Kottke, W. M. O'Fallon, J. P. Whisnant. 1991. Predictors of intracranial carotid artery atherosclerosis: Duration of cigarette smoking and hypertension are more powerful than serum lipid levels. *Arch. Neurol.* 48:687–691.

841. Kim, Y. S., J. W. Hong, W. S. Jung, S. U. Park, J. M. Park, S. I. Cho, Y. M. Bu, S. K. Moon. 2011. Gender differences in risk factors for intracranial cerebral atherosclerosis among asymptomatic subjects. *Gend. Med.* 8:14–22.

842. Vrselja, Z., H. Brkic, S. Mrdenovic, R. Radic, G. Curic. 2014. Function of circle of Willis. *J. Cereb. Blood Flow Metab.* 34:578–584.

843. Routsonis, K. G., E. Stamboulis, M. Christodoulaki. 1973. Anomalies of the circle of Willis and athero-sclerosis. *Vasc. Surg.* 7:141–145.
844. Hartkamp, M. J., J. van Der Grond, K. J. van Everdingen, B. Hillen, W. P. Mali. 1999. Circle of Willis collateral flow investigated by magnetic resonance angiography. *Stroke* 30:2671–2678.
845. Eftekhar, B., M. Dadmehr, S. Ansari, M. Ghodsi, B. Nazparvar, E. Ketabchi. 2006. Are the distributions of variations of circle of Willis different in different populations? Results of an anatomical study and review of literature. *BMC Neurol.* 6:22.
846. López-Cancio, E. et al. 2012. Biological signatures of asymptomatic extra- and intracranial atheroscle-rosis: The Barcelona-AsIA (Asymptomatic Intracranial Atherosclerosis) study. *Stroke* 43:2712–2719.
847. Gorelick, P. B., L. R. Caplan, D. B. Hier, D. Patel, P. Langenberg, M. S. Pessin, J. Biller, D. Kornack. 1985. Racial differences in the distribution of posterior circulation occlusive disease. *Stroke* 16:785–790.
848. Sato, S., T. Uehara, M. Hayakawa, K. Nagatsuka, K. Minematsu, K. Toyoda. 2013. Intra- and extracranial atherosclerotic disease in acute spontaneous intracerebral hemorrhage. *J. Neurol. Sci.* 332:116–120.
849. Park, J. H., K. S. Hong, E. J. Lee, J. Lee, D. E. Kim. 2011. High levels of apolipoprotein B/AI ratio are associated with intracranial atherosclerotic stenosis. *Stroke* 42:3040–3046.
850. Qian, Y., Y. Pu, L. Liu, D. Z. Wang, X. Zhao, C. Wang, Y. Wang, G. Liu, Y. Pan, Y. Wang. 2013. Low HDL-C level is associated with the development of intraCranial Artery stenosis: Analysis from the Chinese IntraCranial AtheroSclerosis (CICAS) study. *PLoS One* 8:e64395.
851. Uekita, K., N. Hasebe, N. Funayama, H. Aoyama, K. Kuroda, H. Aizawa, R. Kataoka, K. Kikuchi. 2003. Cervical and intracranial atherosclerosis and silent brain infarction in Japanese patients with coronary artery disease. *CerebroVasc. Dis.* 16:61–68.
852. Wong, K. S., H. Li. 2003. Long-term mortality and recurrent stroke risk among Chinese stroke patients with predominant intracranial atherosclerosis. *Stroke* 34:2361–2366.
853. Arenillas, J. F., J. Candell-Riera, G. Romero-Farina, C. A. Molina, P. Chacón, S. Aguadé-Bruix, J. Montaner, G. de León, J. Castell-Conesa, J. Alvarez-Sabín. 2005. Silent myocardial ischemia in patients with symptomatic intracranial atherosclerosis: Associated factors. *Stroke* 36:1201–1206.
854. Adams, R. J., M. I. Chimowitz, J. S. Alpert, I. A. Awad, M. D. Cerqueria, P. Fayad, K. A. Taubert. 2003. Coronary risk evaluation in patients with transient ischemic attack and ischemic stroke: A scientific statement for healthcare professionals from the Stroke Council and the Council on Clinical Cardiology of the American Heart Association/American Stroke Association. *Circulation* 108:1278–1290.
855. Seo, W. K., H. S. Yong, S. B. Koh, S. I. Suh, J. H. Kim, S. W. Yu, J. Y. Lee. 2008. Correlation of coronary artery atherosclerosis with atherosclerosis of the intracranial cerebral artery and the extracranial carotid artery. *Eur. Neurol.* 59:292–298.
856. Yoo, J. H., C. S. Chung, S. S. Kang. 1998. Relation of plasma homocyst(e)ine to cerebral infarction and cerebral atherosclerosis. *Stroke* 29:2478–2483.
857. Werner, M. H., P. C. Burger, E. R. Heinz, A. H. Friedman, E. C. Halperin, S. C. Schold Jr. 1988. Intracranial atherosclerosis following radiotherapy. *Neurology* 38:1158–1160.
858. Pfister, H. W., W. Feiden, K. M. Einhäupl. 1993. Spectrum of complications during bacterial meningitis in adults: Results of a prospective clinical study. *Arch. Neurol.* 50:575–581.
859. Ueno, M., A. Oka, T. Koeda, R. Okamoto, K. Takeshita. 2002. Unilateral occlusion of the middle cere-bral artery after varicella-zoster virus infection. *Brain Dev.* 24:106–108.
860. Palacio, S., R. G. Hart, D. G. Vollmer, K. Kagan-Hallet. 2003. Late-developing cerebral arteropathy after pyogenic meningitis. *Arch. Neurol.* 60:431–433.
861. Suri, M. F., S. C. Johnston. 2009. Epidemiology of intracranial stenosis. *J. Neuroimaging* 19(Suppl. 1):11S–16S.
862. Urowitz, M. B. et al.; Systemic Lupus International Collaborating Clinics. 2010. Atherosclerotic vas-cular events in a multinational inception cohort of systemic lupus erythematosus. *Arthritis Care Res. (Hoboken)* 62:881–887.
863. Filosa, J. A., J. A. Iddings. 2013. Astrocyte regulation of cerebral vascular tone. *Am. J. Physiol. Heart Circ. Physiol.* 305:H609–H619.
864. Fathi, A. R., C. Yang, K. D. Bakhtian, M. Qi, R. R. Lonser, R. M. Pluta. 2011. Carbon dioxide influ-ence on nitric oxide production in endothelial cells and astrocytes: Cellular mechanisms. *Brain Res.* 1386:50–57.
865. Andresen, J., N. I. Shafi, R. M. Bryan Jr. 2006. Endothelial influences on cerebrovascular tone. *J. Appl. Physiol.* 100:318–327.
866. Rea, W. J. 1996. *Chemical Sensitivity. Tools for Diagnosis and Methods of Treatment*, 1st ed., Vol. 4. Boca Raton, FL: CRC Press..

867. Viadro, C. I. 2013. Sulfate, sleep and sunlight: The disruptive and destructive effects of heavy metals and glyphosate. *Wise Traditions.* 14(4):23–31.
868. Seneff, S., N. Swanson, C. Li. 2015. Aluminum and glyphosate can synergistically induce pineal gland pathology: Connection to gut dysbiosis and neurological disease. *Agric. Sci.* 6:42–70.
869. Pearson, B. L., M. J. Corley, A. Vasconcellos, D. C. Blanchard, R. J. Blanchard. 2013. Heparan sulfate deficiency in autistic postmortem brain tissue from the subventricular zone of the lateral ventricles. *Behav. Brain Res.* 243:138–145.
870. Mercier, F., Y. C. Kwon, V. Douet. 2012. Hippocampus/amygdala alterations, loss of heparan sulfates, fractones and ventricle wall reduction in adult BTBR T+ tf/J mice, animal model for autism. *Neurosci. Lett.* 506(2):208–213.
871. Tricoire, H., A. Locatelli, P. Chemineau, B. Malpaux. 2002. Melatonin enters the cerebrospinal fluid through the pineal recess. *Endocrinology* 143(1):84–90.
872. Kern, J. K., B. E. Haley, D. E. Geier, L. K. Sykes, P. G. King, M. R. Geier. 2013. Thimerosal exposure and the role of sulfation chemistry and thiol availability in autism. *Int. J. Environ. Res. Public Health* 10(8):3771–3800.
873. Seneff, S., R. M. Davidson, J. Liu. 2012. Empirical Data Confirm Autism Symptoms Related to Aluminum and Acetaminophen Exposure. *Entropy* 14:2227–2253.
874. Chen, L., B. Zhang, M. Toborek. 2013. Authophagy is involved in Nanoalumina-induced cerebrovascular toxicity. *Nanomedicine.* 9(2):212–221.
875. Rea, W. J. 1994. *Chemical Sensitivity. Sources of Total Body Load,* 1st ed., Vol. 2. Boca Raton, FL: Lewis.
876. Goldner, W. S., D. P. Sandler, F. Yu, J. A. Hoppin, F. Kamel, T. D. Levan. 2010. Pesticide use and thyroid disease among women in the agricultural health study. *Am. J. Epidemiol.* 171(4):455–464.
877. EWG. Dirty Dozen Endocrine Disruptors. October 28, 2013. Accessed January 20, 2016.
878. Liu, S., D. Knewski, Y. Shi, Y. Chen, R. T. Burnett. 2003. Association between gaseous ambient air pollutants and adverse pregnancy outcomes in Vancouver, British Columbia. *Environ. Health Perspect.* 111:1773–1778.
879. Lin, M., H. F. Chui, H. S. Yu, S. S. Tsai, B. H. Cheng, T. N. Wu, F. C. Sung, C. Y. Yang. 2001. Increased risk of preterm delivery in areas with air pollution from a petroleum refinery plant in Taiwan. *J. Toxic Environ. Health A* 64:637–644.
880. Yang, C. Y., H. H. Cheng, T. Y. Hsu, H. Y. Chuang, T. N. Wu, P. C. Chen. 2002. Association between petrochemical pollution and adverse pregnancy outcomes in Taiwan. *Arch. Environ. Health* 57:461–465.
881. Loomis, D., M. Castillejos, D. R. Gold, W. McDonnel, V. H. Borja-Abutro. 1999. Air pollution and infant mortality in Mexico City. *Epidemiology* 10:118–123.
882. Bobak, M., D. A. Leon. 1999. The effect of air pollution on infant mortality appears specific for respiratory causes in the postneonatal period. *Epidemiology* 10:666–670.
883. Woodruff, T. J., J. Grillo, K. C. Schoendorf. 1997. The relationship between selected causes of postneonatal infant mortality and particulate air pollution in the US. *Environ. Health Perspect.* 105:608–612.
884. Klonoff-Cohen, H., P. K. Lam, A. Lewis. 2005. Outdoor carbon monoxide, nitrogen dioxide, and sudden infant death syndrome. *Arch. Dis. Child.* 90:750–753.
885. Vassilev, Z., M. G. Robson, J. B. Klotz. 2001. Outdoor exposure to airborne polycyclic organic matter and adverse reproductive outcomes. *Am. J. Ind. Med.* 40:255–262.
886. Sagiv, S. K., P. Mendola, D. Loomis, A. H. Herring, L. M. Neas, D. A. Savitz, C. Poole. 2005. A time-series analysis of air pollution and preterm birth in Pennsylvania, 1997–2001. *Environ. Health Perspect.* 113:602–606.
887. Gilboa, S. M., P. Mendola, A. P. Olshan, P. H. Langois, D. A. Savitz, D. Loomis, A. H. Herring, D. E. Fixler. 2005. Relation between ambient air quality and selected birth defects, Seven County Study, Texas, 1997–2000. *Am. J. Epidemiol.* 162:236–252.
888. Feschenko, S. P., H. C. Schroder, Wem Muller, G. I. Lazjuk. 2002. Congenital malformations and developmental abnormalities among human embryos in Belarus after the Chernobyl accident. *Cell Mol. Biol.* 48:423–426.
889. Ritz, B., F. Yu, S. Fruin, G. Chapa, G. W. Shaw, J. A. Harris. 2002. Ambient air pollution and risk of birth defects in southern California. *Am. J. Epidemiol.* 155:17–25.
890. Smrcka, V., D. Leznarova. 1998. Environmental pollution and the occurrence of congenital defects in a 15 year period in a South Moravian District. *Acta. Chir. Plast.* 40:112–114.
891. Cordier, S., C. Chevrier, E. Robert-Gnansia, C. Lorene, P. Brula, M. Hours. 2004. Risk of congenital anomalies in the vicinity of solid waste incinerators. *Occup. Environ. Med.* 61:8–15.

892. Jarup, L. 2003. Hazards of heavy metal contamination. *Br. Med. Bull.* 68(1):167–182.
893. Pie, C. 2013. Environmental pollution and allergy: Immunological mechanisms. *Rev. Pneumol. Clin.* 69(1):18–25.
894. West, A. P., G. S. Shadel, S. Ghosh. 2011. Mitochondria in innate immune responses. *Nat. Rev. Immunol.* 11(6):389–402.
895. Hayden, M. S., A. P. West, S. Ghosh. 2006. NF-κB and the immune response. *Oncogene* 25:6758–6780.
896. West, A. P., A. A. Koblansky, S. Ghosh. 2006. Recognition and signaling by Toll-like receptors. *Annu. Rev. Cell Dev. Biol.* 22:409–437.
897. Kerrigan, A. M., G. D. Brown. 2010. Syk-coupled C-type lectin receptors that mediate cellular activation via single tyrosine based activation motifs. *Immunol. Rev.* 234:335–352.
898. Bonawitz, N. D., D. A. Clayton, G. S. Shadel. 2006. Initiation and beyond: Multiple functions of the human mitochondrial transcription machinery. *Mol. Cell* 24:813–825.
899. Ryan, M. T., N. J. Hoogenraad. 2007. Mitochondrial–nuclear communications. *Annu. Rev. Biochem.* 76:701–722.
900. Soubannier, V., H. M. McBride. 2009. Positioning mitochondrial plasticity within cellular signaling cascades. *Biochim. Biophys. Acta* 1793:154–170.
901. Hamanaka, R. B., N. S. Chandel. 2010. Mitochondrial reactive oxygen species regulate cellular signaling and dictate biological outcomes. *Trends Biochem. Sci.* 35:505–513.
902. Arnoult, D., L., Carneiro, I. Tattoli, S. E. Girardin. 2009. The role of mitochondria in cellular defense against microbial infection. *Semin. Immunol.* 21:223–232.
903. Ohta, A., Y. Nishiyama. 2011. Mitochondria and viruses. *Mitochondrion* 11:1–12.
904. Takeuchi, O., S. Akira. 2009. Innate immunity to virus infection. *Immunol. Rev.* 227:75–86.
905. Brennan, K., A. G. Bowie. 2010. Activation of host pattern recognition receptors by viruses. *Curr. Opin. Microbiol.* 13:503–507.
906. Satoh, T., H. Kato, Y. Kumagai, M. Yoneyama, S. Sato, K. Matsushita, T. Tsujimura, T. Fujita, S. Akira, O. Takeuchi. 2010. LGP2 is a positive regulator of RIG-I- and MDA5-mediated antiviral responses. *Proc. Natl. Acad. Sci. U.S.A.* 107:1512–1517.
907. Michallet, M. C. et al. 2008. TRADD protein is an essential component of the RIG-like helicase antiviral pathway. *Immunity* 28:651–661.
908. Kawai, T., K. Takahashi, S. Sato, C. Coban, H. Kumar, H. Kato, K. J. Ishii, O. Takeuchi, S. Akira. 2005. IPS-1, an adaptor triggering RIG-I- and Mda5-mediated type I interferon induction. *Nat. Immunol.* 6:981–988.
909. Meylan, E., J. Curran, K. Hofmann, D. Moradpour, M. Binder, R. Bartenschlager, J. Tschopp. 2005. Cardif is an adaptor protein in the RIG-I antiviral pathway and is targeted by hepatitis C virus. *Nature* 437:1167–1172.
910. Lin, R. et al. 2006. Dissociation of a MAVS/IPS-1/VISA/Cardif-IKKε molecular complex from the mitochondrial outer membrane by hepatitis C virus NS3-4A proteolytic cleavage. *J. Virol.* 80:6072–6083.
911. Wang, Y. Y., L.-J. Liu, B. Zhong, T.-T. Liu, Y. Li, Y. Yang, Y. Ran, S. Li, P. Tien, H.-B. Shu. 2010. WDR5 is essential for assembly of the VISA-associated signaling complex and virus-triggered IRF3 and NF-κB activation. *Proc. Natl. Acad. Sci. U.S.A.* 107:815–820.
912. Neupert, W., J. M. Herrmann. 2007. Translocation of proteins into mitochondria. *Annu. Rev. Biochem.* 76:723–749.
913. Chan, D. C. 2006. Mitochondrial fusion and fission in mammals. *Annu. Rev. Cell Dev. Biol.* 22:79–99.
914. Detmer, S. A., D. C. Chan. 2007. Functions and dysfunctions of mitochondrial dynamics. *Nat. Rev. Mol. Cell Biol.* 8:870–879.
915. de Brito, O. M., L. Scorrano. 2008. Mitofusin 2 tethers endoplasmic reticulum to mitochondria. *Nature* 456:605–610.
916. Jin, L., L. Lenz, J. Cambier. 2010. Cellular reactive oxygen species inhibit MPYS induction of IFNβ. *PLoS One* 5:e15142.
917. Soucy-Faulkner, A., E. Mukawera, K. Fink, A. Martel, L. Jouan, Y. Nzengue, D. Lamarre, C. Vande Velde, N. Grandvaux. 2010. Requirement of NOX2 and reactive oxygen species for efficient RIG-Imediated antiviral response through regulation of MAVS expression. *PLoS Pathog.* 6:e1000930.
918. Tal, M. C., M. Sasai, H. K. Lee, B. Yordy, G. S. Shadel, A. Iwasaki. 2009. Absence of autophagy results in reactive oxygen species-dependent amplification of RLR signaling. *Proc. Natl. Acad. Sci. U.S.A.* 106:2770–2775. An important study showing that mROS can augment RLR signalling and that autophagy and mitophagy regulate antiviral responses by limiting mROS production.

919. Jounai, N. et al. 2007. The Atg5–Atg12 conjugate associates with innate antiviral immune responses. *Proc. Natl. Acad. Sci. U.S.A.* 104:14050–14055.

920. Lambeth, J. D. 2004. NOX enzymes and the biology of reactive oxygen. *Nat. Rev. Immunol.* 4:181–189.

921. Underhill, D. M., A. Ozinsky. 2002. Phagocytosis of microbes: Complexity in action. *Annu. Rev. Immunol.* 20:825–852.

922. Matyniak, J. E., S. L. Reiner. 1995. T helper phenotype and genetic susceptibility in experimental Lyme disease. *J. Exp. Med.* 181:1251–1254.

923. Sigal, L. H. 1997. Lyme disease: A review of aspects of its immunology and immunopathogenesis. *Annu. Rev. Immunol.* 15:63–92.

924. Keshavarzian A., G. Morgan, S. Sedghi, J. H. Gordon, M. Doria. 1990. Role of reactive oxygen metabolites in experimental colitis. *Gut* 31:786–790.

925. Grisham, M. B. 1991. *Role of Neutrophil Derived Oxidants in the Pathogenesis of Inflammatory Bowel Disease. Progress in Inflammatory Bowel Disease. Crohns and Colitis Foundation of America.* Research Report No. 1. 12:6–8.

926. Simmonds, N. J., R. E. Allen, T. R. Stevens, R. N. Van Somerren, D. R. Blake, D. S. Rampton. 1992. Chemiluminescence assay of mucosal reactive oxygen metabolites in inflammatory bowel disease. *Gastroenterology* 103:186–196.

927. Pekoe, G., K. Van Dyke, H. Mengoli, D. Peden, English. 1982. Comparison of the effects of antioxidant non-steroidal anti-inflammatory drugs against myeloperoxidase and hypochlorous acid luminol-enhanced chemiluminescence. *Agents. Actions* 12:1–2.

928. Karyalcin, S. S., W. Sturbaum, J. T. Wachasman, J. H. Cha, D. W. Powell. 1990. Hydrogen peroxide stimulates rat colonic prostaglandin production and alters electrolyte transport. *J. Clin. Invest.* 86:60–78.

929. Vangossum, A., J. Decuyper. 1989. Breath alkanes as an index of lipid peroxidation. *Eur. Respir. J.* 2:787–791.

930. Babior, B. M., R. S. Kipness, J. T. Curnutte. 1973. The production by leukicytes of superoxide, a potential bactericidal agent. *J. Clin. Invest.* 52:741–744.

931. Riely, C. A., G. Cohen, M. Lieberman. 1974. Ethane evolution: A new index of lipid peroxidation. *Science* 183:205–210.

932. Kessler, W., H. Remmer. 1990. Generation of volatile hydrocarbons from amino acids and proteins by an iron/ascorbate/GSH system. *Biochem. Pharmacol.* 39:1347–1351.

933. Princemail, J., C. Deby, A. Dethier. 1987. Pentane measurement in man as an index of lipoperoxidation. *Bioelectrochem. Bioeng.* 18:117–125.

934. Humad, S., E. J. Zarling, M. Clapper, J. Skosey. 1988. Breath pentane excretion as a marker of disease activity in rheumatoid arthritis. *Free Radic. Res.* 5:101–106.

935. Sobotka, P. A., M. D. Brottman, Z. Weitz, A. J. Birmbaum, J. L. Skosey, E. J. Zarling. 1993. Elevated breath pentane in heart failure reduced by free radical scavenger. *Free Radic. Biol. Med.* 14:643–647.

936. Ondrula, D., R., L., Nelson, G. Andrianopoulos, D. Schwartz, H. Abcarian, A. Birnbaum, J. Skosey. 1993. Quantitative determination of pentane in exhaled air correlates with colonic inflammation in the rat colitis model. *Dis. Colon. Rectum* 36:457–462.

937. Kokoszka, J., R. L. Nelson, W. I. Swedler, J. Skosey, H. Abcarian. 1993. Determination of inflammatory bowel disease activity by breath pentane analysis. *Dis. Colon. Rectum* 36:597–601.

938. Borowitz, S. M., C. Montgomery. 1989. The role of phospholipase A2 in microsomal lipid peroxidation induced witht-butyl hydroperoxide. *Biochem. Biophys. Res. Commun.* 158:1021–1028.

939. Samsel, A., S. Seneff. 2013. Glyphosate, pathways to modern diseases II: Celiac sprue and gluten intolerance. *Interdiscip. Toxicol.* 6(4):159–184.

940. Green, P. H. R., C. Cellier. 2007. Celiac disease. *N. Engl. J. Med.* 357:1731–1743.

941. Rubio-Tapia A. et al. 2009. Increased prevalence and mortality in undiagnosed celiac disease. *Gastroenterology* 137(1):88–93.

942. Lorand, L., R. M. Graham. 2003. Transglutaminases: Crosslinking enzymes with pleiotropic functions. *Nat. Rev. Mol. Cell Biol.* 4:140–156.

943. Esposito, C. et al. 2002. Anti-tissue transglutaminase antibodies from coeliac patients inhibit transglutaminase activity both *in vitro* and *in situ. Gut* 51(2):177–181.

944. Williams, G. M., R. Kroes, I. C. Munro. 2000. Safety evaluation and risk assessment of the herbicide Roundup and its active ingredient, glyphosate, for humans. *Regul. Toxicol. Pharmacol.* 31(2):117–165.

945. de María, N., J. M. Becerril, J. I. Garca-Plazaola, A. H. Hernandez, M. R. de Felipe, M. Fernández-Pascual. 1996. New insights on glyphosate mode of action in nodular metabolism: Role of shikimate accumulation. *J. Agric. Food Chem.* 54:2621–2628.

946. Franz, J. E., M. K. Mao, J. A. Sikorski. 1997. *Glyphosate: A Unique Global Herbicide*. Washington, DC: American Chemical Society.

947. Monsanto International Sàrl. 2010. *The Agronomic Benefits of Glyphosate in Europe. Review of the Benefits of Glyphosate Per Market Use*. Monsanto Europe SA. Accessed September 4, 2013. www.monsanto.com/products/Documents/glyphosate-background-materials/Agronomic%20benefits%20of%20glyphosate%20in%20Europe.pdf

948. Senapati, T., A. K. Mukerjee, A. R. Ghosh. 2009. Observations on the effect of glyphosate based herbicide on ultrastructure (SEM) and enzymatic activity in different regions of alimentary canal and gill of Channa punctatus (Bloch). *J. Crop. Weed* 5(1):236–245.

949. Hershko, C., J. Patz. 2008. Ironing out the mechanism of anemia in celiac disease. *Haematologica* 93(12):1761–1765.

950. Fasano, A. 2011. Zonulin and its regulation of intestinal barrier function: The biological door to inflammation, autoimmunity, and cancer. *Physiol. Rev.* 91:151–175.

951. Fasano A., T. Not, W. Wang, S. Uzzau, I. Berti, A. Tommasini, S. E. Goldblum. 2000. Zonulin, a newly discovered modulator of intestinal permeability, its expression in coeliac disease. *Lancet* 358:1518–1519.

952. Tursi, A., G. Brandimarte, G. Giorgetti. 2003. High prevalence of small intestinal bacterial overgrowth in celiac patients with persistence of gastrointestinal symptoms after gluten withdrawal. *Am. J. Gastroenterol.* 98:839–843.

953. Shehata, A. A., W. Schrödl, A. A. Aldin, H. M. Hafez, M. Krüger. 2013. The effect of glyphosate on potential pathogens and beneficial members of poultry microbiota *in vitro*. *Curr. Microbiol.* 66:350–358.

954. Krüger, M., W. Schrödl, J. Neuhaus, A. A. Shehata. 2013. Field investigations of glyphosate in urine of Danish dairy cows. *J. Environ. Anal. Toxicol.* 3(5):100186.

955. Carman, J. A., H. R. Vlieger, L. J. Ver Steeg, V. E. Sneller, G. W. Robinson, C. A. Clinch-Jones, J. I. Haynes, J. W. Edwards. 2013. A long-term toxicology study on pigs fed a combined genetically modified (GM) soy and GM maize diet. *J. Organic Syst.* 8(1):38–54.

956. Krüger, M., A. A. Shehata, W. Schrödl, A. Rodloff. 2013. Glyphosate suppresses the antagonistic effect of *Enterococcus* spp. on *Clostridium botulinum*. *Anaerobe* 20:74–78.

957. Sanz, Y., G. De Palma, M. Laparra. 2011. Unraveling the ties between celiac disease and intestinal microbiota. *Int. Rev. Immunol.* 30(4):207–218.

958. Di Cagno, R. et al. 2011. Duodenal and faecal microbiota of celiac children: Molecular, phenotype and metabolome characterization. *BMC Microbiol.* 11:219.

959. Collado, M. C., M. Calabuig, Y. Sanz. 2007. Differences between the fecal microbiota of coeliac infants and healthy controls. *Curr. Issues Intest. Microbiol.* 8(1):9–14.

960. Nada, L. I., E. Donat, C. Ribes-Koninckx, M. Calabuig, Y. Sanz. 2007. Imbalance in the composition of the duodenal microbiota of children with coeliac disease. *J. Med. Microbiol.* 56:1669–1674.

961. Tamm, A. O. 1984. Biochemical activity of intestinal microflora in adult coeliac disease. *Nahrung* 28(6–7):711–715.

962. D'Ari, L., H. A. Barker. 1985. p-Cresol formation by cell free extracts of *Clostridium difficile*. *Arch. Microbiol.* 143:311–312.

963. Kelly, C. P., C. Pothoulakis, J. T. LaMont. 1994. *Clostridium difficile* colitis. *N. Engl. J. Med.* 330:257–262.

964. Gobbetti, M., C. Giuseppe Rizzello, R. Di Cagno, M. De Angelis. 2007. Sourdough lactobacilli and celiac disease. *Food Microbiol.* 24(2):187–196.

965. Famularo, G., De C. Simone, V. Pandey, A. R. Sahu, G. Minisola. 2005. Probiotic lactobacilli: An innovative tool to correct the malabsorption syndrome of vegetarians? *Med. Hypotheses* 65(6):11325.

966. Cavallaro, R., P. Iovino, F. Castiglione, A. Palumbo, M. Marino, S. Di Bella, F. Sabbatini, F. Labanca, R. Tortora, G Mazzacca, C. Ciacci. 2004. Prevalence and clinical associations of prolonged prothrombin time in adult untreated coeliac disease. *Eur. J. Gastroenterol. Hepatol.* 16(2):219–223.

967. Smecuol, E. et al. 2013. Exploratory, randomized, doubleblind, placebo-controlled study on the effects of *Bifidobacterium infantis* natren life start strain super strain in active celiac disease. *J. Clin. Gastroenterol.* 47(2):139–147.

968. Whorwell, P. J., L. Altringer, J. Morel, Y. Bond, D. Charbonneau, L. O'Mahony, B. Kiely, F. Shanahan, E. M. Quigley. 2006. Efficacy of an encapsulated probiotic *Bifidobacterium infantis* 35624 in women with irritable bowel syndrome. *Am. J. Gastroenterol.* 101(7):1581–1590.

969. Medina, M., G. De Palma, C. Ribes-Koninckx, M. Calabuig, Y. Sanz. 2008. Bifidobacterium strains suppress *in vitro* the pro-inflammatory milieu triggered by the large intestinal microbiota of coeliac patients. *J. Infl. Amm. (Lond.)* 5:19.

970. Lindfors, K., T. Blomqvist, K. Juuti-Uusitalo, S. Stenman, J. Venalainen, M. Maki, K. Kaukinen. 2008. Live probiotic *Bifidobacterium lactis* bacteria inhibit the toxic effects induced by wheat gliadin in epithelial cell culture. *Clin. Exp. Immunol.* 152(3):552–558.

971. Lamb, D. C., D. E. Kelly, S. Z. Hanley, Z. Mehmood, S. L. Kelly. 1998. Glyphosate is an inhibitor of plant cytochrome P450: Functional expression of *Thlaspi arvensae* cytochrome P45071B1/reductase fusion protein in *Escherichia coli*. *Biochem. Biophys. Res. Commun.* 244:110–114.

972. Hietanen, E., K. Linnainmaa, H. Vainio. 1983. Effects of phenoxyherbicides and glyphosate on the hepatic and intestinal biotransformation activities in the rat. *Acta Pharmacol. Toxicol. (Copenh.)* 53(2):103–112.

973. Lindros, K. O. 1997. Zonation of cytochrome P450 expression, drug metabolism and toxicity in liver. *Gen. Pharmacol.* 28(2):191–196.

974. El-Shenawy, N. 2009. Oxidative stress responses of rats exposed to Roundup and its active ingredient glyphosate. *Environ. Toxicol. Pharmacol.* 28(3):379–385.

975. Cupp, M. J., T. S. Tracy. 1998. Cytochrome P450: New nomenclature and clinical implications. *Am. Fam. Physician.* 57(1):107–116.

976. Lang, C. C., R. M. Brown, M. T. Kinirons, M. A. Deathridge, F. P. Guengerich, D. Kelleher, D. S. O'Briain, F. K. Ghishan, A. J. Wood. 1996. Decreased intestinal CYP3A in celiac disease: Reversal after successful gluten-free diet: A potential source of interindividual variability in first-pass drug metabolism. *Clin. Pharmacol. Ther.* 59(1):41–46.

977. Colombato, L. O., H. Parodi, D. Cantor. 1977 Biliary function studies in patients with celiac sprue. *Am. J. Dig. Dis.* 22(2):96–98.

978. Dickey, W., S. A. McMillan, M. E. Callender. 1997. High prevalence of celiac sprue among patients with primary biliary cirrhosis. *J. Clin. Gastroenterol.* 25(1):328–329.

979. Lorbek, G., M. Lewinska, D. Rozman. 2012. Cytochrome P450s in the synthesis of cholesterol and bile acids—From mouse models to human diseases. *FEBS J.* 279(9):1516–1533.

980. Wikvall, K. 2001. Cytochrome P450 enzymes in the bioactivation of vitamin D to its hormonal form (review). *Int. J. Mol. Med.* 7(2):201–209.

981. Kemppainen, T., H. Kröger, E. Janatuinen, I. Arnala, V. M. Kosma, P. Pikkarainen, R. Julkunen, J. Jurvelin, E. Alhava, M. Uusitupa. 1999. Osteoporosis in adult patients with celiac disease. *Bone* 24(3):249–255.

982. Brown, A. M., M. J. Bradshaw, R. Richardson, J. G. Wheeler, R. F. Harvey. 1987. Pathogenesis of the impaired gall bladder contraction of coeliac disease. *Gut* 28(11):1426–1432.

983. Benini, F., A. Mora, D. Turini, S. Bertolazzi, F. Lanzarotto, C. Ricci, V. Villanacci, G. Barbara, V. Stanghellini, A. Lanzini. 2012. Slow gallbladder emptying reverts to normal but small intestinal transit of a physiological meal remains slow in celiac patients during gluten-free diet. *Neurogastroenterol. Motil.* 24(2):100–107, e79–80.

984. Patel, R. S., F. C. Johlin Jr., J. A. Murray. 1999. Celiac disease and recurrent pancreatitis. *Gastrointest. Endosc.* 50(6):823–827.

985. Ejderhamn, J., K. Samuelson, B. Strandvik. 1992. Serum primary bile acids in the course of celiac disease in children. *J. Pediatr. Gastroenterol. Nutr.* 14(4):443–449.

986. Deprez, P., C. Sempoux, B. E. Van Beers, A. Jouret, A. Robert, J. Rahier, A. Geubel, S. Pauwels, P. Mainguet. 2002. Persistent decreased plasma cholecystokinin levels in celiac patients under gluten-free diet: Respective roles of histological changes and nutrient hydrolysis. *Regul. Pept.* 110(1):55–63.

987. Maton, P. N., A. C. Selden, M. L. Fitzpatrick, V. S. Chadwick. 1985. Defective gallbladder emptying and cholecystokinin release in celiac disease. Reversal by gluten-free diet. *Gastroenterology* 88(2):391–396.

988. Sunergren, K. P., R. P. Fairman, G. G. deBlois, F. L. Glauser. 1987. Effects of protamine, heparinase and hyaluronidase on endothelial permeability and surface charge. *J. Appl. Physiol.* 63:1987–1992.

989. Klein, N. J., G. I. Shennan, R. S. Heyderman, M. Levin. 1992. Alteration in glycosaminoglycan metabolism and surface charge on human umbilical vein endothelial cells induced by cytokines, endotoxin and neutrophils. *J. Cell Sci.* 102:821–832.

990. Vernier, R. L., D. J. Klein, S. P. Sisson, J. D. Mahan, T. R. Oegema, D. M. Brown. 1983. Heparan sulphate-rich anionic sites in the human glomerular basement membrane: Decreased concentration in congenital nephrotic syndrome. *N. Engl. J. Med.* 309:1001–1009.

991. Murch, S. H., T. T. MacDonald, J. A. Walker-Smith, M. Levin, P. Lionetti, N. J. Klein. 1993. Disruption of sulphated glycosaminoglycans in intestinal inflammation. *Lancet* 341:711–714.

992. Murch, S. H. 1995. Sulphation of proteoglycans and intestinal function. *J. Gastroenterol. Hepatol.* 10:210–212.

993. Murch, S. H., P. J. Winyard, S. Koletzko, B. Wehner, H. A. Cheema, R. A. Risdon, A. D. Phillips, N. Meadows, N. J. Klein, J. A. Walker-Smith. 1996. Congenital enterocyte heparan sulphate deficiency with massive albumin loss, secretory diarrhoea, and malnutrition. *Lancet* 347(9011):1299–1301.

994. Tieri, P., A. Termanini, E. Bellavista, S. Salvioli, M. Capri, C. Franceschi. 2012. Charting the NF-κB pathway interactome map. *PLoS One* 7(3):e32678.

995. Bhatia, M. 2012. Role of hydrogen sulfide in the pathology of inflammation. *Scientifica* 2012: Article ID 159680, 12 pages.

996. Iwasaki, Y., M. Asai, M. Yoshida, T. Nigawara, M. Kambayashi, N. Nakashima. 2004. Dehydroepiandrosterone-sulfate inhibits nuclear factor-κBdependent transcription in hepatocytes, possibly through antioxidant effect. *J. Clin. Endocrinol. Metab.* 89(7):3449–3454.

997. Li, L., P. Rose, P. K. Moore. 2011. Hydrogen sulfide and cell signaling. *Annu. Rev. Pharmacol. Toxicol.* 51:169–187.

998. Módis, K., C. Coletta, K. Erdélyi, A. Papapetropoulos, C. Szabo. 2013. Intramitochondrial hydrogen sulfide production by 3-mercaptopyruvate sulfurtransferase maintains mitochondrial electron flow and supports cellular bioenergetics. *FASEB J.* 27(2):601–611.

999. Ingenbleek, Y., H. Kimura. 2013. Nutritional essentiality of sulfur in health and disease. *Nutr. Rev.* 71(7):413–432.

1000. Hildebrandt, T. M., M. K. Grieshaber. 2008. Three enzymatic activities catalyze the oxidation of sulfide to thiosulfate in mammalian and invertebrate mitochondria. *FEBS J.* 275(13):3352–3361.

1001. Goubern M., M. Andriamihaja, T. Nubel, F. Blachier, F. Bouillaud. 2007. Sulfide, the first inorganic substrate for human cells. *FASEB J.* 21(8):1699–1706.

1002. Seneff, S., A. Lauritzen, R. Davidson, L. Lentz-Marino. 2012. Is endothelial nitric oxide synthase a moonlighting protein whose day job is cholesterol sulfate synthesis? Implications for cholesterol transport, diabetes and cardiovascular disease. *Entropy* 14:2492–2530.

1003. Ziolkowski, A. F., S. K. Popp, C. Freeman, C. R. Parish, C. J. Simeonovic. 2012. Heparan sulfate and heparanase play key roles in mouse cell survival and autoimmune diabetes. *J. Clin. Invest.* 122(1):132–141.

1004. Ito, N., Y. Iwamori, K. Hanaoka, M. Iwamori. 1998. Inhibition of pancreatic elastase by sulfated lipids in the intestinal mucosa. *J. Biochem.* 123:107–114.

1005. Lucendo, A. J., M. Sánchez-Cazalilla. 2012. Adult versus pediatric eosinophilic esophagitis: Important differences and similarities for the clinician to understand. *Expert Rev. Clin. Immunol.* 8(8):733–745.

1006. Mishra, A., M. E. Rothenberg. 2003. Intratracheal IL-13 induces eosinophilic esophagitis by an IL-5, eotaxin-1, and STAT6 dependent mechanism. *Gastroenterology* 125:1419–1427.

1007. Leslie, C., C. Mews, A. Charles, M. Ravikumara. 2010. Celiac disease and eosinophilic esophagitis: A true association. *J. Pediatr. Gastroenterol. Nutr.* 50(4):397–399.

1008. Gross, S., R. L. van Wanrooij, P. Nijeboer, K. A. Gelderman, S. A. G. M. Cillessen, G. A. Meijer, C. J. J. Mulder, G. Bouma, B. M. E. von Blomberg, H. J. Bontkes. 2013. Differential IL-13 production by small intestinal leukocytes in active coeliac disease versus refractory coeliac disease. *Mediat. Inflamm.* 2013:939047, ISSN: 1466-1861.

1009. Furuta, G. T., C. A. Liacouras, M. H. Collins, S. K. Gupta, C. Justinich, P. E. Putnam, P. Bonis, E. Hassall, A. Straumann, M. E. Rothenberg; First International Gastrointestinal Eosinophil Research Symposium (FIGERS) Subcommittees. 2007. Eosinophilic esophagitis in children and adults: A systematic review and consensus recommendations for diagnosis and treatment. *Gastroenterology* 133:1342–1363.

1010. Prasad, G. A., J. A. Alexander, C. D. Schleck, A. R. Zinsmeister, T. C. Smyrk, R. M. Elias, G. R. Locke 3rd, N. J. Talley. 2009. Epidemiology of eosinophilic esophagitis over three decades in Olmsted County, Minnesota. *Clin. Gastroenterol. Hepatol.* 7:1055–1061.

1011. Chang, C. Y., Y. C. Peng, D. Z. Hung, W. H. Hu, D. Y. Yang, T. J. Lin. 1999. Clinical impact of upper gastrointestinal tract injuries in glyphosate-surfactant oral intoxication. *Hum. Exp. Toxicol.* 18:475–478.

1012. Zouaoui, K., S. Dulaurent, J. M. Gaulier, C. Moesch, G. Lachâtre. 2013. Determination of glyphosate and AMPA in blood and urine from humans: About 13 cases of acute intoxication. *Forensic Sci. Int.* 226(1–3):e20–e25.

1013. Blanchard, C., M. E. Rothenberg. 2008. Basics pathogenesis of eosinophilic esophagitis. *Gastrointest. Endosc. Clin. N. Am.* 18(1):133–143.

1014. Li, H., X. Liu, H. Cui, Y.-R. Chen, A. J. Cardounel, J. L. Zweier. 2006. Characterization of the mechanism of cytochrome P450 reductase-cytochrome P450-mediated nitric oxide and nitrosothiol generation from organic nitrates. *JBC* 281(18):12546–12554.

1015. Förstermann, U., T. Münzel. 2006. Endothelial nitric oxide synthase in vascular disease: From marvel to menace. *Circulation* 113:1708–1714.

1016. Zenjari, T., A. Boruchowicz, P. Desreumaux, E. Laberenne, A. Cortot, J. F. Colombel. 1995. Association of coeliac disease and portal venous thrombosis. *Gastroenterol. Clin. Biol.* 19:953–954.

1017. Marteau, P., J. F. Cadranel, B. Messing, D. Gargot, D. Valla, J. C. Rambaud. 1994. Association of hepatic vein obstruction and coeliac disease in North African subjects. *J. Hepatol.* 20:650–653.

1018. Grigg, AP. 1999. Deep venous thrombosis as the presenting feature in a patient with coeliac disease and homocysteinaemia. *Aust. N. Z. J. Med.* 29:566–567.

1019. Halfdanarson, T. R., M. R. Litzow, J. A. Murray. 2007. Hematologic manifestations of celiac disease. *Blood* 109:412–421.

1020. Jabri, B., L. M. Sollid. 2009. Tissue-mediated control of immunopathology in coeliac disease. *Nat. Rev. Immunol.* 9(12):858–870.

1021. Mora, J. R., M. Iwata, U. H. von Andrian. 2008. Vitamin effects on the immune system: Vitamins A and D take centre stage. *Nat. Rev. Immunol.* 8(9):685–698.

1022. Coombes, J. L., K. R. Siddiqui, C. V. Arancibia-Cárcamo, J. Hall, C. M. Sun, Y. Belkaid, F. Powrie. 2007. A functionally specialized population of mucosal CD103+ DCs induces Foxp3+ regulatory T cells via a TGF-beta and retinoic acid-dependent mechanism. *J. Exp. Med.* 204(8):1757–1764.

1023. Mucida, D., Y. Park, G. Kim, O. Turovskaya, I. Scott, M. Kronenberg, H. Cheroutre. 2007. Reciprocal TH17 and regulatory T cell differentiation mediated by retinoic acid. *Science* 317(5835):256–260.

1024. Nanda, S. 2011. Celiac disease: Retinoic acid and IL-15 jointly implicated in reversal of oral tolerance. *Nat. Rev. Gastroenterol. Hepatol.* 8:181.

1025. DePaolo, R. W. et al. 2011. Co-adjuvant effects of retinoic acid and IL-15 induce inflammatory immunity to dietary antigens. *Nature* 471(7337):220–224.

1026. Putcha, G. V. et al. 2003. JNK-mediated BIM phosphorylation potentiates BAX-dependent apoptosis. *Neuron* 38(6):899–914.

1027. Thacher, S. M., E. L. Coe, R. H. Rice. 1985. Retinoid suppression of transglutaminase activity and envelope competence in cultured human epidermal carcinoma cells: Hydrocortisone is a potent antagonist of retinyl acetate but not retinoic acid. *Differentiation* 29(1):82–87.

1028. Sulik, K. K., C. S. Cook, W. S. Webster. 1988. Teratogens and craniofacial malformations: Relationships to cell death. *Development* 103:213–231.

1029. Clotman, F., G. van Maele-Fabry, L. Chu-Wu, J. J. Picard. 1998. Structural and gene expression abnormalities induced by retinoic acid in the forebrain. *Reprod. Toxicol.* 12:169–176.

1030. Freeman, H. J. 2010. Reproductive changes associated with celiac disease. *World J. Gastroenterol.* 16(46):5810–5814.

1031. Martinelli, P., R. Troncone, F. Paparo, P. Torre, E. Trapanese, C. Fasano, A. Lamberti, G. Budillon, G. Nardone, L. Greco. 2000. Coeliac disease and unfavourable outcome of pregnancy. *Gut* 46(3):332–335.

1032. Dickey, W., F. Stewart, J. Nelson, G. McBreen, S. A. McMillan, K. G. Porter. 1996. Screening for coeliac disease as a possible maternal risk factor for neural tube defect. *Clin. Genet.* 49(2):107–108.

1033. Collin, P., S. Vilska, P. K. Heinonen, O. Hällström, P. Pikkarainen. 1996. Infertility and coeliac disease. *Gut* 39(3):382–384.

1034. Taimi, M., C. Helvig, J. Wisniewski, H. Ramshaw, J. White, M. Amad, B. Korczak, M. Petkovich. 2004. A novel human cytochrome P450, CYP26C1, involved in metabolism of 9-cis and all-trans isomers of retinoic acid. *J. Biol. Chem.* 279:77–85.

1035. Paganelli, A., V. Gnazzo, H. Acosta, S. L. López, A. E. Carrasco. 2010. Glyphosate-based herbicides produce teratogenic effects on vertebrates by impairing retinoic acid signaling. *Chem. Res. Toxicol.* 23:1586–1595.

1036. Relyea, R. A. 2005. The lethal impact of Roundup on aquatic and terrestrial amphibians. *Ecol. Appl.* 15:1118–1124.

1037. Carrasco, A. 2013. Teratogenesis by glyphosate based herbicides and other pesticides: Relationship with the retinoic acid pathway. In *GM-Crop Cultivation Ecological Effects on a Landscape Scale.* Theorie in der kologie 17. B. Breckling, R. Verhoeven, Eds. Frankfurt: Peter Lang, pp. 113–117.

1038. Benítez-Leite, S., M. L. Macchi, M. Acosta. 2009. Malformaciones congenítas asociadas a agrotóxicos. *Archivos de Pediatría del Uruguay* 80:237–247.

1039. Gasnier, C., C. Dumont, N. Benachour, E. Clair, M.-C. Chagnon, G.-E. Seralini. 2009. Glyphosate-based herbicides are toxic and endocrine disruptors in human cell lines. *Toxicology* 262:184–191.

1040. Russell, R. M. 2000. The vitamin A spectrum: From deficiency to toxicity. *Am. J. Clin. Nutr.* 71:878–884.

1041. Krasinski, S. D., J. S. Cohn, E. J. Schaefer, R. M. Russell. 1990. Postprandial plasma retinyl ester response is greater in older subjects compared with younger subjects. *J. Clin. Invest.* 85:883–892.

1042. Ellis, J. K., R. M. Russell, F. L. Makrauer, E. J. Schaefer. 1986. Increased risk of vitamin A toxicity in severe hypertriglyceridemia. *Ann. Intern. Med.* 105:877–879.

1043. Jetten, A. M., M. A. George, G. R. Pettit, C. L. Herald, J. I. Rearick. 1989. Action of phorbol esters, bryostatins, and retinoic acid on cholesterol sulfate synthesis: Relation to the multistep process of differentiation in human epidermal keratinocytes. *J. Invest. Dermatol.* 93:108–115.

1044. Meloni, G. F., S. Dessole, N. Vargiu, P. A. Tomasi, S. Musumeci. 1999. The prevalence of coeliac disease in infertility. *Hum. Reprod.* 14(11):2759–2761.

1045. Farthing, M. J. G., C. R. W. Edwards, L. H. Rees, A. M. Dawson. 1982. Male gonadal function in coeliac disease: 1. Sexual dysfunction, infertility, and semen quality. *Gut* 23(7):608–614.

1046. de Liz Oliveira Cavalli, V. L., D. Cattani, C. E. Heinz Rieg, P. Pierozan, L. Zanatta, E. Benedetti Parisotto, D. Wilhelm Filho, F. R. Mena Barreto Silva, R. Pessoa-Pureur, A. Zamoner. 2013. Roundup disrupts male reproductive functions by triggering calcium-mediated cell death in rat testis and Sertoli cells. *Free Radic. Biol. Med.* 65:335–346.

1047. Saibeni, S., A. Lecchi, G. Meucci, M. Cattaneo, L. Tagliabue, E. Rondonotti, S. Formenti, R. De Franchis, M. Vecchi. 2005. Prevalence of hyperhomocysteinemia in adult gluten-sensitive enteropathy at diagnosis: Role of B12, folate, and genetics. *Clin. Gastroenterol. Hepatol.* 3:574–580.

1048. Dickey, W., M. Ward, C. R. Whittle, M. T. Kelly, K. Pentieva, G. Horigan, S. Patton, H. McNulty. 2008. Homocysteine and related B-vitamin status in coeliac disease: Effects of gluten exclusion and histological recovery. *Scand. J. Gastroenterol.* 43:682–688.

1049. Rossi, M., A. Amaretti, S. Raimondi. 2011. Folate production by probiotic bacteria. *Nutrients* 3(1):118–134.

1050. Dahele, A., S. Ghosh. 2001. Vitamin B12 deficiency in untreated celiac disease. *Am. J. Gastroenterol.* 96(3):745–750.

1051. Refsum, H. et al. 2001. Hyperhomocysteinemia and elevated methylmalonic acid indicate a high prevalence of cobalamin deficiency in Asian Indians. *Am. J. Clin. Nutr.* 74:233–241.

1052. Hadithi, M., C. J. J. Mulder, F. Stam, J. Azizi, J. B. A. Crusius, A. S. Peña, C. D. A. Stehouwer, Y. M. Smulders. 2009. Effect of B vitamin supplementation on plasma homocysteine levels in celiac disease. *World J. Gastroenterol.* 15(8):955–960.

1053. Herrmann, W., R. Obeid. 2012. Cobalamin deficiency. *Subcell. Biochem.* 56:301–322.

1054. Cusiel, A. L. 2005. The Synthesis and Reactivity of Novel Co(L)(PMG).n+ Complexes. MS Thesis, University of Canterbury, April.

1055. Ganson, R. J., R. A. Jensen. 1988. The essential role of cobalt in the inhibition of the cytosolic lsozyme of 3-deoxy-D-arabino-heptulosonate-7-phosphate synthase from Nicotiana silvestris by glyphosate. *Arch. Biochem. Biophys.* 260(1):85–73.

1056. Bode, R., C. Melo, D. Birnbaum. 1984. Mode of action of glyphosate in *Candida maltosa*. *Arch. Microbiol.* 140(1):83–85.

1057. Hoagland, R. E., S. E. Duke. 1982. Biochemical effects of glyphosate. In *Biochemical Responses Induced by Herbicides*, D. E. Moreland, J. B. St. John, F. D. Hess, Eds., pp. 175–205 (ACS Symposium Series 181). Washington, DC: American Chemical Society.

1058. Bottaro, G., F. Cataldo, N. Rotolo, M. Spina, G. R. Corazza. 1999. The clinical pattern of subclinical/silent celiac disease: An analysis on 1026 consecutive cases. *Am. J. Gastroenterol.* 94:691–696.

1059. Eker, S., L. Ozturk, A. Yazici, B. Erenoglu, V. Romheld, I. Cakmak. 2006. Foliar-applied glyphosate substantially reduced uptake and transport of iron and manganese in sunflower (*Helianthus annuus L.*) plants. *J. Agric. Food Chem.* 54(26):10019–10025.

1060. Bellaloui, N., K. N. Reddy, R. M. Zablotowicz, H. K. Abbas, C. A. Abel. 2009. Effects of glyphosate application on seed iron and root ferric (III) reductase in soybean cultivars. *J. Agric. Food. Chem.* 57(20):9569–9574.

1061. Bergamaschi, G., K. Markopoulos, R. Albertini, A. Di, Sabatino, F. Biagi, R. Ciccocioppo, E. Arbustini, G. R. Corazza. 2008. Anemia of chronic disease and defective erythropoietin production in patients with celiac disease. *Haematologica* 93(12):1785–1791.

1062. Jasper, R., G. O. Locatelli, C. Pilati, C. Locatelli. 2012. Evaluation of biochemical, hematological and oxidative parameters in mice exposed to the herbicide glyphosate-Roundup. *Interdiscip. Toxicol.* 5(3):133–140.

1063. Cakal, B., Y. Beyazit, S. Koklu, E. Akbal, I. Biyikoglu, G. Yilmaz. 2010. Elevated adenosine deaminase levels in celiac disease. *J. Clin. Lab. Anal.* 24(5):323–326.

1064. Allen, R. H., S. P. Stabler, D. G. Savage, J. Lindenbaum. 1993. Metabolic abnormalities in cobalamin (vitamin B12) and folate deficiency. *FASEB J.* 7:1344–1353.

1065. Boss, G. R. 1985. Cobalamin inactivation decreases purine and methionine synthesis in cultured lymphoblasts. *J. Clin. Invest.* 76:213–218.

1066. Boles, R. G., L. R. Ment, M. S. Meyn, A. L. Horwich, L. E. Kratz, P. Rinaldo. 1993. Short-term response to dietary therapy in molybdenum cofactor deficiency. *Ann. Neurol.* 34(5):742–744.

1067. Beswick, E., J. Millo. 2011. Fatal poisoning with glyphosate-surfactant herbicide. *JICS* 12(1):37–39.
1068. Lu, W., L. Li, M. Chen, Z. Zhou, W. Zhang, S. Ping, Y. Yan, J. Wang, M. Lin. 2013. Genome-wide transcriptional responses of *Escherichia coli* to glyphosate, a potent inhibitor of the shikimate pathway enzyme 5-enolpyruvylshikimate-3-phosphate synthase. *Mol. Biosyst.* 9:522–530.
1069. Peixoto, F. 2005. Comparative effects of the Roundup and glyphosate on mitochondrial oxidative phosphorylation. *Chemosphere* 61(8):1115–1122.
1070. Haderlie, L. C., J. M. Widholm, F. W. Slife. 1977. Effect of glyphosate on carrot and tobacco cells. *Plant Physiol.* 60:40–43.
1071. Ali, A., R. A. Fletcher. 1977. Phytotoxic action of glyphosate and amitrole on corn seedlings. *Can. J. Bot.* 56:2196–2202.
1072. Jansson, E. A. et al. 2008. A mammalian functional nitrate reductase that regulates nitrite and nitric oxide homeostasis. *Nat. Chem. Biol.* 4(7):411–417.
1073. Högberg, L., C. Webb, K. Fälth-Magnusson, T. Forslund, K. E. Magnusson, L. Danielsson, A. Ivarsson, O. Sandström, T. Sundqvist. 2011. Children with screening-detected coeliac disease show increased levels of nitric oxide products in urine. *Acta Paediatr.* 100(7):1023–1027.
1074. Collin, P., K. Kaukinen, M. Valimaki, J. Salmi. 2002. Endocrinological disorders and celiac disease. *Endocrine Rev.* 23(4):464–483.
1075. Valentino, R., S. Savastano, M. Maglio, F. Paparo, F. Ferrara, M. Dorato, G. Lombardi, R. Troncone. 2002. Markers of potential coeliac disease in patients with Hashimoto's thyroiditis. *Eur. J. Endocrinol.* 146:479–483.
1076. Hinks, L. J., K. D. Inwards, B. Lloyd, B. E. Clayton. 1984. Body content of selenium in coeliac disease. *Br. Med. J.* 288:1862–1863.
1077. Sher, L. 2000. Selenium and human health. *Lancet* 356:233–241.
1078. Chanoine, J. P., J. Neve, S. Wu, J. Vanderpas, P. Bourdoux. 2001. Selenium decreases thyroglobulin concentrations but does not affect the increased thyroxine-to-triiodothyronine ratio in children with congenital hypothyroidism. *J. Clin. Endocrinol. Metab.* 86:1160–1163.
1079. Köhrle, J. 2013. Selenium and the thyroid. *Curr. Opin. Endocrinol. Diabetes Obes.* 20(5):441–448.
1080. Papp, L. V., J. Lu, A. Holmgren, K. K. Khanna. 2007. From selenium to selenoproteins: Synthesis, identity, and their role in human health. *Antiox. Redox Signal.* 9:775–806.
1081. Prabhakar, R., K. Morokuma, D. G. Musaev. 2006. Peroxynitrite reductase activity of selenoprotein glutathione peroxidase: A computational study. *Biochemistry* 45:6967–6977.
1082. Huggins, D. R., J. P. Reganold. 2008. No till: The quiet revolution. *Sci. Am.* 99(1):70–77.
1083. Zhao, F. J., F. J. Lopez-Bellido, C. W. Gray, W. R. Whalley, L. J. Clark, S. P. McGrath. 2007. Effects of soil compaction and irrigation on the concentrations of selenium and arsenic in wheat grains. *Sci. Total Environ.* 372(2–3):433–439.
1084. Saes Zobiole, L. H., R. S. de Oliveira Jr., R. J. Kremer, A. S. Muniz, A. de Oliveira, Jr. 2010. Nutrient accumulation and photosynthesis in glyphosate-resistant soybeans is reduced under glyphosate use. *J. Plant Nutr.* 33:1860–1873.
1085. Pessione, E. 2012. Lactic acid bacteria contribution to gut microbiota complexity: Lights and shadows. *Front Cell Infect. Microbiol.* 2:86.
1086. Iglesias, P., J. J. Díez. 2009. Thyroid dysfunction and kidney disease. *Eur. J. Endocrinol.* 160:503–515.
1087. Tsatsoulis, A. 2002. The role of apoptosis in thyroid disease. *Minerva Med.* 93:169–180.
1088. Nafziger, E. D., J. M. Widholm, H. C. Steinrücken, J. L. Killmer. 1984. Selection and characterization of a carrot cell line tolerant to glyphosate. *Plant Physiol.* 76(3):571–574.
1089. Welander, A., K. G. Prütz, M. Fored, J. F. Ludvigsson. 2012. Increased risk of end-stage renal disease in individuals with coeliac disease. *Gut* 61(1):64–68.
1090. Tonelli, M., F. Sacks, M. Pfeffer, G. S. Jhangri, G. Curhan; Cholesterol and Recurrent Events (CARE) Trial Investigators. 2005. Biomarkers of inflammation and progression of chronic kidney disease. *Kidney Int.* 68:237–245.
1091. Bash, L. D., T. P. Erlinger, J. Coresh, J. Marsh-Manzi, A. R. Folsom, B. C. Astor. 2009. Inflammation, hemostasis, and the risk of kidney function decline in the Atherosclerosis Risk in Communities (ARIC) Study. *Am. J. Kidney Dis.* 53:596–605.
1092. Rodríguez-Iturbe, B., G. Garca Garca. 2010. The role of tubulointerstitial inflammation in the progression of chronic renal failure. *Nephron. Clin. Pract.* 116:c81–c88.
1093. Sun, C. Y., H. H. Hsu, M. S. Wu. 2012. p-Cresol sulfate and indoxyl sulfate induce similar cellular inflammatory gene expressions in cultured proximal renal tubular cells. *Nephrol. Dial. Transplant.* 28(1):70–78.

1094. Dou, L., E. Bertrand, C. Cerini, V. Faure, J. Sampol, R. Vanholder, Y. Berland, P. Brunet. 2004. The uremic solutes p-cresol and indoxyl sulfate inhibit endothelial proliferation and wound repair. *Kidney Int.* 65:442–451.

1095. Banoglu, E., R. S. King. 2002. Sulfation of indoxyl by human and rat aryl (phenol) sulfotransferases to form indoxyl sulfate. *Eur. J. Drug Metab. Pharmacokinet.* 27(2):135–140.

1096. Niwa, T. 2010. Indoxyl sulfate is a nephro-vascular toxin. *J. Ren. Nutr.* 20(Suppl. 5):S2–S6.

1097. Cañal, M. J., R. S. Tamés, B. Fernández. 1987. Glyphosate-increased levels of indole-3-acetic acid in yellow nutsedge leaves correlate with gentisic acid levels. *Physiol. Plantar.* 71(3):384–388.

1098. Samsel, A., S. Seneff. 2013. Glyphosate's suppression of cytochrome P450 enzymes and amino acid biosynthesis by the gut microbiome: Pathways to modern diseases. *Entropy* 15:1416–1463.

1099. Lee, J. H., J. Lee. 2010. Indole as an intercellular signal in microbial communities. *FEMS Microbiol. Rev.* 34:426–444.

1100. Roe, D. A. 1971. Effects of methionine and inorganic sulfate on indole toxicity and indican excretion in rats. *J. Nutr.* 101(5):645–653.

1101. Drexler, J. 1958. Effect of indole compounds on vitamin B12 utilization. *Blood* 13(3):239–244.

1102. Furukawa, S., K. Usuda, M. Abe, S. Hayashi, I. Ogawa. 2007. Indole-3-acetic acid induces microencephaly in mouse fetuses. *Exp. Toxicol. Pathol.* 59(1):43–52.

1103. Bostwick, H. E., S. H. Berezin, M. S. Halata, R. Jacobson, M. S. Medow. 2001. Celiac disease presenting with microcephaly. *J. Pediatr.* 138(4):589–592.

1104. Lapunzina, P. 2002. Celiac disease and microcephaly. *J. Pediatr.* 140(1):141–142.

1105. Uggla, C., T. Moritz, G. Sandberg, B. Sundberg. 1996. Auxin as a positional signal in pattern formation in plants. *Proc. Natl. Acad. Sci. U.S.A.* 93(17):9282–9286.

1106. Hallert, C., C. Grant, S. Grehn, C. Granno, S. Hultén, G. Midhagen, M. Ström, H. Svensson, T. Valdimarsson. 2002. Evidence of poor vitamin status in celiac patients on a gluten-free diet for 10 years. *Aliment. Pharmacol. Ther.* 16:1333–1339.

1107. Hernanz, A., I. Polanco. 1991. Plasma precursor amino acids of central nervous system monoamines in children with coeliac disease. *Gut* 32:1478–1481.

1108. Koyama, T., H. Y. Melzter. 1986. A biochemical and neuroendocrine study of the serotonergic system in depression. In *New Results in Depression Research*, H. Hippius, G. L. Klerman, N. Matussek, Eds., pp. 164–188. New York: Springer-Verlag.

1109. Saad, R. J., W. D. Chey. 2006. Review article: Current and emerging therapies for functional dyspepsia. *Aliment. Pharmacol. Ther.* 24(3):475–492.

1110. Manocha, M., W. I. Khan. 2012. Serotonin and GI disorders: An update on clinical and experimental studies. *Clin. Transl. Gastroenterol.* 3:e13.

1111. Kim, M., H. J. Cooke, N. H. Javed, H. V. Carey, F. Christofi, H. E. Raybould. 2001. D-glucose releases 5-hydroxytryptamine from human BON cells as a model of enterochromaffin cells. *Gastroenterology* 121:1400–1406.

1112. Chin, A., B. Svejda, B. I. Gustafsson, A. B. Granlund, A. K. Sandvik, A. Timberlake, B. Sumpio, R. Pfragner, I. M. Modlin, M. Kidd. 2012. The role of mechanical forces and adenosine in the regulation of intestinal enterochromaffin cell serotonin secretion. *Am. J. Physiol. Gastrointest. Liver Physiol.* 302:G397–G405.

1113. Fukumoto, S., M. Tatewaki, T. Yamada, M. Fujimiya, C. Mantyh, M. Voss, S. Eubanks, M. Harris, T. N. Pappas, T. Takahashi. 2003. Short-chain fatty acids stimulate colonic transit via intraluminal 5-HT release in rats. *Am. J. Physiol. Regul. Integr. Comp. Physiol.* 284:R1269–R1276.

1114. Grider, J. R., B. E. Piland. 2007. The peristaltic reflex induced by short-chain fatty acids is mediated by sequential release of 5-HT and neuronal CGRP but not BDNF. *Am. J. Physiol. Gastrointest. Liver Physiol.* 292:G429–G437.

1115. Wheeler, E. E., D. N. Challacombe. 1984. Quantification of enterochromaffin cells with serotonin immunoreactivity in the duodenal mucosa in coeliac disease. *Arch. Dis. Child* 59:523–527.

1116. Challacombe, D. N., P. D. Dawkins, P. Baker. 1977. Increased tissue concentrations of 5-hydroxy-tryptamine in the duodenal mucosa of patients with coeliac disease. *Gut* 18:882–886.

1117. Erspamer, V. 1986. Historical introduction: The Italian contribution to the discovery of 5-hydroxytryptamine (enteramine, serotonin). *J. Hypertens. Suppl.* 4(1):S3–S5.

1118. Coleman, N. S. et al. 2006. Abnormalities of serotonin metabolism and their relation to symptoms in untreated celiac disease. *Clin. Gastroenterol. Hepatol.* 4:874–881.

1119. Madsen, H. E. L., H. H. Christensen, C. Gottlieb-Petersen. 1978. Stability constants of copper (II), zinc, manganese (II), calcium, and magnesium complexes of N-(phosphonomethyl) glycine (glyphosate). *Acta Chem. Scand.* 32:79–83.

1120. Motekaitis, R. J., A. E. Martell. 1985. Metal chelate formation by N-phosphonomethylglycine and related ligands. *J. Coord. Chem.* 14:139–149.

1121. Undabeytia, T. S., E. Morillo, C. Maqueda. 2002. FTIR study of glyphosate-copper complexes. *J. Agric. Food Chem.* 50:1918–1921.

1122. Cakmak, I., A. Yazici, Y. Tutus, L. Ozturk. 2009. Glyphosate reduced seed and leaf concentrations of calcium, manganese, magnesium, and iron in nonglyphosate resistant soybean. *Eur. J. Agron.* 31(3):114–119.

1123. Singhal, N., S. Alam, R. Sherwani, J. Musarrat. 2008. Serum zinc levels in celiac disease. *Indian Pediatr.* 45(4):319–321.

1124. Halfdanarson, T. R., N. Kumar, W. J. Hogan, J. A. Murray. 2009. Copper deficiency in celiac disease. *J. Clin. Gastroenterol.* 43(2):162–164.

1125. Goldman, A. S., D. D. Van Fossan, E. E. Baird. 1962. Magnesium deficiency in celiac disease. *Pediatrics* 29(6):948–952.

1126. Rude, R. K., M. Olerich. 1996. Magnesium deficiency: Possible role in osteoporosis associated with gluten-sensitive enteropathy. *Osteoporos. Int.* 6(6):453–461.

1127. Lerner, A., Y. Shapira, N. Agmon-Levin, A. Pacht, D. Ben-Ami Shor, H. M. López, M. Sanchez-Castanon, Y. Shoenfeld. 2012. The clinical significance of 25OH-vitamin D status in celiac disease. *Clin. Rev. Allergy Immunol.* 42(3):322–330.

1128. Ponchon, G., A. L. Kennan, H. F. DeLuca. 1969. Activation of vitamin D by the liver. *J. Clin. Invest.* 48(11):2032–2037.

1129. Sakaki, T., N. Kagawa, K. Yamamoto, K. Inouye. 2005. Metabolism of vitamin D3 by cytochromes P450. *Front. Biosci.* 10:119–134.

1130. Holick, M. F. 2005. The Vitamin D Epidemic and its Health Consequences. *J. Nutr.* 135(11):2739S–2748S.

1131. Glass, R. L. 1984. Metal complex formation by glyphosate. *J. Agric. Food Chem.* 32:1249–1253.

1132. Homann, P. E. 1967. Studies on the manganese of the chloroplast. *Plant Physiol.* 42:997–1007.

1133. Thompson, W. W., T. E. Weier. 1962. The fine structure of chloroplasts from mineral-deficient leaves of *Phaseolus vulgaris. Am. J. Bot.* 49:1047–1056.

1134. Ames, B. N., M. K. Shigenaga, T. M. Hagen. 1993. Oxidants, antioxidants, and the degenerative diseases of aging. *Proc. Natl. Acad. Sci. U.S.A.* 90:7915–7922.

1135. Coussens, L. M., Z. Werb. 2002. Inflammation and cancer. *Nature* 420:860–867.

1136. Nielsen, O. H., O. Jacobsen, E. R. Pedersen, S. N. Rasmussen, M. Petri, S. Laulund, S. Jarnum. 1985. Non-tropical sprue. Malignant diseases and mortality rate. *Scand. J. Gastroenterol.* 20:13–18.

1137. Logan, R. F., E. A. Rifkind, I. D. Turner, A. Ferguson. 1989. Mortality in celiac disease. *Gastroenterology* 97:265–271.

1138. Pricolo, V. E., A. A. Mangi, B. Aswad, K. I. Bland. 1998. Gastrointestinal malignancies in patients with celiac sprue. *Am. J. Surg.* 176:344–347.

1139. Cottone, M. et al. 1999. Mortality and causes of death in celiac disease in a Mediterranean area. *Dig. Dis. Sci.* 44:2538–2541.

1140. Corrao, G. et al.; Club del Tenue Study Group. 2001. Mortality in patients with coeliac disease and their relatives: A cohort study. *Lancet* 358:356–361.

1141. Green, P. H., A. T. Fleischauer, G. Bhagat, R. Goyal, B. Jabri, A. I. Neugut. 2003. Risk of malignancy in patients with celiac disease. *Am. J. Med.* 115(3):191–195.

1142. Matheus-Vliezen, E. M. E., H. Van Halteran, G. N. J. Tylgut. 1994. Malignant lymphoma in coeliac disease: Various manifestations with distinct symptomatology and prognosis? *J. Intern. Med.* 236(1):43–49.

1143. Egan, L. J., S. V. Walsh, F. M. Stevens, C. E. Connolly, E. L. Egan, C. F. McCarthy. 1995. Celiac associated lymphoma: A single institution experience of 30 cases in the combination chemotherapy era. *J. Clin. Gastroenterol.* 21(2):123–129.

1144. Nelson, M. A., B. W. Porterfield, E. T. Jacobs, L. C. Clark. 1999. Selenium and prostate cancer prevention. *Semin. Urol. Oncol.* 17(2):91–96.

1145. Björnstedt, M., P. Aristi. A. P. Fernandes. 2010. Selenium in the prevention of human cancers. *EPMA J.* 1:389–395.

1146. Szaflarska-Poplawska, A., A. Siomek, M. Czerwionka-Szaflarska, D. Gackowski, R. Rozalski, J. Guz, A. Szpila, E. Zarakowska, R. Olinski. 2010. Oxidatively damaged DNA/oxidative stress in children with celiac disease. *Cancer Epidemiol. Biomarkers Prev.* 19(8):1960–1965.

1147. Rivabene, R., E. Mancini, M. Vincenzi. 1999. In vitro cytotoxic effect of wheat gliadin-derived peptides on the Caco-2 intestinal cell line is associated with intracellular oxidative imbalance: Implications for coeliac disease. *Biochim. Biophys. Acta* 1453:152–160.

1148. Miteva L., S. Ivanov, V. Alexieva, E. Karanov. 2003. Effect of herbicide glyphosate on glutathione levels, glutathione-S-transferase and glutathione reductase activities in two plant species. *C. R. Acad. Bulg. Sci.* 56:79–84.

1149. Negri, E. 2010. Sun exposure, vitamin D, and risk of Hodgkin and non-Hodgkin lymphoma. *Nutr. Cancer* 62(7):878–882.

1150. Vigfusson, N. V., E. R. Vyse. 1980. The effect of the pesticides, Dexon, Captan and Roundup, on sister-chromatid exchanges in human lymphocytes *in vitro*. *Mutat. Res.* 79:53–57.

1151. Pavkov, K. L., J. C. Turnier. 1986. *2-Year Chronic Toxicity and Oncogenicity Dietary Study with SCm-0224 in Mice. T-11813.* Farmington: Stauffer Chemical Company, pp. 159–184.

1152. Hardell, L., M. Eriksson. 1999. A case-control study of non-Hodgkin lymphoma and exposure to pesticides. *Cancer* 85(6):1353–1360.

1153. McDuffie, H. H., P. Pahwa, J. R. McLaughlin, J. J. Spinelli, S. Fincham, J. A. Dosman, D. Robson, L. F. Skinnider, N. W. Choi. 2001. Non-Hodgkins lymphoma and specific pesticide exposures in men: Cross-Canada study of pesticides and health. *Cancer Epidemiol. Biomarkers Prev.* 10(11):1155–1163.

1154. De Roos, A. J., S. H. Zahm, K. P. Cantor, D. D. Weisemburger, F. F. Holmes, L. F. Burmeister, A. Blair. 2003. Integrative assessment of multiple pesticides as risk factors for non-Hodgkins lymphoma among men. *Occup. Environ. Med.* 60(9):e11.

1155. Nalewaja, J. D., R. Matysiak. 1993. Influence of diammonium sulfate and other salts on glyphosate phytotoxicity. *Pestic. Sci.* 38:77–84.

1156. Dørum, S., M. Ø. Arntzen, S.-W. Qiao, A. Holm, C. J. Koehler, B. Thiede, L. M. Sollid, B. Fleckenstein. 2010. The preferred substrates for transglutaminase 2 in a complex wheat gluten digest are peptide fragments harboring celiac disease T-cell epitopes. *PLoS One* 5(11):e14056.

1157. Qiao, S.-W., E. Bergseng, Ø. Molberg, G. Jung, B. Fleckenstein, L. M. Solli. 2005. Refining the rules of gliadin T cell epitope binding to the disease-associated DQ2 molecule in celiac disease: Importance of proline spacing and glutamine deamidation. *J. Immunol.* 175(1):254–261.

1158. Selvapandiyan, A., K. Majumder, F. A. Fattah, S. Ahmad, N. Arora, R. K. Bhatnagar. 1995. Point mutation of a conserved arginine (104) to lysine introduces hypersensitivity to inhibition by glyphosate in the 5-enolpyruvylshikimate-3-phosphate synthase of Bacillus subtilis. *FEBS Lett.* 374(2):253–256.

1159. Sammons, R. D., K. J. Gruys, K. S. Anderson, K. A. Johnson, J. A. Sikorski. 1995. Reevaluating glyphosate as a transition-state inhibitor of EPSP synthase: Identification of an EPSP synthase EPSP glyphosate ternary complex. *Biochemistry* 34(19):6433–6440.

1160. Cabrera-Chávez, F., A. R. Islas-Rubio, O. Rouzaud-Sández, N. Sotelo-Cruz, A. M. Calderón de la Barcaa. 2010. Modification of gluten by methionine binding to prepare wheat bread with reduced reactivity to serum IgA of celiac disease patients. *J. Cereal Sci.* 52(2):310–313.

1161. Lai, T. S., A. Hausladen, T. F. Slaughter, J. P. Eu, J. S. Stamler, C. S. Greenberg. 2001. Calcium regulates S-nitrosylation, denitrosylation, and activity of tissue transglutaminase. *Biochemistry* 40(16):4904–4910.

1162. Hoppe, H. W. 2013. *Determination of Glyphosate Residues in Human Urine Samples from 18 European Countries.* Report Glyphosate MLHB-2013-06-06. Medical Laboratory Bremen, Haferwende 12, 28357 Bremen, Germany, March, December 6, 2013.

1163. Kaplan, M. M., A. Ohkubo, E. G. Quaroni, D. Sze-Tu. 1983. Increased synthesis of rat liver alkaline phosphatase by bile duct ligation. *Hepatology* 3(3):368–376.

1164. Beuret, C. J., F. Zirulnik, M. S. Gimenez. 2005. Effect of the herbicide glyphosate on liver lipoperoxidation in pregnant rats and their fetuses. *Reprod. Toxicol.* 19:501–504.

1165. Nomura, N. S., H. W. Hilton. 1977. The adsorption and degradation of glyphosate in five Hawaiian sugarcane soils. *Weed Res.* 17:113–121.

1166. Vencill, W. K. (Ed.). 2002. *Herbicide Handbook*, 8th ed. Lawrence, KS: Weed Science Society of America.

1167. O'Keeffe, M. G. 1980. The control of Agropyron repens and broad-leaved weeds pre-harvest of wheat and barley with the isopropylamine salt of glyphosate. *Proceedings of British Crop Protection Conference—Weeds*, 53–60.

1168. O'Keeffe, M. G. 1981. The control of perennial grasses by pre-harvest applications of glyphosate. *Proceedings of the Conference on Grass Weeds in Cereals in the United Kingdom.* Association of Applied Biologists, Warwick, UK, 137–144.

1169. Stride, C. D., R. V. Edwards, J. C. Seddon. 1985. Sward destruction by application of glyphosate before cutting or grazing. *British Crop Protection Conference—Weeds 7B–6*, 771–778.

1170. Darwent, A. L., K. J. Kirkland, L. Townley-Smith, K. N. Harker, A. J. Cessna, O. M. Lukow, L. P. Lefkovitch. 1994. Effect of preharvest applications of glyphosate on the drying, yield and quality of wheat. *Can. J. Plant Sci.* 74(2):221–230.

1171. Orson, J. H., D. K. H. Davies. 2007. Pre-harvest glyphosate for weed control and as a harvest aid in cereals. Research Review No. 65. HGCA.

1172. Waltz, E. 2010. Glyphosate resistance threatens Roundup hegemony. *Nat. Biotechnol.* 28:537–538.

1173. Culpepper, A. S., A. C. York, R. B. Batts, K. M. Jennings. 2000. Weed management in glufosinate- and glyphosate-resistant soybean (glycine max). *Weed Technol.* 14(1):77–88.

1174. Ramirez-Rubio, O., D. R. Brooks, J. J. Amador, J. S. Kaufman, D. E. Weiner, M. K. Scammell. 2013. Chronic kidney disease in Nicaragua: A qualitative analysis of semi-structured interviews with physicians and pharmacists. *BMC Public Health* 13:350.

1175. Trabanino, R. G., R. Aguilar, C. R. Silva, M. O. Mercado, R. L. Merino. 2002. End-stage renal disease among patients in a referral hospital in El Salvador. *Rev. Panam. Salud Publica* 12:202–206. (Article in Spanish).

1176. Cerdas, M. 2005. Chronic kidney disease in Costa Rica. *Kidney Int. Suppl.* 97:31–33.

1177. Torres, C., A. Aragon, M. Gonzalez, I. Lopez, K. Jakobsson, C. G. Elinder, I. Lundberg, C. Wesseling. 2010. Decreased kidney function of unknown cause in Nicaragua: A community-based survey. *Am. J. Kidney Dis.* 55:485–496.

1178. Peraza, S., C. Wesseling, A. Aragon, R. Leiva, R. A. Garca-Trabanino, C. Torres, K. Jakobsson, C. Elinder, C. Hogstedt. 2012. Decreased kidney function among agriculture workers in El Salvador. *Am. J. Kidney Dis.* 59:531–540.

1179. Sanoff, S. L., L. Callejas, C. D. Alonso, Y. Hu, R. E. Colindres, H. Chin, D. R. Morgan, S. L. Hogan. 2010. Positive association of renal insufficiency with agriculture employment and unregulated alcohol consumption in Nicaragua. *Ren. Fail.* 32:766–777.

1180. Agúndez, J. A., E. García-Martín, C. Martínez. 2009. Genetically based impairment in CYP2C8- and CYP2C9-dependent NSAID metabolism as a risk factor for gastrointestinal bleeding: Is a combination of pharmacogenomics and metabolomics required to improve personalized medicine? *Expert Opin. Drug Metab. Toxicol.* 5(6):607–620.

1181. Katz, A., R. F. Dyck, R. A. Bear. 1979. Celiac disease associated with immune complex glomerulonephritis. *Clin. Nephrol.* 11(1):39–44.

1182. Peters, U., J. Askling, G. Gridley, A. Ekbom, M. Linet. 2003. Causes of death in patients with celiac disease in a population-based Swedish cohort. *Arch. Intern Med.* 163(13):1566–1572.

1183. Richard, E. P Jr., C. D. Dalley. 2009. Effects of glyphosate ripener timing and rate on cane and sugar yields. *J. Am. Soc. Sugarcane Technol.* 29:81–82.

1184. Orgeron, A. J. 2012. Sugarcane Growth, Sucrose Content, and Yield Response to the Ripeners Glyphosate and Trinexapacethyl. PhD Dissertation, School of Plant, Environmental, and Soil Sciences, Louisiana State University.

1185. State-Specific Trends in Chronic Kidney Failure—United States. 1990–2001. http://www.cdc.gov/mmwr/preview/mmwrhtml/mm5339a3.htm [Accessed September 3, 2013].

1186. Network Coordinating Council. 2013. *2012 Annual Report. End Stage Renal Disease Network 13.* http://www.network13.org/PDFs/NW13 Annual Report 2012 Final.pdf [Accessed September 3, 2013].

1187. Legendre, B. L., K. A. Gravois, K. P. Bischoff, J. L. Griffin. 2005. Timing of glyphosate applications, alternatives to the use of glyphosate and response of new varieties to glyphosate in maximizing the yield of sugar per acre of Louisiana sugarcane in 2005. *LSUAgCenter Sugarcane Ann. Rep.* 182–191.

1188. Subiros, J. F. 1990. The effect of applying glyphosate as ripener in three varieties. *Turrialba* 40(4):527–534.

1189. Shapira, Y., N. Agmon-Levina, Y. Shoenfeld. 2010. Defining and analyzing geoepidemiology and human autoimmunity. *J. Autoimmun.* 34:J168–J177.

1190. Grube, A., D. Donaldson, T. Kiely, L. Wu. 2011. *Pesticide Industry Sales and Usage: 2006 and 2007 Market Estimates.* Washington, DC: U.S. Environmental Protection Agency.

1191. Kiely, T., D. Donaldson, A. Grube. 2004. *Pesticides Industry Sales and Usage—2000 and 2001 Market Estimates.* Washington, DC: U.S. Environmental Protection Agency.

1192. Kimmel, G. L., C. A. Kimmel, A. L. Williams, J. M. DeSesso. 2013. Evaluation of developmental toxicity studies of glyphosate with attention to cardiovascular development. *Crit. Rev. Toxicol.* 43(2):79–95.

1193. Duke, S. O., S. B. Powles. 2008. Glyphosate: A once-in-a-century herbicide. *Pest Manag. Sci.* 64:319–325.

1194. Koning, F. 2005. Celiac disease: Caught between a rock and a hard place. *Gastroenterology* 129(4):1294–1301.

1195. Fasano, A. et al. 2003. Prevalence of celiac disease in at-risk and not-at-risk groups in the United States a large multicenter study. *Arch. Intern Med.* 163:286–292.

1196. Sonnenberg, A., D. J. McCarty, S. J. Jacobsen. 1991. Geographic variation of inflammatory bowel disease within the United States. *Gastroenterology* 100:143e9.
1197. Bernfield, M., M. Götte, P.-W. Park, O. Reizes, M.L. Fitzgerald, J. Lincecum, M. Zako. 1999. Functions of cell surface heparan sulfate proteoglycans. *Annu. Rev. Biochem.* 68:729–777.
1198. Turnbull, J., A. Powell, S. Guimond. 2001. Heparan sulfate: Decoding a dynamic multifunctional cell regulator. *Trends Cell Biol.* 11:75–82.
1199. Collins, D., R. Wilcox, M. Nathan, R. Zubarik. 2012. Celiac disease and hypothyroidism. *Am. J. Med.* 125(3):278–282.
1200. Laurin, P., K. Fälth-Magnusson, T. Sundqvist. 2003. Increase in nitric oxide urinary products during gluten challenge in children with coeliac disease. *Scand. J. Gastroenterol.* 38(1):55–60.
1201. Jaya, B., L. Hu, J. W. Bauman, S. C. Fu, A. S. Reddi. 1993. Effect of galactose regimen on glomerular heparan sulfate synthesis and albumin excretion in diabetic rats. *Res. Commun. Chem. Pathol. Pharmacol.* 80(2):143–152.
1202. Gopee, E., E. L. van den Oever, F. Cameron, M. C. Thomas. 2013. Coeliac disease, gluten-free diet and the development and progression of albuminuria in children with type 1 diabetes. *Pediatr. Diabetes* 14(6):455–458.
1203. Barbosa, E. R., M. D. Leiros da Costa, L. A. Bacheschi, M. Scaff, C. C. Leite. 2001. Parkinsonism after glycine-derivate exposure. *Mov. Disord.* 16(3):565–568.
1204. Baizabal-Carvallo, J. F., J. Jankovic. 2012. Movement disorders in autoimmune diseases. *Mov. Disord.* 27(8):935–946.
1205. Roels, H., R. Lauwerys, J. Konings, J. P. Buchet, A. Bernard, S. Green, D. Bradley, W. Morgan, D. Chettle. 1994. Renal function and hyperfiltration capacity in lead smelter workers with high bone lead. *Occup. Environ. Med.* 51(8):505–512.
1206. Jarup, L., M. Berglund, C. G. Elinder, G. Nordberg, M. Vahter. 1998. Health effects of cadmium exposure—A review of the literature and a risk estimate. *Scand. J. Work Environ. Health* 24(Suppl. 1):1–51.
1207. Hambach, R., D. Lison, P. C. D'Haese, J. Weyler, E. De Graef, A. De Schryver, L. V. Lamberts, M. Van Sprundel. 2013. Co-exposure to lead increases the renal response to low levels of cadmium in metallurgy workers. *Toxicol. Lett.* 222(2):233–238.
1208. Tomakh, IuF. 1993. The physicochemical and biochemical signs of nephrolithiasis. *Urol. Nefrol. (Mosk)* 6:19–21.
1209. Bogolepova, A. E., A. A. Kuznetsova, B. G. Lukichev, Iu V. Natochkin, Olu Parshukova, N. P. Prutskova, El. Shakhmatova. 2000. Mechanism F Kidney Participation in Maintaining Osmotic and Ion Homeostasis in Chronic Renal Failure. *Urologiia* 3:5–8.
1210. Corradi, M., A. Mutti. 2011. Metal ions affecting the pulmonary and cardiovascular systems. *Metal Ions Life Sci.* 8:81–105.
1211. Bernier, J., P. Brousseau, K. Krzystyniak, H. Tryphonas, M. Fournier. 1995. Immunotoxicity of heavy metals in relation to Great Lakes. *Environ. Health Perspect.* 103:23.
1212. Nordberg, G. F., R. A. Goyer, T. W. Clarkson. 1985. Impact of effects of acid precipitation on toxicity of metals. *Environ. Health Perspect.* 63:169.
1213. Shukla, G. S., R. L. Singhal. 1984. The present status of biological effects of toxic metals in the environment: Lead, cadmium, and manganese. *Can. J. Physiol. Pharmacol.* 62(8):1015–1031.
1214. Suntharalingam, K., O. Mendoza, A. A. Duarte, D. J. Mann, R. Vilar. 2013. A platinum complex that binds non-covalently to DNA and induces cell death via a different mechanism than cisplatin. *Metallomics* 5(5):514.
1215. Purchase, R. 2013. The link between copper and Wilson's disease. *Sci. Prog.* 96(3):213–223.
1216. Kamunde, C., C. M. Wood. 2003. The influence of ration size on copper homeostasis during sublethal dietary copper exposure in juvenile rainbow trout, *Oncorhynchus mykiss. Aquat. Toxicol.* 62(3):235–254.
1217. Clearwater, S. J., A. M. Farag, J. S. Meyer. 2002. Bioavailability and toxicity of dietborne copper and zinc to fish. *Comp. Biochem. Physiol. C Toxicol. Pharmacol.* 132(3):269–313.
1218. Chou, S., J. Colman, C. Tylenda, C. De Rosa. 2007. Chemical-specific health consultation for chromated copper arsenate chemical mixture: Port of Djibouti. *Toxicol. Ind. Health* 23(4):183–208.
1219. Sun, S., J. Qin, N. Yu, X. Ge, H. Jiang, L. Chen. 2013. Effect of dietary copper on the growth performance, non-specific immunity and resistance to *Aeromonas hydrophila* of juvenile Chinese mitten crab, *Eriocheir Sinensis. Fish Shellfish Immunol.* 34(5):1195–1201.
1220. Zhu, Y. Z., D. W. Liu, Z. Y. Liu, Y. F. Li. 2013. Impact of aluminum exposure on the immune system: A mini review. *Environ. Toxicol. Pharmacol.* 35(1):82–87.
1221. Vota, D. M., R. L. Crisp, A. B. Nesse, D. C. Vittori. 2012. Oxidative Stress due to aluminium exposure induces eryptosis which is prevented by erythropoietin. *J. Cell. Biochem.* 113(5):1581–1589.

1222. Niemoeller, O. M., V. Kiedaisch, P. Dreischer, T. Wieder, F. Lang. 2006. Stimulation of eryptosis by aluminium ions. *Toxicol. Appl. Pharmacol.* 217(2):168–175.

1223. Asuma, K. 2007. *Publications of the Astronomical Society of the Pacific* 119(862):1488–1497.

1224. Wang, R., T. King, M. DeFelcie, W. Guo, M. H. Ossipov, F. Porreca. 2013. Descending facilitation maintains long-term spontaneous neuropathic pain. *J. Pain* 14(8):845–853.

1225. Burgess, S. E., C. R. Gardell, M. H. Ossiprov, T. P. Malan Jr., T. W. Vanderah, J. Lai, F. Porreca. 2002. Time-dependent descending facilitation from the rostral ventromedial medulla maintains, but does not initiate, neuropathic pain. *J. Neurosci.* 22(12):5129–5136.

1226. Paoletti, P., J. Neyton. 2007. NMDA receptor subunits: Function and pharmacology. *Curr. Opin. Pharmacol.* 7(1):39–47.

1227. Qiu, C., M. Kivipelto, E. von Strauss. 2009. Epidemiology of Alzheimer's disease: Occurrence, determinants, and strategies toward intervention. *Dialogues Clin. NeuroSci.* 11:111–128.

1228. Phillips, M., K. Gleeson, J. M. Hughes, J. Greenberg, R. N. Cataneo, L. Baker, W. Patrick Mcvay. 1999. Volatile organic compounds in breath as markers of lung cancer: A cross-sectional study. *Lancet* 353(9168):1930–1933.

1229. Barger, A. C., R. Beeuwkes 3rd, L. L. Lainey, K. J. Silverman. 1984. Hypothesis: Vasa vasorum and neovascularization of human coronary arteries. A possible role in the pathophysiology of atherosclerosis. *N. Engl. J. Med.* 310:175–177.

1230. Liu, R., Y. Jin, W. H. Tang, L. Qin, X. Zhang, G. Tellides, J. Hwa, J. Yu, K. A. Martin. 2013. Ten-eleven translocation-2 (TET2) is a master regulator of smooth muscle cell plasticity. *Circulation* 128:2047–2057.

1231. Colditz, G. A., P. Martin, M. J. Stampfer, W. C. Willett, L. Sampson, B. Rosner, C. H. Hennekens, F. E. Speizer. 1986. Validation of questionnaire information on risk factors and disease outcomes in a prospective cohort study of women. *Am. J. Epidemiol.* 123:894–900.

1232. Cross, C. E., B. Halliwell, E. T. Borish, W. A. Pryor, B. N. Ames, R. L. Saul, J. M. McCord, D. Harman. 1987. Oxygen radicals and human disease. *Ann. Intern. Med.* 107:526–545.

1233. Liacouras, C. A. et al. 2011. Eosinophilic esophagitis: Updated consensus recommendations for children and adults. *J. Allergy Clin. Immunol.* 128:3–20.

1234. Rea, W. J. 1976. Environmentally triggered thrombophlebitis. *Ann. Allergy* 37:101–109.

1235. Triggiani, V., E. Tafaro, V. A. Giagulli, C. Sabbà, F. Resta, B. Licchelli, E. Guastamacchia. 2009. Role of iodine, selenium and other micronutrients in thyroid function and disorders. *Endocr. Metab. Immune Disord. Drug Targets* 9(3):277–294.

1236. Kitchen, L. M., W. W. Witt, C. E. Rieck. 1981. Inhibition of chlorophyll accumulation by glyphosate. *Weed Sci.* 29:513–516.

1237. Soderland, P., S. Lovekar, D. E. Weiner, D. R. Brooks, J. S. Kaufman. 2010. Chronic kidney disease associated with environmental toxins and exposures. *Adv. Chronic Kidney Dis.* 17(3):254–264.

3 Evaluation of Water and Its Contaminants

GENERAL INTRODUCTION

Water contains minerals, toxic and nontoxic inorganic and organic chemicals, particulate matter (molds, algae, bacteria, viruses, and parasites), and radiation. It is an important conduit through which these nutrients and contaminants enter and affect the human organism. It is especially important in the onset, exacerbation, and treatment of chemical sensitivity and chronic degenerative disease. Following ingestion, since all of its components must be anabolized, catabolized, or compartmentalized, water, when contaminated, can contribute to gross increases in total body pollutant load, exacerbating chemical sensitivity and chronic degenerative disease. In contrast, they have seen in many cases that less contaminated water greatly benefits individual health by not only contributing valuable nutrients and/or by not adding to the total body pollutant load, but also by significantly reducing this pollutant load.

A voluminous body of the literature indicates that in developed nations, the incidence of many chronic diseases, particularly cardiovascular, neurological, and bronchopulmonary diseases in the general population, is associated with various water characteristics including purity, mineral, and pollutant content.[1] At the EHC-Dallas and Buffalo, we have observed that water quality also affects our chemically and food sensitive patients, many of whom react both acutely and chronically to the pollutant and mineral content. This is because the chemically sensitive are unable to tolerate most kinds of water contamination. Pure water is essential to the proper management of their illnesses. This is not used usually in medical and hospitals in the United States and most of the world clinics.

OCEAN ACIDIFICATION

Change in ocean pH is important because so many people as well as sea life are dependent on the ocean.

Unlike many areas of global change, there is no argument that rising CO_2 emissions will make the world's oceans more acidic. Average pH in surface waters is now 8.1, a 30% increase in acidity since the start of the industrial revolution and forecasters say it could drop to 7.8 by 2100, if carbon emissions continue unabated. How fisheries and other marine life will respond is far from clear. It is even more unclear how the humans, especially the chemically sensitive, will respond.

Many species suffer; for example, fish and shellfish larvae exposed to more acidic waters often fail to thrive. They do not grow as big or live as long as those born in more alkaline waters. But some species show substantial resilience. After they used acidic water to completely dissolve the shells of developing sea urchins, for instance, the urchins were able to regrow them and live normally once they were returned to normal seawater.[2]

Such limited studies, however, cannot really tell you whether a species has the capacity to adapt to acidification or how pH changes affect a larger ecosystem.

To evaluate acidification's potential impact on modern ecosystems, researchers are also seeking out rare places where the future has already arrived, such as natural seafloor seeps, where bubbling carbon dioxide gas dramatically lowers the pH of surrounding seawater. Studies of seeps off Papua New Guinea have already shown that tropical coral reefs in acidified waters have fewer species and slower growth rates than nearby reefs.[2]

Similar changes are apparent on rocky bottoms at seeps in the more temperate Mediterranean waters. Off the coast of Italy, studies on shallow-water seeps nestled beneath a tower medieval castle are being performed. There small, fast-growing invertebrates and weedy filamentous algae are displacing an array of larger, flashier shell-building species.[2]

Bacteria in the acidified tanks greatly stepped up their nitrogen fixing activity over time. They did not revert to lower activity when moved back into the less acidic tanks, suggesting true adaptive changes. Genetic studies backed up that idea. Acidification could have major implications for the future of the marine nitrogen cycle by altering bacterial populations. Thus, influencing the effects on the chemically sensitive and chronic degenerative disease patients in a variety of ways, including the food chain.

WORLD WATER QUALITY FACTS AND STATISTICS

Every day, 2 million tons of sewage and industrial and agricultural waste are discharged into the world's water,[3] the equivalent of the weight of the entire human population of 6.8 billion people. This discharge makes it impossible to get clean seawater and, thus, foods from the sea to eat for the chemically sensitive and chronic degenerative disease patients.

The UN estimates that the amount of wastewater produced annually is approximately 1500 km[3], six times more water than that exists in all the rivers of the world.[3]

Lack of adequate sanitation contaminates water courses worldwide and is one of the most significant forms of water pollution. Worldwide, 2.5 billion people live without improved sanitations.[4]

Over 70% of these people who lack sanitation, or 1.8 billion people, live in Asia.

Sub-Saharan Africa is the slowest of the world's regions in achieving improved sanitation: Only 31% of residents had access to improved sanitation in 2006.

In addition, 18% of the world's population, or 1.2 billion people (1 out of 3 in rural areas), defecate in the open. Open defecation significantly compromises quality in nearby water bodies and poses an extreme human health risk.[4]

In Southern Asia, 63% of rural people—778 million people—practice open defecation.

Worldwide, infectious diseases such as waterborne diseases are the number one killer of children under five years of age and more people die from unsafe water annually than from all forms of violence, including war.[5] Public water supply is toxic to the chemically sensitive in the developed countries of the world. It can trigger and propagate chemical sensitivity and chronic degenerative disease.

Unsafe or inadequate water, sanitation, and hygiene cause approximately 3.1% of all deaths worldwide and 3.7% of DALYs (disability adjusted life years) worldwide.[5]

Unsafe water causes 4 billion cases of diarrhea each year, and results in 2.2 million deaths, mostly of children under five. This means that 15% of the child deaths each year are attributable to diarrhea, a child dying every 15 seconds. In India alone, the single largest cause of ill health and death among children is diarrhea, which kills nearly half a million children each year.[6]

There has been a widespread decline in biological health in inland (noncoastal) water. Globally, 24% of mammals and 12% of birds connected to inland waters are considered threatened.[3]

In some regions, more than 50% of native freshwater fish species and nearly one-third of the world's amphibians are at risk of extinction.[7]

Freshwater species face an estimated extinction rate five times greater than that of terrestrial species.[8]

Freshwater ecosystems sustain a disproportionately large number of identified species, including a quarter of known vertebrates. Such systems provide more than US$75 billion worth of goods and ecosystem services for people, but are increasingly threatened by a host of water quality problems.[7]

Freshwater ecosystems provide marshes in particular, which aid in water purification and the assimilation of wastes, and are valued at US$ 400 billion worldwide.[9] These ecosystems are so full that they cannot be cleaned now.

Point-of-use drinking water treatment through chlorine and safe storage of water could result in 122.2 million avoided DALYs (Disability Adjusted Life Years, a measure of morbidity), at a total cost of US$ 11.4 billion.[3] They could sterilize the water from bacteria, virus, and parasites, but contaminate it further with chemicals, which can trigger chemical sensitivity and chronic degenerative disease.

Nearly 70 million people living in Bangladesh are exposed to groundwater contaminated with natural arsenic beyond the WHO recommended limits of 10 µg/L.[10] The naturally occurring arsenic pollution in groundwater now affects nearly 140 million people in 70 countries on all continents.[10]

In developing countries, 70% of industrial wastes are disposed of untreated into waters, where they contaminate the existing water supplied.[11] An estimated 500,000 abandoned mines in the United States will cost $20 billion in management and remediation of pollution; many of these sites will require management in perpetuity. In the U.S. state of Colorado alone, some 23,000 abandoned mines have polluted 2300 km of streams.[12] Chlorinated solvents were found in 30% of groundwater supplies in 15 Japanese cities, sometimes traveling as much as 10 km from the source of pollution.[14]

Roughly one unit of mercury is emitted into the environment for every unit of gold produced by small-scale miners, adding up to a total of as much as 1000 tons of mercury emitted each year.[13] 200 tons of Hg rains down on earth through the melting of the polar ice cap each year.

In a recent comparison of domestic, industrial, and agricultural sources of pollution from the coastal zone of Mediterranean countries, agriculture was the leading source of phosphorous compounds and sediment.[14] Nutrient enrichment, most often associated with nitrogen and phosphorus from agricultural runoff, can deplete oxygen levels and eliminate species with higher oxygen requirements, affecting the structure and diversity of ecosystems.

Nitrate is the most common chemical contaminant in the world's groundwater aquifers.[15,718] Mean nitrate levels have risen by an estimated 36% in global waterways since 1990 with the most dramatic increases observed in the Eastern Mediterranean and Africa, where nitrate contamination has more than doubled.[16]

According to various surveys in India and Africa, 20%–50% of wells contain nitrate[1] levels greater than 50 mg/L and, in some cases, as high as several hundred milligrams per liter.

In Chennai, India, over-extraction of groundwater has resulted in saline groundwater nearly 10 km inland from the sea and similar problems can be found in populated coastal areas around the world.[14]

Sixty percent of the world's 227 biggest rivers have interrupted stream flows due to dams and other infrastructure. Interruptions in stream flow dramatically decrease sediment and nutrient transport to downstream stretches, reducing water quality and nutrient transport to downstream stretches, reducing water quality and impairing ecosystem health.[3] Eighty-five percent of the world population lives in the driest half of the planet. Furthermore, 783 million people do not have access to clean water and almost 2.5 billion do not have access to adequate sanitation. Annually, 6–8 million people die from the consequences of disasters and water related diseases. Various estimates indicate that, based on business as usual, 3.5 planets Earth would be needed to sustain a global population achieving the current lifestyle of the average European or North American. Global population growth projections of 2–3 billion people over the next 40 years, combined with changing diets, could result in a predicted increase in food demand of 70% by 2050.

With the expected increases in population, by 2030, food demand is predicted to increase by 50% (70% by 2050),[17] while energy demand from hydropower and other renewable energy resources will rise by 60%.[18] These issues are interconnected—increasing agricultural output, for example, will substantially increase both water and energy consumption, leading to increased competition for water between water-using sectors.

Pollution of surface water is a problem of over half of our planet's population. Each year, 250 million documented cases of water-borne diseases are documented, with approximately 5–10 million deaths. Fifty percent of worldwide groundwater is unsuitable for drinking because of pollution and only approximately 0.007% of the water on earth is accessible for human use. The world water pollution and sanitation crisis claims more lives through disease than anyone can claim through the use of weapons. Every 20 seconds, a child dies from a water-related disease. Children in polluted environments often carry approximately 1000 parasitic worms in their bodies at any time.

There is 20 times more lead in rivers in industrialized countries.[19] In Ireland, approximately 30% of the rivers are polluted with fertilizers and sewage, which make them too polluted for swimming, fishing, or aquatic life.[19] One of the most polluted rivers in the world is the King River in Australia.[19] Over 1 million sea birds and 100,000 marine mammals and other creatures have died from the toxins and acidity in this river.

The United Nation estimates that by 2025, 48 nations, with combined populations of 2.8 billion, will face freshwater scarcity.

It is clear that our problems as physicians is to get nonpolluted food and water to treat the environmentally wounded individual.

Spatial and temporal variations of groundwater arsenic occur in South and Southeast Asia. This has become a devastating problem for Public Health as well as the creation of chemical sensitivity and chronic degenerative disease.

For example, over the past decades, groundwater wells were installed in rural areas throughout the major river basin draining the Himalayas. These supplied drinking water for millions of people. Even though this water contained less bacteria and viruses, it contained hazardous amounts of arsenic. The arsenic became the largest mass poisioning in history according to Smith et al.[20] This occurred in many parts of Bangladesh. Arsenic levels that were toxic covered over 100 million people in India, China, Myanmar, Pakistan, Vietnam, Nepal, and Cambodia.[21] Studies have shown a doubling of mortality risks for liver, bladder, and lung cancer.[22,23] Groundwater containing As also causes cardiovascular disease and inhibits mental development of children.[24,25] Wells containing 10 µg/L of As are considered contaminated.

Arsenic is released from Fe oxides into groundwater as a result of two potentially concurrent processes under the anoxic conditions that prevail in the subsurface. First, field and laboratory evidence suggests that microbial reduction of Fe(III) oxides liberates As into the dissolved phase.[26,27] Reduction of As(V) to more labile As(III) probably contributes to this release but is hard to distinguish from the reduction of Fe oxides under natural conditions, given the rates of groundwater flow. Second, dissolution of Fe oxides is accompanied by the release of other ligands, such as phosphate, that compete with As for adsorption on the remaining Fe oxide surface sights (Figure 3.1).

CHEMICAL LEAKS INTO WATER

Water can be contaminated by industrial leaks, sewage, and pesticides into the water source supply; for example; Jilin chemical plant disaster, in the Songhua River dumped 100 tons of benzene and nitrobenzene into the Songhua River on November 13, 2005.

The Jilin chemical plant explosions were a series of explosions that occurred on November 13, 2005 in the No. 101 Petrochemical plant in Jilin City, Jilin Province, China.

Ok Tedi disaster (1984–2003): Two billion tons of mine water were discharged into the Fly river, New Guinea, and the copper was 30 times above the standard level.

Environmental Impact

In 1999, the Broken Hill Proprietary Company Limited (BHP) reported that 90 million tons of mine waste were annually discharged into the river for more than 10 years and destroyed downstream villages, agriculture, and fisheries. As of 2006, mine operators continued to discharge 80 million tons of tailings, overburden and mine-induced erosion into the river system each year. Approximately 1588 square kilometers (613 sq mi) of forest have died or are under stress. As many as 3000 square kilometers (1200 sq mi) may eventually be harmed, an area equal to the U.S. state of Rhode Island or the Danish island of Funen.[28]

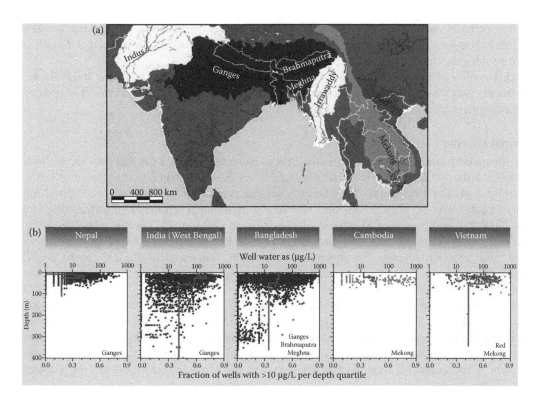

FIGURE 3.1 Distribution of arsenic in groundwater of South and Southeast Asia. (a) Map of four major river basins draining the Himalayas. (b) Depth distribution of As in groundwater determined for five affected countries. Concentrations of As are shown on a logarithmic scale. Symbols are color-coded according to the major river basins shown in (a). The pink line depicts the fraction of wells that exceed the WHO As guideline of 10 µg/L for each depth, quartile of the available data (data sources and methods are available on Science Online). (From Fendorf, S. et al. 2010. *Science* 32(5982):1123–1127. doi: 10.1126/science.1172974; Used with permission from Science AAAS Spatial and Temporal Variations of Groundwater Arsenic in South and Southeast Asia.)

Other disasters have occurred damaging clean water. For example, the Minamata Disaster (1956) resulted in release of methylmercury in the industrial wastewater, Minamata bay and Shiranui sea Japan. Minamata disease resulted in a neurological syndrome caused by severe mercury poisoning. Symptoms included ataxia, numbness in the hands and feet, general muscle weakness, narrowing of the field of vision, and damage to hearing and speech. In extreme cases, insanity, paralysis, coma, and death followed within weeks of the onset of symptoms. A congenital form of the disease can also affect fetuses in the womb.

As of March 2001, 2265 victims had been officially recognized (1784 of whom had died)[29] and over 10,000 had received financial compensation from Chisso. By 2004, Chisso Corportion had paid $86 million in compensation, and in the same year was ordered to clean up its contamination.[30] On March 29, 2010, a settlement was reached to compensate as-yet uncertified victims.[31]

A second outbreak of Minamata disease occurred in Niigata Prefecture in 1965. The original Minamata disease and Niigata Minamata disease are considered two of the four Big Pollution Diseases of Japan.

In 2000, the Baia Mare Cyanide Spill Occurred in Romania

The 2000 Baia Mare cyanide spill was a leak of cyanide near Baia Mare, Romania, into the Somes River by the gold mining company Aurul, a joint-venture of the Australian company Esmeralda Exploration and the Romanian government.

The polluted waters eventually reached the Tisza and then the Danube, killing large numbers of fish in Hungary and Yugoslavia. The spill has been called the worst environmental disaster in Europe since the Chernobyl disaster.[32]

On the night of January 30, 2000, a dam holding contaminated waters burst and 100,000 cubic meters of cyanide-contaminated water (containing an estimated 100 tons of cyanides[33]) spilled over some farmland and then into the Somes river.[32,34]

Bhopal Disaster

The Bhopal disaster, also referred to as the Bhopal gas tragedy, was a gas leak incident in India, considered the world's worst industrial disaster.[35] Over 500,000 people were exposed to methyl isocyanate gas and other chemicals. The toxic substance made its way in and around the shanty towns located near the plant.[36] Estimates vary on the death toll. The official immediate death toll was 2259. The government of Madhya Pradesh confirmed a total of 3787 deaths related to the gas release.[37] Others estimate that 8000 died within two weeks and another 8000 or more have since died from gas-related diseases.[38] A government affidavit in 2006 stated that the leak caused 558,125 injuries including 38,478 temporary partial injuries and approximately 3900 severely and permanently disabling injuries.[39]

Civil and criminal cases are pending in the District Court of Bhopal, India, involving UCC and Warren Anderson, UCC CEO at the time of the disaster.[40,41] In June 2010, seven ex-employees, including the former UCIL chairman, were convicted in Bhopal of causing death by negligence and sentenced to two years imprisonment and a fine of about $2000 each, the maximum punishment allowed by Indian law. An eighth former employee was also convicted but died before the judgment was passed.[35]

Amoco Cadiz Disaster (1978)

The Amoco Cadiz, an VLCC owned by the company Amoco (now merged with BP) sank near the Northwest Coasts of France, resulting in the spilling of 68,684,000 U.S. Gallons of crude oil (1,635,000 barrels). This is the largest oil spill of its kind (spill from an oil tanker) in history.

A huge crude carrier bearing the flag of Liberia split into three parts and sank, releasing 1,604,500 barrels (219,97 tons) of light crude oil and 4000 tons of fuel oil, making it the largest oil spill of its kind at that time and resulted in the largest loss of marine life ever recorded from an oil spill.

Tiete River, Brazil (1992)

The authority has spent more than 1.5 billion since 1992 to clean up the 14 mi Tiete river with 13,000 L factory waste. Acid rain accompanied the disaster at the Tiete River in Sao Paulo.

The process of degradation of the river by industrial pollution and household debris along the stretch of Grand Sao Paulo takes its origin mainly in the process of industrialization and of the uncoordinated urban expansion from the 1940s to the 1970s. This was accompanied by the expansion of the population during that period, such that the city's population grew from 2 million inhabitants in the 1940s to more than 6 million in the 1960s.

Although the Tiete River is said to be one of the most important rivers, economically, for the state of Sao Paulo and for the country, the Tiete River is best known for its environmental problems, especially for the stretch through the City of Sao Paulo.

The pollution of the Tiete River did not start long ago. Even in the 1960s, the river still had fish in the stretch within the capital. However, the environmental degradation of the Tiete River started subtly in the 1920s with the construction of the Guarapiranga Reservoir, for the generation of electrical energy in the hydroelectric power stations. This intervention altered the regime of the waters in the capital and was accompanied by some rectification works, which left the bed of the river less winding, creating more pollution.

Novaya Zemlya, Russia

Nuclear reactor dumping ground, Novaya Zemlya, Russia—unknown because the communists did not reveal any data of the water being contaminated.

Ganga River, India: Pollution of the Ganges

With the hope of cleansing their sins, 100 million Hindus take a pilgrimage to Allahabad, where the Ganges and the Yamuna meet, and immerse themselves in the water.

The Ganges is the largest river in India, with an extraordinary religious importance for Hindus. Along its banks are some of the world's oldest inhabited places such as Varanasi and Patna. It provides water to approximately 40% of India's population in 11 states,[42] an estimated 500 million people or more,[43,44] which is larger than any other river in the world. Today, it is the fifth most polluted river in the world.[45]

Recently, a drive was undertaken, in which the river was reported to have been cleaned, and the municipal commissioner urged people to refrain from polluting.

In addition, the polluted river contained 100 million fecal coliform per 100 mL, and organisms causing cholera, hepatitis A, typhoid, and dysentery, along with extremely high levels of mercury and arsenic.

Yamuna River, India

In 1909, the waters of the Yamuna were distinguishable as "clear blue," as compared to the silt-laden yellow waters of the Ganges.[46] However, owing to the high density population growth and rapid industrialization, today Yamuna is one of the most polluted rivers in the world, especially around New Delhi, the capital of India, which dumps approximately 58% of its waste into the river.

Causes of pollution: New Delhi generates 1900 million liter per day (MLD) of sewage. Though numerous attempts have been made to process it, the efforts have proven to be futile. Although the government of India has spent nearly $500 million to clean up the river, the Yamuna continues to be polluted with garbage, while most sewage treatment facilities are underfunded to malfunctioning. In addition, the water in this river remains stagnant for almost 9 months in a year, aggravating the situation. Delhi alone contributes around 3296 MLD of sewage in the river.

The river is flushed with 500,000,000 gallons of peshades and insecticides (Lindane) waste.

The percentage of pollution contributed in Yamuna is 20% by agriculture waste and 70% by waste from cities, especially Delhi city.

Pasig River, Philippines (1989)

This 15.5 mi river connects Laguna Bay to Manila Bay. Since 1989, authority has been trying to fix it, but the results are futile.

Danube River (2010)

Toxic sludge of 180 million tons leaked from a Hungarian aluminum company into the Danube River, the second longest river in Europe after the Volga, with 30 tributaries. Ten million euros were spent trying to neutralize the alkalinity of the water of pH 14.

Beirut River, Lebanon 2010: Every 2 Months, the River Turns Red

Bandung, Indonesia: PH 14 highest possible levels of alkalinity capable of burning.

Nonylphenol ethoxylate, Tributyl phosphate antimony from 800 textile companies waste.

Jakarta, Indonesia: Pollution level: 450,000,000 m^3/y. Every day, 400.00 L of waste are dumped into the water. Excess of nitrates and phosphates cleaning canal project 63.5 million.

Yellow River, China

Yellow River is the second longest river in Asia (3.395 mi). Nov. 25, 2008. Level 5 according to the UNEP 4.29 tons of whatever should be waste and sewage.

Fuhe River, China (2013): 100,000 Tons of Dead Fish (Ammonia): September 4, 2013

Thousands of fish were killed on a 25 mile stretch of the Fuhe River in central China. The Hubei province environmental protection blamed the local Fuhe River company Hubei Shvanghvan Science and Technology Stock Co. for the disaster (soda ash, ammonium chloride, and industrial salt).

Samples taken at a water outlet from the plant indicated that ammonia density reached 196 mg/L. The WHO natural ammonia level in water is 0.2 mg/L, whereas the ammonia level found in the tested sample was 196 mg/L.

Yangtze River, China

Longest river in Asia, 3.988 mi, and 62 billion was spent on a project to clean it up in a 12-year plan. Consequences of proposed and completed hydropower dams on Yangtze fish and cetaceans were shown. Another important but largely ignored concern is water pollution (1); rising contamination and hydrological changes in the Yangtze are accelerating species losses.

A good example of these endangered Yangtze species is the finless porpoise (*Neophocaena phocaenoides*), which has declined by more than 5% annually for nearly 20 years.[47,48] The Yangtze water is heavily polluted by organic and inorganic compounds (such as metals, persistent organic pollutants, and agro-fertilizers) from new large-scale industrial, agricultural, and domestic developments.[49] Hydropower impoundment reservoirs (such as the Three Gorges Reservoir) have exacerbated water pollution by trapping water and sediment and by increasing eutrophication, resulting in oxygen depletion.[50] Heavy metal concentrations, including lead, copper, and cadmium, in Three Gorges Reservoir water have generally increased.[51] Mercury is of particular concern because of contaminated land inundated by rising water.[52] Mercury in suspended sediment now exceeds the European Union recommendations by a factor of four.[53]

In the Yangtze River (Chongqing, China), 16,000 dead pigs were recovered from the tributaries of the city's river. The Hvangpu, a tributary of the Yangtze, is a source of tap water. In Jiaxing, 7 M pigs are raised with a mortality rate of 2–4, which means up to 300,000 carcasses need to be disposed of each year. In a livestock company, 70,000 pigs died by presumptive Porcine eircovirus and extreme temperature; thus, 16,000 pigs were found in the river.

Nyos Lake (196 mi)

In Cameroon (1986), large-scale emission of CO_2 suffocated and killed 1700 people (Hydrogen, Sulfur). Lake Nyos is one of only three lakes in the world known to be saturated with CO_2, while the others are Lake Monoun, also in Cameroon, and Lake Kivu in the Democratic Republic of Congo. A magma chamber beneath the region is an abundant source of carbon dioxide, which seeps up through the lake bed, charging the waters of Lake Nyos with an estimated 90 million tons of CO_2.

Lake Nyos is thermally stratified, with layers of warm, less dense water near the surface floating on the colder, denser water layers near the lake's bottom. Over long periods, carbon dioxide gas seeping into the cold water at the lake's bottom is dissolved in great amounts.

Most of the time, the lake is stable and the CO_2 remains in solution in the lower layers. However, over time the water becomes supersaturated, and if an event such as an earthquake or landslide occurs, large amounts of CO_2 may suddenly come out of the solution.

Lake Nyos is a crater lake in the Northwest Region of Cameroon, located at 315 km (196 mi) north of Yaounde.[54] Nyos is a deep lake high on the flank of an inactive volcano in the Oku volcanic plain along the Cameroon line of volcanic activity. A volcanic dam impounds the lake waters.

It is not known what triggered the catastrophic outgassing. Most geologists suspect a landslide, but some believe that a small volcanic eruption may have occurred on the bed of the lake. A third possibility is that cool rainwater falling on one side of the lake triggered the overturn. Others still believe there was a small earthquake, but as witnesses did not report feeling any tremors on the ground.

Today, the lake also poses a threat because its natural wall is weakening. A geological tremor could cause this natural dike to give way, not only allowing water to rush into downstream villages all the way into Nigeria but also allowing much carbon dioxide to escape.

Onondaga Lake Northwest of Syracuse, New York, USA (4.5 mi): Ammonia Phosphorus, Algae, Benzene BTEC, CBS, PAHS, 165,000 Pounds of Mercury by Honeywell (1940–1973)

With the industrialization of the region, much of the lake's shoreline was developed; domestic and industrial waste, owing to industrialization and urbanization, led to the severe degradation of the lake. Unsafe levels of pollution led to the banning of ice harvesting as early as 1901. In 1940, swimming was banned and, in 1977, fishing was banned due to mercury contamination.[55,56] Mercury pollution is still a problem for the lake today.[57] Despite the passage of the Clean Water Act in 1973 and the closing of the major industrial polluter in 1986, Onondaga Lake is still one of the most polluted lakes in the United States.

Lake Peigneur Empty Mining, Drilling Disaster, 1980, Louisiana

Lake Peigneur was a 10-foot (3 m) deep freshwater body popular with sportsmen until an unusual man-made disaster changed its structure and the surrounding land.[58–60]

On November 20, 1980, when the disaster took place, the Diamond Crystal Salt Company was operating the Jefferson Island salt mine under the lake, while a Texaco oil rig was drilling down from the surface of the lake searching for petroleum. Owing to a miscalculation, the 14 inch (36 cm) drill bit entered the mine, starting a chain of events which turned the lake from freshwater to salt water, with a deep hole.[61]

Lake Kjaracky, Russia 120 million Curies of Radioactivity
Lethal Dose after Merely an Hour of Exposure

The lake accumulated some 4.44 exabecquerels (EBq) of radioactivity over less than 1 sq mi of water,[62] including 3.6 EBq of cesium 173 and 0.74 EBq of strontium 90. For comparison, the Chernobyl disaster released from 5 to 12 EBq of radioactivity over thousands of square miles. The sediment of the lake bed is estimated to be composed almost entirely of high level radioactive waste deposits to a depth of approximately 11 ft.

The radiation level in the region near where radioactive effluent was discharged into the lake was 600 rontgens per hour (approximately 6 Sv/h) in 1990, according to the Washington D.C. based Natural Resources Defense Council,[63,64] sufficient to give a lethal dose to a human within an hour.

The reports of this worldwide contamination by various toxic exposures shows how early water can be contaminated. The hope of clean drinking water gets dimmer every day.

WATER SUPPLY TERRORISM

Water supply terrorism involves intentional sabotage of a water supply system, through chemical or biological warfare or infrastructural sabotage. Throughout military history and the history of terrorism, water supply attacks have been perpetrated by eco-terrorist and political groups intending to scare, cause death, or drought. It has added to the difficulty of cleaning up our drinking water.

Chemical and Biological Attacks Which Damaged Drinking Water

In 1984, members of the Rajneeshee religious cult contaminated a city water supply tank in The Dalles, Oregon, using Salmonella and infecting 750 people.[65]

In 1992, the Kurdish Workers Party PKK put lethal concentrations of potassium cyanide in the water tanks of a Turkish Air Force compound in Istanbul.

In 2000, workers at the Cellatex chemical plant in northern France dumped 5000 L of sulfuric acid into a tributary of the Meuse River when they were denied workers' benefits.[65]

In 2000, Queensland, Australia, police arrested a man for using a computer and radio transmitter to take control of the Maroochy Shire wastewater system and release sewage into parks, rivers, and property.

LSD Threats to the Water supply

Despite the fact that it is impractical and very unlikely to produce any effect on a large scale, during the 1960s a great deal of attention was paid to the idea that counter-culture figures could intoxicate a whole city by putting a small dose of LSD in the water supply.

On March 19, 1966, London Life ran an interview claiming that anyone could take control of London in under eight hours by putting acid in the water system. It is quite feasible that LSD could be used to take over a city or even a country. It is agreed that if it were put into reservoirs, it would disable people sufficiently for an enemy to take control.[66]

The counter-culture threatened to put LSD in Chicago's water supply to protest against the Vietnam War during the Democratic convention.[67]

In Lusaka, Zambia in 1999, a bomb destroyed the main water pipeline, cutting off water for the city with a population of 3 million.

In 2001, water flow to Kumanovo (with a population of 100,000) was cut off for 12 days in the conflict between ethnic Albanians and Macedonian forces.[65]

The Revolutionary Armed Forces of Colombia (FARC) detonated a bomb inside a tunnel in the Chingaza Dam, which provides most of Bogota's water.[65]

Four incendiary devices were found in the pumping station of a Michigan water-bottling plant. The Earth Liberation Front (ELF) claimed responsibility, accusing the Ice Mountain Water Company of stealing water for profit.

In 2003, Jordanian authorities arrested Iraqi agents in connection with a failed plot to poison the water supply that serves American troops in the eastern Jordanian desert near the border with Iraq.

In 2006, Tamil Tiger rebels cut the water supply to government-held villages in northeastern Sri Lanka. Sri Lankan government forces then launched attacks on the reservoir, declaring the Tamil actions to be terrorism.

The draining of the Mesopotamian Marshes occurred in Iraq and, to a smaller degree, in Iran between the 1950s and 1990s to clear large areas of the marshes in the Tigris-Euphrates river system. Formerly covering an area of around 20,000 km^2 (7700 sq mi), the main sub-marshes, the Hawizeh, Central, and Hammar Marshes and all three were drained at different times for different reasons. Initial draining of the Central Marshes was intended to reclaim land for agriculture, but later all three marshes would become a tool of war and revenge.

Many international organizations such as the U.N. Human Rights Commission, the Supreme Council of the Islamic Revolution in Iraq (SCIRI), the International Wildfowl and Wetlands Research Bureau, and Middle East Watch have described the draining as a political attempt to force the Ma'dan people out of the area through water diversion tactics.[68]

Clearly, water sabotage can be a problem in contaminating water worldwide and should be stopped at all costs if possible.

It is clear that toxic leaks and terrorism contamination really have contaminated our clean water supply. This contamination is the harbinger of chronic disease which can create chemical sensitivity and chronic degenerative disease.

U.S. WATER POLLUTION FACTS

Over two-thirds of U.S. estuaries and bays are severely degraded because of nitrogen and phosphorus pollution. Water quality reports indicate that 45% of U.S. streams, 47% of lakes, and 32% of bays are polluted. Forty percent of America's rivers are too polluted for fishing, swimming, or aquatic life. The lakes are even worse as over 46% are too polluted for fishing, swimming, or aquatic life. Every year, almost 25% of U.S. beaches are closed at least once because of water pollution. Americans use over 2.2 billion pounds of pesticides every year, which eventually washes into our rivers and lakes. Over 73 different kinds of pesticides have been found in U.S. groundwater that eventually ends in drinking water unless it is adequately filtered. Even then, it is not totally clean and adds to the body's total pollutant load. The Mississippi River, which drains over 40% of the continental U.S., carries an estimated 1.5 million metric tons of nitrogen pollution into the Gulf of Mexico every year. This resulting pollution is the cause of a coastal dead zone the size of Massachusetts every summer.

Septic systems are failing all around the country, causing untreated waste materials to flow freely into streams, rivers, and lakes. Annually, 1.2 trillion gallons of untreated sewage, groundwater, and industrial waste are discharged into U.S. waters. The 5-minute daily shower most Americans take uses more water than a typical person in a developing country uses in a whole day (Table 3.1).

DRINKING WATER CONTAMINATION

The mineral content of drinking water, along with its source and treatment, determines water hardness or softness, both of which appear to have a highly significant effect on human health. They are involved in heart disease, hypertension, and stroke, particularly if the water is soft. Hard water that is rich in magnesium and calcium has been shown to decrease heart disease and reduce the occurrence of heart attacks and fatal heart attacks.[69] In contrast, soft water that is low in magnesium may contribute to fatal heart attacks. Schroeder[70] found that death rates from cardiovascular diseases (particularly from coronary heart attacks in white men 45–64 years old) were significantly higher in states with soft water than in states with hard water. Since vasospasm, which is one of the hallmarks of chemical sensitivity and chronic degenerative disease, can at times be prevented and corrected with calcium and magnesium supplementation, both minerals are essential for the prevention of further vascular damage. Thus, water rich in these minerals can be beneficial not only in managing this illness but also in maintaining health.

Not only does hard water appear to benefit the person with chemical sensitivity or chronic degenerative disease by eliminating vasospasm, but the lithium, sodium, potassium, calcium, magnesium and zinc, and other trace minerals it contains also help to stabilize pollutant damaged membranes and enhance detoxification mechanisms. This membrane stabilization is particularly true for cardiac and brain membranes but is necessary to obtain homeostasis in any part of the body.

Most water pollution problems stem from land-based activities within drainage basins. However, water based activities, such as boating, are also becoming a problem, as is generalized dumping of toxics, oil shale fracking, and oil spills.

Rainwater

Most water, other than a few springs, is contaminated. Rainwater derives the pollutants from contaminated clouds, which originate from the fumes of cars and trucks, industry, factory farming, and so on. As a result, it contains a whole gamut of dissolved acids, organic compounds, pesticide, and heavy metals. For example, 200 tons of mercury rains down on earth each year from melting of the polar ice caps.[71] Surface basins, in which potable water is draining, such as lakes, rivers, streams, and lakes, accumulate ground level pollutants in addition to those carried by rain. Underground sources such as oil and gas wells, mining, toxic dumps wells, and so on further contaminate the water.

Lake and ocean waters are contaminated by both rains and waste runoff oil spill, dumps, factory, farming, and industry. For example, it has now been shown that Beluga whales have Teflon, scotchgard, and other fluorinated compounds in their blood. They also have high levels of lead, aluminum, cadmium, silver, mercury, and titanium in their tissue. These examples were taken from 1000 whales.

The source of water determines its quality. For example, one source may be a spring from a granite vault that will be chemically pure but perhaps a bit radioactive. A riverbed that has given way to

TABLE 3.1
Nonpoint Sources of Pollution and Results

Pollutant	Sources	Some Possible Results
Ammonia nitrogen	Decaying organic material	Reduces amount of dissolved oxygen endangering fish. Produces nitrogen which may stimulate growth of algae or undesirable plants which can overload the ecological system.
Nitrates	Agricultural fertilizers, sewage, industrial wastes, drainage from feedlots, farm manures, and legumes	Large amount in drinking water can cause methemoglobinemia (blue babies). Stimulate growth of algae which can reduce dissolved oxygen when they die and decompose.
Phosphates	Excessive drainage from agricultural areas	Eutrophication. Algal blooms which result in oxygen depletion and fish kills. Rapid decomposition of algae can produce odors associated with hydrogen sulfide gas.
Sediment	Agriculture, forestry, urban runoff, construction, mining	Decreases water clarity and light transmission which can interfere with fish populations. Acts as substrate for organic pollutants. Decreases recreational commercial values of streams. Decreases quality of drinking water.
Salts (salinity— including halides and bicarbonate being converted to carbonate)	Agriculture, mining, urban runoff	Decreases species diversity by favoring salt tolerant species. Reduces crop yield. Impacts stream habitats and plants that are food sources for other species. Decreases quality of drinking water.
Pesticide, herbicides	Agriculture, forestry	Kills aquatic organisms. Adversely affects reproduction, growth respiration, and development in other aquatic species. Decreases food supply and destroys habitat of aquatic species. Bioaccumulate in tissues of plants, macroinvertebrates, and fish. Some are carcinogenic and/or mutagenic. Decreases photosynthesis in aquatic plants. Reduces recreational and commercial activities.
Polycyclic aromatic hydrocarbons (PAHs)	Urban runoff	Bioaccumulate, biomagnify, and are toxic to aquatic life. Can produce carcinogenic metabolites when digested.
Polychlorinated biphenyls (PCBs)	Urban runoff, landfills	Toxic to aquatic organisms; can bioaccumulate, biomagnify, and be stored in fat deposits. Adsorb to sediments. Persist in environment longer than most chlorinated compounds.
Petroleum hydrocarbons	Urban runoff	Water soluble components can be toxic to life. Portions may adsorb to particulate organic matter, be deposited in sediment, and may adversely affect biological functions
Silica	Decomposition of alumina silicate minerals in the drainage basin through which the water flows	Forms a hard, dense scale (which is resistant to heat transfer) in boilers. Causes loss of turbine efficiency due to deposit of insoluble silica deposits on turbine blades.
Sulfates	Mining, industrial runoff	Lower pH in streams which stresses aquatic animals and leaches toxic metals out of sediment and rocks. High acidity and concentrations of heavy metals can be lethal to aquatic organisms and eliminate entire aquatic communities.
Sulfides	Sewage, industrial runoff, paper manufacturing	In the form of hydrogen sulfide cause noticeable odor. Hydrogen sulfide is toxic; acts as a respiratory depressant in humans and fish.
Radionuclides	Mining/ore processing, nuclear power plant wastes, commercial and industry.	Some are toxic, carcinogenic, or mutagenic. Some degenerate into other substances (e.g., radium, lead) which are toxic and carcinogenic to aquatic organisms. When ingested, they can bioconcentrate in tissues, bones, and organs, where they emit radiation for a long time.

Source: Agriculture Pollution. http://protectingwater.com/agriculture.html.

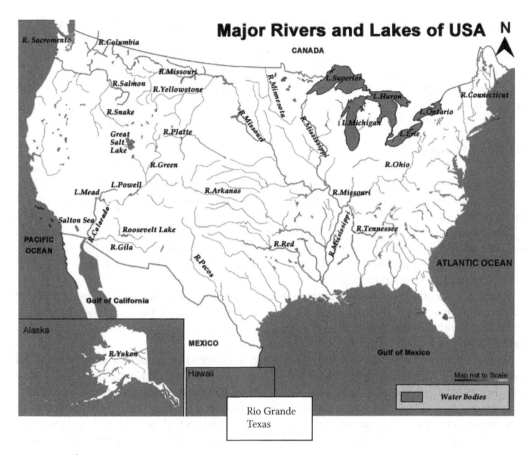

FIGURE 3.2 This map shows the major rivers of the United States. Most are contaminated in one way or another. This occurs by natural and man-made pollution. (From ideagirlseverestormpredictionswarnings.wordpress.com https://ideagirlseverestormpredictionswarnings.wordpress.com/2012/11/12/hurricane-circle-pattern-geomagnetic-storm-cells-cuba-to-chicago-12-nov-2012-353-pm-est-high-wind-network/major-rivers-and-lakes-of-usa-sept-2012-2/.)

dolomite rock may be another source; it will have increased calcium and magnesium content as well as increased water hardness. However, it may be contaminated due to sewer effluent, toxic wastes and dumps, road runoff, and so on (Figure 3.2).

Toxins Found in Whales Bode Ill for Humans

According to Max,[73] sperm whales feeding even in the most remote reaches of Earth's oceans have a buildup of high levels of toxics and heavy metals.

They also noted high levels of cadmium, aluminum, chromium, lead, silver, mercury, and titanium in tissue samples taken by a dart gun from nearly 1000 whales over 5 years. From polar areas to equatorial waters, the whales ingested pollutants that may have been produced by humans thousands of miles away. These contaminants are threatening the human food supply.

The studies found mercury to be as high as 16 parts per million in the whales. Fish, such as shark and swordfish, are high in mercury. These typically have levels of approximately 1 part per million.

The whales studies averaged 2.4 parts of mercury per million. The entire ocean life is just loaded with a series of contaminants, most of which have been released by human beings.

According to Payne,[73] sperm whales, which occupy the top of the food chain, absorb the contaminants and pass them on to the next generation, when a female nurses her calf. What this whale is actually doing is dumping her lifetime accumulation of that fat-soluble stuff into her baby and each generation passes on more to the next.

Sperm whales are toothed whales that eat all kinds of fish and even sharks. Dozens of whales have been taken by whaling ships in the past decade. Most of the whales hunted by the whaling countries of Japan, Norway, and Iceland are minke whales, which are baleen whales that feed largely on tiny krill.

Chromium was found in all but two of the 361 sperm whale samples that were tested for it.[71]

For Human Consumption

Contaminant Samples found in New Orleans Drinking Water are presented. These can obviously compromise the health of the chemically sensitive as well as the average person (Tables 3.2 and 3.3).

Water Pollution of the U.S. as compared with the New Orleans drinking water (Tables 3.4 through 3.6).

The microbial profile of water sources before filtration is also quite revealing and shows organisms that can cause ill health not only in well humans but also the chemically sensitive (Tables 3.7 and 3.8).

This is compared with Dallas drinking water in 2015, which has 22 chemicals in it. Therefore, no improvement is observed in 35 years.

Reservoirs are often built in farm areas or in the middle of cities. They usually have streams or water running into them. Therefore, they are depositories for pollution from rain containing nitric and sulfuric acid, solvents, pesticides, and radioactivity and from runoff originating from manufacturing, dumps, municipal wastes, and agricultural wastes.

Wells in polluted industrial and farm areas are contaminated by groundwater infiltration. All wells of less than 200 ft in the state of Iowa are polluted with pesticides and herbicides.[74] This is now true over most of the Midwest. Low birth weight babies have been observed in these areas along with an incidence of leukemia and recurrent infections that occur when the water is contaminated with trichloroethylene, tetrachloroethylene, and 1,2-transdichloroethylene.[75] Also, these substances have effects on the liver, the brain (anesthetic effects and cardiovascular system (arrhythmias, bacterial, and myocardial infarctions).

Rainwater cisterns become contaminated by toxic rain. In cities, cloud tainted by contaminants from car exhaust and factory emissions may form, while in farm areas nitrates and pesticides from various land and plant treatments may be absorbed into the clouds. Rainwater that is released from these clouds is then collected into cisterns, since there is clearly much cross contamination due to rain, runoff, sewage, and dumping, and contamination of underground water (Figure 3.3). Most drinking water today is a product of someone's waste. Although sources of water vary, all man-made contaminations are theoretically preventable. It is clear that there is little to no public drinking water that is free of chemicals in the United States.

Man-made contaminants are either inorganic or organic chemicals, particulates, and heat or radiation (EMF and ionize). Sources of man-made water contamination occur in four major categories: (1) municipal sewage, (2) agricultural wastes, (3) industrial wastes, and (4) waste from pharmaceuticals (Table 3.9; EPA 2003 Environmental Report—Appendix B—Types of Waste and Contaminated Lands).

Rivers originating in, or passing through, swamps or marshes are usually somewhat acidic and discolored because they pick up organic acids that are generated from decomposing microorganisms and vegetation. Sulfur springs can lead to sulfur contamination of rivers. Rivers that flow from melting glaciers become full of finely ground-up rock that can prevent the proliferation of aquatic life and cause intestinal disorders in humans. Gas and oil may contaminate springs and wells located near gas and oil fields. Fracking of oil and gas shale will contaminate whole water areas. Areas with a high population of wild or domestic animals may experience problems with microbial contamination. Gaitan[76] has shown that water coming from wells in areas of oil shale and coal contains high levels of resorcinol (phenol), which is a strong goitrogen. Algae and fungi can also contaminate a source naturally. Natural Arsenic has contaminated many wells around the world and has contributed to much

TABLE 3.2
Common Ground, June 2006—Five Samples

Total phenols
Arsenic
Barium
Cadmium
Chromium
Lead
Mercury
Selenium
Silver
Cyanide
1,1,2-Tetrachloroethane
1,1,1-Trichloroethane
1,1,2,2-Tetrachloroethane
1,1,2-Trichloroethane
1,1-Dichloroethane
1,1-Dichloroethene
1,2-Dibromo-3-chloropropane
1,2-Dibromoethane (ethylene dibromide)
1,2-Dichlorobenzene
1,2-Dichloroethane
1,2-Dichloropropane
1,3-Dichlorobenzene
1,4-Dichlorobenzene
1,4-Dioxane
2-Butanone (MEK)
2-Chloroethyl vinyl ether
2-Hexanone
4-Methyl-2-pentanone (MIBK)
Acetone (2-propanone)
Acetonitrile
Acrolein
Acrylonitrile
Benzene
Bromobenzene
Bromodichloromethane
Bromoform (tribromomethane)
Broomethane (methyl bromide)
Carbon disulfide
Carbon tetrachloride
Chlorobenzene
Chloroethane
4-Bromophenyl phenyl ether
4-Chloro-3-methylphenol
4-Chloroaniline (p-chloroaniline)
4-Chlorophenylo phenyl ether4-nitroaniline
4-Nitrophenol
7,12-Dimethylbenz[a]anthracene
Acenaphthene
Acenaphthylene

Chloroform (trichloromethane)
Chloromethane (methyl chloride)
cis-1,2-dichloroethene
cis-1,3-dichloropropene
Dibromochloromethane
Dibromomethane (methylene bromide)
Dichlorodifluoromethane
Ethylbenzene
Iodomethane (methyl iodide)
m,p-Xylenes
Mehylene chloride (dichloromethane)
o-Xylene
Styrene
Tetrachloroethene (perchlorethylene)
Toluene
trans-1,2-dichloroethene
trans-1,3-dichloropropene

Trichlorofluoromethane
Vinyl acetate
Vinyl chloride
1,2,4-Trichlorobenzene
1,2-Diphenylhydrazine
1-Methylnaphthalene
2,4,6-Trichlorophenol
2,4-Dichlorophenol
2,4-Dimethylphenol
2,4-Dinitrophenol
2,4-Dinitrotoluene
2,6-Dichlorophenol
2,6-Dinitrotoluene
2-Chloronaphthalene
2-Chlorophenol
2-Methylnaphthalene
2-Methylphenol
2-Nitroaniline
2-Nitrophenol
3,4 Methylphenol (m,p-cresol)
3,3′-Dichlorobenzidine
3-Nitroaniline
4,6-Dinitro-2-methylphenol
Pentachlorophenol
Phenanthrene
Phenol
Pyrene
Pyridine
Quinoline
Benzenethiol/TIC
4,4′-DDD

(Continued)

TABLE 3.2 (*Continued*)

Common Ground, June 2006—Five Samples

Aniline	
Anthracene	4,4'-DDT
Benzidine	Aldrin
Benzoic acid	alpha-BHC (alpha-Hexachlorocyclohexane)
Benzo[a] anthracene	alpha-Chlordane (cis-Chlordane)
Benzo[a] pyrene	beta-BHC (beta-hexachlorocyclohexane)
Benzo[b] fluoranthene	delta-BHC (delta-hexachlorocylohexane)
Benzo[ghi]perylene	Dieldrin
Benzo[jk]fluoranthene	Endosulfan I
Benzyl alcohol	Endosulfan II
bis(2-chloroethoxy)methane	Endosulfan sulfate
bis(2-chloroethy)ether	Endrin
bis(2-chloroisopropyl)ether	Endrin aldehyde
bis(2-ethylhexyl)phthalate	gamma-chlordane (trans-chlordane)
Butyl benzyl phthalate	Heptachlor
Chrysene	Heptachlor epoxide
Di-n-butyl phthalate (dibutylphthalate)	Lindane (gamma-Hexachlorocyclohexane)
Di-n-octylphthalate (dioctylphthalate)	Methoxychlor
Dibenzofuran	Toxaphene
Dibenz[1h] acridine	2,4,5,6-Terrachloro-m-xylene
Dibenz[1h] anthracene	Decachlorobiphenyl
Diethylphthalate	1,2-Dichloroethane
Dimethylphthalate	4-Bromofluorobenzene
Fluoranthene	Toluene
Fluorene	2,4,6-Tribromophenol
Hexachlorobenzene	2-Fluorobiphenyl
Hexachlorobutadiene	2-Fluorophenol
Hexachlorocyclopentadiene (HCCPD)	Nitrobenzene
Hexachloroethane	Phenol
Indene	Terphenyl
Indeno [1,2,3-cd]pyrene	
Isophorone	
Methylchrysene	
N-nitrosodi-n-propylamine	
N-nitrosodimethylamine	
N-nitrosodiphenylamine naphthalene	
Nitrobenzene	

Source: Solomon, G. M. 2006. *Drinking Water Quality in New Orleans*. Natural Resources Defense Council. https://www.nrdc.org/health/effects/katrinadata/water.pdf. Used with permission of NRDC Drinking Water Quality in New Orleans, June–October 2006.

chemical sensitivity and chronic degenerative disease; all of the aforementioned has the possibility of triggering chemical sensitivity and chronic degenerative disease.

Society has not been adept at stopping water pollution at its source. For example, horse manure and garbage used to be collected from the streets and dumped into the nearest river. When this dumping was stopped, refuse was dumped into oceans and lakes causing beach contamination. There is now a dead area the size of the state of Louisiana at the bottom of the Mississippi river delta in the Gulf of Mexico. This dead area is due to the nitrogen runoff from farms into the tributaries

TABLE 3.3

Retesting of Three Samples of New Orleans Water, October 2006

Contaminant	No. of Samples	Units	Average	Range	Regulatory or Guideline Limit
Heterotrophic plate count	3	Present or not present	281	4–740	500 (guideline) colonies
Total coliform bacteria	3	Present or not present	Not	Negative at two sites, positive at one site.	0 colonies
E. coli bacteria	3	Present or not present	Not	Negative at all three sites	0 colonies
Residual chlorine	3	mg/L	2.34	1.63–3.34	Between 0.5 and 4.0

Source: Solomon, G. M. 2006. *Drinking Water Quality in New Orleans.* Natural Resources Defense Council. https://www. nrdc.org/health/effects/katrinadata/water.pdf. Used with permission of NRDC Drinking Water Quality in New Orleans, June–October 2006.

of the Mississippi as well as chemical contamination by factories, cities, and so on. This nitrogen runoff is similar to other rivers, such as the Columbia (100,000 tons in the 1990s), the Susquehanna (50,000 tons), and the St. Lawrence (50,000 tons), all of which dump nitrogen into oceans and contaminate their estuaries. Figure 3.4 illustrates the EPA picture of this area.

Eventually, the use of landfills replaced this latter dumping but landfills created a runoff problem and contributed to severe contamination of public drinking water. This type of biological contamination often created large epidemics of waterborne diseases throughout the world. There are thousands of landfills in the U.S. and other parts of the world. There are 12,000–24,000 tons of plastic that deep-dwelling North Pacific fish ingest each year, based on findings from the Scripps Environmental Accumulation of Plastic Expedition known as SEAPLEX.

Some springs are contaminated by sewage and chemical dump runoff or underground gas and oil wells, while lakes may be contaminated by runoff from agriculture or manufacturing. For example, areas that are designated for rural agricultural activities, including cultivation, and areas that accumulate urban industrial wastes may become saturated with pollutants that then run off to lakes and rivers. Also, lakes and rivers may be contaminated by exhaust and bilge from boat motors. At one time, the Cuyahoga River in Cleveland, Ohio caught fire due to too much industrial runoff which was going to Lake Erie. The lake became devoid of fish at one time due to the severe industrial runoff. Simultaneously, there were massive polio epidemics in these areas.

TABLE 3.4

Naturally Occurring Pollutants in U.S. Drinking Water

Hexavalent chromium	Uranium-238
Lithium	Total radium
Phosphorus	Radium-226
Chloromethane	Radium-228
Alpha particle activity (excluding radon and uranium)	Alpha particle activity (suspended)
Radon	Gross beta particle activity (dissolved)
Total uranium	Gross beta particle activity (suspended)
Uranium-234	Potassium-40
Uranium-235	Gross beta particle and photon emitters (man-made)

Source: Used by permission from *Science Direct.* Human toxicology of chemical mixtures, pp. 100–109. Zeliger, H. I. 2008. ISBN: 978-0-8155-1589-0.

TABLE 3.5
Contaminants in U.S. Drinking Water for Which No MCLs Exist

Ammonia	Vanadium
Bromide	Oil and grease (total)
Chlorate	Phosphorus
Hydrogen sulfide	Carbon disulfide
Phosphate	Desisopropylatazine
Orthophosphate	Carbaryl
Strontium	Methomyl
Lithium	Baygon (propoxur)
Molybdenum	Methiocarb
Acetochlor	Butyl acetate
Papaquat	Ethyl ether
Prometon	Isopropyl alcohol
p-Isopropyltoluene	Bromacil
Aldicarb	Dacthal
Aldicarb sulfoxide	Diuron
Aldicarb sulfone	2,4-DB
Metolachlor	2,4,5-T
1.4-Dioxane	Chloramben
Eptam	Dichloprop
Sutan	Chloromethane
Cyanazine	Bromomethane
Trifluralin	Dichlorodifluoromethane
Ethion	Chloroethane
3-Hydroxycarbofuran	Trichlorofluoromethane
Endosulfan I	n-Nitrosodiphenylamine
Dieldrin	Aniline
DDT	1,2-Dibromoethylene
Butachlor	Acrylonitrile
Propachlor	Acetone
Isopropyl ether	Butyl benzylphthalate
Hexachlorobutadiene	Methyl methacrylate
Methyl ethyl ketone	Chrysene
Naphthalene	Benzo[a] anthracene
Methyl isobutyl ketone	Benzo [b] fluoranthene
Methyl t-butyl ether	Benzo [k] fluoranthene
Nitrobenzene	Indino [1,2,3-cd]pyrene
Acenaphthylene	Dibenz[ah]anthracene
Acenaphthene	Benzo[g,h,i]perylene
Isophorone	Aldrin
Tetrahydrofuran	n-Hexane
Fluorine	Dibromomethane
2-Hexanone	1,1-Dichloropropene
2,4-Dinitrotoluene	1,3-Dichloropropane
Phenanthrene	1,2,3-Trichloropropane
Anthracene	n-Butylbenzene
Dimethylphthalate	1,3,5-Trimethylbenzene

(Continued)

TABLE 3.5 (*Continued*)
Contaminants in U.S. Drinking Water for Which No MCLs Exist

Diethylphtalate	t-Butylbenzene
Fluoranthrene	sec-Butylbenzene
Pyrene	Bromochloromethane
Di-n-butylphthalate	
Dicamba	1,1-Dichloroethane
Bromochloroacetic acid	1,1,1,2-Tetrachloroethane
Iodomethane	1,1,2,2-Tetrachloroethane
Dichloroacetonitrile	Bromobenzene
1,1-Dichloropropanone	Isopropylbenzene
Chloropicrin	n-Propylbenzene
2-Nitropropane	Potassium-40
Gyloxal	Tritium
Metribuzin	Manganese-54
Bentazon	Strontium-90
Molinate	Perchlorate
Thiobencarb	Total aldicarbs
Trichlorotrifluoroethane	Bromodichloroacetic acid
Phenols	Chlor dibromoacetic acid
Formaldehyde	Tribromoacetic acid
o-Chlorotoluene	Alpha chlordane
p-Chlorotoluene	Ethyl-t-butyl
m-Dichlorobenzene	Dichlorofluoromethane
Dichloroiodomethane	

Source: Used by permission from *Science Direct.* Human toxicology of chemical mixtures, pp. 100–109. Zeliger, H. I. 2008. ISBN: 978-0-8155-1589-0.

TABLE 3.6
Test Results for Contaminants in New Orleans Water, June 2006

Contaminant	No. of Samples	Units	Average	Range	Regulatory or Guideline Limit
Bromodichloromethane	5	μg/L	7.0	6.4–7.3	0 (guideline)
Dibromochloromethane	5	μg/L	2.2	1.3–2.6	60 (guideline)
Bromnoform	5	μg/L	<1.0	–	0 (guideline)
Chloroform	5	μg/L	12.7	1.7–18.0	None
Total Trihalomethanes	5	μg/L	26.0	22.2–27.6	80
Barium	5	μg/L	57.5	55.5–63.1	2000
Selenium	5	μg/L	14.2	13.1–16.3	50
Lead	5	μg/L	6.9	<LOD[a]–14.3	0 (guideline)
15 μg/L (action level)					
Total Phenols	5	μg/L	4.2	<LOD–5.4	None

Source: Solomon, G. M. 2006. *Drinking Water Quality in New Orleans.* Natural Resources Defense Council. https://www.nrdc.org/health/effects/katrinadata/water.pdf. Used with permission of NRDC Drinking Water Quality in New Orleans, June–October 2006.

[a] LOD = limit of detection.

TABLE 3.7

Microbial Profile of Water Sources before Filtration

Organism	Number of Samples Contaminated with Target Pathogenic Bacteria Using Culture Based Methods (6 Trials)			
	SWL[a]	SWH[a]	GWL	GWH
Presumptive *Shigella* spp.	6(100%)	6(100%)	0	0
Presumptive *Salmonella* spp.	6(100%)	6(100%)	0	0
Presumptive *Vibrio* spp.	6(100%)	6(100%)	0	0

Average concentration of organisms spiked in synthetic and groundwater sources before filtration (CFU/100 mL $\pm$ SD)

Organisms	Synthetic (5 Trials) Spiked Sterile Saline Water (0.9%)	GWL (6 Trials)	GWH (6 Trials)
S. dysenteriae	3.98×10^6	$1,0 \times 10^5$	3.2×10^3
	$(\pm 3.7 \times 10^4)$	$(\pm 1.72 \times 10_2)$	$(\pm 1.93 \times 10^1)$
S. typhimurium	2.02×10^6	5.6×10^3	1.4×10^4
	$(\pm 1.4 \times 10^4)$	$(\pm 3.86 \times 10^2)$	$(\pm 1.82 \times 10^2$
V. cholera	4.12×10^6	2.4×10^3	8.0×10^3
	$(\pm 3.06 \times 10^4)$	$(\pm 1.57 \times 10^2)$	$(\pm 1.57 \times 10^3)$

Source: Mwabi, J. K., B. B. Mamba, M. N. B. Momba. Removal of waterborne bacteria from surface water and groundwater by cost-effective household water treatment systems (HWTS): A sustainable solution for improving water quality in rural communities of Africa. http://www.scielo.org.za/pdf/wsa/v39n4/02.pdf.

Note: All values are an average of triplicate samples with the $\pm$ standard deviation (SD) presented in parentheses.

[a] Presence of target pathogenic bacteria in surface water samples after enrichment steps.

The toxic red mud that spilled from an alumina tailings reservoir in Hungary last year could make the soil too salty for plants to grow, according to a new report. The commission says the red mud was incorrectly classified as nonhazardous. The catastrophe killed 10 people as the pH spill poured over more than 15 sq mi of the Hungarian landscape.

Researchers went to Hungary to collect samples of the red mud contaminated soil which they then used to grow barley plants in the lab.

TABLE 3.8

Volatile Organic Constituents Identified in New Orleans Drinking Water

Acetaldehyde	Dichlormethane
Acetone	Dichloropropane
Benzene	Dichloropropene[a]
Bromodichloromethane	Diethyl ether
Tert-butyl alcohol	3-Methylbutan-1-al
Carbon tetrachloride	Tetrachloroethylene
Chloroform	Trichloroethylene
1-Chloropropene	Toluene
Dibromochloromethane	Xylene
Dichlorethane	
Dichlorodiomethane	

Source: Laseter, J. L., B. J., Dowtry. 1977. Association of biorefractories in drinking water and body burden in people. *Ann. N.Y. Acad. Sci.* 298:547–556. With permission.

[a] Several isomers observed.

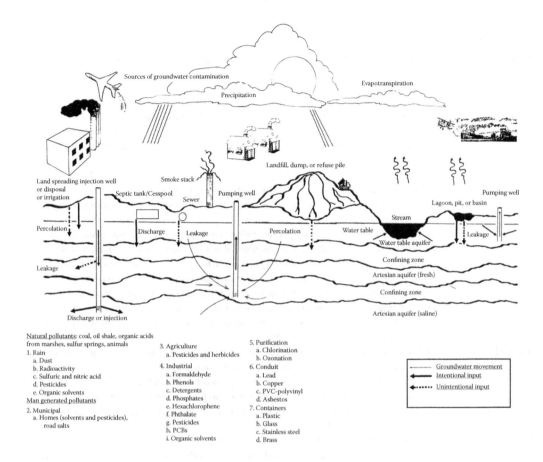

Natural pollutants: coal, oil shale, organic acids
from marshes, sulfur springs, animals
1. Rain
   a. Dust
   b. Radioactivity
   c. Sulfuric and nitric acid
   d. Pesticides
   e. Organic solvents
Man generated pollutants
2. Municipal
   a. Homes (solvents and pesticides),
      road salts

3. Agriculture
   a. Pesticides and herbicides
4. Industrial
   a. Formaldehyde
   b. Phenols
   c. Detergents
   d. Phosphates
   e. Hexachlorophene
   f. Phthalate
   g. Pesticides
   h. PCBs
   i. Organic solvents

5. Purification
   a. Chlorination
   b. Ozonation
6. Conduit
   a. Lead
   b. Copper
   c. PVC-polyvinyl
   d. Asbestos
7. Containers
   a. Plastic
   b. Glass
   c. Stainless steel
   d. Brass

——— Groundwater movement
◄——— Intentional input
◄····· Unintentional input

FIGURE 3.3 Water cycle of contamination able to affect adversely the chemically sensitive. (Modified from *Drinking Water: A Community Action Guide*, p. 2. Washington, DC: Concern, Inc.; Publication 1 CCC Republication Taylor and Francis Group LLC Books. Chemical Sensitivity 1/1/1994 Water Pollution Chapter 7, pp. 544–56. With permission from Taylor & Francis.)

Yields of barley grown in soil with red mud concentrations of 5% were 25% lower than those of crops grown in untainted soil. The researchers also grew barley in soil tainted only with sodium hydroxide, a caustic agent in red mud that increases salt concentrations in soil. The NaOH-spiked soil slowed the growth of barley plants as much as the Hungarian red mud did.

"People were very afraid because red mud contains toxic trace elements." Adding gypsum (hydrated calcium sulfate) to the landscape, as Hungarian authorities have done, can reduce the pH and improve the soil's porosity, allowing rain to flush away the salt.

If a source of water has been contaminated by softeners, soaps, and detergents that are used in the cleaning process to counteract water hardness, then water quality may also be diminished. Man has intentionally contaminated good water sources. Some of these substances add phosphates to the water and yield downstream pollution.

According to the EPA report on the Environment,[77] eutrophication is a natural process characterized by a high rate of algal production. In recent years, human activities have substantially increased the delivery rate of nutrients to most coastal waters, resulting in greater algal production than would have occurred naturally. A National Oceanic and Atmospheric Administration (NOAA) survey between 1992 and 1998 assessed symptoms of eutrophication, including high levels of algae and toxic algal blooms, lack of oxygen, and loss of aquatic plants that provide shelter and habitat for many species of bottom-living organism.[77] Although the assessments were more a subjective

TABLE 3.9

Types of Waste and Contaminated Lands (EPA 2003 Environmental Report)

Type: Waste	Description
Municipal solid waste	Municipal Solid Waste (MSW) is the waste discarded by households, hotels/motels, and commercial, institutional, and industrial sources. MSW typically consists of everyday items such as product packaging, grass clippings, furniture, clothing, bottles, food scraps, newspapers, appliances, paints, and batteries. It does not include waste water. In 2000, 232 million tons of MSW were generated.
RCRA hazardous waste	The term "RCRA hazardous waste" applies to certain types of hazardous wastes that appear on EPA's regulatory listing (RCRA) or that exhibit specific characteristics of ignitability, corrosiveness, reactivity, or excessive toxicity. More than 40 million tons of RCRA hazardous waste were generated in 1999.
Radioactive waste	Radioactive waste is the garbage, refuse, sludge, and other discarded material including solid, liquid, semi-solid, or contained gaseous material that must be managed for its radioactive content. The technical names for the types of waste that are considered "radioactive waste" for this report are high-level waste, spent nuclear fuel, transuranic waste, low-level waste, mixed low-level waste, and contaminated media. Fallout from the Fukushima nuclear disaster in Japan.
Extraction wastes	Extraction activities such as mining and mineral processing are large contributors to the total amount of waste generated and land contaminated in the U.S. EPA estimates that 5 billion tons of mining wastes were generated in 1988.
Industrial nonhazardous waste	Industrial nonhazardous waste is process waste associated with electric power generation and manufacturing of materials such as pulp and paper, iron and steel, glass, and concrete. This waste usually is not classified as either municipal waste or RCRA hazardous waste by federal or state laws. State, tribal, and some local governments have regulatory programs to manage industrial waste. EPA estimated that 7.6 billion tons of industrial nonhazardous wastes were generated in 1988.
Household hazardous Waste	Most household products that contain corrosive, toxic, ignitable, or reactive ingredients are considered household hazardous waste. Examples include most paints, stains, varnishes, solvents, and household pesticides. Special disposal of these materials is necessary to protect human health and the environment, but some amount of this type of waste is improperly disposed of by pouring the waste down the drain, on the ground, in storm sewers, or by discarding the waste with other household waste as part of municipal solic waste. EPA estimates that Americans generate 1.6 million tons of household hazardous waste per year, with the average home accumulating up to 100 pounds annually.
Agricultural waste	Agricultural solid waste is waste generated by the rearing of animals and the production and harvest of crops or trees. Animal waste, a large component of agricultural waste, includes waste from livestock, dairy, milk, and other animal-related agricultural and farming practices. Some of this waste is generated at sites called Confined Animal Feeding Operations (CAFOs). The waste associated with CAFOs results from congregating animals, feed, manure, dead animals, and production operations on a small land area. Animal waste and wastewater can enter water bodies from spills or breaks of waste storage structures (due to accidents or excessive rain), and nonagricultural application of manure to crop land. National estimates are not available.
Construction and demolition waste	Construction and demolition debris is waste generated during construction, renovation, and demolition projects. This type of waste generally consists of materials such as wood, concrete, steel, brink, and gypsum. National estimates are not available.
Medical waste	Medical waste is any solid waste generated during the diagnosis, treatment, or immunization of human beings or animals, in research, production, or testing. National estimates are not available.
Oil and gas waste	Oil and gas production wastes are the drilling fluids, produced waters, and other wastes associated with the exploration, development, and production of crude oil or natural gas that are conditionally exempt from regulation as hazardous wastes. National estimates are not available.
Sludge	Sludge is the solid, semisolid, or liquid waste generated from municipal, commercial, or industrial wastewater. National estimates are not available.

(Continued)

TABLE 3.9 (*Continued*)
Types of Waste and Contaminated Lands (EPA 2003 Environmental Report)

Type: Contaminated Lands	Description
Superfund national priorities list sites	Congress established the Superfund Program in 1980 to clean up abandoned hazardous waste sites throughout the U.S. The most seriously contaminated sites are on the National Priorities List (NPL). As of October 2002, there were 1498 sites on the NPL.
RCRA correction action sites	EPA and authorized states have identified 1714 hazardous waste management facilities that are the most seriously contaminated and may pose significant threats to humans or the environment. Some RCRA corrective Action sites are also identified by the Superfund Program as NPL sites.
Leaking underground storage tanks	Many petroleum and hazardous substances are stored in underground storage tanks (USTs). EPA regulates many categories of UST systems, including those at gas stations, convenience stores, and bus depots. USTs that have failed due to faulty materials, installation, operating procedures, or maintenance systems are categorized as leaking underground storage tanks (LUSTs). LUSTs can contaminate soil, groundwater, and sometimes drinking water. Vapors from UST releases can lead to explosions and other hazardous situations if those vapors migrate to a confined area such as a basement. LUSTs are the most common source of groundwater contamination, and petroleum is the most common groundwater contaminant. According to EPA's corrective action reports, in 1996, there were 1,064,478 active tanks located at approximately 400,000 facilities. In 2002, there were 697,966 active tanks (a 34% decrease) and 1,525,402 closed tanks (a 42% increase). The number of national USTs within each area of the U.S. has not fluctuated significantly between 1996 and 2001. As of the fall of 2002, 427,307 UST releases (LUSTs) were confirmed.
Accidental spill sites	Each year, thousands of oil and chemical spills occur on land and in water. Oil and gas materials that have spilled include drilling fluids, produced waters, and other wastes associated with the exploration, development, and production of crude oil or natural gas. Accurate national spill data are not available.
Land contaminated with radioactive and other hazardous materials	Approximately 0.54 million acres of land spanning 129 sites over 30 states are contaminated with radioactive and other hazardous materials as a result of activities associated with nuclear weapons production and research. Although DOE is the landlord at most of these sites, other parties including other federal agencies, private parties, and one public university also have legal responsibilities over these lands.
Brownfields	Brownfields are real property, the expansion, redevelopment of reuse of which may be complicated by the presence of potential presence of a hazardous substance, pollutant, or contaminate. Brownfields are often found in and around exonomically depressed neighborhoods. As brownfields are cleaned and redeveloped, surrounding communities benefit from a reduction in health and environmental risks, more functional space, and improved economic conditions. A complete inventory of brownfields does not exist. According to the General Accounting Office (1987), there are approximately 450,000 brownfields nationwide. The EPA's national Brownfield tracking system includes a large volume of data on brownfields across the nation, but does not track all of them. EPA's Brownfield Assessment Pilot Program includes data collected from over 400 communities.
Some military bases	Some (exact number or percentage unknown) military bases are contaminated as a result of a variety of activities. A national assessment of land contaminated at military bases has not been conducted. However, under the Base Realignment and Closure (BRAC) laws, closed military bases undergo site investigation processes to determine the extent of possible contamination and the need for site cleanup. Currently, 204 military installations that have been closed or realigned are undergoing environmental cleanup. These installations collectively occupy over 400,00 acres, though not all of this land is contaminated. Thirty-six of these installations are on the Superfund NPL list, and, of these, 32 are being cleaned up under the Fast Track program to make them available for other uses as quickly as possible.

(Continued)

TABLE 3.9 (*Continued*)

Types of Waste and Contaminated Lands (EPA 2003 Environmental Report)

Type: Contaminated Lands	Description
Waste management sites that were poorly designed or poorly managed	Prior to the 1970s, untreated waste was typically placed in open pits or directly onto the land. Some of these early waste management sites are still contaminated. In other cases, improper management of facilities (that were typically used for other purposes such as manufacturing) resulted in site contamination. Federal and state cleanup efforts are not addressing those early land disposal units and poorly managed sites that are still contaminated.
Illegal dumping sites	Also known as "open dumping" or "midnight dumping," illegal dumping of such materials as construction waste, abandoned automobiles, appliances, household waste, and medical waste raises concerns for safety, property values, and quality of life. People tend to dump illegally because legal dumping costs money and/or is inconvenient. While a majority of illegally dumped waste is not hazardous, some of it is, creating contaminated lands.
Abandoned mine lands	Abandoned mine lands are sites that have historically been mined and have not been properly cleaned up. These abandoned or inactive mine sites may include disturbances or features ranging from exploration holes and trenches to full-blown, large-scale mine opening, pits, waste dumps, and processing facilities. The Department of the Interior's (DOI) Bureau of Land Management (BLM) is presently aware of approximately 10,200 abandoned hard rock mines located within the roughly 264 million acres under its jurisdiction. Various government and private organizations have made estimates over the years about the total number of abandoned and inactive mines in the United States, including estimates for the percentage land management agencies, and state and privately owned lands. Those estimates range from about 80,000 to hundreds of thousands of small to medium-sized sites. The BLM is attempting to identify, prioritize, and take appropriate actions on those historic mine sites that pose safety risks to the public or present serious threats to the environment.

Source: EPA's Draft Report on the Environment 2003, Appendix B-Types of Waste and Contaminated LandsB-2-5.

determination of expert opinion than a systematic data analysis, they suggest that 40% of U.S. estuarine waters—as measured by surface area—are degraded by excess nutrients. That condition can lead to high levels of algae and eventually to lower levels of oxygen in the water. The heat of summer also promotes algae. For example, in the Southwest of United States in the months of June, July, and August, the ponds and lakes are so filled with blue, green, and red algae that one can see them with the naked eye.

Preventive action by stopping initial source contamination would be a far less costly and healthier practice than attempting to repair damaged areas after the fact, as is done now with chlorination. Seldom is such cleanup ever totally or satisfactorily accomplished.

Lakes contain whatever contaminants happen to run off from the area surrounding them, whether these be agricultural residues, city street pollutants, or landfill contaminants. The drinking water in the city of Toronto, for example, comes from the Great Lakes.[92] Figure 3.4 shows the overall condition of waters, lakes, and estuaries in North America. This source is a virtual chemistry laboratory due to contaminants generated mostly by man.

These substances will increase the total environment and then the total individual pollutant load that the chemically sensitive and chronic degenerative patient has to cope with. This increase in environmental load puts a strain on the homeostatic mechanism and, thus, the neurological, vascular, and immune systems. This strain can lead to the development of hypersensitivity and/or chronic degenerative disease.

The overall condition of estuaries in the great lakes is shown in Figure 3.4. As one can observe, none obtain a good rating, while most are rated from fair to poor.

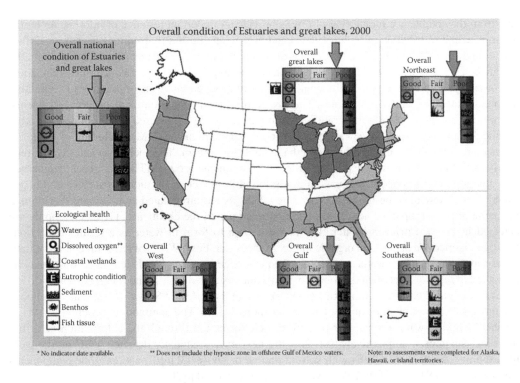

FIGURE 3.4 EPA report, September 2001. National Coastal Canadian report modified. No area ranked good. All rated from fair to poor. They are clearly swimming in dirty water all over the North American continent.

VOLATILE ORGANIC CHEMICALS

According to Moran et al.,[78,87] volatile organic chemicals (VOCs) in drinking water supplied by community water systems (CWSs) are available for 12 Northeast and Mid-Atlantic States from 1993 to 1998. The data are from 2110 CWSs, representing a 20% random selection of the total 10,749 active CWSs in the region. The data were collected for compliance monitoring under the Safe Drinking Water Act from both surface and groundwater sources and largely represent samples of finished drinking water collected prior to distribution. Overall, 39% of the 2110 randomly selected CWSs reported a detection of one or more VOCs at or above 1.0 µg/L (micrograms per liter).

Individually, the THMs were the most frequently detected VOCs ranging 33%.

VOCs were more frequently detected in drinking water from systems that are supplied by surface water sources, or both surface and groundwater sources, than in systems that are supplied exclusively by groundwater, and from systems serving very large populations (serving >3300 people) compared to systems serving medium and small populations (serving ≤3300 people).

Contamination of drinking water supplies by VOCs is a human health concern because many are toxic or are known or suspected to be human carcinogens.[79] The occurrence of VOCs in surface and groundwater resources is widespread,[80–83] and the occurrence of VOCs in public drinking water has been noted for some time.[84] In a recent national survey of community water systems (CWSs), 38% of CWSs identified VOCs as potential contaminants in their source waters.[85] In that same survey, 23% of CWSs with exclusively surface water sources and 27% of CWSs with exclusively groundwater sources indicated that they used some type of treatment in at least one facility to remove organic contaminants.[85]

Under the Safe Drinking Water Act (SDWA), the U.S. Environmental Protection Agency (USEPA) has established Maximum Contaminant Levels (MCLs for 21 VOCs in drinking water supplied by CWSs. Drinking water supplied by CWSs is required to be monitored for compounds with MCLs. The data from the compliance monitoring of CWSs provide an important resource of information on the occurrence and distribution of both regulated and unregulated VOCs in drinking water from surface and groundwater sources. For example, Dallas drinking water has 22 different chemicals (individually) that are below the toxic threshold, but the question is regarding the toxicity of chemicals in combination.

For purposes of comparison, individual VOCs were grouped into categories generally reflecting the predominant use of the compounds. The five groups based on predominant use are: (1) solvents, (2) gasoline components, (3) refrigerants, (4) fumigants, and (5) VOCs used in the synthesis of other chemicals; another group also was included (6) trihalomethanes (THM), including chloroform, bromodichloromethane, chlorodibromomethane, and bromoform. The fuel oxygenate methyl tert-butyl ether (MTBE) was included in the gasoline components group. MTBE has recently emerged as a contaminant of concern that is commonly found at low concentrations in surface and group water[86,87] and now must be monitored in some CWSs as an unregulated contaminant.[88] Although the name of this group does not reflect a predominant use of the chemicals, THMs commonly are detected in finished drinking water. THMs are known to form in water as a result of reactions between disinfection agents and organic matter in the water. For CWSs that have some or all of their water supplied by surface water sources, the frequent occurrence of THMs in treated water may be attributed to reactions between disinfection agents and organic matter in the water. Although differences in analytical coverage complicate comparisons, in the 1543 CWSs with THM data at or above 1.0 µg/L, 42% reported an occurrence of one or more THMs. The common detection of THMs in finished drinking water probably is related to their formation through the chlorination of drinking water supplies. Comparatively, solvents, the next most frequently detected VOC group, were reported in 9.8% of 2097 CWSs with solvent data at or above 1.0 µg/L, and gasoline components were detected in 9.0% of 2098 CWSs with data at or above 1.0 µg/L.

Of the 2110 randomly selected CWSs, 39% had a detection of one or more VOCs at or above 1.0 µg/L. The distribution of surface and groundwater sources from CWSs with and without a detection of any VOC is shown in Figure 3.5. The sources indicated as having a detection of any

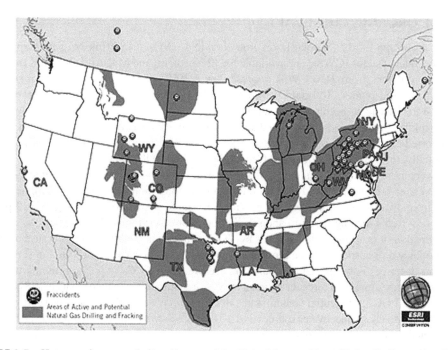

FIGURE 3.5   Hot areas for gas and oil wells around the United States. (From Hydraulic Fracturing Causing 'Fraccidents' All Across United States. 2011. http://www.treehugger.com/energy-disasters/hydraulic-fractur-ing-causing-fraccidents-all-across-united-states.html.)

TABLE 3.10

Volatile Organic Compounds (VOCs; µg/L, Micrograms Per Liter)

VOC Group	Number of Systems with Analyses of One or More VOCs in Group	Number of Systems with Detection of One or More VOCs in Group at 1.0 µg/L	Frequency of Detection
Trihalomethanes	1543	644	41.7
Solvents	2097	206	9.8
Gasoline components	2098	188	9.0
Refrigerants	1669	36	2.2
Organic synthesis	2098	24	1.1
Fumigants	2102	18	0.9

Source: Moran, M., S. Grady, J. Zogorski. 2001. Occurrence and Distribution of Volatile Organic Compounds in Drinking Water Supplied by Community Water Systems in the Northeast and Mid-Atlantic Regions of the United States, 1993–1998.

Note: Number of systems with analyses of one or more compounds in groups of volatile organic compounds, number of systems with a detection of one or more compounds in groups of volatile organic compounds at or above 1.0 micrograms per liter, and frequency of detection of groups of volatile organic compounds in drinking water from randomly selected community water systems in the study area.

VOC in Figure 3.5 include all of the sources for a system with a detection and do not indicate the specific source that had the detection.

The pattern of detection of VOCs by group was statistically significant at the 95% confidence interval (p = 0.001). In general, VOCs in groups that are more widely used, such as solvents and gasoline components, were detected more frequently than VOCs in groups that are not as widely used, such as organic synthesis compounds, refrigerants, and fumigants (Table 3.10).

The detection of VOCs at or above 1.0 µg/L in water supplied by CWSs was fairly common. Since some drinking water has been affected by the occurrence of VOCs from various groups, it would be beneficial for purveyors of drinking water to consider strengthening or enhancing plans for protecting source waters from contamination, in addition to treatment, as a means of further enhancing the quality of drinking water. Although only a relatively small percentage of CWSs had one or more samples with a concentration of a VOC above a health standard, some compounds such as total THMs, tetrachloroethene, and trichloroethene exceeded standards fairly frequently. Since health standards or criteria have been exceeded in some drinking water, a better understanding of the sources, transport, and receptors of VOCs that exceed these values would help in developing plans for better protecting source waters from contamination.

VOLATILE ORGANIC COMPOUNDS IN THE NATION'S DRINKING WATER SUPPLY WELLS

When volatile organic compounds (VOCs) are detected in samples from drinking water supply wells, it is important to understand what these results may mean to human health. As a first step toward understanding VOC occurrence in the context of human health, a screening level assessment was conducted by comparing VOC concentrations to human health benchmarks. One sample from each of 3497 domestic and public wells was analyzed for 55 VOCs; samples were collected prior to treatment or blending. At least one VOC was detected in 623 well samples (approximately 18% of all well samples) at a threshold of 0.2 part per billion. Eight of the 55 VOCs had concentrations greater than human health benchmarks in 45 well samples (approximately 1% of all well samples); these concentrations may be of potential human health concern if the water were to be ingested without treatment for many years. VOC concentrations were less than human health benchmarks in most well samples with VOC detections (Figure 3.3), indicating that adverse effects are unlikely to occur, even if water with such concentrations were to be ingested over a lifetime. Seventeen VOCs may warrant further investigation because their concentrations were greater than, or approached, human health benchmarks. Of course, no one knows the safe levels of VOC in water. Certainly, our studies at the EHC-Dallas on VOC show that hypersensitivity and chronic degenerative disease occur in the long term when exposure is chronic.

VOCs CONTAMINATION OF GROUNDWATER

When VOCs are spilled or dumped, a portion will evaporate but some usually soak into the ground. In soil, the VOCs can be carried deeper with percolating rainwater or melting snow. If they reach the water table, they can persist for years because the cool, dark, low-bacterial environment does not promote decomposition. If the VOCs in the groundwater migrate to nearby wells, they can end up in someone's drinking water.

The Department of Natural Resources has been conducting a great deal of VOC testing since 1982. All community wells and surface water sources have now been tested for a wide range of VOCs, as have approximately 1500 noncommunity public and private wells.

Of the 2230 community wells sampled in Wisconsin, 113 (5.1%) have shown the presence of at least one VOC. Some of these are bare traces, one or two parts per billion. However, 28 community wells exceed state health advisory levels for drinking water.

Of the 1500 private and noncommunity public wells which have been tested, 355 show the presence of at least one VOC. Many of the private wells were selected for sampling because they were especially vulnerable to contamination, were near other contaminated wells, or were delivering water with strange tastes or odors.

Several factors increase a well's vulnerability to VOC contamination. These include: (1) The distance between the well and source of contamination; (2) the amount of chemical dumped or spilled; (3) the depth of the well; (4) local geology; and (5) the amount of groundwater.

The first factor is the distance between the well and the source or sources of contamination. Many of the VOC-contaminated wells are located near industrial or commercial areas, gas stations, landfills, or railroad tracks.

A second factor is the amount of VOC which has been dumped or spilled. VOC contamination is often caused by local spills or dumping and is confined to a rather small geographical area (although there may often be more than one suspected source of VOCs in the area). When a large quantity of contaminant is released, as sometimes occurs with industrial spills or leaking underground storage tanks, a large geographical area can be affected.

A third factor is the depth of the well casing. Since contaminants are seeping from the ground surface, a shallow well will be affected sooner than a deep well.

A fourth factor is the local geology. Areas with highly porous or "thin" soils and shallow depths to groundwater are most vulnerable. On the other hand, areas with thick layers of certain types of soil can absorb and significantly slow down the movement of some contaminants. This is particularly important because many organic chemicals can be broken down by soil bacteria, if they are held near the ground surface long enough for the bacteria to work.

A fifth factor is time. Groundwater typically moves very slowly, and it can sometimes take a year for a spilled contaminant to reach nearby wells. The time and distance contaminants must travel are extremely important because many wells which presently show no contamination may eventually become contaminated by spills which have already occurred. In other words, they would not know the full impacts of the contamination they have already caused for many years to come. This is why they cannot be complacent, and must continue to test our water supplies.

At the EHC-Dallas, they have determined some of the victims of these water contamination sites and have found that their blood contained some of the same toxic volatile substances as were in the drinking water. These toxic substances appeared to trigger their chemical sensitivity. Pathology appears to be related, as shown in the following two cases.

Case Study: A 66-year-old teacher with symptoms of esophagitis with bleeding, vomiting, and multiple food and chemical sensitivities was assessed in the environmental control unit. He had a history of exposure to groundwater that was contaminated by a toxic waste dump site that was used to dispose of a number of solvents and other chemicals. He also had a past history of prostate carcinoma, incontinence secondary to a prostatectomy, hypocomplementemia, and Gilbert's disease. He had experienced esophageal reflux, gastritis, gastric polyps, and chronic constipation. Medications were Zantac, 150 mg, and Reglan, one at bedtime. His family history included parents, who had allergies, and a son and daughter, who had multiple food and chemical sensitivities.

Abnormal blood analysis for chemicals showed the following: Hgb, 13.7 g/dL (C = 14–18 g/dL); Hct, 41.5% (C = 42–52%); RBC, 4.49 × 10^6/mm^3 (C = 4.7–6.1 × 10^6/mm^3); chloride, 96 mEq/L (C = 100–112 mEq/L; bilirubin, 1.32 mg/dL (C < 1.0 mg/dL); creatinine, 1.5 mg/dL (C = 0.8–1.4 mg/dL); calcium, 11.0 mg/dL (# = 7.5–10.1 mg/dL); BUN, 22.6 mg/dL (C = 7–21 mg/dL); Total hemolytic serum complement (CH$_{100}$) was 20 U/L (normal = 70–150 U/L).

Blood analysis for chemicals showed the presence of significant levels of benzene, dichlorobenzene, toluene, trimethylbenzene, bromoform, trichloroethane, trichloroethylene, and tetrachloroethylene. These were the same as had been found in the patient's drinking water from the public water supply of Tucson, AZ. The chlorinated pesticides β-BHC, β-BHC, DDE, dieldrin, heptachlor, epoxide, and hexachlorobenzene were also found in his blood. Ambient doses and double-blind challenges with toxic chemicals of this type led to reproduction of symptoms.

The patient's symptoms cleared in the environmental control unit after two weeks. His blood levels of chlorinated solvents decreased as he recovered.

The wide variety of chemicals found in this patient gives a graphic example of what may happen when a person is exposed to contaminated water. No doubt there are multiple factors in the induction of illness or malignancy, but this toxic load could certainly contribute to the pathogenesis of disease states, especially in susceptible individuals (Table 3.11).

The degree of reaction in this patient upon exposure to tetrachloroethylene was dramatic, especially at the somewhat higher concentration. Virtually all of the symptoms that he had experienced

---

TABLE 3.11

Inhaled Double-Blind Challenge after 4 days Deadaptation in the ECU with Total Load Reduced

Exposures	Symptoms	Signs
Tetrachloroethylene (5 ppm)	Muscle and joint pains; lightheadedness	Tachycardia
Tetrachloroethylene (50 ppm)	Severe malaise and joint pains; lightheadedness; nausea	Pallor, sweating, skin rash, tachycardia
	Wandering paresthesia; irritability; poor concentration; depression	Cognitive impairment on objective measurement

Chemical	ppb	Symptoms	Signs
Ethanol (petroleum derived)	<0.5	+	+
Phenol	<0.002	+	+
Formaldehyde	<0.20	+	+
Pesticide (2,3, DNP)	<0.0034	+	+
Chlorine	<0.33	+	+
Xylene	<0.17	+	+
Placebo	saline	n	n

Source: Environmental Health Center-Dallas; Rea, W. J. 1992. *Chemical Sensitivity Vol II: Sources of Total Body Load.* Boca Raton, FL: CRC Press, p. 554 Table 7.

over the several years of exposure to contaminated drinking were reproduced. Moreover, his symptoms reached their peak of intensity not with the initial exposure, but several hours later.

This case illustrates the compounding effect of environmental factors that are inherent in medical practice, wherein the physician was made substantially worse by exposures to disinfectants, anesthetic gases, and other potential toxins in the operating room. He became especially ill after exposure to methyl methacrylate cement, while assisting at total hip replacements. Eventually, he had to give up operating room work, which was a component of his practice that he had previously found very gratifying.

With treatment including environmental control, avoidance of exposures, and dietary and nutritional therapy, the physician has improved substantially, and after 5 years of disability, he is continuing to recover. He took a fellowship and is practicing environmental medicine vigorously.

Along with examination of the effects of contamination of surface and groundwater used for drinking and bathing, the effects of water pollution on the production of food must also be considered. Each category of potential food production and water supply will be discussed separately.

Industrial Waste

EWG's analysis of the water supplier's tap water test results shows that water contaminated with 166 industrial pollutants, including plasticizers, solvents, and propellants, is served to 210,528,000 people in 42 states. Fifty-six percent of those people were served water with one or more industrial contaminants present at levels above nonenforceable, health-based limits. Ninety-four of the industrial chemicals detected in tap water are unregulated, without a legal health-based limit in tap water. No one knows the effects of these combinations. However, good sense would tell you that the combinations of most would cause adverse effects.

On the previous pages, they discussed individual waste contaminants which will be further elicited here. Aluminum is high in many public water supplies because it is used as a flocculant in the purification process. Lead, cadmium, copper, and zinc tend to be found in higher concentrations in soft water due to the lack of calcium and magnesium and will exacerbate chemical sensitivity through damage to the aforementioned detoxification mechanisms.

Water pollution is now a problem worldwide. Officials in New Mexico have identified 25 cities where hydrocarbons and solvents contaminated the groundwater.[89] Analysis of the drinking water in New Orleans revealed the presence of 13 halogenated hydrocarbons.[90] In addition, conditions for the spontaneous creation of new toxic chemicals from the ones present in the water have been observed. See Table 3.8 again (Ref. CSII p.541 Table 3—Volatile Organic Constituents Identified in New Orleans Drinking Water). This kind of contamination apparently occurs all over the world. Australia's great inland river system is largely regulated to irrigate agricultural areas upstream of Adelaide, and the intensive use of agricultural chemicals that have the potential to pollute water sources with a very diverse range of synthetic organic compounds is causing concern. Contamination with organic compounds from industrial sources is mainly relevant to the potential pollution of groundwater supplies in Perth.[91] The Rhine River in Germany has been severely contaminated from near its source in Switzerland as well as down river by other industries. Similar pollution problems are also occurring in the rivers of Asia, South America, and Africa (Tables 3.12 and 3.13).[92]

Large spills happen. For instance, the water provider West Virginia American Water has issued a DO NOT USE WATER NOTICE for all West Virginia American Water customers in Kanawha, Boone, Putnam, Lincoln, Logan, Clay, Roane, and Jackson counties, as well as customers in Culloden in Cabell County due to the chemical spill.

The spill occurred at a Freedom Industries storage facility 1.5 miles upstream from West Virginia American's water intake along the Elk River in Charleston.

The station said that the chemical leaked from a tank at Freedom Industries in Charleston. The leaked product is 4-methylcyclohexane methanol, which is used in the froth flotation process of coal washing and preparation according to WSAZ.

TABLE 3.12

Industrial Pollutants in U.S. Drinking Water

Aluminum	Arochlor 1221
Ammonia	Arochlor 1232
Bromide	Arochlor 1242
Arsenic	Arochlor 1248
Chlorate	Arochlor 1252
Barium	Arochlor 1260
Cadmium	1,1-Dichloropropene
Chromium	1,3-Dichloropropane
Cyanide	1,2,3-Trichloropropane
Hydrogen sulfide	2,2-Dichloropropane
Lead	1,2,4-Trimethylbenzene
Manganese	1,2,3-Trichloropropane
Mercury	2,2-Dichloropropane
Nitrate and nitrite (mix)	1,2,4-Trimethylbenzene
Nitrate	1,2,3-Trichlorobenzene
Nitrite	n-Butylbenzene
Phosphate	sec-Butylbenzene
Selenium	tert-Butylbenzene
Silver	1,3,5-Trimethylbenzene
Strontium	Bromochloromethane
Sulfate	Chloropicrin
Antimony	2-Nitropropane
Beryllium	Glyoxal
Chromium (hexavalent)	Trichlorotrifluoroethane
Lithium	Foaming agents
Molybdenum	Phenols
Thallium	Ethylene dibromide
Vanadium	Xylenes (total)
MBAS	o-Xylene
Oil and grease (total)	m-Xylene
Phosphorus	p-Xylene
Carbon disulfide	Meta and para xylene (mix)
Lindane	Formaldehyde
p-Isopropyltoluene	Methylene chloride
Di(2-ethylhexyl)adipate	o-Chlorotoluene
Di(2-ethylhexyl)phthalate	p-Chlorotoluene
Hexachlorocylcopentadiene	o-Dichlorobenzene
1,4-Dioxane	m-Dichlorobenzene
Endosulfan I	p-Dichloroethane
Butyl acetate	Vinyl chloride
Ethyl ether	1,1-Dichloroethylene
Ispropyl alcohol	1,2-Dichloroethane
Chloromethane	Trichloroethylene
Trichlorofluoromethane	1,1,1,2-Trichloroethane
n-Nitrosodiphenylamine	1,1,2,2-Tetrachloroethane
Aniline	Chlorobenzene
1,2-Dibromoethane	Benzene
Acrylonitrile	Toluene
Acetone	Ethylbenzene

(Continued)

TABLE 3.12 (*Continued*)
Industrial Pollutants in U.S. Drinking Water

Isopropyl ether	Bromobenzene
Hexachlorobutadiene	Ispropylbenzene
Methylethyl ketone	Styrene
Naphtalene	n-Propylbenzene
Methyl isobutyl ketone	Perchlorate
Methyl tertiary butyl ether	Ethyl-t-butyl ether
Nitrobenzene	Dichlorofluoromethane
Acenaphthylene	Alpha particle activity (including radon and uranium)
Acenaphthylene	Alpha particle activity (excluding radon and uranium)
Dimethylphthalate	Uranium (total
Diethylphthalate	Uranium-234
Fluoranthene	Uranium-235
Pyrene	Uranium-238
Di-n-butyl phthalate	Radium (total)
Butyl benzyl phthalate	Radium-226
Methyl methacrylate	Radium-228
Chrysene	Alpha particle activity (suspended)
Indeno [1,2,3-cd]pyrene	Gross beta activity (dissolved)
Dibenz[a,h] anthracene	Gross beta activity (suspended)
Pentachlorophenol	Potassium-40
n-Hexane	Tritium
1,2,4-Trichlorobenzene	Gross beta particles and photon emitter (man-made)
Cis-1,2-dichloroethylene	Manganese-54
Total PCBs	Strontium-90
Arochlor 1016	

Source: Used by permission from *Science Direct.* Human toxicology of chemical mixtures, pp. 100–109. Zeliger, H. I. 2008. ISBN: 978-0-8155-1589-0.

TABLE 3.13
Water Treatment and Distribution By-Product Pollutants in U.S. Drinking Water

Chloramine	Fluoranthene
Chlorate	Benzo[1] anthracene
Chlorine dioxide	Benzo[b] fluoranthene
Chlorite	Benzo[k]fluoranthene
Bromate	Benzo[a]pyrene
Cadmium	Benzo[g,h,I,]perylene
Orthophosphate	Dibromomethane
Asbestos	Bromochloromethane
Di(2-ethylhexyl)phthalate	Monochloroacetic acid
Chloromethane	Dichloroacetic acid
Methyl ethyl ketone	Trichloroacetic acid
2-Hexanone	

Source: Used by permission from *Science Direct.* Human toxicology of chemical mixtures, pp. 100–109. Zeliger, H. I. 2008. ISBN: 978-0-8155-1589-0.

Methylcyclohexanol's production and use as a solvent for cellulose esters and ethers and for lacquers resins, oils, and waxes, an antioxidant for lubricants, and a blending agent for special textile soaps and detergents may result in its release to the environment through various waste streams. Methylcyclohexanol is a commercial mixture that contains isomers of 2-,3-, and 4-methylcyclohexanol, which are expected to behave in a similar manner in the environment. If released in air, a vapor pressure of 1.2 mm Hg at 25°C indicates that trans-2-cyclohexanol will exist solely as a vapor in the atmosphere. A list of Industrial Contaminants and their potential health effects follows (Table 3.14).

POLLUTION'S EFFECTS ON THE GREAT LAKES ECOSYSTEM

With over 20% of the world's freshwater supply residing in them, the North American Great Lakes are the world's largest freshwater system.[93] Including Lake Erie, Michigan, Huron, Superior, and Ontario, the five lakes are an important source of fresh water and are home to many species of wildlife. However, with the belief that water could dilute any substance, the lakes also became a destination of dumping grounds for many different types of pollutants. Ranging from point source pollution such as industrial waste from drainage pipes to nonpoint source pollution such as pesticide and fertilizer runoff from farms, these pollutants and others have had adverse effects on the lakes. Such adverse effects include reducing the water quality, contaminating soils, and damaging the lake ecosystems. This damage produces harmful repercussions on the fish and wildlife stocks, as well as on the humans surrounding the Great Lakes region as well.

SOURCES OF POLLUTION IN THE GREAT LAKES

Point source pollution refers to a direct source of pollution, such as a pipe or other vessel. Early industries such as pulp and paper companies located in the Great Lakes region believed that anything could be dissolved in water, and thus neutralized. As a result, many wastes (such as mercury) were dumped into the Great Lakes. There have also been observations of fecal matter pollution from sewage, which results in harmful bacteria such as *E. coli* and enterococci.[94] Both sewage and other organic and inorganic wastes cause the water quality to decline and bacteria growth to increase.[95]

Nonpoint source pollution is pollution that does not come from specific locations. Many of these pollutants found in the Great Lakes are air-bound and many others are from fertilizer and pesticide runoff. One of the categories of chemical pollutants is organic contaminants, which are discovered by testing the tissue of fish and mussels found in the Great Lakes. Polychlorinated biphenyls (PCBs) have been found in the Great Lakes and are a result of synthetic fertilizers and pesticides.[96] Chlorodiphenyl-tichloroethane, commonly known as DDT, was found in all mussel tissue testing sites and is the most common chemical pollutant in the Great Lakes. According to the results from the mussel testing, dieldrin is the second most prevalent pollutant in the Great Lakes, behind DDT. Lindane is also a very harmful insecticide which was found in the tissues of Great Lake trout and walleye.[97] Another detrimental insecticide, toxaphene, breaks down very slowly in water, so it is still found in the lakes today, even though it was banned in 1990.[98]

The majority of the pollutants that contaminate the Great Lakes are harmful to the ecosystem in a variety of ways. Many times, pollutants move up the food chain, affecting not only the organisms that utilize chemical nutrients such as phytoplankton, protozoa, and crustaceans but also the animals that feed upon the smaller organisms. Predators higher along on the food chain tend to accumulate more pollutant residues, which can have harmful effects on humans.[99] This would include not only such animals as rainbow, smelt, walleye, and mussels but humans themselves. As shown in Figure 3.6 below, fish stocks have been decreasing in recent years, which they suspect is due to the increased abundance of pollutants.

Some of the common organic chemicals from pesticides such as DDT polluting the Great Lakes have been known to be toxic and cause major health problems in fish and other fauna. Fertilizers, phosphate detergents, and other pollutants that contain important nutrients have caused major algae

TABLE 3.14

List of Industrial Contaminants and Potential Health Effects in Addition to Chemical Sensitivity

Contaminant	MCLG[1] (mg/L)[2]	MCL or TT[1] (mg/L)[2]	Potential Health Effects from Long-Term Exposure above the MCL	Sources of Contaminant in Drinking Water
Bromate	Zero	0.010	Increased risk of cancer	By-product of drinking water disinfection
Chlorite	0.8	1.0	Anemia; infants, young children: nervous system	By-product of drinking water disinfection
Haloacetic acids (HAA5)	n/a[6]	0.060[7]	Increased risk of cancer	By-product of drinking water disinfection
Total trihalomethanes (TTHMs)	→	→	Liver, kidney dysfunction, CNS; increased risk of cancer	By-product of drinking water disinfection
	n/a[6]	0.080[7]		By-product of drinking water disinfection
Disinfectants				
Chloramines (as Cl[2])	MRDLG = 4[1]	MRDL = 4.0[1]	Eye/nose irritation; stomach discomfort, anemia	Water additive used to control microbes
Chlorine (as Cl[2])	MRDLG = 4[1]	MRDL = 4.0[1]	Eye/nose irritation; stomach discomfort	Water additive used to control microbes
Chlorine dioxide (as ClO[2])	MRDLG-0.8[1]	MRDL = 0.8[1]	Anemia; infants, young children: effects	Water additive used to control microbes
Inorganic Chemicals				
Antimony	0.006	0.006	Increase in blood cholesterol; decreased blood sugar	Discharge from petroleum refineries; fire retardants; ceramics; electronics; solder
Arsenic	0	0.010 as of 01/23/06	Skin damage or circulatory systems, increased risk of cancer	Erosion of natural deposits; runoff from orchards, runoff from glass and electronics production wastes
Asbestos (fiber >10 micrometers	7 million fibers per liter (MFL)	7 MFL	Increased risk of developing benign intestinal polyps	Decay of asbestos cement in water mains; erosion of natural deposits
Barium	2	2	Increase in blood pressure	Discharge of drilling wastes; metal refineries; erosion of natural deposits
Beryllium	0.004	0.004	Intestinal lesions	Discharge from metal refineries coal-burning factories; electrical, aerospace, defense industries

(Continued)

TABLE 3.14 (Continued)
List of Industrial Contaminants and Potential Health Effects in Addition to Chemical Sensitivity

Contaminant	MCLG[1] (mg/L)[2]	MCL or TT[1] (mg/L)[2]	Potential Health Effects from Long-Term Exposure above the MCL	Sources of Contaminant in Drinking Water
Cadmium	0.005	0.005	Kidney damage	Corrosion of galvanized pipes; erosion of natural deposits; discharge from metal refineries; runoff from waste batteries, paints.
Chromium (total)	0.1	0.1	Allergic dermatitis term exposure: Gastrointestinal distress Long-term exposure: Liver or kidney damage	Discharge from steel, pulp mills; erosion of natural deposits
Copper	1.3	TT[2]; Action Level = 1.3	Wilson's Disease	Corrosion of household plumbing systems; erosion of natural deposits
Cyanide (as free cyanide)	0.2	0.2	Nerve damage or thyroid problems	Discharge from steel/metal factories; plastic fertilizer
Fluoride	4.0	4.0	Bone disease (pain and tenderness of the bones); mottled teeth	Water additive which promotes strong teeth; erosion of natural deposits; fertilizer aluminum factories
Lead	Zero	TT[7], Action Level = 0.015	Children: Delays in physical or mental development; deficits in attention span learning abilities Adults: Kidney dysfunction; high blood pressure	Corrosion of household plumbing systems; erosion of natural deposits
Mercury (inorganic)	0.002	0.002	Kidney damage	Erosion of natural deposits; discharge from refineries and factories: runoff from landfills and croplands
Nitrate (measured as Nitrogen)	10	10	Infants below the age of six months who drink water containing nitrate in excess of the MCL could become seriously ill and, if untreated, may die. Symptoms include shortness of breath (blue-baby) syndrome	Runoff from fertilizer use; leaking from septic tanks, sewage; erosion of natural deposits.

(Continued)

TABLE 3.14 (Continued)
List of Industrial Contaminants and Potential Health Effects in Addition to Chemical Sensitivity

Contaminant	MCLG[1] (mg/L)[2]	MCL or TT[1] (mg/L)[2]	Potential Health Effects from Long-Term Exposure above the MCL	Sources of Contaminant in Drinking Water
Nitrite (measured as Nitrogen)	1	1	Infants below the age of six months, who drink water containing nitrite in excess of the MCLean, if untreated, may die. Symptoms: shortness of breath (blue baby) syndrome.	Runoff from fertilizer use; leaking from septic tanks, sewage; erosion of natural deposits
Selenium	0.05	0.05	Hair or fingernail loss; numbness in fingers or toes;	Discharge from petroleum refineries; erosion of natural deposits; discharge from mines
Thallium	0.0005	0.002	Hair loss; changes in blood; kidney, intestine, liver problems	Leaching from ore-processing sites; discharge from electronics, glass, and drug factories
Organic Chemicals				
Acrylamide	Zero	TT[8]	Nervous system or blood problems; Increased risk of cancer	Added to water during sewage/wastewater treatment
Alachlor	Zero	0.002	Eye, liver, kidney, or spleen problems; anemia; Increased risk of cancer	Runoff from herbicide used on row crops
Atrazine	0.003	0.003	Cardiovascular system or reproductive problems	Runoff from herbicide used on row crops
Benzene	Zero	0.005	Anemia; Decrease in blood platelets; Increased risk of cancer	Discharge from factories; leaching from gas storage tanks and landfills
Benzo(a)pyrene(PAHs)	Zero	0.0002	Reproductive difficulties; increased risk of cancer	Leaching from linings of water storage tanks and distribution lines
Carbofuran	0.04	0.04	Dysfunction blood, nervous or reproductive system	Leaching of soil fumigant used on rice and alfalfa
Carbon tetrachloride	Zero	0.005	Liver dysfunction; Increased risk of cancer	Discharge chemical plants industrial activities
Chlordane	Zero	0.002	Liver or nervous system dysfunctions; increased risk of cancer	Residue of banned termiticide
Chlorobenzene	0.1	0.1	Liver or kidney dysfunction	Discharge from chemical, agricultural chemical factories
2,4-D	0.07	0.07	Kidney, liver, or adrenal gland dysfunction	Runoff from herbicide used on row crops

(Continued)

TABLE 3.14 (Continued)
List of Industrial Contaminants and Potential Health Effects in Addition to Chemical Sensitivity

Contaminant	MCLG[1] (mg/L)[2]	MCL or TT[1] (mg/L)[2]	Potential Health Effects from Long-Term Exposure above the MCL	Sources of Contaminant in Drinking Water
Dalapon	0.2	0.2	Minor kidney changes	Runoff from herbicide used on rights of way
1,2-Dibromo-3-chloropropane (DBCP)	Zero	0.0002	Reproductive difficulties; Increased risk of cancer	Runoff/leaching from soil fumigant used on soybeans, cotton, pineapples, orchards
o-Dichlorobenzene	0.6	0.6	Liver, kidney, or circulatory system dysfunction	Discharge from industrial chemical factories
p-Dichlorobenzene	0.075	0.075	Anemia; liver, kidney, or spleen damage: Δ's in blood	Discharge from industrial chemical factories
1,2-Dichloroethane	Zero	0.005	Increased risk of cancer	Discharge from industrial chemical factories
1,1-Dichloroethylene	0.007	0.007	Liver dysfunction	Discharge from industrial chemical factories
Cis-1,2-Dichloroethylene	0.7	0.07	Liver dysfunction	Discharge from industrial chemical factories
Trans-1,2-Dichloroethylene	0.1	0.1	Liver dysfunction	Discharge from industrial chemical factories
Dichloromethane	Zero	0.005	Liver dysfunction; Increased risk of cancer	Discharge from drug and chemical factories
1,2-Dichloropropane	Zero	0.005	Increased risk of cancer	Discharge from industrial chemical factories
Di(2-ethylhexyl) adipate	0.4	0.4	Weight loss, liver dysfunction, reproductive difficulties	Discharge from chemical factories
Di(2-ethylhexyl)phthalate	Zero	0.006	Reproductive difficulties; liver dysfunction; Increased risk of cancer	Discharge from rubber and chemical factories
Dinoseb	0.007	0.007	Reproductive difficulties	Runoff from herbicide used on soybeans and vegetables
Dioxin (2,3,7,8-TCDDE)	Zero	0.00000003	Reproductive difficulties; increased risk of cancer	Emissions from waste incineration combustion; discharge from chemical factories
Diquat	0.02	0.02	Cataracts	Runoff from herbicide
Endothall	0.1	0.1	Stomach and intestinal upset	Runoff from herbicide use
Endrin	0.002	0.002	Liver dysfunction	Residue of banned insecticide
Epichlorohydrin	Zero	TT[8]	Increased cancer risk, over a long period. G.I. upset	Discharge from industrial chemical factories; impurity water chemicals
Ethylbenzene	0.7	0.7	Liver kidneys dysfunction	Discharge from petroleum refineries

(Continued)

TABLE 3.14 (Continued)
List of Industrial Contaminants and Potential Health Effects in Addition to Chemical Sensitivity

Contaminant	MCLG[1] (mg/L)[2]	MCL or TT[1] (mg/L)[2]	Potential Health Effects from Long-Term Exposure above the MCL	Sources of Contaminant in Drinking Water
Ethylene dibromide	Zero	0.00005	Problems with liver, stomach, reproductive system, or kidneys; Increased cancer risk	Discharge from petroleum refineries
Glyphosate	0.7	0.7	Kidney; reproductive difficulties	Runoff from herbicide use
Heptachlor	Zero	0.0004	Liver damage; Increased risk of cancer	Residue of banned termiticide
Heptachlor epoxide	Zero	0.0002	Liver damage; Increased risk of cancer	Breakdown of heptachlor
Hexachlorobenzene	Zero	0.001	Liver, kidney; reproductive difficulties; Increased cancer	Discharge from metal refineries and agricultural chemical factories
Hexachlorocyclopentadiene	0.05	0.05	Kidney or stomach problems	Discharge from chemical factories
Lindane	0.0002	0.0002	Liver or kidney dysfunction	Runoff/leaching from insecticide used on cattle, lumber, gardens
Methoxychlor	0.04	0.04	Reproductive difficulties	Runoff/leaching from insecticide used on fruits, vegetables, alfalfa, livestock
Oxamyl (vydate)	0.2	0.2	Slight nervous system effects	Runoff/leaching from insecticide used on apples, potatoes, tomatoes
Polychlorinated biphenyls (PCBs)	Zero	0.0005	Skin changes; thymus gland, immune deficiencies; reproductive or nervous system difficulties; increased risk of cancer	Runoff from landfills; discharge of waste chemicals
Pentachlorophenol	Zero	0.001	Liver or kidney dysfunction; increased cancer risk	Discharge from wood preserving factories
Picloram	0.5	0.5	Liver dysfunction	Herbicide runoff
Simazine	0.004	0.004	Problems with blood	Herbicide runoff
Styrene	0.1	0.1	Liver, kidney, or circulatory system dysfunctions	Discharge from rubber and plastic factories; leaching from landfills
Tetrachloroethylene	Zero	0.005	Liver dysfunction; increased risk of cancer	Discharge from factories and dry cleaners
Toluene	1	1	Nervous system, kidney, or liver dysfunctions	Discharge from petroleum factories
Toxaphene	Zero	0.003	Kidney, liver, thyroid dysfunctions; increased risk of cancer	Runoff/leaching from insecticide used on cotton and cattle
2,4,5-TP (Silvex)	0.05	0.05	Liver dysfunction	Residue of banned herbicide

(Continued)

TABLE 3.14 (Continued)
List of Industrial Contaminants and Potential Health Effects in Addition to Chemical Sensitivity

Contaminant	MCLG[1] (mg/L)[2]	MCL or TT[1] (mg/L)[2]	Potential Health Effects from Long-Term Exposure above the MCL	Sources of Contaminant in Drinking Water
1,2,4-Trichlorobenzene	0.07	0.07	Changes in adrenal glands	Discharge from textile finishing factories
1,1,1-Trichloroethane	0.20	0.2	Liver, nervous system, circulatory dysfunction	Discharge from metal degreasing sites and other factories
1,1,2-Trichloroethane	0.003	0.005	Liver, kidney, immune system dysfunctions	Discharge from industrial chemical factories
Trichloroethylene	Zero	0.005	Liver dysfunction; increased risk of cancer	Discharge from metal degreasing sites and other factories
Vinyl chloride	Zero	0.002	Increased risk of cancer	Leaching from PVC pipes; discharge from plastic factories
Xylenes (total)	10	10	Nervous system damage	Discharge from petroleum, chemical factories
Radionuclides				
Alpha particles	None[7] Zero	15 Picocuries per Liter (pCi/L)	Increased risk of cancer	Erosion of natural deposits of certain minerals that are radioactive emit of radiation alpha radiation
Beta particles and photon emitters	None[7] Zero	–4 millirems per year	Increased risk of cancer	Decay of natural and man-made deposits radioactive minerals, radiation known as photons and beta radiation
Radium 226 and radium 228 (combined)	None[7] Zero	5 pCi/L	Increased risk of cancer	Erosion of natural deposits
Uranium	Zero	30 µg/L as of 123/08/03	Increased risk of cancer, kidney toxicity	Erosion of natural deposits

Source: Drinking Water Contaminants. http://water.epa.gov/drink/contaminants/index.cfm

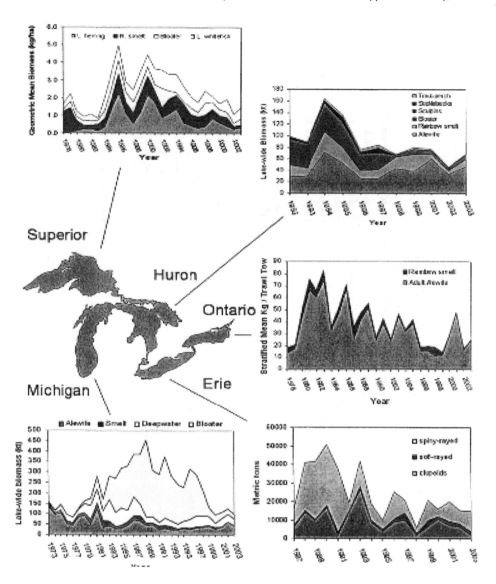

FIGURE 3.6   Graphs of fish prey population stocks.

blooms that lead to nutrient imbalance and lack of oxygen in the water, reducing fish populations and other wildlife.[95] Levels of PCBs from point source industrial dumping that were higher than the legal limit approved by the FDA were consistently found in fish in the Great Lakes.[99]

Sewage is another common pollutant of the Great Lakes, and studies have shown that two kinds of bacteria *(Enterococcus and E. coli),* which are indicators of human fecal matter, were present in 20% of the samples taken from Lake Michigan beaches in 2004.[95] If ingested by humans, these bacteria could cause such illnesses as extreme as typhoid fever.[95] Infections, gastrointestinal diseases, and parasites are other possible risks from coming into contact with these bacteria as well.[94] As a result of fecal matter pollution that has been plaguing beaches on the Great Lakes, there was a 32% increase in the number of Great Lakes beach closings and advisories in 2003.[94]

Mercury, a heavy metal that is known for its toxicity in even small amounts, has been known to affect the lakes as well, and even substances that are not chemically toxic are contributing to the problems of the Great Lakes as well. Tiny particles of solids of pollutants suspended in the water may block sunlight from the water and become breeding grounds for bacteria.[94]

Heterotrophic plate count (HPC) is a measurement of mixed bacteria in water. This test provides a quantitative assessment of the viable bacteria in a water sample that are able to grow under standardized test conditions. HPC testing may be used to monitor changes in the quality of water throughout a distribution system, thus giving an indication of the effectiveness of chlorination or other disinfection in the system as well as the possible existence of cross-connections, sediment accumulation, and other problems within the distribution lines. Although industry and several government agencies state that HPC poses no health risk, that statement remains somewhat controversial. HPC includes some opportunistic pathogens that may pose risks to immunocompromised people such as the chemically sensitive with T cell and gamma globulin deficiency. Examples of bacteria that may be included in HPC include *Aeromonas, Acinetobacter, Corynebacterium, Klebsiella Legionella, Morazella, Mycobacteria, Pseudomonas, Staphylococcus,* and *Vibro*. Bacteria in all of these areas can affect humans under certain circumstances. Also, HPC levels that are high can interfere with coliform testing and may mask fecal or total coliform.[99]

CHEMICAL INTEGRITY OF THE GREAT LAKES: MERCURY

The chemical integrity of the Great Lakes is dynamic. The waters of the Great Lakes are continuously changing through the addition, interaction, and loss of both natural and man-made substances. Natural geophysical processes change these substances' spatial and temporal distribution within the Great Lakes system. While much is known, considerable uncertainty remains concerning the chemical integrity of the Great Lakes and the impacts of various chemicals, and combinations of chemicals, on the basin's human and other inhabitants.

Mercury, a persistent bioaccumulative toxic metal, provides an excellent example of the challenges inherent in understanding impacts on the chemical integrity of the Great Lakes. It occurs widely in nature, both in concentrated form in cinnabar (ore) and in small amounts in fossil fuels such as coal industry.[100]

Mercury reaches the waters of the Great Lakes directly, through discharges into the waters, and indirectly, through disturbances in previous mercury deposition and through atmospheric deposition, especially by the melting of the polar ice caps which yields 200 tons per year.

Mercury can be released into the air by human activities such as metallurgical processing, municipal and medical waste incineration, and electrical power generation such as from coal combustion. It is also released to the atmosphere by various natural phenomena, including volcanic eruptions, forest fires, and the weathering of geological formations.[100]

Reactive gaseous mercury (or the ionic form of mercury) is both substantially more soluble in water and more reactive than elemental mercury. It remains in the *atmosphere from 1 to 10 days,* and therefore tends to be deposited locally and regionally from a few miles to a few hundred miles from its source. Its limited range of travel, solubility, and high reactivity contribute to its ultimate presence in biota on a regional basis.[101,102]

Mercury particulate is mercury bound to airborne particles. Mercury particulate can remain in the atmosphere for 1 to 10 days, comparable to reactive gaseous mercury, and thus is deposited regionally and locally. However, it is less available to living organisms than the reactive gaseous form.[101,102]

Once deposited in or discharged to water bodies, mercury can be converted by bacteria into organic mercury compounds, such as methylmercury, that accumulate in the food chain. Human exposure to methylmercury is predominantly through fish consumption.

Methylmercury compounds can cross biological membranes, are soluble in lipids and adipose tissues, and can bind to various cell receptors and enzyme sites. Methylmercury has not been found to be a carcinogen and has not been conclusively established as a teratogen. Without cancer as a complicating factor, scientists have been able to conduct relatively straightforward analyses of the risks posed by human exposure to mercury compounds. At sufficient levels of accumulation of methylmercury compounds, toxic effects occur. Serious toxic effects include neurotoxicity and nephrotoxicity. These toxic effects can impact organisms from birds to mammals, including humans.

At very high levels of methylmercury contamination, such as was observed in Minamata Bay, Japan, in the 1950s, serious health effects occur.[103] Recently, scientists have been exploring the effects of chronic low doses of methylmercury, particularly for higher risk populations including children, fetuses, and women of child-bearing age. Mercury can create and propagate chemical sensitivity. Developing damaged fetuses may be at greater risk because of methylmercury's ability to pass through the placenta.

Several cohort studies have been conducted on children who were exposed to methylmercury before and after birth in the Seychelles Islands and in the Faroe Islands. No neurodevelopmental deficits were identified in the Seychelles Islands children, while some neuropsychological effects were identified in the Faroe Islands children. Notable differences exist between the two populations that may explain the differing results, including diet (ocean fish in the Seychelles versus the higher levels of methylmercury in pilot whale meat in the Faroe Islands).[104] The studies also raise questions concerning the complicating factor of selenium, its interaction with mercury, and subsequent health effects.[105,106] Selenium, which is found in some ocean fish, provides a substitute for sulfur that permits a weaker bond with mercury, allowing the human body to remove mercury more easily and excrete mercury in greater quantities, reducing both the exposure period and the dose.[107] No comparable studies to these international efforts have been undertaken in the Great Lakes area. However, recent work intended to investigate the effects of PCB levels on the development of children whose mothers consumed large amounts of fish during pregnancy in the Oswego, New York, area, have also raised questions concerning effects of mercury.[107]

Studies reviewed by the U.S. National Academy of Sciences associate chronic low-dose prenatal methylmercury exposure with poor performance by children on neurobehavioral tests that measure such things as attention, language, ability, fine motor skills, and intelligence.[108] Further research is required to investigate methylmercury exposure and coronary disease.

Eating fish offers many nutritional benefits, including protein and omega-3 polyunsaturated fatty acids. However, caution must be exercised to avoid eating too much fish containing excessive levels of methylmercury or other persistent toxic substances. The primary human exposure to methylmercury is through fish consumption.

Complications of Chemical Mixtures

Fish advisories are often concerned with mercury and PCBs for the same species in the same water bodies. PCBs affect the thyroid which controls brain development.[109] Mercury binds to brain tissue and may cause other problems. Both PCBs and mercury can pass throughout the placenta.[109] Therefore, their combination may pose a greater risk to a developing fetus than either alone.

The U.S. Environmental Protection Agency cites rough estimates showing that 20% of global mercury emissions are from natural emissions, 40% from global recycling of previous anthropogenic activity, and 0% from current anthropogenic emissions.[110] As shown in Table 3.15, North America contributed approximately 11% of the total global anthropogenic mercury emissions in 1995.

With their later industrialization, mercury emissions are now increasing in developing countries. Preliminary findings from the U.S. Environmental Protection Agency and Environment Canada indicate that the increases in global anthropogenic mercury emissions reaching North America, largely from Asia, offset anthropogenic mercury reductions achieved within the United States and Canada. With respect to Lake Superior, the lake most remote from regional industrial sources, the majority of specific sources of mercury deposition were located at a distance greater than 700 kilometers away. Although global emissions are largely of the unreactive form, the sheer volume and increasing proportion of the global mercury balance warrants attention.

In the United States, significant mercury reductions came principally from emission controls on municipal and medical waste incinerators, as well as improved screening and removal from the waste stream of commercial products such as batteries and paint. In Canada, significant reductions were achieved largely through controls and process alterations in the metal smelting industry, the near complete closure of the chlor-alkali industry, and further control and restrictions on waste

TABLE 3.15

Global Emissions of Total Mercury from Major Anthropogenic Sources in the Year 1995

Continent	Stationary Combustion	Nonferrous Metal Production	Pig Iron and Steel Production	Cement Production	Waste Disposal	Total	%
Europe	185.5 (204)	15.4 (17)	10.2 (11)	26.2 (29)	12.4 (14)	249.7 (275)	13.1
Africa	197 (217)	7.9 (9)	0.5 (0.6)	5.2 (6)		210.6 (232)	11
Asia	860.4 (948)	87.4 (96)	12.1 (13)	81.8 (90)	332.6 (36)	1074.3 (1184)	56.1
North America	104.8 (116)	25.1 (28)	4.6 (5)	12.9 (13)	66.1 (73)	213.5 (235)	11.2
South America	26.9 (30)	25.4 (28)	1.4 (2)	5.5 (6)		59.2 (65)	3.1
Australia and Oceania	99.9 (110)	4.4 (5)	0.3 (0.3)	0.8 (0.9)	0. 1 (0.1)	105.5 (116)	5.5
Total Year 1995	1474.5 (1625)	165.6 (183)	29.1 (32)	132.4 (146)	111.2 (123)	1912.8 (2108)	
Total Year 1990[a]	1295.1 (1428)	394.4 (435)	28.4 (31)	114.5 (126)	139 (153)	2143.1[b] (2362)	

Source: E. G. Pacyna and J. M. Pacyna. 1995. 12th Biennal Report on Great Lakes Water Quality.

[a] Estimates of maximum values, which are regarded as close to the best estimate value.

[b] The total emission estimates for the year 1990 include also 171.1 tons (189 tons) of mercury emission from chlor-alkali production and other less significant sources.

incineration. In 1999, U.S. mercury emissions were estimated at approximately 174 tons; further detail verification of these data now indicate total 1999 emissions were 116 tons. Canadian mercury emissions were approximately 12.1 tons. Coal-fired utilities account for approximately 35% and 2% of mercury emissions in the U.S. and Canada, respectively.

CHEMICAL CONTAMINANTS

The tests done by Common Ground in June 2006 for 170 chemical contaminants did not detect pesticides, polycyclic aromatic hydrocarbons, or most chemical contaminants at quantifiable concentrations. Trihalomethanes (THMs) were the only contaminants that were detected in all five samples, and the concentrations were well below regulatory limits, averaging about 25 micrograms per liter (µg/L) of total THMs in comparison with the EPA regulatory limit of 80 µg/L. The other contaminants found at quantifiable concentrations included barium, selenium, total phenols, and lead. The concentrations of barium and selenium were far below regulatory limits. Phenols were detected in three out of five samples, but there is no regulatory limit with which to compare them. However, they are well-known toxics to the chemically sensitive patients. Lead was detected in one sample at 14.3 µg/L, which is above the guideline level of zero. Lead is a contaminant that can leach from old drinking water pipes and especially from old household plumbing. A number of contaminants were detected at trace levels in one or more samples. However, the levels were so low that the laboratory was unable to quantify the concentration in the water. These included acetone, benzadine, chloromethane, xylene, nitrophenol, 4,4′-DDE, arsenic, methoxychlor, delta BHC, and heptachlor. Table 3.6 summarizes the quantifiable results from the June 2006 independent sampling. However, breath and blood analysis do show some of them in the chemically sensitive patients.

SHIPWRECKS HAVE BEEN KNOWN TO CONTAMINATE WATERS AS THEY HAVE IN THE GREAT LAKES AND OCEANS AROUND THE WORLD

The SS Edmund Fitzgerald, a 729 foot freighter, was the largest ship on the Great Lakes. Launched in June 1958, it transported iron ore from mines near Duluth, Minnesota to the major iron works around Lake Superior. Over time, the ship had become popular due to its size, record breaking performance, and captain who was known for blaring music over the ship's intercom system while passing through the St. Clair and Detroit Rivers. On November 9, 1975 the ship departed for Detroit loaded with more than 26,000 tons of iron. The Edmund Fitgerald ran into a storm early the next morning, and by mid-afternoon reported encountering 25-foot waves with 50-knot winds. In mid-afternoon, the ship radioed that it was taking on water.

The SS Edmund Fitzgerald sank minutes later in Canadian waters 17 miles Northwest of Whitefish Bay, Michigan.

Top 10 Shipwrecks and Maritime Disasters in U.S. History

(1) USS Arizona, (2) SS Sultana, (3) PS General Slocum, (4) SS Eastland, (5) Texas City Disaster, (6) SS Central, (7) USS Tresher, America, (8) Andrea Doria, (9) SS Edmund Fitzgerald, and (10) Exxon Valdez.

Operation Chase Munitions

Operation Chase (Cut Holes and Sink 'Em) was a United States Department of Defense program that involved the disposal of unwanted munitions at sea from May 1964 into the early 1970s.[111,112]

The disposal program involved loading old munitions onto ships which were then slated to be scuttled once they were up to 250 miles off shore.[113,114] While most of the sinkings involved ships loaded with conventional weapons, there were four which involved chemical weapons.[113] The chemical weapons disposal site was a three mile (5 km) area of the Atlantic Ocean between the coast of the U.S. state of Florida and the Bahamas.[115] The CHASE program was predated by the United States Army disposal of 8000 tons of mustard and lewisite chemical warfare gas aboard the scuttled SS William C. Ralston in April 1958.[111,116] These ships were sunk by having Explosive Ordnance Demolition (EOD) teams open seacocks on the ship after arrival at the disposal point.[111] The typical Liberty ship sank about three hours after the seacocks were opened.[111]

Operations: CHASE 1–12

CHASE 1: The mothballed C-3 Liberty ship John F. Shafroth was taken from the National Defense Reserve Fleet at Suisun Bay and towed to the Concord Naval weapons Station for stripping and loading.[111] A major fraction of the munitions in CHASE 1 was Bofors 40 mm gun ammunition from the Naval Ammunition Depot at Hastings, Nebraska.[111] CHASE 1 also included bombs, torpedo warheads, naval mines, cartridges, projectiles, fuzes, detonators, boosters, overage UGM-27 Polaris motors, and a quantity of contaminated cake mix that an army court had ordered dumped at sea.[111] Shafroth was sunk 47 miles off San Francisco on July 23, 1964 with 9799 tons of munitions.[111]

CHASE 2: Village was loaded with 7348 short tons of munitions at the Naval weapons Station Earle and towed to a deep-water dump site on September 17, 1964.[111] There were three large and unexpected detonations five minutes after Village slipped beneath the surface.[111] An oil slick and some debris appeared on the surface.[111]

CHASE 3: Coastal Mariner was loaded with 4040 short tons of munitions at the Naval weapons Station Earle.[111] The munitions included 512 tons of actual explosives.[111] Four SOFAR bombs were packed in the explosives cargo hold with booster charges of 500 pounds of TNT to detonate the cargo at a depth of 1000 feet (300 meters). The detonation created a 600-foot (200 meter) water spout, but was not deep enough to be recorded on seismic instruments.[111]

CHASE 4: Santiago Iglesias was loaded with 8715 tons of munitions at the Naval weapons Station Earle, rigged for detonation at 1000 feet (300 meters), and detonated 31 seconds after sinking on *September 16, 1965.*[111]

CHASE 5: Isaac Van Zandt was loaded with 8000 tons of munitions (including 400 tons of high explosives) at the Naval Base Kitsap and rigged for detonation at 4000 feet (1.2 kilometers).[111]

CHASE 6: Horace Greeley was loaded at the Naval weapons Station Earle, rigged for detonation at 4000 feet (1.2 kilometers), and detonated on July 28, 1966.[111]

CHASE 7: Michael J. Monahan was loaded with overage UGM-27 Polaris motors at the Naval Weapons Station Charleston and sunk without detonation on April 30, 1967.[111]

CHASE 8: The first chemical weapons disposal via the program was in 1967 . Chase 8 disposed of mustard gas and GB-filled M-55 rockets.

CHASE 9: Eric C. Gibson was sunk on June 15, 1967.[111]

CHASE 10: CHASE 10 dumped 3000 tons of United States Army nerve agent filled rockets encased in concrete vaults.[113]

CHASE 11: It occurred in June 1968 and disposed of United States Army GB and VX, all sealed in tin containers.

CHASE 12: In August 1968, again disposed of United States Army mustard agent, and was numerically (although not chronologically) the final mission to dispose of chemical weapons.

TOXIC DISCHARGE US 2010 (TABLE 3.16)

MISSISSIPPI RIVER (TABLE 3.17)

Accidents Releasing Toxics into U.S. Water

Three Mile Island Accident—1979 Release of 40,000 gallons of radioactive waste and iodine directly in the Susquehanna river, Pennsylvania. The three mile island accident was a partial nuclear meltdown which occurred in one of the two United States nuclear reactors on March 28, 1979.

Love Canal disaster—1970 21.00 tons of toxic waste by on Niagara river and Lake Ontario.

Love Canal was a neighborhood in Niagara Falls, New York, located in the LaSalle section of the city. Love Canal had formerly been used to bury 21,000 tons of toxic waste by Hooker Chemical (now Occidental Petroleum Corporation).

Cuyahoga River, Ohio, USA is known as the river which caught fire in 1952. The Cuyahoga River and its tributaries drain 813 square miles (2110 km²) of land in portions of six counties. At its terminus into Lake Erie was multiple factories that dumped all their waste into the river.

The BP Deep water horizon (BP) oil spill 2013 (also referred to as the BP oil Spill) in the Gulf of Mexico is considered the largest accidental marine oil spill in the history of the petroleum industry. The oil spill was a direct result of the explosion and sinking of the deepwater horizon oil rig which claimed 11 lives. The total oil wasted is estimated at 4.9 million barrels.

TABLE 3.16

Top 10 Waterways for Total Toxic Discharges

Waterway	Toxic Discharges (lb)
Ohio River (IL, IN, KY, OH, PA, WV)	32,111,718
Mississippi River (AR, IA, IL, KY, LA, MN, MO, MS, N, WI)	12,739,749
New River (NC, VA)	12,529, 948
Savannah River (GA, SC)	9,624,090
Delaware River (DE, NJ, PA)	6,719,436
Muskingum River (OH)	5,754,118
Missouri River (IA, KA, MO, ND, NE)	4,887,971
Shonka Ditch (N)	4,614,722
Tricounty Canal (NE)	3,386,162
Rock River (IL,WI)	3,370,39

Source: America's Top 10 Most-Polluted Waterways. 2012. http://www.motherjones.com/ blue-marble/2012/03/top-10-polluted-rivers-waterways

---

TABLE 3.17

Organic Compounds Measured to Evaluate Wastewater Contamination of the Mississippi River, 1987–1992

Contaminant	Abbreviation	Compounds and Sources
Dissolved Organic carbon	DOC	All natural and synthetic organic compounds; regional-scale natural sources.
Fecal coliform bacteria	None	Bacteria derived predominantly from human and livestock fecal wastes; from unchlorinated sewage effluents and feedlot and agricultural runoff.
Methylene blue-active substances	MBAS	Composite measure of synthetic and natural anionic surfactants; predominantly from municipal sewage-wastewater discharges.
Linear alkylbenzenesulfonate	LAS	Complex mixture of specific anionic surfactant compounds used in soap and detergent products; primary source is domestic sewage effluent.
Nonionic surfactants	NP,PEG	Complex mixture of compounds derived from nonionic surfactants that includes nonylphenol (NP) and polyethylene glycol (PEG) residues; from sewage and industrial sources.
Adsorbable organic halogen	AOX	Adsorbable halogen-containing organic compounds, including by-products from chlorination of DOC and synthetic organic compounds, solvents, and pesticides; from multiple natural and anthropogenic sources.
Fecal sterols	None	Natural biochemical compounds found predominantly in human and livestock wastes; primary source is domestic sewage and feedlot runoff.
Polynuclear aromatic hydrocarbons	PNA	Complex mixture of compounds, many of which are priority pollutants; from multiple sources associated with combustion of fuels.
Caffeine	None	Specific component of beverages, food products, and medications specifically for human consumption; most significant source is domestic sewage effluent.
Ethylenediaminetetraacetic acid	EDTA	Widely used synthetic chemical for complexing metals; from a variety of domestic, industrial, and agricultural sources.
Volatile organic compounds	VOC	A variety of chlorinated solvents and aromatic hydrocarbons; predominantly from industrial and fuel sources.
Semivolatile organic compounds	TTT,THAP	Wide variety of synthetic organic chemicals including priority pollutants and compounds such as trimethyltriazinetrione (TTT) and trihaloalkylphosphates (THAP); predominantly from industrial sources.

Source: http://pubs.usgs.gov/circ/circ1133/

Mayflower was an Exxon Mobil Pipeline Spill Mayflower, AR March 29, 2013.

The Exxon Valdez Oil Spill (1989). On March 24, 1989, from 260,000 to 750,000 barrels of crude oil was spilled in Prince William Sounds, Alaska by the oil tanker after it ran into Bligh Reef. It is considered to be one of the most devastating human caused environmental disasters with both the long-term and short-term effects of the oil spill having been studied. Immediate effects included the deaths of 100,000 to as many as 250,000 seabirds, at least 2800 sea otters, 300 harbor seals, 247 Bald Eagles, and 22 Orcas, and an unknown number of salmon and herring (Table 3.18).

TABLE 3.18

Polycyclic Aromatic Hydrocarbons Average Recoveries (Rec), Standard Deviations (SD) and Limits of Detections (LODs), Calibration Equations and R^2 Values from Sediment and Water Samples

	Sediment			Water				
	Rec (%)	SD	LOD	Rec (%)	SD	LOD		
	(n = 9)		(μg kg^1)	(n = 15)		(μg L^4)	Calibration Curves	R^2
Naphthalene	80	2.7	0.30	70	1.4	0.01	$Y = 0.799X + 0.0620$	0.9992
Acenaphthylene	69	1.6	0.10	73	1.1	0.03	$Y = 0.8371X - 0.1433$	0.9980
Acenaphthene	74	2.2	0.30	78	1.8	0.03	$Y = 1.2966X - 0.2363$	0.9947
Fluorene	62	7.3	0.03	94	0.3	0.06	$Y = 0.0688X + 0.0202$	0.9985
Phenanthrene	78	6.1	0.03	75	0.1	0.06	$Y = 1.736X - 0.0873$	0.9957
Anthracene	75	2.5	0.01	65	0.1	0.03	$Y = 0.9367X - 0.0099$	0.9995
Fluoranthene	71	5.5	0.06	72	0.3	0.06	$Y = 0.2335X + 0.0466$	0.9850
Pyrene	62	5.2	0.40	73	0.1	0.03	$Y = 0.2408X + 0.0256$	0.9975
Chrysene	75	1.2	0.10	92	0.1	0.09	$Y = 0.2225X + 0.0842$	0.9984
Benzo[a]anthracene	81	1.1	0.09	80	0.1	0.06	$Y = 0.098X + 0.0298$	0.9896
Benzo[b]fluoranthene	92	6.2	0.30	74	0.2	0.03	$Y = 0.5688X - 0.0035$	0.9974
Benzo[k]fluoranthene	79	2.2	0.70	88	0.2	0.03	$Y = 0.1249X + 0.086$	0.9983
Benzo[a]pyrene	108	7.4	0.30	74	0.1	0.06	$Y = 0.4222X + 0.0071$	0.9864
Dibenzo[a,h]anthracene	74	7.8	0.03	81	0.1	0.03	$Y = 0.1524X + 0.0363$	0.9979
Benzo[g,h,j]perylene	67	8.1	0.40	71	0.2	0.03	$Y = 0.1413X + 0.0818$	0.9970
Indeno[1,2,3-cd]pyrene	83	3.1	0.50	72	0.2	0.03	$Y = 0.1844X + 0.0443$	0.9790

Source: da Silva, T. F. de Almeida Azevedo, D., de Aquino Neto, F. R. 2007. Distribution of polycyclic aromatic hydrocarbons in surface sediments and waters from Guanabara Bay, Rio de Janeiro, Brazil. *J. Braz. Chem. Soc.* 18 (3): 628–637.

DEAD ZONE

Dead zones are hypoxic (low-oxygen) areas in the world's oceans and large lakes, caused by "excessive nutrient pollution from human activities coupled with other factors that deplete the oxygen required to support most marine life in bottom and near-bottom water. (NOAA)."[117] In the 1970s, oceanographers began noting increased instances of dead zones. These occur near inhabited coastlines, where aquatic life is most concentrated. The vast middle portions of the oceans, which naturally have little life, are not considered "dead zones."

In March 2004, 146 dead zones were reported in the world's oceans where marine life could not be supported due to depleted oxygen levels. Some of these were as small as a square kilometer (0.4 mi^2), but the largest dead zone covered 70,000 square kilometers (27,000 mi^2). A 2008 study counted 405 dead zones worldwide.[118,119]

Aquatic and marine dead zones can be caused by an increase in chemical nutrients (particularly nitrogen and phosphorus) in the water, known as *eutrophication*. These chemicals are the fundamental building blocks of single-celled, plant-like organisms that live in the water column, and whose growth is limited in part by the availability of these materials. Eutrophication can lead to rapid increases in the density of certain types of these phytoplankton, a phenomenon known as an algal bloom.

The fish-killing blooms that devastated the Great Lakes in the 1960s and 1970s have not gone away; they have moved West into an arid world in which people, industry, and agriculture are increasingly taxing the quality of what little freshwater there is to be had here. This is not just a prairie problem. Global expansion of dead zones caused by algal blooms is rising rapidly.[120]

The major groups of algae are Cyanobacteria, Green Algae, Dinoflagellates, Coccolithophores, and Diatom Algae. Increase in input of nitrogen and phosphorus generally causes Cyanobacteria to bloom and this cause the Dead Zones. Cyanobacteria are not good food for zooplankton and fish and hence accumulate in water, die, and then decompose. Other algae are consumed and hence do not accumulate to the same extent as Cyanobacteria.[121] Dead zones can be caused by natural and anthropogenic factors. Use of chemical fertilizers is considered the major human-related cause of dead zones around the world. Natural causes include coastal upwelling and changes in wind and water circulation patterns. Runoff from sewage, urban land use, and fertilizers can also contribute to eutrophication.[122]

Notable dead zones in the United States include the northern Gulf of Mexico region,[123] surrounding the outfall of the Mississippi River, and the coastal regions of the Pacific Northwest, and the Elizabeth River in Virginia Beach, all of which have been shown to be recurring events over the last several years.

In addition, natural oceanographic phenomena can cause deoxygenation of parts of the water column. For example, enclosed bodies of water, such as fjords or the Black Sea, have shallow sills at their entrances, causing water to be stagnant there for a long time. The eastern tropical Pacific Ocean and northern Indian Ocean have lowered oxygen concentrations which are thought to be in regions where there is minimal circulation to replace the oxygen that is consumed (e.g., Pickard and Emery 1982, p 47).[124] These areas are also known as oxygen minimum zones (OMZ). In many cases, OMZs are permanent or semipermanent areas.

Remains of organisms found within sediment layers near the mouth of the Mississippi River indicate four hypoxic events before the advent of artificial fertilizer. In these sediment layers, anoxia-tolerant species are the most prevalent remains found. The periods indicated by the sediment record correspond to historic records of high river flow recorded by instruments at Vicksburg, Mississippi. Changes in ocean circulation triggered by ongoing climate change could also add or magnify other causes of oxygen reductions in the ocean.[125] Low oxygen levels recorded along the Gulf Coast of North America have led to reproductive problems in fish involving decreased size of reproductive organs, low egg counts, and lack of spawning.

In a study by the Southeastern Louisiana University done in three bays along the Gulf Coast, fish living in bays where the oxygen levels in the water dropped to 1 to 2 parts per million (ppm) for three or more hours per day were found to have smaller reproductive organs. The male gonads were 34% to 50% as large as males of similar size in bays where the oxygen levels were normal (6–8 ppm). Females were found to have ovaries that were half as large as those in normal oxygen levels. The number of eggs in females living in hypoxic waters were only one-seventh the number of eggs in fish living in normal oxygen levels.[126] Fish raised in laboratory-created hypoxic conditions showed extremely low sex hormone concentrations and increased elevation of activity in two genes triggered by the hypoxia-inductile factor (HIF) protein. Under hypoxic conditions, HIF pairs with another protein, ARNT. The two then bind to DNA in cells, activating genes in those plant cells.

Under normal oxygen conditions, ARNT combines with estrogen to activate genes. Hypoxic cells *in vitro* did not react to estrogen placed in the tube. HIF appears to render ARNT unavailable to interact with estrogen, providing a mechanism by which hypoxic conditions alter reproduction in fish.[127]

It might be expected that fish would flee this potential suffocation, but they are often quickly rendered unconscious and doomed. Slow-moving bottom-dwelling creatures such as clams, lobsters, and oysters are unable to escape. All colonial animals are extinguished. The normal remineralization and recycling that occurs among benthic life-forms is stifled.

Mora et al.[128] showed that future changes in oxygen could affect most marine ecosystems and have socioeconomic ramifications due to human dependency on marine goods and services.

In the 1970s, marine dead zones were first noted in areas where intensive economic use stimulated "first-world" scientific scrutiny: in the U.S. East Coast's Chesapeake Bay, in Scandinavia's strait called the Kattegat, which is the mouth of the *Baltic Sea*, and in other important Baltic Sea fishing grounds, in the Black Sea, which may, however, have been anoxic in its deepest levels for millennia, and in the northern Adriatic.

Other marine dead zones have appeared in coastal waters of South America, China, Japan, and New Zealand. A 2008 study counted 405 dead zones worldwide.[118,119,129]

LAKE ERIE

A dead zone exists in the central part of Lake Erie from east of Point Pelee to Long Point and stretches to shores in Canada and the United States. The zone has been noticed since the 1950s to 1960s, but efforts since the 1970s have been made by Canada and the US to reduce runoff pollution into the lake as a means to reverse the dead zone growth. Overall, the lake's oxygen level is poor with only a small area to the east of Long Point that has better levels. The biggest impact of the poor oxygen levels is on marine life and the fisheries industry.

LOWER ST. LAWRENCE ESTUARY

A dead zone exists in the Lower St. Lawrence River area from east of the Saguenay River to east of Baie Comeau, greatest at depths over 275 m (902 ft) and has been noticed since the 1930s.[130] The main concerns for Canadian scientists is the impact on the fish found in the area.

OREGON

Off the coast of Cape Perpetua, Oregon, there is also a dead zone with a 2006 reported size of 300 square miles (780 km^2).[131] This dead zone only exists during the summer, perhaps due to wind patterns.

Gulf of Mexico "Dead Zone"

Currently, the Gulf of Mexico's dead zone, off the coast of Louisiana and Texas,[132] is the largest hypoxic zone in the United States.[133] The Mississippi River, which is the drainage area for 41% of the continental United States, dumps high-nutrient runoff such as nitrogen and phosphorus into the Gulf of Mexico. According to a 2009 fact sheet created by NOAA, "seventy percent of nutrient loads that cause hypoxia are a result of this vast drainage basin,"[134] which includes the heart of U.S. agribusiness, the Midwest. The discharge of treated sewage from urban areas (pop. c 12 million in 2009) combined with agricultural runoff deliver c. 1.7 million tons of potassium and nitrogen into the Gulf of Mexico every year.[133]

The frequency of occurrence of hypoxia in the Gulf of Mexico hypoxic zone was mapped annually every summer from 1985 through 1999. The size varies annually from a record high in 2002 when it encompassed more than 21,756 sq kilometers (8400 square miles) to a record low in 1988 of 39 sq kilometers (15 square miles).[132] In 2010, it was the size of New Jersey.[135] Rabalais of the Louisiana Universities Marine Consortium in Cocodrie predicted that the dead zone or hypoxic zone in 2012 will cover an area of 17,353 sq kilometers (6700 square miles), which is larger than Connecticut. In 2011, it was approximately 17,521 sq kilometers (6765 square miles).[123]

In the late summer of 1988, the dead zone disappeared as the great drought caused the flow of Mississippi to fall to its lowest level since 1933. During times of heavy flooding in the Mississippi River Basin, as in 1993, "the 'dead zone' dramatically increased in size, approximately 5000 km (3107 mi) larger than the previous year."[136]

On average, the dead zone doubled in size since the late 1980s. "Hypoxia in bottom waters covered an average of 8000–9000 km^2 in 1985–92, but it increased to 16,000–20,000 km^2 in 1993–99."[137] In March 1998, the National Science and Technology Council's Committee on Environment and Natural Resources and The Mississippi River/Gulf of Mexico (MR/GM) Watershed Nutrient Task Force developed and approved an assessment plan calling for six teams of experts from inside and outside of government to perform in-depth studies examining the issue of hypoxia and the watershed–Gulf system including oceanographic, hydrologic, agricultural, and economic factors.[138]

There is some concern that the Deepwater Horizon oil spill from April to July 2010 may have significantly affected the dead zone. However, Hazen, a microbial ecologist with the Lawrence Berkeley National Laboratory, has suggested that the oil released from the spill did not travel far enough West in appreciable quantities to affect the current size of the dead zone.

History of Gulf of Mexico "Dead Zone"

Shrimp trawlers first reported a "dead zone" in the Gulf of Mexico in 1950, but it was not until 1970, when the size of the hypoxic zone had increased, that people began to investigate.[139]

The conversion of forests and wetlands for agricultural and urban developments accelerated after 1950. "Missouri River Basin has had hundreds of thousands of acres of forests and wetlands (66,000,000 acres) replaced with agriculture activity [...] In the Lower Mississippi one third of the valley's forests were converted to agriculture between 1950 and 1976."[139]

A dead zone off the coast of Texas, where the Brazos River empties into the Gulf, was also discovered in July 2007.[140]

Dead zones are reversible. The Black Sea dead zone, previously the largest in the world, largely disappeared between 1991 and 2001 after fertilizers became too costly to use following the collapse of the Soviet Union and the demise of centrally planned economies in Eastern and Central Europe. Fishing has again become a major economic activity in the region.[141]

While the Black Sea "cleanup" was largely unintentional and involved a drop in hard-to-control fertilizer usage, the U.N. has advocated other cleanups by reducing large industrial emissions.[141] From 1985 to 2000, the North Sea dead zone had nitrogen reduced by 37% when policy efforts by countries on the Rhine River reduced sewage and industrial emissions of nitrogen into the water. Other cleanups have taken place along the Hudson River[142] and San Francisco Bay.[118] The chemical aluminum sulfate can be used to reduce phosphates in water (Figures 3.7 and 3.8).[143]

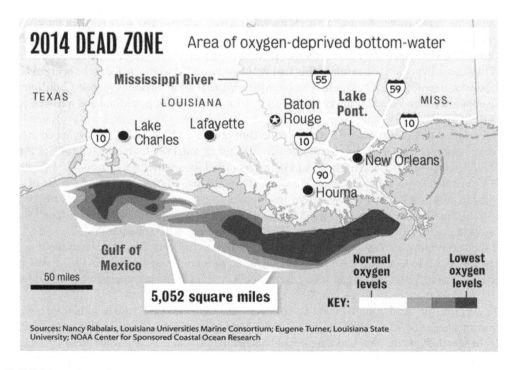

FIGURE 3.7   Area of oxygen-deprived bottom-water.

DEAD ZONES THROUGH THE YEARS

This year's area of oxygen-deprived bottom-water smaller than 2013

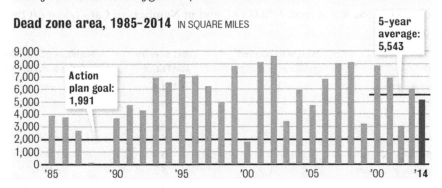

Dead zone area, 1985–2014 IN SQUARE MILES

5-year average: 5,543

Action plan goal: 1,991

FIGURE 3.8 EPA data of dead area in the Gulf of Mexico (2014).

CHEMICALS FROM SPRAWL AND URBAN AREAS: RECYCLING

In a national assessment of tap water quality, the Environmental Working Group (EWG's) analysis of water suppliers' tap water test results shows that water contaminated with 59 pollutants linked to sprawl and urban areas, including plasticizers, solvents, and propellants, are served to 202,697,000 people in 42 states.[144] Fifty-three percent of those people were served water with one or more of these contaminants present at levels above nonenforceable, health-based limits. Forty-one of the urban and sprawl chemicals detected in tap water are unregulated, without a legal, health-based limit in tap water.[144] This fact can make the water more toxic for the public. The chemically sensitive cannot drink this water.

The same drainage-basin waste activities that pollute surface water pollute groundwater, including landfills, agriculture, septic tanks, and industrial wastes.

One solution to the problem of microbial contamination of drinking water has been the chlorination of water. This kind of "purification," which is really a misnomer for microbial decontamination, has resulted in an even greater long-term problem when combined with organic matter.

The U.S. Environmental Protection Agency (EPA) has collected and reported data on the generation and disposal of waste in the United States for more than 30 years. They use this information to measure the success of waste reduction and recycling programs across the country. These facts and figures are current through calendar year 2011.[145]

In 2011, Americans generated about 250 million tons of trash and recycled and composted almost 87 million tons of this material, equivalent to a 34.7% recycling rate. On average, they recycled and composted 1.53 pounds out of our individual waste generation of 4.40 pounds per person per day.[145]

Trash, or municipal solid waste (MSW), is made up of the things commonly used and then thrown away. These materials include items such as packaging, food waste, grass clippings, sofas, computers, tires, and refrigerators. MSW does not include industrial, hazardous, or construction waste.

In 2011, Americans recovered over 66 million tons of MSW (excluding composting) through recycling. Composting recovered over 20 million tons of waste. They combusted about 29 million tons for energy recovery (approximately 12%). Subtracting out what was recycled and composted, was combusted (with energy recovery) or discarded amounted to 2.9 pounds per person per day.

In 2011, newspaper/mechanical papers recovery was about 73% (6.6 million tons), and over 57% of yard trimmings were recovered (Figure 3.3). Metals were recycled at a rate of approximately 34%. By recycling, instead of landfilling and combustion, about 7.5 million tons of metals (which includes aluminum, steel, and mixed metals), they eliminated greenhouse gas (GHG) emissions

TABLE 3.19

Greenhouse Gas Benefits Associated with Recovery of Specific Materials, 2011[a]
(In Millions of Tons Recovered, MMTCO$_2$E and in Numbers of Cars Taken off the
Road per Year)[b]

Material	Weight Recovered (millions of tons)	GHG Benefits MMTCO$_2$E	Numbers of Cars Taken off the Road per Year
Paper and paperboard	45.9	134.5	28 million
Glass	3.17	1	210 thousand
Metals			
Steel	5.45	9	1.9 million
Aluminum	0.72	6.4	1.3 million
Other nonferrous metals[c]	1.34	5.2	1 million
Total metals	7.51	20.6	4.2 million
Plastics	2.65	3.1	640 thousand
Rubber and leather[d]	1.31	0.6	130 thousand
Textiles	2	5.1	1 million
Wood	2.38	4.2	1 million
Other Wastes			
Food, other[e]	1.40	1.1	230 thousand
Yard trimmings	19.3	0.8	170 thousand

Source: WARM model (www.epa.gov/warm, www.epa.gov/epawaste/nonhaz/municipal/msw99.htm, www.epa.
            gov/recycle).

[a]   Includes materials from residential, commercial, and institutional sources.
[b]   These calculations do not include an additional 1.28 million tons of MSW recovered that could not be addressed
      in the WARM model. MMTCO$_2$E is a million metric tons of the carbon dioxide equivalent.
[c]   Includes lead from lead-acid batteries. Other nonferrous metals calculated in WARM as mixed metals.
[d]   Recovery only includes rubber from tires.
[e]   Includes recovery of other MSW organics for composting.

totaling more than 20 million metric tons of carbon dioxide equivalent (MMTCO2E). This is equivalent to removing more than 4 million cars from the road for one year. Approximately 134 million
tons of MSW (53.6%) were discarded in landfills in 2011.

Over the past few decades, the generation, recycling, composting, and disposal of MSW have
changed substantially. Solid waste generation per person per day peaked in 2000 while the 4.40
pounds per person per day is the lowest since the 1980s. The recycling rate has increased from
less than 10% of MSW generated in 1980 to over 34% in 2011. Disposal of waste to a landfill has
decreased from 89% of the amount generated in 1980 to under 54% of MSW in 2011 (Tables 3.19
through 21).

WATER TREATMENT

Material chlorination creates trichlormethanes and other toxic by-products (Table 3.20).

Speciation of trihalomethane mixtures for the Mississippi, Missouri, and Ohio Rivers (Table 3.22).

Trihalomethane formation potentials were determined for the chlorination of water samples
from the Mississippi, Missouri, and Ohio Rivers. Samples were collected during the summer and
fall of 1991 and the spring of 1992 at 12 locations on the Mississippi from New Orleans, LA to
Minneapolis, MN and on the Missouri and Ohio 1.6 km upstream from their confluences with the

TABLE 3.20

Generation, Recovery, and Discards of Products in MSW, 2011[a] (In Millions of Tons and Percent of Generation of Each Product)

Products	Weight Generated	Weight Recovered	Recovery as Percent of Generation	Weight Discarded
Durable goods				
Steel	14.34	3.88	27.1%	10.46
Aluminum	1.43	Negligible	Negligible	1.43
Other nonferrous metals[b]	1.96	1.34	68.4%	0.62
Glass	2.19	Negligible	Negligible	2.19
Plastics	11.42	0.74	6.5%	10.68
Rubber and leather	6.44	1.31	20.3%	5.13
Wood	6.03	Negligible	Negligible	6.03
Textiles	3.84	0.52	13.5%	3.32
Other materials	1.69	1.28	75.7%	0.41
Total durable goods	**49.34**	**9.07**	**18.4%**	**40.27**
Nondurable goods				
Paper and paperboard	31.99	17.24	53.9%	14.75
Plastics	6.52	0.11	1.7%	6.41
Rubber and leather	1.05	Negligible	Negligible	1.05
Textiles	8.95	1.48	16.5%	7.47
Other materials	3.10	Negligible	Negligible	3.10
Total nondurable goods	**51.61**	**18.83**	**36.5%**	**32.78**
Containers and packaging				
Steel	2.18	1.57	72.0%	0.61
Aluminum	1.85	0.72	38.9%	1.13
Glass	9.28	3.17	34.2%	6.11
Paper and paperboard	38.02	28.66	75.4%	9.36
Plastics	13.90	1.80	12.9%	12.10
Wood	10.00	2.38	23.8%	7.62
Other materials	0.35	Negligible	Negligible	0.35
Total containers and packaging	**75.58**	**38.30**	**50.7%**	**37.28**
Other wastes				
Food, other[c]	36.31	1.40	3.9%	34.91
Yard trimmings	33.71	19.30	57.3%	14.41
Miscellaneous inorganic wastes	3.87	Negligible	Negligible	3.87
Total other wastes	73.89	20.70	28.0%	53.19
Total municipal solid waste	**250.42**	**86.90**	**34.7%**	**163.52**

Details might not add to totals due to rounding

Negligible = less than 5000 tons or 0.05%

[a] Includes waste from residential, commercial, and institutional sources.

[b] Includes lead from lead-acid batteries.

[c] Includes recovery of other MSW organics for composting.

Mississippi. Formation potentials were determined as a function of pH and initial free-chlorine concentration.

Water treatment plants along the East Coast are struggling to recover from Superstorm Sandy, whose torrential rains washed tens of millions of gallons of raw or partially treated sewage into waterways.

The less dramatic but equally urgent story: inside those waterworks, and others across the nation, chlorine, added as a disinfectant to kill disease-causing microorganisms in dirty source water, is

TABLE 3.21

Generation, Materials Recovery, Composting, Combustion with Energy Recovery, and Discards of MSW, 1960 to 2011 (in millions of tons)

Activity	1960	1970	1980	1990	2000	2005	2007	2009	2010	2011
Generation	88.1	121.1	151.6	208.3	243.5	253.7	256.5	244.3	250.5	250.4
Recovery for recycling	5.6	8.0	14.5	29.0	53.0	59.2	63.1	61.6	65.0	66.2
Recovery for composting[a]	Negligible	Negligible	Negligible	4.2	16.5	20.6	21.7	20.8	20.2	20.7
Total materials recovery	5.6	8.0	14.5	33.2	69.5	79.8	84.8	82.4	85.2	86.9
Discards after recovery	82.5	113.1	137.1	175.1	174.0	173.9	171.7	161.9	165.3	163.5
Combustion with energy recovery[b]	0.0	0.4	2.7	29.7	33.7	31.6	32.0	29.0	29.3	29.3
Discards to landfill, other disposal[c]	82.5	112.7	134.4	145.3	140.3	142.3	139.7	132.9	136.0	134.2

Details might not add to totals due to rounding.

[a] Composting of yard trimmings, food waste, and other MSW organic material. Does not include backyard composting.

[b] Includes combustion of MSW in mass burn or refuse-derived fuel form, and combustion with energy recovery of source separated materials in MSW (e.g., wood pallets and tire-derived fuel).

[c] Discards after recovery minus combustion with energy recovery. Discards include combustion without energy recovery.

reacting with rotting organic matter such as sewage, manure from livestock, dead animals, and fallen leaves to form toxic chemicals that are potentially harmful to people.

This unintended side effect of chlorinating water to meet federal drinking water regulations creates a family of chemicals known as trihalomethanes.

The EPA regulates four members of the trihalomethane family, the best known of which is chloroform, once used as an anesthetic. Today, the U.S. government classifies chloroform as a "probable" human carcinogen. Three other regulated trihalomethanes are bromodichloromethane, bromoform, and dibromochloromethane. Hundreds more types of toxic trash are unregulated. Chloroform concentrations decreased with distance downstream and approximately paralleled the decrease in the dissolved organic-carbon concentration. This anesthetic substance will cause brain, liver, and cardiac dysfunction. It is no wonder that many people in our society have brain dysfunction. They observed this brain dysfunction in chemically sensitive and chronic degenerative disease patients, who frequently drink chemicals and brominated and fluorinated water. Bromide concentrations were 3.7–5.7 times higher for the Missouri and 1.4–1.6 times higher for the Ohio than for

TABLE 3.22

Total Trihalomethanes Found as Water Goes Down The Mississippi from the First City to the Last City

Minneapolis	14.5 ppb
East St. Louis	108 ppb
New Orleans	156 ppb

Source: Laseter, J. L. 1985. Personal communication; Rea, W. J. 1992. *Chemical Sensitivity, Vol II: Sources of Total Body Load.* Boca Raton, FL : CRC Press. p. 565 Table 3. Publication 1 CCC Republication Taylor and Francis Group LLC Books. Chemical Sensitivity 1/1/1994 Water Pollution, Chapter 7, pp. 544–556. With permission of Taylor & Francis.

the Mississippi above their confluences, resulting in an overall increase in the bromide concentration with distance downstream. Variations in the concentrations of the brominated trihalomethanes with distance downstream approximately paralleled the variation in the bromide concentration. Concentrations of all four trihalomethanes increased as the pH increased. Concentrations of chloroform and bromodichloromethane increased slightly.

The concentration of bromoform decreased as the initial free-chlorine concentration increased; the chlorodibromomethane concentration had little dependence on the free-chlorine concentration.

Evidence now shows that many forms of ill health, including cancer of the colon, may be related to the chlorination of drinking water.[146] Chlorinated water exacerbates chemical sensitivity and chronic degenerative disease. Chlorinated city water contains from 100 to 10,000 times as many synthetic compounds as natural spring water.[147] Reports reveal that other sources of contamination include drinking water disinfectants and by-products.[148]

The variety of toxic halogenated compounds found before and after water processing is presented in Table 3.18.

Trihalomethanes are Just the Tip of the Iceberg

Studies have shown that there are more than 600 unwanted chemicals created by the interaction of water treatment disinfectants and pollutants in source water.[149] Most of these water treatment contaminants have not been studied in depth. Among them are haloacetonitriles, haloaldehydes, haloketones, halohydroxyfuranones, haloquinones, aldehydes, haloacetamides, halonitriles, halonitromethanes, nitrosamines, organic N-chloramines, iodoacids, ketones, and carboxylic acids.[150–153] Some of these compounds are suspected carcinogens.[147] Notably, some believe that hundreds more water treatment contaminants are present in drinking water but have not yet been identified.[149] Many of these will exacerbate chemical sensitivity.

Besides the four regulated trihalomethanes, the EPA regulates five other contaminants in a family of chemicals known as haloacetic acids—monochloroacetic acid, dichloroacetic acid, trichloroacetic acid, monobromoacetic acid, and dibromoacetic acid.[154] The current EPA legal limit for these five chemicals is 60 parts per billion. Of course, these levels are meaningless except for acute toxicity because they disrupt the function of the chemically sensitive and those with chronic degenerative disease.

While there have been relatively few epidemiological studies on the potential health effects of haloacetic acids, there is evidence suggesting that exposure to these chemicals during the second and third trimesters of pregnancy may be linked to intrauterine growth retardation and low birth weight[153–157] as well as disruption of chemical sensitivity.

Haloacetic acids have been classified by the EPA as possibly carcinogenic to humans because of evidence of carcinogenicity in animals. According to the EPA, long-term consumption of water that contains haloacetic acid concentrations in excess of the legal limit of 60 parts per billion is associated with an increased risk of cancer.[158] A technical bulletin released by the Oregon Department of Human Services in 2004 warned that long-term exposure to haloacetic acids at or above 60 parts per billion may cause injury to the brain, nerves, liver, kidneys, eyes, and reproductive systems. Acetic acid when combined with pine terpenes gives camphor, which can be extremely toxic to the chemically sensitive; add chlorine to it and one can have a brew that will be extremely toxic, yet no one makes a supreme effort to eliminate it at its source.

Some studies point to concerns with specific haloacetic acids. Dibromoacetic acid has been shown to disturb the balance of the intestinal tract and to cause disease, especially in people with weakened immune systems[159] such as the chemically sensitive patient. They often see G.I. dysfunction in chemically sensitive patients who drink public water. This particular haloacetic acid compound is toxic to the sperm of adult rats at concentrations as low as 10 parts per billion. At high doses, it has caused a range of neurological problems in test animals, including awkward gait, tremors, and immovable hind limbs.[160] Two members of the haloacetic acid family—dichloroacetic acid and trichloroacetic acid—have been shown to cause severe skin and eye irritations in humans.

WASTES: MUNICIPAL SOLID WASTE

Landfills are engineered areas where waste is placed into the land. Landfills usually have liner systems and other safeguards to prevent pollution of groundwater. Energy Recovery from Waste is the conversion of nonrecyclable waste materials into usable heat, electricity, or fuel. Combustion MSW is done to reduce the amount of landfill space needed. Transfer Stations are facilities where municipal solid waste is unloaded from collection vehicles and briefly held while it is reloaded onto larger long-distance transport vehicles for shipment to landfills or other treatment or disposal facilities (Figure 3.9).

Source reduction, or waste prevention, is designing products to reduce the amount of waste that will later need to be thrown away and also to make the resulting waste less toxic.

Recycling is the recovery of useful materials, such as paper, glass, plastic, and metals, from the trash to use for making new products, reducing the amount of virgin raw materials needed.

Composting involves collecting organic waste, such as food scraps and yard trimmings, and storing it under conditions designed to help it break down naturally. This resulting compost can then be used as a natural fertilizer.

Currently, in the United States, 33.8% is recovered and recycled or composted, 11.9% is burned at combustion facilities, and the remaining 54.3% is disposed of in landfills.

Recycling and composting prevented 82 million tons of material from being disposed of in 2009, up from 15 million tons in 1980. This prevented the release of approximately 178 million metric tons of carbon dioxide equivalent into the air in 2009, equivalent to taking 33 million cars off the road for a year (Figures 3.10 through 3.12).

Government studies show that each new person joining the ranks of the U.S. population spurs development that consumes an average of just over an acre of countryside for new housing, businesses, and infrastructure.[161,162]

Development degrades water supplies in unexpected ways. When the U.S. Geological Survey set out to study insecticides in U.S. streams and rivers, they found the highest concentrations not only in the heavily sprayed farm belt, but in urban streams and rivers. When homeowners use insecticides, rainwater and groundwater carry those chemicals to local waters. Scientists found more than half of all streams tainted with insecticides that exceeded levels set to protect health and the environment, in 10%–40% of all samples. Ten percent of tested streams contained at least two neurotoxic,

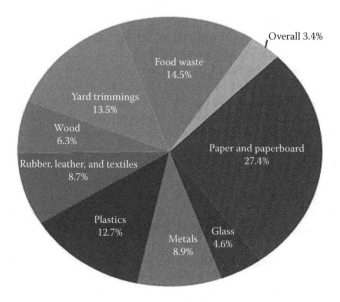

FIGURE 3.9   Total MSW generation (by material), 2009, is 243 million tons (before recycling). (From http://www3.epa.gov/epawaste/nonhaz/municipal/pubs/msw2009-fs.pdf)

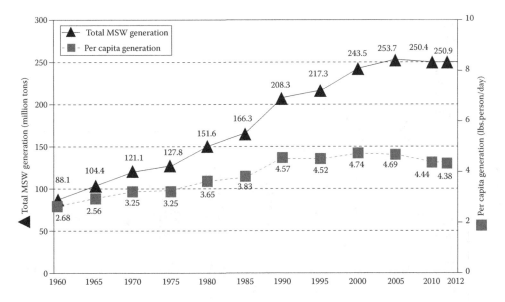

FIGURE 3.10 MSW generation rates, 1960–2009.

organophosphate insecticides in combination with at least four herbicides.[163] Interestingly, recent studies using breath analyses at the EHC- Dallas found somewhat similar ratios.

New studies of urban and sprawl pollutants reveal more than just pesticides, though. USGS scientists have detected 82 pharmaceuticals, hormones, medications, and other residues of consumer products in streams from 30 states.

Synthetic musk fragrances which are used in personal care and cleaning products and pharmaceuticals are among the eight classes of chemicals that are emerging contaminants in the Great Lakes, according to a report from the International Joint Commission. The organization, which oversees issues affecting waters shared by the U.S. and Canada, says an antiepileptic drug, carbamazepine, was the

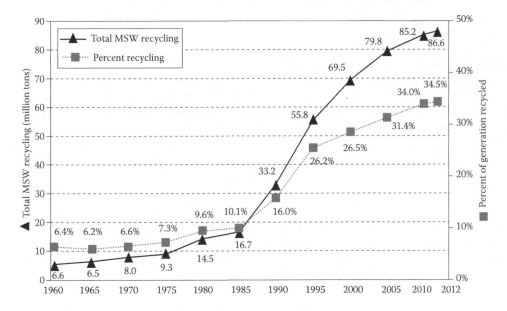

FIGURE 3.11 MSW recycling rates, 1960–2009. (From http://www3.epa.gov/epawaste/nonhaz/municipal/pubs/msw2009-fs.pdf.)

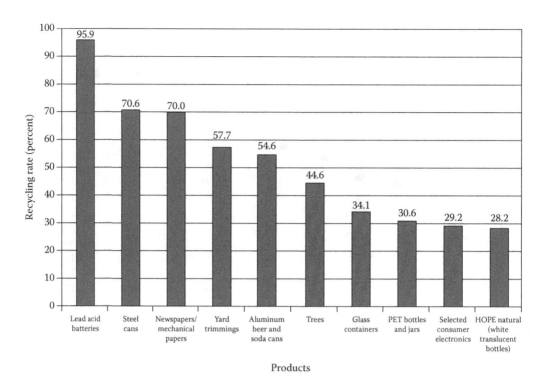

FIGURE 3.12 Recycling rates of selected products, 2009. (From http://www3.epa.gov/epawaste/nonhaz/municipal/pubs/msw2009-fs.pdf.)

pharmaceutical most frequently detected coming into drinking water filtration plants in the Great Lakes region. Pesticides are another category of concern, noting that studies have consistently detected atrazine, metolachlor, and mecoprop in the basin's waterways. Another group of contaminants consists of brominated and chlorinated flame retardants and chlorinated paraffin. The other classes are perfluorinated surfactants, notably perfluorooctane sulfonate and perfluorooctanoic acid; alkylphenolic substances including the surfactants nonylphenol and octylphenol; plasticizers, especially bisphenol A; and polycyclic aromatic hydrocarbons. Eighty percent of streams contained at least one synthetic chemical, and the most contaminated stream contained detectable levels of 38 chemicals. Scientists found the antidepressant Prozac, anti-microbial hand soap and toothpaste chemicals (triclosan and triclocarban); active ingredients in oral contraceptives and thyroid hormone treatments; and hormone-mimicking detergents called alkylphenols.[164] Interestingly, many of these substances are found in the breath of the chemically sensitive patients who never had chemotherapy, including birth control chemicals.

Many of these chemicals are excreted in human urine or are washed down the drain. Many toxics resist standard treatment regimens at wastewater treatment plants causing the public to reject digest them in their drinking water. In a landmark study released in November 2005, it appears that many of these chemicals also resist removal downstream, at tap water treatment plants. In first-time tests in tap water of Organic Wastewater Contaminants, or OWCs, as they are called, USGS scientists found prescription and nonprescription drugs and their metabolites, fragrance compounds, flame retardants and plasticizers, and cosmetic compounds (between 11 and 17 compounds) in each sample. Stackleberg et al.[165] noted deficiencies in current safety standards revealed by their findings (WWN CEN online. Org., September 26, 2011).

The U.S. population is growing at a rate of one person every 10 seconds. If they fail to undertake a national, coordinated initiative to control pollution from growth and sprawl, consumers can expect ever-growing loads of these pollutants in tap water supplies. If they fail to modernize health protections for drinking water exposures, they can expect health risks to increase.

TABLE 3.23

Sprawl and Urban Pollutants in U.S. Drinking Water

Ammonia	Dimethylphthalate
Arsenic	Diethylphthalate
Cadmium	Fluoranthene
Copper	Pyrene
Hydrogen sulfide	di-n-butylphthalate
Lead	Butyl benzylphthalate
Mercury	Benzo[a]anthracene
Nitrate and nitrite mix	Benzo[b]fluoranthene
Nitrate	Benzo[k]fluoranthene
Nitrite	Benzo[a]pyrene
Phosphate	Indeno[1,2,3-cd]pyrene
Antimony	Dibenz[a,h]anthracene
Lithium	Benzo[g,h,i]perylene
Molybdenum	Alpha-lindane
Oil and grease total	Beta-lindane
Phosphorus	Tert-butylbenzene
Lindane	Sec-butylbenzene
Baygon (Propoxur)	Chloropicrin
Paraquat	Trichlorofluoroethane
Glyphosate	Phenols
Trifluralin	Xylenes (total)
Isopropyl alcohol	p-Xylene
Trichlorofluoromethane	o-Xylene
Acetone	m-Xylene
Naphthalene	Tetrachloroethylene
Methyl tertiary butyl ether	Benzene
Fluorine	Bromobenzene
Phenanthrene	n-Propylbenzene
Anthracene	Ethyl-t-butyl ether

Source: Used by permission from *Science Direct*. Human toxicology of chemical mixtures, pp. 100–109. Zeliger, H. I. 2008. ISBN: 978-0-8155-1589-0.

One of the main disasters that have occurred is the Gulf of Mexico oil spill. This spill has contaminated a large area in the eastern Gulf of Mexico. It has contaminated areas from Pensicola, Florida to west of New Orleans. Much sea life and humans have been made ill by the spill. They are just beginning to see the long-term effects relating to the spill with many patients developing chemical sensitivity and chronic degenerative disease (see Chapter 2 for more details).

Another example of water contamination is the marine base at Camp Lejune in eastern North Carolina. This camp suffered decades of contamination on a 156,000 area base. The potable water had tri and tetrachloroethylene, PCB, benzene, and many other volatile organic chemicals. Many marines got sick years later with maliorganics and neurological diseases.

According to Zilger, the U.S. drinking water confirms this contamination (Table 3.23).

AGRICULTURAL WASTES

Agricultural wastes from soil erosion, livestock, and toxic chemicals are significant contributors to water pollution. If these wastes contaminate the water supply of the chemically sensitive person, they can have detrimental effects, including causing easy triggering of symptoms. In farmland, various pollutants run off into the groundwater, resulting in contamination of wells, springs, and surface water. These sources then drain into rivers and lakes, further propagating pollution.

Commercial chicken raising factories use arsenic as growth promoters. Inorganic substances such as arsenic from pesticides used as growth promoters, nitrates from nitrogen fertilizers, and mercury from seed preservation and germination can be found in the groundwater. In one Mexican village, for example, the cause of various forms of arthritis in almost the whole population was high, though sublethal, levels of arsenic that had contaminated the entire village well water supply.[92] Bangladesh has created new wells with natural arsenic in them as previously mentioned in this chapter. This contamination has created a severe health problem.[92] Beef and other animal feed lots will contribute to contamination.

Other sources of agricultural contamination are organic compounds found in agricultural wastes, including animal wastes, pesticides, and herbicides. These include chlorinated, brominated, and phosphate compounds. Some of these toxic chemicals, all of which have at times been found to be detrimental to the chemically sensitive individual, are listed in Table 3.18 (Ref: CS II p.546–547, Table 3.48). Since agricultural wastes from toxic substances are diffuse and therefore difficult to control, their use will have to be stopped in order to prevent further drinking water contamination. It is not improbable that failure to prevent further water contamination could result in a significant lack of available safe bathing and drinking water regardless of the employment of a variety of water depollution methods. In fact, they have seen such an outcome with some severely chemically sensitive patients who live in highly polluted areas.

Agricultural Chemicals in Tap Water

Analysis shows that water contaminated with 83 agricultural pollutants, including pesticides and fertilizer ingredients, are served to 201,955,000 people in 41 states. Fifteen percent of those people were served water with one or more agricultural contaminants present at levels above nonenforceable, health-based limits. Fifty-four of the agricultural chemicals detected in tap water are unregulated, without a legal, health-based limit in tap water.

According to the U.S. Department of Agriculture figures, in 2002 the agriculture industry spread commercial fertilizer over one-eighth of the continental U.S., 110 billion pounds of fertilizer over 248 million acres altogether.[166,167]

Crop production on those lands was supported by pesticide and herbicide applications spread over literally one-tenth of the lower 48 states.[166] Between farmed land tracts are what EPA estimates to be 238,000 concentrated feed lots for cattle and pigs, the equivalent of 75 in every U.S. county, that collectively produce 500 million tons of contaminated manure yearly.[168]

Runoff from these farms and feed lots can be laden with sediment, disease-causing microorganisms, pesticides, growth promoters, and fertilizer ingredients that can widely contaminate water supplies. In fact, in its most recent in a series of mandated biannual investigations on national water quality, EPA found that agricultural pollutants impair nearly one of every five miles of rivers and streams across the country.[167]

In 2009, the Pesticide Data Program (PDP) analyzed 612 drinking water samples, including 306 finished drinking water samples and 306 untreated (raw intake) drinking water samples. PDP detected 53 different residues (including metabolites), representing 42 pesticides, in finished drinking water and 49 different residues (including metabolites), representing 38 pesticides, in the untreated intake water; most of the detections were herbicides.

As one can see, there are some very toxic chemicals which can disturb the chemically sensitive and chronic degenerative disease patients. This is particularly true for the farm states in the Midwest where the state of Iowa is tied for number 1 with the state of New Jersey (manufacturing wastes) for cancer (Table 3.24).

TABLE 3.24
Distribution of Residues by Pesticide in Drinking Water

Pesticide/Commodity	Pest Type	Number of Samples	Samples with Defects	% of Samples with Defects	Range of Values Detected, ppt	Range of LODs, ppt	EPA MCL, ppt[1]	EPA HA[2] ppt[1]	EPA FAO[3], ppt[1]
2,4-D	H								
Water, finished		306	249	81.4	1.1–180	0.65–3.6	70,000		
Water, untreated		305	250	82.0	1.1–690	0.65–3.6			
Acetochlor	H								
Water, finished		306	12	3.9	15.3[a]	9.2–49.5			
Water, untreated		306	34	11.1	15.3–210	9.2–49.5			
Acetochlor thanesulfonic acid	HM								
Water, finished		306	119	38.9	2.7–960	1.6–4.8			
Water, untreated		305	127	41.6	2.7–1000	1.6–4.8			
Acetochlor oxanilic acid (OA)	HM								
Water, finished		306	120	39.2	2.3–1300	1.4–4.8			
Water, untreated		305	128	42.0	2.3–1300	1.4–4.8			
Alachlor	H								
Water, finished		306	2	0.7	13[a]	7.8–9.8	2000		
Water, untreated		306	4	1.3	13–16.3	7.8–9.8			
Alachlor ethanesulfonic acid (ESA)	HM								
Water, finished		306	135	44.1	2.8–110	1.7–4.8			
Water, untreated		305	143	46.9	2.8–110	1.7–4.8			
Alachlor oxanilic acid (OA)	HM								
Water, finished		306	109	35.6	1.0–61	0.61–4.8			
Water, untreated		305	116	38.0	1.0–81	0.61–4.8			
Atrazine	H								
Water, finished		306	269	87.9	1.1–1248	0.66–2.3	3000		
Water, untreated		306	273	89.2	1.1–1832	0.66–2.2			
Bentazon	H								
Water, finished		306	76	24.8	0.30–7.1	0.18–1.2		200,000	
Water, untreated		305	120	39.3	0.30–13	0.18–1.2			

(Continued)

TABLE 3.24 (Continued)
Distribution of Residues by Pesticide in Drinking Water

Pesticide/Commodity	Pest Type	Number of Samples	Samples with Defects	% of Samples with Defects	Range of Values Detected, ppt	Range of LODs, ppt	EPA MCL, ppt[1]	EPA HA[2] ppt[1]	EPA FAO[3], ppt[1]
Bromacil	H							70,000	
Water, finished		306	2	0.7	27–45	2.5–9.6			
Water, untreated		305	22	7.2	4.2–41	2.5–9.6			
Carbaryl	I								
Water, finished		306	2	0.7	20–100	12–23			
Water, untreated		305	2	0.7	38–92	12–23			
Carbendazim (MBC)	F								
Water, finished		119		12.7	3.0–5.2	1.8a			
Water, untreated		118	15			1.8a			
Carbofuran	I								
Water, finished		306	3	1.0	2.0a	0.60–1.0	40,000		
Water, untreated		305	2	0.7	2.0–7.7	0.60–1.0			
Chlorimuron ethyl	H								
Water, finished		298	17	5.7	22–52	8.4–13			
Water, untreated		297	22	7.4	22–57	8.4–13			
Clopyralid	H								
Water, finished		226	27	11.9	5.7–92	3.4–30			
Water, untreated		225	32	14.2	5.7–38	3.4–30			
Desethyl atrazine	HM								
Water, finished		306	234	76.5	0.72–540	0.43–24.8			
Water, untreated		306	245	80.1	0.72–520	0.43–24.8			
Desisopropyl atrazine	HM								
Water, finished		306	164	53.6	5.2–333	3.1–9.8			
Water, untreated		306	182	59.5	5.2–310	3.1–9.8			
Dimethenamid	H								
Water, finished		119	4	3.4	1.0a	0.60a			
Water, untreated		118	18	15.3	1.0–4.2	0.60a			

(Continued)

TABLE 3.24 (Continued)
Distribution of Residues by Pesticide in Drinking Water

Pesticide/Commodity	Pest Type	Number of Samples	Samples with Defects	% of Samples with Defects	Range of Values Detected, ppt	Range of LODs, ppt	EPA MCL, ppt[1]	EPA HA[2] ppt[1]	EPA FAO[3], ppt[1]
Dimethenamid oxanilic acid	HM								
Water, finished		187	23	12.3	1.0–21	0.63[a]			
Water, untreated		187	67	35.8	1.0–61	0.63[a]			
Dimethenamid/Dimethenamid P	H								
Water, finished		187	13	7.0	4.2–17	2.5[a]			
Water, untreated		187	43	23	4.2–510	2.5[a]			
Dimethoate	I								
Water, finished		306	2	0.7	7.5–68	4.5–7.5			
Water, untreated		306				4.5–7.5			
Dinoseb	H								
Water, finished		306	2	0.7	1.0–1.3	0.70–0.78	7000	7000	
Water, untreated		305				0.60–0.78			
Diuron	H								
Water, finished		306	40	13.1	5.8–62	3.5–9.6			
Water, unfinished		305	70	23.0	5.8–309	3.5–9.6			
Fludioxonil	F								
Water, finished		119	1	0.8	62.4[a]	37.5–125			
Water, untreated		119				37.5–125			
Flufenacet oxanilic acid	HM								
Water, finished		187	24	12.8	3.3–7.7	0.75[a]			
Water, untreated		187	24	12.8	2.5–5.7	0.75[a]			
Hydroxy atrazine	HM								
Water, finished		187	139	74.3	2.0–350	1.2[a]			
Water, untreated		187	133	71.1	2.0–360	1.2[a]			
Imazamethabenz methyl	H								
Water, finished		306	2	0.7	19–23	0.31–2.0			
Water, untreated		305				0.31–2.0			

(Continued)

TABLE 3.24 (Continued)
Distribution of Residues by Pesticide in Drinking Water

Pesticide/Commodity	Pest Type	Number of Samples	Samples with Defects	% of Samples with Defects	Range of Values Detected, ppt	Range of LODs, ppt	EPA MCL, ppt[1]	EPA HA[2], ppt[1]	EPA FAO[3], ppt[1]
Imazapic	H								
Water, finished		306	3	1.0	1.5[a]	0.90–2.4			
Water, untreated		305	2	0.7	1.5[a]	0.90–2.4			
Imazapyr	H								
Water, finished		306	108	35.3	1.5–110	0.90–1.0			
Water, untreated		305	102	33.4	1.5–55	0.90–1.0			
Imazaquin	H								
Water, finished		306	2	0.7	1.8[a]	1.1–2.4			
Water, untreated		305	1	0.3	1.8[a]	1.1–2.4			
Imazethapyr	H								
Water, finished		306	18	5.9	2.0–3.9	1.0–2.4			
Water, untreated		305	14	4.6	2.0–5.5	1.0–2.4			
Imidacloprid	I								
Water, finished		306	22	7.2	2.5–21	1.5–6.2			
Water, untreated		305	52	17.0	2.5–29	1.5–6.2			
MCPA	H								
Water, finished		306	47	15.4	1.3–47	0.78–7.2		30,000	
Water, untreated		305	66	21.6	1.3–69	0.78–7.2			
Metalaxyl	F								
Water, finished		306	17	5.6	5.0–11	3.0–22.5			
Water, untreated		306	21	6.9	5.0–37.5	3.0–22.5			
Metolachlor	H								
Water, finished		306	175	57.2	2.5–295	1.5–3.0		700.000	
Water, untreated		306	200	65.4	2.5–603	1.5–3.0			
Metolachlor ethanesulfonic acid	HM								
Water, finished		306	253	82.7	0.60–887	0.36–4.8			
Water, untreated		305	255	83.6	0.60–1023	0.36–4.8			

(Continued)

TABLE 3.24 (Continued)
Distribution of Residues by Pesticide in Drinking Water

Pesticide/Commodity	Pest Type	Number of Samples	Samples with Defects	% of Samples with Defects	Range of Values Detected, ppt	Range of LODs, ppt	EPA MCL, ppt[1]	EPA HA[2] ppt[1]	EPA FAO[3], ppt[1]
Metolachlor oxanilic acid	HM								
Water, finished		306	171	55.9	5.3–394	3.2–4.8			
Water, untreated		305	104	73.6	5.3–370	3.2–4.8			
Metsulfuron methyl	H								
Water, finished		298	2	0.7	2.5[a]	1.5–8.4			
Water, untreated		297	2	0.7	2.5–6.0	1.5–8.4			
Neburon	H								
Water, finished		306	2	0.7	61–100	1.2–9.4			
Water, untreated		305				1.2–9.4			
Nicosulfuron	H								
Water, finished		306	1		11[a]	1.7–4.8			
Water, untreated		305		0.3		1.7–4.8			
Nurflurazon	H								
Water, finished		119	11	9.2	31.3–96	18.8[a]			
Water, untreated		119	11	9.2	321.3–100	18.8[a]			
Omethoate	IM								
Water, finished		187	3	1.6	0.50–3.6	0.30[a]			
Water, untreated		187				0.30[a]			
Picioram	H								
Water, finished		306	5	1.6	37–84	22–30	500,000		
Water, untreated		305	3	1.0	37–89	22–30			
Prometon	H								
Water, finished		306	270	88.2	0.28–19	0.17–1.5		400,000	
Water, untreated		306	275	89.9	0.28–36	0.17–1.5			
Prometryn	H								
Water, finished		306	3	1.0	0.28–76	0.17–24			
Water, untreated		306	21	6.9	0.28–0.98	0.17–24			

(Continued)

TABLE 3.24 (Continued)
Distribution of Residues by Pesticide in Drinking Water

Pesticide/Commodity	Pest Type	Number of Samples	Samples with Defects	% of Samples with Defects	Range of Values Detected, ppt	Range of LODs, ppt	EPA MCL, ppt[1]	EPA HA[2] ppt[1]	EPA FAO[3], ppt[1]
Propanil	H								
Water, finished		306	3	1.0	11.2–170	6.7–24.8			
Water, untreated		306				6.7–24.8			
Propazine	H								
Water, finished		306	44	14.4	5.5–16	3.3–4.5		10,000	
Water, untreated		306	70	22.9	5.5–28	3.3–4.5			
Propiconazole	F								
Water, finished		306	2	0.7	5.7[a]	3.4–6.0			
Water, untreated		305	9	3.0	10[a]	3.4–6.0			
Siduron	H								
Water, finished		306	2	0.7	23–25	2.1–2.4			
Water, untreated		305	2	0.7	4.0[a]	2.1–2.4			
Simazine	H								
Water, finished		306	180	58.8	1.2–484	0.71–3.8	4000		
Water, untreated		306	210	68.6	1.2–1143	0.71–3.8			
Sulfometuron methyl	H								
Water, finished		306	5	1.6	3.2–9.1	1.9–12			
Water, untreated		305	24	7.9	3.2–59	1.9–12			
Tebuconazole	F								
Water, finished		306	2	0.7	150[a]	3.5–4.8			
Water, untreated		305				3.5–4.8			
Tebuthiuron	H								
Water, finished		306	164	53.6	0.35–16	0.21–0.60		500,000	
Water, untreated		305	204	66.9	0.35–16	0.21–0.60			
Tetraconazole	F								
Water, finished		306	1	0.3	3.2[a]	1.8–1.9			
Water, untreated		305				1.8–1.9			

(Continued)

TABLE 3.24 (Continued)
Distribution of Residues by Pesticide in Drinking Water

Pesticide/Commodity	Pest Type	Number of Samples	Samples with Defects	% of Samples with Defects	Range of Values Detected, ppt	Range of LODs, ppt	EPA MCL, ppt[1]	EPA HA[2] ppt[1]	EPA FAO[3], ppt[1]
Thifensulfuron	H								
Water, finished		187	1	0.5	14.8[a]	8.9[a]			
Water, untreated		187				8.9[a]			
Thiobencarb	H								
Water, finished		306	2	0.7	71–190	7.7–18			
Water, untreated		305				7.7–18			
Triasulfuron	H								
Water, finished		187	1	0.5	5.2[a]	3.1[a]			
Water, untreated		187				3.1[a]			
Triclopyr	H								
Water, finished		306	115	37.6	2.7–76	1.6–6.0			
Water, untreated		305	122	40.0	2.7–100	1.6–6.0			

Source: Pesticide Data Control Program. 2009. USDA Agricultural Marketing Service, Washington, DC.

Pesticide Types: F = Fungicide, FM = Fungicide Metabolite, H = Herbicide, HM = Herbicide Metabolite, I = Insecticide, IM = Insecticide Metabolite, P = Plant Growth Regulator.

[a] Only one distinct detected concentration or LOD value was reported for the pair.

Over 140 toxics tested were negative. However, there were more than 50 different pesticides, fungicides, herbicides, and growth promotors found in drinking water. This is a staggering amount. Even if they were not found in many of the final products, they do not know the final effects because they may have been present at below threshold levels. They also could be additive with the chlorine and fluoride levels and have created other toxic substances. Not only are the cancer rates high, but so are the cardiovascular and neurological dysfunctions. They do cause and trigger chemical sensitivity.

AGRICULTURE WASTE

Distribution of Residues by Pesticide in Groundwater

This section shows residue detections for all compounds tested in groundwater, including the range of values detected and range of Limits of Detection (LODs) for each pair in parts per trillion (ppt).

In 2009, the Pesticide Data Program (PDP) analyzed 278 groundwater samples from 278 different collection sites, including 95 from agricultural wells, 113 from school/daycare wells, and 70 from private residential wells. PDP detected 29 different residues (including metabolites), representing 19 pesticides, in the groundwater samples. Most of the detections were for herbicides. The samples with detectable residues came from 152 different sites.

As one can see, there are some extremely high incidence of toxics found in many wells. Ethane sulfonic acids, atrazine, and glyphosate compounds and bromocide were the most common. All these can be detrimental to an individual's health as well as some of the other chemicals that were found.

The incidence of malignancy in the state of Iowa (a farm area) and that of New Jersey (chemical dump area) is tied for number one in the United States.

Iowa is due to farm chemical excess while New Jersey is due to industrial chemical waste (Tables 3.25 and 3.26).

AGRICULTURAL WASTEWATER TREATMENT

Agricultural wastewater treatment relates to the treatment of wastewaters produced in the course of agricultural activities. Nonpoint source pollution from farms is caused by surface runoff from fields during rain storms. Agricultural runoff is a major source of pollution, in some cases the only source, in many watersheds.[170]

Soil washed off fields is the largest source of agricultural pollution in the United States. Excess sediment causes high levels of turbidity in water bodies, which can inhibit growth of aquatic plants, clog fish gills, and smother animal larvae.[170]

Farmers may utilize erosion controls to reduce runoff flows and retain soil on their fields. Common techniques include: contour ploughing,[171] crop mulching,[172] crop rotation, planting perennial crops, and installing riparian buffers.[173]

NUTRIENT RUNOFF

Nitrogen and phosphorus are key pollutants found in runoff, and they are applied to farmland in several ways, such as in the form of commercial fertilizer, animal manure, or municipal or industrial wastewater (effluent) or sludge. These chemicals may also enter runoff from crop residues, irrigation water, wildlife, and atmospheric deposition.[173]

Farmers can develop and implement nutrient management plans to mitigate impacts on water quality by: mapping and documenting fields, crop types, soil types, and water bodies; developing realistic crop yield projections; conducting soil tests and nutrient analyses of manures and/or sludges applied; identifying other significant nutrient sources (e.g., irrigation water); evaluating significant field features such as highly erodible soils, subsurface drains, and shallow aquifers; applying fertilizers, manures, and/or sludges based on realistic yield goals; and using precision agriculture techniques.[173,174]

TABLE 3.25

Distribution of Residues by Pesticide in Groundwater

Pesticide/Commodity/Well Type	Pest Type	Number of Samples	Samples with Detections	% of Samples with Detections	Range of Values Detected, ppt	Range of LODs, ppt
2,4-D	H					
Groundwater—agricultural/farm wells		95	2	2.9	4.2[a]	2.5[a]
Groundwater—private residence wells		70	6	5.3	4.2–24.9	2.5[a]
Groundwater—school/daycare wells		113				2.5[a]
Acetochlor ethanesulfonic acid (ESA)	HM					
Groundwater—agricultural/farm wells		95	4	4.2	15–57.3	9.0[a]
Groundwater—private residence wells		70	30	42.9	15–600	9.0[a]
Groundwater—school/daycare wells		113	4	3.5	15–91.2	9.0[a]
Acetochlor oxanilic acid (OA)	HM					
Groundwater—agricultural/farm wells		95	6	8.6	17–63.9	10[a]
Groundwater—private residence wells		70	2	1.8	17–46	10[a]
Groundwater—school/daycare wells		113				10[a]
Alachlor	H					
Groundwater—agricultural/farm wells		95	1	1.1	17[a]	10[a]
Groundwater—private residence wells		70				10[a]
Groundwater—school/daycare wells		113				10[a]
Alachlor ethanesulfonic acid (ESA)	HM					
Groundwater—agricultural/farm wells		95	21	22.1	20.8–3920	12.5[a]
Groundwater—private residence wells		70	52	74.3	20.8–2630	12.5[a]
Groundwater—school/daycare wells		113	18	15.9	20.8–294	12.5[a]
Alachlor oxanilic acid	HM					
Groundwater—agricultural/farm wells		95	18	18.9	17–3900	10[a]
Groundwater—private residence wells		70	15	21.4	17–2160	10[a]
Groundwater—school/daycare wells		113	3	2.7	17–80.3	10[a]
Atrazine	H					
Groundwater—agricultural/farm wells		95	32	45.7	17–172	10[a]
Groundwater—private residence wells		70	3	2.7	17–231	10[a]
Groundwater—school/daycare wells		113				10[a]
Bentazon	H					
Groundwater—agricultural/farm wells		6	6	100	0.30–19.3	0.30[a]
Groundwater—private residence wells		2	2	100	0.53–2.2	0.30[a]
Bromacil	H					
Groundwater—agricultural/farm wells		95	19	20.0	6.2–21800	6.0[a]
Groundwater –private residence wells		70	2	2.9	10–50.2	6.0[a]
Groundwater—school/daycare wells		113				6.0[a]
Chlorimuron ethyl	H					
Groundwater—agricultural/farm wells		95	1	1.4	10[a]	6.0[a]
Groundwater—private residence wells		70				6.0[a]
Groundwater—school/daycare wells		113				6.0[a]
Cloyralid	H					
Groundwater—agricultural/farm wells		95	1	1.4	20.8[a]	12.5[a]
Groundwater—private residence wells		70				12.5[a]
Groundwater—school/daycare wells		113				12.5[a]

(Continued)

TABLE 3.25 (*Continued*)

Distribution of Residues by Pesticide in Groundwater

Pesticide/Commodity/Well Type	Pest Type	Number of Samples	Samples with Detections	% of Samples with Detections	Range of Values Detected, ppt	Range of LODs, ppt
Desethyl atrazine	HM					
Groundwater—agricultural/farm wells		95	41	58.6	17–1070	10[a]
Groundwater—private residence wells		70	9	8.0	17–767	10[a]
Groundwater—school/daycare wells		113				10[a]
Desethyl-desisopropyl atrazine	HM					
Groundwater—agricultural/farm wells		95	2	2.1	25[a]	15[a]
Groundwater—private residence wells		70	36	51.4	25–990	15[a]
Groundwater—school/daycare wells		113	2	1.8	25–334	15[a]
Desisopropyl atrazine	HM					
Groundwater—agricultural/farm wells		95	19	27.1	83–202	50[a]
Groundwater—private residence work		70	1	0.9	83[a]	50[a]
Groundwater—school/daycare wells		113				50[a]
Dimethenamid ethanesulfonic acid (ESA)	HM					
Groundwater—agricultural/farm wells		95	6	8.6	3.0–80.3	2.0[a]
Groundwater—private residence wells		70				2.0[a]
Groundwater—school/daycare wells		113				2.0[a]
Dimethenamid oxanilic acid (OA)	HM					
Groundwater—agricultural/farm wells		95	2	2.9	5.0–15.4	3.0[a]
Groundwater—private residence wells		70				3.0[a]
Groundwater—school/daycare wells		113				3.0[a]
Diuron	H					
Groundwater—agricultural/farm wells		95	4	4.2	7.0–26.3	4.0[a]
Groundwater—private residence wells		70	1	1.4	89.1[a]	4.0[a]
Groundwater—school/daycare wells		113	2	1.8	7.0	4.0[a]
Hydroxy atrazine	HM					
Groundwater—agricultural/farm wells		95	2	2.1	3.0[a]	2.0[a]
Groundwater—private residence wells		70	41	58.6	3.0–50.8	2.0[a]
Groundwater—school/daycare wells		113	2	1.8	19.4–35.4	2.0[a]
Imazapic	H					
Groundwater—agricultural/farm wells		95	1	1.1	5.0[a]	3.0[a]
Groundwater—private residence wells		70				3.0[a]
Groundwater—school/daycare wells		113				3.0[a]
Imazapyr	H					
Groundwater—agricultural/farm wells		95	5	5.3	14.8–414	2.5[a]
Groundwater—private residence wells		70	1	0.9	8.4[a]	2.5[a]
Groundwater—school/daycare wells		113				2.5[a]
Imazaquin	H					
Groundwater—agricultural/farm wells		95	1	1.4	8.0[a]	5.0[a]
Groundwater—private residence wells		70				5.0[a]
Groundwater—school/daycare wells		113				5.0[a]
Imazethapyr	H					
Groundwater—agricultural/farm wells		95	3	4.3	3.0[a]	2.0[a]
Groundwater—private residence wells		70				2.0[a]
Groundwater—school/daycare wells		113				2.0[a]

(*Continued*)

TABLE 3.25 (*Continued*)

Distribution of Residues by Pesticide in Groundwater

Pesticide/Commodity/Well Type	Pest Type	Number of Samples	Samples with Detections	% of Samples with Detections	Range of Values Detected, ppt	Range of LODs, ppt
Metalaxyl	F					
Groundwater—agricultural/farm wells		95	24	25.3	4.2–955	2.5[a]
Groundwater—private/residence wells		70	1	1.4	4.2[a]	2.5[a]
Groundwater—school/daycare wells		113				2.5[a]
Metolachlor	H					
Groundwater—agricultural/farm wells		95	2	2.1	25[a]	15[a]
Groundwater—private residence wells		70	7	10.0	25–11900	15[a]
Groundwater—school/daycare wells		113	1	0.9	25[a]	15[a]
Metolachlor ethanesulfonic acid (ESA)	HM					
Groundwater—agricultural/farm wells		95	13	13.7	5.0–97.1	3.0[a]
Groundwater—private residence wells		70	55	78.6	5.0–15900	3.0[a]
Groundwater—school/daycare wells		113	40	35.4	5.0–1360	3.0[a]
Metolachlor oxanilic acid (OA)	HM					
Groundwater—agricultural/farm wells		95	3	3.2	5.0–102	3.0[a]
Groundwater—private residence wells		70	49	70.0	5.0–3760	3.0[a]
Groundwater—school/daycare wells		113	14	12.4	5.0–109	3.0[a]
Myclobutanil	F					
Groundwater—agricultural/farm wells		95	1	1.1	83[a]	50[a]
Groundwater—private residence wells		70				50[a]
Groundwater—school/daycare wells		113				50[a]
Picioram	H					
Groundwater—agricultural/farm wells		95	1	1.4	20.8[a]	12.5[a]
Groundwater—private residence wells		70	1	0.9	20.8[a]	12.5[a]
Groundwater—school/daycare wells		113				12.5[a]
Tebuthiuron	I					
Groundwater—agricultural/farm wells		95	1	1.1	50[a]	30[a]
Groundwater—private residence wells		70	1	1.4	333[a]	30[a]
Groundwater—school/daycare wells		113				30[a]

Source: Pesticide Data Control Program. 2009.

Pesticide Types: F = Fungicide. H = Herbicide, HM = Herbicide Metabolite. I = Insecticide, IM = Insecticide Metabolite.

[a] Only one distinct detected concentration or LOD value was reported for the pair.

PESTICIDES

Pesticides are widely used by farmers to control plant pests and enhance production, but chemical pesticides can also cause water quality problems. Pesticides may appear in surface water due to: direct application (e.g., aerial spraying or broadcasting over water bodies), runoff during rain storms, and aerial drift (from adjacent fields).[173]

Some pesticides have also been detected in groundwater.[173]

Farmers may use Integrated Pest Management (IPM) techniques (which can include biological pest control) to maintain control over pests, reduce reliance on chemical pesticides, and protect water quality.[175,176]

There are few safe ways of disposing of pesticide surpluses other than through containment in well managed landfills or by incineration. In some parts of the world, spraying on land is a permitted method of disposal.

TABLE 3.26
Agricultural Pollutants in U.S. Drinking Water

Ammonia	Trifluralin
Chlorate	Ethion
Nitrate and Nitrite Mix	Hepatochlor
Nitrate (alone)	3-Hydroxycarbofuran
Nitrite (alone)	Hepatochlor epoxide
Phosphate	Endosulfan
Sulfate	Dieldrin
Thallium	DDT
MBAS (surfactants)	Butachlor
Phosphorus	Propachlor
Endrin	Bromacil
Desethylatrazine	Dacthal
Desisopropyatrazine	Diuron
Lindane	2,4-D
Methoxychlor	2,4-DB
Toxaphene	2,4,5-TP (Silvex)
Carbaryl	2,4,5-T
Methomyl	Chloramben
Baygon (Propoxur)	Dichloroprop
Methiocarb	Bromomethane
Acetochlor	Isophorone
Paraquat	Alpha-lindane
Prometon	Beta-lindane
2,4-bis 6 (Isopropylamino)	Aldrin
Dalapon	1,3-Dichloropropene
Diquat	Dicamba
Endothal	Iodomethane
Glyphosate	Chloropicrin
Oxamyl (Vydate)	Metribuzin
Simazine	Bentazon (Basagran)
Pichloram	Molinate (Ordram)
Dinoseb	Thiobencarb (Bolero)
Aldicarb sulfoxide	Foaming agents
Aldicarb sulfone	Phenols
Metolachlor	1.2-Dibromo-3-chloropropane
Carbofuran	Ethylene dibromide
Aldicarb	Chlordane
Atrazine	m-Dichlorobenzene
Alaclor	Ethylbenzene
EPTC (Eptam)	Perchlorate
Butylate (Sutan)	Total aldicarbs
Cyanazine (Bladex)	Alpha chlordane

Source: U.S. Environmental Protection Agency. *Protecting Water Quality from Agricultural Runoff.* March 2005. Available at http://www.epa.gov/owow/nps/Ag_Runoff_Fact_Sheet.

Wastewater generated from agricultural and food operations has distinctive characteristics that set it apart from common municipal wastewater managed by public or private sewage treatment plants throughout the world: It is biodegradable and nontoxic but has high concentrations of biochemical oxygen demand (BOD) and suspended solids (SS).[177] The constituents of food and agriculture wastewater are often complex to predict due to the differences in BOD and pH in effluents from vegetables, fruit, and meat products and due to the seasonal nature of food processing and postharvesting.

Processing of food from raw materials requires large volumes of high grade water. Vegetable washing generates waters with high loads of particulate matter and some dissolved organic matter. It may also contain surfactants.

Animal slaughter and processing produces very strong organic waste from body fluids, such as blood, and gut contents. This wastewater is frequently contaminated by significant levels of antibiotics and growth hormones from the animals and by a variety of pesticides used to control external parasites. Insecticides residues in fleeces is a particular problem in treating waters generated in wool processing.

Processing food for sale produces wastes generated from cooking which are often rich in plant organic material and may also contain salt, flavorings, coloring material, and acids or alkali. Very significant quantities of oils or fats may also be present.

FOOD INDUSTRY

Farms with large livestock and poultry operations, such as factory farms, can be a major source of point source wastewater. In the United States, these facilities are called *concentrated animal feeding operations* or *confined animal feeding operations* and are being subject to increasing government regulation.[178]

The constituents of animal wastewater typically contain:[179] strong organic content—much stronger than human sewage—high solids concentration, high nitrate and phosphorus content, antibiotics, synthetic hormones, and often high concentrations of parasites and their eggs, Spores of *Cryptosporidum* (a protozoan) resistant to drinking water treatment processes, Spores of *Giardia*, and Human pathogenic bacteria such as *Brucella* and *Salmonella*.

Animal wastes from cattle can be produced as solid or semisolid manure or as a liquid slurry. The production of slurry is especially common in housed dairy cattle.

While solid manure heaps outdoors can give rise to polluting wastewaters from runoff, this type of waste is usually relatively easy to treat by containment and/or covering of the heap.

Animal slurries require special handling and are usually treated by containment in lagoons before disposal by spray or trickle application to grassland. Constructed wetlands are sometimes used to facilitate treatment of animal wastes, as are anaerobic lagoons. Excessive application or application to sodden land or insufficient land area can result in direct runoff to water sources, with the potential for causing severe pollution. Application of slurries to land overlying aquifers can result in direct contamination or, more commonly, elevation of nitrogen levels as nitrite or nitrate.

The disposal of any wastewater containing animal waste upstream of a drinking water intake can pose serious health problems to those drinking the water because of the highly resistant spores present in many animals that are capable of causing disabling disease in humans. This risk exists even for very low-level seepage via shallow surface drains or from rainfall runoff.

Some animal slurries are treated by mixing with straws and composted at high temperature to produce a bacteriologically sterile and friable manure for soil improvement.

PIGGERY WASTE

Piggery waste is comparable to other animal wastes and is processed as for general animal waste, except that many piggery wastes contain elevated levels of copper that can be toxic in the natural environment. The liquid fraction of the waste is frequently separated off and reused in the piggery to avoid the prohibitively expensive costs of disposing of copper-rich liquid. Ascaris worms and their eggs are also common in piggery waste and can infect humans if wastewater treatment is ineffective.

SILAGE LIQUOR

Fresh or wilted grass or other green crops can be made into a semi-fermented product called silage which can be stored and used as winter forage for cattle and sheep. The production of silage often involves the use of an acid conditioner such as sulfuric acid or formic acid. The process of silage making frequently produces a yellow-brown strongly smelling liquid which is very rich in simple sugars, alcohol, short-chain organic acids, and silage conditioner. This liquor is one of the most polluting organic substances known. The volume of silage liquor produced is generally in proportion to the moisture content of the ensiled material.

Silage liquor is best treated through prevention by wilting crops well before silage making. Any silage liquor that is produced can be used as part of the food for pigs. The most effective treatment is by containment in a slurry lagoon and by subsequent spreading on land following substantial dilution with slurry. Containment of silage liquor on its own can cause structural problems in concrete pits because of the acidic nature of silage liquor.

MILKING PARLOR (DAIRY FARMING) WASTES

Although milk has a deserved reputation as an important and valuable food product, its presence in wastewaters is highly polluting because of its organic strength, which can lead to very rapid deoxygenation of receiving waters. Milking parlor wastes also contain large volumes of wash-down water, some animal waste together with cleaning and disinfection chemicals.

Treatment

Milking parlor wastes are often treated in admixture with human sewage in a local sewage treatment plant. This ensures that disinfectants and cleaning agents are sufficiently diluted and amenable to treatment. Running milking wastewaters into a farm slurry lagoon is a possible option, although this tends to consume lagoon capacity very quickly. Land spreading is also a treatment option. *See also Industrial wastewater treatment.*

Slaughtering Waste

Wastewater from slaughtering activities is similar to milking parlor waste (see above), although considerably stronger in its organic composition and therefore potentially much more polluting. Treatment is similar to the milking parlor waste treatment method.

Vegetable Washing Water

Washing of vegetables produces large volumes of water contaminated by soil and vegetable pieces. Low levels of pesticides used to treat the vegetables may also be present together with moderate levels of disinfectants such as chlorine.

Treatment

Most vegetable washing waters are extensively recycled with the solids removed by settlement and filtration. The recovered soil can be returned to the land.

Firewater

Although few farms plan for fires, fires are nevertheless more common on farms than on many other industrial premises. Stores of pesticides, herbicides, fuel oil for farm machinery, and fertilizers can all help promote fire and can all be present in environmentally lethal quantities in firewater from firefighting at farms.

Treatment

All farm environmental management plans should allow for containment of substantial quantities of firewater and for its subsequent recovery and disposal by specialist disposal companies.[180]

The concentration and mixture of contaminants in firewater make them unsuited to any treatment method available on the farm. Even land spreading has produced severe taste and odor problems for downstream water supply companies in the past.

CONTAMINATION: UNREGULATED CONTAMINANTS IN TAP WATER

The first ever nationwide compilation of tap water testing results from drinking water utilities shows widespread contamination of drinking water with scores of contaminants for which there are no enforceable health standards. Examples include the gasoline additive MTBE, the rocket fuel component perchlorate, and a variety of industrial solvents. The pollution affects more than one hundred million people in 42 states.

Serves 290,000 people—test data available: 2004–2008.

The drinking water quality report shows results of tests conducted by the water utility and provided to the Environmental Working Group (EWG) by the Texas Commission on Environmental Quality. It is part of EWG's national database that includes 47,667 drinking water utilities and 20 million test results. Water utilities nationwide detected more than 300 pollutants between 2004 and 2009. More than half of these chemicals are unregulated, legal in any amount which of course means nothing except to the federal bureaucracy. Despite this widespread contamination, the federal government invests few resources to protecting rivers, reservoirs, and groundwater from pollution in the first place. The information below summarizes test results for this utility and lists potential health concerns (Tables 3.27 and 3.28).

Of course, whether contaminants are regulated or unregulated to the clinician is unimportant. This is because neither should be there. No one knows the significance of the combination and whether there is or how much the combinations make the individual worse. Therefore, whether the government says they are unregulated is immaterial and a false category of concern.

There were several contaminants observed (Table 3.29).

Fort Worth, TX alone serves 501,954 people—Test data available: 2004–2008.

Of the 260 contaminants detected in tap water from 42 states, for only 114 has EPA set enforceable health limits (called Maximum Contaminant Levels, or MCLs), and for 5 others the Agency has set nonenforceable goals called secondary standards.[181]

The 141 remaining chemicals without health-based limits contaminate water served to 195,257,000 people in 22,614 communities in 42 states. Of the 141 unregulated contaminants found in tap water, 40 were detected in tap water served to at least one million people while 20 unregulated contaminants were detected in just one system, only one time. Nineteen unregulated contaminants were detected above health-based limits[182] in tap water served to at least 10,000 people. Forty-eight unregulated contaminants were not detected above health-based limits anywhere, and seventy lack health-based limits, which have yet to be developed by EPA (Figure 3.13).

The Agency's own scientists have identified 600 chemicals in tap water formed as by-products of disinfection,[183–186] tracked some 220 million pounds of 650 industrial chemicals discharged into rivers and streams each year[187] (EPA 2003-ref below), and spearheaded research on emerging contaminants after the U.S. Geological Survey found 82 unregulated pharmaceuticals and personal care product chemicals in rivers and streams across the country that provide drinking water for millions of Americans.[186–189] The EPA has set safety standards for fewer than 20% of the many hundreds of chemicals that it has identified in tap water. In the opinion of the physicians and scientists at the EHC- Dallas and Buffalo and AAEM, the safety standards are not adequate since no one knows the effects of the combination of these chemicals. Most chemically sensitive and chronic degenerative disease cannot drink the public water supply in the U.S. They rapidly become ill after ingesting the water. Also, in contracts, the nonchemically sensitive may develop chronic debilitating disease or malignancy years later.

TABLE 3.27

Contaminants Above Maximum Health and Legal Limits

Contaminant	Average/ Maximum Result	Health Limit Exceeded	Legal Limit Exceeded
Dichloroacetic acid	6.41 ppb	Yes	No
	13.38 ppb	MCLG: 0 ppb	60 ppb
Bromodichloromethane	8.12 ppb	Yes	No
	14.83 ppb	MCLG: 0 ppb	80 ppb
Dibromochloromethane	5.12 ppb	Yes	No
	10.85 ppb	0.4 ppb	80 ppb
Total trihalomethanes (TTHMs)	22.62 ppb	Yes	No
	40.35 ppb	9.8 ppb	80 ppb
Chloroform	8.94 ppb	Yes	No
	19.43 ppb	5.7 ppb	80 ppb
Total haloacetic acids (HAAs)	11.86 ppb	Yes	No
	23.98 ppb	0.7 ppb	60 ppb
Bromoform	0.45 ppb	Yes	No
	1.74 ppb	MCLG: 0 ppb	80 ppb
Bromochloroacetic acid	3.65 ppb	No	Legal at
	7.07 ppb		any level
Trichloroacetic acid	2.14 ppb	No	No
	7.13 ppb	20 ppb	60 ppb
Dibromoacetic acid	1.11 ppb	No	No
	3.13 ppb		60 ppb
Monochloroacetic acid	2.3 ppb	No	No
	13.56 ppb	70 ppb	60 ppb
Nitrate	0.24 ppm	No	No
	0.34 ppm	10 ppm	10 ppm
Atrazine	0.02 ppb	No	No
	0.11 ppb	0.15 ppb	3 ppb
Nitrite	0.01 ppm	No	No
	0.01 ppm	1 ppm	1 ppm
Gross beta particle activity (pCi/L)	6.03 pCi/L	No	No
	6.03 pCi/L		50 pCi/L

Source: Environmental Working Group (EWG) by the Texas Commission on Environmental Quality.

Note: Water utilities are noted as exceeding the legal limit if any test is above the maximum contaminant level (MCL). Most MCLs are based on annual averages, so exceeding the MCL for one test does not necessarily indicate that the system is out of compliance.

By failing to clean up rivers and reservoirs that provide drinking water for hundreds of millions of Americans, EPA and the Congress have forced water utilities to decontaminate water that is polluted with industrial chemicals, factory farm waste, sewage, pesticides, fertilizer, and sediment. In its most recent national Water Quality Inventory, EPA found that 45% of lakes and 39% of streams and rivers are "impaired," unsafe for drinking, fishing, or even swimming, in some cases.[169] Even after water suppliers filter and disinfect the water, scores of contaminants remain, with conventional treatment regimens removing less than 20% of some contaminants.[190] New and more precise filters should be developed and instituted so as to deliver clean water. If and when they can stop water contamination at the source, they might find a massive decrease in disease processes and much more vigor in the population.

TABLE 3.28

Pollution Summary

15	Total Contaminants Detected (2004–2008)
	Nitrate, nitrite, atrazine, monochloroacetic acid, dichloroacetic acid, trichloroacetic acid, dibromoacetic acid, bromochloroacetic acid, total haloacetic acids (HAAs), chloroform, bromoform, bromodichloromethane, dibromochloromethane, total trihalomethanes (TTHMs), gross beta particle activity (pCi/L)
3	Agricultural pollutants
	(pesticides, fertilizer, factory farms)
	Nitrate, nitrite, atrazine
2	Sprawl and urban pollutants
	(road runoff, lawn pesticides, human waste)
	Nitrate, nitrite
3	Industrial pollutants
	Nitrate, nitrite, gross beta particle activity (pCi/L)
11	Water treatment and distribution by-products
	(pipes and fixtures, treatment chemicals, and by-products)
	Total trihalomethanes (TTHMs), total haloacetic acids (HAAs), chloroform, bromodichloromethane, dibromochloromethane, dichloroacetic acid, trichloroacetic acid, bromoform, dibromoacetic acid, monochloroacetic acid, bromochloroacetic acid
3	Naturally Occurring
	Naturally present but increased for lands denuded by sprawl, agriculture, or industrial development

Source: Environmental Working Group (EWG) by the Texas Commission on Environmental Quality.

By failing to set tap water safety standards expeditiously or require and fund comprehensive testing, EPA allows widespread exposures to chemical mixtures posing unknown risks to human health.

Of the 141 unregulated contaminants utilities detected in water supplies between 1998 and 2003, 52 are linked to cancer, 41 to reproductive toxicity, 36 to developmental toxicity, and 16 to immune system damage, according to chemical listings in seven standard government and industry toxicity references. These findings are only touching the surface. Unfortunately, no studies have been conducted on biologic risks for the population or the chemically sensitive. Despite the potential health risks, any concentration of these chemicals in tap water is legal, no matter how high. The combinations of the chemicals definitely can cause chemical sensitivity and chronic degenerative disease. These tumors and arteriosclerosis effects of the combinations are totally unknown.

For 46 of these chemicals, no health information whatsoever is available in standard government and academic references.

Altogether, the unregulated chemicals that pollute public tap water supplies include the gasoline additive MTBE; the rocket fuel component perchlorate; at least 15 chemical by-products of water disinfection; four industrial plasticizers such as phthalates linked to birth defects and reproductive toxicity; 78 chemicals used in industrial and consumer products; and 20 chemical pollutants from gasoline, coal, and other fuel combustion. Many of the pollutants are known to cause cancer, arteriosclerosis, and chemical sensitivity. The neurological effects of these pollutants can cause neuropathy as well as anesthetic effects on the general population as well as the chemically sensitive and chronic degenerative disease and can account for short-term memory loss, confined to dull thinkings.

It was found that between 1998 and 2003, water suppliers collectively identified in treated tap water 83 agricultural pollutants, including pesticides and chemicals from fertilizer- and manure-laden runoff; 59 contaminants linked to sprawl and urban areas from polluted runoff and wastewater treatment plants; 166 industrial chemicals from factory waste and consumer products; and 44

TABLE 3.29

Contaminants Seen Above Legal Limits

Contaminant	Average/ Maximum Result	Health Limit Exceeded	Legal Limit Exceeded
Dibromochloromethane	2.99 ppb	Yes	No
	4.2 ppb	0.4 ppb	80 ppb
Bromodichloromethane	2.05 ppb	Yes	No
	4.33 ppb	MCLG: 0 ppb	80 ppb
Dichloroacetic acid	2.33 ppb	Yes	No
	4.35 ppb ppb	MCLG: 0 ppb	60 ppb
Bromoform	0.53 ppb	Yes	No
	2.4 ppb	MCLG: 0 ppb	80 ppb
Total haloacetic acids (HAAs)	2.25 ppb	Yes	No
	6.3 ppb	0.7 ppb	60 ppb
Total trihalomethanes (TTHMs)	6.75 ppb	Yes	No
	11.8 ppb	9.8 ppb ppb	80 ppb
Atrazine	0.09 ppb	Yes	No
	0.28 ppb	0.15 ppb	3 ppb
Dibromoacetic acid	1.18 ppb	No	No
	2.25 ppb		60 ppb
Chloroform	0.96 ppb	No	No
	4.02 ppb	5.7 ppb	80 ppb
Bromochloroacetic acid	1.63 ppb	No	Legal at
	3.25 ppb		any level
Nitrate	0.38 ppm	No	No
	0.51 ppm	10 ppm	10 ppm
Monochloroacetic acid	0.26 ppb	No	No
	2.8 ppb	70 ppb	60 ppb
Monobromoacetic acid	0.05 ppb	No	No
	0.75 ppb		60 ppb
Gross beta particle activity (pCi/L)	2.4 pCi/L	No	No
	4.8 pCi/L		50 pCi/L
Nitrite	0.01 ppm	No	No
	0.01 ppm	1 ppm	1 ppm

Source: Environmental Working Group (EWG) by the Texas Commission on Environmental Quality.

Note: Water Utilities are Noted as Exceeding the Legal Limit if Any Test is Above the Maximum Contaminant Level (MCL). Most MCLs are Based on Annual Averages, So Exceeding the MCL for One Test Does Not Necessarily Indicate That the System is Out of Compliance.

pollutants that are by-products of the water treatment process or that leach from pipes and storage tanks.[144] Since then, there are epidemics of cancer and cardiovascular disease.

The water cycle can be and is probably contaminated at every level. Rain and Fog are radioactive, containing many toxics, especially those coming from the Fukushima nuclear plant in Japan. Areas west of the Rockies are now 200–300 times more than they used to be spewing radiation all over especially California, Oregon, Washington, and Idaho states.

An outbreak of gastroenteritis occurred among two patrons at a golf course (Minnesota, *1979*). Acute illness occurred within minutes of consuming water from a water cooler located next to the

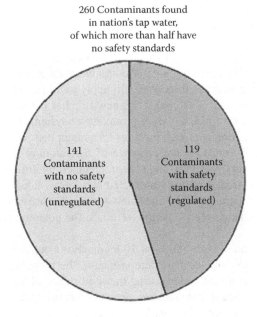

260 Contaminants found
in nation's tap water,
of which more than half have
no safety standards

141
Contaminants
with no safety
standards
(unregulated)

119
Contaminants
with safety
standards
(regulated)

FIGURE 3.13 EPA has set enforceable safety standards (called maximum contaminant levels or MCLs) for 80 chemicals or chemical groups, which are present in tap water tests analyzed by EWG as 114 individual chemicals or chemical variants called isomers. It has also established 15 guidelines called National Secondary Drinking Water Regulations (NSDWRs), five of which are represented in tap water tests analyzed by EWG. (EWG analysis of water utility test data for 1998–2003, compiled and provided to EWG by state drinking water offices.)

golf course. The water dispenser had become contaminated after a bucket with detergent residues was used to fill the water container.

During September–November *1995*, a hepatitis A outbreak involved eight persons in a community (Tennessee, 1995). All ill persons reported consuming untreated drinking water from groundwater sources. Water testing revealed fecal contamination in multiple wells from this community.

One outbreak of gastroenteritis (Tennessee, October *1988*) involved an unidentified etiologic agent. The outbreak report implicated *water and ice* served at a restaurant as the cause of gastroenteritis in 89 persons. Filtered and chlorinated stream water was used for drinking water and ice. Three days before the onset of illnesses, the sewage system at an upstream campground overflowed, which presumably overwhelmed the restaurant's water-treatment system.

One outbreak of *Pseudomonas folliculitis* among 27 persons occurred in an industrial facility (Louisiana, 2002) and was linked with the use of recycled water in the manufacturing process.[191] Although this closed water system was chemically treated, substantially high concentrations of *P. aeruginosa* were detected in multiple water samples at the facility.

Surface water: Only one (12.5%) of the eight outbreaks with deficiencies 1–3 was associated with consumption of inadequately treated surface water. In this outbreak (Oregon, 2005), chronically inadequate chlorination and inadequate filtration of the river water supplying the camp were cited as the underlying reasons for illness among camp attendees. Since the early 1990s, the percentage of reported WBDOs associated with inadequately treated surface water has been declining.

Groundwater: Seven (87.5%) of the eight outbreaks with deficiencies 1–3 were associated with consumption of contaminated groundwater, either from wells or springs. Among these seven outbreaks, four (57.1%) involved consumption of untreated groundwater (deficiency 2), and three (42.9%) involved treatment deficiencies associated with contaminated groundwater (deficiency 3). These seven groundwater-associated outbreaks indicate that groundwater contamination is a continuing problem. Wells and springs must be protected from contamination, even if disinfection is provided, because groundwater can become contaminated with pathogens that are not easily disinfected, and source water conditions might overwhelm the disinfection process (e.g., highly turbid water as a result of excessive rainfall).

Five of the seven outbreaks associated with contaminated groundwater during the 2005–2006 surveillance period occurred in noncommunity or community water systems that will be subject to EPA's new GWR. Beginning in 2009, the GWR will apply to all public systems that use groundwater as a source of drinking water. Although this new rule has not yet been fully implemented, it will establish a risk-based approach to target groundwater systems that are vulnerable to fecal contamination. The risk-targeting approach includes four major components: (1) sanitary surveys, (2) source water monitoring to test for the presence of indicators of fecal contamination in the groundwater source, (3) corrective action, and (4) compliance-monitoring to ensure that the treatment technology installed to treat drinking water reliably achieves at least 99.99% (4-log) inactivation or removal of viruses. Operators of groundwater systems that are identified as being at risk for fecal contamination must take corrective action to reduce the potential for illness from exposure to microbial pathogens.

During 2005–2006, a total of eight (80%) of 10 legionellosis outbreaks associated with drinking water occurred in health-care settings, demonstrating the propensity for *Legionella* spp. to colonize potable water systems and underscoring the importance of maintaining a high index of suspicion for legionellosis in health-care settings. Seven outbreaks occurred in acute care hospitals and one in a long-term care facility. *Legionella* spp. colonize the biofilm layer frequently found inside the large, complex plumbing systems of hospitals.[192] This biofilm protects *Legionella* from biocides and allows the bacteria to amplify to levels sufficient to be transmitted and/or cause disease. Patients in hospitals or long-term care facilities typically are older and have underlying illness factors that increase the risk for disease (e.g., chronic lung disease, diabetes, and immunocompromising conditions).

Superheating and superchlorination are the traditional methods for remediation; however, *Legionella* might regrow in the distribution system.[193] Other remediation options are under investigation. Monochloramine might be an effective biocide for *Legionella* control; hospitals supplied with drinking water containing monochloramine were less likely to have a reported outbreak of LD than those that used water with free chlorine as a residual disinfectant.[194] Each health-care facility should develop a plan for legionellosis prevention to address predisposing conditions for *Legionella* growth in the potable water supply. Guidelines for reducing the risk for legionellosis associated with building water systems are available.[193]

Deficiencies involving drinking water that occur at points not under the jurisdiction of a water utility or at the point-of-use have been presented. During the 2005–2006 surveillance period, only two reported non-*Legionella* WBDOs involving deficiencies in this category were reported. Both WBDOs involved point-of-use contamination. One outbreak of giardiasis was associated with contamination of a 5-gallon drinking water ceramic crock dispenser at a gym (California, August 2005). Epidemiologic evidence linked all the cases to the dispenser, although the mechanism of contamination of the dispenser could not be determined. An outbreak of norovirus G1 at a camp (Maryland 2006) involved water treatment and distribution system deficiencies in addition to contamination at the point-of-use. Garden hoses stored improperly on the ground were used to fill large water containers from which campers filled their cups and water bottles. These point-of-use contamination events illustrate the vulnerability of shared water containers and the importance of practicing good hygiene.

During the 2005–2006 surveillance period, eight WBDOs occurred that were associated with WNID or WUI. Five of these outbreaks were associated with *Legionella* spp. Three of these outbreaks were in health-care settings and attributed to cooling towers. Although the building potable water system is more frequently implicated in health-care-associated outbreaks, community sources should also be considered. Aerosols containing *Legionella* can travel great distances; an investigation of an outbreak among residents of a long-term care facility implicated a cooling towers that were 0.4 km from the facility.[195]

The other three non-*Legionella* WNID/WUI outbreaks were associated with bacterial and parasitic diseases. An outbreak caused by *E. coli* O157:H7 occurred at a sports camp (Tennessee 2005). The primary water exposure associated with illness could not be identified. Illness was associated with swimming in one of the outdoor pools, dining at pool picnic tables, and attending a tennis camp. Unlabeled irrigation faucets drawing water from a nonpotable well were located at multiple points around the tennis courts. Sampling of this water system detected fecal contamination. The remaining two WBDOs involved cases of giardiasis that developed after exposure to WNID. One outbreak involved a family which had canal water piped into their home to use for bathing, dish washing, house cleaning, and laundry (California, July 2005). The second outbreak involved a school trip to a state forest (Colorado, 2006). Six of 26 campers became ill. The epidemiologic data indicated that inadequate treatment of river water before consumption was a risk factor. Adding a sports drink powder to river water while concurrently adding iodine for disinfection was a statistically significant risk factor for becoming ill. The relative risk for boiling water <3 minutes could not be defined because none of the persons who boiled water for a longer period became ill. Both of these giardiasis outbreaks illustrate the risks associated with consuming untreated surface water, even water that might appear pristine.

A team of U.S. Geological Survey (USGS) and academic scientists are analyzing samples of coral and surrounding sediments from an area damaged near the Deepwater Horizon site in the Gulf of Mexico. These samples are being used to investigate how and why the corals on these reefs died.

The cruise revisited MC 338, the site where dead and dying corals were found covered by an unknown brown substance in November 2010. The collected samples of the animals living on the seafloor show how deep-sea reefs in the Gulf of Mexico have been affected by the Deepwater Horizon oil spill.

OTHER SOURCES OF INDUSTRIAL WASTEWATER

MINES AND QUARRIES

The principal wastewaters associated with mines and quarries are slurries of rock particles in water.[196] Hundreds of these are in the state of Colorado. These arise from rainfall washing, exposed surfaces, and haul roads and also from rock washing and grading processes. Volumes of water can be very high, especially rainfall-related arising on large sites. Some specialized separation operations, such as coal washing to separate coal from native rock using density gradients, can produce wastewater contaminated by fine particulate hematite and surfactants. Oils and hydraulic oils are also common contaminants.

Wastewater from metal mines and ore recovery plants are inevitably contaminated by the minerals present in the native rock formations.[196] Following crushing and extraction of the desirable materials, undesirable materials may become contaminated in the wastewater. For metal mines, this can include unwanted metals such as zinc and other materials such as arsenic.[196] Extraction of high value metals such as gold and silver may generate slimes containing very fine particles in which physical removal of contaminants becomes particularly difficult.

IRON AND STEEL INDUSTRY

The production of iron from its ores involves powerful reduction reactions in blast furnaces. Cooling waters are inevitably contaminated with products, especially ammonia *and* cyanide. Production of coke from coal in coking plants also requires water cooling and the use of water in by-products separation.[196] Contamination of waste streams includes gasification products such as benzene, naphthalene, anthracene, cyanide, ammonia, phenols, and cresols together with a range of more complex organic compounds such as polycyclic aromatic hydrocarbons (PAH).[196]

The conversion of iron or steel into sheet, wire, or rods requires hot and cold mechanical transformation stages frequently employing water as a lubricant and coolant. Contaminants include hydraulic oils, tallow, *and* particulate solids. Final treatment of iron and steel products before onward sale into manufacturing includes pickling in strong mineral acid to remove rust and prepare the surface for tin or chromium plating or for other surface treatments such as galvanization or painting. The two acids commonly used are hydrochloric acid and sulfuric acid. Wastewaters include acidic rinse waters together with waste acid. Although many plants operate acid recovery plants (particularly those using hydrochloric acid), where the mineral acid is boiled away from the iron salts, there remains a large volume of highly acid ferrous sulfate or ferrous chloride to be disposed of. Many steel industry wastewaters are contaminated by hydraulic oil, also known as *soluble oil* (Table 3.30).

ARSENIC AND SELENIUM

Adjusted mean values of [^{3}H] methyl incorporation and As variables by category of plasma Se are presented into genomic DNA generally increased with increasing plasma Se categories, although there appeared to be little difference between the second and third categories. Adjusted mean values of total uAs decreased with increasing categories of plasma Se. For total bAs and blood %MMA, there appeared to be a threshold effect; adjusted mean values in the first three categories of plasma Se were similar and higher than the values in the two highest categories. There also appeared to be a threshold in the association between plasma Se and blood %DMA, such that the adjusted mean values in the three lowest categories of plasma Se were similar and lower than the values in the two highest categories.

In this cross-sectional study of 287 Bangladeshi adults, Pilsner et al.[224] observed that plasma Se is inversely associated with genomic methylation of leukocyte DNA, with and without adjustment for covariates including plasma folate concentrations and water As. In addition, they found inverse associations between plasma Se and both total uAs and bAs concentrations. Plasma Se was also inversely associated with %MMA and positively associated with %DMA in blood.

PLASMA SE AND GENOMIC DNA METHYLATION

Their findings, which suggest that plasma Se concentrations are inversely related to genomic DNA methylation, are contrary to their original hypothesis that Se deficiency would be associated with genomic hypomethylation of DNA. Previous animal and *in vitro* studies examining the influence of Se on DNA methylation have been inconsistent. A series of animal studies indicate that dietary Se deficiency caused genomic hypomethylation of liver and colon DNA,[197,198] whereas supplementation with Se^{IV} increased DNMT activity and DNA methylation in the liver and colon, respectively. *In vitro* studies using Friend erythroleukemic and HCT116 colon carcinoma cells, however, have shown that Se^{IV} exposure caused a decrease in DNMT activity concomitant with DNA hypomethylation.[199,200] Additional data indicate that Se^{IV} treatment induced genomic DNA hypomethylation and was associated with the downregulation of DNMT 1 and DNMT 3a expression and histone deacetylase activity in the LNCaP human prostate cancer cell line.[201] Although speculative, their results are consistent with the *in vitro* assays, suggesting that the inverse association between plasma Se concentrations and genomic DNA methylation in and heir study could reflect a decrease in DNMT expression and/ or activity.

Previous work has suggested that the association between As exposure and clinical outcomes may be modified by Se nutritional status.[202] This hypothesis is supported by experimental studies indicating that As and Se each mutually facilitate biliary excretion of the other.[203] An Se–As–glutathione complex, seleno-bis(S-glutathionyl) arsinium ion, [(GS)$_2$AsSe]$^-$, has been detected in biliary excretion of rabbits, suggesting that one potential mechanism whereby Se

TABLE 3.30

General Characteristics of the Study Sample (n = 287)

Variable	Mean ± SD (Range) or Percent
Age (years)	37.9 ± 10.4 (18–66)
Male	48
BMI (kg/m²M	19.8 ± 3.2 (13.3–30.5)
Ever Smoking	37.0
Ever betel nut use	33.8
Education (Years)	3.3 ± 3.5 (0–16)
Type of housing	
Thatched	3.1
Corrugated tin	88.5
Other	8.4
Plasma measures	
Plasma Se (µg/L)	87.6 ± 1.8 (45.4–148.8)
Se deficient[a]	16
Plasma B_{12} (pmol/L)	276.3 ± 115.1 (86.1–920)
B_{12} deficient[b]	23
Plasma folate (mmol/L)	8.8 ± 4.3 (3.0–44.7)
Folate deficient[c]	63
Plasma homocysteine (umol/L)	10.9 ± 5.2 (0.24–49.8)
Water As (µg/L)	113.6 ± 108.0 90.1–716)
Urinary measures	
uAs (µg/L)	172.6 ± 172.4 (8.0–1519.0)
Urinary Cre (mg/dl)	60.5 ± 43.6 (5.6–334.8)
uAs/g Cre	339.0 ± 302.2 (21.0–2018.0)
%InAs	15.1 ± 6.1 (6.0–60.1)
%MMA	12.6 ± 4.2(3.8–26.9)
%DMA	72.4 ± 7.8 (36.2–87.9)
Blood measures[d]	
bAs (µg/L)	9.9 ± 6.3 (0.89–30.7)
%InAs	26.0 ± 3.9 (16.2–40.2)
%MMA	40.3 ± 6.3 (15.9–68.5)
%DMA	33.4 ± 6.5 (7.6–48.0)
[³H]Methyl incorporation	42,270 ± 3984 (27,256–56,940)

Source: Pilsner, J. R. et al. 2007. *Am. J. Clin. Nutr.* 86 (4):1179–1186.
Abbreviations: Cre, creatinine, Incorp, incorporation.
[a] Plasma Se <70.0 µg/L.
[b] Plasma cobalamin <184 pmol/L.
[c] Plasma folate <90 nmol/L.
[d] n = 223.

intake may reduce the body burden of As is by increasing its loss through biliary excretion,[204] although this complex has not yet been definitively identified in humans. In this cross-sectional analysis, it is not possible to determine the temporal nature of the relationship between plasma Se and uAs/bAs or whether this is a causal relationship. An additional possibility is that As in the environment may adversely affect Se nutritional status. For example, a recent study reported that high concentrations of As in rice in Bangladesh are associated with lower levels of Se and other trace minerals in rice.[205]

In the present study, Pilsner et al.[224] observed a significant inverse association between plasma Se and uAs, a finding that is in agreement with the results from a previous case–cohort study from an other study area where higher blood Se concentrations were associated with lower uAs and reduced risk for As-induced premalignant skin lesions.[206] Pilsner et al.[224] also observed an inverse association between plasma Se and bAs concentrations as well, despite the fact that they previously detected no association between whole-blood Se and bAs concentrations.[206] The explanation for these discrepant findings is unclear. One difference between the studies is that they measured plasma Se in this study, as opposed to whole-blood Se in the previous study.

Arsenic methylation and the toxicity of its metabolites have undergone considerable investigation in recent years. Compelling evidence from experimental data suggests that trivalent arsenical intermediates, in particular MMA^{III}, are more toxic than their pentavalent counterparts.[207–209] In agreement with the experimental data, population-based studies indicate that individuals with lower relative proportions of urinary DMA (and higher MMA) exhibit a greater risk for skin cancers[210–212] and bladder cancers,[213] as well as peripheral vascular disease.[214] These results suggest that individuals who have a reduced capacity to fully methylate InAs to DMA^V, the less toxic metabolite, are at heightened risk for As-induced health outcomes and as chemical sensitivity and chronic degenerative diseases.

Antagonism between As and Se, whereby each reduces the toxicity of the other, has long been documented.[215,216] It is possible that As and Se may cause alterations in the biotransformation, distribution, and excretion of each other.[217,218] For example, mice fed diets with excess Se^{IV} excreted significantly higher proportions of InAs than of methylated arsenicals in urine compared with mice fed Se-adequate diets.[218] Experimental studies have shown that Se^{IV} exposure reduced the methylation of InAs in rat cytosol.[219] In a subsequent study, those authors also found Se^{IV} to be a potent inhibitor of recombinant arsenic methyltransferase.[220] Furthermore, experiments in rat hepatocytes revealed that exposure to both Se^{IV} and As^{III} decreased the ratio of DMA to MMA, suggesting that the second As methylation step is more sensitive to Se than the first.[221] Conversely, in rats injected with either As^V or As^{III}, Se^{IV} (10 μmol/kg, intravenous) lowered tissue concentrations of MMA^{III} and MMA^V but increased the concentration of DMA^V.[217] However, the effect of supplementation with selenomethionine (commonly found in food and commercial Se supplements) on As methylation has not been tested, and the direct relevance of these studies employing inorganic forms of Se to the metabolism and toxicity of As in humans is unclear.

In this study, Pilsner et al.[224] observed significant associations between plasma Se and proportions of As metabolites in blood. Plasma Se was associated with lower blood %MMA and higher blood %DMA. They observed no significant associations between Se and the individual proportions of As metabolites in urine. These results are not consistent with those of the animal studies. This may be due to the use of inorganic forms of Se in the animal studies and/or to important differences in As metabolism across species.[222] A potential mechanism by which Se may influence As metabolism is via the Trx/TR system. Trx can provide reducing equivalents for the reduction of MMA^V to MMA^{III}, a prerequisite for the generation of DMA^V. Se deficiency results in decreased activity of TR, a selenoprotein, thereby limiting the regeneration of Trx.[223] Pilsner's data are consistent with the possibility that Se sufficiency may be permissive for the reduction of MMA^V to MMA^{III}, consequently facilitating the methylation of MMA^{III} to DMA^V.

In conclusion, Pilsner et al.'s[224] results indicate that plasma Se concentrations are inversely related to total bAs and uAs concentrations, inversely related to %MMA in blood, and positively associated with %DMA in blood. Collectively, the data suggest that Se may reduce the body burden of As and, moreover, may help to reduce concentrations of blood MMA, the most toxic metabolite in the As methylation pathway. The cross-sectional design of this study limits our ability to determine the temporal nature of our observed associations. Ongoing studies in Bangladesh are exploring the efficacy of Se supplementation in reducing As-induced health outcomes. The underlying mechanisms and biological implications of the inverse association between Se and genomic DNA methylation are unclear and warrant further investigation.

An Emerging Role for Epigenetic Dysregulation in Arsenic Toxicity and Carcinogenesis

The International Agency for Research on Cancer (IARC) classified arsenic, a toxic metalloid, as a group 1 carcinogen >20 years ago[225] (IARC, 1987). It is widely accepted that exposure to arsenic is associated with lung, bladder, kidney, liver, and nonmelanoma skin cancers.[226–229] High levels of arsenic have also been associated with the development of several other diseases and deleterious health effects in humans, such as skin lesions (dyspigmentation, keratosis), peripheral vascular diseases, reproductive toxicity, and neurological effects.[230]

Exposure to arsenic typically results from either oral arsenic consumption through contaminated drinking water, soil, and food, or arsenic inhalation in an industrial work setting. Arsenic-contaminated drinking water has been associated with increased mortality of bladder and lung cancer in Chile[231] and with increased mortality from both noncancerous causes and cancers in Bangladesh.[232] In the human arsenic metabolic pathway, inorganic pentavalent arsenic (As^V) is converted to trivalent arsenic (As^{III}), with subsequent methylation to monomethylated and dimethylated arsenicals (MMA and DMA, respectively).[233] The general scheme is as follows:

$$As^V O_4{}^{3-} + 2e \rightarrow As^{III} O_3{}^{3-} + Me^+$$
$$\rightarrow MMA^V O_3{}^{2-} + 2e$$
$$\rightarrow MMA^{III} O_2{}^{2-} + Me^+$$
$$\rightarrow DMA^V O_2{}^- + 2e \rightarrow DMA^{III} O^-.$$

Methylated arsenicals, especially MMA^{III}, are considered more toxic than inorganic As^{III} both *in vivo* (in animals)[208] and *in vitro* (human cell lines).[234] Several mechanisms by which arsenical compounds induce tumorigenesis have been proposed, including oxidative stress,[235] genotoxic damage and chromosomal abnormalities,[236,237] and cocarcinogenesis with other environmental toxicants;[238] epigenetic mechanisms, in particular, have been reported to alter DNA methylation.[239]

It is generally believed that arsenic does not induce point mutations, based on negative findings in both bacterial and mammalian mutagenicity assays.[240,241] Arsenic does induce deletion mutations, but arsenical compounds vary in their potency.[242] With respect to arsenic's ability to induce chromosomal alterations in humans, studies in the early 1990s showed that the cell micronucleus assay could be used as a biological marker of the genotoxic effects of arsenic exposure.[243] Later studies validated this assay and demonstrated higher frequencies of micronuclei in individuals who were chronically exposed to arsenicals.[236] Analysis of chromosomal alterations in DNA from bladder tumors of 123 patients who had been exposed to arsenic in drinking water showed that tumors from patients with higher estimated levels of arsenic exposure had higher levels of chromosomal instability than did tumors from patients with lower estimated levels of exposure, suggesting that bladder tumors from arsenic-exposed patients may behave more aggressively than tumors from unexposed patients.[244] On the basis of these overall findings, a plausible and generally accepted mechanism for arsenic carcinogenicity is the induction of structural and numerical chromosomal abnormalities through indirect effects on DNA. However, as has been demonstrated for several tumors, including urothelial and hematological malignancies,[245,246] it is likely that interrelated genetic and epigenetic mechanisms together contribute to the toxicity and carcinogenicity of arsenic.[239,247]

Epigenetic Modifications Induced by Arsenic

Epigenetic alteration, which is not a genotoxic effect, leads to heritable phenomena that regulate gene expression without involving changes in the DNA sequence and thus could be considered a form of potentially reversible DNA modification. Recent mechanistic studies of arsenic carcinogenesis have directly or indirectly shown the potential involvement of altered epigenetic regulation in gene expression changes induced by arsenic exposure. They showed that urinary defensin, beta 1 (DEFB1) protein levels were significantly decreased among men highly exposed to arsenic in studies conducted in Nevada (USA) and in Chile.[248] DNA methylation is thought to play a role in regulating *DEFB1* expression.[249] Follow-up studies are under way in their laboratory to determine if reduced levels of DEFB1 in exposed populations are due to arsenic-induced targeted gene silencing. Several studies have observed extensive changes in global gene expression in individuals after arsenic exposure.[250–253] Further, maternal exposure to arsenic has been shown to alter expression of transcripts in the mouse fetus[254] and human newborn.[255] Since epigenetic processes are major regulators of gene expression, these findings suggest that dysregulation of epigenetic processes could contribute mechanistically to arsenic-induced changes in gene expression and cancer, affecting both people exposed to arsenic directly and those of future generations in a heritable manner, without directly altering the genome. Dysregulation of epigenetic processes could also contribute to vascular disease[256] and neurological disorders, and if this is the case, it will also contribute to chemical sensitivity and vaculitis.[257]

Three major epigenetic mechanisms proposed to play roles in arsenic-induced carcinogenesis are: altered DNA methylation, histone modification, and microRNA (miRNA) expression. They also propose future directions that can further inform our understanding of the epigenetic and overall mechanisms underlying the effects of arsenic.

Arsenic Exposure and DNA Methylation

DNA methylation is tightly regulated in mammalian development and is essential for maintaining the normal functioning of the adult organism.[258] Altered DNA methylation has been associated with several human diseases.[259] Global genomic DNA hypomethylation is a hallmark of many types of cancers,[260] resulting in illegitimate recombination events and causing transcriptional deregulation of affected genes.[259] In mammalian systems, DNA methylation occurs predominantly in cytosine-rich gene regions, known as CpG islands, and serves to regulate gene expression and maintain genome stability.[261] DNA methyltransferases (DNMTs) are responsible for transferring a methyl group from the S-adenosyl methionine (SAM) cofactor to the cytosine nucleotide, producing $5'$-methylcytosine and S-adenosyl homocysteine (Figure 3.14).[262] Three different families of *DNMT* genes have been identified so far: *DNMT1*, *DNMT2*, and *DNMT3*.[263]

Mechanisms of Arsenic-Induced Changes in DNA Methylation

An association between arsenic-induced carcinogenesis and DNA methylation was proposed because arsenic methylation and DNA methylation both use the same methyl donor, SAM (Figure 3.14). SAM is a coenzyme involved in >40 metabolic reactions that require methyl group transfers.[264–266] Since SAM is the unique methyl group donor in each conversion step of biomethylation of arsenic, long-term exposure to arsenic may lead to SAM insufficiency and global DNA hypomethylation.[239,267,268] Further, since SAM synthesis requires methionine, an essential amino acid in humans, dietary methyl insufficiency could exacerbate effects of arsenic on DNA methylation (Figure 3.14).[269] Indeed, human exposure to arsenic often occurs in relatively resource-poor populations in developing countries that also may have low dietary intakes of methionine.[270] In addition to its effect on SAM availability, arsenic can directly interact with DNMTs and inhibit their activities. Several studies have shown that arsenic exposure leads to a dose-dependent reduction of mRNA levels and activity of DNMTs both in vitro and in vivo, including DNMT1, DNMT3A, and DNMT3B.[266,271–273]

Arsenic and Global DNA Hypomethylation

Global DNA hypomethylation is expected to result from arsenic exposure through both SAM insufficiency and reduction of *DNMT* gene expression.[266] Arsenic exposure has been reported to induce DNA hypomethylation *in vitro* and in animal studies (Figure 3.14). For example, rats[274] and mice[275–277] exposed to As^III for several weeks displayed global hepatic DNA hypomethylation.

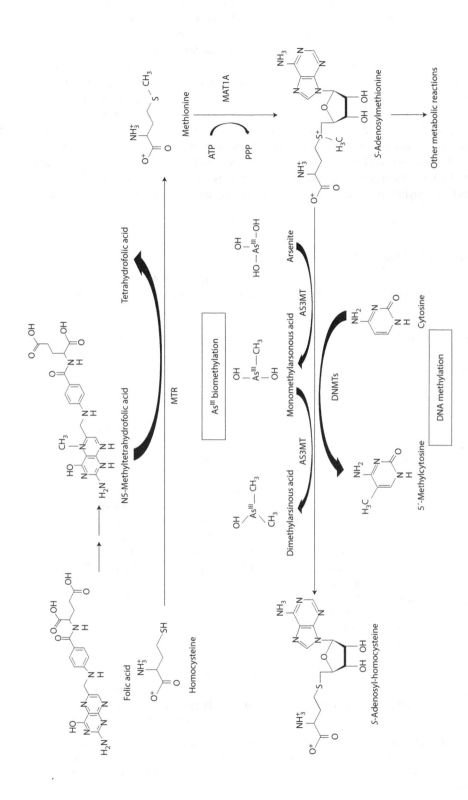

FIGURE 3.14 Simplified scheme of SAM synthesis and its involvement in arsenic and DNA methylation. The human arsenic metabolic pathway involves a series of methylation reactions; both arsenic metabolism and DNA methylation require SAM as the methyl donor. Here, they show the intermediate steps of SAM synthesis and its involvement in the methylation of DNA and arsenic. Abbreviations: AS3MT: arsenic (+3 oxidation state) methyltransferase; ATP: Adenosine-t'-triphosphate; MAT1A: methionine adenosyltransferase 1; MTR: 5–methyltetrahydrofolate-homocysteine methyltransferase; PPP: tripolyphosphate. (From Razin A., Riggs A. D. 1980. *Science* 210 (4470):604–610.)

Similarly, exposure of fish to As[III] for 1, 4, or 7 days resulted in sustained DNA hypomethylation compared with nonexposed fish.[281] Studies in cell lines *in vitro* yielded similar results, with a reduction in global genomic DNA methylation resulting from As[III] exposure (Table 3.31).[239,266,267,279,280] In contrast to the animal and *in vitro* findings, there are limited human population studies available. A cross-sectional study of 64 people reported by Majumdar et al.[281] indicated that exposure to arsenic-contaminated water (250–500 μg/L) was associated with global DNA hypermethylation. However, the participants in the highest estimated exposure group (>500 μg/L) had methylation levels that were comparable with those in the two lowest groups. The one possible reason for this inconsistency may be that the actual intake of arsenic into the body is different in the participants whose exposures were estimated based on the concentrations in their drinking water. In another well-designed nested case–control study, Pilsner et al.[224] assessed the relationship between arsenic and DNA methylation in 294 participants and observed a positive association between urinary arsenic and DNA hypermethylation. Plasma folate level apparently has a significant effect on the level

TABLE 3.31
Arsenic Exposure and Global DNA Methylation

Model	Arsenical	Dose	Time (weeks)	Global DNA Methylation	References
Human cells					
Prostate epithelial cell line RWPE—1	As[III]	5 μM	16	Hypo	Coppin et al.[267]
Prostate epithelial cell line RWPE-1	As[III]	5 μM	29	Hypo	Benbrahim-Tallaa et al.[279]
HaCaT keratinocytes	As[III]	0.2 μM	4	Hypo	Reichard et al.[266]
Animal cells					
TRL 1215 rat liver Epithelial cell line	As[III]	125–500 nM	18	Hypo	Zhao et al.[239]
V79-C13 Chinese hamster Cells	As[III]	10 μM	8	Hypo	Sciandrello et al.[280]
Animal studies					
Goldfish	As[III]	200 μM	1	Hypo	Bagnyukova et al.[278]
Fisher 344 rat	As[III]	450 μg/g body weight	12	Hypo	Uthus and Davis[274]
129/SvJ mice	As[III]	45 ppm	49	Hypo	Chen et al.[275]
C3H mice	As[III]	85 ppm	1.5	Hypo	Waalkes et al.[283]
C57BL/6J mice	As[III]	2.6–14.6 μg/g body weight	18.5	Hypo	Okoji et al.[276]
Homozygous TgAC mice	As[III]	150 ppm	17	Hypo	Xie et al.[277]
	As[v]	200 ppm			
	MMA[v]	1500 ppm			
	DMA[v]	1200 ppm			
Human subjects					
	As[III]	2–250 μg/L	NA	Hyper	Pilsner et al.[224]; Majumdar et al.[281]
	As[III]	2–250 μg/L	NA	Hypo (in skin lesion patients)	Pilsner et al.[282]

Source: Pilsner, J. R. et al. 2009. Folate deficiency, hyperhomocysteinemia, low urinary creatinine, and hypomethylation of leukocyte DNA are risk factors for arsenic-induced skin lesions. *Environ. Health Perspect.* 117:254–260.

Abbreviations: Hyper, hypermethylated; Hypo, hypomethylated; NA, not available. See text for additional information on human subjects.

of DNA methylation because a dose–response relation was evident only among participants with adequate folate levels (≥9 nmol/L) when estimates were stratified according to plasma folate level after controlling for other factors. In a separate but closely related nested case-control study, Pilsner et al.[282] found that individuals with hypomethylation of peripheral blood leukocyte (PBL) DNA were 1.8 (95% confidence interval, 1.2–2.8) times more likely to have skin lesions 2 years later after adjusting for age, urinary arsenic, and other factors. Pilsner et al.[282] speculated that

> adequate folate may be permissive for an adaptive increase in genomic methylation of PBL DNA associated with [arsenic] exposure, and that individuals who are similarly exposed but in whom the increase in genomic DNA methylation does not occur (or cannot be sustained) are at elevated risk for skin lesions.

Further studies are required to determine if exposure to As[III] has differential effects on the status of DNA methylation across tissues, cells, and species (Table 3.32).

Arsenic and Gene Promoter Methylation

Although the effects of arsenic exposure on global genomic DNA methylation remain unclear, DNA hypomethylation or hypermethylation of promoters of some genes has been reported in human skin cancer[285] and bladder cancer[286,287] associated with arsenic exposure. It has also been observed in human cell lines,[288–291] animal cell lines,[295,298] animals,[276,283,293] and humans[285–287,292] exposed to arsenic (Table 3.32). Although the gene-specific effect observed in these studies could be due to study bias, since researchers examined only a small group of genes, the similar methylation pattern repeatedly reported in the same genes after arsenic exposure might also suggest that arsenic could selectively target specific genes. However, little is known about how DNA methylation is targeted to specific regions.[294] Hypo- and hypermethylation of genes could mediate carcinogenesis through upregulation of oncogene expression or downregulation of tumor suppressor genes, respectively. Both observations have been reported. Hypomethylation of the promoter region of oncogenic *Hras1* and an elevated *Hras1* mRNA level was demonstrated in mice treated with sodium arsenite.[276] Similar results on mRNA expression and promoter hypomethylation of *Hras1* and *c-myc* were also observed *in vitro*.[295,298] The evidence has linked overexpression of *Esr1* (estrogen receptor 1) gene with estrogen-induced hepatocellular carcinoma in mice.[296] Arsenic exposure leads to overexpression of the *Esr1* gene resulting from hypomethylation of its promoter region, indicating an association between overexpression of *Esr1* and arsenic hepatocarcinogenesis.[275,283]

Dose-dependent hypermethylation at the promoter region of several tumor suppressor genes [e.g., *p15*, *p16*, *p53*, and death-associated protein kinase (*DAPK*)] was induced by arsenic exposure *in vitro* and *in vivo*.[284,285,289,291,292] In a population-based study of human bladder cancer in 351 patients, *RASSF1A* and *PRSS3* promoter hypermethylation was positively associated with toenail arsenic concentrations, and promoter hypermethylation in both genes also was associated with invasive (vs. noninvasive low grade) cancer.[297] This outcome was recapitulated in arsenic-induced lung cancer in A/J mice, in which the arsenic exposure reduced the expression of *RASSF1A* resulting from hypermethylation of its promoter region and was associated with arsenic-induced lung carcinogenesis.[293] DAPK is a positive mediator of γ-interferon–induced programmed cell death and a tumor suppressor candidate. In a study of 38 patients with urothelial carcinoma, Chen et al.[286] reported hypermethylation of *DAPK* in 13 of 17 tumors in patients living in arsenic-contaminated areas compared with 8 of 21 tumors from patients living in areas not contaminated with arsenic. This hypermethylation of *DAPK* was also observed in an *in vitro* study when immortalized human uroepithelial cells were exposed to arsenic.[288] The increase in DNA hypermethylation of promoter in *p16* was observed in arseniasis patients compared with people with no history of arsenic exposure.[292] In another study, Chanda et al.[285] examined the methylation status of promoters in *p53* and *p16* in DNA extracted from peripheral lymphocytes and observed an increase in methylation in both

TABLE 3.32

Arsenic Exposure and Gene-Specific (Promoter) Methylation Status

Mode	Arsenical	Dose	Time (weeks)	Genes Hyper	Genes Hypo	Reference
Human cells						
UROtsa urothelial cells	As[III]	1 μM	9	DBC1, FAM183A		Jensen et al.[290]
	MMA[III]	50 nM		ZSCAN12, C1QTNF6 DAPK		
Urothelial SV-HUC-1 cells	As[III]	2, 4, 10 μM	24 or 52	P16		Chai et al.[288]
Myeloma cell line U266	As[III]	1.2 μM	0.4			Fu and Shen[289]
Lung adenocarcinoma A549	As[III]	0.08–2 μM	0.3	P53		Mass and Wang[291]
Cells	As[III]	30–300 μM	0.3			
Animal cells						
Syrian hamster embryo cells	As[III]	3–10 μM	0.3	c-myc, c-Ha-ras		Takahashi et al.[295]
	As[v]	50–150 μM	0.3			
Trl 1215 rat liver epithelial Cells	As[III]	125–500 nM	8–18	c-myc		Chen et al.[298]
Animal studies						
C57BL/6J mice	As[III]	2.6–14.6 μg body weight	18.5		c-Ha-ras	Okoji et al.[276]
A/J mice	As[v]	100 ppm	74	P16,RASSF1		Cui et al.[293] Waalkes et al.[283]
C3H mice	As[III]	85 ppm	1.4		ER[06]	
Human subjects						
	As[III]	NA	NA	DAPK		Chen et al.[286]
	As[III]	Variable[a]	NA	053,P16		Chanda et al.[285]
	As[III]	NA	NA	P16		Zhang et al.[292]
	As[III]	Variable[b]	NA	RASSF1A,PRS3		Marsit et al.[297]

Source: Pilsner, J. R. et al. 2009. *Environ. Health Perspect.* 117: 254–260.

Abbreviations: ERa, estrogen receptor a; Hyper, hypermethylated; Hypo, hypomethylated; NA not available.

[a] Study subjects were grouped based on historical arsenic concentration in drinking water, and the range of arsenic concentration in drinking water was <50 μg/L and >300 μg/L.

[b] The estimated toenail arsenic concentration of study subjects was <0.01 μg/L and >50 μg/L.

p53 and *p16* associated with an estimated arsenic exposure in a dose-dependent manner. However, this same study also showed that the subjects from the highest arsenic exposure group exhibited hypomethylation of both *p53* and *p16*. Chronic exposure to arsenic *in vitro* has been shown to induce malignant transformation in several human cell types[239,279] in which the alteration of DNA methylation level has been shown to be involved.[239,290,299]

Manganese Intellectual Impairment in School-Age Children Exposed to Manganese from Drinking Water

Manganese is an essential nutrient involved in the metabolism of amino acids, proteins, and lipids, but in excess can be a potent neurotoxicant. Occupational and environmental exposure to airborne manganese has been associated with neurobehavioral deficits in adults and children.[300,301] In exposed workers, neurobehavioral deficits have been shown to correlate with manganese deposition in the brain observed by magnetic resonance imaging.[302]

Manganese is commonly found in groundwater because of the weathering and leaching of manganese-bearing minerals and rocks into the aquifers; concentrations can vary by several orders of magnitude.[303] Since homeostatic mechanisms regulate manganese concentration in the organism, notably low absorption levels and a high rate of presystemic elimination by the liver,[304] it is generally believed that the oral route poses no significant toxic risk.[305] Moreover, exposure to manganese from water consumption has been of little concern, because the intake of manganese from ingestion of water is small compared with that from foods, except for infants.[306]

Few data are available on the risks from exposure to manganese from drinking water. One study in adults[307] and three studies in children[308-310] suggest that high manganese levels in water can be neurotoxic. In the Chinese province of Shanxi, 92 children 11–13 years of age, exposed to 240–350 μg manganese/L in water, had elevated hair manganese concentration (MnH), impaired manual dexterity and speed, short-term memory, and visual identification when compared with children from a control area.[309] In Bangladesh, higher manganese concentration in water (MnW) was significantly associated with lower intelligence quotient (IQ) in 142 children 10 years of age; the mean MnW was 800 μg/L.[310] In Quebec (Canada), our pilot study on 46 children 6–15 years of age showed that those exposed to higher MnW had significantly higher MnH, and the latter was associated with teacher-reported hyperactive and oppositional behaviors.[308] Finally, two case reports show child manganese intoxication from water containing >1000 μg manganese/L, one presenting with attention and memory impairments[311] and the other with neurologic symptoms including a repetitive stuttered speech, poor balance, coordination, and fine motor skills.[312]

Manganese concentration in drinking water is not regulated in the United States or Canada. Health-based guidelines for the maximum level of manganese in drinking water are set at 300 μg/L by the U.S. Environmental Protection Agency (EPA)[718] and at 400 μg/L by the World Health Organization (WHO).[313]

They conducted this cross-sectional study in southern Quebec (Canada) between June 2007 and June 2009. Municipalities were considered as potential study sites if their aqueduct was supplied by groundwater. They selected eight municipalities to achieve a gradient of Mn manganese. Recruitment was restricted to children who had lived in the same house for >3 months, to ensure continuous exposure to the same source of water for this minimum period of time; 362 children (age 6–13 years) participated in the study.

They collected a hair sample from the occiput of each child, cutting as close as possible to the root. They used the 2 cm closest to the scalp and washed samples to minimize external contamination, using the method described by Wright et al.[314] In a test phase, they photographed hair strands with an electronic microscope and observed that the washing procedure effectively removed all particulates from the surface of the hair strand without compromising its structural integrity. They measured metals (manganese, lead [Pb], iron [Fe], arsenic [As], zinc [Zn], and copper [Cu]) by inductively coupled plasma-mass spectrometry (ICP-MS). Details of the analyses are in the Supplemental Material (doi:10.1289/ehp.1002321 via http://dx.doi.org/).

When manganese concentrations for certified hair material were outside of the designated concentrations, they excluded the measures from the analyses. Nine children who reported using hair dye in the preceding 5 months were also excluded, because hair dye could influence manganese hair content.[315] Children who reported use of hair dye had higher Mn compared with the others (geometric mean [GM], 1.1 μg/g, and 0.7 μg/g, respectively). A total of 302 children were included in the analyses of Mn.

During the home visit, a parent responded to an interview-administered questionnaire about the source of the domestic tap water (private well/public well), residential history, and changes to domestic water treatments. They collected a water sample from the kitchen tap and a second sample when there was a point-of-use filter (filter attached to the tap). They used the following procedure to standardize tap water sampling (van den Hoven and Slaats[316]): (a) open the tap for

5 minutes, (b) close and leave untouched for 30 minutes, and (c) collect first draw samples. They added 0.15 mL nitric acid (50%) to the 50-mL water sample and stored samples at 4°C. They measured metals (manganese, Pb, Fe, As, Zn, and Cu) by ICP-MS. Calibration curves were run every 30 samples, along with field and laboratory blanks and quality controls (CRM TM-26.3; Environment Canada, Laboratory for Environmental Testing, Burlington, ON, Canada) every 15 samples.

For a subsample of participating families (n = 20), they sampled tap water on three occasions over a 1-year period to examine time-dependent variability.

During the home visit, they orally administered a semiquantitative food frequency questionnaire to the parent and the child to assess manganese intake from the diet and water consumption. They used 3-dimensional models of portion size to obtain more precise estimates for all sites except the first site; thus, data for these participants (n = 16) were not included in the analyses on dietary intake. They estimated manganese intake from water consumption for direct water ingestion and for water incorporated in food preparations. They estimated water consumption from different sources—bottled, tap, tap filtered with a pitcher, and tap with an attached filter. For each water source, the amount consumed was multiplied by the measured or estimated concentration of manganese, yielding a total intake in micrograms per month. Further methodological details can be found in the Supplemental Material (doi:10.1289/ehp.1002321 via http://dx.doi.org/).

They used the Wechsler Abbreviated Scale of Intelligence (WASI) to assess general cognitive abilities.[317] This standardized test yields a Verbal IQ score (based on the subtests Vocabulary and Similarities), a Performance IQ score (Block Design and Matrix Reasoning), and a Full Scale IQ score. Throughout the study, three psychometricians administered the WASI, but all scoring was performed by the same person. They administered the WASI within 1 week of tap water sampling.

They collected information from the mother on factors that might confound the association between manganese exposure and cognitive abilities of the child, such as socioeconomic status indicators (i.e., maternal education, family income, and structure), parity, and alcohol and tobacco consumption during pregnancy. They assessed maternal nonverbal intelligence with Raven's Progressive Matrices Test,[318] home cognitive stimulation with a modified version of the Short-Form HOME (Home Observation for Measurement of the Environment) interview,[319] and maternal symptoms of depression with the Beck Depression Inventory-II.[320] Data on family income were missing for four families, and the Raven score was missing for one mother; for missing data, they assigned the mean value of individuals with data.

The distributions of manganese concentrations in hair and water, as well as manganese intakes, were considerably skewed. They thus employed log_{10} transformation to normalize residuals. Similarly, they log-transformed the concentrations of other elements measured in water. Manganese intakes from consumption of water and from the diet were divided by the weight of the child for use in the analyses (micrograms per kilogram per month). They used generalized estimating equations (GEE) to examine relationships between exposure to manganese and children's IQ scores. GEE is an extension of generalized linear models for nonindependent data.[321] These analyses were used to account for the community- and family-clustered data in our study. Some of the advantages of using GEE, instead of the more common approach of mixed models with random intercepts, include more efficient estimators of regression parameters and reasonably accurate standard errors (i.e., confidence intervals [Cis] with the correct coverage rates). With GEE, the computational complexity is a function of the size of the largest cluster rather than of the number of clusters—an advantage and a source of reliable estimates when there are many small clusters,[322] such as in the present study (i.e., the 251 families). CIs were calculated with Wald statistics. An exchangeable working covariance matrix was used, with a robust estimator providing a consistent estimate of the covariance even when the working correlation matrix is misspecified.

Changes in IQ were examined in relation to four manganese exposure metrics reflecting different assumptions for exposure pathways and toxicokinetics: MnW, MnH, manganese intake from water consumption, and dietary manganese intake. The change in IQ (β) associated with a 10-fold increase in manganese exposure indicators was examined with adjustments for two sets of covariates. The first set of covariates (model A) was chosen based on the examination of directed acyclic graphs[323] and included several socioeconomic indicators. Since manganese causes aesthetic problems, families which have the means might treat water domestically to remove it. The second set of covariates (model B) included the same variables as model A, as well as variables significantly associated with IQ or MnW, to reduce the unexplained variance, thus diminishing type 2 error.[324] They conducted sensitivity analyses on inclusion of additional covariates in the models. They used 0.05 as the threshold for statistical significance (two-sided tests). They examined residuals for normality and homoscedasticity and detected no problem.

This study included 362 children from 251 families. Most children (85%) had resided for >12 months in their present home. The mean ($\pm$ SD) age of the children was 9.3 ± 1.8 years; range, 6.2–13.4 years, and 99% of children were white. Seventy-eight percent of mothers had at least some college education (Table 3.33). Tap MnW ranged from 1 to 2700 μg/L (Table 3.34), with an arithmetic mean of 98 μg/L and a GM of 20 μg/L. MnW from repeated sampling in the same residence for over a period of 1 year had an intraclass correlation coefficient of 0.91.

MnW was not associated with socioeconomic or other family characteristics such as family income, family structure, home stimulation score, nonverbal maternal intelligence, or maternal education (Table 3.33). MnW was lower in houses with a private well (GM, 8 μg/L) than in those on a public well (GM, 55 μg/L). The concentration distribution for elements other than manganese in residential tap water is in the Supplemental Material (doi:10.1289/ehp.1002321 via http://dx.doi.org/). The Pearson correlation of MnW with other elements was 0.68 (Fe), 0.26 (Zn), 0.11 (Cu), 0.06 (As), and -0.02 (Pb).

The median of estimated manganese intakes from direct consumption of water (1.6 μg/kg/month) was similar to the median of intakes from water incorporated into food preparations (1.9 μg/kg/month) (Table 3.34). The estimated dietary manganese intakes were much higher than the intakes from water consumption, with a median of 2335 μg/kg/month (Table 3.34).

Children's MnH increased with MnW and estimated manganese intake from water consumption (Figure 3.15a), but not from the estimated dietary manganese intake (Figure 3.15b). In a multivariate model, MnH was significantly associated with manganese intake from water consumption ($p < 0.001$) but not with dietary intake ($p = 0.76$). In this multivariate model, there was no difference in MnH between boys and girls ($p = 0.46$; GM for both, 0.7 μg/g), and age was not associated with MnH ($p = 0.88$) (Table 3.35).

MANGANESE EXPOSURE AND CHILDREN'S IQ

Estimated dietary manganese intake was not significantly associated with IQ scores in unadjusted or adjusted analyses (results not shown). MnW, estimated manganese intake from water consumption, and MnH were significantly associated with lower full scale IQ scores in unadjusted analyses. Adjustment for covariates, with either model A or model B, did not considerably change the point estimates. Higher MnW was significantly associated with lower full scale IQ scores in model A (change in scores for a 10-fold increase in concentration (β) = -1.9 [95% CI, -3.1 to -0.7]) and model B ($\beta = -2.4$ [95% CI, -3.9 to -0.9]). Higher MnW was also significantly associated with lower performance IQ scores in model A ($\beta = -2.3$ [95% CI, -3.7 to -0.8]) and model B ($\beta = -3.1$ [95% CI, -4.9 to -1.3]). Higher MnW was associated with lower verbal IQ scores, significantly for model A but not for model B. (The point estimates were similar for both models but the 95% CI was larger for model B.) Higher estimated manganese intake from water consumption was significantly associated with lower full scale and performance IQ, both in model A and model B. Sex-stratified analyses on MnW and full scale IQ resulted in a higher point estimate for girls (using model B, $\beta = -3.2$ [95% CI, -5.0 to -1.5]) than for boys ($\beta = -2.3$ [95% CI, -4.8 to 0.2]), but the term for interaction with sex was not significant ($p = 0.14$).

TABLE 3.33
Manganese Concentrations in Domestic Tap Water (μg/L) by Characteristics of Participant

Characteristic	Frequency	Percent	MnW (GM)	p-Value[a]
Sex of child[b]				0.71
Male	168	46	19	
Female	194	54	21	
Child drinks tap water[b]				0.41
No	121	33	23	
Yes	241	67	19	
Maternal smoking during pregnancy[b]				0.13
No	265	73	18	
Yes	97	27	27	
Maternal alcohol consumption during pregnancy[b]				0.10
No	310	86	22	
Yes	52	14	13	
Home tap water source[c]				<0.001
Private well	117	47	8	
Public well	134	53	55	
Family income[c]				0.28
≤Can$50,000	106	42	27	
>Can$50,000	145	58	20	
Family structure[c]				0.87
Two biological parents	189	75	22	
One biological and one nonbiological parent	37	15	21	
Single parent	25	10	28	
Maternal education[c]				0.86
Less than high school	11	4	13	
High school diploma	44	18	24	
Some college	116	46	24	
Some university	80	32	21	
Nonverbal maternal intelligence (Raven)[c]				0.71
<23	94	38	110	
23–25	94	38	84	
>25	63	25	123	
Maternal depressive symptoms (Beck-II scorer)[c]				0.08
Normal range	206	82	24	
Mild symptoms	34	14	11	
Moderate or severe symptoms	11	4	40	

Source: Bouchard, M. F. et al. 2011. *Environ. Health Perspect.* 119: 138–143. http://dx.doi.org/10.1289/ehp.1002321 [online September 20, 2010].

[a] Difference in MnW, from univariato general linear models.

[b] One measure per child (n = 382).

[c] One measure per family (n = 251).

When MnH was examined as the predictor of IQ in unadjusted analyses, it was significantly associated with lower full scale IQ scores but not performance or verbal IQ scores (Table 3.35). In adjusted analyses, higher MnH was associated with lower full scale IQ scores, both in model A ($\beta = -3.7$ [95% CI, -6.5 to -0.8]) and in model B ($\beta = -3.3$ [95% CI, -6.1 to -0.5]). MnH was also associated with lower performance and verbal IQ scores, although these relations did not reach statistical significance except for verbal IQ in model A ($\beta = -3.1$ [95% CI, -5.9 to -0.3]).

TABLE 3.34
Distribution of Concentrations for Manganese in Drinking Water and Children's Hair, as well as Manganese Intakes from Water Consumption and Dietary Sources

			Percentile					
Manganese Exposure Indicators	**n**	**Min**	**5th**	**25th**	**50th**	**75th**	**95th**	**Max**
Manganese concentrations								
Tap water manganese (μg/L)	362	0.1	0.5	2.5	30.8	128	255	2,700
Hair manganese (μg/g)	302	0.1	0.2	0.3	0.7	1.6	4.7	21
Manganese intakes (μg/kg/month)								
From drinking water	362	0.0	0.0	0.0	1.6	22.9	160	566
From water used in food preparations	362	0.0	0.0	0.2	1.9	14.5	149	480
Total intake from water consumption	362	0.0	0.0	1.0	8.0	59.6	286	945
From dietary sources	346	311	840	1,632	2,335	3,487	6,418	13,159

Source: Bouchard, M. F. et al. 2011. Environ. Health Perspect. 119:138–143. http://dx.doi.org/10.1289/ehp.1002321 [online September 20, 2010].
Abbreviations: Max, maximum; Min, minimum.

Sex-stratified analyses resulted in higher point estimates for the association between MnH and full scale IQ for girls ($\beta = -4.8$ [95% CI, −8.1 to −1.6]) than for boys ($\beta = -3.5$ [95% CI, −8.7 to 1.6]), but the term for interaction with sex was not significant ($p = 0.55$).

IQ scores decrease steadily with increasing MnW (Figure 3.16a). Children in the highest MnW quintile (median, 216 μg/L) scored 6.2 points below those in the lowest quintile (median, 1 μg/L). For estimated manganese intake from water ingestion (Figure 3.16b), children in the lowest quintile had the highest IQ scores, and those in the highest quintile had the lowest scores, but point estimates in the middle quintiles did not show a consistent pattern of increasing or decreasing trend. There was a steeper decrease for children in the highest quintile. A similar plot for dietary manganese intake showed no association, even in the higher range of intakes (data not shown).

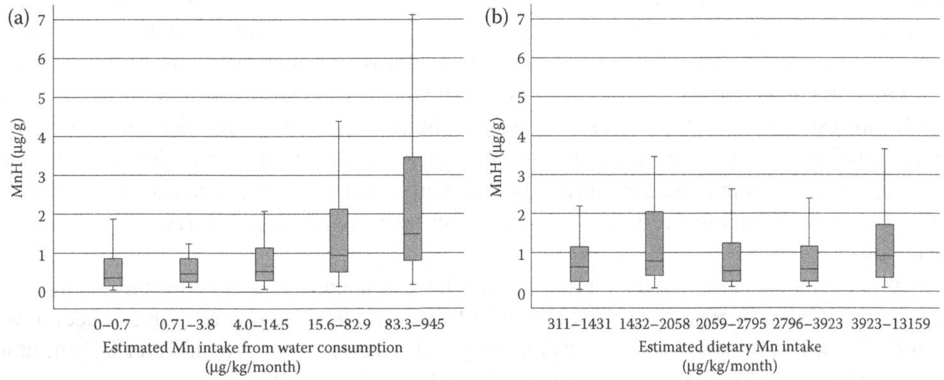

FIGURE 3.15 Distribution of MnH by quintiles of (a) estimated manganese intake from water consumption ($n = 302$), and (b) estimated manganese intake from the diet ($n = 288$). (Central bar: 50th percentile; lower and upper bounds of the rectangle: 25th and 75th percentiles; lower and upper tails: 5th and 95th percentiles. Observations outside the 95% CIs are not shown.). (From Bouchard, M. F. et al. 2011. *Environ. Health Perspect.* 119:138–143. http://dx.doi.org/10.1289/ehp.1002321 [online September 20, 2010].)

TABLE 3.35

Unadjusted and Adjusted Changes in Children's IQ for a 10-fold Increase in Indicators of Manganese Exposure (β [95% CIs])

Model	MnW (n = 362)	Manganese Intake from Water Consumption (n = 362)	MnH (n = 302)
Unadjusted model			
Full Scale IQ	−2.1(−3.5 to −0.8)**	−1.3 (−2.5 to −0.2)*	−3.2 (−6.2 to−0.2)*
Performance IQ	−2.4(−4.0 to −0.7)**	−1.6(−3.0 to −0.3)*	−2.5 (−5.7 to 0.8)
Verbal IQ	−1.4(−2.6 to −0.2)*	−0.7 (−1.7 to 0.3)	−2.8 (−5.6 to 0.5)
Adjusted model A[a]			
Full Scale IQ	−1.9(−3.1 to −0.7)**	−1.2 (−2.3 to −0.1)*	−3.7 (−6.5 to−0.8)*
Performance IQ	−2.3(−3.7 to −0.8)**	−1.6 (−2.9 to −0.3)*	−3.0 (−6.1 to 0.1)
Verbal IQ	−1.5(−2.6 to −0.3)*	−0.6 (−1.6 to 0.3)	−3.1(−5.9 to−0.3)*
Adjusted model B[b]			
Full Scale IQ	−2.4(−3.9 to −0.9)**	−1.2(−2.3 to −0.1)*	−3.3(−6.1 to −0.5)*
Performance 10	−3.1 (−4.9 to −1.3)**	−1.9 (−3.3 to −0.4)*	−2.8(−5.9 to 0.4)
Verbal IQ	−1.2(−2.7 to 0.3)	−0.3 (−1.4 to 0.7)	−2.7 (−5.4 to 0.1)

Source: Bouchard, M. F. et al. 2011. *Environ. Health Perspect.* 119:138–143. http://dx.doi.org/10.1289/ehp. 1002321 [online September 20, 2010].

[a] Adjusted for maternal education (less than high school/high school diploma/some college/some university) and nonverbal intelligence, family income, home stimulation score, and family structure (two biological parents/one biological and one nonbiological parent/single parent).

[b] Adjusted for same variables as above, and sex and age of child, IQ testing session (started at 0900/1300/1500), source of water (private well/public well), and Fe concentration in tap water.

*p < 0.05. **p < 0.01.

They conducted sensitivity analyses on the inclusion of additional covariates in the models: birth weight of the child, rank of the child in the family, maternal smoking or alcohol consumption during pregnancy, maternal depressive symptoms, psychometrician, and concentration of Pb, As, Cu, and Zn in tap water. They did not retain these covariates, because they did not change point estimates by >10% and were not significantly associated with IQ scores (p > 0.2).

This study shows that children exposed to a higher concentration of manganese in tap water had lower IQ scores. This finding was robust to adjustment for socioeconomic status indicators and other metals present in water. The association between MnW and IQ scores was strong, with a 6.2 full scale IQ point difference between the children exposed to water with 1 and 216 µg manganese/L (median of lowest and highest quintiles). Manganese intake from water ingestion, but not from the diet, was significantly associated with elevated manganese concentration in children's hair. These findings suggest that manganese exposure from drinking water is metabolized differently than that from the diet and can lead to overload and subsequent neurotoxic effects expressed by intellectual impairments in children.

In New England, 45% of wells for public use have manganese concentrations >30 µg/L.[303] Throughout the United States, approximately 5% of domestic household wells have concentrations >300 µg/L[325] (U.S. Geological Survey, 2009). Elevated manganese in groundwater is common in several countries including Sweden,[719] Vietnam,[336] and Bangladesh.[310]

The present findings are consistent with those of the two previous studies examining drinking water manganese-related cognitive deficits in children, although in the present study the mean manganese concentration was considerably lower than in the others: 100 µg/L versus approximately 300 µg/L[309] and 800 µg/L.[310] Similar to our findings, Wasserman et al.[310] observed a stronger association of water manganese level with performance IQ than with verbal IQ.

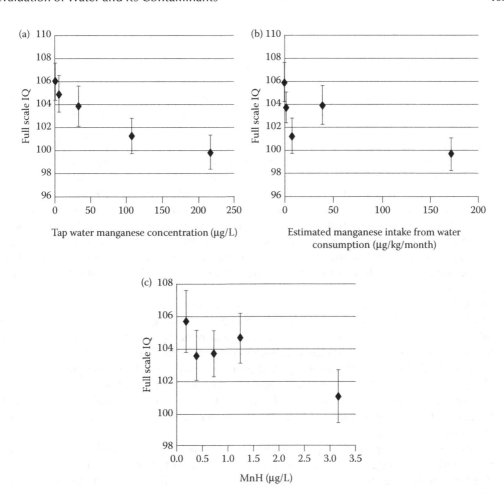

FIGURE 3.16 Mean full scale IQ (±SE), with respect to manganese exposure indicators, adjusted for covariates in model B. (a) IQ is plotted by median of tap water manganese concentration (μg/L) quintiles. The medians and ranges of MnW are as follows: 1st quintile (lowest), 1 (0–2); 2nd, 6 (3–19); 3rd, 34 (20–66); 4th, 112 (67–153); and 5th (highest), 216 (154–2,700). (b) IQ is plotted by median of manganese intake from water consumption (μg/kg/month) quintiles. The medians and ranges of manganese intakes are as follows: 1st quintile (lowest), 0.1 (0–0.7); 2nd, 1.6 (0.71–3.8), 3rd, 7.6 (4.0–14.6), 4th, 39.4 (15.6–82.9), and 5th (highest), 172 (83.3–945). (c) IQ is plotted by median of MnH (μg/g) quintiles. The medians and ranges of MnH are as follows: 1st quintile (lowest), 0.2 (0.1–0.3); 2nd, 0.4 (0.31–0.5); 3rd, 0.7 (0.51–0.9); 4th, 1.2 (0.91–1.9); and 5th (highest), 3.2 (1.91–20.7). (From Bouchard, M. F. et al. 2011. *Environ. Health Perspect.* 119:138–143. http://dx.doi.org/10.1289/ehp.1002321 [online September 20, 2010].)

The different manganese exposure indicators showed consistent associations with lower IQ scores, although the shape of the dose–response curve differed by exposure indicators. Full scale IQ scores decreased steadily with increasing MnW, but a discernible diminution in IQ was present only at higher concentrations of MnH. Interestingly, tap water manganese concentration was a better predictor of children's IQ scores than the estimated intake from water ingestion, possibly because of error measurement in intakes. However, there may be pathways of exposure not captured by assessment of the ingested dose, such as inhalation of aerosols containing manganese ions in the shower,[326] although this hypothesis is debated.[327] More studies are needed on manganese toxicokinetics and neurotoxicity to better understand these findings.

Their study does not address the mechanisms involved in manganese-related cognitive impairments, but an extensive body of literature shows perturbation of neurotransmitter activities,[328] notably disruption of the striatal dopaminergic system. Studies also reported data suggestive of perturbations of gamma-aminobutyric acid and serotonin.[329,330] Manganese effects can be persistent; adult mice exposed by gavage as juveniles had decreased striatal dopamine activity.[331] In nonhuman primates, chronic manganese exposure causes accumulation of the metal in the basal ganglia, white matter, and cortical structures, with signs of neuronal degeneration.[332,333] Perturbations in the regulation of other metals in the brain could also be implicated in the cognitive impairment associated with manganese exposure.[334]

In this study, dietary manganese intake was similar to the recommended dietary allowance of 1.5–1.9 mg/day for children 6–13 years of age.[335] Manganese intake from ingestion of water was very small compared with the amount ingested from foods (by more than two orders of magnitude), yet only intake from water was significantly associated with MnH content. Previous studies have likewise reported a relation between the concentration of manganese in drinking water and hair.[307–309,336] This suggests that there might be differences in the regulation of manganese present in food and water. The chemical form of manganese, notably the valence state and solubility, might modify its toxicity, perhaps because of changes in toxicokinetic properties.[337] Moreover, manganese absorption is decreased in the digestive system with concurrent intake of dietary fiber, oxalic acids, tannins, and phytic acids.[338]

Currently, no consensus has emerged as to the optimal biomarker of exposure to manganese.[720] Even at very high MnW, no relation was observed between water manganese and blood manganese in children[310] or adults.[307] Blood manganese can vary widely in the short term and thus might not reflect long-term exposure. For instance, in a case report of suspected manganese intoxication, three consecutive blood samples for plasma manganese on a single day showed large variability: 0.6, 2.2, and 2.4 µg/L.[312] In contrast, the manganese content in hair will reflect the metal uptake averaged over the duration of the follicle formation. The mechanism of manganese uptake into hair is not well understood, but its affinity for melanin, a protein present in hair, skin, and the central nervous system, could be involved.[339]

Manganese intake from water ingestion, but not from the diet, was significantly associated with elevated MnH, suggesting that homeostatic regulation of manganese does not prevent overload upon exposure from water. The findings from this study support the hypothesis that low-level, chronic exposure to manganese from drinking water is associated with significant intellectual impairments in children. These findings should be replicated in another population. Owing to the common occurrence of this metal in drinking water and the observed effects at low MnW, they believe that national and international guidelines for safe manganese in water should be revisited.

HAZARDOUS WASTE

The waste production from the nuclear and radio-chemicals industry is dealt with under radioactive waste. Radioactive waste comes from nuclear power plants, nuclear weapons, production sites, hospitals, and research laboratories.

The term "RCRA hazardous waste" applies to hazardous waste (waste that is ignitable, corrosive, reactive, or toxic) that is regulated under the RCRA. In 1999, EPA estimated that 20,000 businesses generating large quantities—more than 2200 pounds each per month—of hazardous waste collectively generated 40 million tons of RCRA hazardous waste. Comparisons of annual trends in hazardous waste generation are difficult because of changes in the types of data collected (e.g., exclusion of wastewater over the past several years). However, the amount of a specific set of priority toxic chemicals found in hazardous waste and tracked in the Toxics Release Inventory is declining. In 1999, approximately 69% of the RCRA hazardous waste was disposed of on land by one of four disposal methods: deep well/underground injection, landfill disposal, surface impoundment, or land treatment/application farming. These technologies may give us a short-term respite, but what about the long-term consequences?

NUCLEAR EXPOSURES THAT HAVE LED TO CHRONIC ILLNESSES

Los Alamos, New Mexico

The first atomic bomb was set off in the Los Alamos area of New Mexico. Residents of this area know that the water is contaminated with radioactive waste. The residents we have seen from this area with chemical sensitivity all seem to have a residual of radioactive signs in their hair analysis. They have also developed chemically sensitivity in parallel or as a result of this overexposure.

Hiroshima and Nagasaki

The United States dropped an atomic bomb on each of these cities and there were many deaths, as well as acute and chronic injuries that presented. Thyroiditis and dysfunction was one of the main chronic problems. Many other debilitating entities occurred during the next 30 years.

Chernobyl

The first peacetime disaster occurred in the Ukraine in the old Soviet Union. Until recently, the short- and long-term data were not available, but now this disaster can be reported and there are many increases in illness.

With the two nuclear disasters of Chernobyl and Fukushima, there are a lot more radioactive wastes dumped into the groundwater, rivers, and oceans. This drainage will again increase the radioactivity of water.

PULP AND PAPER INDUSTRY

Effluent from the pulp and paper industry is generally high in SS and BOD. Stand-alone paper mills using imported pulp may only require simple primary treatment, such as sedimentation or dissolved air flotation. Increased BOD or chemical oxygen demand (COD) loadings, as well as organic pollutants, may require biological treatment such as activated sludge or upflow anaerobic sludge blanket reactors. For mills with high inorganic loadings such as salt, tertiary treatments may be required, either general membrane treatments such as ultrafiltration or reverse osmosis or treatments to remove specific contaminants, such as nutrients.

WATER TREATMENT OF INDUSTRIAL WASTE WATER

Many industries have a need to treat water to obtain very high quality water for demanding purposes. Water treatment produces organic and mineral sludges from filtration and sedimentation. Ion exchange using natural or synthetic resins removes calcium, magnesium, and carbonate ions from water, replacing them with hydrogen and hydroxyl ions. Regeneration of ion exchange columns with strong acids and alkalis produces a wastewater rich in hardness ions which are readily precipitated out, especially when in admixture with other wastewater.

The various types of contamination of wastewater require a variety of strategies to remove the contamination.[340,341]

1. *Brine treatment*: Brine treatment involves removing dissolved salt ions from the waste stream. Although similarities to seawater or brackish water desalination exist, industrial brine treatment may contain unique combinations of dissolved ions, such as hardness ions or other metals, necessitating specific processes and equipment.

   Brine management examines the broader context of brine treatment and may include consideration of government policy and regulations, corporate sustainability, environmental impact, recycling, handling and transport, containment, centralized compared to on-site treatment, avoidance and reduction, technologies, and economics. Brine management also shares some issues with leachate management and more general waste management.

2. *Solids removal*: Most solids can be removed using simple sedimentation techniques with the solids recovered as slurry or sludge. Very fine solids and solids with densities close to the density of water pose special problems. In such cases, filtration or ultrafiltration may be required, although flocculation may be used, using alum salts or the addition of polyelectrolytes.

   Oils and grease removal: Many oils can be recovered from open water surfaces by skimming devices. Considered a dependable and cheap way to remove oil, grease, and other hydrocarbons from water, oil skimmers can sometimes achieve the desired level of water purity. At other times, skimming is also a cost-efficient method to remove most of the oil before using membrane filters and chemical processes. Skimmers will prevent filters from blinding prematurely and keep chemical costs down because there is less oil to process.

   Since grease skimming involves higher viscosity hydrocarbons, skimmers must be equipped with heaters powerful enough to keep grease fluid for discharge. If floating grease forms into solid clumps or mats, a spray bar, aerator, or mechanical apparatus can be used to facilitate removal.[342]

   However, hydraulic oils and the majority of oils that have degraded to any extent will also have a soluble or emulsified component that will require further treatment to eliminate. Dissolving or emulsifying oil using surfactants or solvents usually exacerbates the problem rather than solving it, producing wastewater that is more difficult to treat.

   The wastewaters from large-scale industries such as oil refineries, petrochemical plants, chemical plants, and natural gas processing plants commonly contain gross amounts of oil and SS. Those industries use a device known as an API oil–water separator which is designed to separate the oil and SS from their wastewater effluents. The name is derived from the fact that such separators are designed according to standards published by the American Petroleum Institute (API).[341,343]

   The API separator is a gravity separation device designed by using Stokes Law to define the rise velocity of oil droplets based on their density and size. The design is based on the specific gravity difference between the oil and the wastewater because that difference is much smaller than the specific gravity difference between the SS and water. The SS settle to the bottom of the separator as a sediment layer, the oil rises to the top of the separator, and the cleansed wastewater is the middle layer between the oil layer and the solids.[341]

   Typically, the oil layer is skimmed off and subsequently reprocessed or disposed of, and the bottom sediment layer is removed by a chain and flight scraper (or similar device) and a sludge pump. The water layer is sent for further treatment consisting usually of an electroflotation module for additional removal of any residual oil and then to some type of biological treatment unit for removal of undesirable dissolved chemical compounds.

   Parallel plate separators[344] are similar to API separators but they include tilted parallel plate assemblies (also known as parallel packs). The parallel plates provide more surface for suspended oil droplets to coalesce into larger globules. Such separators still depend upon the specific gravity between the suspended oil and the water. However, the parallel plates enhance the degree of oil–water separation. The result is that a parallel plate separator requires significantly less space than a conventional API separator to achieve the same degree of separation.

3. *Removal of biodegradable organics*: Biodegradable organic material of plant or animal origin is usually possible to treat using extended conventional sewage treatment processes such as activated sludge or trickling filter.[337,340] Problems can arise if the wastewater is excessively diluted with washing water or is highly concentrated such as undiluted blood or milk. The presence of cleaning agents, disinfectants, pesticides, or antibiotics can have detrimental impacts on treatment processes.

4. *Activated sludge process*: Activated sludge is a biochemical process for treating sewage and industrial wastewater that uses air (or oxygen) and microorganisms to biologically oxidize organic pollutants, producing a waste sludge (or floc) containing the oxidized

material. In general, an activated sludge process includes: an aeration tank where air (or oxygen) is injected and thoroughly mixed into the wastewater; and a settling tank (usually referred to as a clarifier or "settler") to allow the waste sludge to settle. Part of the waste sludge is recycled to the aeration tank and the remaining waste sludge is removed for further treatment and ultimate disposal.

5. *Trickling filter process*: A trickling filter consists of a bed of rocks, gravel, slag, peat moss, or plastic media over which wastewater flows downward and contacts a layer (or film) of microbial slime covering the bed media.

6. *Complex organic chemicals industry treatment*: A range of industries manufacture or use complex organic chemicals. These include pesticides, pharmaceuticals, paints and dyes, petrochemicals, detergents, plastics, paper pollution, and so on. Waste waters can be contaminated by feedstock materials, by-products, product material in soluble or particulate form, washing and cleaning agents, solvents, and added value products such as plasticizers. Treatment facilities that do not need control of their effluent typically opt for a type of aerobic treatment, that is, aerated lagoons.[343]

   Treatment of other organics: Synthetic organic materials including solvents, paints, pharmaceuticals, pesticides, coking products, and so forth can be very difficult to treat. Treatment methods are often specific to the material being treated. Methods include advanced oxidation processing, distillation, adsorption, vitrification, incineration, chemical immobilization, or landfill disposal. Some materials such as some detergents may be capable of biological degradation, and in such cases a modified form of wastewater treatment can be used.

7. *Treatment of acids and alkalis*: Acids and alkalis can usually be neutralized under controlled conditions. Neutralization frequently produces a precipitate that will require treatment as a solid residue that may also be toxic. In some cases, gases may be evolved requiring treatment for the gas stream. Some other forms of treatment are usually required following neutralization.

   Waste streams rich in hardness ions as from deionization processes can readily lose the hardness ions in a buildup of precipitated calcium and magnesium salts. This precipitation process can cause severe *furring* of pipes and can, in extreme cases, cause the blockage of disposal pipes. A 1-meter diameter industrial marine discharge pipe serving a major chemicals complex was blocked by such salts in the 1970s. Treatment is by concentration of deionization waste waters and disposal to landfill or by careful pH management of the released wastewater.

8. *Treatment of toxic materials*: Toxic materials including many organic materials, metals (such as zinc, silver, cadmium, thallium, etc.), acids, alkalis, and nonmetallic elements (such as arsenic or selenium) are generally resistant to biological processes unless very dilute. Metals can often be precipitated out by changing the pH or by treatment with other chemicals. Many, however, are resistant to treatment or mitigation and may require concentration followed by landfilling or recycling. Dissolved organics can be *incinerated* within the wastewater by the advanced oxidation process.

HAZARDOUS ACTIVITIES AND INDUSTRIES LIST (HAIL)

The HAIL is a compilation of activities and industries that are considered likely to cause land contamination resulting from hazardous substance use, storage, or disposal. The HAIL has grouped similar industries together, which typically use or store hazardous substances that could cause contamination if these substances escaped from safe storage, were disposed of on the site, or were lost to the environment through their use. Similar industries together, which typically use or store hazardous substances that could cause contamination if these substances escaped from safe storage, were disposed of on the site, or were lost to the environment through their use. The HAIL is intended to identify most situations in New Zealand where hazardous substances could cause and, in many cases, have caused land contamination.

1. Chemical manufacture, application, and bulk storage
   a. Agrichemicals including commercial premises used by spray contractors for filling, storing, or washing out tanks for agrichemical application
   b. Chemical manufacture, formulation, or bulk storage
   c. Commercial analytical laboratory sites
   d. Corrosives including formulation or bulk storage
   e. Dry-cleaning plants including dry-cleaning premises or the bulk storage of dry-cleaning solvents
   f. Fertilizer manufacture or bulk storage
   g. Gasworks including the manufacture of gas from coal or oil feedstocks
   h. Livestock dip or spray race operations
   i. Paint manufacture or formulation (excluding retail paint stores)
   j. Persistent pesticide bulk storage or use including sport turfs, market gardens, orchards, glass houses, or spray sheds
   k. Pest control including the premises of commercial pest control operators or any authorities that carry out pest control where bulk storage or preparation of pesticide occurs, including preparation of poisoned baits or filling or washing of tanks for pesticide application
   l. Pesticide manufacture (including animal poisons, insecticides, fungicides, or herbicides) including the commercial manufacturing, blending, mixing, or formulating of pesticides
   m. Petroleum or petrochemical industries including a petroleum depot, terminal, blending plant or refinery, or facilities for recovery, reprocessing, or recycling petroleum-based materials, or bulk storage of petroleum or petrochemicals above or below ground
   n. Pharmaceutical manufacture including the commercial manufacture, blending, mixing or formulation of pharmaceuticals, including animal remedies or the manufacturing of illicit drugs with the potential for environmental discharges
   o. Printing including commercial printing using metal type, inks, dyes, or solvents (excluding photocopy shops)
   p. Skin or wool processing including a tannery or fellmongery, or any other commercial facility for hide curing, drying, scouring, or finishing or storing wool or leather products
   q. Storage tanks or drums for fuel, chemicals, or liquid waste
   r. Wood treatment or preservation including the commercial use of antisapstain chemicals during milling, or bulk storage of treated timber outside
2. Electrical and electronic works, power generation, and transmission
   a. Batteries including the commercial assembling, disassembling, manufacturing, or recycling of batteries (but excluding retail battery stores)
   b. Electrical transformers including the manufacturing, repairing, or disposing of electrical transformers or other heavy electrical equipment
   c. Electronics including the commercial manufacturing, reconditioning, or recycling of computers, televisions, and other electronic devices
   d. Power stations, substations, or switchyards
3. Explosives and ordinances production, storage, and use
   a. Explosive or ordinance production, maintenance, dismantling, disposal, bulk storage, or repackaging
   b. Gun clubs or rifle ranges, including clay targets clubs that use lead munitions outdoors
   c. Training areas set aside exclusively or primarily for the detonation of explosive ammunition

4. Metal extraction, refining and reprocessing, storage and use
   a. Abrasive blasting including abrasive blast cleaning (excluding cleaning carried out in fully enclosed booths) or the disposal of abrasive blasting material
   b. Foundry operations including the commercial production of metal products by injecting or pouring molten metal into moulds
   c. Metal treatment or coating including polishing, anodizing, galvanizing, pickling, electroplating, or heat treatment or finishing using cyanide compounds
   d. Metalliferous ore processing including the chemical or physical extraction of metals, including smelting, refining, fusing, or refining metals
   e. Engineering workshops with metal fabrication
5. Mineral extraction, refining and reprocessing, storage and use
   a. Asbestos products manufacture or disposal including sites with buildings containing asbestos products known to be in a deteriorated condition
   b. Asphalt or bitumen manufacture or bulk storage (excluding single-use sites used by a mobile asphalt plant)
   c. Cement or lime manufacture using a kiln including the storage of wastes from the manufacturing process
   d. Commercial concrete manufacture or commercial cement storage
   e. Coal or coke yards
   f. Hydrocarbon exploration or production including well sites or flare pits
   g. Mining industries (excluding gravel extraction) including exposure of faces or release of groundwater containing hazardous contaminants, or the storage of hazardous wastes including waste dumps or dam tailings
6. Vehicle refueling, service, and repair
   a. Airports including fuel storage, workshops, wash-down areas, or fire practice areas
   b. Brake lining manufacturers, repairers, or recyclers
   c. Engine reconditioning workshops
   d. Motor vehicle workshops
   e. Port activities including dry docks or marine vessel maintenance facilities
   f. Railway yards including goods-handling yards, workshops, refueling facilities, or maintenance areas
   g. Service stations including retail or commercial refueling facilities
   h. Transport depots or yards including areas used for refueling or the bulk storage of hazardous substances
7. Cemeteries and waste recycling, treatment, and disposal
   a. Cemeteries
   b. Drum or tank reconditioning or recycling
   c. Landfill sites
   d. Scrap yards including automotive dismantling, wrecking, or scrap metal yards
   e. Waste disposal to land (excluding where biosolids have been used as soil conditioners)
   f. Waste recycling or waste or wastewater treatment
8. Any land that has been subject to the migration of hazardous substances from adjacent land in sufficient quantity that it could be a risk to human health or the environment
9. Any other land that has been subject to the intentional or accidental release of a hazardous substance in sufficient quantity that it could be a risk to human health or the environment

WORST OIL SPILLS

An oil spill is the release of a liquid petroleum hydrocarbon into the environment, especially marine areas, due to human activity, and is a form of pollution (Figure 3.17). The term is usually applied to marine oil spills, where oil is released into the ocean or coastal waters, but spills may also occur on

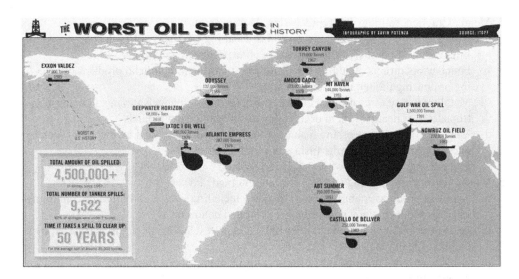

FIGURE 3.17   Worst oil spills.

land. Oil spills may be due to releases of crude oil from tankers, offshore platforms, drilling rigs and wells, as well as spills of refined petroleum products (such as gasoline, diesel) and their by-products, heavier fuels used by large ships such as bunker fuel, or the spill of any oily refuse or waste oil.

Spilled oil penetrates into the structure of the plumage of birds and the fur of mammals, reducing its insulating ability, and making them more vulnerable to temperature fluctuations and much less buoyant in the water. Cleanup and recovery from an oil spill is difficult and depends upon many factors, including the type of oil spilled, the temperature of the water (affecting evaporation and bio-degradation), and the types of shorelines and beaches involved.[345] Spills may take weeks, months, or even years to clean up.

This is a reverse chronological list of oil spills that have occurred throughout the world and spill(s) that are currently ongoing. Quantities are measured in tons of crude oil with one ton being roughly equal to 308 U.S. gallons, or 7.33 barrels, or 1165 L. This calculation uses a median value of 0.858 for the specific gravity of light crude oil; actual values can range from 0.816 to 0.893, so the amounts shown below are inexact. They are also estimates, because the actual volume of an oil spill is difficult to measure exactly (Table 3.36, Figure 3.18).

The *Deepwater Horizon* oil spill (also referred to as the BP oil spill, the BP oil disaster, the Gulf of Mexico oil spill, and the Macondo blowout) began on April 20, 2010 in the Gulf of Mexico on the BP-operated Macondo Prospect. It claimed eleven lives[407–411] and is considered the largest accidental marine oil spill in the history of the petroleum industry, an estimated 8%–31% larger in volume than the previously largest, the Ixtoc I oil spill. Following the explosion and sinking of the *Deepwater Horizon* oil rig, a seafloor oil gusher flowed for 87 days, until it was capped on July 15, 2010.[408,412] The U.S. Government estimated the total discharge at 4.9 million barrels (210 million U.S. gal; 780,000 m³).[721]

A massive response ensued to protect beaches, wetlands, and estuaries from the spreading oil uti-lizing skimmer ships, floating booms, and controlled burns and 1.84 million U.S. gallons (7000 m³) of Corexit oil dispersant.[413] Owing to the months-long spill, along with adverse effects from the response and cleanup activities, extensive damage to marine and wildlife habitats and fishing and tourism industries was reported.[414,415] In Louisiana, 4.6 million pounds of oily material was removed from the beaches in 2013, over double the amount collected in 2012. Oil cleanup crews worked four days a week on 55 miles of the Louisiana shoreline throughout 2013.[416] Oil continued to be found as far from the Macondo site as the waters off the Florida Panhandle and Tampa Bay, where scientists said the oil and dispersant mixture is embedded in the sand.[417] In 2013, it was reported that dolphins and other marine life continued to die in record numbers with infant dolphins dying at six times the

TABLE 3.36

Oil Spills throughout the World

Spill/Vessel	Location	Dates	Min Tons	Max Tons	Link(s)
North Dakota pipeline spill	North Dakota, Tioga	September 25, 2013–September 29, 2013	2810	2810	346,347
Cushing storage terminal spill	Oklahoma, Cushing	May 18, 2013	340	340	348,349
2013 Mayflower oil spill	Arkansas, Mayflower	March 30, 2013	680	950	350
Magnolia refinery spill	Arkansas, Magnolia	March 9, 2013	680	760	351,352
Arthur Kill storage tank spill (Hurricane Sandy)	New Jersey, Sewaren	October 29, 2012	1090	1130	353,354
2011 Yellowstone River oil spill	Billings, Montana, Yellowstone River	July 1, 2011	105	140	355
Barataria Bay oil spill	Barataria Bay, Gulf of Mexico	July 27, 2010–August 1, 2010	23	45	356,357,358
Kalamazoo River oil spill	Kalamazoo River, Calhoun County, Michigan	July 26, 2010	2800	3250	359,360
Red Butte Creek oil spill	Salt Lake City, Utah	June 11, 2010–June 12, 2010	65	107	361,362
Trans-Alaska Pipeline spill	Anchorage, Alaska	May 25, 2010	400	1200	363
Deepwater Horizon	Gulf of Mexico	April 20, 2010–July 15, 2010	492,000	627,000	364
2010 Port Arthur oil spill	Port Arthur, Texas	January 23, 2010	1500	1500	365
2008 New Orleans oil spill	New Orleans, Louisiana	July 28, 2008	8800	8800	366
COSCO Busan oil spill	San Francisco, California	November 7, 2007	188	188	367
Citgo refinery oil spill	Lake Charles, Louisiana	June 19, 2006	6500	6500	368
Prudhoe Bay oil spill	Alaska North Slope, Alaska	March 2, 2006	653	689	369
Bass Enterprises (Hurricane Katrina)	Cox Bay, Louisiana	August 30, 2005	12,000	12,000	370
Shell (Hurricane Katrina)	Pilottown, Louisiana	August 30, 2005	3400	3400	370
Chevron (Hurricane Katrina)	Empire, Louisiana	August 30, 2005	3200	3200	370
Murphy Oil USA refinery spill (Hurricane Katrina)	Meraux and Chalmette, Louisiana	August 30, 2005	2660	3410	370,371
Bass Enterprises (Hurricane Katrina)	Pointe a la Hache, Louisiana	August 30, 2005	1500	1500	370
Chevron (Hurricane Katrina)	Port Fourchon, Louisiana	August 30, 2005	170	170	370
Venice Energy Services Company (Hurricane Katrina)	Venice, Louisiana	August 30, 2005	81	81	370
Shell Pipeline Oil (Hurricane Katrina)	Nairn, Louisiana	August 30, 2005	44	44	370
Sundown Energy (Hurricane Katrina)	West Potash, Louisiana	August 30, 2005	42	42	370

(Continued)

TABLE 3.36 (*Continued*)
Oil Spills throughout the World

Spill/Vessel	Location	Dates	Min Tons	Max Tons	Link(s)
MV Selendang Ayu	Unalaska Island, Alaska	December 8, 2004	1560	1560	372
Athos 1	Delaware River, Paulsboro, New Jersey	November 26, 2004	860	860	373
MP-80 Delta 20″ pipeline (Hurricane Ivan)	Louisiana	September 16, 2004–September 19, 2004	963	963	374
MP-69 nakika 18″ & MP-151 Nakika 18″ pipeline (Hurricane Ivan)	Louisiana	September 16, 2004–October 6, 2004	618	618	374
Chevron-Texaco tank collapse (Hurricane Ivan)	Louisiana	September 16, 2004–September 17, 2004	423	423	374
Bouchard No. 120	Buzzards Bay, Bourne, Massachusetts	April 27, 2003	320	320	375
Trans-Alaska Pipeline gunshot spill	Alaska	October 4, 2001	932	932	376
Julie N.	Portland, Maine	September 27, 1996	586	586	377
North Cape	Rhode Island	January 19, 1996	2500	2500	378
Mega Borg	Gulf of Mexico, 57 mi (92 km) SE of Galveston, Texas	June 8, 1990	16,499	16,501	379
American Trader	Bolsa Chica State Beach, California	February 7, 1990	979	981	372,380
Arthur Kill pipeline spill	New Jersey, Sewaren	January 1, 1990	1840	1840	381,382
Presidente Rivera	Delaware River, Marcus Hook, Pennsylvania	June 24, 1989	993	993	383
Exxon Valdez	Prince William Sound, Alaska	March 24, 1989	37,000	104,000	384,385
Ashland oil spill	Floreffe, Pennsylvania	January 2, 1988	10,000	10,000	386,387
Grand Eagle	Delaware River, Marcus Hook, Pennsylvania	September 28, 1985	1400	1400	388
SS Mobil Oil	Columbia River, Longview Washington	March 19, 1984	550	650	389,390
Burnah Agate	Galveston Bay, Texas	November 1, 1979	8440	8440	391
Trans-Alaska Pipeline sabotage by explosives	Alaska	February 15, 1978	2162	2162	392
Hawaiian Patriot	300 nmi (560 km; 350 mi) off Honolulu, Hawaii	February 26, 1977	95,000	95,000	372,384
Argo Merchant	Nantucket Island, Massachusetts	December 15, 1976	25,000	28,000	393,394
NEPCO 140 oil spill	Saint Lawrence River	June 23, 1976	1000	1000	395,396
Corinthos	Delaware River, Marcus Hook, Pennsylvania	January 31, 1975	36,000	36,000	395,396

(Continued)

TABLE 3.36 (Continued)
Oil Spills throughout the World

Spill/Vessel	Location	Dates	Min Tons	Max Tons	Link(s)
Arizona Standard/Oregon Standard collision	San Francisco Bay	January 17, 1971	2700	2700	397,398,399
1969 Santa Barbara oil spill	Santa Barbara, California	January 28, 1969	10,000	14,000	400
African Queen oil spill	Ocean City, Maryland	December 30, 1958	21,000	21,000	401,402
Avila Beach pipeline	Avila Beach, California	1950s–1996	1300	1300	403
Guadalupe Oil Field	Guadalupe, California	1950s–1994	29,000	29,000	403
Greenpoint, Brooklyn oil spill	Newtown Creek, Greenpoint, Brooklyn, New York	1940s–1950s	55,200	97,400	404
SS Frank H. Buck/SS President Coolidge collision	San Francisco Bay, California	March 6, 1937	8870	8870	397,405
Lakeview Gusher	Kern County, California	March 14, 1910–September 10, 1911	1,230,000	1,230,000	406

Spill/Vessel	Location	Dates	Estimated Flow Rate (Tons/Day)	Full Cargo (Tons)	Spilled (Min Tons)	Spilled (Max Tons)
Taylor Energy wells Platform 2301	Gulf of Mexico	September 16, 2004 to present (3400 days)	0.03–0.05	n/a	70	109

Source: https://en.wikipedia.org/wiki/List_of_oil_spills.

Note: The "flow rate" column applies to leaking wells, pipelines, and so on, and is often used to estimate the total amount of oil spilled. The "full cargo" column applies to vessels, vehicles, and so on, and represents the maximum amount of oil that could be spilled. The "spilled" columns indicate the total amount of oil that has been released to the environment so far, and should be based on official estimates found in referenced sources whenever possible. When official estimates vary, use the "min tons" and "max tons" columns to show the range of estimates (minimum and maximum) in metric tons (i.e., 1 ton = 1000 kg).

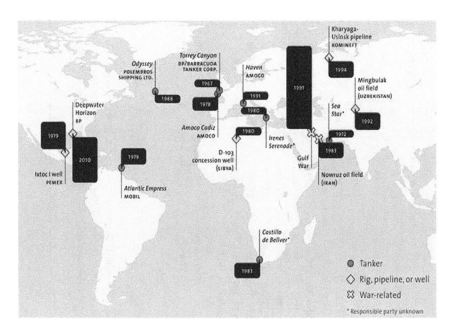

FIGURE 3.18 Historical oil spill. (From http://www.motherjones.com/environment/2010/09/bp-ocean-15-biggest-oil-spills, illustration: Nicholas Felton.)

normal rate.[418] One study released in 2014 reported that tuna and amberjack that were exposed to oil from the spill developed deformities of the heart and other organs that would be expected to be fatal or at least life-shortening and another study found that cardiotoxicity might have been widespread in animal life exposed to the spill.[419,420]

Numerous investigations explored the causes of the explosion and record-setting spill. Notably, the U.S. government's September 2011 report pointed to defective cement on the well, faulting mostly BP, but also rig operator Transocean and contractor Halliburton.[421,422]

BACKGROUND

Deepwater Horizon Drilling Rig

The *Deepwater Horizon* was a 9-year-old semi-submersible, mobile, floating, dynamically positioned drilling rig that could operate in waters up to 10,000 feet (3000 m) deep (Figure 3.19).[423] Built by the South Korean company Hyundai Heavy Industries[424] and owned by Transocean, the rig operated under the Marshallese flag of convenience, and was chartered to BP from March 2008 to September 2013.[425] It was drilling a deep exploratory well, 18,360 feet (5600 m) below sea level, in approximately 5100 feet (1600 m) of water. The well is situated in the Macondo Prospect in Mississippi Canyon Block 252 (MC252) of the Gulf of Mexico, in the United States' exclusive economic zone. The Macondo well is located roughly 41 miles (66 km) off the Louisiana coast.[426–428] BP was the operator and principal developer of the Macondo Prospect with a 65% share, while 25% was owned by Anadarko Petroleum Corporation, and 10% by MOEX Offshore 2007, a unit of Mitsui.[428]

At approximately 9:45 pm CDT, on April 20, 2010, high-pressure methane gas from the well expanded into the drilling riser and rose into the drilling rig, where it ignited and exploded, engulfing the platform.[429,430]

An oil leak was discovered when a large oil slick began to spread at the former rig site.[431] The oil flowed for 87 days. BP originally estimated a flow rate of 1000–5000 barrels per day (160–790 m³/d). The Flow Rate Technical Group (FRTG) estimated the flow rate at 62,000 barrels per

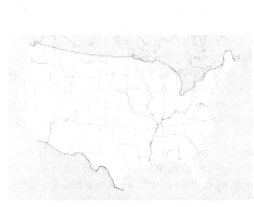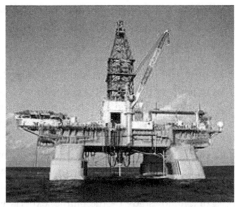

FIGURE 3.19 Deepwater horizon. Parts of the rig providing buoyancy are not visible below the waterline in this picture. (From https://en.wikipedia.org/wiki//Deepwater_Horizon_il_spill#/media/File:Deepwater_Horizon/jpg.)

day (9900 m³/d).[432–434] The total estimated volume of leaked oil approximated 4.9 million barrels (210,000,000 U.S. gal; 780,000 m³) with plus or minus 10% uncertainty,[412] including oil that was collected,[435] making it the largest accidental oil spill in history.

According to the satellite images, the spill directly impacted 68,000 square miles (180,000 km²) of ocean, which is comparable to the size of Oklahoma.[436,437] By early June 2010, oil had washed up on 125 miles (201 km) of Louisiana's coast and along the Mississippi, Florida, and Alabama coastlines.[438,439] Oil sludge appeared in the Intracoastal Waterway and on Pensacola Beach and the Gulf Islands National Seashore.[440] In late June, oil reached Gulf Park Estates, its first appearance in Mississippi.[441] In July, tar balls reached Grand Isle and the shores of Lake Pontchartrain.[442,443] In September, a new wave of oil suddenly coated 16 miles (26 km) of the Louisiana coastline and marshes west of the Mississippi River in Plaquemines Parish.[444] In October, weathered oil reached Texas.[445] As of July 2011, about 491 miles (790 km) of coastline in Louisiana, Mississippi, Alabama, and Florida were contaminated by oil and a total of 1074 miles (1728 km) had been oiled since the spill began.[446] As of December 2012, 339 miles (546 km) of coastline remain subject to evaluation and/or cleanup operations.[447]

Two weeks after the wellhead was capped on July 15, 2010, the surface oil appeared to have dissipated, while an unknown amount of subsurface oil remained.[448] Estimates of the residual ranged from a 2010 NOAA report that claimed that about half of the oil remained below the surface to independent estimates of up to 75%.[449–451] That means that over 100 million U.S. gallons (2.4 Mbbl) remained in the Gulf.[447] As of January 2011, tar balls, oil sheen trails, fouled wetlands marsh grass, and coastal sands were still evident. Subsurface oil remained offshore and in fine silts.[452] In April 2012, oil was still found along as much as 200 miles (320 km) of Louisiana coastline and tar balls continued to wash up on the barrier islands.[453] In 2013, some scientists at the Gulf of Mexico Oil Spill and Ecosystem Science Conference said that as much as one-third of the oil may have mixed with deep ocean sediments, where it risks damage to ecosystems and commercial fisheries.[454]

In 2013, more than 2.7 million pounds of "oiled material" were removed from the Louisiana coast. In the same year, tar balls were being reported almost every day on the Alabama and Florida beaches.[455]

Containment booms stretching over 4,200,000 feet (1300 km) were deployed, either to corral the oil or as barriers to protect marshes, mangroves, shrimp/crab/oyster ranches, or other ecologically sensitive areas. Booms extended 18–48 inches (0.46–1.22 m) above and below the water surface and were effective only in relatively calm and slow-moving waters. Including one-time use of sorbent booms, a total of 13,300,000 feet (4100 km) of booms were deployed.[456] Booms were criticized for washing up on the shore with the oil, allowing oil to escape above or below the boom, and for ineffectiveness in more than 3–4-ft waves.[457–459]

The spill was also notable for the volume of Corexit oil dispersant used and for application methods that were "purely experimental."[456] Altogether, 1.84 million U.S. gallons (7000 m³) of dispersants were used; of this, 771,000 U.S. gallons (2920 m³) were released at the wellhead.[413]

A 2011 analysis showed that the dispersant could contain cancer-causing agents, hazardous toxins, and endocrine-disrupting chemicals.[460] Corexit EC9500A and Corexit EC9527A were the principal variants.[461]

Underwater injection of Corexit into the leak may have created the oil plumes which were discovered below the surface.[462] Since the dispersants were applied at depth, much of the oil never rose to the surface.[463] One plume was 22 miles (35 km) long, more than a mile wide, and 650 feet (200 m) deep.[464] In a major study on the plume, experts were most concerned about the slow pace at which the oil was breaking down in the cold, 40°F (4°C) water at depths of 3000 feet (910 m).[465]

Two years after the spill, a study found that Corexit had increased the toxicity of the oil by up to 52 times.[466]

The three basic approaches for removing the oil from the water were: combustion, offshore filtration, and collection for later processing. USCG said 33 million U.S. gallons (120,000 m³) of tainted water was recovered, including 5 million U.S. gallons (19,000 m³) of oil. BP said 826,800 barrels (131,450 m³) had been recovered or flared.[467] It is calculated that about 5% of leaked oil was burned at the surface and 3% was skimmed.[468] On the most demanding day, 47,849 people were assigned to the response works.[412]

Owing to the use of Corexit, the oil was too dispersed to collect, according to a spokesperson for ship owner TMT.[469] In mid-June 2010, BP ordered 32 machines that separate oil and water, with each machine capable of extracting up to 2000 barrels per day (320 m³/d).[470,471] After one week of testing, BP began to proceed[472] and by 28 June had removed 890,000 barrels (141,000 m³).[473]

After the well was captured, the cleanup of the shore became the main task of the response works. Two main types of affected coast were sandy beaches and marshes. On beaches, the main techniques were sifting sand, removing tar balls, and digging out tar mats manually or by using mechanical devices.[412] For marshes, techniques such as vacuum and pumping, low-pressure flush, vegetation cutting, and bioremediation were used.[456]

OIL EATING MICROBES

Dispersants are said to facilitate the digestion of the oil by microbes. Mixing dispersants with oil at the wellhead would keep some oil below the surface and, in theory, allow microbes to digest the oil before it reaches the surface. Various risks were identified and evaluated, in particular that an increase in microbial activity might reduce subsea oxygen levels, threatening fish and other animals.[474]

Several studies suggest that microbes successfully consumed part of the oil.[447,475] By mid-September, other research claimed that microbes mainly digested natural gas rather than oil.[476,477] Valentine[476] said that the oil-gobbling properties of microbes had been grossly overstated.[475]

Some experts suggested that the bacteria may have caused health issues for Gulf residents, such as an outbreak of skin rashes. Genetically modified *Alcanivorax borkumensis* was added to the water to speed digestion.[478,479] The delivery method of microbes to oil patches was proposed by the Russian Research and Development Institute of Ecology and the Sustainable Use of Natural Resources.[480]

ENVIRONMENTAL IMPACT

The greatest impact was on marine species. The spill area hosts 8332 species, including more than 1200 fish, 200 birds, 1400 mollusks, 1500 crustaceans, 4 sea turtles, and 29 marine mammals.[481,482] In addition to the 14 species under federal protection, the spill threatened 39 more ranging from "whale sharks to seagrass." Damage to the ocean floor especially endangered the Louisiana pancake batfish whose range is entirely contained within the spill-affected area.[483] The oil contained approximately 40% methane by weight, compared with about 5% found in typical oil deposits.[484] Methane can potentially suffocate marine life and create "dead zones" where oxygen is depleted.[484] In March 2012, a definitive link was found between the death of a Gulf coral community and the spill.[485–488] During a January 2013 flyover, former NASA physicist Schumaker noted a "dearth of marine life in a radius 30–50 miles (48–80 km) around the well."[489]

Between May and June 2010, the spill waters contained 40 times more PAHs than before the spill.[490,491] PAHs are often linked to oil spills and include carcinogens and chemicals that pose various health risks to humans and marine life. The PAHs were most concentrated near the Louisiana Coast, but levels also jumped twofold to threefold in areas off Alabama, Mississippi, and Florida.[491] PAHs can harm marine species directly and microbes used to consume the oil can reduce marine oxygen levels.[492] Estimates state that only 2% of the carcasses of killed mammals were recovered. In the first birthing season for dolphins after the spill, dead baby dolphins washed up along Mississippi and Alabama shorelines at about 10 times the normal number.[493]

Fifteen of the 406 dolphins that washed ashore in the first 14 months had oil on their bodies; the oil found on eight was linked to the spill.[494] A NOAA/BP study in the summer of 2011 found that "many of the 32 dolphins studied were underweight, anemic and suffering from lung and liver disease, while nearly half had low levels of a hormone that helps the mammals deal with stress as well as regulating their metabolism and immune systems."[495] Other conditions included drastically low weight and low blood sugar.[496] By 2013, over 650 dolphins had been found stranded in the oil spill area, a fourfold increase over the historical average.[497] NWF scientist Inkley noted that the death rates are unprecedented,[497] and occurring high in the food chain strongly suggest that there is "something amiss with the Gulf ecosystem."[498]

USGS ecologists collected tissue samples from corals known as Madrepora and gorgonians at the damaged reefs. The samples are being used to examine the health of coral tissues including damage at the genetic level. Cell structure in corals can change in response to stress, such as by increasing the number of mucus-producing cells. Corals may also upregulate certain genes in response to stressors, comparing the proteins expressed in certain genes of the corals found at the MC 338 site with coral from control areas. Using push cores, they collected sediments at the damage site. They also suctioned the unknown brown material off the corals.

Scientists also visited a nearby chemosynthetic tubeworm community for similar analyses. There are numerous chemosynthetic communities throughout the Gulf of Mexico, and organisms that live there are also vulnerable to impacts from the oil spill. Although they live in a seemingly hostile environment, chemosynthetic animals still need oxygen to survive. Any material that clogs their tissues or limits their respiration can be deadly. The following is the Tap Water Quality Report for the State of Texas representing 6110 water systems serving 23,045,518 people (Table 3.37, Figure 3.20).

The health-based limits included in this analysis include enforceable drinking water limits (maximum contaminant limits, or MCLs) as well as governmental nonenforceable health guidelines, such as maximum contaminant limit goals (MCLGs), lifetime health advisory levels, 1-day and 10-day advisory levels to protect children from noncancer health end points, and other government-established health guidelines for tap water contaminants.

The federal government has set standards for 80 chemical pollutants in tap water, balancing health concerns and treatment costs. None of these should be in tap water; therefore, if a significant and unconceivable amount is found, these can cause chemical sensitivity and chronic degenerative disease. These are ridiculous set up standards that are compromised by severe chemical contamination.

TABLE 3.37

Analysis of Tap Water Tests from 1998 through 2003 for 6110 Communities across Texas Shows 105 Pollutants Found in Drinking Water across the State

105	Total Contaminants Detected (1998–2003)
15	**Agricultural pollutants**
	(pesticides, fertilizer, factory farms)
	Nitrate and nitrite, nitrate, nitrite, sulfate, thallium (total), prometon (2,4-bis-6-(isopropylamino)), simazine, metolachlor, atrazine, alachlor (lasso), bromacil, bromomethane, iodomethane, ethylbenzene, perchlorate
25	**Sprawl and urban pollutants**
	(road runoff, lawn pesticides, human waste)
	Arsenic (total), cadmium (total), copper, lead (total), mercury (total inorganic), nitrate and nitrite, nitrate, nitrite, antimony (total), isopropyl alcohol, acetone, naphthalene, MTBE, fluorene, phenanthrene, diethylphthalate, pyrene, di-n-butylphthalate, benzo[a]anthracene, benzo[b]fluoranthene, benzo[k]fluoranthene, benzo[a]pyrene, tetrachloroethylene, benzene, o-xylene
79	**Industrial pollutants**
	Aluminum, arsenic (total), barium (total), cadmium (total), chromium (total), lead (total), manganese, mercury (total inorganic), nitrate and nitrite, nitrate, nitrite, selenium (total), silver (total), sulfate, antimony (total), beryllium (total), thallium (total), carbon disulfide, di(2-ethylhexyl) adipate, di(2-ethylhexyl) phthalate, hexachlorocyclopentadiene, butyl acetate, isopropyl alcohol, chloromethane, bromomethane, chloroethane, aniline, acetone, hexachlorobutadiene, methyl ethyl ketone, naphthalene, methyl isobutyl ketone, MTBE, acenaphthene, tetrahydrofuran, fluorene, 2-hexanone, phenanthrene, diethylphthalate, pyrene, di-n-butylphthalate, methyl methacrylate, chrysene, n-hexane, 1,2,4-trichlorobenzene, cis-1,2-dichloroethylene, 1,2,4-trimethylbenzene, n-butylbenzene, 1,3,5-trimethylbenzene, bromochloromethane, dichloromethane (methylene chloride), p-dichlorobenzene, vinyl chloride, 1,1-dichloroethylene, 1,1-dichloroethane, 1,2-dichloroethane, 1,1,1-trichloroethane, carbon tetrachloride, 1,2-dichloropropane, trichloroethylene, tetrachloroethylene, monochlorobenzene (chlorobenzene), benzene, toluene, ethylbenzene, styrene, o-xylene, m- and p-xylene, alpha particle activity (excluding radon and uranium), combined uranium (mg/L), uranium-234, uranium-235, uranium-238, combined radium (-226 and -228), radium-226, radium-228, alpha particle activity, perchlorate, gross beta particle activity (pCi/L)
25	**Water treatment and distribution by-products**
	(pipes and fixtures, treatment chemicals, and by-products)
	cadmium (total), di(2-ethylhexyl) phthalate, chloromethane, methyl ethyl ketone, 2-hexanone, benzo[a]anthracene, benzo[b]fluoranthene, benzo[k]fluoranthene, benzo[a]pyrene, dibromomethane, bromochloromethane, monochloroacetic acid, dichloroacetic acid, trichloroacetic acid, monobromoacetic acid, dibromoacetic acid, total haloacetic acids, chloroform, bromoform, bromodichloromethane, dibromochloromethane, total trihalomethanes (TTHMs), dichloroiodomethane, vinyl chloride, dichloroacetonitrile
24	**Naturally occurring**
	(naturally present but increased for lands denuded by sprawl, agriculture, or industrial development)
	Aluminum, arsenic (total), chromium (total), copper, lead (total), manganese, mercury (total inorganic), nitrate and nitrite, nitrate, nitrite, selenium (total), silver (total), sulfate, chloromethane, alpha particle activity (excluding radon and uranium), combined uranium (mg/L), uranium-234, uranium-235, uranium-238, combined radium (-226 and -228), radium-226, radium-228, alpha particle activity, gross beta particle activity (pCi/L)
40	**Unregulated contaminants**
	EPA has not established a maximum legal limit in tap water for these contaminants.
	Carbon disulfide, prometon (2,4-bis-6-(isopropylamino)), metolachlor, butyl acetate, isopropyl alcohol, bromacil, chloromethane, bromomethane, chloroethane, aniline, acetone, hexachlorobutadiene, methyl ethyl ketone, naphthalene, methyl isobutyl ketone, MTBE, acenaphthene, tetrahydrofuran, fluorene, 2-hexanone, phenanthrene, diethylphthalate, pyrene, di-n-butylphthalate, methyl methacrylate, chrysene, benzo[a]anthracene, benzo[b]fluoranthene, benzo[k] fluoranthene, n-hexane, dibromomethane, 1,2,4-trimethylbenzene, n-butylbenzene, 1,3,5-trimethylbenzene, bromochloromethane, iodomethane, dichloroacetonitrile, dichloroiodomethane, 1,1-dichloroethane, perchlorate

Source: National Drinking Water Database. Environmental Working Group. http://www.ewg.org/tap-water/TexasDrinking WaterQualityReport/.

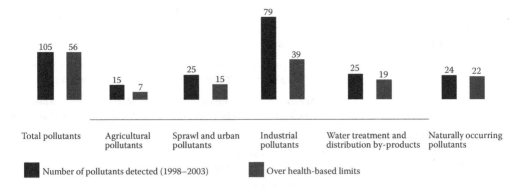

FIGURE 3.20 Pollution summary.

HEALTH SUMMARY TEXAS

Contaminants found above health-based limits (Tables 3.38 and 3.39, Figure 3.21): 56.

Health effects or target organs of contaminants found were cardiovascular or blood toxicity, cancer, developmental toxicity, endocrine toxicity, immunotoxicity, kidney toxicity, gastrointestinal or liver toxicity, neurotoxicity, reproductive toxicity, respiratory toxicity, and skin sensitivity.

These data show how drinking so-called clean tap water is severely contaminated. It is an initiator and propagator of chemical sensitivity.

Contaminants listed may not have exceeded legal limits, which are set to balance cost and benefits and are often higher than health-based limits (Tables 3.40 and 3.41).

MEDICATIONS FOUND IN PUBLIC WATER SUPPLY

According to Kohls,[499] the tests on public drinking water have consistently found measurable levels of prescription drugs, including arthritis drugs, contraceptives, psychostimulants, tranquilizers, and antidepressants such as Prozac, as well as cosmetics and synthetic food additives such as dyes and preservatives that are excreted down the drain through the pill-popping public's kidneys. These are all unregulated and potentially dangerous.

Psychotropic drugs can cross the placental barrier into the fetal circulation. The umbilical cord blood contains hundreds of toxic chemicals, many of which are known to be carcinogens. The ubiquitous effluent from our industrialized society is poisoning bodies of pregnant women and thus is contaminating the previously sacrosanct blood of fetuses and innocent newborn babies. There is an epidemic of congenital abnormalities and so-called "mental illnesses" and attention and other behavioral abnormalities among children. These illnesses are neurological poisonings and not mental illnesses of "unknown origin."

Chemicals enter public water supplies mostly through human urination and defecation, although flushing unused pills down the toilet or tossing them into landfills that are upstream from aquifers or streams is also a significant source of water contamination.

When humans defecate, urinate, sweat, or bathe, their organ systems are simultaneously getting rid of toxic substances. Ingested material first goes into the intestinal tract which attempts, through extensive enzyme systems, to break down the large molecule foodstuffs into smaller, more efficiently absorbed molecules of essential nutrients such as amino acids, simple sugars, and fatty acids, along with essential minerals and vitamins. These digested molecules mainly pass directly into the bloodstream (the "enterohepatic circulation") that flows directly into the liver, which, among other functions, attempts to metabolize, detoxify, and excrete poisonous substances into the biliary system (back into the intestines, however), although many of the metabolized substances go into

TABLE 3.38

Fifty-Six Contaminants of Concern in Texas

Rank	Contaminant Name	Population Exposed (of 23,045,518 Total)		Number of Water Systems (of 6110) Total	
		At Any Level	Above Health Limits	With Detected	Above Health Limits
1	Dibromochloromethane	17,663,613	12,869,413	2232	1665
	Disinfection by-product				
2	Bromodichloromethane	16,975,548	11,939,797	1834	1191
	Disinfection by-product				
3	Arsenic (total)	8,145,634	8,145,634	1267	1267
	Metal that enters water by erosion of natural deposits, runoff from glass, and electronics processing. Chicken raising				
4	Total trihalomethanes (TTHMs)	15,767,878	3,282,891	2566	847
	Measure of four disinfection by-products				
5	Combined Uranium (mg/L)	3,038,726	3,038,726	95	95
	Radioactive element commonly found in most rocks; processed ore used for power generation and weapons manufacture.				
6	Chloroform	16,756,094	3,024,193	1801	387
	Disinfection by-product				
7	Tetrachloroethylene	1,233,301	1,231,701	16	13
	Pollutant from dry cleaning and various industrial factories				
8	Lead (total)	4,875,274	1,126,631	1256	417
	Metal that enters water by corrosion of household plumbing systems; industrial pollutant; erosion of natural deposits.				
9	Bromoform	16,134,704	998,773	1995	318
	Disinfection by-product				
10	Total haloacetic acids	2,715,574	870,911	51	21
	Measure of disinfection by-products; refers to the sum of the concentrations of dichloroacetic acid, trichloroacetic acid, monochloroacetic acid, monobromoacetic acid, and dibromoacetic acid in a water sample				
11	Atrazine	3,447,217	359,941	105	38
	Herbicide used on row crops				
12	Manganese	10,154,614	284,677	1816	299
	Element from natural deposits as well as industrial use				
13	Alpha particle activity (exclradon and uranium)	5,180,533	199,418	1316	109
	From mining waste pollutants and natural sources				
14	Perchlorate	111,850	111,850	2	2
	Perchlorate is an oxygen additive in solid fuel propellant or rockets, missiles, and fireworks				
15	Alpha particle activity	3,785,884	104,327	1127	96
	From mining waste pollutants and natural sources				
16	Trichloroacetic acid	2,351,946	99,104	39	3
	Disinfection by-product				
17	Combined Radium (−226 and −228)	3,061,506	68,832	800	36
	Radioactive element usually found around uranium deposits				
18	Di(2-ethylhexyl)phthalate	580,501	62,588	28	11
	Pollutant from rubber and industrial chemical factories; leachate from PVC pipes				

(Continued)

TABLE 3.38 (*Continued*)
Fifty-Six Contaminants of Concern in Texas

Rank	Contaminant Name	Population Exposed (of 23,045,518 Total)		Number of Water Systems (of 6,110) Total	
		At Any Level	Above Health Limits	With Detected	Above Health Limits
19	Copper	13,764,908	56,418	2171	15
		Contaminant that enters water by corrosion of household plumbing systems; erosion of natural deposits			
20	Radium-226	6,203,908	50,747	848	40
		Radioactive element usually found around uranium deposits			
21	Thallium (total)	50,388	50,388	17	17
		Widely used as a rodenticide and ant killer; home use has been banned; used for speciality glass manufacture			
22	Nitrate	17,387,944	48,336	2782	46
		Chemical that enters water from fertilizer runoff, leaching septic tanks, and erosion of natural deposits			
23	Aluminum	10,139,828	43,956	735	21
		Metal from metal refineries and mining operations			
24	Nitrate and nitrite	13,969,387	33,869	1302	32
		Chemical that enters water from fertilizer runoff, leaching septic tanks, an erosion of natural deposits			
25	Carbon tetrachloride	55,839	28,391	16	12
		Pollutant from various chemical plants			
26	Dibromoacetic acid	2,715,574	28,326	51	1
		Disinfection by-product			
27	Cadmium (total)	28,284	19,773	23	21
		Metal from corrosion of galvanized pipes; runoff from metal refineries, waste batteries, and paints; erosion of natural deposits.			
28	Radium-228	2,253,832	19,058	527	13
		Radioactive element usually found around uranium deposits			
29	Chrysene	14,862	14,862	1	1
		Pollutant from the incomplete combustion of fossil fuels			
30	Benzo(a)anthracene	14,862	14,862	1	1
		Pollutant from combustion of organic matter, including fossil fuel and wood; research chemical			
31	Benzo(b)fluoranthene	14,862	14,862	1	1
		Pollutant from combustion of organic matter, including fossil fuel and wood; research chemical			
32	Benzo(k)fluoranthene	14,862	14,862	1	1
		Chemical from water distribution system tanks and pipes lined with coal tar or asphalt; pollutant from combustion of organic matter, including fossil fuel and wood; no commercial uses			
33	Benzo(a)pyrene	14,862	14,862	1	1
		Chemical from leaching water distribution and storage liners; product of combustion			
34	Benzene	23,463	11,823	9	7
		Chemical from factory pollution, leaching landfills, and gas storage tanks			
35	Barium (total)	19,210,829	2,442	3893	7
		Mineral from drilling and mining waste runoff; erosion of natural deposits			

(*Continued*)

TABLE 3.38 (*Continued*)
Fifty-Six Contaminants of Concern in Texas

		Population Exposed (of 23,045,518 Total)		Number of Water Systems (of 6,110) Total	
Rank	Contaminant Name	At Any Level	Above Health Limits	With Detected	Above Health Limits
36	1,1-Dichloroethylene	2,438	2,438	1	1
	Pollutant from producing adhesives; synthetic fibers, refrigerants, and plastic wraps				
37	Selenium (total)	10,659,438	1,257	1114	6
	Metal from mining or petroleum refining pollution; erosion of natural deposits.				
38	Dichloromethane (methylene chloride)	344,410	537	22	1
	Pollutant from drug and industrial chemical factories				
39	Chloromethane	1,158,851	511	421	3
	Chloromethane is a by-product of water disinfection and an EPA top priority for testing and study in tap water based on toxicity concerns. It is also an industrial chemical used in manufacture of silicone rubber, pesticides, and more; was formerly used as refrigerant, now banned; is an industry and municipal wasterwater pollutant; and is produced naturally in small quantities				
40	1,2-Dichloropropane	474	474	1	1
	Pollutant from various industrial chemical factories				
41	Nitrite	5,708,988	255	228	1
	Chemical that enters water from fertilizer runoff, leaching septic tanks, and erosion of natural deposits				
42	Mercury (total inorganic)	73,814	105	24	1
	Metal from refinery and factory pollution; coal burning; landfill and agricultural runoff, erosion of natural deposits				
43	Beryllium (total)	165	63	2	1
	Metal from metal refineries and coal burning; pollution from electrical, aerospace, and defense industries				
44	1,2-Dichloroethane	50	50	1	1
	Pollutant from various industrial chemical factories				
45	Sulfate	19,012,322	0	3682	0
	Substance from natural deposits, industrial processes, and agriculture				
46	Hexachlorobutadiene	22,500	0	1	0
	Hexachlorobutadiene is an intermediate in the manufacture of rubber compounds and fluoriantede lubricants, and is used in numerous industrial applications, including as a solvent for elastomers and as a heat transfer liquid.				
47	MTBE	195,007	0	11	0
	MTBE is a fuel additive used as an octane enhancer in unleaded gasoline; its ban or phaseout is in progress in 16 states as of December 2005.				
48	Monochloroacetic acid	1,164,215	0	24	0
	>Disinfection by-product				
49	Dichloroacetic acid	2,647,048	0	47	0
	Disinfection by-product				
50	Monobromoacetic acid	1,039,683	0	19	0
	Disinfection by-product				

(Continued)

TABLE 3.38 (*Continued*)
Fifty-Six Contaminants of Concern in Texas

		Population Exposed (of 23,045,518 Total)		Number of Water Systems (of 6,110) Total	
Rank	Contaminant Name	At Any Level	Above Health Limits	With Detected	Above Health Limits
51	Vinyl chloride	148	0	1	0
		Leachate from PVC pipes; pollutant from plastic factories			
52	Trichloroethylene	2,794	0	7	0
		Pollutant from metal degreasing sites			
53	Uranium-234	12,600	0	9	0
		Radioactive element commonly found in most rocks; processed ore used for power generation and weapons manufacture			
54	Uranium-235	1,606	0	9	0
		Radioactive element commonly found in most rocks; processed ore used for power generation and weapons manufacture			
55	Uranium-238	8,993	0	3	0
		Radioactive element commonly found in most rocks; processed ore used for power generation and weapons manufacture			
56	Gross beta particle activity (pCi/L)	11,733,194	0	1744	0
		Mainly pollutants from nuclear testing and industrial and medical instruments.			

Source: National Drinking Water Database. Environmental Working Group. http://www.ewg.org/tap-water/TexasDrinking WaterQualityReport/.

Note: The top contaminants of concern based on government health limits: bromodichloromethane; dibromochloromethane

the bloodstream and thus to the rest of the body. Many of the partially detoxified drugs are still pharmacologically active and may still be toxic.

In this highly poisoned planet, with the tens of thousands of synthetic chemicals virtually everywhere (and almost none of them have been tested for safety), the liver's detoxifying capacity can be easily overwhelmed which probably explains why Americans are among the sickest, if not the sickest, group of people in the developed world.

This situation is especially problematic in people who take a lot of drugs, frequently get vaccinated with the highly toxic metals aluminum and mercury (plus a variety of toxic adjuvants in the shots), eat a lot of long shelf-life junk foods that are laden with preservatives, drink a lot of nutritionally deficient soda pop that has synthetic sweeteners in or are simply living and breathing downwind from polluting smokestacks or living downstream from corporate facilities that are polluting the water.

Male alligators in Florida are developing micropenises—and probably infertility—from the estrogen-mimicking pollutants in the water of the Everglades.

The famous mutant (and disappearing) frogs in Minnesota were being turned into sterile hermaphrodites by the estrogen mimic, Atrazine, which is ubiquitous in the runoff water from the farming industry. Atrazine has been found in the majority of drinking water supplies in the farming regions in southern Minnesota.

Environmental toxicologists from Texas have found high levels of Prozac in the brains, livers, and muscle tissue of bluegills, channel catfish, and black crappies from a stream in a Dallas suburb that receives effluent from the city's wastewater treatment plant. Prozac (fluoxetine)

TABLE 3.39

Pollution Summary of Local Water System Report from Fort Worth, TX, Which Serves 534,695 People

Total Contaminants Detected (1998–2003)

11   Barium (total), nitrate and nitrite, nitrate, sulfate, atrazine, chloroform, bromoform, bromodichloromethane, dibromochloromethane, radium-228, gross beta particle activity (pCi/L)

Agricultural Pollutants

4   (pesticides, fertilizer, factory farms)
Nitrate and nitrite, nitrate, sulfate, atrazine

Sprawl and Urban Pollutants

2   (road runoff, lawn pesticides, human waste)
Nitrate and nitrite, nitrate

Industrial Pollutants

6   Barium (total), nitrate and nitrite, nitrate, sulfate, radium-228, gross beta particle activity (pCi/L)

Water Treatment and Distribution By-Products

4   (pipes and fixtures, treatment chemicals and byproducts)
Chloroform, bromoform, bromodichloromethane, dibromochloromethane

Naturally Occurring

5   (naturally present but increased for lands denuded by sprawl, agriculture, or industrial development)
Nitrate and nitrite, nitrate, sulfate, radium-228, gross beta particle activity (pCi/L)

Source: National Drinking Water Database. http://www.ewg.org/tap-water/whatsinyourwater/TX/Fort-Worth-Water-Department/2200012/.

and the iver-metabolized form of the drug norfluoxetine (which is as pharmacologically active as Prozac itself!) were found in alarming concentrations in every tissue sample examined in the fish.

Prozac works by artificially—and very potently—"goosing" serotonin nerve transmission at the level of the serotonin synapses in brain cells (as well as other cells, especially intestinal cells). We

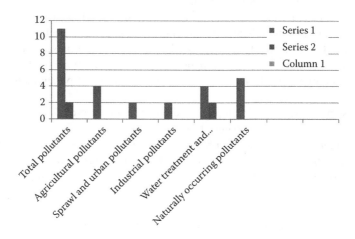

FIGURE 3.21   Health effects or target organs of contaminants.

TABLE 3.40

Contaminants Found above Health-Based Limits

Contaminant Name	Average Result	Maximum Result	Health Limit Exceeded	Has Legal Limit	Legal Limit Exceeded
Bromodichloromethane	1.03 ppb	23 ppb	Yes	Yes	No
	Disinfection by-product				
Dibromochloromethane	0.66 ppb	20 ppb	Yes	Yes	No
	Disinfection by-product				

Source: National Drinking Water Database. http://www.ewg.org/tap-water/whatsinyourwater/TX/Fort-Worth-Water-Department/2200012/.

use serotonin intradermal neutralization often to quell reaction of the chemically sensitive. Prozac affects other nonserotonin neurotransmitter systems in other parts of the body as well and is therefore not "selective" for serotonin, despite its class name, SSRI—selective serotonin reuptake pump inhibitor. Serotonin, incidentally, is the most important antidepressant neurotransmitter in the brain and is known to elevate mood, enhance impulse control, enhance sleep quality, relieve anxiety, and produce satiety. However, it also has major effects on other organ systems such as the intestinal tract, platelets, and the heart.

SSRI drugs such as Prozac artificially prevent serotonin nerves (as well as dopamine and norepinephrine nerves) from reabsorbing, recycling, reusing, and therefore storing serotonin for future use (and this affects dopamine and norepinephrine recycling as well), thus providing a temporary increase in the level and activity of the neurotransmitter in the synapse. However, the action of these drugs is ultimately serotonin-depleting because of the "reuptake inhibition" action.

Since the costs of high-tech filtering systems are out of the reach of every financially strapped municipality in this nation, the only solution for the problem of brain- and body-altering drugs in the water is by prevention, however, that must come about.

As shown in Chapter 6, serotonin neutralization is one of the prime intradermal neutralization treatments for many chemically sensitive and chronic degenerative disease patients. People often are afraid or reluctant to get off these drugs because of mental abbreviations. However, neutralization of the serotonin is often achieved and the patient improves markedly. Many other intradermal antigen

TABLE 3.41

Water Testing Summary

Contaminant reported as tested by this water supplier:	168
Contaminants with federal legal limit in tap water, with testing required for most water systems:	73
Regulated contaminants tested (chemicals with federal legal limits in tap water):	131
Unregulated contaminants tested (chemicals without federal legal limits in tap water):	37

Source: National Drinking Water Database. http://www.ewg.org/tap-water/whatsinyourwater/TX/Fort-Worth-Water-Department/2200012/.

medications can cause other disruptions in the physiology of the chemically sensitive, resulting in many of the derangements in bodily function.

Of the 62 major water providers contacted, the drinking water for only 28 was tested. Of the 28 major metropolitan areas where tests were performed on drinking water supplies, only the Albuquerque, Austin, Texas, and Virginia Beach tests were negative.

At the Orange County Sanitation District, a settling basin is used to filter water as part of the advanced secondary treatment, before the water is diverted into the ocean, in Fountain Valley, California. Pharmaceuticals in waterways are damaging wildlife across the nation and around the globe.

A vast array of pharmaceuticals, including antibiotics, anticonvulsants, mood stabilizers, and sex hormones, have been found in the drinking water supplies of at least 41 million Americans.

The concentrations of these pharmaceuticals are measured in quantities of parts per billion or trillion, far below the levels of a medical dose. Also, therefore, utilities insist their water is safe. This is nonsense since they do not protect the total body pollutant load.

However, the presence of so many prescription drugs and over-the-counter medicines such as acetaminophen and ibuprofen in so much of the drinking water is heightening worries of long-term consequences to human health.

Testing in Philadelphia discovered 56 pharmaceuticals or by-products in treated drinking water, including medicines for pain, infection, high cholesterol, asthma, epilepsy, mental illness, and heart problems. Sixty-three pharmaceuticals or by-products were found in the city's watersheds. Antiepileptic and antianxiety medications were detected in a portion of the treated drinking water for 18.5 million people in Southern California.

Researchers at the USGS analyzed a Passaic Valley Water Commission drinking water treatment plant, which serves 850,000 people in Northern New Jersey, and found a metabolized angina medicine and the mood-stabilizing carbamazepine in drinking water. A sex hormone was detected in San Francisco's drinking water. The drinking water for Washington, D.C. and surrounding areas tested positive for six pharmaceuticals. Three medications, including an antibiotic, were found in drinking water supplied to Tucson.

The AP's (Associated Press) investigation also indicates that watersheds, the natural sources of most of the nation's water supply, also are contaminated. Tests were conducted in the watersheds of 35 of the 62 major providers surveyed by the AP, and pharmaceuticals were detected in 28.

The New York state health department and the USGS tested the source of the city's water, upstate. They found trace concentrations of heart medicine, infection fighters, estrogen, anticonvulsants, a mood stabilizer, and a tranquilizer.

A Tulane University researcher and his students have published a study that found the pain reliever naproxen, the sex hormone estrone, and the anticholesterol drug by-product clofibric acid in treated drinking water.[500]

Rural consumers who draw water from their own wells are not in the clear either. The Stroud Water Research Center, in Avondale, Pennsylvania, has measured water samples from New York City's upstate watershed for caffeine, a common contaminant that scientists often look for as a possible signal for the presence of other pharmaceuticals. Though more caffeine was detected at suburban sites, researcher Anthony Aufdenkampe was struck by the relatively high levels even in less populated areas.

Even users of bottled water and home filtration systems do not necessarily avoid exposure. Bottlers, some of whom simply repackage tap water, do not typically treat or test for pharmaceuticals, according to the industry's main trade group. The same goes for the makers of home filtration systems. They have seen this at EHC-Dallas where the filters are not only inadequate but also put out noxious incitants.

Studies have detected pharmaceuticals in waters throughout Asia, Australia, Canada, and Europe—even in Swiss lakes and the North Sea.[500]

For example, in Canada, a study of 20 Ontario drinking water treatment plants by a national research institute found nine different drugs in water samples. Japanese health officials in December 2008 called for human health impact studies after detecting prescription drugs in drinking water at seven different sites.[500]

In the United States, the problem is not confined to surface waters. Pharmaceuticals also permeate aquifers deep underground, the source of 40% of the nation's water supply. Federal scientists who drew water in 24 states from aquifers near contaminant sources such as landfills and animal feed lots found minuscule levels of hormones, antibiotics, and other drugs.[500]

One technology, reverse osmosis, removes virtually all pharmaceutical contaminants but is very expensive for large-scale use and leaves several gallons of polluted water for every one that is made drinkable.[500] It is one of the safer waters if double filtered. One pass is not enough for the chemically sensitive.

Another issue is that there is evidence that adding chlorine, a common process in conventional drinking water treatment plants, makes some pharmaceuticals more toxic.[500]

Other veterinary drugs also play a role. Pets are now treated for arthritis, cancer, heart disease, diabetes, allergies, dementia, and even obesity—sometimes with the same drugs as humans. The inflation-adjusted value of veterinary drugs rose by 8%, to $5.2 billion, over the past 5 years, according to an analysis of data from the Animal Health Institute.

Recent laboratory research has found that small amounts of medication have affected human embryonic kidney cells, human blood cells, and human breast cancer cells. The cancer cells proliferated too quickly; the kidney cells grew too slowly; and the blood cells showed biological activity associated with inflammation.[500]

Also, pharmaceuticals in waterways are damaging wildlife across the nation and around the globe. Notably, male fish are being feminized, creating egg yolk proteins, a process usually restricted to females. Pharmaceuticals also are affecting sentinel species at the foundation of the pyramid of life—such as earthworms in the wild and zooplankton in the laboratory, studies show.

Our bodies may shrug off a relatively big one-time dose, yet suffer from a smaller amount delivered continuously over a half century, perhaps subtly stirring allergies or nerve damage. Pregnant women, the elderly, and the very ill might be more sensitive.

Many concerns about chronic low-level exposure focus on certain drug classes: chemotherapy that can act as a powerful poison; hormones that can hamper reproduction or development; medicines for depression and epilepsy that can damage the brain or change behavior; antibiotics that can allow human germs to mutate into more dangerous forms; pain relievers, and blood pressure diuretics.

Pesticides, lead, PCBs, which are present in higher concentrations, clearly pose a health risk.

However, some experts say medications may pose a unique danger because, unlike most pollutants, they were crafted to act on the human body.

These are chemicals that are designed to have very specific effects at very low concentrations. That is what pharmaceuticals do.

While drugs are tested to be safe for humans, the time frame is usually over a matter of months, not a lifetime. Pharmaceuticals also can produce side effects and interact with other drugs at normal medical doses. That is why, aside from therapeutic doses of fluoride injected into potable water supplies, pharmaceuticals are prescribed to people who need them, not delivered to everyone in their drinking water (Figure 3.22).

Pharmaceuticals and their metabolites undergo natural attenuation by adsorption, dilution, or degradation in the environment, depending on their hydrophobicity and biodegradability and on the temperature. Therefore, pharmaceuticals in water sources and drinking water are often present at trace concentrations, as these compounds would have undergone metabolism and removal through natural processes and, if applicable, wastewater and drinking water treatment processes.

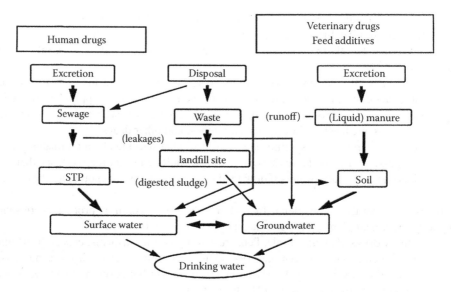

FIGURE 3.22   Fate of pharmaceuticals in the environment. (Modified from Ternes, T. 1998. *Water Res.* 32:3245–3260; Used by permission from World Health Organization Pharmaceuticals in Drinking Water, Figure 1.)

It was demonstrated that the presence of pharmaceuticals in the environment occurred more than 30 years ago, with studies in the United States in the 1970s that reported the presence of heart medications, pain relievers, and birth control medications in wastewater.[501–503] The most cited reference in the peer-reviewed literature on the occurrence of pharmaceuticals in surface waters is the survey by the USGS, in which more than 50 pharmaceuticals in 139 streams across 30 states in the United States were investigated during 1999 and 2000.[504]

Many peer-reviewed and published studies have shown that the primary sources of pharmaceuticals entering surface water are from excretion and bathing through treated or untreated municipal wastewater effluent discharges into receiving surface water bodies[504–511] and improper disposal of pharmaceutical waste and excess medication by consumers and health-care and veterinary facilities into sewers and drains. Table 3.42 illustrates several classes of pharmaceuticals found in wastewater influent in a study conducted by the Drinking Water Inspectorate in the United Kingdom.

A monitoring program in the United Kingdom focused on 12 pharmaceutical compounds or their metabolites in surface waters.[514] The results showed that a range of pharmaceuticals from different therapeutic classes were present in both effluents from sewage treatment works and receiving waters in England. The values reported were within the same range as those reported in continental Europe and the United States, where more extensive monitoring has been conducted. Results in the published literature for studies conducted in the United States and Europe also suggest that usage data are positively associated with concentrations of pharmaceuticals measured in effluent and in surface water bodies receiving the treated effluent. Tables 3.43 and 3.44 show additional illustrative examples of pharmaceuticals that have been found in the United Kingdom and other European countries, respectively.

Studies in the United States have detected very low levels of pharmaceuticals in finished drinking water. The highest concentration reported was 40 ng/L for meprobamate.[521] Studies have also found several pharmaceuticals in tap water at concentrations ranging from nanograms to low micrograms per liter in several countries in Europe, including Germany, the Netherlands, and Italy.[522] Two separate studies in Germany[511,523] found phenazone and propyphenazone (an analgesic and an antipyretic drug, respectively) in Berlin drinking water, with the highest concentration being 400 ng/L for phenazone. This high value was largely attributed to groundwater, used as a drinking

TABLE 3.42

Excretion Rates of Unmetabolized Active Ingredients for Selected Pharmaceuticals

Compound	Pharmaceutical Product Group	Parent Compound Excreted (%)	Reference
Amoxicillin	Antibiotic	60	Bound and Voulvoulis[512]
Atenolol	Beta blocker	90	Bound and Voulvoulis[512]
Bezafibrate	Lipid regulator	50	Bound and Voulvoulis[512]
Carbamazepine	Antiepileptic	3	Bound and Voulvoulis[512]
Cetirizine	Antihistamine	50	Bound and Voulvoulis[512]
Clofibric acid	Active metabolite	6	Alder et al.[513]
Diclofenac	Anti-inflammatory	15	Alder et al.[513]
Erythromycin	Antibiotic	25	Bound and Voulvoulis[512]
Felbamate	Antiepileptic	40–50	Bound and Voulvoulis[512]
Ibuprofen	Analgesic	10	Bound and Voulvoulis[519]

Source: DWI. 2007. Desk based review of current knowledge on pharmaceuticals in drinking water and estimation of potential levels. Final report prepared by Watts and Crane Associates for Drinking Water Inspectorate, Department for Environment, Food and Rural Affairs (Defra Project Code: CSA 7184/WT02046/DWI70/2/213). http://dwi.defra. gov.uk/research/completed-research/reports/dwi70-2-213.pdf; Used with permission of World Health Organization. Pharmaceuticals in Drinking Water, Table 1.

water source, contaminated with sewage.[524] In the Netherlands, traces of antibiotics, antiepileptics, and beta blockers were detected in the drinking water supply at concentrations below 100 ng/L, with most concentrations below 50 ng/L.[525]

To date, between 15 and 25 pharmaceuticals have been detected in treated drinking water worldwide, as reported in the peer-reviewed scientific literature.[521,524] More pharmaceutical compounds have been detected in untreated water sources, such as wastewater, surface waters, and groundwaters,[526,527] in the water cycle, largely attributable to pharmaceuticals of very high usage, including antihyperlipidemic compounds and nonsteroidal anti-inflammatory drugs (NSAIDs).

The occurrence of pharmaceuticals in the environment, including the water cycle, at concentrations ranging from nanograms to low micrograms per liter has been widely discussed and published in the literature in the past decade.[510,523,524,527–538]

The published literature and national studies have shown that concentrations of pharmaceuticals in surface water and groundwater sources impacted by wastewater discharges are typically less than 0.1 μg/L (or 100 ng/L), and concentrations in treated drinking water are usually well below 0.05 μg/L (or 50 ng/L).

There are few comprehensive, systematic monitoring studies on pharmaceuticals in drinking water, and limited occurrence data are a challenge in assessing potential human health risks from exposure to trace concentrations of pharmaceuticals in drinking water. In addition, there is no standardized protocol for the sampling and analytical determination of pharmaceuticals. More systematic studies, using comparable methods, will help further research on the transport, occurrence, and fate of these compounds in various environmental media, and standardization of protocols for their sampling and analytical determination would help to facilitate the comparison of data.

Concern has been raised, however, because exposure to pharmaceuticals through drinking water is an unintended and involuntary exposure over potentially long periods of time. Moreover, there are few scientific risk assessments of exposure to low levels of pharmaceuticals, both as individual species or as mixtures, in drinking water.

Health risks from pharmaceuticals in water have been most frequently assessed but using crude and unrealistic parameters.

TABLE 3.43

Measured Concentrations of Selected Pharmaceuticals in the Aquatic Environment in the United Kingdom

Compound	Median (Maximum) Concentration (ng/L)		References
	Sewage Treatment Works Effluent	Stream or River Waters	
Bleomycin	11 (19)	nd (17)	Aherne, Hardcastle and Nield[515]
Clotrimazole	14 (27)	21 (34)	Roberts and Thomas[516]
		7 (22)	Thomas and Hilton[517]
Diclofenac	424 (2349)	<LOQ (568)	Ashton, Hilton and Thomas[514]
	2389(598	<LOQ	Roberts and Thomas[516]
	–	<LOQ (195)	Thomas and Hilton[517]
Dextropropoxyphene	195 (585)	58 (682)	Ashton, Hilton and Thomas[514]
	37 (64)	12 (98)	Roberts and Thomas[516]
Erythromycin	–	<LOQ (80)	Thomas and Hilton[517]
	<LOQ (1842)	<LOQ (1022)	Ashton, Hilton and Thomas[514]
Fluoxetine	202 (290)	5 (70)	Roberts and Thomas[516]
	7.6–52.9	2–43.7	Boucard and Gravell[518]
Ibuprofen	3086 (27,256)	826 (5044)	Ashton, Hilton and Thomas[514]
	2972 (4239)	297(2370)	Roberts and Thomas[516]
		48 (930)	Thomas and Hilton[517]
Mefenamic acid	133 (1440)	62 (366)	Ashton, Hilton and Thomas[514]
	340 (396)	<LOQ	Roberts and Thomas[516]
	–	<LOQ(196)	Thomas and Hilton[517]
Norfluoxetine	5.2–30.7	4.5–83.0	Boucard and Gravell[518]
Paracetamol	<20	–	Roberts and Thomas[516]
	–	555	Bound and Voulvoulis[519]
Propanolol	76 (284)	29 (215)	Ashton, Hilton and Thomas[514]
	304 (373)	61 (107)	Roberts and Thomas[516]
	–	<LOQ (56)	Thomas and Hilton[517]
Sulfamethoxazole	<LOQ (132)	<LOQ	Ashton, Hilton and Thomas[514]
Tamoxifen	<LOQ (42)	<LOQ	Ashton, Hilton and Thomas[514]
Tetracycline	–	−1000	Watts et al.[520]
Theophylline	–	−1000	Watts et al.[520]
Trimethoprim	70 (1288)	<LOQ (42)	Ashton, Hilton and Thomas[514]
	271 (322)	9 (19)	Roberts and Thomas[516]
	–	7 (569)	Thomas and Hilton[517]

Source: DWI. 2007. Desk based review of current knowledge on pharmaceuticals in drinking water and estimation of potential levels. Final report prepared by Watts and Crane Associates for Drinking Water Inspectorate, Department for Environment, Food and Rural Affairs (Defra Project Code: CSA 7184/WT02046/DWI70/2/213). http://dwi. defra.gov.uk/research/completed-research/reports/dwi70-2-213.pdf; Used with permission of World Health Organization. Pharmaceuticals in Drinking Water, Table 2.

LOQ, limit of quantification; nd, not detected (below the detection limit).

TABLE 3.44

Concentrations of Selected Pharmaceuticals Found in European Surface Water

Compound	Median (Maximum) Concentrations (ng/L)				
	Austria	Finland	France	Germany	Switzerland
Bezafibrate	20 (160)	5 (25)	102 (430)	350 (3100)	–
Carbamazepine	75 (294)	70 (370)	78 (800)	25 (110)	30–150
Diclofenac	20 (64)	15 (40)	18 (41)	150 (1200)	20–150
Ibuprofen	nd	10 (65)	23 (120)	70 (530)	ng (150)
Iopomide	91 (211)	–	7 (17)	100 (1910)	–
Roxithromycin	nd	–	9 (37)	<LOQ (560)	–
Sulfamethoxazole[a]	nd	–	25 (133)	30 (480)	–

Source: Used by permission from World Health Organization. Pharmaceuticals in Drinking Water Table 3; Ternes et al., 2005. Assessment of technologies for the removal of pharmaceuticals and personal care products in sewage and drinking water to improve the indirect potable water reuse. POSEIDON project detailed report (EU Contract No. EVK1-CT-2000-00047).

[a] Includes the human metabolite N-acetyl-sulfamethoxazole.

LOQ, limit of quantification; nd, not detected (below the detection limit).

Notwithstanding this, especially in cases where the margins of exposure (MOEs) are substantial, use of the maximum tolerated dose (MTD) could be considered a pragmatic and sensible method to broadly assess and screen risks.

The main challenges in assessing risks include the limited occurrence data available for pharmaceuticals in drinking water, the diverse range of pharmaceuticals in use, the wide variation in the use of individual pharmaceuticals between countries, the limited number of data in the public domain, and technical limitations relating to assessing risks from chronic exposure to low dose of pharmaceuticals and mixtures (Table 3.45).

The Awwa Research Foundation commissioned a study to provide critical information regarding the occurrence of and risk assessment for pharmaceuticals and potential endocrine disrupting chemicals (EDCs) in drinking water. The study examined 62 chemicals, including 20 pharmaceuticals and active metabolites, 26 potential EDCs, 5 steroid hormones, and 11 phytoestrogens (natural estrogens from plants). The health value applied in this study was the acceptable daily intake (ADI), and a conservative approach was taken in the process of developing the ADI values, as illustrated in Table 3.46.

Even with the use of advanced and highly sensitive analytical procedures (with reporting limits in the nanograms per liter or parts per trillion range), none of the pharmaceuticals tested in this study were detected in finished drinking water above the calculated health risk thresholds. Adopting a conservative worst-case scenario approach, the maximum detected concentrations in finished and piped drinking water were used to calculate drinking water equivalent levels (DWELs) for each of the target pharmaceuticals. It was found that none of the pharmaceuticals detected in drinking water exceeded their corresponding ADI (Tables 3.46 and 3.47).

In the course of a 5-month inquiry, it was discovered that drugs have been detected in the drinking water supplies of 24 major metropolitan areas, from Southern California to Northern New Jersey, from Detroit to Louisville.

Water providers rarely disclose results of pharmaceutical screenings, unless pressed. Bodies absorb some of the medication, but the rest of it passes through and is flushed down the toilet. The wastewater is treated before it is discharged into reservoirs, rivers, or lakes. Then, some of the water is cleansed again at drinking water treatment plants and piped to consumers. But most treatments do not remove all drug residues.

TABLE 3.45

Probabilistic Modeling Data for the Top 24 Drugs from Worst-Case Deterministic Modeling

Drug Name	Mean PEC$_{dw}$ (µg/L)	MTD (mg)	MOE	Comments
Total NSAIDs	2.74	7.5	2737	Combination of 19 anti-inflammatory drugs
Cannabis (tetrahydrocannabinol)	1.377	1	726	Illegal drug
Oseltamivir carboxylate (Tamiflu active metabolite)	107	52	486	Used under pandemic conditions
LSD	0.997	1	10,309	Illegal drug
Cocaine (methylbenzoylecgonine)	0.029	1	34,483	Illegal drug
Aminophylline	0.15	1	6667	Smooth muscle relaxant
Beclometasone	0.005	0.05	10,000	Anti-asthmatic
Zidovudine	0.057	0.5	8772	Antiviral
Ecstasy	0.487	1	2053	Illegal drug
Acamprosate	0.435	1	2299	Alcoholism treatment
Total statins	1.27	5	3937	Cholesterol reduction
Nitroglycerine	0.035 4	0.15	4234	Vasodilator
Heroin (diamorphine)	0.00449	1	222,717	Illegal drug
Simvastatin	1.18	5	4227	Cholesterol reduction
Codeine	0.0157	20	1,277,139	Narcotic analgesic
Ramipril	0.153	1.25	8177	Diuretic
Lisinopril	0.396	2.5	6316	Angiotensin converting enzyme inhibitor
Methadone	0.0822		1	12,173
Furosemide	1.74	20		11,507
Amphetamine	0.0174		1	57,405
Norethisterone	0.0236		0.35	14,824
Doxazosin	0.00681	1	146,843	α-Blocker
Bendroflumethiazide	0.275		2.5	9094
Cyclosporin	0.0008		2	2,500,000

Source: Used with permission from World Health Organization 2011. Pharmaceuticals in drinking water, Table 4, Page 11; DWI. 2007. Desk based review of current knowledge on pharmaceuticals in drinking water and estimation of potential levels. Final report prepared by Watts and Crane Associates for Drinking Water Inspectorate, Department for Environment, Food and Rural Affairs (Defra Project Code: CSA 7184/WT02046/DWI70/2/213). http://dwi.defra.gov.uk/research/completed-research/reports/dwi70-2-213.pdf.

LSD, lysergic acid diethylamide; PEC$_{dw}$, predicted concentration in drinking water.

Persistent exposures of random combinations of low levels of pharmaceuticals have gone unnoticed for decades until recent studies showed alarming effects on human cells and wildlife.

They are certainly part of the total environmental pollutant load and thus will be part of the total body load of pollutant intake of the population and the chemically sensitive. Also, homeopathic doses are known to alter EMF frequencies and may change the individual functionally (Table 3.48).

MUNICIPAL SEWAGE

In order to prevent flooding, large storm pipes empty into the nearest rivers and lakes. Thus, during a rainstorm, large volumes of toxic substances such as animal and human wastes (hydraulic fluids, oils, a large variety of pesticides, radiants, mycotoxins, and coolants) are washed into drinking

TABLE 3.46
MOEs Calculated for Compounds Considered in the Awwa Research Foundation Study

Compound	MOE
Atenolol	2700
Diazepam	110,000
Fluoxetine	41,000
Meprobamate	6000
Norfluoxetine	44,000
Sulfamethoxazole	6,000,000
Triclosan	2,200,000

Source: Used with permission from World Health Organization 2011. Pharmaceuticals in drinking water, Table 6, Page 12.

TABLE 3.47
Conventional and Advanced Wastewater Treatment Processes and Their Expected Range of Removal Efficiency for Pharmaceuticals

Treatment Process	Removal Range (%)	Water Source	Areas Studied	Reference
Conventional Wastewater Treatment Processes				
Activated sludge	11–99	Raw sewage	Australia	Watkinson, Murby and Costanzo[539]
	7–100	Primary settled sewage	Europe, Japan DWI[541]	
	<20–80	Primary settled sewage	France	Gabet-Giraud et al.[541]
	−193 to 86	Primary settled sewage	Europe	Vieno, Tuhkanen and Kronberg[542]
	8–98	Not specified	Brazil, Europe, Japan	Ziylan and Ince[543]
Biological filtration	6–71	Primary settled sewage	Europe	DWI[540]
Primary settling	3–45	Not specified	Brazil, Europe, Japan	Ziylan and Ince[543]
Coagulation, filtration, and settling	5–36	Not specified		
Sand filtration	0–99	Activated sludge Effluent		
Advanced Wastewater Treatment Processes				
Ozonation	1–99	Activated sludge effluent	Brazil, Europe, Japan	Ziylan and Ince[543]
	86–100	Secondary effluent	France	Gabet-Giraud et al.[541]
Ozonation/ultrasound and sonocatalysis	23–45	Not specified	Europe, India, Japan, Turkey, USA	Ziylan and Ince[543]
Ozonation and catalytic ozonation	>9–100			
UV irradiation	29	Not specified	Brazil, Europe, Japan	Ziylan and Ince[543]
Photolysis (UV/hydrogen peroxide)	52–100	Not specified	Europe, India Japan, Turkey, USA	Ziylan and Ince[543]
Dark and light fenton	80–100			
UV/TIO$_2$	>95			
Biomembrane	23–99	Treated effluent	Brazil, Europe, Japan	Ziylan and Ince[543]
Microfiltration and reverse osmosis	91–100	Secondary treated effluent	Australia	Watkinson, Murby and Costanzo[539]

Source: Ternes, T.A. et al. 1999. *Sci. Tot. Environ.* 225:91–99; Vieno, N. et al. 2007. *Water Res.* 41:1001–1012.

TABLE 3.48

Organic Compounds Present in Some Drinking Water Able to Affect Blood Concentrations, Half-Life Estimates in the General Population, Perhaps Longer in the Chemically Sensitive

Compound	Arithmetic Mean	Frequency of Occurrence Per 100	Body Half-Life (Single Exposure) Estimates	Common Environmental Sources
Chlorinated Pesticides				
Aldrin	0.02	1.6		Agricultural insecticide
Dieldrin	0.17	66.8	50–266 days (humans)	Metabolite of aldrin
α-BHC	0.02	3.3		Agriculture-lindane termite control
γ-BHC	1.20	71.5		Termite control
DDT	0.28	54.3	2+ years (humans)	Illegal use; inert ingredient; contaminated imports
DDE	5.64	97.3	2+ years (humans)	Metabolite of DDT
DDD	0.02	2.8	2+ years (humans)	Metabolite of DDT
γ-Chlordane	0.01	1.4	21–88 days (humans)	Agriculture, termite control
Heptachlor	0.01	0.5	21–88 days (humans)	Agriculture, termite Control
Heptachlor epoxide	0.43	78.5	21–88 days (humans)	Metabolite of heptachlor
Trans-Nonachlor	0.21	80.7	21–88 days (humans)	Termite control
Endosulfan I	0.01	2.8	235 hours (rabbits)	Agriculture
Endosulfan II	0.01	1.1	597 hours (rabbits)	
HCB	0.54	95.3	Up to 3 years (Rhesus monkeys)	Fungicide, by product of chlorinated solvent
Mirex	0.01	1.1	3–4 months (rats)	Fire ant insecticide
Endrin	0.01	3.7	3–4 days (rats)	Agriculture crops
Chlorinated Phenols				
Penta	13.5	92.9	Approx. 8 days (humans)	Fungicide, bacteriocide, herbicide, packaging, shoe leather, etc.
2,3,5,6-Tetra	0.1	0.6		
2,3,4,5-Tetra	0.1	2.4		Fungicide, insecticide, contaminants of penta
2,3,4,5,6-Tri	0.1	0.6		Biocide, germicide
Total dichloro	0.10	0.30		
Polychlorinated Biphenyls (PCBs)	2.01	100.00	(humans)	Herbicide 2,4-D insulating coolants in electrical transformers, paints, coatings, and lubricants

Source: Adapted from Davies, K. 1986. *Human Exposure to Selected Persistent Toxic Chemical in the Great Lakes Basin: A Case Study of Toronto and Southern Ontario Region.* Toronto: Department of Public Health.

Notes: Time in the body may be much longer in the chemically sensitive. These are, in most cases, only gross estimates of the half-life of the parent chemical. There is increased evidence that the parent and/or metabolites may persist for considerably long periods of time in the tissues of the exposed animal or human. Recurrent symptoms (of subclinical symptoms) may occur for much longer than expected based on simple half-life calculations.
Major source is residence of United States.

water sources, markedly increasing their level of contamination. The aforementioned New Orleans floods and hurricanes are an example. Additionally, salts composed of either calcium or sodium chloride and asbestos become pollutants from road runoff not only in areas of the country where there is snow and ice but also in hot areas where the asbestos melts. Phosphorus from detergents also increases sewage contamination. Generally, the pollutants in municipal sewage waste are not greater than one-tenth of 1% of the total weight of pollutants, but they contain many toxic substances such as solvents, detergents, paints, pesticides, cleansers, petroleum products, medications, and so on, which are harmful to the individual with dyshomeostasis.

This volume of pollutants makes it extremely difficult to deliver less polluted water, both drinking and bathing, to the chemically sensitive person. "Purification" has to be accomplished not only through antimicrobial decontamination but also in the home with multiple series of filters.

SEWAGE TREATMENT

Sewage treatment is the process of removing contaminants from wastewater, including household sewage and runoff (effluents), domestic, commercial, and institutional. It includes physical, chemical, and biological processes to remove physical, chemical, and biological contaminants. Its objective is to produce an environmentally safe fluid waste stream (or treated effluent) and a solid waste (or treated sludge) suitable for disposal or reuse (usually as farm fertilizer). Using advanced technology, it is now possible to reuse sewage effluent for drinking water, although Singapore is the only country to implement such technology on a production scale in its production of NEWater (Figures 3.23 and 3.24).

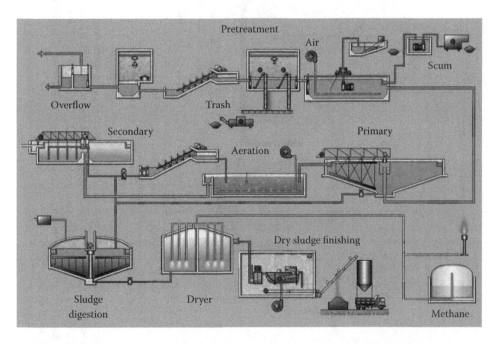

FIGURE 3.23 Simplified process flow diagrams for a typical large-scale treatment plant. (From https://www.google.com/search?q=Simplified+process+flow+diagrams+for+a+typical+large-scal e+treatment+plant&biw=1280&bih=929&tbm=isch&imgil=3_ShfwR7tjjNyM%253A%253B5dY-d6381cuilM%253Bhttps%25253A%25252F%25252Fen.wikipedia.org%25252Fwiki%25252FSewage_treatment&source=iu&pf=m&fir=3_ShfwR7tjjNyM%253A%252C5dY-d6381cuilM%252C_&usg=___6PU pv2l0s4I2hTLQpuDWePR_jA%3D&ved=0ahUKEwjuy-K8xqXLAhXFlYMKHc6SAx0QyjclJQ&ei=p7jY Vq7cGcWrjgTOpY7oAQ#imgrc=3_ShfwR7tjjNyM%3A.)

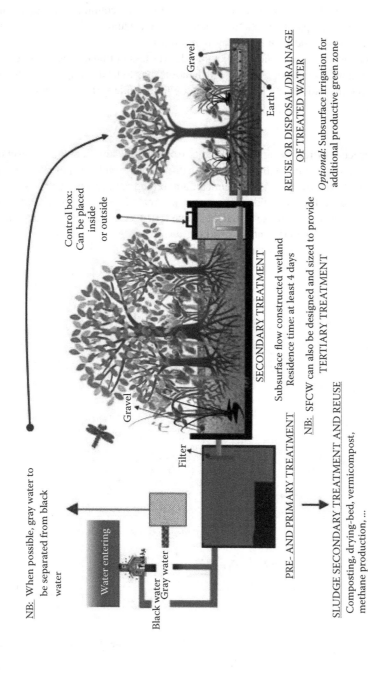

FIGURE 3.24 Process flow diagram for a typical treatment plant *via* subsurface flow constructed wetlands (SFCW). (From https://www.google.com/search?q=Simplified+process+flow+diagrams+for+a+typical+large-scale+treatment+plant&biw=1280&bih=929&tbm=isch&imgil=3_ShfwR7tjiNyM%253A%253B5dY-d6381cuilM%253Bhttps%25253A%25252F%25252Fen.wikipedia.org%25252Fwiki%25252FSewage_treatment&source=iu&pf=m&fir=3_ShfwR7tjiNyM%253A%252C5dY-d6381cuilM%252C_&usg=__6PUpv210s4I2hTLQpuDWePR_jA%3D&ved=0ahUKEwjuy-K8xqXLAhXFlYMKHc6SAx0QyjcIJQ&ei=p7jYVq7cGcWrjgTOpY7oAQ#imgrc=2WRliMaByByecM%3A.)

WASTEWATER

Wastewater is any water that has been adversely affected in quality by anthropogenic influence. Municipal wastewater is usually conveyed in a combined sewer or sanitary sewer, and treated at a wastewater treatment plant. Treated wastewater is discharged into receiving water via an effluent sewer. Wastewaters generated in areas without access to centralized sewer systems rely on on-site wastewater systems. These typically comprise a septic tank, a drain field, and optionally an on-site treatment unit.

Sewage is the subset of wastewater that is contaminated with feces or urine, but is often used to mean any wastewater. It includes domestic, municipal, or industrial liquid waste products disposed of, usually via a pipe or sewer (sanitary or combined), sometimes in a cesspool emptier.

Sewage is the physical infrastructure, including pipes, pumps, screens, channels, and so on, used to convey sewage from its origin to the point of eventual treatment or disposal. It is found in all types of sewage treatment, with the exception of septic systems, which treat sewage on site.

CYANOBACTERIA AND CYANOTOXINS: THE INFLUENCE OF NITROGEN VERSUS PHOSPHORUS

The importance of nitrogen (N) versus phosphorus (P) in explaining total cyanobacterial biovolume, the biovolume of specific cyanobacterial taxa, and the incidence of cyanotoxins was determined for 102 north German lakes, using methods to separate the effects of joint variation in N and P concentration from those of differential variation in N versus P. While the positive relationship between total cyanobacteria biovolume and P concentration disappeared at high P concentrations, cyanobacteria biovolume increased continually with N concentration, indicating potential N limitation in highly P-enriched lakes. The biovolumes of all cyanobacterial taxa were higher in lakes with above average joint NP concentrations, although the relative biovolumes of some Nostocales were higher in less enriched lakes. Taxa were found to have diverse responses to differential N versus P concentration, and the differences between taxa were not consistent with the hypothesis that potentially N_2-fixing Nostocales taxa would be favored in low N relative to P conditions. In particular, *Aphanizomenon gracile* and the subtropical invasive species *Cylindrospermopsis raciborskii* often reached their highest biovolumes in lakes with high nitrogen relative to phosphorus concentration. Concentrations of all cyanotoxin groups increased with increasing TP and TN, congruent with the biovolumes of their likely producers. Microcystin concentration was strongly correlated with the biovolume of *Planktothrix agardhii* but concentrations of anatoxin, cylindrospermopsin, and paralytic shellfish poison were not strongly related to any individual taxa. Cyanobacteria should not be treated as a single group when considering the potential effects of changes in nutrient loading on phytoplankton community structure and neither should the N_2-fixing Nostocales. This is of particular importance when considering the occurrence of cyanotoxins, as the two most abundant potentially toxin-producing Nostocales in our study were found in lakes with high N relative to P enrichment.[544]

Anthropogenic loading of nitrogen (N) and phosphorus (P) to freshwaters and coastal marine systems is a global environmental problem[545,546] that generates social and financial costs for human populations.[547,548] One of the more unpleasant consequences of eutrophication is an increase in the occurrence of unsightly, odorous, and sometimes toxic cyanobacterial blooms.[549,550] Control of cyanobacteria is thus a major concern in freshwater management.

The observation that cyanobacteria increase with eutrophication has been recognized for several decades.[551–556] For a long time, phosphorus was considered the primary nutrient limiting the development of cyanobacterial biovolumes,[557,558] despite there being considerable evidence that N limitation is a common and widespread phenomenon in lakes.[559,560] Nitrogen consequently received less attention than phosphorus and there is less known about the role nitrogen may play in controlling eutrophication and, in particular, its influence on the taxonomic composition of phytoplankton.[561,562]

There has been a great deal of research into the various traits, such as buoyancy regulation and colony formation, that allow cyanobacteria to become dominant in the phytoplankton assemblages of highly eutrophic lakes.[563,564] One such trait is the ability of some cyanobacteria to fix atmospheric nitrogen (N_2), giving them a competitive advantage when the ratio of N to P is low and N availability is limiting phytoplankton growth rates.[565] Given the tendency of more eutrophic lakes to have a lower ratio of N to P,[566] this has been suggested as one reason why cyanobacteria tend to dominate the phytoplankton in eutrophic lakes.[567] More common is the claim that cyanobacteria become dominant in lakes with a low N to P ratio in general and that reducing nitrogen inputs as a means of controlling phytoplankton would be a waste of effort because cyanobacteria could readily replace the missing nitrogen through fixation.[568,569] Thus, legislation governing inputs to water systems and recommendations to water managers have in the past focused on P reduction.

The cyanobacteria are highly diverse and the traits that may help them to dominate are not shared by all taxa. For example, N_2 fixation can only be done by the Nostocales and a small number of non-heterocystous taxa such as the marine *Trichodesmium*. However, most studies examining the response of phytoplankton composition to changes in nutrient concentrations across a large number of lakes treat cyanobacteria as a single response group (e.g., References 555, 556, 566, and 570). Many studies have examined compositional changes in individual lakes during eutrophication (or abatement) (e.g., References 571–573) or have examined the ecology of specific taxa (e.g., Reference 574), but there have been surprisingly few comprehensive studies of how functional groups of cyanobacteria change along eutrophication gradients and fewer still along gradients of both P and N (but see Reference 575).

The occurrence of particular cyanotoxins is dependent on the composition of cyanobacteria communities because different species can produce different toxins. For example, microcystins are mainly produced by *Microcystis, Planktothrix,* or *Anabaena* species[576]; cylindrospermopsin by *Cylindrospermopsis* and *Aphanizomenon*[577]; and anatoxin and paralytic shellfish poison by various *Anabaena* and *Aphanizomenon* species.[578–580] Furthermore, there are some taxa, such as the *Limnothrix*, for which no toxic substances have yet been identified. In addition, it is known that toxigenic and nontoxigenic strains coexist within populations of the same species and that the proportion of toxigenic and nontoxigenic cells in a population can be quite variable.[581,582] Total toxin concentrations in the water column also depend on the cellular toxin content of the producing taxa, which can be affected by environmental parameters such as light, temperature, and nutrients (Figure 3.25).[583–585]

Plant Nutrients

If excessive quantities of plant nutrients are discharged into lakes, ocean bays, and rivers from any possible sources of human activity, the natural aging processes of a waterway accelerate. The essential nutrients of aquatic plants are phosphorus from phosphates and nitrogen from nitrates. With an excess of these, plant life such as algae increases which causes the oxygen supply to decrease. The plants die, the water becomes contaminated, and finally the fish are killed. Nitrates used in fertilizers and organophosphates used in insecticides are major contributors to rural contamination. Contributing to an increase in total body load is domestic sewage containing phosphate detergents and urban runoff containing nitrogen and phosphorus from lawn fertilizers, animals, leaves, dust, combustion products, and phosphorus mining.

Toxic Substances

Toxic substances disrupt aquatic organisms because they alter the metabolism of the organism as a result of ingestion or contact. If the immediate effects of toxic pollutants are not lethal, there is a long-term bioaccumulation throughout the food chain that eventually results in an increase in the pollutant levels of humans, exacerbating chemical sensitivity and chronic degenerative disease. The organisms that reach the highest trophic levels are exposed to the highest levels of pollutants. This bioaccumulation means that humans, who are at the top of the food chain, take in the most contaminants. The food chain of water organisms has four to six levels, whereas terrestrial organisms have only two or three, and generally more pollutants occur in waterborne foods for humans. This bioaccumulation of toxic chemicals

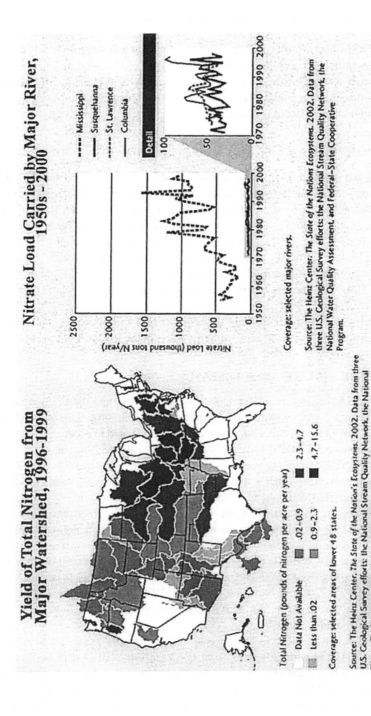

FIGURE 3.25 Yield of total nitrogen from major watershed and nitrate load carried by major river. (From EPA Draft Report on the Environment 2003. Chapter 5, Ecological Condition, pp. 5–11.)

is one of the reasons for the increased levels of these found in some chemically sensitive patients. One example is the levels of benzene found at Camp Lejeune Marine base where they found 380 ppb in the drinking water. These levels can result in acute dizziness, vomiting, sleepiness, convulsions, and death. Long-term exposure results in bone marrow damage, anemia, and leukemia.[545]

Another example is the fact that many wells are contaminated with arsenic which often makes the public ill.[545]

However, newer data from California arsenic rick from Mono Lake shows arsenic incorporated into DNA sequences and certain other proteins and major metabolites such as glucose and phosphate.[545]

They frequently find arsenic in the hair and blood analysis of the chemically sensitive and chronic degenerative disease patient and always assume it to be detrimental; however, more data on its biological function may modify our opinion.

POLLUTANTS FROM WATER TREATMENT, STORAGE, AND DISTRIBUTION

EWG's analysis of water suppliers' tap water test results shows that water contaminated with 44 pollutants that are residues of water treatment, storage, and distribution, including chemical by-products of water disinfection, is served to 178,679,000 people in 41 states. Of those, 79% people were served water with one or more of these contaminants present at levels above nonenforceable, health-based limits. Twenty-four of these chemicals detected in tap water are unregulated, without a legal, health-based limit in tap water. Again, whether regulated or unregulated, these toxics are combined and surely in many cases can have a synergistic effect on the individuals whose consequence is unknown. However, they are detrimental in the chemically sensitive and chronic degenerative disease patient.

Tap water disinfection is crucial for controlling waterborne infectious disease, but the chemicals used for disinfecting can form harmful chemical by-products in the treated water.[545]

MICROBIOLOGICAL WATERBORNE DISEASE

Since 1971, CDC, the U.S. Environmental Protection Agency (EPA), and the Council of State and Territorial Epidemiologists have maintained a collaborative Waterborne Disease and Outbreak Surveillance System (WBDOSS) for collecting and reporting data related to occurrences and causes of waterborne-disease outbreaks (WBDOs) and cases of waterborne disease. This surveillance system is the primary source of data concerning the scope and effects of waterborne disease in the United States.

Data presented summarize 28 WBDOs that occurred during January 2005 and December 2006 and four previously unreported WBDOs that occurred during 1979–2002.

The surveillance system includes data on waterborne disease occurrence and outbreak. Surveillance system WBDOs associated with recreational water, drinking water, water not intended for drinking (WNID) (excluding recreational water), and water use of unknown intent.

Fourteen states reported 28 WBDOs that occurred during 2005–2006: a total of 20 were associated with drinking water, six were associated with WNID, and two were associated with water of unknown intent (WUI). The 20 drinking water-associated WBDOs caused illness among an estimated 612 persons and were linked to four deaths. Etiologic agents were identified in 18 (90.0) of the drinking water-associated WBDOs.

Among the 18 WBDOs with identified pathogens, 12 (66.7%) were associated with bacteria, 3 (16.7%) with viruses, 2 (11.1%) with parasites, and 1 (5.6%) mixed WBDO with both bacteria and viruses. In both WBDOs where the etiology was not determined, norovirus was the suspected etiology.

Of the 20 drinking water WBDOs, 10 (50%) were outbreaks of acute respiratory illness (ARI), 9 (45%) were outbreaks of acute gastrointestinal illness (AGI), and 1 (5.0%) was an outbreak of hepatitis. All WBDOs of ARI were caused by *Legionella*, and this is the first reporting period in which the proportion of ARI WBDOs has surpassed that of AGI WBDOs since the reporting of *Legionella* WBDOs was initiated in 2001.[586]

A total of 23 deficiencies were cited in the 20 WBDOs associated with drinking water: 12 (52.2%) deficiencies fell under the classification NWU/POU (deficiencies occurred at points not under the jurisdiction of a water utility or at the point of use), 10 (43.5%) deficiencies fell under the classification SWTDs (contamination at or in the source water, treatment facility, or distribution system), and for 1 (4.3%) deficiency, the classification was unknown. Among the 12 NWU/POU deficiencies, 10 (83.3%) involved *Legionella* spp. in the drinking water system. The most frequently cited SWTD deficiencies were associated with a treatment deficiency (n = 4 [40.0%]) and untreated groundwater (n = 4 [40.0%]). Three of the four WBDOs with treatment deficiencies used groundwater sources.

Approximately half (52.2%) of the drinking water deficiencies occurred outside the jurisdiction of a water utility. The majority of these WBDOs were associated with *Legionella* spp., which suggests that increased attention should be targeted toward reducing illness risks associated with *Legionella* spp. Nearly all of the WBDOs associated with SWTD deficiencies occurred in systems using groundwater. EPA's new Ground Water Rule (GWR) might prevent similar outbreaks in the future in public water systems.

The majority of drinking water deficiencies are now associated with contamination at points outside the jurisdiction of public water systems (e.g., regrowth of *Legionella* spp. in hot water systems) and water contamination that might not be regulated by EPA (e.g., contamination of tap water at the point of use). Improved education of consumers and plumbers might help address these risk factors.

Of the 20 drinking water-associated WBDOs, 12 (60.0%) were caused by bacteria, 3 (15.0%) were caused by viruses, 2 (10.0%) were caused by parasites, and 1 (5.0%) was caused by more than one etiologic agent type. Two (10.0%) were of unknown etiology (Figure 3.29).

Bacteria: Twelve WBDOs affecting 135 persons were attributed to bacterial infections: 10 outbreaks caused by *Legionella*; one outbreak caused by *Campylobacter*; and one outbreak (Oregon, 2005) in which persons had multiple stool specimens that tested positive for *C. jejuni*, *Escherichia* O157:H7, and *E. coli* O145. Illnesses from these 12 WBDOs resulted in four deaths, all of which were associated with *Legionella* spp.

Viruses: Three WBDOs affecting 212 persons were attributed to viral infections: two outbreaks caused by norovirus G1 and one outbreak caused by hepatitis A. No deaths were reported.

Parasites: Two WBDOs affecting 51 persons were attributed to parasites: one outbreak caused by *Giardia intestinalis* and one outbreak caused by *Cryptosporidium*. No deaths were reported.[586]

Mixed agent types: One WBDO was attributed to more than one type of etiologic agent; no deaths were reported. This outbreak affected 139 persons and involved two viruses (norovirus G1 and norovirus G2) and one bacterium (*C. jejuni*).[587]

Unidentified etiologic agents: Two WBDOs involving AGI of unidentified etiology affected 75 persons; no deaths were reported. No viral testing was attempted in one of the outbreaks (Ohio 2005). In the other outbreak (New York 2006), norovirus, enterovirus, and rotavirus were isolated from water samples. In both of the outbreaks, norovirus was the suspected etiology on the basis of incubation period, symptoms, and duration of illness.[586]

During 2005–2006, five drinking water-related WBDOs associated with water-treatment deficiencies were reported; all were associated with inadequate chlorination. One WBDO was associated with a malfunctioning chlorine feeder (Indiana, 2006). Two outbreaks occurred because existing water treatment was overwhelmed. Heavy rain might have overwhelmed a camp surface water treatment system in one outbreak (Oregon, 2005), and remnants of Hurricane Katrina might have created surface water runoff into a spring supplying drinking water to a restaurant in the other outbreak (Ohio, 2005).

Although treatment deficiencies (deficiency 3) made up the greatest proportion (50.0%) of SWTD deficiencies during the 2005–2006 surveillance period, the majority (80.0%) of these treatment deficiencies were associated with failures to adequately treat contaminated groundwater. When these deficiencies are considered with deficiency 2, contaminated groundwater becomes the single largest contributing factor to SWTD-related outbreaks, underscoring the need for the GWR previously described.

Distribution system deficiencies make up the smallest proportion of the SWTD deficiencies during this surveillance period. During 2005–2006, two drinking water-related WBDOs involving distribution system deficiencies occurred. Before one outbreak (Indiana, 2006), a new water main was installed without a valid permit. The water main was pressure tested and was left under pressure with nonpotable water, resulting in a cross-contamination hazard. In the second outbreak, backflow prevention devices were absent on water distribution lines to toilet facilities in a camp (Maryland, 2006). Drinking water quality within the distribution systems of public water supplies is regulated under EPA's Total Coliform Rule, which is currently undergoing revisions to better protect public health.

Legionella in water intended for drinking: Legionellosis includes two clinically distinct syndromes: Legionnaires' disease (LD), characterized by severe pneumonia, and Pontiac fever (PF), a febrile cough illness that does not progress to pneumonia. Legionellosis outbreaks accounted for 50% of all drinking water-associated WBDOs reported during 2005–2006 and 83.3% of all NWU/POU deficiencies, indicating that *Legionella* is a serious public health threat. When outbreaks of legionellosis occur in the setting of contaminated drinking water, they typically manifest as cases of LD rather than PF. Approximately 8000–18,000 cases of LD occur each year in the United States.[588] Regardless of the syndrome, the source of legionellosis outbreaks typically share common features (e.g., warm stagnant water, inadequate biocide concentrations, and aerosolization, which provide the mechanism for inhalation).

The outbreaks of legionellosis highlight the challenges related to its detection and prevention. LD is underdiagnosed because the majority of patients with community-acquired pneumonia are treated empirically with broad-spectrum antibiotics.[589] However, since *Legionella* spp. are not transmitted from person to person and are always acquired from an environmental source, even a single case of LD implies the presence of a contaminated aquatic source to which others can be exposed. Certain host factors (e.g., underlying lung disease and immunodeficiencies) influence the development and severity of legionellosis. Typically, the attack rate during documented LD outbreaks is quite low (i.e., <5%). Not everyone who is exposed to *Legionella*-contaminated water is susceptible to symptomatic illness. Identification of two or more cases of LD in association with a potential source is adequate justification for an investigation. All of the legionellosis outbreaks described in this report involved 10 or fewer cases. Nonetheless, in all instances but one, the epidemiologic and laboratory data were compelling enough to implicate point sources that were subsequently remediated.[586]

During 2005–2006, a total of 8 (80%) of 10 legionellosis outbreaks associated with drinking water occurred in health-care settings, demonstrating the propensity of *Legionella* spp. to colonize potable water systems and underscoring the importance of maintaining a high index of suspicion for legionellosis in health-care settings. Seven outbreaks occurred in acute care hospitals and one in a long-term care facility. *Legionella* spp. colonize the biofilm layer frequently found inside the large, complex plumbing systems of hospitals.[590] This biofilm protects *Legionella* from biocides and allows the bacteria to amplify to levels sufficient to be transmitted and/or cause disease. Patients in hospitals or long-term care facilities typically are older and have underlying illness factors that increase the risk for disease (e.g., chronic lung disease, diabetes, and immunocompromising conditions).[586]

Two primary trends can be observed from the 2005–2006 surveillance period data. Since it was first included in WBDOSS in 2001, *Legionella* has become the single most common cause of reported outbreaks in WBDOSS. This does not mean that *Legionella* is a more important cause of waterborne disease than other agents (e.g., norovirus), and nor does it mean that legionellosis outbreaks are increasing because they have only been included in the WBDOSS since 2001. Therefore, there is a limited basis for historical comparison. However, outbreaks associated with other agents are not being reported as frequently as outbreaks caused by *Legionella*. Whether this is a result of barriers to laboratory confirmation of non-*Legionella* pathogens in clinical specimens and environmental samples, lack of detection of non-*Legionella* pathogens as a result of different incubation periods or milder illness, use of adequate water treatment technologies for non-*Legionella* pathogens, or other factors that might be responsible for fewer outbreaks associated with non-*Legionella* is not clear (Table 3.49, Figures 3.26 through 3.29).

During 1999–2000, a total of 44 outbreaks (18 from private wells, 1 from noncommunity systems, and 12 from community systems) associated with drinking water were reported by 25 states. Nicholson[591] has found mycoplasma infections in many cases of autistic and chronic fatigue cases in the children and veterans from the Gulf War (Tables 3.50 and 3.51, Figure 3.30).[591]

Despite advances in water management and sanitation, waterborne disease outbreaks continue to occur in the United States. CDC collects data on waterborne disease outbreaks submitted from all states and territories through the WBDOSS. During 2009–2010, the most recent years for which

TABLE 3.49

Waterborne Disease Outbreaks Associated with Drinking Water (n = 12), by State—United States, 2006

State	Month	Class	Etiologic Agent	Predominant Illness[a]	No. of Cases (Deaths)[b] (n = 432)	Type of System[c]	Deficiency[d]	Water Source	Setting
Indiana	Feb	I	Campylobacter	AGI	32	Com	3, 4	Well	Community
Maryland	Jul	III	Norovirus G1	AGI	148	Ncom	3, 4, 11B	Well	Camp
North Carolina	Jul	I	Hepatitis A	Hep	16	Ind	2	Spring	Private residence
New York	Aug	III	Unidentified[e]	AGI	16	Ind	2	Well	Bed and Breakfast
New York	Jun	III	Legionella[f]	ARI	4	Com	5A	Lake[g]	Hospital
New York	Jan	III	L. pneumophila serogroup 3	ARI	2	Com	5A	Reservoir[g]	Hospital
Ohio	Sep	III	Cryptosporidium	AGI	10	Com	99A	Well	Church
Ohio	Aug	III	L. pneumophila serogroup 1	ARI	3	Com	5A	Lake[g]	Hospital
Oregon	Dec	III	Norovirus G1	AGI	48	Ncom	2	Well	Restaurant
Pennsylvania	Apr	III	L. pneumophila serogroup 1	ARI	4	Ncom	5A	Well[g]	Hotel
Texas	Apr	III	L. pneumophila[f]	ARI	10(3)	Com	5A	Unknown[g]	Hospital
Wyoming	Jun	I	Norovirus G1, C. jejuni, Norovirus G2[h]	AGI	139	Ncom	2	Well	Camp

Source: Yoder, J. et al. 2011. *Surveillance for Waterborne Disease and Outbreaks Associated with Drinking Water and Water Not Intended for Drinking—United States, 2005–2006.* U.S. Department of Health and Human Services, Washington, DC, 60(12):38–68; CDC. 2007. Gastroenteritis among attendees at a summer camp—Wyoming, June–July 2006. *MMWR* 56:368–370.

[a] AGI: acute gastrointestinal illness; ARI: acute respiratory illness; and Hep: viral hepatitis.

[b] Deaths are indicated in parentheses if they occurred.

[c] Com: community; Ncom: noncommunity; and Ind: individual. Community and noncommunity water systems are public water systems.

[d] Deficiency classification for drinking water, water not intended for drinking (excluding recreational water), and water of unknown intent.

[e] Etiology unidentified: norovirus suspected baed upon incubation period, symptoms, and duration of illness. Norovirus, enterovirus and rotavirus were isolated from the well.

[f] Environmental testing detected *L. pneumophilia* serogroup 1. *L. pneumophilia* other than serogroup 1, and non-pneumophila *Legionella* species.

[g] Transmission of *Legionella* thought to be as a result of building-specific factors and not related to water source.

[h] Eight persons had stool specimens that tested positive for norovirus G1, six persons had stool specimens that tested positive for C. jejuni, and three persons had stool specimens that tested positive for norovirus G2.

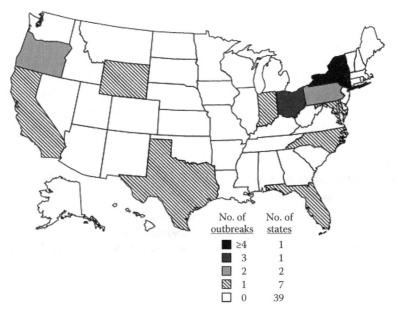

No. of outbreaks	No. of states
≥4	1
3	1
2	2
1	7
0	39

* n=20; numbers are dependent on reporting and surveillance activities in individual states and do not necessarily indicate that more outbreaks occurred in a given state.

FIGURE 3.26 Number of waterborne-disease outbreaks associated with drinking water—United States, 2005–2006. (From Yoder, J. et al. 2011. *Surveillance for Waterborne Disease and Outbreaks Associated with Drinking Water and Water Not Intended for Drinking—United States, 2005–2006.* U.S. Department of Health and Human Services, Washington, DC, 60(12):38–68.)

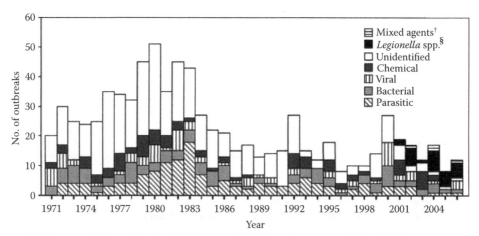

* Single cases of disease related to drinking water (n=16) have been removed from this figure; therefore, it is not comparable to figures in previous *Surveillance Summaries.*
† Beginning in 2003, mixed agents of more than one etiologic agent type were included in the surveillance system. However, the first observation is a previously unreported outbreak in 2002.
§ Beginning in 2001, Legionnaires' disease was added to the surveillance system, and *Legionella* species were classified separately in this figure.

FIGURE 3.27 Number of waterborne disease outbreaks associated with drinking water (n = 814) *by year and etiologic agent)—United States, 1971–2006. (From Yoder, J. et al. 2011. *Surveillance for Waterborne Disease and Outbreaks Associated with Drinking Water and Water Not Intended for Drinking—United States, 2005–2006.* U.S. Department of Health and Human Services, Washington, DC, 60(12):38–68.)

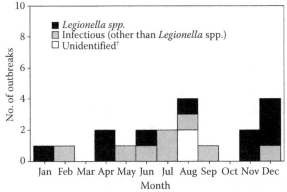

* n=20.
† Unidentified etiology includes suspected etiologies not confirmed during
  the outbreak investigation.

FIGURE 3.28 Number* of waterborne disease outbreaks associated with drinking water, by etiologic agent and month—United States, 2005–2006. (From Yoder, J. et al. 2011. *Surveillance for Waterborne Disease and Outbreaks Associated with Drinking Water and Water Not Intended for Drinking—United States, 2005– 2006.* U.S. Department of Health and Human Services, Washington, DC, 60(12):38–68.)

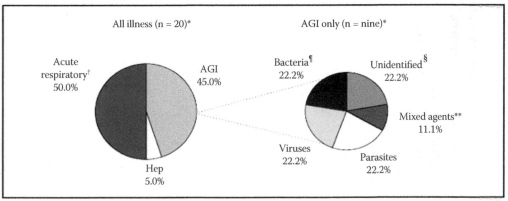

* AGI: acute gastrointestinal illness; ARI: acute respiratory illness; Hep: viral hepatitis.
† All acute respiratory illness was attributed to *Legionella* spp.
§ Norovirus suspected based upon incubation period, symptoms, and duration of illness.
¶ Including one outbreak that involved multiple bacterial agents.
** One outbreak that involved bacterial and viral agents.

FIGURE 3.29 Percentage of waterborne-disease outbreaks (WBDOs) associated with drinking water, by illness and etiology—United States, 2005–2006. (From Yoder, J. et al. 2011. *Surveillance for Waterborne Disease and Outbreaks Associated with Drinking Water and Water Not Intended for Drinking—United States, 2005–2006.* U.S. Department of Health and Human Services, Washington, DC, 60(12):38–68.)

finalized data are available, 33 drinking water-associated outbreaks were reported, comprising 1040 cases of illness, 85 hospitalizations, and 9 deaths. *Legionella* accounted for 58% of outbreaks and 7% of illnesses, and *Campylobacter* accounted for 12% of outbreaks and 78% of illnesses. The most commonly identified outbreak deficiencies in drinking water-associated outbreaks were *Legionella* in plumbing systems (57.6%), untreated groundwater (24.2%), and distribution system deficiencies (12.1%), suggesting that efforts to identify and correct these deficiencies could prevent many outbreaks and illnesses associated with drinking water. In addition to the drinking water outbreaks,

TABLE 3.50

Characteristics of Waterborne Disease Outbreaks Associated with Drinking Water (N = 33) and Other Nonrecreational Water[a] (N = 12), but State Jurisdiction—Waterborne Disease and Outbreak Surveillance System, United States, 2011–2012

State/ Jurisdiction	Month	Year	Etiology[a]	Predominant Illness[b]	No. Cases	No. Hospitalization[c]	No. Deaths[d]	Water System[e]	Water Source	Setting
Alaska	Jun	2012	*Giardia intestinalis*	AGI	21	0	0	Transient noncommunity	Spring, Well, River/Stream[f]	Camp/Cabin
Arizona	Mar	2011	Unknown	AGI	3	0	0	Nontransient noncommunity	Spring	Outdoor workplace
Colorado	Oct	2012	Propylene glycol suspected[g]	AGI	7	0	0	Community	Lake/Reservoir/ Impoundment	Hospital/Health care
Florida	Aug	2009[h]	*L. pneumophila* serogroup 1	ARI	10	4	1	Community	Unknown	Hotel/Motel/Lodge/Inn
Florida	Jul	2011	*Shigella sonnei* subgroup D	AGI	22	0	0	Commercially bottled	Unknown	Indoor workplace/Office
Florida	Mar	2012	Unknown[i]	AGI	3	0	0	Commercially bottled	Well	Indoor workplace/Office
Idaho	May	2012	*Campylobacter Giardia intestinalis*	AGI	7	0	0	Community	River/Stream/Well	Community/Municipality
Illinois	Aug	2012	*Pantoea agglomerans*[j]	Other	12	0	0	Community	Lake/Reservoir/ Impoundment	Hospital/Health care
Maryland	May	2011	*L. pneumophila* serogroup 1	ARI	7	6	1	Community	Well	Hotel/Motel/Lodge/Inn
Maryland	May	2012	*L. pneumophila* serogroup 1	ARI	3	2	1	Community	Lake/Reservoir/ Impoundment	Hospital/Health care
New Mexico	Jun	2011	Norovirus	AGI	119	0	0	Transient noncommunity	Spring[k]	Camp/Cabin
New York	Apr	2009[l]	*L. pneumophila* serogroup 1	ARI	4	4	0	Community	Lake/Reservoir/ Impoundment	Apartment/Condo
New York	Jun	2011	*L. pneumophila* serogroup 1	ARI	2	2	0	Community	River/Stream	Hospital/Health care
New York	Sep	2011	*L. pneumophila* serogroup 1	ARI	12	10	0	Community	Lake/Reservoir/ Impoundment	Hotel/Motel/Lodge/Inn
New York	Sep	2011	*L. pneumophila* serogroup 1	ARI	3	0	0	Community	Lake/Reservoir/ Impoundment	Hospital/Health care
New York	Jan	2012	*L. pneumophila* serogroup 1	ARI	3	0		Community	Lake/Reservoir/ Impoundment	Hotel/Motel/Lodge/Inn

(Continued)

TABLE 3.50 (Continued)

Characteristics of Waterborne Disease Outbreaks Associated with Drinking Water (N = 33) and Other Nonrecreational Water[a] (N = 12), but State Jurisdiction—Waterborne Disease and Outbreak Surveillance System, United States, 2011–2012

State/Jurisdiction	Month	Year	Etiology[a]	Predominant Illness[b]	No. Cases	No. Hospitalization[c]	No. Deaths[d]	Water System[e]	Water Source	Setting
New York	Mar	2012	L. pneumophila serogroup 1	ARI	2	1	0	Community	Lake/Reservoir/Impoundment	Hospital/Health care
New York	Apr	2012	L. pneumophila serogroup 1	ARI	2	2		Community	Lake/Reservoir/Impoundment	Apartment/Condo
New York	Oct	2012	L. pneumophila serogroup 1	ARI	2	1	0	Community	Lake/Reservoir/Impoundment	Hospital/Health care
New York	Nov	2012	L. pneumophila serogroup 1	ARI	2	2	0	Community	Lake/Reservoir/Impoundment	Hospital/Health care
Ohio	Jan	2011	L. pneumophila serogroup 1	ARI	11	11	1	Community	Well	Hospital/Health care
Ohio	Mar	2011	L. pneumophila serogroup 1	ARI	8	7	0	Community	Lake/Reservoir/Impoundment	Hospital/Health care
Ohio	Aug	2011	L. pneumophila	ARI	10	4	2	Community	Lake/Reservoir/Impoundment	Hospital/Health care
Ohio	Nov	2012	L. pneumophila serogroup 1	ARI	2	2	0	Community	Lake/Reservoir/Impoundment	Hospital/Health care
Pennsylvania	Feb	2011	L. pneumophila serogroup 1	ARI	22	22	5	Community	Lake/Reservoir/Impoundment	Hospital/Health care[m]
Pennsylvania	May	2011	L. pneumophila serogroup 1	ARI	2	2	0	Community	Well	Long-term care facility
Pennsylvania	Aug	2011	L. pneumophila serogroup 1	ARI	6	5	1	Community	Well	Hospital/Health care
Pennsylvania	Mar	2012	L. pneumophila	ARI	2	2	1	Community	Lake/Reservoir/Impoundment	Hospital/Health care
Pennsylvania	Nov	2012	L. pneumophila serogroup 1	ARI	4	4	1	Community	River/Stream	Apartment/Condo
Utah	Aug	2011	STEC O121, STEC O157:H7	AGI[n]	56	2	0	Transient noncommunity	Spring	Camp/Cabin
Utah	Jul	2012	L. pneumophila serogroup 1	ARI	3	3	0	Community	Lake/Reservoir/Impoundment	Hotel/Motel/Lodge/Inn
Utah	Aug	2012	Giardia intestinalis	AGI	28	0	0	Community	Well	Subdivision/Neighborhood
Washington	Jan	2011	L. pneumophila serogroup 1	ARI	3	3	1	Community	Well	Hospital/Healthcare

(Continued)

TABLE 3.50 (Continued)

Characteristics of Waterborne Disease Outbreaks Associated with Drinking Water (N = 33) and Other Nonrecreational Water[a] (N = 12), but State Jurisdiction—Waterborne Disease and Outbreak Surveillance System, United States, 2011–2012

State/Jurisdiction	Month	Year	Etiology[a]	Predominant Illness[b]	No. Cases	No. Hospitalization[c]	No. Deaths[d]	Water System[e]	Water Source	Setting
Wisconsin	Aug	2012	Norovirus Genogroup1.2	AGI	19	0	0	Transient noncommunity	Well[o]	Hall/Meeting facility

Source: Beer, K. D. et al., 2015. Surveillance for waterborne disease outbreaks associated with drinking water—United States, *2011–2012 Morbidity and Mortality Weekly Report*, 64(31):842–848.

Alternate Text: The figure above shows the number of waterborne disease outbreaks associated with drinking water (N = 851), by year and etiology, in the United States during 1971–2010. The outbreaks resulted in 1040 illnesses, 85 hospitalizations (8.2% of cases), and nine deaths. At least one etiologic agent was identified in all but one drinking water outbreak; *Legionella* was implicated in 19 outbreaks, 72 illnesses, 58 hospitalizations, and eight deaths, and *Campylobacter* was implicated in four single-etiology outbreaks involving 812 illnesses, 17 hospitalizations, and no deaths, as well as two multiple-etiology outbreaks resulting in 17 illnesses.

Abbreviations: AGI = acute gastrointestinal illness; ARI = acute respiratory illness; *L. pneumophila* = *Legionella pneumophila*; other = undefined, illnesses, conditions, or symptoms that cannot be categorized as gastrointestinal, respiratory, ear-related, eye-related, skin-related, neurologic, hepatitis, or caused by leptospirosis; STEC = Shiga toxin-producing *Escherichia coli*.

a　Etiologies listed are confirmed, unless indicated "suspected." For multiple-etiology outbreaks, etiologies are listed in alphabetical order.

b　The category of illness reported by ≥50% of ill respondents. All legionellosis outbreaks were categorized as ARI.

c　Value was set to "missing" in reports where zero hospitalizations were reported and the number of people for whom information was available was also zero.

d　Value was set to "missing" in reports where zero deaths were reported and the number of people for whom information was available was also zero.

e　Community and noncommunity water systems are public water systems that have ≥15 service connections or serve an average of ≥25 residents for ≥60 days/year. A community water system serves year-round residents of a community, subdivision, or mobile home park. A noncommunity water system serves an institution, industry, camp, park, hotel, or business and can be nontransient or transient. Nontransient systems serve ≥25 of the same persons for ≥6 months of the year but not year-round (e.g., factories and schools), whereas transient systems provide water to places in which persons do not remain for long periods of time (e.g., restaurants, highway rest stations, and parks). Water systems in this table include community, noncommunity, and bottled.

f　Spring water source contaminated during temporary connection with contaminated surface water source (stream).

g　Skin and eye symptoms in addition to AGI; other possible chemical exposures from cross-contamination between drinking water and boiler water.

h　The first case of illness in this outbreak occurred before 2011–2012, but the outbreak was reported later and not previously described in a surveillance report.

i　Chemical contamination suspected due to short incubation period; three bottled water samples tested, no chemical contamination detected.

j　Outbreak of *Pantoea agglomerans* bloodstream infection in a health-care facility linked to the drinking water system. Oncology clinic patients received infusions contaminated with *P. agglomerans* via a central line, and environmental samples from the clinic and pharmacy where infusions were prepared shared the PFGE pattern found in patient blood samples. *P. agglomerans* was isolated from the pharmacy sink where the infusates were prepared, as well as from the oncology clinic icemaker. This is the first report of a *Pantoea* infection outbreak in a health-care facility, and in a drinking water–associated outbreak surveillance report.

k　Outbreak occurred at the same venue with the same etiology and water source as an outbreak previously reported in 1999; contamination by surface water was suspected, based on the 1999 investigation.

l　The first ill cases were identified in 2009, and were linked by molecular subtyping in 2012 to additional ill individuals living in the same apartment complex with onset dates in 2011 and 2012.

m　Hospital had a copper/silver ionization system, with concentrations at manufacturer-recommended levels, in place to control *Legionella* at the time of the outbreak.

n　No outbreak-associated cases of hemolytic uremic syndrome (HUS) were reported.

o　Setting was a meeting facility, where owner was unaware of and not maintaining septic system; system overflowed and contaminated the well.

TABLE 3.51
Rank Order (Most to Least Common) of Etiology, Water System, Water Source, Predominant Illness, and Deficiencies Associated with 32 Drinking Water Outbreaks and 431 Outbreak-Related Cases—United States 2011–1012

Characteristic	Rank	Outbreaks (N = 32)			Cases (N = 431)		
		Category	No.	(%)	Category	No.	(%)
Etiology	1	Bacteria, *Legionella*	21	(65.6)	Viruses	138	(32.0)
	2	Bacteria, non-*Legionella*	3	(9.4)	Bacteria, *Legionella*	111	(25.8)
	3	Parasites	2	(6.3)	Bacteria, non-*Legionella*	90	(20.9)
	4	Viruses	2	(6.3)	Parasites	49	(11.4)
	5	Unknown	2	(6.3)	Chemical[a]	26	(6.0)
	6	Chemical[a]	1	(3.1)	Unknown	10	(2.3)
	7	Multiple[b]	1	(3.1)	Multiple[b]	7	(1.6)
Water System[c]	1	Community	25	(78.1)	Noncommunity	222	(51.5)
	2	Noncommunity	5	(15.6)	Community	184	(42.7)
	3	Bottled	2	(6.3)	Bottled	25	(5.8)
Water source	1	Surface water	18	(56.3)	Ground water	261	(60.6)
	2	Ground water	11	(34.4)	Surface water	120	(27.8)
	3	Mixed[d]	2	(6.3)	Unknown	22	(5.1)
	4	Unknown	1	(3.1)	Mixed[d]	28	(6.5)
Predominant Illness[e]	1	ARI	21	(65.6)	AGI	308	(71.5)
	2	AGI	10	(31.3)	ARI	111	(25.8)
	3	Other[f]	1	(3.1)	Other[f]	12	(2.8)
Deficiency[g]	1	*Legionella spp.* in drinking water system[h]	21	(65.6)	Untreated ground water[i]	201	(46.6)
	2	Untreated ground water[i]	4	(12.5)	*Legionella spp.* in drinking water system[h]	111	(25.8)
	3	Premise plumbing system[j]	2	(6.3)	Premise plumbing system	33	(7.7)

(Continued)

TABLE 3.51 *(Continued)*
Rank Order (Most to Least Common) of Etiology, Water System, Water Source, Predominant Illness, and Deficiencies Associated with 32 Drinking Water Outbreaks and 431 Outbreak-Related Cases—United States 2011–1012

Characteristic	Rank	Outbreaks (N = 32) Category	No.	(%)	Cases (N = 431) Category	No.	(%)
	4	Unknown/Insufficient information	2	(6.3)	Distribution system[k]	28	(6.5)
	5	Distribution system[k]	1	(3.1)	Point of use, bottled[l]	22	(5.1)
	6	Multiple[m]	1	(3.1)	Multiple[m]	21	(4.9)
	7	Point of use, bottled[l]	1	(3.1)	Unknown/Insufficient information	15	(3.5)

Source: Beer, K. D. et al., 2015. Surveillance for waterborne disease outbreaks associated with drinking water—United States, *2011–2012 Morbidity and Mortality Weekly Report,* 64(31):842–848.

Abbreviations: AGI = acute gastrointestinal illness; ARI = acute respiratory illness.

a   Propylene glycol detected in drinking water after cross-connection with the HVAC water system.

b   One outbreak had multiple etiologic agent types: *Campylobacter* spp. (i.e., non-*Legionella* bacterium) and *Giardia intestinalis* (i.e., parasite).

c   Community and noncommunity water systems are public water systems that have ≥15 service connections or serve an average of ≥25 residents for ≥60 days a year. Community water systems serve year-round residents of a community, subdivision, or mobile home park. Noncommunity water systems serve an institution, industry, camp, park, hotel, or business.

d   Includes outbreaks with mixed water sources (i.e., groundwater and surface water). Two giardiasis outbreaks were associated with mixed source community water systems.

e   The category of illness reported by ≥50% of ill respondents; all legionellosis outbreaks were categorized as ARI.

f   Symptoms for one outbreak caused by *Pantoea agglomerans* bloodstream infection were categorized as "other."

g   Outbreaks are assigned one or more deficiency classifications. (*Source:* Brunkard, J. M. et al. 2011. Surveillance for waterborne disease outbreaks associated with drinking water—United States, 2007–2008. *MMWR Surveill. Summ.* 60:38–68.)

h   Deficiency 5A. Drinking water, contamination of water at points not under the jurisdiction of a water utility or at the point of use: *Legionella* spp. in water system, drinking water.

i   Deficiency 2. Drinking water, contamination of water at/in the water source, treatment facility, or distribution system: untreated groundwater.

j   Deficiency 6. Drinking water, contamination of water at points not under the jurisdiction of a water utility or at the point of use: Plumbing system deficiency after the water meter or property line (e.g., cross-connection, backflow, or corrosion products).

k   Deficiency 4. Drinking water, contamination of water at/in the water source, treatment facility, or distribution system: Distribution system deficiency, including storage (e.g., cross-connection, backflow, contamination of water mains during construction or repair).

l   Deficiency 11C. Drinking water, contamination of water at points not under the jurisdiction of a water utility or at the point of use: Contamination at point of use, commercially bottled water.

m   Multiple deficiencies were assigned to one giardiasis outbreak which contributed 21 cases: Deficiency 1, untreated surface water; and deficiency 2, untreated groundwater.

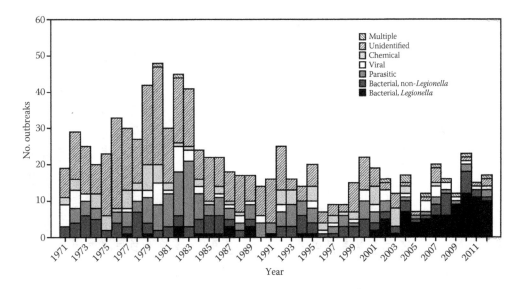

FIGURE 3.30 Number of waterborne disease outbreaks associated with drinking water by year and etiology—United States, 1971–2010. (From Beer, K. D. et al., 2015. Surveillance for waterborne disease outbreaks associated with drinking water—United States, 2011–2012 *Morbidity and Mortality Weekly Report*, 64(31):842–848.)

12 outbreaks associated with other nonrecreational water were reported, comprising 234 cases of illness, 51 hospitalizations, and 6 deaths. *Legionella* accounted for 58% of these outbreaks, 42% of illnesses, 96% of hospitalizations, and all deaths. Public health, regulatory, and industry professionals can use this information to target prevention efforts against pathogens, infrastructure problems, and water sources associated with waterborne disease outbreaks.

Surface Water Pollution—Microbial

Many infectious agents can cause disease. The following are some major infections that have been found (Table 3.52, Figure 3.31).

HARMFUL ALGAL BLOOMS

A *harmful algal bloom* (HAB) is an algal bloom that causes negative impacts to other organisms via production of natural toxins, mechanical damage to other organisms, or by other means (Figures 3.32 and 3.33). HABs are often associated with large-scale marine mortality events and have been associated with various types of shellfish poisonings.[592] They can also harm humans, especially the chemically sensitive and chronic degenerative disease patients.

In the marine environment, single-celled, microscopic, plant-like organisms naturally occur in the well-lit surface layer of any body of water. These organisms, referred to as phytoplankton or microalgae, form the base of the food web upon which nearly all other marine organisms depend. Of the 5000+ species of marine phytoplankton that exist worldwide, about 2% are known to be harmful or toxic.[593] Blooms of harmful algae can have large and varied impacts on marine ecosystems, depending on the species involved, the environment where they are found, and the mechanism by which they exert negative effects.

HABs have been observed to cause adverse effects to a wide variety of aquatic organisms, most notably marine mammals, sea turtles, seabirds, and finfish. The impacts of HAB toxins on these groups can include harmful changes to their developmental, immunological, neurological, or

TABLE 3.52

Infections

Disease and Transmission	Microbial Agent	Sources of Agent in Water Supply	General Symptoms
		Protozoal Infections	
Amoebiasis (hand-to-mouth)	Protozoan (*Entamoeba histolytica*) (Cyst-like appearance)	Sewage, nontreated drinking water, flies in water supply	Abdominal discomfort, fatigue, weight loss, diarrhea, bloating, fever
Cryptosporidiosis (oral)	Protozoan (*Cryptosporidium parvum*)	Collects on water filters and membranes that cannot be disinfected, animal manure, seasonal runoff of water	Flu-like symptoms, watery diarrhea, loss of appetite, substantial loss of weight, bloating, increased gas, nausea
Cyclosporiasis	Protozoan parasite (*Cyclospora cayetanensis*)	Sewage, nontreated drinking water	Cramps, nausea, vomiting, muscle aches, fever, and fatigue
Giardiasis (fecal-oral) (hand-to-mouth)	Protozoan (*Giardia lamblia*), most common intestinal parasite	Untreated water, poor disinfection, pipe breaks, leaks, groundwater contamination, campgrounds where humans and wildlife use same source of water. Beavers and muskrats create ponds that act as reservoirs for *Giardia*.	Diarrhea, abdominal discomfort, bloating, and flatulence
Microsporidiosis	Protozoan phylum (*Microsporidia*), but closely related to fungi	*Encephalitozoon intestinalis* has been detected in groundwater, the origin of drinking water	Diarrhea and wasting in immunocompromised individuals
		Parasitic Infections (Kingdom Animalia)	
Disease and Species	Microbial Agent	Sources of Agent in Water Supply	General Symptoms
Schistosomiasis (immersion)	Members of the genus *Schistosoma*	Fresh water contaminated with certain types of snails that carry schistosomes	Blood in urine (depending on the type of infection), rash or itchy skin. Fever, chills, cough, and muscle aches
Dracunculiasis (guinea worm disease)	*Dracunculus medinensis*	Stagnant water containing larvae, generally in parasitized Copepoda	Allergic reaction, urticaria rash, nausea, vomiting, diarrhea, asthmatic attack
Taeniasis	Tapeworms of the genus *Taenia*	Drinking water contaminated with eggs	Intestinal disturbances, neurologic manifestations, loss of weight, cysticercosis
Fasciolopsiasis	*Fasciolopsis buski*	Drinking water contaminated with encysted metacercaria	Gastrointestinal disturbance, diarrhea, liver enlargement, cholangitis, cholecystitis, obstructive jaundice
Hymenolepiasis (dwarf tapeworm infection)	*Hymenolepis nana*	Drinking water contaminated with eggs	Abdominal pain, severe weight loss, itching around the anus, nervous manifestation

(Continued)

TABLE 3.52 (Continued)
Infections

Disease and Transmission	Microbial Agent	Sources of Agent in Water Supply	General Symptoms
Echinococcosis (hydatid disease)	*Echinococcus granulosus*	Drinking water contaminated with feces (usually canid) containing eggs	Liver enlargement, hydatid cysts press on bile duct and blood vessels; if cysts rupture, they can cause anaphylactic shock
Coenurosis	*Multiceps multiceps*	Contaminated drinking water with eggs	Increases intracranial tension
Ascariasis	*Ascaris lumbricoides*	Drinking water contaminated with feces (usually canid) containing eggs	Mostly, disease is asymptomatic or accompanied by inflammation, fever, and diarrhea. Severe cases involve Löffler's syndrome in lungs, nausea, vomiting, malnutrition, and underdevelopment
Enterobiasis	*Enterobius vermicularis*	Drinking water contaminated with eggs	Perianal itch, nervous irritability, hyperactivity, and insomnia
Bacterial Infections			
Botulism	*Clostridium botulinum*	Bacteria can enter an open wound from contaminated water sources. Can enter the gastrointestinal tract through consumption of contaminated drinking water or (more commonly) food	Dry mouth, blurred and/or double vision, difficulty swallowing, muscle weakness, difficulty breathing, slurred speech, vomiting, and sometimes diarrhea. Death is usually caused by respiratory failure
Campylobacteriosis	Most commonly caused by *Campylobacter jejuni*	Drinking water contaminated with feces	Produces dysentery-like symptoms along with a high fever. Usually lasts 2–10 days
Cholera	Spread by the bacterium *Vibrio cholerae*	Drinking water contaminated with the bacterium	In severe forms, it is known to be one of the most rapidly fatal illnesses. Symptoms include very watery diarrhea, nausea, cramps, nosebleed, rapid pulse, vomiting, and hypovolemic shock (in severe cases), at which point death can occur in 12–18 hours
E. coli infection	Certain strains of *Escherichia coli* (commonly *E. coli*)	Water contaminated with the bacteria	Mostly diarrhea. Can cause death in immunocompromised individuals, the very young, and the elderly due to dehydration from prolonged illness

(Continued)

TABLE 3.52 (Continued)
Infections

Disease and Transmission	Microbial Agent	Sources of Agent in Water Supply	General Symptoms
Mycobacterium marinum infection	*Mycobacterium marinum*	Naturally occurs in water; most cases from exposure in swimming pools or, more frequently, aquariums; rare infection since it mostly infects immunocompromised individuals	Symptoms include lesions typically located on the elbows, knees, and feet (from swimming pools) or lesions on the hands (aquariums). Lesions may be painless or painful
Dysentery	Caused by a number of species in the genera *Shigella* and *Salmonella* with the most common being *Shigella dysenteriae*	Water contaminated with the bacterium	Frequent passage of feces with blood and/or mucus and in some cases vomiting of blood.
Legionellosis (two distinct forms: Legionnaires' disease and Pontiac fever)	Caused by bacteria belonging to the genus *Legionella* (90% of cases caused by *Legionella pneumophila*)	Contaminated water: the organism thrives in warm aquatic environments	Pontiac fever produces milder symptoms resembling acute influenza without pneumonia. Legionnaires' disease has severe symptoms such as fever, chills, pneumonia (with cough that sometimes produces sputum), ataxia, anorexia, muscle aches, malaise, and occasionally diarrhea and vomiting
Leptospirosis	Caused by bacterium of genus *Leptospira*	Water contaminated by the animal urine carrying the bacteria	Begins with flu-like symptoms, then resolves. The second phase then occurs involving meningitis, liver damage (causes jaundice), and renal failure
Otitis externa (swimmer's ear)	Caused by a number of bacterial and fungal species	Swimming in water contaminated by the responsible pathogens	Ear canal swells, causing pain and tenderness to the touch
Salmonellosis	Caused by many bacteria of genus *Salmonella*	Drinking water contaminated with the bacteria. More common as a foodborne illness	Symptoms include diarrhea, fever, vomiting, and abdominal cramps
Typhoid fever	*Salmonella typhi*	Ingestion of water contaminated with feces of an infected person	Characterized by sustained fever up to 40°C (104°F), profuse sweating; diarrhea may occur. Symptoms progress to delirium, and the spleen and liver enlarge if untreated. In this case, it can last up to 4 weeks and cause death. Some people with typhoid fever develop a rash called "rose spots," small red spots on the abdomen and chest

(Continued)

TABLE 3.52 (*Continued*)
Infections

Disease and Transmission	Microbial Agent	Sources of Agent in Water Supply	General Symptoms
Vibrio illness	*Vibrio vulnificus, Vibrio alginolyticus,* and *Vibrio parahaemolyticus*	Can enter wounds from contaminated water. Also gets by drinking contaminated water or eating undercooked oysters	Symptoms include abdominal tenderness, agitation, bloody stools, chills, confusion, difficulty paying attention (attention deficit), delirium, fluctuating mood, hallucination, nosebleeds, severe fatigue, slow, sluggish, lethargic feeling, weakness
Viral Infections			
SARS (severe acute respiratory syndrome)	Coronavirus	Manifests itself in improperly treated water	Symptoms include fever, myalgia, lethargy, gastrointestinal symptoms, cough, and sore throat
Hepatitis A	Hepatitis A virus (HAV)	Can manifest itself in water (and food)	Symptoms are only acute (no chronic stage to the virus) and include fatigue, fever, abdominal pain, nausea, diarrhea, weight loss, itching, jaundice, and depression
Poliomyelitis (Polio)	Poliovirus	Enters water through the feces of infected individuals	About 90–95% of patients show no symptoms, 4–8% have minor symptoms (comparatively) with delirium, headache, fever, and occasional seizures, and spastic paralysis, while 1% have symptoms of nonparalytic aseptic meningitis. The rest have serious symptoms resulting in paralysis or death
Polyomavirus infection	Two of Polyomavirus: JC virus and BK virus	Very widespread, can manifest itself in water, ~80% of the population has antibodies to Polyomavirus	BK virus produces a mild respiratory infection and can infect the kidneys of immunosuppressed transplant patients. JC virus infects the respiratory system, kidneys, or can cause progressive multifocal leukoencephalopathy in the brain (which is fatal)

Source: Nwachcuku, N., and Gerba, C. 2004. Emerging waterborne pathogens: Can we kill them all? *Curr. Opin. Biotechnol.,* 15(3), 175–180.

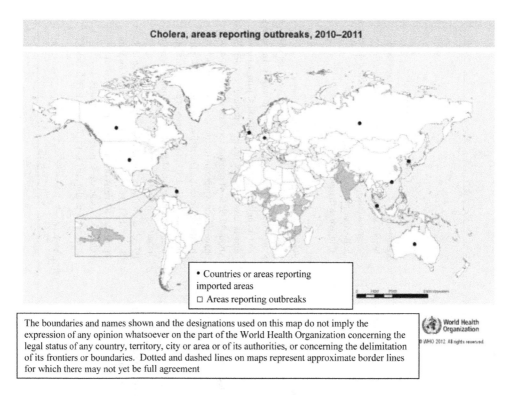

FIGURE 3.31   Cholera, areas reporting outbreaks, 2010–2011. (Data from the World Health Organization. Map Production: Public Health Information and Geographic Information Systems (GIS) World Health Organization.)

reproductive capacities. The most conspicuous effects of HABs on marine wildlife are large-scale mortality events associated with toxin-producing blooms. For example, a mass mortality event of 107 bottlenose dolphins occurred along the Florida panhandle in the spring of 2004 due to ingestion of contaminated menhaden with high levels of brevetoxin.[594] Manatee mortalities have also been attributed to brevetoxin but unlike dolphins, the main toxin vector was endemic seagrass species

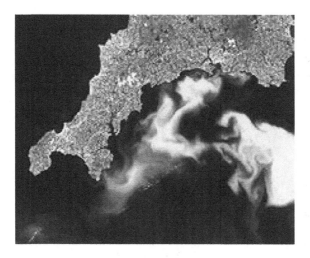

FIGURE 3.32   An algal bloom off the southern coast of Devon and Cornwall in England in 1999. (From https://upload.wikimedia.org/wikipedia/commons/8/86/Cwall99_lg.jpg.)

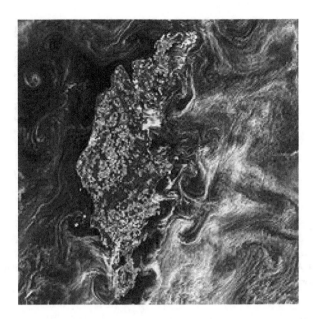

FIGURE 3.33   Satellite image of phytoplankton swirling around the Swedish island of Gotland in the Baltic Sea in 2005. (From https://upload.wikimedia.org/wikipedia/commons/c/c5/Van_Gogh_from_Space.jpg. A harmful algal bloom (HAB) is an algal bloom that causes negative impacts to others.)

(*Thalassia testudinum*) in which high concentrations of brevetoxins were detected and subsequently found as a main component of the stomach contents of manatees.[594]

HABs are caused by high concentrations of certain types of algae that produce toxic compounds. These blooms can cause sickness and death in humans, pets, and livestock who come in contact with or drink the water. Oregon has several documented cases of dogs dying and humans becoming ill. The Oregon Health Authority (OHA) is the agency responsible for posting warnings and educating the public about HABs. Once a waterbody is identified as having an HAB, Department of Environmental Quality (DEQ) is responsible for investigating the causes, identifying sources of pollution, and writing a pollution reduction plan.

HABs have occurred in a number of Oregon's lakes, reservoirs, and rivers. The blooms look different depending on local conditions. They can appear green, blue-green, or reddish brown and form foam, slicks, scum, or mats (Figures 3.34 and 3.35).

An algal bloom is a rapid increase or accumulation in the population of algae (typically microscopic) in an aquatic system. Typically, only one or a small number of phytoplankton species are involved, and some blooms may be recognized by discoloration of the water resulting from the high density of pigmented cells. Although there is no officially recognized threshold level, algae can be considered to be blooming at concentrations of hundreds to thousands of cells per milliliter, depending on the severity. Algal bloom concentrations may reach millions of cells per milliliter. Algal blooms are often green, but they can also be other colors such as yellow-brown or red, depending on the species of algae (Figure 3.36).

Bright green blooms are a result of cyanobacteria (colloquially known as blue-green algae) such as *Microcystis*. Blooms may also consist of macroalgal (nonphytoplanktonic) species. These blooms are recognizable by large blades of algae that may wash up onto the shoreline.

Of particular note are HABs, which are algal bloom events involving toxic or otherwise harmful phytoplankton such as dinoflagellates of the genus *Alexandrium* and *Karenia*, or diatoms of the genus *Pseudo-nitzschia*. Such blooms often take on a red or brown hue and are known colloquially as red tides.

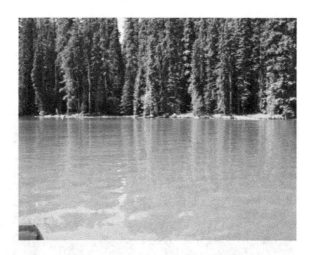

FIGURE 3.34   2004 Anabaena bloom, a type of cyanobacteria, in Odell Lake (photo by Joe Eilers). (From http://www.deq.state.or.us/wq/algae/algae/htm.)

Freshwater Algal Blooms

Freshwater algal blooms are the result of an excess of nutrients, particularly some phosphates.[595,596] The excess of nutrients may originate from fertilizers that are applied to land for agricultural or recreational purposes. They may also originate from household cleaning products containing phosphorus.[597] These nutrients can then enter watersheds through water runoff.[598] Excess carbon and nitrogen have also been suspected as causes. The presence of residual sodium carbonate acts as a catalyst for the algae to bloom by providing dissolved carbon dioxide for enhanced photosynthesis in the presence of nutrients.

When phosphates are introduced into water systems, higher concentrations cause increased growth of algae and plants. Algae tend to grow very quickly under high nutrient availability, but each alga is short-lived, and the result is a high concentration of dead organic matter which starts to decay. The decay process consumes dissolved oxygen in the water, resulting in hypoxic conditions. Without sufficient dissolved oxygen in the water, animals and plants may die off in large numbers.

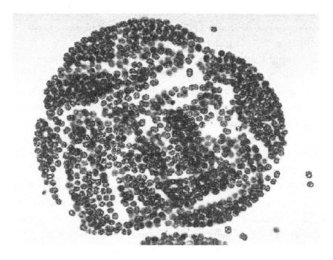

FIGURE 3.35   Microscopic image of *Microcystis*, a type of cyanobacteria. (From http:www-canosie.bio.purdue.edu/.)

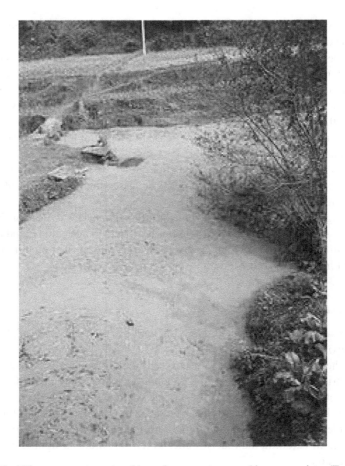

FIGURE 3.36 Algal blooms can present problems for ecosystems and human society. (From Felix Andrews (Floybix).)

Blooms may be observed in freshwater aquariums when fish are overfed and excess nutrients are not absorbed by plants. These are generally harmful for fish, and the situation can be corrected by changing the water in the tank and then reducing the amount of food given.

Causes of HABs

It is unclear what causes HABs; their occurrence in some locations appears to be entirely natural,[599] while in others they appear to be a result of human activities.[600] Furthermore, there are many different species of algae that can form HABs, each with different environmental requirements for optimal growth. The frequency and severity of HABs in some parts of the world have been linked to increased nutrient loading from human activities. In other areas, HABs are a predictable seasonal occurrence resulting from coastal upwelling, a natural result of the movement of certain ocean currents.[601] The growth of marine phytoplankton (both nontoxic and toxic) is generally limited by the availability of nitrates and phosphates, which can be abundant in coastal upwelling zones as well as in agricultural runoff. The type of nitrates and phosphates available in the system are also a factor, since phytoplankton can grow at different rates depending on the relative abundance of these substances (e.g., ammonia, urea, nitrate ion). A variety of other nutrient sources can also play an important role in effecting algal bloom formation, including iron, silica, or carbon. Coastal water pollution produced by humans and systematic increase in seawater temperature have also been suggested as possible contributing factors in HABs.[602] Other factors such as iron-rich dust influx from large desert areas such as the Sahara are thought to play a role in causing HABs.[603] Some algal blooms on the Pacific coast have also been linked to natural occurrences of large-scale climatic oscillations such as El Niño events. While HABs in the Gulf of Mexico have been occurring since the time of early explorers such as Cabeza de Vaca,[604] it is unclear what initiates these blooms and how large a role anthropogenic and natural factors play in their development. It is also unclear whether the apparent increase in frequency and severity of HABs in various parts of the world is in fact a real increase or is due to increased observation effort and advances in species identification technology.[605,606]

The decline in filter-feeding shellfish populations, such as oysters, likely contribute to HAB occurrence.[607] As such, numerous research projects are assessing the potential of restored shellfish populations to reduce HAB occurrence.[608–610]

Since many Algal blooms are caused by a major influx of nutrient-rich runoff into a water body, programs to treat wastewater, reduce the overuse of fertilizers in agriculture, and reducing the bulk flow of runoff can be effective for reducing severe algal blooms at river mouths, estuaries, and the ocean directly in front of the river's mouth.

Notable Occurrences

1. In 1972, a red tide was caused in New England by a toxic dinoflagellate *Alexandrium (Gonyaulax) tamarense*.[611]
2. In 2005, the Canadian HAB was discovered to have come further south than it has in years prior by a ship called The Oceanus, closing shellfish beds in Maine and Massachusetts and alerting authorities as far south as Montauk (Long Island, NY) to check their beds.[612] Experts who discovered the reproductive cysts in the seabed warn of a possible spread to Long Island in the future, halting the area's fishing and shellfish industry and threatening the tourist trade, which constitutes a significant portion of the island's economy.
3. In 2009, Brittany, France, experienced recurring algal blooms caused by the high amount of fertilizer discharging in the sea due to intensive pig farming, causing lethal gas emissions that have led to one case of human unconsciousness and three animal deaths.[613]
4. In 2010, dissolved iron in the ash from the Eyjafjallajökull volcano triggered a plankton bloom in the North Atlantic.[614]
5. In 2013, an algal bloom was caused in Qingdao, China, by sea lettuce.[615]
6. In 2014, *Myrionecta rubra* (previously known as *Mesodinium rubrum*), a ciliate protist that ingests cryptomonad algae, caused a bloom on the southeastern coast of Brazil.[616]
7. In 2014, a blue-green alga caused a bloom in the western basin of Lake Erie, poisoning the Toledo, Ohio, water system connected to 500,000 people.[617]

Amnesic Shellfish Poison

Amnesic shellfish poisoning (ASP) is caused by consumption of shellfish that have accumulated domoic acid, a neurotoxin produced by some strains of phytoplankton. The neurotoxic properties of domoic acid result in neuronal degeneration and necrosis in specific regions of the hippocampus. A serious outbreak of ASP occurred in Canada in 1987 and involved 150 reported cases, 19 hospitalizations, and 4 deaths after consumption of contaminated mussels. Symptoms ranged from gastrointestinal disturbances, to neurotoxic effects such as hallucinations, memory loss, and coma. Monitoring programs are in place in numerous countries worldwide and closures of shellfish harvesting areas occur when domoic acid concentrations exceed regulatory limits.

Paralytic Shellfish Poisons from Australian Cyanobacterial Blooms

According to Humpage et al.,[618] saxitoxin-group neurotoxins (paralytic shellfish poisons) have been identified in a cultured strain of *Anabaena circinalis* and in natural bloom samples in which this species was the dominant organism collected from widely distributed sites in the Murray-Darling Basin of Australia. These toxins have hitherto been isolated almost exclusively from "red tide" dinoflagellates and contaminated shellfish. Two "aphantoxins," which appear to be identical to two of the paralytic shellfish poisons, have been identified in a cyanobacterium from a small number of sites in New Hampshire, United States. The conclusions are supported by electrophysiological studies and by high-performance liquid chromatographic (HPLC) and fast atom bombardment-mass spectrometric (FAB-MS) analyses.

Paralytic Shellfish Poisoning

Paralytic shellfish poisoning (PSP) is one of the four recognized syndromes of shellfish poisoning that shares some common features and is primarily associated with bivalve mollusks (such as mussels, clams, oysters, and scallops). These shellfish are filter feeders and, therefore, accumulate neurotoxins, called saxitoxin (STX), produced by microscopic algae, such as dinoflagellates, diatoms, and cyanobacteria.[619] Dinoflagellates of the genus *Alexandrium* are the most numerous and widespread STX producers and are responsible for PSP blooms in subarctic, temperate, and tropical locations.[620] The majority of toxic blooms have been caused by the morphospecies *Alexandrium catenella, Alexandrium tamarense*, and *Alexandrium fundyense*,[621] which together comprise the *A. tamarense* species complex.[622] In Asia, PSP is mostly associated with the occurrence of the species *Pyrodinium bahamense*.[623] Human toxicity and mortality can occur after ingestion of these animals, but toxicity is also seen in wild animal populations.

Also, some pufferfish, including Chamaeleon puffer, contain STX, making their consumption hazardous.[624]

The toxins responsible for most shellfish poisonings are water insoluble, heat and acid stable, and ordinary cooking methods do not eliminate the toxins. The principal toxin responsible for PSP is STX. Some shellfish can store this toxin for several weeks after a HAB passes, but others, such as butter clams, are known to store the toxin for up to 2 years. Additional toxins are found, such as neosaxiton and gonyautoxins I to IV. All of them act primarily on the nervous system.

PSP can be fatal in extreme cases, particularly in immunocompromised individuals. Children are more susceptible. PSP affects those who come into contact with the affected shellfish by ingestion.[619] Symptoms can appear 10–30 minutes after ingestion, and include nausea, vomiting, diarrhea, abdominal pain, tingling or burning lips, gums, tongue, face, neck, arms, legs, and toes.[619] Shortness of breath, dry mouth, a choking feeling, confused or slurred speech, and loss of coordination are also possible.

Additional marine mammal species, such as the highly endangered North Atlantic Right Whale, have been exposed to neurotoxins by preying on highly contaminated zooplankton.[625] With the summertime habitat of this species overlapping with seasonal blooms of the toxic dinoflagellate *Alexandrium fundyense*, and subsequent copepod grazing, foraging right whales will ingest large concentrations of these contaminated copepods. Ingestion of such contaminated prey can affect respiratory capabilities, feeding behavior, and ultimately the reproductive condition of the population.[625]

Immune system responses have been affected by brevetoxin exposure in another critically endangered species, the Loggerhead sea turtle. Brevetoxin exposure, via inhalation of aerosolized toxins and ingestion of contaminated prey, can have clinical signs of increased lethargy and muscle weakness in loggerhead sea turtles causing these animals to wash ashore in a decreased metabolic state with increases in immune system responses upon blood analysis.[626] Examples of common harmful effects of HABs include:

1. The production of neurotoxins which cause mass mortalities in fish, seabirds, sea turtles, and marine mammals
2. Human illness or death via consumption of seafood contaminated by toxic algae[627]
3. Mechanical damage to other organisms, such as disruption of epithelial gill tissues in fish, resulting in asphyxiation
4. Oxygen depletion of the water column (hypoxia or anoxia) from cellular respiration and bacterial degradation

Owing to their negative economic and health impacts, HABs are often carefully monitored.[628,629]

HABs occur in many regions of the world, and in the United States are recurring phenomena in multiple geographical regions. The Gulf of Maine frequently experiences blooms of the dinoflagellate *Alexandrium fundyense*, an organism that produces STX, the neurotoxin responsible for PSP. The well-known "Florida red tide" that occurs in the Gulf of Mexico is an HAB caused by *Karenia brevis*, another dinoflagellate which produces brevetoxin, the neurotoxin responsible for neurotoxic shellfish poisoning. California coastal waters also experience seasonal blooms of *Pseudo-nitzschia*, a diatom known to produce domoic acid, the neurotoxin responsible for ASP. Off the west coast of South Africa, HABs caused by *Alexandrium catenella* occur every spring. These blooms of organisms cause severe disruptions in fisheries of these waters as the toxins in the phytoplankton cause filter-feeding shellfish in affected waters to become poisonous for human consumption.[630]

If the HAB event results in a high enough concentration of algae, the water may become discolored or murky, varying in color from purple to almost pink, normally being red or green. Not all algal blooms are dense enough to cause water discoloration.

RED TIDES

Red tide is a term often used to describe HABs in marine coastal areas,[631] as the dinoflagellate species involved in HABs are often red or brown and tint the seawater to a reddish color. Red tides can also be caused by bioluminescent dinoflagellates such as *Noctiluca scintillans*. The more correct and preferred term in use is harmful algal bloom, because:

1. These blooms are not associated with tides.
2. Not all algal blooms cause reddish discoloration of water.
3. Not all algal blooms are harmful, even those involving red discoloration.[632]

Milky seas is a condition on the open ocean where large areas of seawater (up to 6000 square miles) are filled with bioluminescent bacteria causing the ocean to uniformly glow a eerie blue at night. The condition has been present in mariner's tales for centuries. There have been 235 documented sightings of milky seas since 1915—mostly concentrated in the north-western Indian Ocean and near Indonesia (Figure 3.37).

The debate over the cause of red tides is controversial. Red tides occur naturally off coasts all over the world. Not all red tides have toxins or are harmful.[632]

As a technical term, it is being replaced in favor of more precise terminology including the generic term *harmful algal bloom* for harmful species, and *algal bloom* for nonharmful species.

The term *red tide* is also sometimes used to describe HABs on the northern east coast of the United States, particularly in the Gulf of Maine. This type of bloom is caused by another species of dinoflagellate known as *Alexandrium fundyense*. These blooms of organisms cause severe disruptions in fisheries of these waters as the toxins in these organisms cause filter-feeding shellfish in affected waters to become poisonous for human consumption due to STX.[630] The related *Alexandrium monilatum* is found in subtropical or tropical shallow seas and estuaries in the western Atlantic Ocean, the Caribbean Sea, the Gulf of Mexico, and the eastern Pacific Ocean.

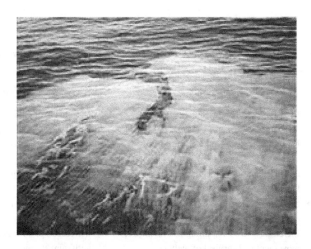

FIGURE 3.37 Red tide (NOAA). (From https://en.wikipedia.org/wiki/Algal_bloom#/media/File:Mar%C3%A9_vermelha.JPG.)

Many phenomena threaten the biological integrity of the Great Lakes. Here, we have highlighted two: the continuing impacts of aquatic alien invasive species and the little-understood threats posed by disease-causing or pathogenic organisms. According to scientists' best estimates, a new aquatic alien invasive species finds its way into the Great Lakes system about every 8 months. The impact of introduced species already in the system, from the sea lamprey to the zebra mussel, serves as harbingers of the economic and environmental costs to come if this crucial threat is not controlled. Similarly, documented surprise outbreaks of gastrointestinal diseases, sometimes with fatal consequences, should serve as a warning that residents of the Great Lakes basin face serious, largely unacknowledged threats from an everyday substance they all tend to assume is safe—the water they depend on for recreation and drinking. Fortunately, options exist to address both of these crucial challenges.

In 2001, it was estimated that 162 invasive species had entered the lakes from all pathways. Today, some have raised that estimate to more than 170 nonindigenous fish, invertebrates, plants, algae, protozoa, and parasites, and predict that one new nonindigenous species will be discovered in the lakes about every 8 months.[633]

Science has shown conclusively that simply exchanging ballast water from ships with highly saline water does not eliminate all aquatic alien invasive species, particularly those benthic and dormant stages of species left behind in residual water and sediment in ballast tanks. Since mandatory ballast water exchange took effect in the Great Lakes over a decade ago (United States Coast Guard 1993),[634] the rate of aquatic alien invasive species introductions has remained approximately the same. What has changed is the species composition, which has shifted to smaller open water forms such as zooplankton and phytoplankton.[634]

Approximately 70% of the ships entering the Great Lakes fall into the No Ballast on Board (NOBOB) category, and have been previously exempted from regulatory requirements. Yet all ships carry some leftover water and sediment in their ballast water tanks, and therefore are never truly "empty." Water and sediment below certain levels in ballast tanks become unpumpable, leaving behind residues that are likely to harbor viable eggs and cysts from invasive species.

The Commission remains concerned about microbial pollution in the Great Lakes basin ecosystem. While major problems occur infrequently, two relatively recent waterborne disease outbreaks in Wisconsin and Ontario make it clear that the potential for tragedy remains if drinking water is inadequately treated or challenged by high pollution loads. In 1993, an apparent failure in water treatment in Milwaukee, Wisconsin, caused an estimated 400,000 cases of diarrheal disease and approximately 100 deaths, most caused by the *Cryptosporidium* parasite. Less than a decade later (2000), in the town of Walkerton, Ontario (located less than 40 km from Lake Huron), over 2300

TABLE 3.53

Factors Associated with the Risk of New Pathogens and Impacts on Water Quality and Health in the Great Lakes Basin

Factor	Environmental Relevance	Outcome
Population growth and aging	• Increased waste, more untreated discharges	• High loads of pathogens, bacteria, parasites, and viruses
Infrastructure	• More runoff from hardened surfaces	• More users of urban beach • Larger sensitive populations
Intensive agriculture	• Greater quantity of manure Generated per land area	• Runoff of pathogens to local water bodies and groundwater
Worldwide transport	• Invasive species from ballast water discharges, products, or packing materials	• Known ecosystem risks, e.g. cholera in South America
Climate Change	• Increased storms and droughts that impact movement and survival of pathogens	• Increased risk of waterborne disease associated with rain, storms, and temperature

Source: Adapted from IJC 2003, Priorities Report. International Joint Commission, 2003. The Status of Restoration Activities in the Great Lakes Areas of Concern. April 2003. 25pp. http://www.ijc.org.

people were sickened and seven died after heavy rains compromised a municipal drinking water well and water treatment processes failed, leading to an outbreak of *Escherichia coli (E. coli.)* 0157 and *Campylobacter jejuni* bacteria.

Microbial infectious disease outbreaks demonstrate the fragility of barriers designed to protect public health. Research suggests that these outbreaks are only a fraction of the actual number of gastrointestinal illnesses caused by microbial pollution each year.[635] The U.S. CDC have reported increasing incidents of waterborne infectious disease in the United States, and it is estimated that 6%–40% of all gastrointestinal illnesses in the United States may be of waterborne origin.[635,636] Similar reports for Canada show that between 1974 and 1996, the last year for collected data, more than 200 reported outbreaks of infectious disease were associated with drinking water.[637]

Several factors that drive microbial contamination and can impact water quality and human health are identified in Table 3.53.

The results of research studies worldwide have demonstrated the importance of environmental factors affecting the viability of microorganisms along transport pathways. Under certain conditions, such as increased rainfall, lower temperatures, and reduced available sunlight, bacteria, viruses, and parasites from manure or sludge spread on land and can remain viable for several weeks to months. Runoff from this material can reach nearby water bodies, contributing to microbial contamination and degraded surface and groundwater quality.

Cyanotoxin

Among cyanotoxins are some of the most powerful natural poisons known, including poisons which can cause rapid death by respiratory failure.[639] The toxins include potent neurotoxins, hepatotoxins, cytotoxins, and endotoxins. Recreational exposure to cyanobacteria can result in gastrointestinal and hay fever symptoms or pruritic skin rashes.[640] It has been suggested that significant exposure to high levels of some species of cyanobacteria neurotoxin may cause Lous Gehrig's disease, but there is no firm evidence. There is also an interest in the military potential of biological neurotoxins such as cyanotoxins, which "have gained increasing significance as potential candidates for weaponization." [641]

The first published report that blue-green algae or cyanobacteria could have lethal effects appeared in *Nature* in 1878. George Francis described the algal bloom he observed in the estuary of the Murray River in Australia as "a thick scum like green oil paint, some two to six inches thick." Wildlife which drank the water died rapidly and terribly.[642] Most reported incidents of poisoning by microalgal toxins have occurred in freshwater environments, and they are becoming more common

TABLE 3.54

Chemical Structure of Cyanotoxins[551]

Structure	Cyanotoxin	Primary Target Organ in Mammals	Cyanobacteria Genera
Cyclic peptides	Microcystins	Liver	*Microcystis, Anabaena, Planktothrix* (Oscillatoria), *Nostoc, Hapalosiphon, Anabaenopsis*
	Nodularins	Liver	*Nodularia*
Alkaloids	Anatoxin-a	Nerve synapse	*Anabaena, Planktothrix* (Oscillatoria), *Aphanizomenon*
	Anatoxin-a(S)	Nerve synapse	*Anabaena*
	Cylindrospermopsins	Liver	*Cylindrospermopsis, Aphanizomenon, Umezakia*
	Lyngbyatoxin-a	Skin, gastrointestinal tract	*Lyngbya*
	Saxitoxins	Nerve axons	*Anabaena, Aphanizomenon, Lyngbya, Cylindrospermopsis*
	Lipopolysaccharides	Potential irritant; affects any exposed tissue	All
Polyketides	Aplysiatoxins	Skin	*Lyngbya, Schizothrix, Planktothrix* (Oscillatoria)
Amino Acid	BMAA	Nervous system	All

Source: Chorus, I., J. Bartram. 1999. *Toxic Cyanobacteria in Water: A Guide to Their Public Health Consequences, Monitoring, and Management.* Taylor & Francis.

Note: Most cyanotoxins have a number of variants (analogues). Altogether, over 84 cyanotoxins are known, although only a small number have been well studied.[550]

and widespread. For example, thousands of ducks and geese died drinking contaminated water in the midwestern United States.[643] In 2010, for the first time, marine mammals were reported to have died from ingesting cyanotoxins.[644]

In freshwater ecosystems, algal blooms are most commonly caused by eutrophication. The blooms can look like foam, scum, or mats or like paint floating on the surface of the water, but they are not always visible. Nor are the blooms always green; they can be blue, and some cyanobacteria species are colored brownish-red. The water can smell bad when the cyanobacteria in the bloom die.[645]

Strong cyanobacterial blooms reduce visibility to 1 or 2 cm. Species which do not need to see to migrate in the water column (such as the cyanobacteria themselves) survive, but species which need to see to find food and partners are compromised. During the day, blooming cyanobacteria saturate the water with oxygen. At night respiring aquatic organisms can deplete the oxygen to the point where sensitive species, such as certain fish, die. This is more likely to happen near the seafloor or a thermocline. Water acidity also cycles daily during a bloom, with the pH reaching 9 or more during the day and dropping to low values at night, further stressing the ecosystem. In addition, many cyanobacteria species produce potent cyanotoxins which concentrate during a bloom to the point where they become lethal to nearby aquatic organisms and any other animals in direct contact with the bloom, including birds, livestock, domestic animals, and sometimes humans.[646]

In 1991, a harmful cyanobacterial bloom affected 1000 km of the Darling-Barwon River in Australia[647] at an economic cost of $10 million AUD.[648] The chemical structure of cyanotoxins falls into three broad groups: cyclic peptides, alkaloids, and lipopolysaccharides (Table 3.54).[550]

Cyclic Peptides

A peptide is a short polymer of amino acids linked by peptide bonds. They have the same chemical structure as proteins, except that they are shorter. In a cyclic peptide, the links link back to the start to form a stable circular chain. In mammals, this stability makes them resistant to the process of digestion and they can bioaccumulate in the liver. Of all the cyanotoxins, the cyclic peptides are of

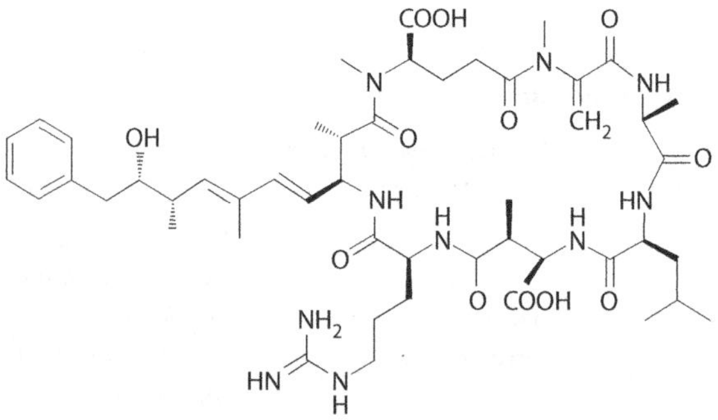

FIGURE 3.38   Microcystin LR. (From https://upload.wikimedia.org/wikipedia/commons/5/51/Microcystin-LR-structure.png.)

most concern to human health. The microcystins and nodularins poison the liver, and exposure to high doses can cause death. Exposure to low doses in drinking water over a long period of time may promote liver and other tumors.[550]

MICROCYSTINS

As with other cyanotoxins, microcystins were named after the first organism discovered to produce them, *Microcystis aeruginosa* (Figure 3.38). However, it was later found that other cyanobacterial genera also produced them.[550] There are about 60 known variants of microcystin, and several of these can be produced during a bloom. The most reported variant is microcystin-*LR*, possible because the earliest commercially available chemical standard analysis was for microcystin-*LR*.[550]

Blooms containing microcystin are a problem worldwide in freshwater ecosystems.[650] Microcystins are cyclic peptides and can be very toxic for plants and animals including humans. They bioaccumulate in the liver of fish, in the hepatopancreas of mussels, and in zooplankton. They are hepatotoxic and can cause serious damage to the liver in humans.[550] In this way, they are similar to the nodularins (below), and together the microcystins and nodularins account for most of the toxic cyanobacterial blooms in fresh and brackish waters.[649] In 2010, a number of sea otters were reported as having been poisoned by microcystin. Marine bivalves were the likely source of hepatotoxic shellfish poisoning. This is the first confirmed example of mammals in a marine environment dying from ingesting a cyanotoxin.[644]

NODULARINS

The first nodularin variant to be identified was nodularin-R, produced by the cyanobacterium *Nodularia spumigena* (Figure 3.39).[651] This cyanobacterium blooms in water bodies throughout the world. In the Baltic Sea, marine blooms of *Nodularia spumigena* are among some of the largest cyanobacterial mass events in the world.[652]

Globally, the most common toxins present in cyanobacterial blooms in fresh and brackish waters are the cyclic peptide toxins of the nodularin family. Like the microcystin family (above), nodularins are potent hepatotoxins and can cause serious damage to the liver. They present health risks for wild and domestic animals as well as humans, and in many areas pose major challenges for the provision of safe drinking water.[651]

ALKALOIDS

Alkaloids are a group of naturally occurring chemical compounds which mostly contain basic nitrogen atoms. They are produced by a large variety of organisms, including cyanobacteria, and are

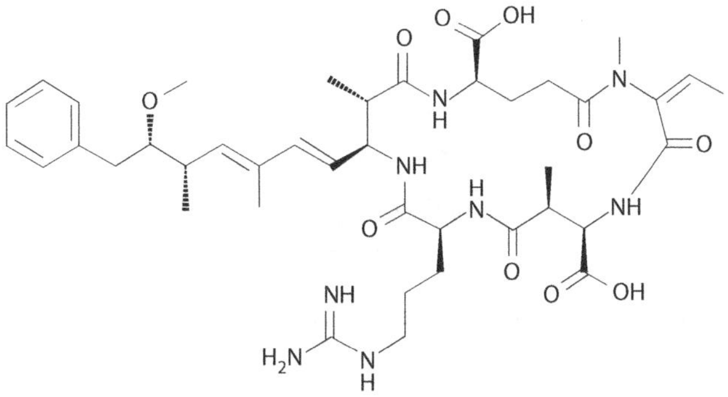

FIGURE 3.39   Nodularin-R. (From https://upload.wikimedia.org/wikipedia/commons/5/53/Nodularin_R. svg.)

part of the group of natural products, also called secondary metabolites. Alkaloids act on diverse metabolic systems in humans and other animals, often with psychotropic or toxic effects. Almost uniformly, they are bitter tasting.[653]

ANATOXIN

Investigations into anatoxin-*a*, also known as "Very Fast Death Factor," began in 1961 following the deaths of cows that drank from a lake containing an algal bloom in Saskatchewan, Canada.[654,655] The toxin is produced by at least four different genera of cyanobacteria and has been reported in North America, Europe, Africa, Asia, and New Zealand.[656]

Toxic effects from anatoxin-*a* progress very rapidly because it acts directly on the nerve cells (neurons) as a neurotoxin. The progressive symptoms of anatoxin-*a* exposure are loss of coordination, twitching, convulsions, and rapid death by respiratory paralysis. The nerve tissues which communicate with muscles contain a receptor called the nicotinic acetylcholine receptor. Stimulation of these receptors causes a muscular contraction. The anatoxin-*a* molecule is shaped so it fits this receptor, and in this way it mimics the natural neurotransmitter normally used by the receptor, acetylcholine. Once it has triggered a contraction, anatoxin-*a* does not allow the neurons to return to their resting state, because it is not degraded by cholinesterase which normally performs this function. As a result, the muscle cells contract permanently, the communication between the brain and the muscles is disrupted, and breathing stops (Figure 3.40).[657,658]

When it was first discovered, the toxin was called the Very Fast Death Factor (VFDF) because when it was injected into the body cavity of mice it induced tremors, paralysis, and death within a few minutes. In 1977, the structure of VFDF was determined as a secondary, bicyclic amine alkaloid, and it was renamed anatoxin-*a*.[659,660] Structurally, it is similar to cocaine.[661] There is continued interest in anatoxin-*a* because of the dangers it presents to recreational and drinking waters, and because it is a particularly useful molecule for investigating acetylcholine receptors in the nervous system.[639] The deadliness of the toxin means that it has a high military potential as a toxin weapon.[641]

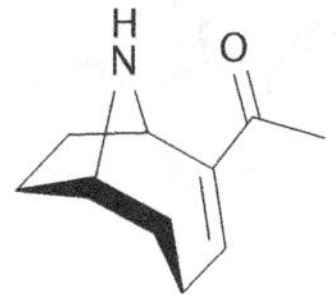

FIGURE 3.40   Anatoxin-a. (From https://en.wikipedia.org/wiki/Cyanotoxin#/media/File:Anatoxin-a.png.)

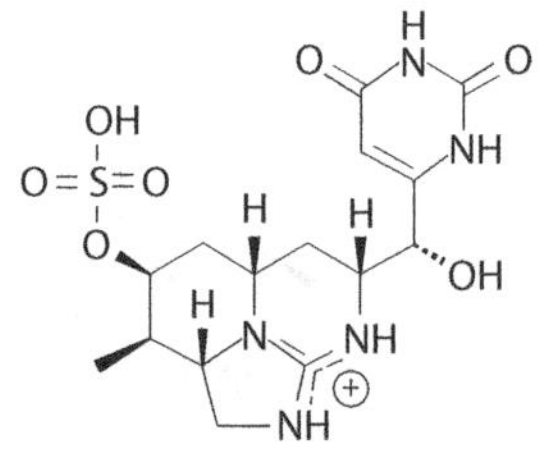

FIGURE 3.41 Cylindrospermopsin. (From https://en.wikipedia.org/wiki/Cyanotoxin#/media/File:Cylindro spermopsin.png.)

CYLINDROSPERMOPSINS

Cylindrospermopsin (abbreviated to CYN or CYL) was first discovered after an outbreak of a mystery disease on Palm Island in Australia (Figure 3.41).[662] The outbreak was traced back to a bloom of *Cylindrospermopsis raciborskii* in the local drinking water supply, and the toxin was subsequently identified. Analysis of the toxin led to a proposed chemical structure in 1992, which was revised after synthesis was achieved in 2000. Several variants of cylindrospermopsin, both toxic and nontoxic, have been isolated or synthesized.[663]

Cylindrospermopsin is toxic to liver and kidney tissue and is thought to inhibit protein synthesis and to covalently modify DNA and/or RNA. There is concern about the way cylindrospermopsin bioaccumulates in freshwater organisms.[664] Toxic blooms of genera which produce cylindrospermopsin are most commonly found in tropical, subtropical, and arid zone water bodies, and have recently been found in Australia, Europe, Israel, Japan, and the United States.[550]

SAXITOXINS

STX is one of the most potent natural neurotoxins known (Figure 3.42). The term saxitoxin originates from the species name of the butter clam (*Saxidomus giganteus*) whereby it was first recognized. STX is produced by the cyanobacteria *Anabaena* spp., some *Aphanizomenon* spp., *Cylindrospermopsis* sp., *Lyngbya* sp., and *Planktothrix* sp.[665] Puffer fish and some marine dinoflagellates also produce STX.[666,667] STXs bioaccumulate in shellfish and certain finfish. Ingestion of STX, usually through shellfish contaminated by toxic algal blooms, can result in PSP.[649]

STX has been used in molecular biology to establish the function of the sodium channel. It acts on the voltage-gated sodium channels of nerve cells, preventing normal cellular function and leading to paralysis. The blocking of neuronal sodium channels which occurs in PSP produces a flaccid paralysis that leaves its victim calm and conscious through the progression of symptoms. Death often occurs from respiratory failure.[668] STX was originally isolated and described by the United States military, which assigned it the chemical weapon designation "TZ." STX is listed in schedule 1 of the Chemical Weapons Convention.[669] According to the book *Spycraft*, U-2 spyplane pilots were provided with needles containing STX to be used for suicide in the event escape was impossible.[670]

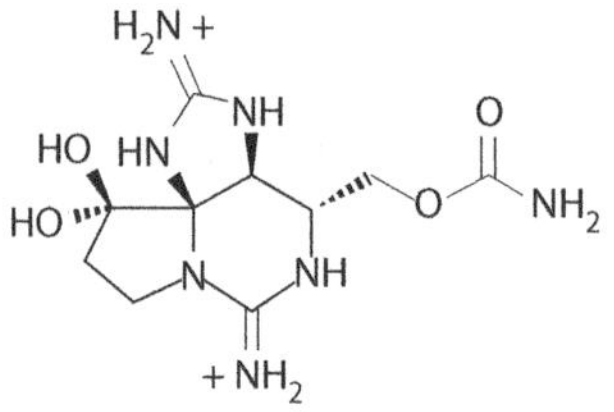

FIGURE 3.42 Saxitoxin. (From https://en.wikipedia.org/wiki/Cyanotoxin#/media/File:Saxitoxin.svg.)

Saxitoxin-Sensitive Na⁺ Channels: Presynaptic Localization in Cerebellum and Hippocampus of Neurological Mutant Mice

The autoradiographic distribution of STX binding sites associated with the voltage-sensitive Na⁺ channel was studied in the cerebellum of the neurological weaver (*wv/wv*), Purkinje cell degeneration (*pcd/pcd*), nervous (*nr/nr*), and reeler (*rl/rl*) mutant mice. The Purkinje cell layer contains the highest density of STX binding sites in normal mice. High densities were observed in the molecular layer. Intermediate and very low densities were present in the granular layer and the white matter, respectively. There was an important decrease in grain density in the molecular layer and Purkinje cell layer of the cerebellum, where a large majority of granular cells had disappeared. A small decrease was observed in the Purkinje cell layer where the Purkinje cells had almost all degenerated. Mutants where all neuronal cells were malpositioned, the compacted molecular layer contained an increased STX binding sites density. Conversely, the labeling of Purkinje cells areas was decreased. The hippocampal formation of mutants presents a homogeneous repartition of the Na⁺ channel protein, in contrast with the laminated distribution observed in normal mice. Our autoradiographic data suggest that a major proportion of STX-sensitive Na⁺ channels are localized in parallel fibers of granular cells and in axons of basket cells in a presynaptic position. In Purkinje cells, the dendritic arborization seems to be devoid of STX binding sites conversely to somata.

Lipopolysaccharides

Lipopolysaccharides are present in all cyanobacteria. Though not as potent as other cyanotoxins, some researchers have claimed that all lipopolysaccharides in cyanobacteria can irritate the skin, while other researchers doubt the toxic effects are that generalized.[671]

BMAA

The nonproteinogenic amino acid BMAA is ubiquitously produced by cyanobacteria in marine, freshwater, brackish, and terrestrial environments.[672,673] The exact mechanisms of BMAA toxicity on neuron cells are being investigated. Research suggests both acute and chronic mechanisms of toxicity.[674,675] BMAA is being investigated as a potential environmental risk factor for neurodegenerative diseases, including amyotrophic lateral sclerosis (ALS), Parkinson's Disease, and Alzheimer's Disease (Figures 3.43 and 3.44).

4-Aminopyridine Antagonizes Saxitoxin- and Tetrodotoxin-Induced Cardiorespiratory Depression

Antagonism of STX- and tetrodotoxin-induced lethality by 4-aminopyridine was studied in urethane-anesthetized guinea pigs instrumented for the concurrent recordings of medullary respiratory-related unit activities (Bötzinger complex and Nu. para-Ambiguus), diaphragmatic electromyogram, electrocorticogram, lead II electrocardiogram, blood pressure, end-tidal CO_2 and arterial $O_2/CO_2/$ pH. The toxin (either STX or tetrodotoxin) was infused at a dose rate of 0.3 μg/kg/min (IV) to

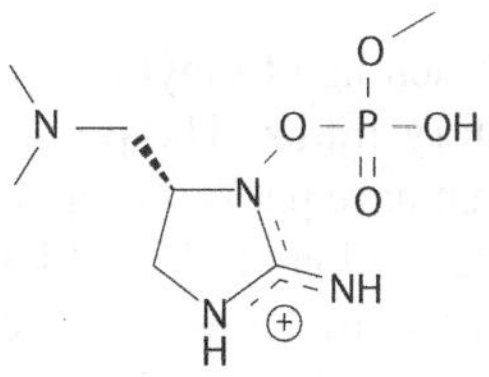

FIGURE 3.43 Anatoxin-a(s). (From https://en.wikipedia.org/wiki/Cyanotoxin#/media/File:Anatoxin-a-S. png.)

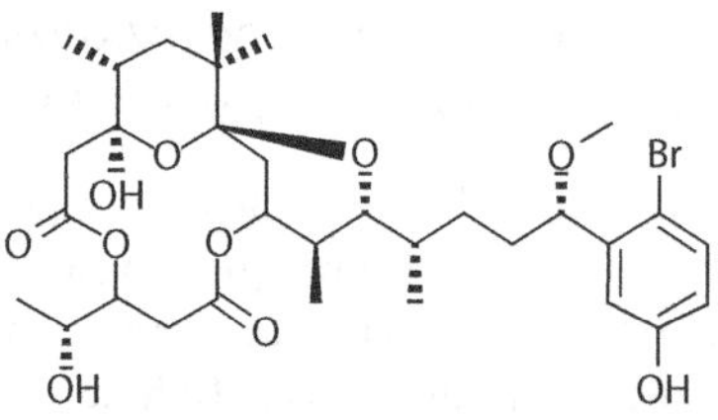

FIGURE 3.44 Aplysiatoxin. (From https://en.wikipedia.org/wiki/Cyanotoxin#/media/File:Aplysiatoxin. svg.)

produce a state of progressive cardiorespiratory depression. The animals were artificially ventilated when the magnitude of integrated diaphragm activities was reduced to 50% of control. Immediately after the disappearance of the diaphragm electromyogram, the toxin infusion was terminated, and 4-aminopyridine (2 mg/kg, IV) was administered. The therapeutic effect of 4-aminopyridine was striking in that the toxin-induced blockade of diaphragmatic neurotransmission, vascular hypotension, myocardial anomalies, bradycardia, and aberrant discharge patterns of medullary respiratory-related neurons could all be promptly restored to a level comparable to that of the control condition. The animals were typically able to breathe spontaneously within minutes after 4-aminopyridine. At the dose level used to achieve the desired therapeutic responses, 4-aminopyridine produced no signs of seizure and convulsion. Although less serious side effects such as cortical excitant/arousal and transient periods of fascicular twitch could be observed, these events were of minor concern, in our opinion, particularly in view of the remarkable therapeutic effects of 4-aminopyridine.

Acrylamide, for instance, a probable human carcinogen, is added to water to aid in coagulation, or the clumping and removal of solids in the water and water tanks and pipes in the distribution system, including pipes in the home, can add pollutants. Lead from pipes and lead-based solder can leach into water. Also, asphalt- or coal tar-lined storage tanks and pipes can leach chemicals linked to cancer (PAHs) into tap water supplies. Critical upgrades to pipes, tanks, and other aging treatment and distribution equipment is part of water utilities' urgent $165 billion current need for infrastructure upgrades.[676]

Polyvinyl chloride pipes now add to significant water contamination.

CONTROLLING VINYL CHLORIDE IN DRINKING WATER DISTRIBUTION SYSTEMS

Drinking water distribution systems containing "early-era" PVC pipe (manufactured prior to 1977) are at risk of vinyl chloride monomer leaching from the pipe into the drinking water in the water distribution system. The majority of the cases of excess vinyl chloride concentrations in drinking water distribution systems have been reported in Kansas, Missouri, Texas, and Arkansas,[677] although the problem may be more widespread.

Vinyl chloride is an odorless, colorless VOC. It is used in the manufacture of numerous products— as well as in many industries. Vinyl chloride is slightly soluble in water.[678] It can cause liver cancer in humans.[679] The MCL is set at 2.0 ig/L (or 0.002 mg/L).[679]

The primary route for vinyl chloride entering a water distribution system is by leaching from an early-era PVC pipe.

Owing to relatively slow rates of leaching of vinyl chloride from PVC pipe, vinyl chloride concentrations rarely exceed the regulatory limits. The problem of elevated vinyl chloride levels is generally limited to dead-end lines that have periods of nonuse or very low flows.

Several factors can affect the concentration of vinyl chloride in the drinking water within a distribution system. First, only pipe manufactured prior to the mid-1970s have been reported to contain vinyl chloride at levels that can lead to problems within a distribution system. After this date, the manufacturing process was controlled to prevent excess levels of vinyl chloride within the pipe. However, they still do not recommend vinyl chloride pipes.

A second factor is the amount of vinyl chloride originally in a PVC pipe. The amount of vinyl chloride in the early-era PVC pipe can vary widely, and therefore the amount of vinyl chloride leaching into the distribution system will also vary from system to system.

A third factor is the temperature of the water and pipe. Higher temperatures lead to higher diffusion rates of vinyl chloride within the PVC pipe, and hence from the pipe into the water. Thus, vinyl chloride may leach from a pipe at much higher rates during the summer months when water temperatures within the pipe are often much higher than in the winter months. This is a critical consideration in adjusting flush frequencies for seasonal temperature swings.

A fourth factor is the pipe diameter. Specifically, excessive concentrations of vinyl chloride will tend to be more of a problem in smaller pipes than in larger pipes. This is because small pipes contain less water to dilute the vinyl chloride that leaches into them. More specifically, a greater pipe surface area leads to a greater mass of vinyl chloride entering the water. Greater water volume within the pipe, however, leads to more dilution of the vinyl chloride and lower vinyl chloride concentrations overall. Therefore, the larger the surface area to volume ratio of a pipe, the greater the vinyl chloride concentration one would expect to find (with all other factors the same). Since smaller pipes have larger surface area-to-volume ratios, vinyl chloride leaching may be a greater problem.

A fifth factor is pipe age. Since there was a finite amount of vinyl chloride within the pipe, eventually most of the vinyl chloride will leach from it. However, calculations show that at the present time, only a small percentage of the vinyl chloride has leached from a typical pipe. Calculations show that for a typical pipe of age 25 versus 40 years, the time it would take to leach sufficient vinyl chloride to exceed the MCL might only vary by approximately 25% (with other factors remaining the same).

Finally, the flow rate of water within the pipe is a critical factor controlling the concentration of vinyl chloride in the water. Vinyl chloride leaches from a PVC pipe at a fixed rate independent of the amount of water flowing through it. When there is a greater flow of water flowing through the pipe, the vinyl chloride is more diluted and the resulting vinyl chloride concentration reaching customers is lower. Thus, the amount of water used (or flushed) is directly related to the maximum vinyl chloride concentration that would be detected in the water.

The utility recognizes that if the occupants leave for some extended period, flushing of the line will be necessary to purge the accumulated vinyl chloride. The utility wants to determine, however, whether the line needs to be flushed on a regular basis and what flush volume to use.

The Missouri Department of Natural Resources often assumes an average use rate of 200 gallons per day per dwelling (gpd) (or 6000 gallons per month per dwelling). More accurate data are available, however, by looking at actual use rates by customers on a dead-end segment. Customers where an elderly person lives alone, the use rate can be 40–50 gallons per day or less. This makes for a good worst-case situation.

In some cases, the daily water usage by a consumer will be more than adequate to control the vinyl chloride concentration within a pipe. A utility manager should, however, educate the consumer on the flushing issue so that if the customer leaves for a sufficient period of time (e.g., on vacation) to cause an unacceptable buildup of vinyl chloride, the line may need to be flushed when the customer returns.

The purpose of the protocol just described is to serve as a guide for estimating the frequency and volume of flushes required to prevent vinyl chloride concentrations from exceeding allowable levels. Owing to the uncertainty associated with the leaching model and the critical need to maintain vinyl chloride concentrations within regulatory limits, it is imperative that utility managers monitor the resulting vinyl chloride concentrations in an appropriate manner (Tables 3.55 through 3.58).

WHAT IS THE SOURCE OF MY DRINKING WATER? SOURCE WATER!

Basic components:

- A well—a hole drilled into an underground aquifer
- A pipe and pump—used to pull water out of the ground

TABLE 3.55

EPA Maximum Contamination Levels (MCLs) for Drinking Water

Contaminant	MCL (mg/L)
Disinfectants and Disinfectant By-Products	
Chloramines	4.0
Chlorine	4.0
Chlorine dioxide	0.8
Bromate	0.010
Chlorite	1.0
Haloacetic acids	0.060
Total trihalomethanes	0.080
Inorganic Chemicals	
Antimony	0.006
Arsenic	0.010
Asbestos	7 million (fibers per liter)
Barium	2
Beryllium	0.004
Cadmium	0.005
Chromium (total)	0.1
Copper	1.3
Cyanide	0.2
Fluoride	4.0
Lead	0.015
Mercury	0.002
Nitrate	10
Selenium	0.05
Thallium	0.002
Organic Chemicals	
Acrylamide	Restricted use by formula
Alachlor	0.002
Atrazine	0.003
Benzene	0.005
Benzo[a]pyrene (PAHs)	0.0002
Carbofuran	0.04
Carbon tetrachloride	0.005
1,2-Dichloropropane	0.005
Di(2-ethylhexyl) adipate	0.4
Di(2-ethylhexyl) phthalate	0.006
Dinoseb	0.007
Dioxin (2,3,7,8-TCDD)	0.00000003

Source: Environmental Protection Agency.

- A screen to filter out unwanted particles
- Some homeowners/landowners install treatment equipment for private wells

Three basic types of wells:

- Bored/shallow wells: Bored into an unconfined water source; generally 50 feet deep or less
- Consolidated/rock wells: Drilled into a formation consisting of a natural rock formation that contains no soil; average depth about 250 feet
- Unconsolidated/sand wells: Drilled into a formation consisting of soil, sand, gravel, or clay material

TABLE 3.56
Disinfection By-Products from Chlorination of Drinking Water and Their K_{ow} Values

	K_{ow}
Trihalomethanes	
Chloroform	1.97
Bromodichloromethane	2.00
Chlorodibromomethane	2.16
Bromoform	2.40
Haloacetic Acids	
Chloroacetic acid	0.22
Dichloroacetic acid	0.92
Trichloroacetic acid	1.33
Bromoacetic acid	0.41
Bromochloroacetic acid	0.61
Dibromoacetic acid	0.70
Haloacetonitriles	
Bromochloroacetontrile	0.38
Dichloroacetontrile	0.29
Haloketones	
1,1-Dichloropropanone	0.20
1,1,1-Trichloropropanone	1.12

Source: Environmental Protection Agency.

PUBLIC DRINKING WATER SYSTEMS

Public water systems are regulated by the EPA. EPA sets standards for drinking water quality and oversees the states, localities, and water suppliers who implement those standards. This illustration shows a public water system with a river as its water source, and shows some sample treatment types (Tables 3.56 and 3.57).

This is a factsheet about a chemical that may be found in some public or private drinking water supplies. It may cause health problems if found in amounts greater than the health standard set by the USEPA.

TABLE 3.57
Water Treatment and Distribution By-Product Pollutants in U.S. Drinking Water

Monobromoacetic acid	Bromodichloromethane
Dibromoacetic acid	Dibromochloromethane
Bromochloroacetic acid	Total trihalomethanes
Haloacetic acids (total)	Formaldehyde
Dichloroacetontrile	m-Dichlorobenzene
1.1-Dichloropropanone	Dichloroiodomethane
Chloropicrin	Vinyl chloride
Glyoxal	Bromodichloroacetic acid
Chloroform	Chlorodibromoacetic acid
Bromoform	Tribromoacetic acid

Source: Environmental Protection Agency.

TABLE 3.58
Naturally Occurring Pollutant in U.S. Drinking Water

Aluminum	Mercury
Ammonia	Nitrate and nitrite mix
Bromine	Nitrate
Arsenic	Nitrite
Chromium	Phosphate
Copper hydrogen sulfide	Selenium
Lead	Silver
Manganese	Sulfate

Source: Environmental Protection Agency.

Antimony is a metal found in natural deposits as ores containing other elements. The most widely used antimony compound is antimony trioxide, used as a flame retardant. It is also found in batteries, pigments, and ceramics/glass.

In 1974, Congress passed the Safe Drinking Water Act. This law requires EPA to determine safe levels of chemicals in drinking water which do or may cause health problems. These nonenforceable levels, based solely on possible health risks and exposure, are called Maximum Contaminant Level Goals (MCLG).

The MCLG for antimony has been set at 6 parts per billion (ppb) because EPA believes this level of protection would not cause any of the potential health problems described below.

On the basis of this MCLG, EPA has set an enforceable standard called a Maximum Contaminant Level (MCL). MCLs are set as close to the MCLGs as possible, considering the ability of public water systems to detect and remove contaminants using suitable treatment technologies (Table 3.55).

The MCL has also been set at 6 ppb because EPA believes, given the present technology and resources, this is the lowest level to which water systems can reasonably be required to remove this contaminant should it occur in drinking water.

These drinking water standards and the regulations for ensuring that these standards are met are called National Primary Drinking Water Regulations. All public water supplies must abide by these regulations (Table 3.58).

Short term: EPA has found antimony to potentially cause the following health effects when people are exposed to it at levels above the MCL for relatively short periods of time: nausea, vomiting, and diarrhea.

Long term: Antimony has the potential to cause the following effects from a lifetime exposure at levels above the MCL: AND/OR—Antimony is a (known/potential drinking water) human carcinogen. OR—No reliable data are available concerning health effects from long-term exposure to antimony in drinking water.

In 1984, 64.5 million lbs of antimony ore were mined and refined. Production of the most commonly used antimony compound, the trioxide, increased during the 1980s to about 31 million lbs, reported in 1985. Industrial dust, auto exhaust, and home heating oil are the main sources in urban air.

From 1987 to 1993, according to the Toxics Release Inventory, antimony and antimony compound releases to land and water totaled over 12 million lbs. These releases were primarily from copper and lead smelting and refining industries. The largest releases occurred in Arizona and Montana. The greatest releases to water occurred in Washington and Louisiana.

Little is known about antimony's fate once it is released to the soil. Some studies indicate that antimony is highly mobile in soils, while others conclude that it strongly adsorbs to soil. In water, it usually adheres to sediments. Most antimony compounds show little or no tendency to accumulate in aquatic life.

The regulation for antimony became effective in 1994. Between 1993 and 1995, EPA required water suppliers to collect water samples every 3 months for 1 year and analyze them to find out if antimony was present above 6 ppb. If it is present above this level, the system must continue to monitor this contaminant.

If contaminant levels are found to be consistently above the MCL, water suppliers must take steps to reduce the amount of antimony so that it is consistently below that level. The following treatment methods have been approved by EPA for removing antimony: coagulation/filtration, reverse osmosis.

If the levels of antimony exceed the MCL, the system must notify the public via newspapers, radio, TV, and other means. Additional actions, such as providing alternative drinking water supplies, may be required to prevent serious risks to public health.

Drinking Water Standards: Table 3.59

MCLG: 6 ppb

MCL: 6 ppb

Consumer Factsheet on: ANTIMONY. http://www.belkraft.com/antimony.htm.

TABLE 3.59
Antimony Releases to Water and Land, 1987 to 1993 (in Pounds)

	Water	Land
Totals	3,30,064	1,20,03,373
Top Ten States[a]		
AZ	505	70,74,128
MT	0	23,38,697
TX	24,817	8,40,392
LA	55,414	3,44,762
WI	1,445	3,92,000
MO	784	1,88,266
WA	63,220	99,915
ID	2,600	1,40,250
TN	687	1,08,325
AL	27,536	69,503
Major Industries*[a]		
Copper smelting, refining	505	70,74,128
Other nonferrous smelt.	17,015	23,83,947
Sec. nonferrous smelt.	1,459	8,03,398
Misc indust. organics	18,424	5,81,465
Porcelain plumb. fixtures	1,445	3,92,000
Petroleum refining	1,11,527	2,02,251
Misc. inorganic chems.	4,962	1,40,250
Plastics, resins	20	60,372
Storage batteries	0	45,952
Synthetic fibers	26,803	12,535

[a] Water/land totals only include facilities with releases greater than a certain amount—usually 1000 to 10,000.

TAP WATER

As one can see from the aforementioned sections, tap water is extremely contaminated. It is the breeder and propagator of disease. It must be cleaned up at the source, which today is a horrendous and nearly impossible but necessary task.

Obviously, any source of water dependent upon rain will be contaminated as previously shown. Examination of our groundwater as well as reservoirs reveals the presence of many hundreds of toxic chemicals,[680] a few of which are identified in Table 3.60 and are detrimental to the person with chemical sensitivity.

Tap water in 42 states is contaminated with more than 140 unregulated chemicals that lack safety standards, according to the Environmental Working Group's (EWG's) two-and-a-half year investigation of water suppliers' tests of the treated tap water served to communities across the country.

In an analysis of more than 22 million tap water quality tests, most of which were required under the federal Safe Drinking Water Act, EWG found that water suppliers across the United States detected 260 contaminants in water served to the public. One hundred forty-one of these detected chemicals, more than half, are unregulated; but this is of little matter since water chlorinate plants do not clear them and add to them with their disinfectants. (1) Contaminants found in state tap water (1998–2003): 105, (2) total population exposed above health-based limits: 17,486,112, and (3) communities served water with contaminants above health-based limits: 2887.

The clinician can see the absurdity of this philosophy since the data are flawed and the effects on each individual are unknown. Individual chemically sensitive and chronic degenerative disease patients emphasize how important it is to depollute the water for these patients.

Health effects or target organs of contaminants found are cardiovascular or blood toxicity, cancer, developmental toxicity, endocrine toxicity, immunotoxicity, kidney toxicity, gastrointestinal or liver toxicity, neurotoxicity, reproductive toxicity, respiratory toxicity, and skin sensitivity.

Potential contaminants to tap water are legion. See Figure 3.13 and Table 3.61.

TABLE 3.60
Fort Worth Rolling Hills (Tap Water: June 1984)—EHC-Dallas

Chemical	Amount (μg/L)	Chemical	Level	2008
pH	8.68	Endrin	0.008 ppm	N.D.
Turbidity	0.18	Lindane	0.006 ppm	N.D.
Total solids	182.0	Methoxychlor	0.030 ppm	N.D.
Carbonates	12.0	Toxaphene	0.041 ppm	N.D.
Bicarbonates	69.0	2,3,5-TP Silvex	0.08 ppm	N.D.
Sulfates	26.0	Chloroform ($CHCl_3$)	0.2618 ppm	2.90–4.2 ppb
Chlorides	34.0	Dichlorobromomethane ($CHCl_2Br$)	26.18 ppb	2.33–4.33 ppb
Hardness	80.0	Dibromochloromethane ($CHBr_2Cl$)	0.02992 ppm	5.33–2.4 ppb
Calcium	37.0	Bromoform	29.92 ppb	1.63–3.25 ppb
Magnesium	<1.0	Atrazine	–	0.02–0.011 ppb
Silica	2.0			
Iron Fe_2O_3	0.03			
Aluminum Al_2O_3	0.02			
Sodium	35.0			
Fluoride	0.51			
Chloramines	1.0			

Source: Environmental Health Center-Dallas, 1984–2008-1.58 chemicals not detected—2014. Modified from Table 5, CS Vol II, p. 548.

TABLE 3.61
Known Health Effects of Contaminants Found in Tap Water

Cardiovascular or Blood Toxicity (Known or Suspected) No. 50

Aluminum	Beryllium (total)	Acetone	Bromodichloromethane
Arsenic (total)	Thallium (total)	Hexachlorobutadiene	Dibromochloromethane
Cadmium (total)	Carbon disulfide	Methyl ethyl ketone	Dichloromethane
Copper	Simazine	Naphthalene	(methylene chloride)
Lead (total)	Alachlor (Lasso)	Tetrahydrofuran	p-Dichlorobenzene
Mercury (total inorganic)	Isopropyl alcohol	Methyl methacrylate	Vinyl chloride
Nitrate and nitrite	Chloromethane	cis-1,2-Dichloroethylene	1,1-Dichloroethylene
Nitrate	Bromomethane	1,2,4-Trimethylbenzene	1,1-Dichloroethane
Selenium (total)	Chloroethane	Monochloroacetic acid	1,2-Dichloroethane
Antimony (total)	Aniline	Chloroform	1,1,1-Trichloroethane
			Carbon tetrachloride

Cancer (Known) No. 37

Arsenic (total)	Naphthalene	Iodomethane	1,1-Dichloroethane
Cadmium (total)	Chrysene	Chloroform	1,2-Dichloroethane
Chromium (total)	Benzo[a]anthracene	Bromoform	Carbon tetrachloride
Lead (total)	Benzo[b]fluoranthene	Bromodichloromethane	1,2-Dichloropropane
Beryllium (total)	Benzo[k]fluoranthene	Dichloromethane	Trichloroethylene
Alachlor (Lasso)	Benzo[a]pyrene	(methylene chloride)	Tetrachloroethylene
Chloroethane	Dibromomethane	p-Dichlorobenzene	Benzene
Aniline	Dichloroacetic acid	Vinyl chloride	Combined uranium (mg/L)

Cancer (Suspected) No. 17

Chromium (total)	Bromacil	Dibromochloromethane
Mercury (total inorganic)	Chloromethane	Total trihalomethanes
Di(2-Ethylhexyl) adipate	Hexachlorobutadiene	(TTHMs)
Simazine	MTBE	1,1-Dichloroethylene
Metolachlor	1,2,4-Trichlorobenzene	Ethylbenzene
Atrazine	Trichloroacetic acid	Styrene

Developmental Toxicity (Known) No. 10

Arsenic (total)	Chloromethane
Cadmium (total)	Bromomethane
Lead (total)	Dibromomethane
Mercury (total inorganic)	Benzene
Carbon disulfide	Toluene

Developmental Toxicity (Suspected) No. 34

Barium (total)	Chloroethane	Tetrahydrofuran	p-Dichlorobenzene
Cadmium (total)	Aniline	Di-n-butylphthalate	Vinyl chloride
Copper	Hexachlorobutadiene	Methyl methacrylate	1,1-Dichloroethylene
Selenium (total)	Methyl ethyl ketone	Benzo[a]pyrene	1,2-Dichloroethane
Hexachlorocyclopentadiene	Naphthalene	n-Hexane	1,1,1-Trichloroethane
Alachlor (Lasso)	Methyl isobutyl ketone	1,2,4-Trichlorobenzene	Carbon tetrachloride
Isopropyl alcohol	MTBE	Chloroform	Trichloroethylene

Endocrine Toxicity (Known or Suspected) No. 25

Arsenic (total)	Di(2-Ethylhexyl) adipate	Hexachlorobutadiene	1,2,4-Trichlorobenzene
Cadmium (total)	Simazine	Tetrahydrofuran	Dibromomethane
Lead (total)	Atrazine	Diethylphthalate	Dibromoacetic acid
Mercury (total inorganic)	Alachlor (Lasso)	Di-n-butylphthalate	Chloroform
Carbon disulfide	Bromacil	Benzo[a]pyrene	Dichloromethane (methylene chloride)

(Continued)

TABLE 3.61 (*Continued*)
Known Health Effects of Contaminants Found in Tap Water

Immunotoxicity (Known or Suspected) No. 16

Cadmium (total)	Atrazine	Benzo[a]pyrene
Chromium (total)	Alachlor (Lasso)	Benzene
Lead (total)	Diethylphthalate	Toluene
Mercury (total inorganic)	Di-n-butylphthalate	Styrene
Beryllium (total)	Methyl methacrylate	o-Xylene
		m- and p-Xylene

Kidney Toxicity (Known or Suspected) No. 49

Arsenic (total)	Beryllium (total)	Acetone	Iodomethane
Cadmium (total)	Thallium (total)	Hexachlorobutadiene	Chloroform
Chromium (total)	Simazine	Methyl ethyl ketone	Bromoform
Copper	Hexachlorocyclopentadiene	Naphthalene	Bromodichloromethane
Lead (total)	Alachlor (Lasso)	Methyl isobutyl ketone	Dibromochloromethane
Mercury (total inorganic)	Isopropyl alcohol	MTBE	Dichloromethane (methylene
Nitrate and nitrite	Chloromethane	Di-n-butylphthalate	chloride)
Nitrate	Bromomethane	Methyl methacrylate	p-Dichlorobenzene
Nitrite	Chloroethane	Dibromomethane	1,1-Dichloroethylene
Selenium (total)	Aniline	Monochloroacetic acid	1,2-Dichloroethane
			Carbon tetrachloride

Gastrointestinal or Liver Toxicity (Known or Suspected) No. 58

Arsenic (total)	Hexachlorocyclopentadiene	Methyl isobutyl ketone	Trichloroacetic acid
Chromium (total)	Atrazine	MTBE	Chloroform
Copper	Butyl acetate	Acenaphthene	Bromoform
Lead (total)	Isopropyl alcohol	Tetrahydrofuran	Bromodichloromethane
Manganese	Chloromethane	Fluorene	Dibromochloromethane
Mercury (total inorganic)	Bromomethane	2-Hexanone	Dichloromethane (methylene
Selenium (total)	Chloroethane	Diethylphthalate	chloride)
Antimony (total)	Aniline	Di-n-butylphthalate	p-Dichlorobenzene
Beryllium (total)	Acetone	Methyl methacrylate	Vinyl chloride
Thallium (total)	Hexachlorobutadiene	Benzo[a]pyrene	1,1-Dichloroethylene
Carbon disulfide	Methyl ethyl ketone	Dibromomethane	1,2-Dichloroethane
Simazine	Naphthalene	Bromochloromethane	1,1,1-Trichloroethane

Neurotoxicity (Known or Suspected) No. 65

Aluminum	Atrazine	Tetrahydrofuran	Iodomethane
Arsenic (total)	Butyl acetate	2-Hexanone	Dichloroacetonitrile
Barium (total)	Isopropyl alcohol	Diethylphthalate	Chloroform
Cadmium (total)	Chloromethane	Pyrene	Bromoform
Lead (total)	Bromomethane	Di-n-butylphthalate	Bromodichloromethane
Manganese	Chloroethane	Methyl methacrylate	Dibromochloromethane
Mercury (total inorganic)	Aniline	n-Hexane	Dichloromethane (methylene
Selenium (total)	Acetone	1,2,4-Trichlorobenzene	chloride)
Antimony (total)	Hexachlorobutadiene	cis-1,2-Dichloroethylene	p-Dichlorobenzene
Thallium (total)	Methyl ethyl ketone	Dibromomethane	Vinyl chloride
Carbon disulfide	Naphthalene	1,2,4-Trimethylbenzene	1,1-Dichloroethylene
Simazine	Methyl isobutyl ketone	1,3,5-Trimethylbenzene	1,1-Dichloroethane
Hexachlorocyclopentadiene	MTBE	Bromochloromethane	1,2-Dichloroethane
			1,1,1-Trichloroethane

(Continued)

TABLE 3.61 (*Continued*)
Known Health Effects of Contaminants Found in Tap Water

Reproductive Toxicity (Known) No. 5

Cadmium (total)
Lead (total)
Carbon disulfide
Dibromomethane
Benzene

Reproductive Toxicity (Suspected) No. 43

Aluminum	Nitrate	Bromomethane	Vinyl chloride
Arsenic (total)	Nitrite	Hexachlorobutadiene	1,1-Dichloroethylene
Barium (total)	Selenium (total)	Methyl ethyl ketone	1,2-Dichloroethane
Cadmium (total)	Antimony (total)	Diethylphthalate	1,1,1-Trichloroethane
Chromium (total)	Beryllium (total)	Di-n-butylphthalate	Carbon tetrachloride
Copper	Thallium (total)	Methyl methacrylate	1,2-Dichloropropane
Manganese	Hexachlorocyclopentadiene	n-Hexane	Trichloroethylene
Mercury (total inorganic)	Atrazine	Chloroform	Tetrachloroethylene
Nitrate and nitrite	Chloromethane	Dichloromethane (methylene chloride)	Toluene

Respiratory Toxicity (Known or Suspected) No. 57

Aluminum	Hexachlorocyclopentadiene	Phenanthrene	Iodomethane
Arsenic (total)	Butyl acetate	Diethylphthalate	Dichloroacetonitrile
Barium (total)	Isopropyl alcohol	Methyl methacrylate	Chloroform
Cadmium (total)	Chloromethane	Benzo[a]pyrene	Bromoform
Chromium (total)	Bromomethane	n-Hexane	Dichloromethane (methylene chloride)
Copper	Chloroethane	1,2,4-Trichlorobenzene	p-Dichlorobenzene
Lead (total)	Aniline	Dibromomethane	Vinyl chloride
Manganese	Acetone	1,2,4-Trimethylbenzene	1,1-Dichloroethylene
Mercury (total inorganic)	Methyl ethyl ketone	1,3,5-Trimethylbenzene	1,2-Dichloroethane
Selenium (total)	Naphthalene	Bromochloromethane	Carbon tetrachloride
Antimony (total)	Methyl isobutyl ketone	Monochloroacetic acid	1,2-Dichloropropane
Beryllium (total)	Tetrahydrofuran	Trichloroacetic acid	

Skin Sensitivity (Known or Suspected) No. 51

Arsenic (total)	Atrazine	Methyl isobutyl ketone	Dibromomethane
Chromium (total)	Alachlor (Lasso)	MTBE	Monochloroacetic acid
Lead (total)	Butyl Acetate	2-Hexanone	Trichloroacetic acid
Mercury (total inorganic)	Isopropyl alcohol	Phenanthrene	Iodomethane
Selenium (total)	Chloromethane	Diethylphthalate	p-Dichlorobenzene
Silver (total)	Bromomethane	Pyrene	Vinyl chloride
Antimony (total)	Aniline	Di-n-butylphthalate	1,1-Dichloroethylene
Beryllium (total)	Acetone	Methyl methacrylate	1,2-Dichloroethane
Thallium (total)	Methyl ethyl ketone	Benzo[a]pyrene	1,1,1-Trichloroethane
Carbon disulfide	Naphthalene	n-Hexane	Carbon tetrachloride
Hexachlorocyclopentadiene			

Source: Environmental Working Group.

IMAGING AGENTS FROM TOXIC PRODUCTS WHICH ARE
ANOTHER KNOWN SOURCE OF CONTAMINATION

Iodinated chemicals safely used as contrast agents for medical imaging of soft tissues form toxic compounds when they go through drinking water disinfection at treatment plants, according to a study.[681] The research explains the presence of iodine-containing disinfection by-products in drinking water where there is no known natural source of iodide. In drinking water treatment plants, iodide can react with chlorine or chloramines, two common disinfectant chemicals, to form iodoacids and iodotrihalomethane by-products, which are among the most toxic disinfection by-products known. Looking for an iodide source, Richardson[681] discovered low concentrations of iodine-containing medical contrast agents such as iopamidol in the drinking water of six of 10 U.S. cities they sampled. The researchers also combined the cities' untreated water, iodinated contrast agents, and chlorine or chloramines, as would happen in a water treatment plant. They confirmed that the chemicals reacted to produce iodoacids and iodotrihalomethanes. The toxic compounds did not form when any one of the three ingredients was absent (Table 3.62).

NATURAL GAS FOUND IN DRINKING WATER NEAR FRACKED WELLS IS ANOTHER NEW SOURCE OF CONTAMINATION

Elevated levels of methane and other stray gases have been found in drinking water near natural gas wells in Pennsylvania's gas-rich Marcellus shale region, according to new research. In the case of methane, concentrations were six times higher in some drinking water found within 1 km of drilling operations.

> The bottom line is strong evidence for gas leaking into drinking water in some cases.
>
> **Jackson (2013)[682]**

In addition to the higher methane concentrations, the new study documented higher ethane and propane concentrations. Ethane concentrations were 23 times higher at homes within a kilometer of a shale gas well. Propane was detected in 10 samples, all from wells within 1 km of drilling.

All the gases appear to be fossil in origin. Those are gases that are not generated by microbes that can live in the ground and affect well water.

The methane contamination may be a result of cracks in the cement that surrounds the outside of the steel tubing and serves as a barrier between the rock that is drilled through the well. An improper cement job could permit gas from a pocket at mid-depth to move into the space outside the well, and move up to the drinking water.

The biggest known risk of high methane concentrations in drinking water is an explosion or fire due to the buildup of the gas in a confined space such as a basement or a shed. However, it is also the number one contaminant in homes of the chemically sensitive emanating from gas appliances.

The EPA's intervention is the latest development in its on-again, off-again involvement in Dimock, where the Pennsylvania Department of Environmental Protection blamed drilling by Cabot Oil and Gas Corp., Houston, for contaminating water wells of 19 homes 3 years ago.

EPA toxicologist Loven, in a memo posted on the agency's website, said well-test results from eight homes showed that four "contained contaminants at levels of potential concern."

The well water of one house, whose occupants include two toddlers, contained arsenic at levels that would pose a long-term cancer risk. Three other houses contained excessive levels of manganese

TABLE 3.62

Biologicals and Disinfectants Found in Drinking Water

Contaminant	MCLG[a] (mg/L)[b]	MCL or TT[a] (mg/L)[b]	Potential Health Effects from Long-Term Exposure Above the MCL (Unless Specified as Short-Term)	Sources of Contaminant in Drinking Water
			Microorganisms	
Cryptosporidium	Zero	TT[c]	Gastrointestinal illness (such as diarrhea, vomiting, and cramps)	Human and animal fecal waste
Giardia lamblia	Zero	TT[c]	Gastrointestinal illness (such as diarrhea, vomiting, and cramps)	Human and animal fecal waste
Heterotrophic plate count (HPC)	n/a	TT[c]	HPC has no health effects; it is an analytic method used to measure the variety of bacteria that are common in water. The lower the concentration of bacteria in drinking water, the better maintained the water system is.	HPC measures a range of bacteria that are naturally present in the environment
Legionella	Zero	TT[c]	Legionnaire's disease, a type of pneumonia	Found naturally in water; multiplies in heating systems
Total coliforms (including fecal coliform and *E. Coli*)	Zero	5.0%[d]	Not a health threat in itself; it is used to indicate whether other potentially harmful bacteria may be present[e]	Coliforms are naturally present in the environment; as well as feces, fecal coliforms and *E. coli* only come from human and animal fecal waste
Turbidity	n/a	TT[c]	Turbidity is a measure of the cloudiness of water. It is used to indicate water quality and filtration effectiveness (such as whether disease-causing organisms are present). Higher turbidity levels are often associated with higher levels of disease-causing microorganisms such as viruses, parasites, and some bacteria. These organisms can cause symptoms such as nausea, cramps, diarrhea, and associated headaches.	Soil runoff
Viruses (enteric)	Zero	TT[c]	Gastrointestinal illness (such as diarrhea, vomiting, and cramps)	Human and animal fecal waste
			Disinfection By-Products	
Bromate	Zero	0.010	Increased Risk of Cancer	By-product of drinking water disinfection
Chlorite	0.8	1.0	Anemia; infants and young children: nervous system effects	By-product of drinking water disinfection

(Continued)

TABLE 3.62 (*Continued*)
Biologicals and Disinfectants Found in Drinking Water

Contaminant	MCLG[a] (mg/L)[b]	MCL or TT[a] (mg/L)[b]	Potential Health Effects from Long-Term Exposure Above the MCL (Unless Specified as Short-Term)	Sources of Contaminant in Drinking Water
Haloacetic acids (HAA5)	n/a[f]	0.060[g]	Increased risk of cancer	By-product of drinking water disinfection
Total Trihalomethanes (TTHMs)	--> n/a[f]	--> 0.080[g]	Liver, kidney or central nervous system problems; increased risk of cancer	By-product of drinking water disinfection
Disinfectants				
Chloramines (as Cl_2)	MRDLG = 4[a]	MRDL = 4.0[a]	Eye/nose irritation; stomach discomfort, anemia	Water additive used to control microbes
Chlorine (as Cl_2)	MRDLG = 4[a]	MRDL = 4.0[a]	Eye/nose irritation; stomach discomfort	Water additive used to control microbes
Chlorine dioxide (as ClO_2)	MRDLG = 0.8[a]	MRDL = 0.8[a]	Anemia; infants and young children: nervous system effects	Water additive used to control microbes
Inorganic Chemicals				
Antimony	0.006	0.006	Increase in blood cholesterol; decrease in blood sugar	Discharge from petroleum refineries; fire retardants; ceramics; electronics; solder
Arsenic	0	0.010 as of 01/23/06	Skin damage or problems with circulatory systems, and may have increased risk of getting cancer	Erosion of natural deposits; runoff from orchards; runoff from glass and electronics production wastes
Asbestos (fiber >10 micrometers)	7 million fibers per liter (MFL)	7 MFL	Increased risk of developing benign intestinal polyps	Decay of asbestos cement in water mains; erosion of natural deposits
Barium	2	2	Increase in blood pressure	Discharge of drilling wastes; discharge from metal refineries; erosion of natural deposits
Beryllium	0.004	0.004	Intestinal lesions	Discharge from metal refineries and coal-burning factories; discharge from electrical, aerospace, and defense industries
Cadmium	0.005	0.005	Kidney damage	Corrosion of galvanized pipes; erosion of natural deposits; discharge from metal refineries; runoff from waste batteries and paints
Chromium (total)	0.1	0.1	Allergic dermatitis	Discharge from steel and pulp mills; erosion of natural deposits

(*Continued*)

TABLE 3.62 (Continued)
Biologicals and Disinfectants Found in Drinking Water

Contaminant	MCLG[a] (mg/L)[b]	MCL or TT[a] (mg/L)[b]	Potential Health Effects from Long-Term Exposure Above the MCL (Unless Specified as Short-Term)	Sources of Contaminant in Drinking Water
Copper	1.3	TT[g]; Action Level = 1.3	Short-term exposure: gastrointestinal distress Long-term exposure: liver or kidney damage People with Wilson's disease should consult their personal doctor if the amount of copper in their water exceeds the action level	Corrosion of household plumbing systems; erosion of natural deposits
Cyanide (as free cyanide)	0.2	0.2	Nerve damage or thyroid problems	Discharge from steel/metal factories; discharge from plastic and fertilizer factories
Fluoride	4.0	4.0	Bone disease (pain and tenderness of the bones); children may get mottled teeth	Water additive which promotes strong teeth; erosion of natural deposits; discharge from fertilizer and aluminum factories
Lead	Zero	TT[g]; Action Level = 0.015	Infants and children: Delays in physical or mental development; children could show slight deficits in attention span and learning abilities Adults: Kidney problems; high blood pressure	Corrosion of household plumbing systems; erosion of natural deposits
Mercury (inorganic)	0.002	0.002	Kidney damage	Erosion of natural deposits; discharge from refineries and factories; runoff from landfills and croplands
Nitrate (measured as nitrogen)	10	10	Infants below the age of 6 months who drink water containing nitrate in excess of the MCL could become seriously ill and, if untreated, may die. Symptoms include shortness of breath and blue-baby syndrome	Runoff from fertilizer use; leaking from septic tanks, sewage; erosion of natural deposits
Nitrite (measured as nitrogen)	1	1	Infants below the age of 6 months who drink water containing nitrite in excess of the MCL could become seriously ill and, if untreated, may die. Symptoms include shortness of breath and blue-baby syndrome	Runoff from fertilizer use; leaking from septic tanks, sewage; erosion of natural deposits
Selenium	0.05	0.05	Hair or fingernail loss; numbness in fingers or toes; circulatory problems	Discharge from petroleum refineries; erosion of natural deposits; discharge from mines
Organic Chemicals				
Acrylamide	Zero	TT[h]	Nervous system or blood problems; increased risk of cancer	Added to water during sewage/wastewater treatment

(Continued)

TABLE 3.62 (Continued)
Biologicals and Disinfectants Found in Drinking Water

Contaminant	MCLG[a] (mg/L)[b]	MCL or TT[a] (mg/L)[b]	Potential Health Effects from Long-Term Exposure Above the MCL (Unless Specified as Short-Term)	Sources of Contaminant in Drinking Water
Alachlor	Zero	0.002	Eye, liver, kidney, or spleen problems; anemia; increased risk of cancer	Runoff from herbicide used on row crops
Atrazine	0.003	0.003	Cardiovascular system or reproductive problems	Runoff from herbicide used on row crops
Benzene	Zero	0.005	Anemia; decrease in blood platelets; increased risk of cancer	Discharge from factories; leaching from gas storage tanks and landfills
Benzo(a)pyrene (PAHs)	Zero	0.0002	Reproductive difficulties; increased risk of cancer	Leaching from linings of water storage tanks and distribution lines
Carbofuran	0.04	0.04	Problems with blood, nervous system, or reproductive system	Leaching of soil fumigant used on rice and alfalfa
Carbon tetrachloride	Zero	0.005	Liver problems; increased risk of cancer	Discharge from chemical plants and other industrial activities
Chlordane	Zero	0.002	Liver or nervous system problems; increased risk of cancer	Residue of banned termiticide
Chlorobenzene	0.1	0.1	Liver or kidney problems	Discharge from chemical and agricultural chemical factories
2,4-D	0.07	0.07	Kidney, liver, or adrenal gland problems	Runoff from herbicide used on row crops
Dalapon	0.2	0.2	Minor kidney changes	Runoff from herbicide used on rights of way
1,2-Dibromo-3-chloropropane (DBCP)	Zero	0.0002	Reproductive difficulties; increased risk of cancer	Runoff/leaching from soil fumigant used on soybeans, cotton, pineapples, and orchards
o-Dichlorobenzene	0.6	0.6	Liver, kidney, or circulatory system problems	Discharge from industrial chemical factories
p-Dichlorobenzene	0.075	0.075	Anemia; liver, kidney, or spleen damage; changes in blood	Discharge from industrial chemical factories
1,2-Dichloroethane	Zero	0.005	Increased risk of cancer	Discharge from industrial chemical factories
1,1-Dichloroethylene	0.007	0.007	Liver problems	Discharge from industrial chemical factories
cis-1,2-Dichloroethylene	0.07	0.07	Liver problems	Discharge from industrial chemical factories
trans-1,2-Dichloroethylene	0.1	0.1	Liver problems	Discharge from industrial chemical factories
Dichloromethane	Zero	0.005	Liver problems; increased risk of cancer	Discharge from drug and chemical factories
1,2-Dichloropropane	Zero	0.005	Increased risk of cancer	Discharge from industrial chemical factories

(Continued)

TABLE 3.62 (Continued)
Biologicals and Disinfectants Found in Drinking Water

Contaminant	MCLG[a] (mg/L)[b]	MCL or TT[a] (mg/L)[b]	Potential Health Effects from Long-Term Exposure Above the MCL (Unless Specified as Short-Term)	Sources of Contaminant in Drinking Water
Di(2-ethylhexyl) adipate	0.4	0.4	Weight loss, liver problems, or possible reproductive difficulties	Discharge from chemical factories
Di(2-ethylhexyl) phthalate	Zero	0.006	Reproductive difficulties; liver problems; increased risk of cancer	Discharge from rubber and chemical factories
Dinoseb	0.007	0.007	Reproductive difficulties	Runoff from herbicide used on soybeans and vegetables
Dioxin (2,3,7,8-TCDD)	Zero	0.00000003	Reproductive difficulties; increased risk of cancer	Emissions from waste incineration and other combustion; discharge from chemical factories
Diquat	0.02	0.02	Cataracts	Runoff from herbicide use
Endothall	0.1	0.1	Stomach and intestinal problems	Runoff from herbicide use
Endrin	0.002	0.002	Liver problems	Residue of banned insecticide
Epichlorohydrin	Zero	TT[h]	Increased cancer risk and, over a long period of time, stomach problems	Discharge from industrial chemical factories; an impurity of some water treatment chemicals
Ethylbenzene	0.7	0.7	Liver or kidney problems	Discharge from petroleum refineries
Ethylene dibromide	Zero	0.00005	Problems with liver, stomach, reproductive system, or kidneys; increased risk of cancer	Discharge from petroleum refineries
Glyphosate	0.7	0.7	Kidney problems; reproductive difficulties	Runoff from herbicide use
Heptachlor	Zero	0.0004	Liver damage; increased risk of cancer	Residue of banned termiticide
Heptachlor epoxide	Zero	0.0002	Liver damage; increased risk of cancer	Breakdown of heptachlor
Hexachlorobenzene	Zero	0.001	Liver or kidney problems; reproductive difficulties; increased risk of cancer	Discharge from metal refineries and agricultural chemical factories
Hexachlorocyclopenta-diene	0.05	0.05	Kidney or stomach problems	Discharge from chemical factories
Lindane	0.0002	0.0002	Liver or kidney problems	Runoff/leaching from insecticide used on cattle, lumber, gardens
Methoxychlor	0.04	0.04	Reproductive difficulties	Runoff/leaching from insecticide used on fruits, vegetables, alfalfa, livestock
Oxamyl (Vydate)	0.2	0.2	Slight nervous system effects	Runoff/leaching from insecticide used on apples, potatoes, and tomatoes

(Continued)

TABLE 3.62 (Continued)
Biologicals and Disinfectants Found in Drinking Water

Contaminant	MCLG[a] (mg/L)[b]	MCL or TT[a] (mg/L)[b]	Potential Health Effects from Long-Term Exposure Above the MCL (Unless Specified as Short-Term)	Sources of Contaminant in Drinking Water
Polychlorinated biphenyls (PCBs)	Zero	0.0005	Skin changes; thymus gland problems; immune deficiencies; reproductive or nervous system difficulties; increased risk of cancer	Runoff from landfills; discharge of waste chemicals
Pentachlorophenol	Zero	0.001	Liver or kidney problems; increased cancer risk	Discharge from wood preserving factories
Picloram	0.5	0.5	Liver problems	Herbicide runoff
Simazine	0.004	0.004	Problems with blood	Herbicide runoff
Styrene	0.1	0.1	Liver, kidney, or circulatory system problems	Discharge from rubber and plastic factories; leaching from landfills
Tetrachloroethylene	Zero	0.005	Liver problems; increased risk of cancer	Discharge from factories and dry cleaners
Toluene	1	1	Nervous system, kidney, or liver problems	Discharge from petroleum factories
Toxaphene	Zero	0.003	Kidney, liver, or thyroid problems; increased risk of cancer	Runoff/leaching from insecticide used on cotton and cattle
2,4,5-TP (Silvex)	0.05	0.05	Liver problems	Residue of banned herbicide
1,2,4-Trichlorobenzene	0.07	0.07	Changes in adrenal glands	Discharge from textile finishing factories
1,1,1-Trichloroethane	0.20	0.2	Liver, nervous system, or circulatory problems	Discharge from metal degreasing sites and other factories
1,1,2-Trichloroethane	0.003	0.005	Liver, kidney, or immune system problems	Discharge from industrial chemical factories
Trichloroethylene	Zero	0.005	Liver problems; increased risk of cancer	Discharge from metal degreasing sites and other factories
Vinyl chloride	Zero	0.002	Increased risk of cancer	Leaching from PVC pipes; discharge from plastic factories
Xylenes (total)	10	10	Nervous system damage	Discharge from petroleum factories; discharge from chemical factories
Radionuclides				
Alpha particles	None[g] ------- zero	15 picocuries per liter (pCi/L)	Increased risk of cancer	Erosion of natural deposits of certain minerals that are radioactive and may emit a form of radiation known as alpha radiation
Beta particles and photon emitters	none[g] ------- zero	4 millirems per year	Increased risk of cancer	Decay of natural and man-made deposits of certain minerals that are radioactive and may emit forms of radiation known as photons and beta radiation

(Continued)

TABLE 3.62 (*Continued*)
Biologicals and Disinfectants Found in Drinking Water

Contaminant	MCLG[a] (mg/L)[b]	MCL or TT[a] (mg/L)[b]	Potential Health Effects from Long-Term Exposure Above the MCL (Unless Specified as Short-Term)	Sources of Contaminant in Drinking Water
Radium 226 and radium 228 (combined)	none[g] --------- zero	5 pCi/L	Increased risk of cancer	Erosion of natural deposits
Uranium	Zero	30 μg/L as of 12/08/03	Increased risk of cancer, kidney toxicity	Erosion of natural deposits

Source: Environmental Protection Agency.

[a] Definitions:

Maximum Contaminant Level Goal (MCLG)—The level of a contaminant in drinking water below which there is no known or expected risk to health. MCLGs allow for a margin of safety and are nonenforceable public health goals.

Maximum Contaminant Level (MCL)—The highest level of a contaminant that is allowed in drinking water. MCLs are set as close to MCLGs as feasible using the best available treatment technology and taking cost into consideration. MCLs are enforceable standards.

Maximum Residual Disinfectant Level Goal (MRDLG)—The level of a drinking water disinfectant below which there is no known or expected risk to health. MRDLGs do not reflect the benefits of the use of disinfectants to control microbial contaminants.

Treatment Technique (TT)—A required process intended to reduce the level of a contaminant in drinking water.

Maximum Residual Disinfectant Level (MRDL)—The highest level of a disinfectant allowed in drinking water. There is convincing evidence that addition of a disinfectant is necessary for control of microbial contaminants.

[b] Units are in milligrams per liter (mg/L) unless otherwise noted. Milligrams per liter are equivalent to parts per million (PPM).

[c] EPA's surface water treatment rules require systems using surface water or groundwater under the direct influence of surface water to

Disinfect their water, and

Filter their water or

Meet criteria for avoiding filtration so that the following contaminants are controlled at the following levels:

Cryptosporidium: Unfiltered systems are required to include *Cryptosporidium* in their existing watershed control provisions

Giardia lamblia: 99.9% removal/inactivation.

Viruses: 99.99% removal/inactivation.

Legionella: No limit, but EPA believes that if *Giardia* and viruses are removed/inactivated, according to the treatment techniques in the Surface Water Treatment Rule, *Legionella* will also be controlled.

Turbidity: For systems that use conventional or direct filtration, at no time can turbidity (cloudiness of water) go higher than 1 Nephelometric Turbidity Unit (NTU), and samples for turbidity must be less than or equal to 0.3 NTUs in at least 95% of the samples in any month. Systems that use filtration other than the conventional or direct filtration must follow state limits, which must include turbidity at no time exceeding 5 NTUs.

Heterotrophic Plate Count (HPC): No more than 500 bacterial colonies per milliliter.

(*Continued*)

TABLE 3.62 (Continued)
Biologicals and Disinfectants Found in Drinking Water

Long-Term 1 Enhanced Surface Water Treatment: Surface water systems or groundwater under the direct influence (GWUDI) systems serving fewer than 10,000 people must comply with the applicable Long-Term 1 Enhanced Surface Water Treatment Rule provisions (such as turbidity standards, individual filter monitoring, *Cryptosporidium* removal requirements, updated watershed control requirements for unfiltered systems).

Long-Term 2 Enhanced Surface Water Treatment Rule: This rule applies to all surface water systems or groundwater systems under the direct influence of surface water. The rule targets additional *Cryptosporidium* treatment requirements for higher risk systems and includes provisions to reduce risks from uncovered finished water storage facilities and to ensure that the systems maintain microbial protection as they take steps to reduce the formation of disinfection by-products.

Filter Backwash Recycling: The Filter Backwash Recycling Rule requires systems that recycle to return specific recycle flows through all processes of the system's existing conventional or direct filtration system or at an alternate location approved by the state.

d No more than 5.0% samples total coliform-positive (TC-positive) in a month. (For water systems that collect fewer than 40 routine samples per month, no more than one sample can be total coliform-positive per month.) Every sample that has total coliform must be analyzed for either fecal coliforms or *E. coli* if two consecutive TC-positive samples, and one is also positive for *E.coli* fecal coliforms, system has an acute MCL violation.

e Fecal coliform and *E. coli* are bacteria whose presence indicates that the water may be contaminated with human or animal wastes. Disease-causing microbes (pathogens) in these wastes can cause diarrhea, cramps, nausea, headaches, or other symptoms. These pathogens may pose a special health risk for infants, young children, and people with severely compromised immune systems.

f Although there is no collective MCLG for this contaminant group, there are individual MCLGs for some of the individual contaminants:

  1. *Trihalomethanes*: bromodichloromethane (zero); bromoform (zero); dibromochloromethane (0.06 mg/L); chloroform (0.07 mg/L).
  2. *Haloacetic acids*: dichloroacetic acid (zero); trichloroacetic acid (0.02 mg/L); monochloroacetic acid (0.07 mg/L). Bromoacetic acid and dibromoacetic acid are regulated with this group but have no MCLGs.

g Lead and copper are regulated by a treatment technique that requires systems to control the corrosiveness of their water. If more than 10% of tap water samples exceed the action level, water systems must take additional steps. For copper, the action level is 1.3 mg/L, and for lead it is 0.015 mg/L.

h Each water system must certify, in writing, to the state (using third-party or manufacturer's certification) that when acrylamide and epichlorohydrin are used to treat water, the combination (or product) of dose and monomer level does not exceed the levels specified, as follows:

Acrylamide = 0.05% dosed at 1 mg/L (or equivalent)

Epichlorohydrin = 0.01% dosed at 20 mg/L (or equivalent)

and sodium. Tests also found glycol, at safe levels, and 2-methoxyethanol, a solvent. Those houses are not receiving shipments of water.

POLLUTION SUMMARY (TABLE 3.63)

TABLE 3.63
Drinking Water Quality Report—San Diego, CA Drinking Water Quality Report—San Diego, CA

Total Contaminants Detected (2004–2009)

Aluminum, bromide, barium (total), manganese, nitrate, monochloroacetic acid, dichloroacetic acid, trichloroacetic acid, monobromoacetic acid, dibromoacetic acid, total haloacetic acids (HAAs), chloroform, bromoform, bromodichloromethane, dibromochloromethane, total trihalomethanes (TTHMs), o-Xylene, m- and p-xylene, combined uranium (pCi/L), gross beta particle activity (pCi/L)

Agricultural Pollutants

(pesticides, fertilizer, factory farms)
Nitrate

Sprawl and Urban Pollutants

(road runoff, lawn pesticides, human waste)
Nitrate, m- and p-xylene, o-xylene

Industrial Pollutants

Aluminum, Bromide, Barium (total), Manganese, Nitrate, o-Xylene, m- and p-xylene, combined uranium (pCi/L), gross beta particle activity (pCi/L)

Water Treatment and Distribution By-Products

(pipes and fixtures, treatment chemicals and by-products)
Total trihalomethanes (TTHMs), total haloacetic acids (HAAs), chloroform, bromodichloromethane, dibromochloromethane, dichloroacetic acid, trichloroacetic acid, bromoform, dibromoacetic acid, monochloroacetic acid, monobromoacetic acid

Naturally Occurring

(naturally present but increased for lands denuded by sprawl, agriculture, or industrial development)
Nitrate, barium (total), manganese, gross beta particle activity (pCi/L), combined uranium (pCi/L), aluminum, bromide

Unregulated Contaminants

EPA has not established a maximum legal limit in tap water for these contaminants.
Bromide

Total Contaminants Detected (2004–2008)

Nitrate, monochloroacetic acid, dichloroacetic acid, trichloroacetic acid, dibromoacetic acid, bromochloroacetic acid, total haloacetic acids (HAAs), chloroform, bromoform, bromodichloromethane, dibromochloromethane, total trihalomethanes (TTHMs)

Agricultural Pollutants

(pesticides, fertilizer, factory farms)
Nitrate

Sprawl and Urban Pollutants

(road runoff, lawn pesticides, human waste)
Nitrate

Industrial Pollutants

Nitrate

(Continued)

TABLE 3.63 (*Continued*)

Drinking Water Quality Report—San Diego, CA Drinking Water Quality Report—San Diego, CA

Water Treatment and Distribution By-Products

(pipes and fixtures, treatment chemicals and byproducts)

Total trihalomethanes (TTHMs), total haloacetic acids (HAAs), chloroform, bromodichloromethane, dibromochloromethane, dichloroacetic acid, trichloroacetic acid, bromoform, dibromoacetic acid, monochloroacetic acid, bromochloroacetic acid

Naturally Occurring

(naturally present but increased for lands denuded by sprawl, agriculture, or industrial development)

Nitrate

Unregulated Contaminants

EPA has not established a maximum legal limit in tap water for these contaminants

Bromochloroacetic acid

Total Contaminants Detected (2004–2007)

Aluminum, arsenic (total), barium (total), chromium (total), copper, lead (total), manganese, nitrate, nitrite, selenium (total), dalapon, simazine, metolachlor, atrazine, butane, acetone, methyl isobutyl ketone, pentane, dibromomethane, 1,2,4-trimethylbenzene, monochloroacetic acid, dichloroacetic acid, trichloroacetic acid, monobromoacetic acid, dibromoacetic acid, bromochloroacetic acid, total haloacetic acids (HAAs), chloroform, bromoform, bromodichloromethane, dibromochloromethane, total trihalomethanes (TTHMs), dichloromethane (methylene chloride), benzene, toluene, ethylbenzene, o-xylene, m- and p-xylene, alpha particle activity (incl. radon and uranium), combined uranium (mg/L), radium-226, radium-228, alpha particle activity, combined uranium (pCi/L), uranium-234 (pCi/L), gross beta particle activity (pCi/L)

Agricultural Pollutants

(pesticides, fertilizer, factory farms)

Arsenic (total), nitrate, nitrite, selenium (total), dalapon, simazine, metolachlor, atrazine, ethylbenzene

Sprawl and Urban Pollutants

(road runoff, lawn pesticides, human waste)

Nitrate, copper, lead (total), arsenic (total), nitrite, dalapon, m- and p-xylene, dichloromethane (methylene chloride), o-xylene, benzene, acetone, butane

Industrial Pollutants

Aluminum, arsenic (total), barium (total), chromium (total), lead (total), manganese, nitrate, nitrite, selenium (total), butane, acetone, methyl isobutyl ketone, pentane, dibromomethane, 1,2,4-trimethylbenzene, dichloromethane (methylene chloride), benzene, toluene, ethylbenzene, o-xylene, m- and p-xylene, alpha particle activity (incl. radon and uranium), combined uranium (mg/L), radium-226, radium-228, alpha particle activity, combined uranium (pCi/L), gross beta particle activity (pCi/L)

Water Treatment and Distribution By-Products

(pipes and fixtures, treatment chemicals and byproducts)

Total trihalomethanes (TTHMs), total haloacetic acids (HAAs), chloroform, bromodichloromethane, dibromochloromethane, dichloroacetic acid, trichloroacetic acid, bromoform, dibromoacetic acid, monochloroacetic acid, bromochloroacetic acid, monobromoacetic acid, dibromomethane

Naturally Occurring

(naturally present but increased for lands denuded by sprawl, agriculture, or industrial development)

Nitrate, copper, barium (total), lead (total), arsenic (total), manganese, radium-228, radium-226, alpha particle activity, gross beta particle activity (pCi/L), combined uranium (pCi/L), chromium (total), alpha particle activity (incl. radon and uranium), combined uranium (mg/L), aluminum, selenium (total), nitrite

Unregulated Contaminants

EPA has not established a maximum legal limit in tap water for these contaminants.

Lead (total), metolachlor, butane, acetone, methyl isobutyl ketone, pentane, dibromomethane, 1,2,4-trimethylbenzene, bromochloroacetic acid, uranium-234 (pCi/L)

(Continued)

TABLE 3.63 (*Continued*)

Drinking Water Quality Report—San Diego, CA Drinking Water Quality Report—San Diego, CA

Total Contaminants Detected (2004–2009)

Barium (total), nitrate and nitrite, nitrate, monochloroacetic acid, trichloroacetic acid, monobromoacetic acid, dibromoacetic acid, combined uranium (pCi/L), gross beta particle activity (pCi/L), arsenic (total), dichloroacetic acid, total haloacetic acids (HAAs), 1,2-dibromo-3-chloropropane (DBCP), chloroform, bromoform, bromodichloromethane, dibromochloromethane, total trihalomethanes (TTHMs), tetrachloroethylene, radium-228, alpha particle activity, perchlorate

Agricultural Pollutants

(pesticides, fertilizer, factory farms)

Nitrate and nitrite, nitrate, arsenic (total), 1,2-dibromo-3-chloropropane (DBCP), perchlorate

Sprawl and Urban Pollutants

(road runoff, lawn pesticides, human waste)

Nitrate, nitrate and nitrite, arsenic (total), tetrachloroethylene

Industrial Pollutants

Barium (total), nitrate and nitrite, nitrate, combined uranium (pCi/L), gross beta particle activity (pCi/L), arsenic (total), tetrachloroethylene, radium-228, alpha particle activity, perchlorate

Water Treatment and Distribution By-Products

(pipes and fixtures, treatment chemicals and by-products)

Total trihalomethanes (TTHMs), total haloacetic acids (HAAs), chloroform, bromodichloromethane, dibromochloromethane, dichloroacetic acid, trichloroacetic acid, bromoform, dibromoacetic acid, monochloroacetic acid, monobromoacetic acid

Naturally Occurring

(naturally present but increased for lands denuded by sprawl, agriculture, or industrial development)

Nitrate, nitrate and nitrite, barium (total), arsenic (total), radium-228, alpha particle activity, gross beta particle activity (pCi/L), combined uranium (pCi/L)

Unregulated Contaminants

EPA has not established a maximum legal limit in tap water for these contaminants.

Perchlorate

Source: National Drinking Water Database. http://www.ewg.org/tap-water/whatsinyourwater/CA/San-Diego-Water-Department/3710020/

DRINKING WATER QUALITY REPORT—AUSTIN, TX

This drinking water quality report shows results of tests conducted by the water utility and provided to the Environmental Working Group (EWG) by the Texas Commission on Environmental Quality. It is part of EWG's national database that includes 47,667 drinking water utilities and 20 million test results. Water utilities nationwide detected more than 300 pollutants between 2004 and 2009. More than half of these chemicals are unregulated, legal in any amount. Despite this widespread contamination, the federal government invests few resources to protecting rivers, reservoirs, and groundwater from pollution in the first place. The information below summarizes test results for this utility and lists potential health concerns.

For more information from your water utility, please see their Consumer Confidence Report (Tables 3.64 through 3.66).

DRINKING WATER QUALITY REPORT—HOUSTON, TX

Serum perfluorooctanoic acid (PFOA) concentrations in users of private wells in the area surrounding DuPont's Washington Works facility were much greater than those observed in the general U.S (Table 3.65) population and were comparable to what has been observed in the study area previously.[683–685] Private drinking water wells in the area were contaminated with PFOA, with levels in

TABLE 3.64

Drinking Water System National Average

	This Drinking Water System	National Average
Exceed health guidelines:	7 chemicals	4
Health standard exceedances:	0 chemicals	0.5
Pollutants found:	12 chemicals	8
Tests conducted:	2228 tests	420

Source: Environmental Working Group.

some wells being much greater than those observed in public drinking water supplies in the same area, which ranged from 0.03 µg/L in Mason County to 3.5 µg/L in Little Hocking.[683,684] Using data from private wells, they had a large number of individual exposure levels and were able to assess a wide range of exposures to PFOA via drinking water.

The results of the regression analyses are consistent with a strong association between PFOA levels in serum and PFOA concentrations in drinking water. They found little difference in the association between serum and drinking water PFOA concentrations when they limited the analyses to 67 individuals who were long-term residents.

The serum:drinking-water concentration ratio of 141.5, which was estimated using regression analysis, was similar to ratios obtained in previous partially ecologic analyses.[683–687] In their previous work in the study area, they found serum:drinking-water concentration ratios in public water districts ranging from 59 to 411.[684–687] In Little Hocking, Ohio, near the Washington Works facility,

TABLE 3.65

Contaminants Exceeding Health Guidelines

Contaminant	Average/ Maximum Result	Health Limit Exceeded	Legal Limit Exceeded	Testing History ○-Tested ◐-Detected ◑-Over Health Guidelines ●-Over Legal Limit* (04 05 06 07 08)
Alpha particle activity:	9.17 pCi/L 21.7 pCi/L	Yes MCLG: 0 pCi/L	Yes 15 pCi/L	●——○○——○——○○——●——○-○-○——
Total haloacetic acids (HAAs):	22.22 ppb 70.9 pp	Yes 0.7 ppb	Yes 60 ppb	○○-○—┼——○-●-○——○——○—○-○○—○●●-○——○○○○—○○○○—○-
Gross beta particle activity (pCi/L):	6.55 pCi/L 16.2 pCi/L	Yes	Yes 15 pCi/L	●——◐◐——◑—◑◑-●-◑-◑-◑——————◑
Dibromochlo- romethane:	1.48 ppb 5.85 ppb	Yes 0.4 ppb	No 80 ppb	○○-○——○○-○—○—○○-○——○○○-○—○○-○○—○——○○○○○—○○○○○○-
Bromodichlo- romethane:	4.41 ppb 13.6 ppb	Yes MCLG: 0 ppb	No	

Source: Environmental Working Group. http://www.ewg.org/tap-water/whatsinyourwater/TX/City-of-Houston-Public-Works-/1010013/.

TABLE 3.66

Pharmacokinetic Parameter Values and Sources

Parameter	Symbol	Value	Data Source
Water intake	Q	1.4 L/day	U.S. EPA[710]
Fraction of PFOA absorbed[a]	F	100%	Gibson and Johnson[717]
Half-life	$t_{1/2}$	2.3 years, 840 days	Bartell et al.[691]
Volume of distribution[a]	V_d	Male, 181 mL/kg; female, 198 mL/kg; multiplied by individual body weight	Butenhoff et al.[709]

Source: Hoffman, K. et al. 2011. *Environ. Health Perspect.* 119:92–97. http://dx.doi.org/10.1289/ehp.1002503 [online October 04, 2010].

[a] Based on animal data.

Emmett et al.[683] estimated a water concentration ratio of 105 in an analysis of public water consumers. In addition, in a small sample of private well users (n = 6), serum:water concentration ratios ranged from 142 to 855.[683]

Private drinking water wells in West Virginia and Ohio communities surrounding the DuPont Washington Works facility are contaminated with PFOA. Concentrations in private wells are, in some cases, much greater than those observed in area public water districts. For private well users, adjusted regression analyses indicate that PFOA levels in drinking water are a significant predictor of PFOA levels in serum. The regression analysis predicted a 141.5 µg/L increase in serum levels for each 1 µg/L increase in drinking water PFOA—a very similar result to the 114 µg/L in serum for each 1 µg/L predicted in steady-state pharmacokinetic models. These results may also be applicable in other areas with point-source PFOA contamination.

CHILDREN'S BATH PRODUCTS CONTAMINATED WITH FORMALDEHYDE, 1,4-DIOXANE; CHEMICALS NOT LISTED ON PRODUCT LABELS DUE TO WEAK REGULATORY STANDARDS

Washington: Despite marketing claims such as "gentle" and "pure," dozens of top-selling children's bath products are contaminated with the cancer-causing chemicals formaldehyde and 1,4-dioxane, according to product test results released by the Campaign for Safe Cosmetics. The chemicals were not disclosed on product labels because contaminants are exempt from labeling laws.

This study is the first to document the widespread presence of both formaldehyde and 1,4-dioxane in bath products for children. Many products tested for this study contained both formaldehyde and 1,4-dioxane, including the top-selling Johnson's Baby Shampoo.

Formaldehyde and 1,4-dioxane are known to cause cancer in animals and are listed as probable human carcinogens by the EPA. Formaldehyde can also trigger skin rashes in some children.

Recent data showing that formaldehyde and the formaldehyde-releasing preservative, quaternium-15, are significant sensitizers and causal agents of contact dermatitis in children.

The U.S. government does not limit formaldehyde, 1,4-dioxane, or most other hazardous substances in personal care products sold in the United States, with no required safety assessment. Other nations have stricter standards. Formaldehyde is banned from personal care products in Japan and Sweden. The European Union has banned 1,4-dioxane from personal care products and has recalled products found to contain the chemical. The Campaign for Safe Cosmetics study found both chemicals in baby shampoos, bubble baths, and baby lotions. Parents often use all these products on a child during a single bath session. Children are exposed to toxic chemicals from many sources.

For the study, the Campaign for Safe Cosmetics commissioned an independent laboratory to test 48 top-selling children's products for 1,4-dioxane; 28 of those products were also tested for formaldehyde. The lab found that:

- Seventeen out of 28 products tested (61%) contained both formaldehyde and 1,4-dioxane; these included Johnson's Baby Shampoo, Sesame Street Bubble Bath, Grins & Giggles Milk & Honey Baby Wash, and Huggies Naturally Refreshing Cucumber & Green Tea Baby Wash.
- Twenty-three out of 28 products (82%) contained formaldehyde at levels ranging from 54 to 610 parts per million (ppm). Baby Magic Baby Lotion had the highest levels of formaldehyde.
- Thirty-two out of 48 products (67%) contained 1,4-dioxane at levels ranging from 0.27 to 35 ppm. American Girl shower products had the highest levels of 1,4-dioxane.

PRIVATE DRINKING WATER WELLS AS A SOURCE OF EXPOSURE TO PERFLUOROCTANOIC ACID (PFOA) IN COMMUNITIES SURROUNDING A FLUOROPOLYMER PRODUCTION FACILITY

PFOA or C8 is a synthetic chemical that is used as a processing aid in the manufacture of fluoropolymers. Products made with fluoropolymers possess unique properties, including oil, stain, grease, and water repellency. These properties led to the widespread use of fluoropolymers in a number of products, including nonstick cookware weather- and stain-resistant clothing and textiles, building and construction materials, and electronics.[688]

The chemical structure of PFOA makes the compound extremely resistant to environmental and metabolic degradation. PFOA has been detected globally in the environment.[689] It is well established that PFOA is readily absorbed via inhalation and ingestion. Routes of exposure in the general population remain unclear, although research suggests that diet is a potentially important source.[690] PFOA is detected in the vast majority of serum samples from the U.S. and world populations.[689] Once absorbed, PFOA is eliminated from the human body very slowly. Estimates of the serum half-life of PFOA range from 2.3 years in residents of a contaminated community to 3.8 years in retired fluorochemical workers.[691,692] Some evidence suggests that PFOA concentrations in serum are declining, possibly due to reductions in use; however, the median serum concentrations remain around 4 µg/L in the U.S. population.[692–694] PFOA exposure also has been linked to a variety of health impacts in animals, including increased cancer risk, adverse reproductive outcomes, and liver damage.[689,695] Owing to a lack of data, health impacts of exposure in humans remain largely unknown.[696]

In 2003, the USEPA began an enforceable consent agreement process with industry and other stakeholders to collect additional information for a PFOA risk assessment.[697] The USEPA and DuPont (the maker of Teflon) entered a memorandum of understanding (MOU) in November 2005 as part of the risk assessment. Building on an agreement in place between the West Virginia Department of Environmental Protection and DuPont, the MOU required DuPont to conduct environmental sampling, including the monitoring of groundwater and surface waters around its Washington Works facility in Parkersburg, West Virginia, USA.[698]

DuPont began using PFOA in the manufacture of Teflon at its Washington Works plant in the early 1950s. According to data provided by the company, emissions to air and the Ohio River reached a maximum in the late 1990s.[683,699] The company reported a large reduction in these emissions in recent years.[700] Previous research indicates that the primary source of exposure for individuals in the surrounding communities is contaminated groundwater that is used for drinking.[683,684] The groundwater in the area was contaminated via two main routes: PFOA released into the atmosphere was deposited onto soils and eventually leached downward into groundwater, and PFOA was released directly into the Ohio River, which runs near the facility and is linked to the groundwater supply.[699]

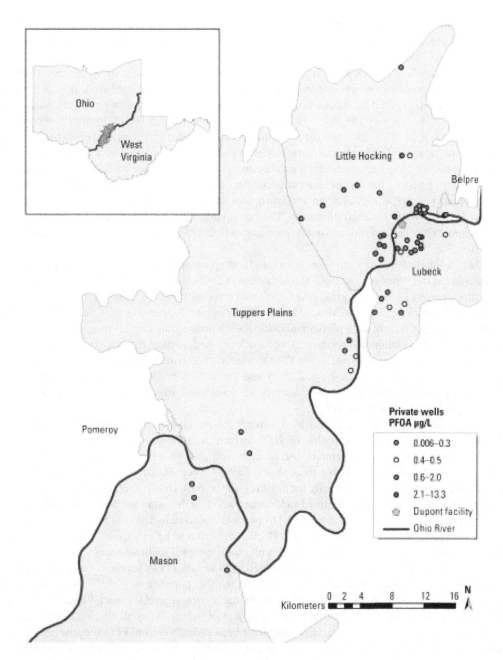

FIGURE 3.45   Water districts included in the C8 Health Project and the locations of private drinking water wells that show the average PFOA concentration for each well. (From Hoffman, K. et al. 2011. *Environ. Health Perspect.* 119:92–97. http://dx.doi.org/10.1289/ehp.1002503 [online 04 October 2010].)

In 2001, a group of residents in communities surrounding the facility filed a class action lawsuit against DuPont alleging health damages after PFOA was detected in public drinking water. The settlement established the C8 Health Project, a baseline survey conducted in 2005–2006 to investigate potential links between PFOA and human disease in the area surrounding the facility.[701] Previous studies showed a significant association between living in an area with contaminated public drinking water and increased PFOA levels in serum using water-district-level data.[683–685,702] These studies are partially ecologic because the exposure variable is assigned at the group level, whereas other variables are assigned at the individual level.[703–705] In particular, previous studies provide information on serum concentration in relation to average exposure for populations serviced by the same water supply, but investigations into the relationship between contaminated private household well water and serum levels are lacking. In the present analyses, they examined the relationship between PFOA concentrations in serum and in drinking water using data collected from private drinking water wells contaminated by industrial emissions. By using data from private drinking water wells, they were able to quantify PFOA levels in the drinking water of C8 Health Project participants at the individual level. They assessed the relationship using standard regression approaches; for comparison, they also used a pharmacokinetic model to explore the association between PFOA in drinking water and in serum levels. Simple, single-compartment, first-order models have been applied previously to estimate the serum concentration after exposure from diet and drinking water.[685,706] In the present analyses, they used updated estimates of pharmacokinetic parameters to predict the serum:drinking-water concentration ratio. They compared the association between drinking-water and serum PFOA concentrations from regression models with those obtained in pharmacokinetic analyses.

The C8 Health Project, a cross-sectional study of approximately 69,000 adults, was conducted by Brookmar Inc. from August 2005 through August 2006.[701] Participants lived in one of six public water districts in West Virginia and Ohio that surround DuPont's Washington Works facility: Belpre, Little Hocking, Lubeck, Mason County, Pomeroy, and Tuppers Plains–Chester (Figure 3.45). Data were collected from each participant using questionnaires and clinical examinations to obtain demographic information and residential, occupational, and medical histories.[701] Concentrations of 10 perfluorinated compounds, including PFOA, were also determined in serum samples taken once from each participant between August 2005 and August 2006. Detailed analytic methods were described previously.[707] Briefly, serum samples were analyzed using automated solid-phase extraction coupled to reversed-phase HPLC.

Water monitoring was conducted by DuPont[708] in public and private wells surrounding the Washington Works facility beginning in 2001. Private well monitoring reports contained PFOA measurements as well as the primary use of each well and the name and address of each well's owner. These reports are available through the EPA.[708] They linked well monitoring data for 62 private wells that were used primarily for drinking water to C8 Health Project participants based on name and address. They also identified individuals who had the same last name and address as the well owner as family members. A total of 115 participants were included in the study. The number of samples taken in each well before the collection of serum samples varied. Although most wells were sampled just once, 11 of the 62 private wells were sampled multiple times.

Age and sex have been previously associated with serum PFOA levels in the population surrounding the Washington Works facility, as well as in other populations.[683,684,702] In addition, working at the Washington Works plant and growing one's own vegetables were linked to increased PFOA levels in serum.[683,684] They included these a priori variables in all statistical models. They also assessed a number of other variables that have been linked to serum PFOA levels: body weight, consuming bottled water (modeled as yes or no), smoking cigarettes, and drinking alcohol.[683,684] Only the a priori variables were included in the final models because the others did not materially alter the association between serum and well-PFOA levels (did not cause a change >10% in the predicted contribution of drinking water to serum).

For wells with multiple PFOA sampling events, they used the arithmetic average PFOA concentration in each well to predict serum levels in regression models. This method provided an estimate of the serum:drinking water concentration ratio that is readily comparable to the results of a steady-state pharmacokinetic model that assumes that the concentration of PFOA in drinking water is constant over time (discussed in the next section). They also performed an analysis using time-weighted water concentrations based on a non-steady-state pharmacokinetic model. In the main analyses, they included all individuals regardless of how long they had lived at their current residence. They also performed analyses investigating the sensitivity of our results to the residential duration at a particular well. By restricting the

TABLE 3.67

Selected Population Characteristics, Serum PFOA Concentrations, and Statistical Significance of Difference

Characteristic	n (%)	Median Serum PFOA (μg/L [interquartile range])	p-Value
Total population	108 (100)	75.7 (31.5–130.5)	
Male	51 (47.2)	82.2 (45.9–164.3)	0.10
Female	57 (52.8)	68.1 (21.0–115.5)	
Grow own vegetables			
No	64 (59.3)	50.7 (24.9–107.3)	<0.001
Yes	44 (40.7)	91.2 (57.0–145.2)	
Employed at DuPont			
No	94 (87.0)	67.6 (72.2–102.4)	0.11
Yes	14 (13.0)	87.1 (27.4–145.1)	
Age (years)			
≤65	63 (58.3)	59.8 (20.6–115.9)	0.35
>65	45 (42.7)	84.9 (49.0–145.1)	
Body weight (kg)			
≤80	50 (46.3)	63.5 (31.5–107.7)	0.64
>80	58 (53.7)	81.2 (30.1–177.4)	

Source: Hoffman, K. et al. 2011. *Environ. Health Perspect.* 119:92–97. http://dx.doi.org/10.1289/ehp.1002503 [online October 04, 2010].

sample to long-term residents (>15 years), they ensured that participants had been exposed to water from a specific well long enough for their serum levels to have reached steady state (Table 3.66).

RESULTS

Linking well-monitoring data to C8 Health Project participants, they were able to identify 115 individuals who used 62 different private wells for drinking water. Of these individuals, 4 (3.5%) were missing data (PFOA levels in serum: n = 1, body weight: n = 2, race/ethnicity: n = 1) and were excluded from the analyses. They also excluded vegetarians (n = 2) and nonwhite participants (n = 1) because the numbers were too small to adequately control for these variables. Our final sample consisted of 108 participants. Serum PFOA levels ranged from 0.9 to 4751.5 μg/L, with a median concentration of 75.7 μg/L (mean ± SD, 177.3 ± 499.7 μg/L). As reported previously in the larger C8 Health Project sample,[684] individuals who grew their own vegetables and who were employed at DuPont had higher median serum PFOA concentrations (Table 3.67). PFOA concentrations were higher among older (>65 years) and heavier (>80 kg) participants, but the differences were not statistically significant (Table 3.67).

The number of participants using each well ranged from 1 to 4. The median PFOA concentration in drinking water wells included in our analyses was 0.2 μg/L (mean ± SD, 0.8 ± 1.9 μg/L). Although the median was below the USEPA provisional health advisory level of 0.4 μg/L, many participants had drinking water levels that exceeded the advisory level.[711] They found considerable variability between wells, with PFOA concentrations ranging from below the limit of quantification (LOQ = 0.006 μg/L) farthest from the Washington Works facility to 13.3 μg/L closest to the facility. One sample was reported below the LOQ and was assigned the LOQ (0.006 μg/L) in the analyses. Multiple samples were taken from 11 wells that were used by 19 study participants. In general, they did not find an overall trend from 2001 to 2005 in the concentrations of PFOA in

TABLE 3.68

Adjusted Robust Regression Model of Serum PFOA

Covariate	β-Coefficient (95% CI)
Intercept	7.4 (−9.8 to 24.4)
Well PFOA	141.5 (134.9 to 148.1)
Males	18.8 (−1.6 to 39.1)
Age >65 years	−4.2 (−24.2 to 15.9)
Grow own vegetables	18.4 (−1.3 to 38.1)
Employed at DuPont	5.9 (−24.1 to 36.2)

Source: Hoffman, K. et al. 2011. *Environ. Health Perspect.* 119:92–97. http://dx.doi. org/10.1289/ehp.1002503 [online October 04, 2010].

Note: The inclusion of other covariates (body weight, bottled water consumption, cigarette smoking, and alcohol consumption) did not alter the main associations.

private drinking water. Although PFOA concentrations in each well appeared to fluctuate by season, these differences may be due to seasonal changes in precipitation. PFOA concentrations measured in 2004 and 2005 for a subset of wells measured seasonally are shown in Supplemental Material, Table 3.68.

Robust regression analyses revealed six outliers (observations for which the standardized residual was >3). For these individuals, the predicted values for serum PFOA concentrations using regression parameters underestimated or overestimated observed concentrations (standardized residuals, 3.0–44.5). In the analyses using GEEs, they observed a small within-family correlation of serum PFOA levels of 0.1. Compared with the results of the robust regression, GEE analyses that excluded outliers produced a very similar estimate of effect (β) for each 1 μg/L increase in PFOA concentration (β = 141.8 μg/L; 95% CI, 134.3–149.4 μg/L) in drinking water. When they included outliers in the GEE, the estimate of the association between PFOA levels in serum and in drinking water was much larger. The inclusion of one participant in particular, with the highest PFOA concentrations in serum and drinking water in the population, increased the estimate of effect to 232.7 μg/L (95% CI, 200.9–264.5 μg/L). They could not identify a plausible explanation for this participant's extreme serum concentration using available data (the participant did not report being employed in the fluorochemical industry). Increased water consumption in this individual may have resulted in the extreme concentration; however, data were not available to evaluate this hypothesis.

When they restricted our analyses to individuals with a residency more than 15 years, our results were similar (β = 140.2 μg/L; 95% CI, 132.1–148.4 μg/L; n = 67). They considered other residential duration restrictions (2, 5, 10, and 20 years), but restrictions had little effect on the magnitude of the association between serum and drinking water. They also excluded participants who were ever employed at the Washington Works facility, because these individuals may have had other significant sources of exposure. Again, the association between drinking water levels and serum was similar when they excluded these individuals. In addition, excluding participants who reported consuming bottled water (n = 6) from analyses had little effect on the magnitude of the association between serum and drinking water.

LESS POLLUTED DRINKING WATER

BOTTLED WATER BRANDS THAT TREAT, TEST, AND TELL

Only 2 of 188 bottled waters surveyed make public three basic facts about their products routinely disclosed by municipal water utilities.

- The water's source
- Purification methods
- Chemical pollutants remaining after treatment

The reason: Bottled water companies enjoy a regulatory holiday under the federal Food, Drug and Cosmetic Act, which grants them complete latitude to decide what, if any, information about their water is divulged to customers.

In contrast, every one of the nation's 52,000 municipal water suppliers produces an annual water quality report detailing both its water source and pollutant testing results, as required under the federal Safe Drinking Water Act. An estimated 58% of these reports also describe water treatment methods. However, these results are open to question since they are clouded by chlorination for biological decontamination. This is very toxic and no chemically sensitive patient has been found who can tolerate this public water.

The Environmental Working Group's 18-month survey of bottled water labels and websites, including top domestic and imported brands, has found that:

1. Just 2 bottled waters—Ozarka Drinking Water and Penta Ultra-Purified Water—list specific water sources and treatment methods on their labels and offer a recent water quality test report on their websites.
2. Major bottled water brands obscure basic data about their products. None of the top 10 U.S. domestic bottled water brands label both their specific water source and treatment method for all their products.
   a. Aquafina Purified Drinking Water "originates from public water sources" but fails to name them on the label. The water is treated through a process called "hydro-7" that is not explained on the label.
   b. Arrowhead Mountain Spring Water lists springs in six California cities or counties as possible sources for the water they obtained, and gives no information on how or if the water is treated.
   c. Crystal Geyser Natural Alpine Spring Water is bottled at "the CG Roxane Source near California's Mount Shasta" but offers no information on treatment methods.
   d. Dasani Purified Water does not name its water source on the label, but notes the water is treated through reverse osmosis.
   e. Dear Park Natural Spring Water lists seven towns in Pennsylvania and Maryland as possible locations for the spring water they obtained. No treatment method is listed.
   f. Ice Mountain Natural Spring Water lists two springs in Michigan as possible sources; on the label, they describe its treatment methods.
   g. Nestle Pure Life Purified Water's label indicates that the water is drawn from either a "deep protected" Pennsylvania well or the public water supply of Allentown, PA, and is treated by either reverse osmosis or distillation.
   h. Ozarka Drinking Water is drawn from the "Houston Municipal Water Supply" and treated using "reverse osmosis, carbon filtration, microfiltration, and ozonation." Ozarka does not label this information on other products. Labels on Ozarka's Natural Spring Water and Aquapod Natural Spring Water list springs in two Texas counties as possible sources but fail to reveal how the water is treated.
   i. Poland Spring Natural Spring Water's label lists six towns in Maine as possible locations for its spring water but does not give treatment methods.
   j. Zephyrhills Natural Spring Water lists springs in three Florida counties as possible sources for its water but provides no information on how or if the water is treated.
3. Some of these 10 brands market their products with vague terms such as "pure" "crisp," and "perfect." These claims are potentially misleading and imply an absence of contamination not possible for the drinking water industry to achieve.

However, there are a few spring waters contained in glass bottles that are safe for the chemically sensitive. These are Mountain Valley, Evian, and San Pellegrino. These have been tested by thousands of chemically sensitive patients.

METHODOLOGY

EWG launched an investigation to learn which brands of bottled water tell their customers basic information about the water—where their water comes from, how it is treated, and what contaminants it contains.

Between February and August 2008, volunteers responded to their published email and website and website requests, and sent to EWG's Washington, D.C. office 163 unique bottled water labels representing 1347 brands from 30 states. They created a database detailing the information listed on each brand's label and website.

On January 1, 2009, bottled water brands marketed in California began posting more label and website information required by a new state labeling law. EWG wanted to know how or if the law and the sustained pressure from consumer and public health advocates had affected labeling in other states. In May and June 2009, volunteers sent 85 unique product labels representing 76 brands from 38 states, responding to their renewed requests distributed via email and published on their website. They supplemented our database with this new information.

They graded bottled water brands on how much they tell consumers about what is in the bottle. They failed brands neglecting to provide consumers with significant information on water source, treatment, and testing. They compared 2008 and 2009 labels and websites to learn how many brands are telling customers more this year than last year. The answer was a heartening 52%, though in nearly every case brands provided less information than tap water suppliers give their customers, even though all municipal waters are toxic if they are chlorinated.

All municipal water systems are required by law to publish water quality test results annually. Only 18% of bottled waters disclose quality reports that include contaminant testing results. Brands that provide this important information to consumers include all eight Nestle domestic brands surveyed (Poland Spring, Nestle Pure Life, Arrowhead, Calistoga, Deer Park, Ice Mountain, Ozarka, and Zephyrhills).

By contrast, Culligan Purified Drinking Water, Refreshe Purified Drinking Water, Giant Acadia Filtered Drinking Water, and 151 other bottled waters offer their customers no water quality test data.

Americans account for less than 5% of the world's population but drink 16% of the bottled water. U.S. bottled water sales rose 85% between 2000 and 2007,[712] driven by finely tuned marketing that has exploited consumer anxieties about tap water pollution.

However, in 2008, bottled water sales declined for the first time in the decade. This modest 1% drop, retrenching from the previous year's 6% increase in sales,[712] may signal consumers realizing that bottled water is not worth premium prices or suggesting that demand may reflect the struggling economy or both.

An increasing number of studies raise concerns about plastic bottlers' environmental impacts and the purity of their contents. Waters contained in plastics are contaminated with hexane 2 and 3 methyl pentanes, benzene, and other solvents. In 2006, Americans threw 36 billion water bottles into trash cans, onto the land as litter or into recycling bins.[713] The substantial waste management challenge presented by discarded plastic water bottles is frequently in the news.

Last year EWG commissioned tests that found bottled water not necessarily any safer than tap water, but they know this is not true by evaluating our chemically sensitive group. Ten brands sampled by EWG contained 38 pollutants ranging from fertilizer residue to industrial solvents. Pollutants in two brands exceeded state and industry health standards.[714]

Daily decisions on what to drink are not easy when bottled water companies fail to divulge what is in the bottle. EWG recommends filtered tap water as a first choice but they do not treat chemically sensitive patients. Also, filters must be in two stages to get the toxics out and not be contaminated in plastic jugs. The EHC-D and other environmental clinics do not use these waters unless double filtration using reverse osmosis and ending with a second ceramic steel filter. Even then, some chemically sensitive patients cannot tolerate this water. However, double filtration saves money, is purer than tap water, and helps solve the global plastic bottle problem.

They also advocate for the consumer's right to know about bottled water—where it comes from, and how and if it is treated, and what contaminants it contains. Bottled water companies should provide this information voluntarily.

WHERE DOES THE WATER COME FROM?

Federal law requires community tap water suppliers to identify their water sources. In Philadelphia's 2008 water quality report, residents learned that "the water comes from the Schuylkill and Delaware rivers. Each river contributes approximately one-half of the City's overall supply. "Davis, California residents learned that they drank water from 20 municipal wells and one private well. These wells tap into aquifers beneath the city at depths from 210 to 1730 feet below ground surface." These areas may be contaminated and especially if fracking is present.

1. "Artesian" and "spring waters" are groundwater under pressure that flows toward the ground surface.
2. "Well water" is pumped from a hole bored, drilled, or otherwise constructed in the ground that taps the water of an aquifer.
3. "Purified water," "deionized water," or other waters named by treatment method are often municipal waters that have undergone additional treatment.

Many drinking water sources are vulnerable to pollution. Community water systems must report to their customers potential sources of pollution to their water sources, from detailed surveys called Source Water Assessments. However, most do not or if contamination occurs they say it may smell bad but is okay to drink. Possibly, but it may just be tap water, therefore, if it smells bad do not drink it.

Few water sources are completely free of detectable contaminants. For example, the estimated 25% of bottled waters that rely on tap water[715] are drawing from supplies that collectively contain at least 260 pollutants, according to EWGs 2002–2005 survey of tap water testing conducted by community water supplies.[716]

Consumers append up to 1900 times more for a bottle of water than the same amount of tap water, yet rarely have basic information about the product.[714]

EWG recommends that bottled water labels and websites disclose the same information that the law requires of municipal water utilities.

Bottled water companies should:

1. Provide easy-to-access water quality reports disclosing all test results and containing the information required in Consumer Confidence Reports for tap water suppliers.
2. List on the label water treatment methods; and clear, specific information on the water source and location.
3. Test for unregulated chemicals that may leach from plastic bottles.

They urge consumers to make their first choice filtered tap water. They should consider bottled water a distant second, and then they should pick ranks that provide full water source, treatment, and quality disclosure and that use advanced treatment methods to remove a broad range of pollutants. We disagree. Glass bottled spring water is still the best. The chemically sensitive has three choices: (1) glass bottled spring water, (2) distilled water in steel and ceramic, and (3) reverse osmosis and the refilter in steel, ceramic, and charcoal filters.

GAPS IN THE FEDERAL STANDARD-SETTING PROCESS

POLLUTION BY SEDIMENTS

Sediments occur from runoff of lands made bare by soil erosion, crop cultivation, timber cutting, overgrazing, strip mining, road building, and other construction activities. Coarse sediments such as sand precipitate first, while fine particles such as clay remain in suspension for months. Not only is vigorous top soil lost, decreasing fertility for high-quality food production, but the fine particles cover bottom-dwelling organisms, eliminating fish spawning areas and reducing light penetration, which is necessary for photosynthesis by aquatic plants.

In 2000, approximately 600,000 m^3 of different types of radioactive waste were generated, and approximately 700,000 m^3 were in storage awaiting disposal. By volume, the most prevalent types of radioactive waste are contaminated environmental media (i.e., soil, sediment, water, and sludge requiring cleanup or further assessment) and low-level waste. Both of these waste types typically have the lowest levels of radioactivity when measured by volume. Additional radioactive wastes in the form of spent nuclear fuel (2467 metric tons of heavy metal) and high-level waste "glass logs" (1201 canisters of vitrified high-level waste) are in storage awaiting long-term disposal. Very small amounts of those wastes are still being generated. For example, less than 1 m^3 of spent nuclear fuel was generated in 2000. The total amount of radioactive waste being generated is expected to drop over the next few decades as cleanup operations are completed.

REFERENCES

1. National Research Council. 1977. *Drinking Water and Health*, pp. 439–447. Washington D.C.: National Academy of Sciences.
2. Malakoff, D. 2012. Researchers struggle to assess responses to ocean acidification. *Science* 338 (6103):27–28. Accessed December 10, 2015. http://c-can.msi.ucsb.edu/articles-of-interest/researchers-struggle-to-assess-responses-to-ocean-acidification
3. UN WWAP. 2003. *United Nations World Water Assessment Programme*. The World Water Development Report 1: Water for People, Water for Life. Paris, France: UNESCOik.
4. UNICEF, WHO. 2008. *UNICEF and World Health Organization Joint Monitoring Programme for Water Supply and Sanitation. Progress on Drinking Water and Sanitation: Special Focus on Sanitation.* New York: UNICEF; Geneva: WHO.
5. World Health Organization (WHO). 2002. World Health Report: Reducing Risks, Promoting Healthy Life. France. Accessed July 14, 2009. http://www.who.int/whr/2002/en/whr02_en.pdf
6. World Health Organization (WHO), United Nations Children's Fund (UNICEF). 2000. *Global Water Supply and Sanitation Assessment 2000 Report.* WHO and UNICEF Joint Monitoring Programme for Water Supply and Sanitation.
7. Vié, J. C, C. Hilton-Taylor, S. N. Stuart. 2009. *Wildlife in a Changing World—An Analysis of the 2008 IUCN Red List of Threatened Species.* Gland, Switzerland: IUCN. 180pp. Accessed August 25, 2017. http://data.iucn.org/dbtw-wpd/edocs/RL-2009-001.pdf
8. Ricciardi, A., J. B. Rasmussen. 1999. Extinction rates of North American freshwater fauna. *Conserv. Biol.* 13:1220–1222.
9. Costanza, R. et al. 1997. The value of the world's ecosystem services and natural capital. *Nature* 387:353–360.
10. UN WWAP. 2009. *United Nations World Water Assessment Programme.* The World Water Development Report 3: Water in a Changing World. Paris, France: UNESCO.
11. UN-Water. 2009. World Water Day brochure. Accessed August 25, 2017. http://www.unwater.org/world-waterday/downloads/wwd09brochureenLOW.pdf

12. Banks, D., P. L. Younger, R. T. Arnesen, E. R. Iversen, S. B. Banks. 1997. Mine-water chemistry: The good, the bad, and the ugly. *Environ. Geol.* 32:157–174.

13. United Nations Environment Programme/GRID-Arendal. Accessed August 25, 2017. http://www.grida.no/publications/vg/waste/page/2858.aspx

14. United Nations Environment Programme (UNEP). 1996. *Groundwater: A Threatened Resource.* UNEP Environment Library No. 15. Nairobi, Kenya: UNEP.

15. Stockholm International Water Institute (SIWI). 2005. Making Water a Part of Economic Development: The Economic Benefits of Improved Water Management and Services. Accessed December 16, 2009. http://www.siwi.org/documents/Resources/Reports/CSD_Making_water_part_of_economic_development_2005.pdf; Spalding, R. F., M. E. Exner. 1993. Occurrence of nitrate in groundwater: A review. *J Environ. Qual.* 22:392–402.

16. United Nations Environment Programme Global Environment Monitoring System (GEMS)/Water Programme (GEMS). 2004. *State of Water Quality Assessment Reporting at the Global Level (R. Robarts).* Presentation at the UN International Work Session on Water Statistics. Accessed July 27, 2009. http://unstats.un.org/unsd/environment/watersess_papers.htm

17. Bruinsma, J. 2009. The Resource Outlook to 2050: By How Much do Land, Water and Crop Yields Need to Increase by 2050? *Prepared for the FAO Expert Meeting on 'How to Feed the World in 2050'*, 24–26 June 2009. Rome, Italy.

18. World Water Assessment Programme (WWAP). 2009. *United Nations World Water Development Report 3: Water in a Changing World.* Paris/London: UNESCO Publishing/Earthscan.

19. Water Pollution. Accessed August 25, 2017. http://vkhelawan.weebly.com/uploads/6/4/7/6/64764791/land_pollution_facts.docx

20. Smith, A. H., E. O. Lingas, M. Rahman. 2000. Contamination of drinking-water by arsenic in Bangladesh: A public health emergency. *Bull. World Health Organ.* 78 (9):1093–1103.

21. Ravenscroft P., H. Brammer, K. Richards. 2009. *Arsenic Pollution: A Global Synthesis.* West Sussex, UK: John Wiley & Sons.

22. Chowdhury, U. K. et al. 2000. *Environ. Health Perspect.* 108:393.

23. Chen, Y. H., H. Ahsan. 2004. Cancer burden from arsenic in drinking water in Bangladesh. *Am. J. Public Health* 94 (5):741–744.

24. Chen, C. J, H. Y. Chiou, M. H. Chiang, L. J. Lin, T. Y. Tai. 1996. Dose-response relationship between ischemic heart disease mortality and long-term arsenic exposure. *Arterioscler. Thromb. Vasc. Biol.* 16:504–510.

25. Wasserman, G. A. et al. 2004. *Environ. Health Perspect.* 112:1329.

26. Islam, F. S., A. G. Gault, C. Boothman, D. A. Polya, J. M. Charnock, D. Chatterjee, J. R. Lloyd. 2004. Role of metal-reducing bacteria in arsenic release from Bengal delta sediments. *Nature* 430 (6995):68–71.

27. Tufano, K. J, C. Reyes, C. W. Saltikov, S. Fendorf. 2008. Reductive processes controlling arsenic retention: Revealing the relative importance of iron and arsenic reduction. *Environ. Sci. Technol.* 42 (22):8283–8289.

28. Arthur, M. 2001. Web. "Key Statistics." Ok Tedi Mining. Archived from the original on August 20, 2006. Accessed November 23, 2016. https://en.wikipedia.org/wiki/Ok_Tedi_environmental_disaster

29. Ministry of the Environment Government of Japan. 2016. *Minamata Disease The History and Measures*, Chapter 2. Japan: MOE. https://www.env.go.jp/en/chemi/hs/minamata2002/ch2.html

30. Hightower, J. 2008. *Diagnosis Mercury: Money, Politics and Poison*, p. 77. Island Press.

31. The Asahi Shimbun. 2016. Accessed November 23, 2016. http://www.asahi.com/ajw/

32. BBC News. 2000. BBC News | EUROPE | Death of a River. Accessed November 23, 2016. http://news.bbc.co.uk/2/hi/europe/642880.stm

33. Shukman, D. 2007. BBC NEWS | Science/Nature | The Most Polluted Town in Europe. *BBC News.* Accessed November 23, 2016. https://www.google.com/search?source=hp&q=BBC+NEWS+%7C+Science%2FNature+%7C+The+Most+Polluted+Town+in+Europe.+BBC+News.+Accessed+November+23%2C+2016.&oq=BBC+NEWS+%7C+Science%2FNature+%7C+The+Most+Polluted+Town+in+Europe.+BBC+News.+Accessed+November+23%2C+2016.&gs_l=psy-ab.3...3902.3902.0.5888.1.1.0.0.0.0.67.67.1.1.0....0...1..64.psy-ab..0.0.0.cSc_7_0y8Ac

34. Monboit, G. 2000. Romania's poison dump. *BBC News.* May 19, 2000. Accessed December 19, 2016. http://news.bbc.co.uk/2/hi/programmes/correspondent/755780.stm

35. Bhopal trial: Eight convicted over India gas disaster. BBC News Archived from the original on June 7, 2010. Accessed June 7, 2010. http://www.bbc.com/news/magazine-32352722

36. Varma, R., D. R. Varma. 2005. The Bhopal disaster of 1984. *Bull. Sci. Technol. Soc.* 25 (1):37–45.

37. Madhya Pradesh Government. Bhopal Gas Tragedy Relief and Rehabilitation Department, Bhopal. Accessed August 28, 2012. http://www.nuhem.com/emlinks/LLSA%20Articles%202017/Toxic%20 Industrial%20Chemicals.pdf.

38. Eckerman, I. 2005. *The Bhopal Saga—Causes and Consequences of the World's Largest Industrial Disaster.* India: Universities Press.

39. Dubey, A. K. 2010. Bhopal gas tragedy: 92% injuries termed "minor". *First 14 News.* Archived from the original on June 26, 2010. Accessed June 26, 2010. https://en.wikipedia.org/wiki/Bhopal_disaster

40. Company Defends Chief in Bhopal Disaster. *New York Times.* Archived on August 3, 2009. Accessed April 26, 2010. https://en.wikipedia.org/wiki/Bhopal_disaster

41. U.S. Exec Arrest Sought in Bhopal Disaster. *CBS News.* 31 July 2009. Accessed April 26, 2010.

42. Ganga receives 2,900 million ltrs of sewage daily. 2012. Retrieved December 20, 2016 http://www.hindustantimes.com/. Retrieved 14 May 2015. https://www.revolvy.com/topic/Pollution%20of%20the%20 Ganges&item_type=topic

43. The WaterHub. Accessed November 28, 2016. https://www.thewaterhub.org/

44. Wax, E. 2007. A sacred river endangered by global warming. The Washington Post. June 17, 2007. Accessed December 20, 2016. http://www.washingtonpost.com/wp-dyn/content/article/2007/06/16/ AR2007061600461.html

45. Most Polluted Rivers in the World. Pure Water Begins Here. 2015. Accessed November 28, 2016. https:// bloomwaterpurifiers.wordpress.com/2015/05/02/11-most-polluted-rivers-in-the-world/

46. The Ganges and the Jumna The Imperial Gazetteer of India. 1909. v. 1, p. 23. Accessed December 20, 2016. https://en.wikisource.org/wiki/The_Imperial_Gazetteer_of_India_(1909_Edition)

47. Wang, D. 2009. Population status, threats and conservation of the Yangtze finless porpoise. *Sci. Bull.* 54 (19):3473–484. doi: 10.1007/s11434-009-0522-7

48. Baillie, J., C. Hilton-Taylor, S. N. Stuart. 2004. *IUCN Red List of Threatened Species: A Global Species Assessment.* Gland, Switzerland: IUCN.

49. Wong, C. M., C. E. Williams, J. Pittock, U. Collier, P. Schelle. 2007. *World's Top 10 Rivers at Risk.* Gland, Switzerland: WWF International.

50. Stone, R. 2011. Hydropower. The legacy of the Three Gorges Dam. *Science* 333 (6044):817.

51. Yang H., P. Xie, L. Ni, R. J. Flower. 2011. Underestimation of CH_4 emmision from freshwater lakes in China. *Environ. Pollut. Control* 45 (10):4203–4204.

52. Ullrich, S. M., T. W. Tanton, S. A. Abdrashitova. 2001. Mercury in the aquatic environment: A review of factors affecting methylation. *Crit. Rev. Environ. Sci. Technol.* 31:241–293.

53. Müller, B., M. Berg, Z. P. Yao, X. F. Zhang, D. Wang, A. Pfluger. 2008. How polluted is the Yangtze river? Water quality downstream from the Three Gorges Dam. *Sci. Total Environ.* 402 (2–3):232–247.

54. August: 1986: Hundreds gassed in Cameroon lake disaster. *BBC News.* Accessed December 19, 2008. http://news.bbc.co.uk/onthisday/hi/dates/stories/august/21/newsid_3380000/3380803.stm

55. Matthews, D. A, S. W. Effler, C. M. Matthews. 2000. Ammonia and toxicity criteria in polluted Onondaga Lake, New York. *Water Environ. Res.* 72 (6):731–741.

56. Upstate Freshwater Institute. Upstate Freshwater Institute (UFI): Water Quality Professionals Conducting Applied Research, Monitoring and Laboratory Analysis. Accessed November 28, 2016. http://www.upstatefreshwater.org/

57. Driscoll, C. T. Background of Onondaga Lake. Mercury in Onondaga Lake. Accessed April 4, 2011. http://www.wow.com/wiki/Onondaga_Lake

58. EPA. 2002. *Lake Peigneur TMDLS for dissolved oxygen and nutrients.* EPA 2002 report. Accessed December 20, 2016. https://ofmpub.epa.gov/waters10/attains_impaired_waters.show_ tmdl_document?p_tmdl_doc_blobs_id=74863

59. Lake Peigneur. Lake Peigneur—Oil Rig Disasters—Offshore Drilling Accidents. Accessed December 20, 2016. http://www.offshore-technology.com/features/feature-the-worlds-deadliest-offshore-oil-rig-disasters-4149812/

60. Lake Peigneur: Lousiana's Original Drilling Disaster. The Basement Geographer. August 10, 2010. Accessed December 20, 2016. http://basementgeographer.com/lake-peigneur-lousianas-original-drilling-disaster/

61. Bellows, A. 2013. Lake Peigneur: The Swirling Vortex of Doom. Accessed August 26, 2013. https:// www.damninteresting.com/?s=Lake+Peigneur%3A+The+Swirling+Vortex+of+Doom

62. Weapons of Mass Destruction (WMD). 2015. Chelyabinsk-65. Accessed December 10, 2015. http:// www.globalsecurity.org/wmd/world/russia/chelyabinsk-65_nuc.htm

63. Cochran, T. B., R. Standish Norris, K. L. Sukko. 2015. Radioactive Contamination at Chelyabinsk-65, Russia (PDF). Natural Resources Defense Council. Accessed August 23, 2015. https://en.wikipedia.org/ wiki/Lake_Karachay

64. Wise International. Imagine a World without Nuclear Power. Accessed December 10, 2015. http://www.wiseinternational.org/

65. Gleick, P. H. 2006. Water and terrorism. *Pacific Institute.* 8 (6):481–503. Accessed March 17, 2013. doi: 10.2166/wp.2006.035

66. Roberts, A. 2010. Reservoir drugs are the CIA spiking your water supply? *Fortean Times.* Accessed November 28, 2016. https://en.wikipedia.org/wiki/Water_supply_terrorism

67. Royko, M. 1989. Abbie Hoffman really an Ok guy. *Chicago Tribune.* Accessed March 17, 2013.

68. ICE Case Studies. 1997. Marsh Arabs. *TED Case Studies.* Accessed December 10, 2015. http://www1.american.edu/ted/marsh.htm

69. Seelig, M. S. 1980. *Magnesium Deficiency in the Pathogenesis of Disease,* pp. 1–24. New York: Plenum Medical Book.

70. Schroeder, H. A. 1966. Municipal drinking water and cardiovascular death rates. *JAMA* 95:125–129.

71. Dommergue, A., F. Sprovieri, N. Pirrone, R. Ebinghaus, S. Brooks, J. Courteaud, C. P. Ferrari. 2010. Overview of mercury measurements in the Antarctic troposphere. *Atmos. Chem. Phys.* 10:3309–3319.

72. Kohls, G. G. 2010. We're All On Prozac Now. Accessed December 10, 2015. http://www.thepeoples-voice.org/TPV3/Voices.php/2010/04/20/we-re-all-on-prozac-now

73. Max, A. 2010. *Toxins Found in Whales Bode Ill for Humans.* U.S. News & World Report. Accessed December 19, 2016. http://www.usnews.com/science/articles/2010/06/25/toxins-found-in-whales-bode-ill-for-humans

74. Hallberg, G. R. 1989. Pesticides pollution of groundwater in the humid United States. *Agric. Ecosyst. Environ.* 26:299–367.

75. Byers, V., A. Levin, D. Ozonoff, R. Baldwin. 1988. Association between clinical symptoms and lymphocyte abnormalities in a population with chronic domestic exposure to industrial solvent-contaminated domestic water supply and a high incidence of leukaemia. *Cancer Immunol. Immunother.* 27:77–81.

76. Gaitan, E. 1984. Endemic goiter in western Colombia. *Ecol. Dis.* 2 (4):295–308.

77. EPA's Draft Report on the Environment. 2003. Accessed December 11, 2015. http://capita.wustl.edu/me449-04/EPAIndicatorRept/dChapter2_PurerWater.pdf

78. Moran, M. J., S. J. Grady, J. S. Zogorski. 2001. Occurrence and distribution of volatile organic compounds in drinking water supplied by community water systems in the Northeast and Mid-Atlantic regions of the United States, 1993–98. *USGS—Science for A Changing World.*

79. U.S. Environmental Protection Agency. 2000. *Drinking Water Standards and Health Advisories.* Washington D.C.: Office of Water, EPA-822-B-00-001, 18 p. Accessed December 27, 2000. http://www.epa.gov/ost/drinking/standards

80. Delzer, G. C, J. S. Zogorski, T. J. Lopes. 1997. Occurrence of the gasoline oxygenate MTBE and BTEX compounds in municipal stormwater in the United States, 1991–95. In *American Chemical Society Division of Environmental Chemistry preprints of papers, 213th,* Vol. 37, no. 1, p. 374–376. San Francisco, California: ACS.

81. Lopes, T. J., S. G. Dionne. 1998. *A review of semivolatile and volatile organic compounds in highway runoff and urban stormwater.* USGS—Open-File Report 98-409, p. 67.

82. Squillace, P. J, M. J. Moran, W. W. Lapham, C. V. Price, R. M. Clawges, J. S. Zogorski. 1999. Volatile organic compounds in untreated ambient groundwater of the United States, 1985–1995. *Environ. Sci. Technol.* 33 (23):4176–4187.

83. Lopes, T. J., J. D. Fallon, D. W. Rutherford, M. H. Hiatt. 2000. Volatile organic compounds in storm water from a parking lot. *J. Environ. Eng.* 126 (12):1137–1143.

84. Westrick, J. J, J. W. Mello, R. F. Thomas. 1984. The groundwater supply survey. *J. Am. Water Works Assoc.* 76:52–59.

85. U.S. Environmental Protection Agency. 1997. *Community Water System Survey, v. 1, Overview.* Washington, D.C.: Office of Water, USEPA 815-R-97- 001a.

86. Zogorski, J. S. et al. 1998. MTBE: Summary of findings and research by the U.S. Geological Survey. In *Annual Conference of the American Water Works Association—Water Quality [Proceedings],* June 21–25, 1998, Dallas, Texas. Denver, Colo.: American Water Works Association, pp. 287–309.

87. Moran, M. J., J. S. Zogorski, P. J. Squillace. 1999. MTBE in ground water of the United States—Occurrence, potential sources, and long-range transport. In *Water Resources conference, American Water Works Association [Proceedings],* Norfolk, Va., Sept. 26–29. Denver, Colo.: American Water Works Association, CD-ROM.

88. U.S. Environmental Protection Agency. 1999. Revisions to the Unregulated Contaminant Monitoring Regulation for Public Water Systems; Final Rule: Washington, D.C., Code of Federal Regulations 40, Parts 9, 141 and 142, pp. 50556–50620.

89. Junk, G. A., R. F. Spalding, J. J. Richard. 1980. Areal, vertical, and temporal differences in ground water chemistry: II. Organic constituents. *J. Environ. Qual.* 479.

90. Dowty, B., D. Carlisle, J. Laseter, J. Storer. 1975. Halogenated hydrocarbons in New Orleans drinking water and blood plasma. *Science* 75–77.

91. Australian Society for Environmental Medicine Symposium. 1988. *The Australian and his Chemical Environment.* pp. 24–27. Melbourne: Bowmer.

92. Rea, W. J. 1994. *Chemical Sensitivity.* Vol. 2, p. 552. Boca Raton FL: Lewis.

93. TEACH: Water Pollution in the Great Lakes. Accessed November 28, 2016. http://www.great-lakes.net/teach/pollution/water/water1.html

94. Liu, L., M. S. Phanikumar, S. L. Molloy, R. L. Whitman, D. A. Shivley, M. B. Nevers, D. J. Shwab, J. B. Rose. 2006. Modeling the transport and inactivation of *E. coli* and *Enterococci* in the near-shore region of Lake Michigan. *Environ. Sci. Technol.* 40:5022–5028.

95. Shear, H. 2006. The Great Lakes, an ecosystem rehabilitated, but still under threat. *Environ. Monit. Assess.* 113:199–225.

96. Agency for Toxic Substances and Disease Registry. ToxFAQs for Polychlorinated Biphenyls (PCBs). February 2001. Accessed October 23, 2006. http://www.atsdr.cdc.gov/tfacts17.html#bookmark02

97. Robertson, A., G. G. Lauenstein. 1998. Distribution of chlorinated organic contaminants in Dreissenid Mussels along the Southern shores of the Great Lakes. *J. Great Lakes Res.* 24 (3):608–619.

98. Agency for Toxic Substances and Disease Registry. ToxFAQs for Toxaphene. Sept. 1997. Accessed October 23, 2006. http://www.atsdr.cdc.gov/tfacts94.html

99. Pavlov, D. 2004. Potentially pathogenic features of heterotrophic plate count bacteria isolated from treated and untreated drinking water. *Nt. J. Food Microbiol.* 92 (3):275–287.

100. Mitra, S. 1986. Duplex structures and imbricate thrust systems: Geometry, structural position, and hydrocarbon potential. *Bulletin AAPG Bulletin.*

101. Lin, D., G. F. Koob, A. Markou. 1999. Differential effects of withdrawal from chronic amphetamine or fluoxetine administration on brain stimulation reward in the rat—Interactions between the two drugs. *Psychopharmacology (Berl.)* 145:283–294.

102. Tokos, J., B. Hall, J. Calhoun, E. Prestbo. 1998. Homogeneous gas-phase reaction of Hg0 with H2O2, O3, CH3I, and (CH3)3S: Implications for atmospheric Hg cycling. *Atmos. Environ.* 32:823–827.

103. Study Group of Minamata Disease. 1968. *Minamata Disease.* Kumamoto City, Japan: Kumamoto University.

104. Yagev, Y. 2002. Eating Fish during Pregnancy: Risk of Exposure to Toxic Levels of Methylmercury. Accessed October 05, 2011. http://www.motherisk.org/updates/oct02.php3

105. Zdansky, G. 1973. Selenoamino acids. In *Organic Selenium Compounds: Their Chemistry and Biology.* D. L. Klayman, W. H. Gunther, Eds., pp. 579–601. New York: John Wiley and Sons.

106. Scott, M. L. 1973. Selenoamino acids. In *Selenium Compounds in Nature and Medicine.* D. L. Klayman, W. H. Gunther, Eds., pp. 629–659. New York: John Wiley and Sons.

107. Jacobson, J. L., S. W. Jacobson. 1996. Intellectual impairment of children exposed to PCBs *in utero. N. Engl. J. Med.* 335 (11):783–789.

108. National Research Council. 2000. *Toxicological Effects of Methylmercury,* p. 344. Washington, DC: National Academy of Sciences, the National Academies Press. August 25, 2017. http://www.nap.edu/books/0309071402/html/

109. Persky, V., M. Turyk, H. A. Anderson, E. Poloerejan, A. M. Sweeny, H. E. G. Humphrey, R. J. McCaffrey. 2001. The effects of PCBs and fish consumption on endogenous hormones. *Environ. Health Perspect.* 109 (6):605–611.

110. Federal Register. 2004. Environmental Protection Agency; Proposed Rules. 69 (20) Friday January 30, 2004. http://www.access.gpo.gov/su_docs/fedreg/a040130c.html

111. Kurak, S. 1967. Operation Chase. *United States Naval Institute Proceedings.* September 1967, pp. 40–46.

112. Chemical Stockpile Disposal Program. Chemical Weapons Movement History Compilation, William R. Brankowitz, 12 JUNE 1987 (PDF). Accessed July 26, 2013. https://www.bing.com/search?q=Chemical+Stockpile+Disposal+Program.+Chemical+Weapons+Movement+History+Compilation,+William+R.+Brankowitz,+12+JUNE+1987+(PDF).&src=IE-SearchBox&FORM=IENTTR&conversationid=

113. Pike, J. 2005. Operation CHASE, 27 April 2005, Globalsecurity.org. Accessed November 26, 2007.

114. Mauroni, A. 2007. The US Army Chemical Corps: Past, Present, and Future, Army Historical Foundation. Accessed November 26, 2007. https://www.bing.com/search?q=Mauroni,+A.+2007.+The+US+Army+Chemical+Corps%3A+Past,+Present,+and+Future,+Army+Historical+Foundation.&src=IE-SearchBox&FORM=IENTTR&conversationid=

115. Wagner, T. 2004. Hazardous waste: Evolution of a national environmental problem. *J. Policy Hist.* 16 (4):306–331.

116. Kraft, J. C. 1997. The last triple expander. In *United States Naval Institute Proceedings*, February, 1977, p. 67.

117. National Oceanic and Atmospheric Administration (NOAA). June 21, 2012. NOAA: Gulf of Mexico 'dead zone' predictions feature uncertainty. Accessed June 23, 2012. https://www.bing.com/search?q= National+Oceanic+and+Atmospheric+Administration+(NOAA).+June+21,+2012.+NOAA%3A+Gulf+o f+Mexico%E2%80%98dead+zone%E2%80%99+predictions+feature+uncertainty.&src=IE-SearchBox &FORM=IENTTR&conversationid=

118. Perlman, D. 2008. Chronicle Science Editor. Scientists Alarmed by Ocean Dead-zone Growth. Accessed August 03, 2010.

119. Diaz, R. J., R. Rosenberg. 2008. Spreading dead zones and consequences for marine ecosystems. *Science* 321 (5891):926–929.

120. Schindler, D. W., J. R. Vallentyne. 2008. *The Algal Bowl: Overfertilization of the World's Freshwaters and Estuaries.* Edmonton, Alberta: University of Alberta Press.

121. Lehman E. M., K. E. McDonald, J. T. Lehman. 2009. Whole lake selective withdrawal experiment to control harmful cyanpbacteria in an urban impoundment. *Water Res.* 43 (5):1187–1198.

122. NBC Universal News Group. 2007. Corn Boom Could Expand 'dead Zone' in Gulf. *NBCNews.com.* December 17. Accessed November 28, 2016.

123. Blooming horrible: Nutrient pollution is a growing problem all along the Mississippi. *The Economist.* Accessed June 23, 2012. https://www.google.com/search?source=hp&q=Blooming+horrible%3A+Nutr ient+pollution+is+a+growing+problem+all+along+the+Mississippi.+The+Economist&oq=Blooming+h orrible%3A+Nutrient+pollution+is+a+growing+problem+all+along+the+Mississippi.+The+Economist &gs_l=psy-ab.3...2703.2703.0.8122.1.1.0.0.0.0.108.108.0j1.1.0....0...1..64.psy-ab..0.0.0....0.7WoFl7lsoGQ

124. Pickard, G. L., W. J. Emery. 1982. *Description Physical Oceanography: An Introduction.* p. 249. Oxford: Pergamon Press.

125. Diaz, R. J., R. J. Diaz, R. Rosenberg. 2008. Supporting online material for spreading dead zones and consequences for marine ecosystems. *Science* 321 (926):926–929.

126. Landry, C. A., S. Manning, A. O. Cheek. 2004. Hypoxia suppresses reproduction in Gulf killifish, Fundulus grandis. *e. hormone 2004 conference.* Oct. 27–30. New Orleans.

127. Johanning, K., J. Lee, T. Wiese, B. Beckman, J. A. McLachlan, B. B. Rees. 2004. Assessment of molecular interaction between low oxygen and estrogen in fish cell culture. *Fourth SETAC World Congress, 25th Annual Meeting in North America.* November 14–18. Portland, Oregon.

128. Mora, C. et al. 2013. Biotic and human vulnerability to projected changes in ocean biogeochemistry over the 21st Century. *PLOS Biology* 11:e1001682.

129. Living on Earth. 2005. Living on Earth: Dead Zones. Accessed December 14, 2015. http://loe.org/ shows/segments.html?programID=05-P13-00040&segmentID=8

130. Griffis, R., J. Howard. 2013. *Oceans and Marine Resources in a Changing Climate: A Technical Input to the 2013 National Climate Assessment.* Washingtonn, DC: Island Press.

131. NOAA. Gulf of Mexico "dead Zone" Predictions Feature Uncertainty. Accessed November 29, 2016. http://www.noaanews.noaa.gov/stories2012/20120621_deadzone.html

132. Hypoxia in the Northern Gulf of Mexico. Hypoxia in the Northern Gulf of Mexico. Accessed November 29, 2016. http://www.gulfhypoxia.net/Overview/

133. Dead Zone: Hypoxia in the Gulf of Mexico (PDF). NOAA. 2009. Retrieved June 23, 2012. http://www. noaanews.noaa.gov/stories2009/pdfs/new%20fact%20sheet%20dead%20zones_final.pdf

134. Lochhead, C. 2010. Dead zone in gulf linked to ethanol production. *San Francisco Chronicle.* Accessed November 29, 2016. http://www.sfgate.com/politics/article/Dead-zone-in-gulf-linked-to-ethanol-production-3183032.php

135. Courtney, M. W., J. M. Courtney. 2013. Predictions Wrong Again on Dead Zone Area—Gulf of Mexico Gaining Resistance to Nutrient Loading. Accessed November 29, 2016. http://arxiv.org/ftp/arxiv/ papers/1307/1307.8064.pd

136. Fairchild, L. M. 2005. *The influence of stakeholder groups on the decision making process regarding the dead zone associated with the Mississippi river discharge (Master of Science).* University of South Florida (USF). p. 14.

137. Sherman, B., K. Capelli. 2012. NOAA: Gulf of Mexico 'dead zone' predictions feature uncertainty. *USGS News.* Accessed November 29, 2016. http://www.noaanews.noaa.gov/stories2012/20120621_ deadzone.html

138. Grimes, C. B. 2001. Fishery production and the Mississippi River discharge. *Fisheries* 26 (8):17–26.

139. Biewald, J., A. Rossetti, J. Stevens, W. Cheih Wong. 2010. The Gulf of Mexico's hypoxic zone. *Lecture.* Accessed November 29, 2016. http://ssc.bibalex.org/classification/list.jsf?aid=a27b8a0840e100df2b906 1afcb6df1f3&cid=e61e30469ffceee26cd485483c3f25f3&cpage=4

140. Cox, T. 2007. Exclusive. Accessed November 29, 2016. Bloomberg.com

141. Mee, L. 2006. Reviving dead zones: How can we restore coastal seas ravaged by runaway plant and algae growth caused by human activities? *SciAm.* 295:79–85. doi: 10.1038/scientificamerican1106-78

142. Nielsen, J. 2008. Dead zones multiplying in world's oceans by John Nielsen. August 15, 2008. *Morning Edition, NPR.*

143. Wisconsin Department of Natural Resources (PDF). Accessed August 10, 2010. http://dnr.wi.gov/topic/ surfacewater/documents/WatershedPlanning_Guidance_final_2013.pdf

144. A National Assessment of Tap Water Quality. EWG Investigation. 2005. Accessed December 14, 2015.

145. US EPA. 2011. Municipal Solid Waste Generation, Recycling, and Disposal in the United States: Facts and Figures for 2011. Accessed December 14, 2015. http://www3.epa.gov/epawaste/nonhaz/municipal/ pubs/MSWcharacterization_508_053113_fs.pdf

146. Crump, K. S., H. A. Guess. 1980. Drinking water and cancer: Review of recent finding and assessment of risk. Prepared for the Council on Environmental Quality, Washington D. C.

147. Glaze, W. E. 1980. Personal communication. Denton, TX: University of North Texas, Environmental Division

148. U.S. Environmental Protection Agency. 1977. *Is Your Drinking Water Safe?* Washington D. C.: U.S. EPA, Office of Public Affairs.

149. Barlow, J. 2004. *Byproduct of Water-Disinfection Process Found to be Highly Toxic.* University of Illinois News Bureau. Accessed November, 2012. http://www.news.illinois.edu/news/04/0914water. html

150. Bond, T, J. Huang, M. R. Templeton, N. Graham. 2011. Occurrence and control of nitrogenous disinfection byproducts in drinking water—A review. *Water Res.* 45 (15):4341–4354.

151. Bull, R. J., D. A. Reckhow, X. Li, A. R. Humpage, C. Joll, S. E. Hrudey. 2011. Potential carcinogenic hazards of non- regulated disinfection by-products: Haloquinones, halo-cyclopentene and cyclohexene derivatives, N-halamines, halonitriles, and heterocyclic amines. *Toxicology* 286 (1–3):1–19.

152. Plewa, M. J., E. D. Wagner, S. D. Richardson, A. D. Thruston, Jr., Y. T. Woo, A. B. McKague. 2004. Chemical and biological characterization of newly discovered iodoacid drinking water disinfection byproducts. *Environ. Sci. Technol.* 38 (18):4713–4722.

153. Yang, X., C. Shang, B. Chen, P. Westerhoff, J. Peng, W. Guo. 2012. Nitrogen origins and the role of ozonation in the formation of halocetonitriles and halonitromethanes in chlorine water treatment. *Environ. Sci. Technol.* 46 (23):12832–12838.

154. EPA. 2012. Chloramines in Drinking Water. Accessed November 2012. http://water.epa.gov/lawsregs/ rulesregs/sdwa/mdbp/chloramines_index.cfm

155. Levallois, P., S. Gingras, S. Marcoux, C. Legay, C. Catto, M. Rodriguez, R. Tardif. 2012. Maternal exposure to drinking-water chlorination by-products and small-for-gestational-age neonates. *Epidemiology* 23 (2):267–276.

156. Hinckley, A. F., A. M. Bachand, J. S. Reif. 2005. Late pregnancy exposures to disinfection by-products and growth-related birth outcomes. *Environ. Health Perspect.* 113 (12):1808–1813.

157. Porter, C. K., S. D. Putnam, K. L. Hunting, M. R. Riddle. 2005. The effect of trihalomethane and haloacetic acid exposure on fetal growth in a Maryland county. *Am. J. Epidemiol.* 162 (4):334–344.

158. EPA. 2002. The Occurrence of Disinfection By-Products (DBPs) of Health Concern in Drinking Water: Results of a Nationwide DBP Occurrence Study. Accessed January 2012. www.epa.gov/athens/publications/reports/EPA_600_R02_068.pdf

159. Rusin, P. A., J. B. Rose, C. N. Haas, C. P. Gerba. 1997. Risk assessment of opportunistic bacterial pathogens in drinking water. *Rev. Environ. Contam. Toxicol.* 152:57–83.

160. Linder, R. E., G. R. Klinefelter, L. F. Strader, M. G. Narotsky, J. D. Suarez, N. L. Roberts, S. D. Perreault. 1995. Dibromoacetic acid affects reproductive competence and sperm quality in the male rat. *Fundam. Appl. Toxicol.* 28 (1):9–17.

161. U.S. Census Bureau (USCB). Population Growth Rate in the U.S. Accessed August 25, 2017. http:// www.census.gov/population/www/popclockus.html

162. U.S. Geological Survey (USGS). 2003. *Projections of Land Use and Land Cover Change.* U.S. Global Change Research Program. http://www.usgcrp.gov/usgcrp/ProgramElements/recent/landrecent.htm

163. U.S. Geological Survey (USGS). 1999. *The Quality of Our Nation's Waters. Nutrients and Pesticides.* U.S. Geological Survey Circular 122. http://pubs.usgs.gov/circ/circ1225/html/wq_urban.html

164. Kolpin, D. W., E. T. Furlong, M. T. Meyer, E. M. Thurman, S. D. Zaugg, L. B. Barber, H. T. Buxton. 2002. Pharmaceuticals, hormones, and other organic wastewater contaminants in U.S. streams, 1999–2000: A national reconnaissance. *Environ. Sci. Technol.* 36 (6):1202–1211.

165. Stackelberg, P. E., E. T. Furlong, M. T. Meyer, S. D. Zaugg, A. K. Henderson, D. B. Reissman. 2004. Persistence of pharmaceutical compounds and other organic wastewater contaminants in a conventional drinking water-treatment plant. *Sci. Total Environ.* 329 (1–3):99–113.

166. U.S. Department of Agriculture (USDA). 2002. National Agricultural Statistics Service (NASS) historical data for 2002. http://www.nass.usda.gov/Data_and_Statistics/index.asp

167. Association of American Plant Food Control Officials (AAPFCO). 2002. *Commercial Fertilizer Database (2002).* AAPFCO Division of Regulatory Services, University of Kentucky.

168. Environmental Protection Agency (EPA). 2004. *Protecting Water Quality from Agricultural Runoff.* EPA 841-F-03-004. Accessed December 13, 2005. http://www.epa.gov/owow/nps/agriculture.html

169. Environmental Protection Agency (EPA). 2000. *2000 National Water Quality Inventory.* National Water Quality Report to Congress under Clean Water Act Section 305(b). Accessed December 13, 2005. http://www.epa.gov/305b/2000report/

170. U.S. Environmental Protection Agency (EPA). Washington, DC: Protecting Water Quality from Agricultural Runoff. March 2005. Document No. EPA 841-F-05-001.

171. U.S. Natural Resources Conservation Service (NRCS). June 2007. *Contour Farming. Code 330.* Fort Worth, TX: National Conservation Practice Standard.

172. NRCS. September 2008. National Conservation Practice Standard: Mulching. Code 484.

173. EPA. July 2003. National Management Measures to Control Nonpoint Source Pollution from Agriculture. Document No. EPA-841-B-03-004.

174. NRCS. August 2006. National Conservation Practice Standard: Nutrient Management. Code 590.

175. NRCS. July 2008. National Conservation Practice Standard: Pest Management. Code 595.

176. EPA. Integrated Pest Management (IPM) Principles. Accessed November 30, 2016. https://www.epa.gov/safepestcontrol/integrated-pest-management-ipm-principles

177. EPA. Oxygen Consuming Substances in Rivers. Oxygen Consuming Substances in Rivers—European Environment Agency. Accessed November 30, 2016. http://www.eea.europa.eu/data-and-maps/indicators/oxygen-consuming-substances-in-rivers/oxygen-consuming-substances-in-rivers-7

178. EPA. Animal Feeding Operations (AFOs). Accessed November 30, 2016. https://www.epa.gov/npdes/animal-feeding-operations-afos

179. Agricultural Waste Storage Tanks. Agricultural Waste Comments. Accessed November 30, 2016. http://usatanksales.com/agriculturalwaste.html

180. Managing Fire water and major spillages—Environment Agency Guidance note PPG18. Accessed November 30, 2016. https://www.sepa.org.uk/media/100544/ppg-18-managing-fire-water-and-major-spillages.pdf

181. Environmental Protection Agency (EPA). 2005. List of Contaminants and Their MCLs. Accessed November 30, 2016. http://www.epa.gov/safewater/mcl.html#mcls

182. Environmental Protection Agency (EPA). 2004. 2004 Edition of the Drinking Water Standards and Health Advisories. EPA 822-R-04-005. Accessed November 30, 2016. http://www.epa.gov/water-science/drinking/standards/dwstandards.pdf

183. Richardson, S. D. 1998. Drinking water disinfection byproducts. In *Encyclopedia of Environmental Analysis and Remediation*, Robert A. Myers, Ed. John Wiley & Sons, Inc.

184. Richardson, S. D., A. D. Thruston, Jr., T. V. Caughran, P. H. Chen, T. W. Collette, T. L. Floyd. 1999. Identification of new drinking water disinfection byproducts formed in the presence of bromide. *Environ. Sci. Technol.* 33 (19):3378–3383.

185. Richardson, S. D., A. D. Thruston Jr., T. V. Caughran, P. H. Chen, T. W. Collette, T. L. Floyd, K. M. Schenck, B. W. Lykins Jr., G. R. Sun, G. Majetich. 1999. Identification for new ozone disinfection byproducts in drinking water. *Environ. Sci. Technol.* 33 (19):3368–3377.

186. Richardson, S. D., A. D. Thruston Jr., C. RavAcha, L. Groisman, I. Popilevsky, O. Juraev, V. Glezer, A. Bruce McKague, M. J. Plewa, E. D. Wagner. 2003. Tribromopyrrole, brominated acids, and other disinfection byproducts produced by disinfection of drinking water rich in bromide. *Environ. Sci. Technol.* 37:3782–3793.

187. Environmental Protection Agency (EPA). 2003. U.S. EPA Toxics Release Inventory—Reporting Year 2003 Public Data Release, Summary of Key Findings. Toxics Release Inventory Program. Accessed December 13, 2005. http://www.epa.gov/tri/tridata/tri03/index.htm

188. Kolpin, D. W., E. T. Furlong, M. T. Meyer, E. M. Thurman, S. D. Zaugg, L. B. Barber, H. T. Buxton. 2002. Pharmaceuticals, hormones, and other organic wastewater contaminants in U.S. streams, 1999–2000: A national reconnaissance. *Environ. Sci. Technol.* 36 (6):1202–1211.

189. Environmental Protection Agency (EPA). 2005. *PPCPs as Environmental Pollutants.* National Exposure Research Laboratory. Environmental Sciences. Accessed December 13, 2005. http://www.epa.gov/esd/chemistry/pharma/new.htm

190. Faust, S. D., M. Aly Osman. 1998. *Chemistry of Water Treatment,* 2nd ed. Ann Arbor, MI: Ann Arbor Press.

191. Hewitt, D. J., D. A. Weeks, G. C. Millner, R. G. Huss. 2006. Industrial *Pseudomonas folliculitis. Amer. J. Ind. Med.* 49:895–899.

192. Fields, B. S., R. F. Benson, R. E. Besser. 2002. Legionella and Legionnaires' disease: 25 years of investigation. *Clin. Microbiol. Rev.* 15:506–526.

193. SHRAE Standard Project Committee. 2000. *Minimizing the Risk of Legionellosis Associated with Building Water Systems.* Atlanta, GA: American Society of Heating, Refrigerating and Air-Conditioning Engineers, Inc.

194. Heffelfinger, J. D., J. L. Kool, S. Fridkin, V. J. Fraser, J. Hageman, J. Carpenter, C. G. Whitney. 2003. Society for Healthcare Epidemiology of America. Risk of hospital-acquired Legionnaires' disease in cities using monochloramine versus other water disinfectants. *Infect. Control Hosp. Epidemiol.* 24:569–574.

195. Phares, C. R., E. Russell, M. C. Thigpen, W. Service, M. B. Crist, M. Salyers, J. Engel, R. F. Benson, B. Fields, M. R. Moore. 2007. Legionnaires' disease among residents of a long-term care facility: The sentinel event in a community outbreak. *Am. J. Infect. Control* 35:319–323.

196. Kashiwaya, M., K. Yoshimoto. 1980. Tannery wastewater treatment by the oxygen activated sludge process. *Journal (Water Pollution Control Federation) (Alexandria, VA: Water Environment Federation)* 52 (5):999–1007.

197. Davis, C. D., E. O. Uthus, J. W. Finley. 2000. Dietary selenium and arsenic affect DNA methylation in vitro in Caco-2 cells and in vivo in rat liver and colon. *J. Nutr.* 130 (12):2903–2909.

198. Uthus, E. O., S. A. Ross, C. D. Davis. 2006. Differential effects of dietary selenium (Se) and folate on methyl metabolism in liver and colon of rats. *Biol. Trace Elem. Res.* 109 (3):201–214.

199. Cox, R., S. Goorha. 1986. A study of the mechanism of selenite-induced hypomethylated DNA and differentiation of Friend erythroleukemic cells. *Carcinogenesis* 7 (12):2015–2018.

200. Fiala, E. S., M. E. Staretz, G. A. Pandya, K. El-Bayoumy, S. R. Hamilton. 1998. Inhibition of DNA cytosine methyltransferase by chemopreventive selenium compounds, determined by an improved assay for DNA cytosine methyltransferase and DNA cytosine methylation. *Carcinogenesis* 19 (4):597–604.

201. Xiang, N., R. Zhao, G. Song, W. Zhong. 2008. Selenite reactivates silenced genes by modifying DNA methylation and histones in prostate cancer cells. *Carcinogenesis* 29 (11):2175–2181.

202. Verret, W. J., Y. Chen, A. Ahmed, T. Islam, F. Parvez, M. G. Kibriya, J. H. Graziano, H. Ahsan. 2005. A randomized, double-blind placebo-controlled trial evaluating the effects of vitamin E and selenium on arsenic-induced skin lesions in Bangladesh. *J. Occup. Environ. Med.* 47 (10):1026–1035.

203. Zeng, H., E. O. Uthus, G. F. Combs Jr. 2005. Mechanistic aspects of the interaction between selenium and arsenic. *J. Inorg. Biochem.* 99 (6):1269–1274.

204. Gailer, J., G. N. George, I. J. Pickering, R. C. Prince, S. C. Ringwald, J. E. Pemberton, R. S. Glass, H. S. Younis, D. W. DeYoung, H. Vasken Aposhian. 2000. A metabolic link between arsenite and selenite: The seleno-bis(S-glutathionyl) arsinium ion. *J. Am. Chem. Soc.* 122:4637–4639.

205. Williams, P. N. et al. 2009. Arsenic limits trace mineral nutrition (selenium, zinc, and nickel) in Bangladesh rice grain. *Environ. Sci. Technol.* 43 (21):8430–8436.

206. Chen, Y., M. Hall, J. H. Graziano, V. Slavkovich, A. van Geen, F. Parvez, H. Ahsan. 2007. A prospective study of blood selenium levels and the risk of arsenic-related premalignant skin lesions. *Cancer Epidemiol. Biomarkers Prev.* 16 (2):207–213.

207. Petrick, J. S., F. Ayala-Fierro, W. R. Cullen, D. E. Carter, H. Vasken Aposhian. 2000. Monomethylarsonous acid (MMA^III) is more toxic than arsenite in Chang human hepatocytes. *Toxicol. Appl. Pharmacol.* 163 (2):203–207.

208. Petrick, J. S., B. Jagadish, E. A. Mash, H. V. Aposhian. 2001. Monomethylarsonous acid (MMA^III) and arsenite: LD_{50} in hamsters and in vitro inhibition of pyruvate dehydrogenase. *Chem. Res. Toxicol.* 14 (6):651–656.

209. Styblo, M., L. M. Del Razo, L. Vega, D. R. Germolec, E. L. LeCluyse, G. A. Hamilton, W. Reed, C. Wang, W. R. Cullen, D. J. Thomas. 2000. Comparative toxicity of trivalent and pentavalent inorganic and methylated arsenicals in rat and human cells. *Arch. Toxicol.* 74 (6):289–299.

210. Chen, Y. C., Y. L. Guo, H. J. Su, Y. M. Hsueh, T. J. Smith, L. M. Ryan, M. S. Lee, S. C. Chao, J. Y. Lee, D. C. Christiani. 2003. Arsenic methylation and skin cancer risk in southwestern Taiwan. *J. Occup. Environ. Med.* 45 (3):241–248.

211. Hsueh, Y. M., H. Y. Chiou, Y. L. Huang, W. L. Wu, C. C. Huang, M. H. Yang, L. C. Lue, G. S. Chen, C. J. Chen. 1997. Serum beta-carotene level, arsenic methylation capability, and incidence of skin cancer. *Cancer Epidemiol. Biomarkers Prev.* 6 (8):589–596.

212. Yu, R. C., K. H. Hsu, C. J. Chen, J. R. Froines. 2000. Arsenic methylation capacity and skin cancer. *Cancer Epidemiol. Biomarkers Prev.* 9 (11):1259–1262.

213. Huang, Y. K., Y. L. Huang, Y. M. Hsueh, M. H. Yang, M. M. Wu, S. Y. Chen, I. H. Ling, J. C. Chien. 2008. Arsenic exposure, urinary arsenic speciation, and the incidence of urothelial carcinoma: A twelve-year follow-up study. *Cancer Causes Control* 19 (8):829–839.

214. Tseng, C. H., Y. K. Huang, Y. L. Huang, C. J. Chung, M. H. Yang, C. J. Chen, Y. M. Hsueh. 2005. Arsenic exposure, urinary arsenic speciation, and peripheral vascular disease in blackfoot disease-hyperendemic villages in Taiwan. *Toxicol. Appl. Pharmacol.* 206 (3):299–308.

215. Levander, O. A. 1977. Metabolic interrelationships between arsenic and selenium. *Environ. Health Perspect.* 19:159–164.

216. Moxon, A. L. 1938. The effect of arsenic on the toxicity of seleniferous grains. *Science* 88 (2273):81.

217. Csanaky, I., Z. Gregus. 2003. Effect of selenite on the disposition of arsenate and arsenite in rats. *Toxicology* 186 (1–2):33–50.

218. Kenyon, E. M., M. F. Hughes, O. A. Levander. 1997. Influence of dietary selenium on the disposition of arsenate in the female B6C3F1 mouse. *J. Toxicol. Environ. Health* 51 (3):279–299.

219. Styblo, M., M. Delnomdedieu, D. J. Thomas. 1996. Mono- and dimethylation of arsenic in rat liver cytosol in vitro. *Chem. Biol. Interact.* 99 (1–3):147–164.

220. Walton, F. S., S. B. Waters, S. L. Jolley, E. L. LeCluyse, D. J. Thomas, M. Styblo. 2003. Selenium compounds modulate the activity of recombinant rat AsIII-methyltransferase and the methylation of arsenite by rat and human hepatocytes. *Chem. Res. Toxicol.* 16 (3):261–265.

221. Styblo, M., D. J. Thomas. 2001. Selenium modifies the metabolism and toxicity of arsenic in primary rat hepatocytes. *Toxicol. Appl. Pharmacol.* 172 (1):52–61.

222. Drobna, Z., F. S. Walton, A. W. Harmon, D. J. Thomas, M. Styblo. 2010. Interspecies differences in metabolism of arsenic by cultured primary hepatocytes. *Toxicol. Appl. Pharmacol.* 245 (1):47–56.

223. Hill, K. E., G. W. McCollum, M. E. Boeglin, R. F. Burk. 1997. Thioredoxin reductase activity is decreased by selenium deficiency. *Biochem. Biophys. Res. Commun.* 234:293–295.

224. Pilsner, J. R., X. Liu, H. Ahsan, V. Ilievski, V. Slavkovich, D. Levy, P. Factor-Litvak, J. H. Graziano, M. V. Gamble. 2007. Genomic methylation of peripheral blood leukocyte DNA: Influences of arsenic and folate in Bangladeshi adults. *Am. J. Clin. Nutr.* 86 (4):1179–1186.

225. International Agency for Research on Cancer (IARC). 1987. Overall evaluations of carcinogenicity: An updating of IARC monographs volumes 1 to 42. *IARC Monogr. Eval. Carcinog. Risks Hum. Suppl.* 7:1–440.

226. International Agency for Research on Cancer (IARC). 2004. Some drinking-water disinfectants and contaminants, including arsenic. *IARC Monogr. Eval. Carcinog. Risk Hum.* 84:1–477.

227. Pershagen, G. 1981. The carcinogenicity of arsenic. *Environ. Health Perspect.* 40:93–100.

228. Smith, A. H., C. Hopenhaynrich, M. N. Bates, H. M. Goeden, I. Hertz-Picciotto, H. M. Duggan, R. Wood, M. J. Kosnett, M. T. Smith. 1992. Cancer risks from arsenic in drinking water. *Environ. Health Perspect.* 97:259–267.

229. Smith, A. H., C. M. Steinmaus. 2009. Health effects of arsenic and chromium in drinking water: Recent human findings. *Annu. Rev. Public Health* 30:107–122.

230. Abernathy, C. O. et al. 1999. Arsenic: Health effects, mechanisms of actions, and research issues. *Environ. Health Perspect.* 107:593–597.

231. Marshall, G., C. Ferreccio, Y. Yuan, M. N. Bates, C. Steinmaus, S. Selvin, J. Liaw, A. H. Smith. 2007. Fifty-year study of lung and bladder cancer mortality in Chile related to arsenic in drinking water. *J. Natl. Cancer Inst.* 99 (12):920–928.

232. Sohel, N., L. A. Persson, M. Rahman, P. K. Streatfield, M. Yunus, E. C. Ekström, M. Vahter. 2009. Arsenic in drinking water and adult mortality: A population-based cohort study in rural Bangladesh. *Epidemiology* 20 (6):824–830.

233. Drobna, Z. et al. 2009. Disruption of the arsenic (+3 oxidation state) methyltransferase gene in the mouse alters the phenotype for methylation of arsenic and affects distribution and retention of orally administered arsenate. *Chem. Res. Toxicol.* 22 (10):1713–1720.

234. Styblo, M., Z. Drobna, I. Jaspers, S. Lin, D. J. Thomas. 2002. The role of biomethylation in toxicity and carcinogenicity of arsenic: A research update. *Environ. Health Perspect.* 110:5767–771.

235. Kitchin, K. T., K. Wallace. 2008. Evidence against the nuclear in situ binding of arsenicals—oxidative stress theory of arsenic carcinogenesis. *Toxicol. Appl. Pharmacol.* 232 (2):252–257.

236. Moore, L. E, A. H. Smith, C. Hopenhayn-Rich, M. L. Biggs, D. A. Kalman, M. T. Smith. 1997. Micronuclei in exfoliated bladder cells among individuals chronically exposed to arsenic in drinking water. *Cancer Epidemiol. Biomarkers Prev.* 6 (1):31–36.

237. Zhang, A. H., H. H. Bin, X. L. Pan, X. G. Xi. 2007. Analysis of p16 gene mutation, deletion and methylation in patients with arseniasis produced by indoor unventilated-stove coal usage in Guizhou, China. *J. Toxicol. Environ. Health A* 70 (11):970–975.

238. Rossman, T. G., A. N. Uddin, F. J. Burns. 2004. Evidence that arsenite acts as a cocarcinogen in skin cancer. *Toxicol. Appl. Pharmacol.* 198 (3):394–404.

239. Zhao, C. Q., M. R. Young, B. A. Diwan, T. P. Coogan, M. P. Waalkes. 1997. Association of arsenic-induced malignant transformation with DNA hypomethylation and aberrant gene expression. *Proc. Natl. Acad. Sci. USA* 94 (20):10907–10912.

240. Jacobson-Kram, D., D. Montalbano. 1985. The reproductive effects assessment group's report on the mutagenicity of inorganic arsenic. *Environ. Mutagen* 7 (5):787–804.

241. Jongen, W. M., J. M. Cardinaals, P. M. Bos, P. Hagel. 1985. Genotoxicity testing of arsenobetaine, the predominant form of arsenic in marine fishery products. *Food Chem. Toxicol.* 23 (7):669–673.

242. Moore, M. M., K. Harrington-Brock, C. L. Doerr. 1997. Relative genotoxic potency of arsenic and its methylated metabolites. *Mutat. Res.* 386 (3):279–290.

243. Smith, A. H., C. Hopenhayn-Rich, M. Warner, M. L. Biggs, L. Moore, M. T. Smith. 1993. Rationale for selecting exfoliated bladder cell micronuclei as potential biomarkers for arsenic genotoxicity. *J. Toxicol. Environ. Health* 40 (2–3):223–234.

244. Moore, L. E. et al. 2002. Arsenic-related chromosomal alterations in bladder cancer. *J. Natl. Cancer Inst.* 94 (22):1688–1696.

245. Fournier, A., A. Florin, C. Lefebvre, F. Solly, D. Leroux, M. B. Callanan. 2007. Genetics and epigenetics of 1q rearrangements in hematological malignancies. *Cytogenet. Genome Res.* 118 (2–4):320–327.

246. Muto, S., S. Horie, S. Takahashi, K. Tomita, T. Kitamura. 2000. Genetic and epigenetic alterations in normal bladder epithelium in patients with metachronous bladder cancer. *Cancer Res.* 60 (15):4021–4025.

247. Hei, T. K., M. Filipic. 2004. Role of oxidative damage in the genotoxicity of arsenic. *Free Radic. Biol. Med.* 37 (5):574–581.

248. Hegedus, C. M. et al. 2008. Decreased urinary beta-defensin-1 expression as a biomarker of response to arsenic. *Toxicol. Sci.* 106 (1):74–82.

249. Sun, C. Q. et al. 2006. Human beta-defensin-1, a potential chromosome 8p tumor suppressor: Control of transcription and induction of apoptosis in renal cell carcinoma. *Cancer Res.* 66 (17):8542–8549.

250. Andrew, A. S., D. A. Jewell, R. A. Mason, M. L. Whitfield, J. H. Moore, M. R. Karagas. 2008. Drinking-water arsenic exposure modulates gene expression in human lymphocytes from a U.S. population. *Environ. Health Perspect.* 116:524–531.

251. Bailey, K., Y. Xia, W. O. Ward, G. Knapp, J. Mo, J. L. Mumford, R. D. Owen, S-F Thai. 2009. Global gene expression profiling of hyperkeratotic skin lesions from Inner Mongolians chronically exposed to arsenic. *Toxicol. Pathol.* 37 (7):849–859.

252. Bourdonnay, E., C. Morzadec, L. Sparfel, M. D. Galibert, S. Jouneau, C. Martin-Chouly, O. Fardel, L. Vernhet. 2009. Global effects of inorganic arsenic on gene expression profile in human macrophages. *Mol. Immunol.* 46 (4):649–656.

253. Xie, Y., J. Liu, L. Benbrahim-Tallaa, J. M. Ward, D. Logsdon, B. A. Diwan, M. P. Waalkes. 2007. Aberrant DNA methylation and gene expression in livers of newborn mice transplacentally exposed to a hepatocarcinogenic dose of inorganic arsenic. *Toxicology* 236 (1–2):7–15.

254. Liu, J., L. Yu, E. J. Tokar, C. Bortner, M. I. Sifre, Y. Sun, M. P. Waalkes. 2008. Arsenic-induced aberrant gene expression in fetal mouse primary liver-cell cultures. *Ann. NY Acad. Sci.* 1140:368–375.

255. Fry, R. C. et al. 2007. Activation of inflammation/NF-κB signaling in infants born to arsenic-exposed mothers. *PLoS Genet.* 3 (11):e207.10.1371/journal.pgen.0030207.

256. Yan, M. S., C. C. Matouk, P. A. Marsden. 2010. Epigenetics of the vascular endothelium. *J. Appl. Physiol.* 109 (3):916–226. 10.1152/japplphysiol.00131.2010.

257. Urdinguio, R. G., J. V. Sanchez-Mut, M. Esteller. 2009. Epigenetic mechanisms in neurological diseases: Genes, syndromes, and therapies. *Lancet Neurol.* 8 (11):1056–1072.

258. Schaefer, C. B., S. K. Ooi, T. H. Bestor, D. Bourc'his. 2007. Epigenetic decisions in mammalian germ cells. *Science* 316 (5823):398–399.

259. Robertson, K. D. 2005. DNA methylation and human disease. *Nat. Rev. Genet.* 6 (8):597–610.

260. Esteller, M. et al. 2001. DNA methylation patterns in hereditary human cancers mimic sporadic tumorigenesis. *Hum. Mol. Genet.* 10 (26):3001–3007.

261. Yoder, J. A., C. P. Walsh, T. H. Bestor. 1997. Cytosine methylation and the ecology of intragenomic parasites. *Trends Genet.* 13 (8):335–340.

262. Razin, A., A. D. Riggs. 1980. DNA methylation and gene function. *Science* 210 (4470):604–610.

263. Robertson, K. D., A. P. Wolffe. 2000. DNA methylation in health and disease. *Nat. Rev. Genet.* 1 (1):11–19.

264. Chiang, P. K., R. K. Gordon, J. Tal, G. C. Zeng, B. P. Doctor, K. Pardhasaradhi, P. P. McCann. 1996. S-Adenosylmethionine and methylation. *FASEB J.* 10 (4):471–480.

265. Loenen, W. A. 2006. S-Adenosylmethionine: Jack of all trades and master of everything? *Biochem. Soc. Trans.* 34 (2):330–333.

266. Reichard, J. F., M. Schnekenburger, A. Puga. 2007. Long term low-dose arsenic exposure induces loss of DNA methylation. *Biochem. Biophys. Res. Commun.* 352 (1):188–192.

267. Coppin, J. F., W. Qu, M. P. Waalkes. 2008. Interplay between cellular methyl metabolism and adaptive efflux during oncogenic transformation from chronic arsenic exposure in human cells. *J. Biol. Chem.* 283 (28):19342–19350.

268. Goering, P. L., H. V. Aposhian, M. J. Mass, M. Cebrian, B. D. Beck, M. P. Waalkes. 1999. The enigma of arsenic carcinogenesis: role of metabolism. *Toxicol. Sci.* 49 (1):5–14.

269. McCabe, D. C., M. A. Caudill. 2005. DNA methylation, genomic silencing, and links to nutrition and cancer. *Nutr. Rev.* 63 (6):183–195.

270. Anetor, J. I., H. Wanibuchi, S. Fukushima. 2007. Arsenic exposure and its health effects and risk of cancer in developing countries: Micronutrients as host defence. *Asian Pac. J. Cancer Prev.* 8 (1):13–23.

271. Ahlborn, G. J. et al. 2008. Dose response evaluation of gene expression profiles in the skin of K6/ODC mice exposed to sodium arsenite. *Toxicol. Appl. Pharmacol.* 227 (3):400–416.

272. Cui, X., T. Wakai, Y. Shirai, N. Yokoyama, K. Hatakeyama, S. Hirano. 2006. Arsenic trioxide inhibits DNA methyltransferase and restores methylation-silenced genes in human liver cancer cells. *Hum. Pathol.* 37 (3):298–311.

273. Fu, H. Y., J. Z. Sheng, S. F. Sheng, H. R. Zhou. 2007. n-MSP detection of p16 gene demethylation and transcription in human multiple myeloma U266 cell line induced by arsenic trioxide. *Zhongguo Shi Yan Xue Ye Xue Za Zhi* 15 (1):79–85.

274. Uthus, E. O., C. Davis. 2005. Dietary arsenic affects dimethylhydrazine-induced aberrant crypt formation and hepatic global DNA methylation and DNA methyltransferase activity in rats. *Biol. Trace Elem. Res.* 103 (2):133–145.

275. Chen, H., S. Li, J. Liu, B. A. Diwan, J. C. Barrett, M. P. Waalkes. 2004. Chronic inorganic arsenic exposure induces hepatic global and individual gene hypomethylation: Implications for arsenic hepatocarcinogenesis. *Carcinogenesis* 25 (9):1779–1786.

276. Okoji, R. S., R. C. Yu, R. R. Maronpot, J. R. Froines. 2002. Sodium arsenite administration via drinking water increases genome-wide and Ha-ras DNA hypomethylation in methyl-deficient C57BL/6J mice. *Carcinogenesis* 23 (5):777–785.

277. Xie, Y., K. J. Trouba, J. Liu, M. P. Waalkes, D. R. Germolec. 2004. Biokinetics and subchronic toxic effects of oral arsenite, arsenate, monomethylarsonic acid, and dimethylarsinic acid in v-Ha-ras transgenic (Tg.AC) mice. *Environ. Health Perspect.* 112:1255–1263.

278. Bagnyukova, T. V., L. I. Luzhna, I. P. Pogribny, V. I. Lushchak. 2007. Oxidative stress and antioxidant defenses in goldfish liver in response to short-term exposure to arsenite. *Environ. Mol. Mutagen.* 48 (8):658–665.

279. Benbrahim-Tallaa, L., R. A. Waterland, M. Styblo, W. E. Achanzar, M. M. Webber, M. P. Waalkes. 2005. Molecular events associated with arsenic-induced malignant transformation of human prostatic epithelial cells: Aberrant genomic DNA methylation and K-ras oncogene activation. *Toxicol. Appl. Pharmacol.* 206 (3):288–298.

280. Sciandrello, G., F. Caradonna, M. Mauro, G. Barbata. 2004. Arsenic-induced DNA hypomethylation affects chromosomal instability in mammalian cells. *Carcinogenesis* 25 (3):413–417.

281. Majumdar, S., S. Chanda, B. Ganguli, D. N. Guha Mazumder, S. Lahiri, U. B. Dasgupta. 2010. Arsenic exposure induces genomic hypermethylation. *Environ. Toxicol.* 25 (3):315–318.

282. Pilsner, J. R., X. Liu, H. Ahsan, V. Ilievski, V. Slavkovich, D. Levy, P. Factor-Litvak, J. H. Graziano, M. V. Gamble. 2009. Folate deficiency, hyperhomocysteinemia, low urinary creatinine, and hypomethylation of leukocyte DNA are risk factors for arsenic-induced skin lesions. *Environ. Health Perspect.* 117:254–260.

283. Waalkes, M. P., J. Liu, H. Chen, Y. Xie, W. E. Achanzar, Y. S. Zhou, M. L. Cheng, B. A. Diwan. 2004. Estrogen signaling in livers of male mice with hepatocellular carcinoma induced by exposure to arsenic in utero. *J. Natl. Cancer Inst.* 96 (6):466–474.

284. Boonchai, W., M. Walsh, M. Cummings, G. Chenevix-Trench. 2000. Expression of p53 in arsenic-related and sporadic basal cell carcinoma. *Arch. Dermatol.* 136 (2):195–198.

285. Chanda, S., U. B. Dasgupta, D. Guhamazumder, M. Gupta, U. Chaudhuri, S. Lahiri, S. Das, N. Ghosh, D. Chatterjee. 2006. DNA hypermethylation of promoter of gene p53 and p16 in arsenic-exposed people with and without malignancy. *Toxicol. Sci.* 89 (2):431–437.

286. Chen, W. T., W. C. Hung, W. Y. Kang, Y. C. Huang, C. Y. Chai. 2007. Urothelial carcinomas arising in arsenic-contaminated areas are associated with hypermethylation of the gene promoter of the death-associated protein kinase. *Histopathology* 51 (6):785–792.

287. Marsit, C. J., M. R. Karagas, A. Schned, K. T. Kelsey. 2006. Carcinogen exposure and epigenetic silencing in bladder cancer. *Ann. NY Acad. Sci.* 1076:810–821.

288. Chai, C. Y., Y. C. Huang, W. C. Hung, W. Y. Kang, W. T. Chen. 2007. Arsenic salts induced autophagic cell death and hypermethylation of DAPK promoter in SV-40 immortalized human uroepithelial cells. *Toxicol. Lett.* 173 (1):48–56.

289. Fu, H. Y., J. Z. Shen. 2005. Hypermethylation of CpG island of p16 gene and arsenic trioxide induced p16 gene demethylation in multiple myeloma. *Zhonghua Nei Ke Za Zhi* 44 (6):411–414.

290. Jensen, T. J., P. Novak, K. E. Eblin, A. J. Gandolfi, B. W. Futscher. 2008. Epigenetic remodeling during arsenical-induced malignant transformation. *Carcinogenesis* 29 (8):1500–1508.

291. Mass, M. J., L. Wang. 1997. Arsenic alters cytosine methylation patterns of the promoter of the tumor suppressor gene p53 in human lung cells: A model for a mechanism of carcinogenesis. *Mutat. Res.* 386 (3):263–277.

292. Zhang, A., H. Feng, G. Yang, X. Pan, X. Jiang, X. Huang, X. Dong. 2007. Unventilated indoor coal-fired stoves in Guizhou province, China: Cellular and genetic damage in villagers exposed to arsenic in food and air. *Environ. Health Perspect.* 115:653–658.

293. Cui, X., T. Wakai, Y. Shirai, K. Hatakeyama, S. Hirano. 2006. Chronic oral exposure to inorganic arsenate interferes with methylation status of p16INK4a and RASSF1A and induces lung cancer in A/J mice. *Toxicol. Sci.* 91 (2):372–381.

294. Jones, P. A., S. B. Baylin. 2002. The fundamental role of epigenetic events in cancer. *Nat. Rev. Genet.* 3 (6):415–428.

295. Takahashi, M., J. C. Barrett, T. Tsutsui. 2002. Transformation by inorganic arsenic compounds of normal Syrian hamster embryo cells into a neoplastic state in which they become anchorage-independent and cause tumors in newborn hamsters. *Int. J. Cancer* 99 (5):629–634.

296. Couse, J. F., V. L. Davis, R. B. Hanson, W. N. Jefferson, J. A. McLachlan, B. C. Bullock, R. R. Newbold, K. S. Korach. 1997. Accelerated onset of uterine tumors in transgenic mice with aberrant expression of the estrogen receptor after neonatal exposure to diethylstilbestrol. *Mol. Carcinog.* 19:236–242.

297. Marsit, C. J., M. R. Karagas, H. Danaee, M. Liu, A. Andrew, A. Schned, H. H. Nelson, K. T. Kelsey. 2006. Carcinogen exposure and gene promoter hypermethylation in bladder cancer. *Carcinogenesis* 27 (1):112–116.

298. Chen H., J. Liu, C. Q. Zhao, B. A. Diwan, B. A. Merrick, M. P. Waalkes. 2001. Association of c-myc overexpression and hyperproliferation with arsenite-induced malignant transformation. *Toxicol. Appl. Pharmacol.* 175 (3):260–268.

299. Jensen, T. J., P. Novak, S. M. Wnek, A. J. Gandolfi, B. W. Futscher. 2009. Arsenicals produce stable progressive changes in DNA methylation patterns that are linked to malignant transformation of immortalized urothelial cells. *Toxicol. Appl. Pharmacol.* 241 (2):221–229.

300. Riojas-Rodríguez, H., R. Solís-Vivanco, A. Schilmann, S. Montes, S. Rodríguez, C. Ríos, Y. Rodríguez-Agudelo. 2010. Intellectual function in Mexican children environmentally exposed to manganese living in a mining area. *Environ. Health Perspect.* 118:1465–1470.

301. Zoni, S., E. Albini, R. Lucchini. 2007. Neuropsychological testing for the assessment of manganese neurotoxicity: A review and a proposal. *Am. J. Ind. Med.* 50:812–830.

302. Chang, Y. et al. 2009. High signal intensity on magnetic resonance imaging is a better predictor of neurobehavioral performances than blood manganese in asymptomatic welders. *Neurotoxicology* 30:555–563.

303. Groschen, G. E., T. L. Arnold, W. S. Morrow, K. L. Warner. 2009. *Occurrence and Distribution of Iron, Manganese, and Selected Trace Elements in Ground Water in the Glacial Aquifer System of the Northern United States.* U.S. Geological Survey Scientific Investigations Report 2009-5006. Accessed August 25, 2017. http://pubs.usgs.gov/sir/2009/5006/.

304. Roth, J. A. 2006. Homeostatic and toxic mechanisms regulating manganese uptake, retention, and elimination. *Biol. Res.* 39:45–57.

305. Boyes, W. K. 2010. Essentiality, toxicity, and uncertainty in the risk assessment of manganese. *J. Toxicol. Environ. Health A* 73:159–165.

306. Deveau, M. 2010. Contribution of drinking water to dietary requirements of essential metals. *J. Toxicol. Environ. Health A* 73:235–241.

307. Kondakis, X. G., N. Makris, M. Leotsinidis, M. Prinou, T. Papapetropoulos. 1989. Possible health effects of high manganese concentration in drinking water. *Arch. Environ. Health* 44:175–178.

308. Bouchard, M., F. Laforest, L. Vandelac, D. Bellinger, D. Mergler. 2007. Hair manganese and hyperactive behaviors: Pilot study of school-age children exposed through tap water. *Environ. Health Perspect.* 115:122–127.

309. He, P., D. H. Liu, G. Q. Zhang. 1994. Effects of high-level-manganese sewage irrigation on children's neurobehavior. *Zhonghua Yu Fang Yi Xue Za Zhi* 28:216–218.

310. Wasserman, G. A. et al. 2006. Water manganese exposure and children's intellectual function in Araihazar, Bangladesh. *Environ. Health Perspect.* 114:124–129.

311. Woolf, A., R. Wright, C. Amarasiriwardena, D. Bellinger. 2002. A child with chronic manganese exposure from drinking water. *Environ. Health Perspect.* 110:613–616.

312. Sahni, V., Y. Leger, L. Panaro, M. Allen, S. Giffin, D. Fury, N. Hamm. 2007. Case report: A metabolic disorder presenting as pediatric manganism. *Environ. Health Perspect.* 115:1776–1779.

313. World Health Organization (WHO). 2008. Chemical aspects. In *Guidelines for Drinking-Water Quality Recommendations*, 3rd ed. Geneva: WHO.

314. Wright, R. O., C. Amarasiriwardena, A. D. Woolf, R. Jim, D. C. Bellinger. 2006. Neuropsychological correlates of hair arsenic, manganese, and cadmium levels in school-age children residing near a hazardous waste site. *Neurotoxicology* 27:210–216.

315. Sky-Peck, H. H. 1990. Distribution of trace elements in human hair. *Clin. Physiol. Biochem.* 8:70–80.

316. van den Hoven, T., N. Slaats. 2006. Lead monitoring. In *Analytical Methods for Drinking Water, Advances in Sampling and Analysis*, P. Quevaullier, K. C. Thompson, Eds. Hoboken, NJ: Wiley.

317. Wechsler, D. 1999. *Wechsler Abbreviated Scale of Intelligence (WASI)*. San Antonio, TX: Harcourt Assessment.

318. Raven, J., J. C. Raven, J. H. Court. 2003. *Manual for Raven's Progressive Matrices and Vocabulary Scales*. San Antonio, TX: Harcourt Assessment.

319. Bradley, R. H., R. F. Convyn, M. Burchinal, H. P. McAdoo, C. G. Coll. 2001. The home environments of children in the United States. Part II: Relations with behavioral development through age thirteen. *Child Dev.* 72:1868–1886.

320. Beck, A. T., R. A. Steer, G. K. Brown. 1996. *Manual for Beck Depression Inventory*, 2nd ed. (BDI-II). San Antonio, TX: Psychological Corporation.

321. Zeger, S. L., K. Y. Liang. 1986. Longitudinal data analysis for discrete and continuous outcomes. *Biometrics* 42:121–130.

322. Hanley, J. A., A. Negassa, M. D. Edwardes, J. E. Forrester. 2003. Statistical analysis of correlated data using generalized estimating equations: An orientation. *Am. J. Epidemiol.* 157:364–375.

323. Greenland, S., B. Brumback. 2002. An overview of relations among causal modelling methods. *Int. J. Epidemiol.* 31:1030–1037.

324. Bellinger, D. C. 2007. Lead neurotoxicity in children: Decomposing the variability in dose-effect relationships. *Am. J. Ind. Med.* 50:720–728.

325. U.S. Geological Survey. 2009. National Water-Quality Assessment Program. Quality of Water from Domestic Wells in the United States. Accessed August 30, 2010. http://water.usgs.gov/nawqa/studies/domestic_wells/table2.html

326. Elsner, R. J., J. G. Spangler. 2005. Neurotoxicity of inhaled manganese: Public health danger in the shower?. *Med. Hypotheses* 65:607–616.

327. Aschner, M. 2006. Manganese in the shower: Mere speculation over an invalidated public health danger. *Med. Hypotheses* 66:200–201.

328. Olanow, C. W. 2004. Manganese-induced parkinsonism and Parkinson's disease. *Ann. NY Acad. Sci.* 1012:209–223.

329. Dobson, A. W., K. M. Erikson, M. Aschner. 2004. Manganese neurotoxicity. *Ann. NY Acad. Sci.* 1012:115–128.

330. Eriksson, H., K. Magiste, L. O. Plantin, F. Fonnum, K. G. Hedstrom, E. Theodorsson-Norheim, K. Kristensson, E. Stalberg, E. Heilbronn. 1987. Effects of manganese oxide on monkeys as revealed by a combined neurochemical, histological and neurophysiological evaluation. *Arch. Toxicol.* 61:46–52.

331. Moreno, J. A., E. C. Yeomans, K. M. Streifel, B. L. Brattin, R. J. Taylor, R. B. Tjalkens. 2009. Age-dependent susceptibility to manganese-induced neurological dysfunction. *Toxicol. Sci.* 112:394–404.

332. Guilarte, T. R., J. L. McGlothan, M. Degaonkar, M. K. Chen, P. B. Barker, T. Syversen, J. S. Schnieder. 2006. Evidence for cortical dysfunction and widespread manganese accumulation in the nonhuman primate brain following chronic manganese exposure: a 1H-MRS and MRI study. *Toxicol. Sci.* 94:351–358.

333. Guilarte, T. R., N. C. Burton, T. Verina, V. V. Prabhu, K. G. Becker, T. Syversen, J. S. Schnieder. 2008. Increased APLP1 expression and neurodegeneration in the frontal cortex of manganese-exposed nonhuman primates. *J. Neurochem.* 105:1948–1959.

334. Fitsanakis, V. A., K. N. Thompson, S. E. Deery, D. Milatovic, Z. K. Shihabi, K. M. Erikson, R. W. Brown, M. Aschner. 2009. A chronic iron-deficient/high-manganese diet in rodents results in increased brain oxidative stress and behavioral deficits in the morris water maze. *Neurotox. Res.* 15:167–178.

335. Food and Nutrition Board. 2004. *Dietary Reference Intake Tables: Elements Table.* Food and Nutrition Board, Institutes of Medicine. Accessed December 8, 2010. www.nutrisci.wisc.edu/NS623/driwatersum.pdf

336. Agusa, T., T. Kunito, J. Fujihara, R. Kubota, T. B. Minh, T. Kim, H. Iwata, A. Subramanian, P. H. Viet, S. Tanabe. 2006. Contamination by arsenic and other trace elements in tube-well water and its risk assessment to humans in Hanoi, Vietnam. *Environ. Pollut.* 139:95–106.

337. Michalke, B., S. Halbach, V. Nischwitz. 2007. Speciation and toxicological relevance of manganese in humans. *J. Environ. Monit.* 9:650–656.

338. Gibson, R. S. 1994. Content and bioavailability of trace elements in vegetarian diets. *Am. J. Clin. Nutr.* 59:1223S–1232S.

339. Lyden, A., B. S. Larsson, N. G. Lindquist. 1984. Melanin affinity of manganese. *Acta Pharmacol. Toxicol. (Copenh)* 55:133–138.

340. Tchobanoglous, G., F. L. Burton, H. D. Stensel. 2003. *Wastewater Engineering: Treatment Disposal Reuse/Metcalf & Eddy, Inc.*, 4th ed. McGraw-Hill Book Company.

341. Beychok, M. R. 1967. *Aqueous Wastes from Petroleum and Petrochemical Plants*, 1st ed. John Wiley & Sons, New York. LCCN 67019834.

342. Hobson, T. 2004. *The Scoop on Oil Skimmers. Environmental Protection (formerly Water and Wastewater News).* Dallas, TX: 1105 Media, Inc.

343. Kashiwaya, M., K. Yoshimoto. 1980. Tannery wastewater treatment by the oxygen activated sludge process. *Journal (Water Pollution Control Federation) (Alexandria, VA: Water Environment Federation)* 52 (5):999–1007. JSTOR 25040825.

344. American Petroleum Institute (API). 1990. *Management of Water Discharges: Design and Operations of Oil-Water Separators*, 1st ed. American Petroleum Institute.

345. Beychok, M. R. 1971. Wastewater treatment. *Hydrocarb. Process.* 109–112.

346. Selam Gebrekidan, R. 2013. Corrosion May Have Led to North Dakota Pipeline Leak, Regulators Say. *NBC News.* Accessed October 15, 2013.

347. MacPherson, J. 2013. ND Farmer Finds Oil Spill While Harvesting Wheat. *ABC News.* Associated Press. Accessed October 15, 2013.

348. Sider, A. 2013. Enbridge Spill at Cushing Terminal Mostly Contained. Enbridge Spill at Cushing Terminal Mostly Contained. May 21, 2013. Accessed December 01, 2016. http://www.hydrocarbonprocessing.com/news/2013/05/enbridge-spill-at-cushing-terminal-mostly-contained

349. Enterprise's Seaway Crude Pipeline System Shut after Cushing, Oklahoma Spill. *Reuters.* 2016. Accessed December 01, 2016. http://www.reuters.com/article/us-pipeline-operations-seaway-oklahoma-idUSKCN12O16D

350. White, S. 2013. Exxon Oil Spill Could Be 40% Larger Than Company Estimates, EPA Figures Show. *InsideClimate News (USA).* Accessed December 1, 2016. https://insideclimatenews.org/news/20130405/exxon-oil-spill-could-be-40-larger-company-estimates-epa-figures-show

351. Olson, B., C. Harvey. 2013. Refiner Delek Cleaning Up 5,000-Barrel Spill in Arkansas Bayou. Bloomberg.com. March 13, 2013. Accessed December 01, 2016. https://www.bloomberg.com/news/articles/2013-03-13/refiner-delek-cleaning-up-5-000-barrel-spill-in-arkansas-bayou

352. Jones, L. 2013. Cause of Mayflower Exxon-Mobil Oil Spill Still a Mystery. *Arkansas Business.* May 28, 2013. Accessed December 01, 2016. http://www.arkansasbusin.com/article/92656/cause-of-mayflower-spill-still-a-mystery

353. Thompson, B., C. Glorioso. 336K Gallons of Diesel Fuel Leak in Arthur Kill. *NBC New York.* October 31, 2012. Accessed December 01, 2016. http://www.nbcnewyork.com/news/local/Arthur-Kill-Oil-Spill-Diesel-Fuel-Motiva-Staten-Island-Woodbridge-NJ-176676451.html

354. Kirkham, C. 2012. Arthur Kill Oil Spill: Hurricane Sandy's Surge Dumps Diesel Into New Jersey Waterway. *The Huffington Post.* November 01, 2012. Accessed December 01, 2016. http://www.huffingtonpost.com/2012/11/01/arthur-kill-oil-spill-new-jersey_n_2054267.html

355. Rogers, R., S. Olp. 2011. Ruptured Pipeline Sends Oil Coursing down the Yellowstone River. *The Billings Gazette*. July 02, 2011. Accessed December 01, 2016. http://billingsgazette.com/news/local/ruptured-pipeline-sends-oil-coursing-down-the-yellowstone-river/article_6a8f2313-4279-542c-95c7-92f04639003f.html

356. Lin II, R-G. 2010. Gulf Oil Spill: New Spill in Gulf Area after Barge Crashes into Abandoned Oil Well. *Los Angeles Times*. July 27, 2010. Accessed December 01, 2016. http://latimesblogs.latimes.com/greenspace/2010/07/gulf-oil-spill-new-spill-in-gulf-after-barge-crashes-into-abandoned-oil-well.html

357. Jaffe, M. 2013. Colorado Floods: 1,900 Oil and Gas Wells Shut as Crews Check Damage. *The Denver Post*. September 17, 2013. Accessed December 01, 2016. http://www.denverpost.com/2013/09/17/colorado-floods-1900-oil-and-gas-wells-shut-as-crews-check-damage/

358. Leaking Barataria Bay Oil Well Capped. CNN. August 02, 2010. Accessed December 01, 2016. http://www.cnn.com/2010/US/08/02/louisiana.barataria.bay.leak/

359. Gallucci, J. 2010. *Michigan Oil Spill: 840,000 Gallons of Oil Leak into Talmadge Creek*. Long Island Press. July 27, 2010. Accessed December 01, 2016. http://archive.longislandpress.com/2010/07/27/michigan-oil-spill-840000-gallons-of-oil-leak-into-talmadge-creek/

360. Carlson, C. 2015. Five Years after Spill, Kalamazoo River's a Different Place. *Battle Creek Enquirer*. Accessed December 01, 2016. http://www.battlecreekenquirer.com/story/news/local/2015/07/24/residents-learning-live-new-life-river/30625933/

361. O'Donoghue, A. J., J. Smith. 2010. Oil Spill in Red Butte Creek Threatens Waters, Wildlife. Accessed December 01, 2016. http://www.deseretnews.com/article/700039797/Oil-spill-in-Red-Butte-Creek-threatens-waters-wildlife.html?pg=all

362. Jensen, D. P. 2010. Chevron: We Won't Be Difficult on Oil-spill Cleanup Costs. *The Salt Lake Tribune*. Accessed December 01, 2016. http://archive.sltrib.com/story.php?ref=/D=g/ci_15320863

363. Goldstein, K. 2010. Alaska Oil Spill: Trans-Alaska Pipeline Shuts Down 800 Mile Area In North Slope. *The Huffington Post*. May 26, 2010. Accessed December 01, 2016. http://www.huffingtonpost.com/2010/05/26/alaska-oil-spill-trans-al_n_589974.html

364. Deepwater Horizon MC252 Gulf Incident Oil Budget (PDF). 2010. National Oceanic and Atmospheric Administration. Accessed December 02, 2016. https://www.bing.com/search?q=Deepwater+Horizon+MC252+Gulf+Incident+Oil+Budget+(PDF).+2010.+National+Oceanic+and+Atmospheric+Administration&src=IE-SearchBox&FORM=IENTTR&conversationid=

365. Gonzalez, A., N. Malik. 2010. Collision Causes Crude Oil Spill in Texas. *The Wall Street Journal*. Accessed December 02, 2016. http://www.wsj.com/articles/SB10001424052748704562504575021540843701582

366. Vargas, R. A., C. Kirkham. 2008. Tugboat Operators Involved in Collision Not Properly Licensed. *The Times-Picayune* 23 Jul. 2008. Accessed August 12, 2009. http://www.nola.com/news/index.ssf/2008/07/ap_collision_closes_mississipp.html

367. Curiel, J., J. Kay, K. Fagan. 2007. Spill Closes Bay Beaches as Oil Spreads, Kills Wildlife. *SFGate*. November 07, 2007. Accessed December 02, 2016. http://www.sfgate.com/bayarea/article/Spill-closes-bay-beaches-as-oil-spreads-kills-3236720.php

368. Fruge Jr., G. 2006. CITGO Oil Spill (PDF). *Louisiana Department of Environmental Quality*. July 25, 2006. Accessed November 16, 2008. http://kplc.images.worldnow.com/images/incoming/Citgo/CitgoIncident.pdf

369. Fineberg, F.A. 2006. BP North Slope Spill Reveals A History of Substandard Environmental Performance (PDF). *Alaska Forum for Environmental Responsibility*. Accessed November 16, 2008. http://www.finebergresearch.com/pdf/Neport060315Rev.pdf

370. Oil Spills Found in Southeast Louisiana. 2005. MSNBC News. September 16, 2005. Accessed December 02, 2016. http://www.truth-out.org/archive/component/k2/item/57269:44-oil-spills-found-in-southeast-louisiana

371. Response and Prevention Branch Oil Team. 2006. *Murphy Oil USA Refinery Spill, Chalmette & Meraux, LA Presentation (PDF)*. U.S. Environmental Protection Agency, Region 6. Accessed December 02, 2016.

372. Oil Spill History. The Mariner Group. Retrieved December 02, 2016. http://www.marinergroup.com/oil-spill-history.htm

373. Athos 1 Oil Spill. 2004. Accessed December 02, 2016. http://www.ceoe.udel.edu/oilspill/index.html

374. Research Planning, Inc. 2005. *The MP-69/Hurricane Ivan Oil Discharges, Mississippi River Delta, Louisiana (pp. 10, 18) (PDF) (Report)*. Preassessment Data Report. Damage Assessment Center, National Oceanic and Atmospheric Administration.

375. Buzzards Bay Oil Spill: Bouchard Barge No. 120. 2010. Buzzards Bay National Estuary Program. April 6, 2010. Accessed December 02, 2016. http://buzzardsbay.org/accidentsummary.htm

376. Trans-Alaska Pipeline Shot By A Drunk. Accessed December 02, 2016. http://www.earthlyissues.com/shotdrunk.htm

377. How Do Oil Spills Impact Casco Bay? 1996. Toxic Pollution in Casco Bay: Sources and Impacts. Accessed December 02, 2016. http://muskie.usm.maine.edu/cascobay/pdfs/Toxics%20Chapter%203.pdf

378. Rhode Island Oil Spill Is More Serious Than Initially Thought. 1996. The New York Times. January 22, 1996. Accessed December 02, 2016. http://www.nytimes.com/1996/01/22/us/rhode-island-oil-spill-is-more-serious-than-initially-thought.html

379. M/V Mega Borg. M/V Mega Borg | IncidentNews | NOAA. Accessed December 02, 2016. https://incidentnews.noaa.gov/incident/6748

380. Hampton, S. 2016. American Trader Oil Spill, California Office of Spill Prevention and Response. Accessed December 02, 2016. https://www.wildlife.ca.gov/OSPR/NRDA/american-trader

381. Dvarskas, A. 2008. Restoring Injured Natural Resources in the Harbor (PDF). *The Tidal Exchange (New York—New Jersey Harbor Estuary Program)* 22: p. 3. Accessed December 02, 2016.

382. Desvousges, W. H., R. W. Dunford, K. E. Mathews. 1992. *Natural Resource Damages Valuation: Arthur Kill Oil Spill (PDF). Association of Environmental and Resource Economists Workshop*, Snowbird, Utah. Accessed December 02, 2016. https://yosemite.epa.gov/ee/epa/eerm.nsf/vwAN/EE-0078-03.pdf/$file/EE-0078-03.pdf

383. Wehner, D. E. 2004. *Presidente Rivera Spill—June 24, 1989.* University of Delaware—College of Earth, Ocean, and Environment. Accessed December 02, 2016. http://www.ceoe.udel.edu/oilspill/PresidenteRiveraSpill.html

384. Roser, M. 2015. Oil Spills. *Our World in Data.* Accessed December 02, 2016. https://ourworldindata.org/oil-spills/

385. Holleman, M. 2014. After 25 Years, Exxon Valdez Oil Spill Hasn't Ended. *CNN.* March 25, 2014. Accessed December 02, 2016. http://www.cnn.com/2014/03/23/opinion/holleman-exxon-valdez-anniversary/

386. Kjellstrom, T., T. McMicheal, G. Ranmuthugala, R. Shrestha, S. Kingsland. 2006. Air and Water Pollution: Burden and Strategies for Control. In *Disease Control Priorities in Developing Countries*, 2nd ed., M. Lodh, Ed. Washington, D.C.: Oxford University Press.

387. Lemonic, M. D. 2001. Nightmare on the Monongahela. *Time Magazine.* June 24, 2001. http://content.time.com/time/magazine/article/0,9171,148444,00.html

388. 1985 Grand Eagle Oil Spill. University of Delaware—College of Earth, Ocean, and Environment. Accessed December 02, 2016. http://www.ceoe.udel.edu/oilspill/Grandeagle.html

389. Oil Spills and Near-Misses in Northwest Waters. Seattle Post Intelligencer (Hearst Seattle Media, LLC). November 21, 2002. Accessed February 04, 2011.

390. Helton, D., T. Penn. 1999. *Putting Response and Natural Resource Damage Costs in Perspective (PDF). International Oil Spill Conference: 21.* Paper ID #114. Accessed February 04, 2011.

391. Kana, T. W., Lt. E. P. Thompson, R. Pavia. 1981. *Burmah Agate—Chronology and Containment Operations. International Oil Spill Conference Proceedings*, pp. 131–138. doi: 10.7901/2169-3358-1981-1-131

392. The Trans-Alaska Pipeline. The Center for Land Use Interpretation. 2009. Accessed December 02, 2016. http://www.clui.org/newsletter/spring-2009/trans-alaska-pipeline

393. Argo Merchant, United States, 1976. ITOPF. 2010. Accessed December 02, 2016. http://www.itopf.com/in-action/case-studies/case-study/argo-merchant-united-states-1976/

394. Merchant, C. J., O. Embury, J. Roberts-Jones, E. Fiedler, C. E. Bulgin, G. K. Corlett, S. Good, A. Mclaren, N. Rayner, S. Morak-Bozzo, C. Donlon. 2014. Sea surface temperature datasets for climate applications from phase 1 of the European Space Agency Climate Change Initiative (SST CCI). *Geosci. Data J.* 1 (2):179–191. doi: 10.1002/gdj3.20

395. Albert, T., V. McKinney. US—30 April 1979. Accessed December 02, 2016. https://www.uscg.mil/legal/CDOA/Commandant_Decisions/S_and_R_1980_2279/2153%20-%20MCKINNEY.pdf

396. Save the River Report. Save the River RSS. Accessed December 02, 2016. http://www.savetheriver.org/

397. The Berkeley Daily Planet. 2001. After 30 Years, Tankers Safer but Spills Still a Threat. January 19, 2001. Accessed December 02, 2016. http://www.berkeleydailyplanet.com/issue/2001-01-19/article/3054

398. Wood, R. H. 2006. When Tankers Collide, a Preview. *AuthorHouse.* Accessed May 28, 2010.

399. Leighty, J. M. 1971. Huge Oil Spill in San Francisco Bay—Tanker Collision under Golden Gate Bridge, California (1971)—Newspapers.com. Newspapers.com. January 18, 1971. Accessed December 02, 2016. https://www.newspapers.com/clip/2684558/huge_oil_spill_in_san_francisco_bay/

400. California Oil Seeps. American Oil & Gas Historical Society. 2014. Accessed December 02, 2016. http://aoghs.org/offshore-history/california-oil-seeps/
401. Rasmussen, F. N. 2002. Shoal Marks Beginning of End for 'African Queen'. *The Baltimore Sun*. 2002. Accessed December 02, 2016. http://articles.baltimoresun.com/2002-07-06/features/0207060081_1_danielsen-african-queen-delaware-bay
402. African Queen. 2007. Delmar DustPan. Accessed December 02, 2016. http://delmardustpan.blogspot.com/2007/12/african-queen.html
403. Phuong, L. 1999. Beach town forced to scrape away oil leak and a chunk of its past. Seattle Post-Intelligencer (Hearst Seattle Media, LLC).
404. Berman, R. 2005. Greenpoint, Maspeth Residents Lobby To Get 55-Year-Old Oil Spill Cleaned Up. *The New York Sun*. Accessed December 02, 2016. http://www.nysun.com/new-york/greenpoint-maspeth-residents-lobby-to-get-55-year/23231/
405. Carter, H. R. 2003. Oil and California's Seabirds: An Overview (PDF). *Mar. Ornithol.* 31:2. Accessed December 02, 2016.
406. Rintoul, W., S. F. Hodgson. 1990. *Drilling through Time: 75 Years with California's Division of Oil and Gas*, pp. 13–15. Sacramento: Department of Conservation, Division of Oil and Gas.
407. Robertson, C., C. Krauss. 2010. Gulf Spill Is the Largest of Its Kind, Scientists Say. *The New York Times*. Accessed August 12, 2010.
408. BP Leak the World's Worst Accidental Oil Spill. The Telegraph. 2010. Accessed December 02, 2016. http://www.telegraph.co.uk/finance/newsbysector/energy/oilandgas/7924009/BP-leak-the-worlds-worst-accidental-oil-spill.html
409. Jervis, R., A. Levin. 2010. Obama, in Gulf, Pledges To Push On Stopping Leak. *USA Today*. Associated Press. Accessed March 03, 2013. http://usatoday30.usatoday.com/news/nation/2010-05-27-oil-spill-news_N.htm?csp=34news
410. Welch, W. M., C. Joyner. 2010. Memorial Service Honors 11 Dead Oil Rig Workers. *USA Today*. Accessed December 02, 2016. http://usatoday30.usatoday.com/news/nation/2010-05-25-oil-spill-victims-memorial_N.htm
411. BP Begins Testing New Oil Well Cap. Al Jazeera English. July 15, 2010. Accessed December 05, 2016. http://www.aljazeera.com/news/americas/2010/07/20107150283268524.html
412. On Scene Coordinator Report on Deepwater Horizon Oil Spill (PDF) (Report). September 2011. Accessed February 22, 2013. https://www.osha.gov/oilspills/dwh_osha_response_0511a.pdf
413. The Use of surface and Subsea Disperants during the BP Deewater Horizon Oil Spill. Draft (PDF) (Report). National Commission on the BP Deepwater Horizon Oil Spill and Offshore Drilling. 2010. Accessed February 17, 2013. http://permanent.access.gpo.gov/gpo184/Working%20Paper.Dispersants.For%20Release.pdf
414. Tangley, L. 2010. Bird Habitats Threatened by Oil Spill. *National Wildlife (National Wildlife Federation)*. Accessed December 05, 2016. http://www.nwf.org/news-and-magazines/national-wildlife/birds/archives/2010/oil-spill-birds.aspx
415. Juhasz, A. 2012. Investigation: Two Years after the BP Spill, a Hidden Health Crisis Festers. *The Nation*. Accessed February 03, 2013. https://www.thenation.com/article/investigation-two-years-after-bp-spill-hidden-health-crisis-festers/
416. Elliott, D. 2013. BP Begins Testing New Oil Well Cap. *NPR*. December 21, 2013. Accessed December 05, 2016. http://www.npr.org/2013/12/21/255843362/for-bp-cleanup-2013-meant-4-6-million-pounds-of-gulf-coast-oil
417. Pittman, C. 2013. Oil from BP Spill Pushed onto Shelf off Tampa Bay by Underwater Currents, Study Finds. *Tampa Bay Times*. August 20, 2013. Accessed December 05, 2016. http://www.tampabay.com/news/environment/water/oil-from-bp-spill-was-pushed-onto-shelf-off-tampa-bay-by-underwater/2137406
418. Viegas, J. 2013. Record Dolphin, Sea Turtle Deaths Since Gulf Spill. Accessed December 05, 2016. http://www.seeker.com/record-dolphin-sea-turtle-deaths-since-gulf-spill-1767378408.html
419. Sahagun, L. 2014. Toxins released by oil spills send fish hearts into cardiac arrest. *Los Angeles Times*. Accessed February 17, 2014. http://articles.latimes.com/2014/feb/13/science/la-sci-sn-tuna-hearts-oil-spill-toxins-20140213
420. Wines, M. 2014. Fish Embryos Exposed to Oil from BP Spill Develop Deformities, a Study Finds. *The New York Times*. Accessed December 05, 2016. http://www.nytimes.com/2014/03/25/us/fish-embryos-exposed-to-oil-from-bp-spill-develop-deformities-a-study-finds.html?_r=0
421. Bureau of Ocean Energy Management, Regulation and Enforcement (BOEMRE)/U.S. Coast Guard Joint Investigation Team (September 14, 2011). Deepwater Horizon Joint Investigation Team Releases Final Report (Press Release). U.S. Government. Accessed December 05, 2016

422. Martin, A. 2011. BP Mostly, But Not Entirely, to Blame for Gulf Spill—National. *The Atlantic Wire.* September 14, 2011. Accessed December 05, 2016. http://www.theatlantic.com/national/archive/2011/09/bp-mostly-not-entirely-blame-gulf-spill/337965/

423. Schuler, M. 2009. Transocean's Deepwater Horizon Drills World's Deepest Oil and Gas Well. *GCaptain.* September 03, 2009. Accessed December 05, 2016. http://gcaptain.com/transoceans-deepwater-horizon/

424. Deepwater Horizon Sinks Offshore Louisiana. NEWS| Deepwater Horizon Sinks Offshore Louisiana | Rigzone. April 22, 2010. Accessed December 05, 2016. http://www.rigzone.com/news/oil_gas/a/91509/Deepwater_Horizon_Sinks_Offshore_Louisiana

425. Deepwater Horizon Marine Casualty Investigation Report (PDF) (Report). Office of the Maritime Administrator. August 17, 2011. Retrieved February 25, 2013. https://www.register-iri.com/forms/upload/Republic_of_the_Marshall_Islands_DEEPWATER_HORIZON_Marine_Casualty_Investigation_Report-Low_Resolution.pdf

426. At Least 11 Missing after Blast on Oil Rig in Gulf. CNN. April 21, 2010. Accessed December 05, 2016. http://www.cnn.com/2010/US/04/21/oil.rig.explosion/

427. BP Confirms that Transocean Ltd Issued the Following Statement Today (Press Release). BP. April 21, 2010. Accessed December 05, 2016. http://www.bp.com/en/global/corporate/press/press-releases/bp-confirms-that-transocean-ltd-issued-the-following-statement-today.html

428. Jervis, R. At least 11 workers missing after La. oil rig explosion. USA Today. Associated Press. Accessed April 21, 2010. http://usatoday30.usatoday.com/news/nation/2010-04-21-louisiana-oil-rig_N.htm

429. Brenner, N., A. Guegel, T. Hwee Hwee, A. Pitt. 2010. Coast Guard Confirms Horizon Sinks. *Upstream Online (NHST Media Group).* Accessed December 05, 2016. http://www.upstreamonline.com/live/article212769.ece

430. Schwartz, N., H. R. Weber. 2010. Bubble of methane triggered rig blast. *Southern California Public Radio.* Associated Press. Accessed June 29, 2010. http://www.independent.co.uk/news/world/americas/bubble-of-methane-triggered-rig-blast-say-workers-1968527.html

431. Coast Guard: Oil Rig That Exploded Has Sunk. *CNN.* April 22, 2010. Accessed December 05, 2016. http://news.blogs.cnn.com/2010/04/22/coast-guard-oil-rig-that-exploded-has-sunk/

432. US Military Joins Gulf of Mexico Oil Spill Effort. *BBC News.* April 29, 2010. Accessed December 05, 2016. http://news.bbc.co.uk/2/hi/8651624.stm

433. Krauss, C., J. Broder, J. Calmes. 2010. White House Struggles as Criticism on Leak Mounts. *The New York Times.* Accessed June 01, 2010. http://www.nytimes.com/2010/05/31/us/31spill.html

434. Henry, R. 2010. Scientists Up Estimate of Leaking Gulf Oil. June 15, 2010. MSNBC. Associated Press. Accessed December 06, 2016. http://www.nbcnews.com/id/37717335/ns/disaster_in_the_gulf/t/scientists-estimate-leaking-gulf-oil/#.WEbXXYWcGUk

435. Kunzelman, M. 2013. BP Seeks Judge's Ruling on Size of Gulf Oil Spill. TBO.com. January 12, 2013. Accessed December 06, 2016. http://www.tbo.com/ap/world/bp-seeks-judges-ruling-on-size-of-gulf-oil-spill-604653

436. BP/Gulf Oil Spill—68,000 Square Miles of Direct Impact (Press Release). *SkyTruth.* July 27, 2010. Accessed December 06, 2016. http://skytruth.org/2010/07/bp-gulf-oil-spill-68000-square-miles-of/

437. Norse, E. A., J. Amos. 2010. Impacts, perception, and policy implications of the bp/deepwater horizon oil and gas disaster (PDF). *Environ. Law Report.* 40 (11):11058–11073.

438. National Park Service. 2010. Response to Oil on Gulf Island Beaches Continues (Press Release). June 04, 2010. Accessed June 13, 2010. http://www.nationalparksgallery.com/park_news/10082

439. Bluestein, G. 2010. BP Has Another Setback as Oil Slick Threatens Florida. *The Plain Dealer.* Associated Press. Accessed February 26, 2011.

440. Kunzelman, M. 2010. Oil Spewing Once Again in the Gulf. *The Sun News.* Associated Press. Accessed December 07, 2016.

441. McConnaughey, J., M. Stacy. 2010. Admiral Back on the Gulf Coast for Spill. *The Sun News.* Associated Press. Archived from the original on March 22, 2012. Accessed December 07, 2016.

442. Lozano, J. A. 2010. BP Spill Spreads to Texas. *The Sun News.* Associated Press. Accessed July 06, 2010.

443. Mui, Y. Q., D. A. Fahrenthold. 2010. Oil in Lake Pontchartrain Stokes Worries in New Orleans. *The Washington Post.* Accessed December 07, 2016.

444. Marshall, B. 2010. New Wave of Oil Comes Ashore West of Mississippi River. *The Times-Picayune.* Accessed September 14, 2010.

445. Massive Stretches of Weathered Oil Spotted in Gulf of Mexico. 2010. The Times-Picayune. Nola.com. October 23, 2010. Accessed December 07, 2016.

446. Polson, J. 2011. BP Oil Still Ashore One Year After End of Gulf Spill. *Bloomberg*. Accessed November 05, 2011.
447. Ramseur, J. L., C. L. Hagerty. 2013. *Deepwater Horizon Oil Spill: Recent Activities and Ongoing Developments (PDF) (Report)*. CRS Report for Congress. Congressional Research Service. R42942. Accessed February 13, 2015.
448. Gillis, J., C. Robertson. 2010. Gulf Surface Oil Vanishing Quickly. *The New York Times*.
449. Bolsatd, E., R. Schoof, M. Talev. 2010. Doubts Follow Rosy Oil Report. *The Sun News*. Accessed December 07, 2016.
450. Zabarenko, D. 2010. Nearly 3/4 of BP Spill Oil Gone from Gulf. *Reuters*. Retrieved August 15, 2010.
451. Scientists Call New Gulf Spill Report 'Ludicrous'—Oneindia News. News.oneindia.in. Accessed December 07, 2016.
452. Foul Waters, Hard Lessons from BP Oil Spill. 2011. CNN. January 13, 2011.
453. Schleifstein, M. 2012. Spilled BP Oil Lingers on Louisiana Coast. *The Times-Picayune*. Accessed December 07, 2016.
454. Schrope, M. 2013. Dirty Blizzard Buried Deepwater Horizon Oil. *Nature*. Accessed February 03, 2015.
455. Schrope, M. 2013. Dirty blizzard buried deepwater horizon oil. *Nature*. Retrieved February 3, 2013. http://www.nature.com/news/dirty-blizzard-buried-deepwater-horizon-oil-1.12304
456. Butler, S. J. 2011. *BP Macondo Well Incident. U.S. Gulf of Mexico. Pollution Containment and Remediation Efforts (PDF). Lillehammer Energy Claims Conference*. BDO Consulting. Accessed February 17, 2013.
457. Containment Boom Effort Comes Up Short in BP Oil Spill. 2010. The Christian Science Monitor. June 11, 2010. Accessed April 07, 2011.
458. Klein, N. 2010. BP Oil Spill Deepwater Horizon, BP (Business), Oil Spills (Environment),Oil and Gas Companies (Business), Oil (Environment), Oil (Business), US News, Conservation (Environment), Pollution (Environment),World News, Environment, Business. *The Guardian (London)*.
459. BP spill response plans severely flawed | MNN – Mother nature network. Wayback Machine. Archived May 17, 2013. http://www.mnn.com/earth-matters/wilderness-resources/stories/bp-spill-response-plans-severely-flawed
460. Blair, K. 2011. Containment boom effort comes up short in BP oil spill. *The Christian Science Monitor* (June 11, 2010). Retrieved April 7, 2011. http://www.csmonitor.com/USA/2010/0611/Containment-boom-effort-comes-up-short-in-BP-oil-spill
461. What are oil dispersants? CNN. May 15, 2010. Accessed 02 July 2010.
462. Guarino, M. 2010. Gulf oil spill: Has BP 'turned corner' with siphon success? *The Christian Science Monitor*.
463. Khan, A. 2010. Gulf Oil Spill: Effects of Dispersants Remain a Mystery. *Los Angeles Times*. Accessed September 05, 2010.
464. 22-Mile-Long Oily Plume Mapped Near BP Site—Disaster in the Gulf. 2010. MSNBC. August 19, 2010. Accessed September 05, 2010.
465. AOL. Major Study Charts Long-Lasting Oil Plume in Gulf. News & latest headlines from AOL. http://www.sandiegouniontribune.com/sdut-major-study-charts-long-lasting-oil-plume-in-gulf-2010aug19-story,amp.html San Diego Tribune
466. Drowning in Oil. http://www.newsweek.com/what-bp-doesnt-want-you-know-about-2010-gulf-spill-63015
467. Schoof, R. 2010. Mother Nature Left to Mop Up Oily Mess. *The Sun News*. Accessed July 17, 2010.
468. Kerr, R.A. 2010. A Lot of Oil on the Loose, Not So Much to Be Found (PDF). *Science* 329 (5993):734–735.
469. Rioux, P. 2010. Giant Oil Skimmer 'A Whale' Deemed a Bust for Gulf of Mexico Spill. *The Times-Picayune*. Accessed December 07, 2016.
470. Gabbatt, A. 2010. BP Oil Spill: Kevin Costner's Oil-Water Separation Machines Help with Clean-up. *The Guardian*.
471. Fountain, H. 2010. Advances in Oil Spill Cleanup Lag Since Valdez. *The New York Times*. Accessed July 05, 2010.
472. Sanchez, C., E. Bonfiles. 2010. BP 'Excited' Over Kevin Costner's Oil Cleanup Machine, Purchases 32. *ABC News Good Morning America*.
473. Deep Water Horizon Unified Command Agency. 2010. Gulf of Mexico Oil Spill Response: Current Operations as of June 28. Accessed December 07, 2016.
474. Kintisch, E. 2010. An Audacious Decision in Crisis Gets Cautious Praise (PDF). *Science* 329 (5993):735–736.

475. Valentine, D. L., I. Mezić, N. Crnjarić-Žic, S. Ivić, P. J. Hogan, V. A. Fonoberov, S. Loire. 2011. Dynamic autoinoculation and the microbial ecology of a deep water hydrocarbon irruption (PDF). *Proc. Natl. Acad. Sci. U. S. A.* 109 (50):20286–20291.

476. Brown, E. 2010. Bacteria in the gulf mostly digested gas, not oil, study finds. *Los Angeles Times.* Accessed December 12, 2016. http://articles.latimes.com/2010/sep/16/science/la-sci-oil-20100917

477. Biello, D. 2015. How Microbes Helped Clean BP's Oil Spill. *Scientific American.* April 28, 2015. Accessed December 12, 2016. https://www.scientificamerican.com/article/how-microbes-helped-clean-bp-s-oil-spill/

478. Dykes, B. M. 2010. Oil-eating Microbes May Not Be All They're Cracked up to Be. *Yahoo! News.* September 17, 2010. Accessed December 12, 2016. https://www.yahoo.com/news/blogs/upshot/oil-eating-microbes-may-not-cracked.html

479. Ott, R. 2011. Bio-Remediation or Bio-Hazard? Dispersants, Bacteria and Illness in the Gulf. *Huffington Post.* Accessed December 07, 2016.

480. West Siberian Research Institute to Help Clean Up Deepwater Horizon Spill. 2010. Moscow. RIA Novosti. July 27, 2010. Accessed August 08, 2013.

481. Biello, D. 2010. The BP Spill's Growing Toll on the Sea Life of the Gulf. *Yale Environment 360.* Yale School of Forestry & Environmental Studies. Accessed December 07, 2016.

482. Shirley, T. C., J. W. Tunnell, Jr., F. Moretzsohn, J. Brenner. 2010. *Biodiversity of the Gulf of Mexico: Applications to the Deep Horizon Oil Spill (PDF) (Press Release).* Harte Research Institute for Gulf of Mexico Studies, Texas A&M University. Accessed December 07, 2016.

483. Smith, L. 2011. Deep Sea Fish Named in World Top Ten New Species. *Fish2Fork.* Accessed December 07, 2016.

484. Oil Spill Full of Methane, Adding New Concerns. NBCNews.com. NBC Universal News Group, June 18, 2010. Retrieved December 12, 2016.

485. Gerken, J. 2012. Gulf Oil Spill: Coral Death 'Definitively' Linked To BP Spill. *Huffington Post.* Accessed June 1, 2012.

486. White, H. K. et al. 2012. Impact of the Deepwater Horizon oil spill on a deep-water coral community in the Gulf of Mexico. *PNAS* 109 (50):20303–20308.

487. BP Oil Spill Seriously Harmed Deep-sea Corals, Scientists Warn. The Guardian. March 26, 2012. Accessed December 13, 2016. https://www.theguardian.com/environment/2012/mar/26/bp-oil-spill-deepwater-horizon

488. Gutman, M., S. Netter. 2010. Submarine Dive Finds Oil, Dead Sea Life at Bottom of Gulf of Mexico. *ABSNews.* Accessed February 26, 2011. http://abcnews.go.com/US/exclusive-submarine-dive-finds-oil-dead-sea-life/story?id=12305709

489. Mystery 'Oil Sheen' Grows Near Site of BP Gulf Disaster, Says Researcher. 2013. NBC News. January 31, 2013. Accessed December 13, 2016. https://www.theguardian.com/environment/2012/mar/26/bp-oil-spill-deepwater-horizon

490. Anderson, K. 2010. *OSU Researchers Find Heightened Levels of Known Carcinogens in Gulf.* Oregon State University. September 30, 2010. Accessed December 13, 2016. http://oregonstate.edu/ua/ncs/archives/2010/sep/osu-researchers-find-heightened-levels-known-carcinogens-gulf

491. Schneyer, J. 2010. U.S. Oil Spill Waters Contain Carcinogens: Report. *Reuters.* September 30, 2010. Accessed December 13, 2016. http://www.reuters.com/article/us-oil-spill-carcinogens-idUSTRE68T6FS20100930

492. Collins, J., J. Dearen. 2010. BP: Mile-long Tube Sucking Oil away from Gulf Well. *The Washington Times.* Associated Press. Accessed December 07, 2016. http://www.washingtontimes.com/news/2010/may/16/huge-underwater-oil-plumes-found-gulf-mexico/

493. Nelson, K. 2011. Spike Reported in Number of Stillborn Dolphins on Coast. SunHerald.com. Accessed December 07, 2016. http://www.sunherald.com/news/article36465768.html

494. Olsson, G. 2012. *Water and Energy: Threats and Opportunities.* The International Water Association. IWA Publishing.

495. Beaumont, P. 2012. Gulf's Dolphins Pay Heavy Price for Deepwater Oil Spill. *The Guardian (London).*

496. Kaufman, L. 2012. Gulf Dolphins Exposed to Oil Are Seriously Ill, Agency Says. *The New York Times (Gulf of Mexico; Louisiana).* Accessed December 07, 2016.

497. Inkley, D. 2013. Restoring a Degraded Gulf of Mexico. *National Wildlife Federation.* April 02, 2013. Accessed December 14, 2016. http://www.nwf.org/News-and-Magazines/Media-Center/Reports/Archive/2013/04-02-13-Restoring-A-Degraded-Gulf-of-Mexico.aspx

498. Gerken, J. 2013. Is The Gulf Still Sick? Huffington Post. Accessed December 14, 2016. http://www.huffingtonpost.com/2013/04/02/gulf-of-mexico-dolphin-deaths-bp_n_3001408.html

499. Kohls, G. 2010. Pharma Invades Water Supplies. Consortiumnews.com. April 20, 2010. Accessed December 14, 2016. https://consortiumnews.com/2010/042010b.html

500. Donn, J., M. Mendoza, J. Pritchard. 2015. The Associated Press: Pharmaceuticals Found in Drinking Water, Affecting Wildlife and Maybe Humans. http://hosted.ap.org/specials/interactives/pharmawater_site/day1_01.html

501. Tabak, H. H., R. L. Bunch. 1970. Steroid hormones as water pollutants. I. Metabolism of natural and synthetic ovulation-inhibiting hormones by microorganisms of activated sludge and primary settled sewage. *Dev. Ind. Microbiol.* 11:367–376.

502. Garrison A. W., J. D. Pope, F. R. Allen. 1976. GC/MS analysis of organic compounds in domestic wastewaters. In *Identification and Analysis of Organic Pollutants in Water*, L. H. Keith, Ed., pp. 517–556. Ann Arbor, MI: Ann Arbor Science Publishers Inc.

503. Hignite, C., D. L. Azarnoff. 1977. Drugs and drug metabolites as environmental contaminants: Chlorophenoxyisobutyrate and salicylic acid in sewage water effluent. *Life Sci.* 20 (2):337–341.

504. Kolpin, D. W., E. T. Furlong, M. T. Meyer, E. M. Thurman, S. D. Zaugg, L. B. Barber, H. T. Buxton. 2002. Pharmaceuticals, hormones, and other organic wastewater contaminants in U.S. streams, 1999–2000: A national reconnaissance. *Environ. Sci. Technol.* 36:1202–1211.

505. Buser, H. R., M. D. Muller, N. Theobald. 1998. Occurrence of the pharmaceutical drug clofibric acid and the herbicide mecoprop in various Swiss lakes and in the North Sea. *Environ. Sci. Technol.* 32 (1):188–192.

506. Ternes, T. 1998. Occurrence of drugs in German sewage treatment plants and rivers. *Water Res.* 32:3245–3260.

507. Buser, H. R., T. Poiger, M. D. Muller. 1999. Occurrence and environmental behavior of the chiral pharmaceutical drug ibuprofen in surface waters and in wastewater. *Environ. Sci. Technol.* 33 (15):2529–2535.

508. Daughton, C. G., T. A. Ternes. 1999. Pharmaceuticals and personal care products in the environment: Agents of subtle change? *Environ. Health Perspect.* 107 (Suppl 6):907–938.

509. Daughton, C. G. 2001. Pharmaceuticals and personal care products in the environment: Overarching issues and overview. *ACS Symp. Ser.* 791:2–38.

510. Heberer, T., B. Fuhrmann, K. Schmidt-Baumler, D. Tsipi, V. Koutsouba, A. Hiskia. 2001. Occurrence of pharmaceutical eesidues in sewage, river, ground, and drinking water in Greece and Berlin (Germany). In *Pharmaceuticals and Personal Care Products in the Environment, Scientific and Regulatory Issues*, C. Daughton, T. Jones-Lepp, Eds. Washington, DC: American Chemical Society.

511. Reddersen, K., T. Heberer, U. Dünnbier. 2002. Identification and significance of phenazone drugs and their metabolites in ground- and drinking water. *Chemosphere* 49:539–544.

512. Bound, A., N. Voulvoulis. 2005. Household disposal of pharmaceuticals as a pathway for aquatic contamination in the United Kingdom. *Environ. Health Perspect.* 113:1705–1711.

513. Alder, A. C., A. Bruchet, M. Carballa. 2006. Consumption and occurrence. In *Human Pharmaceuticals, Hormones and Fragrances: The Challenge of Micropollutants in Urban Water Management*, T. A. Ternes, A. Joss, Eds. London: IWA Publishing. [cited in DWI, 2007].

514. Ashton, D., M. Hilton, K. V. Thomas. 2004. Investigating the environmental transport of human pharmaceuticals to streams in the United Kingdom. *Sci. Total Environ.* 333:167–184. [cited in DWI, 2007].

515. Aherne, G. W., A. Hardcastle, A. H. Nield. 1990. Cytotoxic drugs and the aquatic environment: Estimation of bleomycin in river and water samples. *J. Pharm. Pharmacol.* 42:741–742. [cited in DWI, 2007].

516. Roberts, P. H., K. V. Thomas. 2006. The occurrence of selected pharmaceuticals in wastewater effluent and surface waters of the lower Tyne catchment. *Sci. Total Environ.* 356:143–153. [cited in DWI, 2007].

517. Thomas, K. V., M. J. Hilton. 2004. The occurrence of selected human pharmaceutical compounds in UK estuaries. *Mar. Pollut. Bull.* 49:436–444. [cited in DWI, 2007].

518. Boucard, T., A. Gravell. 2006. Concentrations of fluoxetine and norfluoxetine in UK sewage effluents and river waters. United Kingdom Environment Agency [Personal communication, cited in DWI, 2007].

519. Bound, J. P., N. Voulvoulis. 2006. Predicted and measured concentrations for selected pharmaceuticals in UK rivers: Implications for risk Assessment. *Water Res.* 40:2885–2892. [cited in DWI, 2007].

520. Watts, C. D., B. Crathorne, M. Fielding, P. Steel. 1983. Identification of non-volatile organics in water using field desorption mass spectrometry and high performance liquid chromatography. In *Analysis of Organic Micropollutants in Water*, G. Angeletti, A. Bjørseth, Eds., pp. 120–131. Dordrecht: D. Reidel Publishing Co. [cited in DWI, 2007].

521. Benotti, M. J., R. A. Trenholm, B. J. Vanderford, J. C. Holady, B. D. Stanford, S. A. Snyder. 2009. Pharmaceuticals and endocrine disrupting compounds in U.S. drinking water. *Environ. Sci. Technol.* 43 (3):597–603.

522. Huerta-Fontela, M., M. T. Galceran, F. Ventura. 2011. Occurrence and removal of pharmaceuticals and hormones through drinking water treatment. *Water Res.* 45:1432–1442.

523. Zühlke, S., U. Dünnbier, T. Heberer. 2004. Detection and identification of phenazone-type drugs and their microbial metabolites in ground and drinking water applying solid-phase extraction and gas chromatography with mass spectrometric detection. *J. Chromatogr. A* 1050:201–209.

524. Jones, O. A., J. N. Lester, N. Voulvoulis. 2005. Pharamceuticals: A threat to drinking water? *Trends Biol.* 23 (4):163–167.

525. Mons, M. N., A. C. Hoogenboom, T. H. M. Noij. 2003. *Pharmaceuticals and drinking water supply in the Netherlands.* Nieuwegein, Kiwa Water Research (Kiwa Report No. BTO 2003.040).

526. Focazio, M. J., D. W. Kolpin, K. K. Barnes, E. T. Furlong, M. T. Meyer, S. D. Zaugg, L. B. Barber, M. E. Thurman. 2008. A national reconnaissance for pharmaceuticals and other organic wastewater contaminants in the United States—II) Untreated drinking water sources. *Sci. Total Environ.* 402:201–216.

527. Heberer, T., K. Schmidt-Bäumler, H. J. Stan. 1998. Occurrence and distribution of organic contaminants in the aquatic system in Berlin. Part II: Substituted phenols in Berlin surface water. *Acta Hydrochimica et Hydrobiologica* 26:272–278.

528. Zuccato, E., D. Calamari, M. Natangelo, R. Fanelli. 2000. Presence of therapeutic drugs in the environment. *Lancet* 355 (9217):1789–1790.

529. Heberer, T., A. Mechlinski, B. Fanck, A. Knappe, G. Massmann, A. Pekdeger Birgit Fritz. 2004. Field studies on the fate and transport of pharmaceutical residues in bank filtration. *Ground Water Monit. Remediat.* 24:70–77.

530. Stackelberg, P. E., E. T. Furlong, M. T. Meyer, S. D. Zaugg, A. K. Henderson, D. B. Reissman. 2004. Persistence of pharmaceutical compounds and other organic wastewater contaminants in a conventional drinking-water treatment plant. *Sci. Total Environ.* 329:99–113.

531. Stackelberg, P. E., J. Gibs, E. T. Furlong, M. T. Meye, S. D. Zaugg, R. Lee Lippincot. 2007. Efficiency of conventional drinking-water-treatment processes in removal of pharmaceuticals and other organic compounds. *Sci. Total Environ.* 377 (2–3):255–272.

532. Vieno, N. M., T. Tuhkanen, L. Kronberg. 2005. Seasonal variation in the occurrence of pharmaceuticals in effluents from a sewage treatment plant and in the recipient water. *Environ. Sci. Technol.* 39:8220–8226.

533. Loraine, G. A., M. E. Pettigrove. 2006. Seasonal variations in concentrations of pharmaceuticals and personal care products in drinking water and reclaimed wastewater in Southern California. *Environ. Sci. Technol.* 40:687–695.

534. Snyder, S. A., S. Adham, A. M. Redding, F. S. Cannon, J. DeCarolis, J. Oppenheimer, E. C. Wert, Y. Yoon. 2006. Role of membranes and activated carbon in the removal of endocrine disruptors and pharmaceuticals. *Desalination* 202:156–181.

535. Vanderford, B. J., S. A. Snyder. 2006. Analysis of pharmaceuticals in water by isotope dilution liquid chromatography/tandem mass spectrometry. *Environ. Sci. Technol.* 40:7312–7320.

536. Loos, R., J. Wollgast, T. Huber, G. Hanke. 2007. Polar herbicides, pharmaceutical products, perfluorooctanesulfonate (PFOS), perfluorooctanoate (PFOA), and nonylphenol and its carboxylates and ethoxylates in surface and tap waters around Lake Maggiore in Northern Italy. *Anal. Bioanal. Chem.* 387:1469–1478.

537. Pérez, S., D. Barceló. 2007. Application of advanced MS techniques to analysis and identification of human and microbial metabolites of pharmaceuticals in the aquatic environment. *Trends Analyt. Chem.* 26 (6):494–514.

538. Togola, A., H. Budzinski. 2008. Multi-residue analysis of pharmaceutical compounds in aqueous samples. *J. Chromatogr. A* 1177:150–158.

539. Watkinson, A. J., E. J. Murby, S. D. Costanzo. 2007. Removal of antibiotics in conventional and advanced wastewater treatment: Implications for environmental discharge and wastewater recycling. *Water Res.* 41 (18):4164–4176.

540. DWI. 2007. *Desk based review of current knowledge on pharmaceuticals in drinking water and estimation of potential levels.* Final report prepared by Watts and Crane Associates for Drinking Water Inspectorate, Department for Environment, Food and Rural Affairs (Defra Project Code: CSA 7184/WT02046/DWI70/2/213). Accessed October 10, 2017. http://dwi.defra.gov.uk/research/completed-research/reports/dwi70-2-213.pdf.

541. Gabet-Giraud, V., C. Miège, J. M. Choubert, S. M. Ruel, M. Coquery. 2010. Occurrence and removal of estrogens and beta blockers by various processes in wastewater treatment plants. *Sci. Total Environ.* 408:4257–4269.

542. Vieno, N., T. Tuhkanen, L. Kronberg. 2007. Elimination of pharmaceuticals in sewage treatment plants in Finland. *Water Res.* 41:1001–1012.

543. Ziylan, A., N. H. Ince. 2011. The occurrence and fate of anti-inflammatory and analgesic pharmaceuticals in sewage and fresh water: Treatability by conventional and non-conventional processes. *J. Hazard. Mater.* 187 (1–3):24–36.

544. Dolman, A. M., J. Rücker, F. R. Pick, J. Fastner, T. Rohrlack, U. Mischke, C. Wiedner, S. Bertilsson. 2012. Cyanobacteria and cyanotoxins: The influence of nitrogen versus phosphorus. *PLoS ONE* E38757.

545. Smith, V. H. 2003. Eutrophication of freshwater and coastal marine ecosystems a global problem. *Environ. Sci. Pollut. Res.* 10:126–139. http://www.springerlink.com/content/w32259833027620p/

546. Smith, V. H., S. B. Joye, R. W. Howarth. 2006. Eutrophication of freshwater and marine ecosystems. *Limnol. Oceanogr.* 51:351–355.

547. Pretty, J. N., C. F. Mason, D. B. Nedwell, R. E. Hine, S. Leaf, R. Dils. 2003. Environmental costs of freshwater eutrophication in England and Wales. *Environ. Sci. Technol.* 37:201–208.

548. Dodds, W. K., W. W. Bouska, J. L. Eitzmann, T. J. Pilger, K. L. Pitts, A. J. Riley, J. T. Schloesser, D. J. Thornbrugh. 2009. Eutrophication of US freshwaters: Analysis of potential economic damages. *Environ. Sci. Technol.* 43:12–19.

549. Paerl, H. W., N. S. Hall, E. S. Calandrino. 2011. Controlling harmful cyanobacterial blooms in a world experiencing anthropogenic and climatic-induced change. *Sci. Total Environ.* 409 (10):1739–1745

550. Chorus, I., J. Bartram. 1999. *Toxic Cyanobacteria in Water: A Guide to Their Public Health Consequences, Monitoring, and Management.* Taylor & Francis.

551. Pearsall, W. H. 1932. Phytoplankton in the English Lakes: II. The Composition of the Phytoplankton in Relation to Dissolved Substances. *J. Ecol.* 20:241–262. Accessed October 18, 2011. http://www.jstor.org/stable/2256077

552. Gorham, E., J. W. G. Lund, J. E. Sanger, W. E. Dean Jr. 1974. Some relationships between algal standing crop, water chemistry, and sediment chemistry in the English Lakes. *Limnol. Oceanogr.* 19:601–617.

553. Smith, V. H. 1985. Predictive models for the biomass of blue-green algae in lakes. *J. Am. Water Resour. Assoc.* 21:433–439.

554. Downing, J. A., S. B. Watson, E. McCauley. 2001. Predicting cyanobacteria dominance in lakes. *Can. J. Fish. Aquat. Sci.* 58:1905–1908.

555. Håkanson, L., A. C. Bryhn, J. K. Hytteborn. 2007. On the issue of limiting nutrient and predictions of cyanobacteria in aquatic systems. *Sci. Total Environ.* 379:89–108.

556. Ptacnik, R., L. Lepistö, E. Willén, P. Brettum, T. Andersen, S. Rekolainen, A. Lyche Solheim, L. Carvalho. 2008. Quantitative responses of lake phytoplankton to eutrophication in Northern Europe. *Aquat. Ecol.* 42:227–236.

557. Schindler, D. W. 1974. Eutrophication and recovery in experimental lakes: Implications for lake management. *Science* 184:897–899.

558. Schindler, D. 1977. Evolution of phosphorus limitation in lakes. *Science* 195:260–262.

559. Elser, J. J., E. R. Marzolf, C. R. Goldman. 1990. Phosphorus and nitrogen limitation of phytoplankton growth in the freshwaters of North America: A review and critique of experimental enrichments. *Can. J. Fish. Aquat. Sci.* 47:1468–1477.

560. Elser, J. J., M. E. S. Bracken, E. E. Cleland, D. S. Gruner, W. S. Harpole, H. Hillebrand, J. T. Ngai, E. W. Seabloom, J. B. Shurin, J. E. Smith. 2007. Global analysis of nitrogen and phosphorus limitation of primary producers in freshwater, marine and terrestrial ecosystems. *Ecol. Lett.* 10:1135–1142.

561. Lewis, W. M., W. A. Wurtsbaugh. 2008. Control of lacustrine phytoplankton by nutrients: Erosion of the phosphorus paradigm. *Int. Rev. Hydrobiol.* 93:446–465.

562. Sterner, R. W. 2008. On the phosphorus limitation paradigm for lakes. *Int. Rev. Hydrobiol.* 93:433–445.

563. Shapiro, J. 1990. Current beliefs regarding dominance of blue-greens: The case for the importance of CO_2 and pH. *Verh. Int. Ver. Limnol.* 24:38–54.

564. Dokulil, M. T., K. Teubner. 2000. Cyanobacterial dominance in lakes. *Hydrobiologia* 438:1–12.

565. Tilman, D., S. S. Kilham, P. Kilham. 1982. Phytoplankton community ecology: The role of limiting nutrients. *Annu. Rev. Ecol. Syst.* 13:349–372.

566. Downing, J. A., E. McCauley. 1992. The nitrogen: Phosphorus relationship in lakes. *Limnol. Oceanogr.* 37:936–945.

567. Smith, V. H. 1983. Low nitrogen to phosphorus ratios favor dominance by blue-green algae in lake phytoplankton. *Science* 221:669.
568. Schindler, D. W., R. E. Hecky, D. L. Findlay, M. P. Stainton, B. R. Parker, M. J. Paterson, K. G. Beaty, M. Lyng, S. E. Kasian. 2008. Eutrophication of lakes cannot be controlled by reducing nitrogen input: Results of a 37-year whole-ecosystem experiment. *Proc. Natl. Acad. Sci.* 105:11254–11258.
569. Vrede, T., A. Ballantyne, C. Mille-Lindblom, G. Algesten, C. Gudasz, S. Lindahl, A. Kristina Brunberg. 2009. Effects of N: P loading ratios on phytoplankton community composition, primary production and N fixation in a eutrophic lake. *Freshw. Biol.* 54:331–344.
570. Watson, S. B., E. McCauley, J. A. Downing. 1997. Patterns in phytoplankton taxonomic composition across temperate lakes of differing nutrient status. *Limnol. Oceanogr.* 42:487–495.
571. Edmondson, W., J. T. Lehman. 1981. The effect of changes in the nutrient income on the condition of Lake Washington. *Limnol. Oceanogr.* 26:1–29.
572. Cronberg, G. 1982. Changes in the phytoplankton of Lake Trummen induced by restoration. *Hydrobiologia* 86:185–193.
573. Nõges, P., U. Mischke, R. Laugaste, A. G. Solimini. 2010. Analysis of changes over 44 years in the phytoplankton of Lake Võrtsjärv (Estonia): The effect of nutrients, climate and the investigator on phytoplankton-based water quality indices. *Hydrobiologia* 646:33–48.
574. Scheffer, M., S. Rinaldi, A. Gragnani, L. R. Mur, E. H. van Nes. 1997. On the dominance of filamentous cyanobacteria in shallow, turbid lakes. *Ecology* 78:272–282.
575. Harris, G. 1986. *Phytoplankton Ecology—Structure, Function and Fluctuation.* London; New York: Chapman and Hall.
576. Sivonen, K. 2009. *Cyanobacterial Toxins. Encyclopedia of Microbiology,* pp. 290–307. Oxford: Elsevier.
577. Preußel, K., A. Stüken, C. Wiedner, I. Chorus, J. Fastner. 2006. First report on cylindrospermopsin producing Aphanizomenon flos-aquae (Cyanobacteria) isolated from two German lakes. *Toxicon* 47:156–162.
578. Osswald, J., S. Rellán, A. Gago, V. Vasconcelos. 2007. Toxicology and detection methods of the alkaloid neurotoxin produced by cyanobacteria, anatoxin-a. *Environ. Int.* 33:1070–1089.
579. Ballot, A., J. Fastner, M. Lentz, C. Wiedner. 2010. First report of anatoxin-a-producing cyanobacterium Aphanizomenon issatschenkoi in northeastern Germany. *Toxicon* 56:964–971.
580. Ballot, A., J. Fastner, C. Wiedner. 2010. Paralytic shellfish poisoning toxin-producing cyanobacterium Aphanizomenon gracile in Northeast Germany. *Appl. Environ. Microbiol.* 76:1173–1180.
581. Mbedi, S., M. Welker, J. Fastner, C. Wiedner. 2005. Variability of the microcystin synthetase gene -cluster in the genus Planktothrix (Oscillatoriales, Cyanobacteria). *FEMS Microbiol. Lett.* 245:299–306.
582. Vezie, C., L. Brient, K. Sivonen, G. Bertru, J-C Lefeuvre, M. Salkinoja-Salonen. 1998. Variation of microcystin content of cyanobacterial blooms and isolated strains in Lake Grand-Lieu (France). *Microb. Ecol.* 35:126–135.
583. Sivonen, K. 1990. Effects of light, temperature, nitrate, orthophosphate, and bacteria on growth of and hepatotoxin production by Oscillatoria agardhii strains. *Appl. Environ. Microbiol.* 56:2658–2666.
584. Oh, H-M., S. J. Lee, M-H. Jang, B-D. Yoon. 2000. Microcystin production by Microcystis aeruginosa in a phosphorus-limited chemostat. *Appl. Environ. Microbiol.* 66:176–179.
585. Wiedner, C., P. M. Visser, J. Fastner, J. S. Metcalf, G. A. Codd, L. R. Mur. 2003. Effects of light on the microcystin content of microcystis strain PCC 7806. *Appl. Environ. Microbiol.* 69:1475–1481.
586. Yoder, J. et al. 2011. *Surveillance for Waterborne Disease and Outbreaks Associated with Drinking Water and Water Not Intended for Drinking—United States, 2005–2006.* U.S. Department of Health and Human Services, Washington, DC, 60(12):38–68.
587. CDC. 2007. Gastroenteritis among attendees at a summer camp—Wyoming, June–July 2006. *MMWR* 56:368–370.
588. Marston, B. J., J. F. Plouffe, T. M. File, B. A. Hackman, S. J. Salstrom, H. B. Lipman, M. S. Kolczak, R. F. Breiman. 1997. Incidence of community-acquired pneumonia requiring hospitalization. Results of a population-based active surveillance study in Ohio. The community-based pneumonia incidence study group. *Arch. Intern. Med.* 157:1709–1718.
589. Bartlett, J. G. 2004. Decline in microbial studies for patients with pulmonary infections. *Clin. Infect. Dis.* 39:170–172.
590. Fields, B. S., R. F. Benson, R. E. Besser. 2002. Legionella and Legionnaires' disease: 25 years of investigation. *Clin. Microbiol. Rev.* 15:506–526.
591. Nicolson, G. L., N. L. Nicolson. 1998. Gulf War Illnesses: Complex medical, scientific and political paradox. *Med. Conflict Surviv.* 14:74–83.

592. Harmful Algal Blooms. US Department of Commerce, National Oceanic and Atmospheric Administration. Accessed December 14, 2016. http://oceanservice.noaa.gov/hazards/hab/

593. Landsberg, J. H. 2002. The effects of harmful algal blooms on aquatic organisms. *Rev. Fish. Sci.* 10 (2):113–390.

594. Flewelling, L. J. et al. 2005. Red tides and marine mammal mortalieis. *Nature* 435 (7043):755–756.

595. Diersling, N. 2009. *Phytoplankton Blooms: The Basics (PDF)*. NOAA FKNMS. Accessed December 14, 2016. http://floridakeys.noaa.gov/scisummaries/wqpb.pdf

596. Hochanadel, D. 2010. Limited amount of total phosphorus actually feeds algae, study finds. *Lake Scientist.* http://www.lakescientist.com/limited-amount-of-total-phosphorus-actually-feeds-algae-study-finds/

597. Gilbert, P. A., A. L. Dejong. 1977. The use of phosphate in detergents and possible replacements for phosphate. *Ciba Found. Symp.* 57:253–268.

598. Lathrop, R. C., S. R. Carpenter, J. C. Panuska, P. A. Soranno, C. A. Stow. 1998. Phosphorus loading reductions needed to control blue-green algal blooms in Lake Mendota (PDF). *Can. J. Fish. Aquat. Sci.* 55 (5):1169–1178.

599. Adams, N. G., M. Lesoing, V. L. Trainer. 2000. Environmental conditions associated with domoic acid in razor clams on the Washington coast. *J. Shellfish. Res.* 19:1007–1015.

600. Lam, C. W. Y, K. C. Ho. 1989. Red tides in Tolo Harbor, Hong Kong. In *Red Tides, Biology, Environmental Science and Toxicology*, T. Okaichi, D. M. Anderson, T. Nemoto, Eds., pp. 49–52. New York: Elsevier.

601. Trainer, V. L., N. G. Adams, B. D. Bill, C. M. Stehr, J. C. Wekell, P. Moeller, M. Busman, D. Woodruff. 2000. Domoic acid production near California coastal upwelling zones, June 1998. *Limnol. Oceanogr.* 45 (8):1818–1833.

602. Moore, S., V. L. Trainer, N. J. Mantua, M. S. Parker, E. A. Laws, L. C. Backer, L. E. Fleming. 2008. Impacts of climate variability and future climate change on harmful algal blooms and human health. *Proceedings of the Centers for Oceans and Human Health Investigators Meeting.*

603. Walsh, J. J. et al. 2006. Red tides in the Gulf of Mexico: Where, when, and why. *J. Geophys. Res.* 111: C11003.

604. Cabeza de Vaca, Álvar Núnez. La Relación (1542). Translated by Martin A. Dunsworth and José B. Fernández. Houston, Texas: Arte Público Press (1993).

605. Sellner, K. G., G. J. Doucette, G. J. Kirkpatrick. 2003. Harmful algal blooms: Causes, impacts and detection. *J. Ind. Microbiol. Biotechnol.* 30 (7):383–406.

606. Van Dolah, F. M. 2000. Marine algal toxins: Origins, health effects, and their increased occurrence. *Environ. Health Perspect.* 108 (suppl 1):133–141.

607. Brumbaugh, R. D, M. W. Beck, L. D. Coen, L. Craig, P. Hicks. 2006. *A Practitioners Guide to the Design & Monitoring of Shellfish Restoration Projects: An Ecosystem Approach.* Arlington, VA: The Nature Conservancy. Accessed September 21, 2017. http://www.habitat.noaa.gov/pdf/tncnoaa_shellfish_hotlinks_final.pdf

608. Depleted Bivalve Populations. Shinnecock Bay Restoration Program. Web. December 18, 2015. http://www.shinnecockbay.org/program/current.html

609. YSI Environmental. 2009. Delaware Oyster Gardening and Restoration—A Cooperative Effort. Web. December 21, 2015. http://darc.cms.udel.edu/ibog/YSIarticle.pdf

610. 2012. Web. December 21, 2015. http://masgc.org/oyster/documents/2012OGmanual.pdf

611. Devastating Red Tide Events in World History. https://www.leisurepro.com/blog/ocean-news/3-devastating-red-tide-events-world-history/

612. Moore, K. 2008. Northeast Oysters: The bigger danger, growers assert, would be the label of endangered. *National Fisherman.* Accessed. July 31, 2017. http://www.lakescientist.com/limited-amount-of-total-phosphorus-actually-feeds-algae-study-finds/

613. Chrisafis, A. August 10, 2009. Lethal Algae Take Over Beaches in Northern France. *The Guardian (London).*

614. Iceland Volcano Ash Cloud Triggers Plankton Bloom. *BBC News.* April 10, 2013.

615. Jacobs, A. July 05, 2013. Huge Algae Bloom Afflicts Coastal Chinese City. *The New York Times.*

616. A Dark Bloom in the South Atlantic: Image of the Day. 2014. Web. Accessed Decemeber 21, 2015. http://earthobservatory.nasa.gov/IOTD/view.php?id=82968&src=share

617. George, T. 2014. Toxin leaves 500,000 in northwest Ohio without drinking water. *Reuters.* Accessed March 18, 2017. https://www.reuters.com/article/2014/08/02/us-usa-water-ohio-idUSKBN0G20L120140802

618. Humpage, A., J. Rositano, A. Bretag, R. Brown, P. Baker, B. Nicholson, D. Steffensen. 1994. Paralytic shellfish poisons from Australian cyanobacterial blooms. *Aust. J. Mar. Freshw. Res.* 45:761–771.

619. Clark, R. F., S. R. Williams, S. P. Nordt, A. S. Manoguerra. 1999. A review of selected seafood poisonings. *Undersea Hyperb. Med.* 26 (3):175–184.

620. Taylor, F. J. R., Y. Fukuyo, J. Larsen, G. M. Hallegraeff. 2003. Taxonomy of harmful dinoflagellates. In *Manual on Harmful Marine Microalgae*, G. M. Hallegraeff, D. M. Anderson, A. D. Cembella, Eds., pp. 389–432. Springer Ltd.

621. Cembella, A. D. 1998. Ecophysiology and metabolism of paralytic shellfish toxins in marine microalgae. In *Physiological Ecology of Harmful Algal Blooms*, D. M. Anderson, A. D. Cembella, G. M. Hallegraeff, Eds., pp. 381–403. NATO ASI. Berlin: Springer.

622. Balech, E. 1985. The genus Alexandrium or Gonyaulax of the Tamarensis Group. In *Toxic Dinoflagellates*, D. M. Anderson, A. W. White, D. G. Baden, Eds., pp. 33–38. New York: Elsevier.

623. Azanza, R., V. Max, F. J. R. Taylor. 2001. Are Pyrodinium blooms in the Southeast Asian region recurring and spreading? A view at the end of the millennium. *J. Hum. Environ.* 30 (6):356–364.

624. Ngy, L., K. Tada, C-F. Yu, T. Takatani, O. Arakawa. 2008. Occurrence of paralytic shellfish toxins in Cambodian Mekong pufferfish Tetraodon turgidus: Selective toxin accumulation in the skin. *Toxicon* 51 (2):280–288.

625. Durbin E., G. Teegarden, R. Campbell, A. Cembella, M. F. Baumgartner, B. R. Mate. 2002. North Atlantic right whale, Eubalaena glacialis, exposed to paralytic shellfish poisoning (PSP) toxins via a zooplankton vector, Calanus finmarchicus. *Harmful Algae* 1:243–251.

626. Walsh, C. J., S. R. Leggett, B. J. Carter, C. Colle. 2010. Effects of brevetoxin exposure on the immune system of loggerhead sea turtles. *Aquat. Toxicol.* 97 (4):293–303.

627. Red Tide FAQ—Is It Safe to Eat Oysters during a Red Tide? Accessed August 23, 2009. www.tpwd.state.tx.us

628. Florida Fish and Wildlife Research Institute. Red Tide Current Status Statewide Information. Accessed August 23, 2009. research.myfwc.com

629. Red Tide Index. Accessed August 23, 2009. www.tpwd.state.tx.us

630. Red Tide Fact Sheet—Red Tide (Paralytic Shellfish Poisoning). www.mass.gov. Archived from the original on August 26, 2009. Accessed August 23, 2009.

631. Discover NOAA's Coral Reef Data. Accessed August 22, 2009. www.nos.noaa.gov

632. Langlois, G. W., P. D. Tom. *Red Tides: Questions and Answers.* U.S. Government. Accessed August 23, 2009.

633. Duggan, I. C. et al. 2003. Accessed September 10, 2017. http://www.startribune.com/style/news/metro-region/invaded_waters/invaded.html

634. United States Coast Guard. 1993. Aquatic Nuisance Species Information. Accessed September 10, 2017. http://www.uscg.mil/hq/gm/mso/mso4/old/bwm.html

635. Payment, P., M. S. Riley, 2002. *Resolving the Global Burden of Gastrointestinal Illness: A Call to Action*, pp. 25–32. Washington, DC: American Academy of Microbiology. http://www.asm.org

636. Levin, R. B., R. R. Epstein, T. E. Ford, W. Harrington, E. Olson, E. G. Reichard. 2002. U.S. drinking water challenges in the twenty-first century. *Environ. Health Perspect.* 110 (1):43–52.

637. Todd, E. C. D., P. Chatman, 2001. *Food Borne and Water Borne Disease in Canada.* 1974–1996 in NWRI. Polyscience Publications Inc. http://www.nwri.ca/threats/intro-e.html

638. International Joint Commission. 2003. The Status of Restoration Activities in the Great Lakes Areas of Concern. April 2003. 25pp. http://www.ijc.org

639. Stewart, I., A. A. Seawright, G. R. Shaw. 2008. Cyanobacterial poisoning in livestock, wild mammals and birds—An overview (PDF). Cyanobacterial harmful algal blooms: State of the science and research needs. *Adv. Exp. Med. Biol.* 619:613–637.

640. Stewart, I., P. M. Webb, P. J. Schluter, G. R. Shaw. 2006. Recreational and occupational field exposure to freshwater cyanobacteria—A review of anecdotal and case reports, epidemiological studies and the challenges for epidemiologic assessment. *Environ. Health* 5 (1):6.

641. Dixit, A., R. K. Dhaked, S. I. Alam, L. Singh. 2005. Military potential of biological neurotoxins. *Informa Healthcare* 24 (2):175–207.

642. Francis, G. 1878. Poisonous Australian lake. *Nature* 18 (444):11–12.

643. Edwards, N. *Anatoxin.* University of Sussex at Brighton. Updated 1 September 1999. Accessed January 19, 2011.

644. Miller, M. A. et al. 2010. Evidence for a novel marine harmful algal bloom: Cyanotoxin (Microcystin) transfer from land to sea otters. *PLoS ONE* 5 (9):e12576.

645. Harmful algal blooms event response NOAA, Center of Excellence for Great Lakes and Human Health. Accessed August 06, 2014.

646. Vasconcelos, V. 2006. Eutrophication, toxic cyanobacteria and cyanotoxins: When ecosystems cry for help (PDF). *Limnetica* 25 (1–2):425–432.

647. Forc, N.S.W.B.G.A.T. 1992. *Final Report of the NSW Blue-Green Algae Task Force*. Parramatta: NSW Department of Water Resources.

648. Herath, G. 1995. The algal bloom problem in Australian waterways: An economic appraisal. *Rev. Mark. Agric. Econ.* 63 (1):77–86.

649. Sivonen, K., G. Jones. 1999. Cyanobacterial toxins. In *Toxic Cyanobacteria in Water*, I. Chorus, J. Bartram, Eds., pp. 41–111. Geneva: WHO.

650. Pelaez, M. et al. 2009. Sources and occurrence of cyanotoxins worldwide. In *Xenobiotics in the Urban Water Cycle*, pp. 101–127. Vol. 16. Netherlands: Springer.

651. Sivonen, K., K. Kononen, W. W. Carmichael, A. M. Dahlem, K. L. Rinehart, J. Kiviranta, S. I. Niemela. 1989. Occurrence of the hepatotoxic cyanobacterium Nodularia spumigena in the Baltic Sea and structure of the toxin. *Appl. Environ. Microbiol.* 55 (8):1990–1995.

652. David, P., D. P. Fewer, K. Köykkä, K. Halinen, J. Jokela, C. Lyra, K. Sivonen. 2009. Culture-independent evidence for the persistent presence and genetic diversity of microcystin-producing Anabaena (Cyanobacteria) in the Gulf of Finland. *Environ. Microbiol.* 11 (4):855–866.

653. Rhoades, D. F. 1979. Evolution of plant chemical defense against herbivores. In *Herbivores: Their Interaction with Secondary Plant Metabolites*, G. A. Rosenthal, D. H. Janzen, Eds., p. 41. New York: Academic Press.

654. Carmichael, W. W, P. R. Gorham. 1978. Anatoxins from clones of Anabaena flos-aquae isolated from lakes of western Canada. *Mitt. Infernal. Verein. Limnol.* 21:285–295.

655. Carmichael, W. W, D. F. Biggs, P. R. Gorham. 1975. Toxicology and pharmacological action of Anabaena flos-aquae toxin. *Science* 187 (4176):542–544.

656. Yang, X. 2007. *Occurrence of the Cyanobacterial Neurotoxin, Anatoxin-a, in New York State Waters*. ProQuest.

657. Wood, S. A., J. P. Rasmussen, P. T. Holland, R. Campbell, A. L. M. Crowe. 2007. First report of the cyanotoxin anatoxin-A from Aphanizomenon issatschenkoi (Cyanobacteria). *J. Phycol.* 43 (2):356–365.

658. National Center for Environmental Assessment. Toxicological Reviews of Cyanobacterial Toxins: Anatoxin-a. NCEA-C-1743.

659. Devlin, J. P., O. E. Edwards, P. R. Gorham, N. R. Hunter, R. K. Pike, B. Stavric. 1977. Anatoxin-a, a toxic alkaloid from Anabaena flos-aquae NRC-44h. *Can. J. Chem.* 55 (8):1367–1371.

660. Moore, R. E. 1977. Toxins from blue-green algae. *BioScience* 27 (12):797–802.

661. Metcalf, J. S., G. A. Codd. 2009. Cyanobacteria, neurotoxins and water resources: Are there implications for human neurodegenerative disease? *Informa Healthcare* 10 (s2):74–78.

662. Byth, S. July 1980. Palm Island mystery disease. *Med. J. Aust.* 2 (1):40, 42.

663. Griffiths, D. J, M. L. Saker. 2003. The Palm Island mystery disease 20 years on: A review of research on the cyanotoxin cylindrospermopsin. *Environ. Toxicol.* 18 (2):78–93.

664. Kinnear, S. 2010. Cylindrospermopsin: A decade of progress on bioaccumulation research. *Mar. Drugs* 8:542–564. doi: 10.3390/md8030542

665. Clark, R. F., S. R. Williams, S. P. Nordt, A. S. Manoguerra. 1999. A review of selected seafood poisonings. *Undersea Hyperb. Med.* 26 (3):175–184.

666. Nakamuraa, M., Y. Oshimaa, T. Yasumoto. 1984. Occurrence of saxitoxin in puffer fish. *Toxicon* 22 (3):381–385.

667. Landsberg, J. H. 2002. The effects of harmful algal blooms on aquatic organisms. *Rev. Fish. Sci.* 10 (2):113–390.

668. Kao, C. Y., S. R. Levinson. 1986. *Tetrodotoxin, Saxitoxin, and the Molecular Biology of the Sodium Channel*. New York: Academy of Sciences.

669. *Chemical Weapons Convention: Schedule 1*. The Hague, Netherlands: Organisation for the Prohibition of Chemical Weapons. Accessed January 26, 2011.

670. Wallace, R., H. K. Melton, H. R. Schlesinger. 2009. *Spycraft: The Secret History of the CIA's Spytechs from Communism to Al-Qaeda*. USA: Penguin Group.

671. Stewart, I., P. J. Schluter, G. R. Shaw. 2006. Cyanobacterial lipopolysaccharides and human health—A review. *Environ. Health* 5 (1):7.

672. Cox, P. A., S. A. Banack, S. J. Murch, U. Rasmussen, G. Tien, R. R. Bidigare, J. S. Metcalf, L. F. Morrison, G. A. Codd, B. Bergman. 2005. Diverse taxa of cyanobacteria produce b-N-methylamino-L-alanine, a neurotoxic amino acid. *PNAS* 102 (14):5074–5078.

673. Esterhuizen, M., T. G. Downing. 2008. β-N-methylamino-L-alanine (BMAA) in novel South African cyanobacterial isolates. *Ecotoxicol. Environ. Safety* 71 (2):309–313.

674. Weiss, J. H., J. Koh, D. Choi. 1989. Neurotoxicity of β-N-methylamino-L-alanine (BMAA) and β-N-oxalylamino-L-alanine (BOAA) on cultured cortical neurons. *Brain Res.* 497 (1):64–71.

675. Lobner, D., P. M. Piana, A. K. Salous, R. W. Peoples. 2007. β-N-methylamino-L-alanine enhances neurotoxicity through multiple mechanisms. *Neurobiol. Dis.* 25 (2):360–366.

676. EPA (Environmental Protection Agency). 2005. *Drinking Infrastructure Needs Survey and Assessment.* Third Report to Congress. June 2005. Accessed December 13, 2005. http://www.epa.gov/safewater/needssurvey/pdfs/2003/report_needssurvey_2003.pdf

677. Plastic pipe taints other water sources Texas, Arkansas confirm presence of vinyl chloride. *Kansas City Star,* 21 March, A4.

678. Merck Index. 1996. 12th ed. Whitehouse Station, NJ: Merck and Co., Inc.

679. Letterman, R. 1999. *Water Quality and Treatment,* 5th ed., pp. 2.43–2.46. New York: McGraw Hill, Inc.

680. Cherry, R., F. Cherry. 1974. What's in the water we drink?. *The New York Times Magazine,* p. 38, December 8.

681. Duirk, S. E., C. Lindell, C. C. Cornelison, J. Kormos, T. A. Ternes, M. Attene-Ramos, J. Osiol, E. D. Wagner, M. J. Plewa, S. D. Richardson. 2011. Formation of toxic iodinated disinfection by-products from compounds used in medical imaging. *Environ. Sci. Technol.* 15 (16):6845–6854.

682. Jackson, R. 2013. *Natural gas found in drinking water near fracked wells.* Accessed September 15, 2017. http://science.nbcnews.com/_news/2013/06/24/19117694-natural-gas-found-in-drinking-water-near-fracked-wells?lite

683. Emmett, E. A., F. S. Shofer, H. Zhang, D. Freeman, C. Desai, L. M. Shaw. 2006. Community exposure to perfluorooctanoate: Relationships between serum concentrations and exposure sources. *J. Occup. Environ. Med.* 48 (8):759–770.

684. Steenland, K., C. Jin, J. MacNeil, C. Lally, A. Ducatman, V. Vieira, T. Fletcher. 2009. Predictors of PFOA levels in a community surrounding a chemical plant. *Environ. Health Perspect.* 117:1083–1088.

685. Vieira, V., T. Webster, S. Bartell, K. Steenland, D. Savitz, T. Fletcher. 2008. PFOA community health studies: Exposure via drinking water contaminated by a Teflon manufacturing facility. *Organohalogen Compds.* 70:730–732.

686. Webster, T. F. 2000. Bias in Ecologic and Semi-individual Studies [*PhD dissertation*]. Boston, MA: Boston University.

687. Bartell, S. 2003. Statistical Methods for Nonsteady State Exposure Inference Using Biomarkers [*PhD dissertation*]. Davis, CA: University of California–Davis.

688. Renner, R. 2001. Growing concern over perfluorinated chemicals. *Environ. Sci. Technol.* 35 (7):154A–160A.

689. Lau, C., K. Anitole, C. Hodes, D. Lai, A. Pfahles-Hutchens, J. Seed. 2007. Perfluoroalkyl acids: A review of monitoring and toxicological findings. *Toxicol. Sci.* 99 (2):366–394.

690. Trudel, D., L. Horowitz, M. Wormuth, M. Scheringer, I. T. Cousins, K. Hungerbuhler. 2008. Estimating consumer exposure to PFOS and PFOA. *Risk Anal.* 28 (2):251–269.

691. Bartell, S. M., A. M. Calafat, C. Lyu, K. Kato, P. B. Ryan, K. Steenland. 2010. Rate of decline in serum PFOA concentrations after granular activated carbon filtration at two public water systems in Ohio and West Virginia. *Environ. Health Perspect.* 118:222–228.

692. Olsen, G. W., D. C. Mair, W. K. Reagen, M. E. Ellefson, D. J. Ehresman, J. L. Butenhoff, L. R. Zobel. 2007. Preliminary evidence of a decline in perfluorooctanesulfonate (PFOS) and perfluorooctanoate (PFOA) concentrations in American Red Cross blood donors. *Chemosphere* 68 (1):105–111.

693. Calafat, A. M., Z. Kuklenyik, J. A. Reidy, S. P. Caudill, J. S. Tully, L. L. Needham. 2007. Serum concentrations of 11 polyfluoroalkyl compounds in the U.S. population: Data from the National Health and Nutrition Examination Survey (NHANES). *Environ. Sci. Technol.* 41 (7):2237–2242.

694. Calafat, A. M., L. Y. Wong, Z. Kuklenyik, J. A. Reidy, L. L. Needham. 2007. Polyfluoroalkyl chemicals in the U.S. population: data from the National Health and Nutrition Examination Survey (NHANES) 2003–2004 and comparisons with NHANES 1999–2000. *Environ. Health Perspect.* 115:1596–1602.

695. Lau, C., J. L. Butenhoff, J. M. Rogers. 2004. The developmental toxicity of perfluoroalkyl acids and their derivatives. *Toxicol. Appl. Pharmacol.* 198 (2):231–241.

696. Steenland, K., T. Fletcher, D. A. Savitz. 2010. Epidemiologic evidence on the health effects of perfluorooctanoic acid (PFOA). *Environ. Health Perspect.* 118:1100–1108.

697. U.S. EPA (Environmental Protection Agency). 2010. Perfluorooctanoic Acid (PFOA) and Fluorinated Telomers. Enforceable Consent Agreement (ECA) Process to Generate Additional Information. Accessed August 16, 2010. http://www.epa.gov/opptintr/pfoa/pubs/eca.html

698. U.S. EPA. 2004. *Memorandum of Understanding between the US Environmental Protection Agency and E. I. DuPont De Nemours and Company for a Perfluorooctanoic Acid (PFOA) Site-Related Environmental Assessment Program.* Washington, DC: U.S. Environmental Protection Agency. EPA-HQ-OPPT-2004-0113-0002

699. Paustenbach, D. J., J. M. Panko, P. K. Scott, K. M. Unice. 2007. A methodology for estimating human exposure to perfluorooctanoic acid (PFOA): A retrospective exposure assessment of a community (1951–2003). *J. Toxicol. Environ. Health A* 70 (1):28–57.

700. U.S. EPA (Environmental Protection Agency). 2010. *Perfluorooctanoic Acid (PFOA) and Fluorinated Telomers.* 2009 Annual Progress Reports. Accessed August 16, 2010. http://www.epa.gov/opptintr/pfoa/pubs/stewardship/preports3.html#2008

701. Frisbee, S. J. et al. 2009. The C8 Health Project: Design, methods, and participants. *Environ. Health Perspect.* 117:1873–1882.

702. Hölzer, J., O. Midasch, K. Rauchfuss, M. Kraft, R. Reupert, J. Angerer, P. Kleeschulte, N. Marschall, M. Wilhelm. 2008. Biomonitoring of perfluorinated compounds in children and adults exposed to perfluorooctanoate-contaminated drinking water. *Environ. Health Perspect.* 116:651–657.

703. Björk, J., U. Strömberg. 2002. Effects of systematic exposure assessment errors in partially ecologic case–control studies. *Int. J. Epidemiol.* 31 (1):154–160.

704. Webster, T. F. 2000. Bias in Ecologic and Semi-individual Studies [*PhD dissertation*]. Boston, MA: Boston University.

705. Webster, T. F. 2002. Commentary: Does the spectre of ecologic bias haunt epidemiology? *Int. J. Epidemiol.* 31:161–162.

706. Fromme, H. et al. 2007. Exposure of an adult population to perfluorinated substances using duplicate diet portions and biomonitoring data. *Environ. Sci. Technol.* 41 (22):7928–7933.

707. Kuklenyik, Z., J. A. Reich, J. S. Tully, L. L. Needham, A. M. Calafat. 2004. Automated solid-phase extraction and measurement of perfluorinated organic acids and amides in human serum and milk. *Environ. Sci. Technol.* 38 (13):3698–3704.

708. U.S. EPA. 2004. *DuPont PFOA Site-Related Monitoring and Environmental Assessment at Washington, West Virginia.* Washington, DC: U.S. Environmental Protection Agency. EPA-HQ-OPPT-2004-0113

709. Butenhoff, J. L., G. L. Kennedy Jr., P. M. Hinderliter, P. H. Lieder, R. Jung, K. J. Hansen, G. S. Gorman, P. E. Noker, P. J. Thomford. 2004. Pharmacokinetics of perfluorooctanoate in cynomolgus monkeys. *Toxicol. Sci.* 82 (2):394–406.

710. U.S. EPA. 1997. *Exposure Factors Handbook (Final Report).* Washington, DC: U.S. Environmental Protection Agency. EPA/600/P-95/002F a-c

711. U.S. EPA. 2009. *Provisional Health Advisories for Perfluorooctanoic Acid (PFOA) and Perfluorooctane Sulfonate (PFOS).* Washington, DC: U.S. Environmental Protection Agency. EPA-HQ-OW-2007-1189-0183

712. Rodwan, J. G. Jr. 2009. *Confronting challenges. U.S. and international bottled water developments and statistics for 2008.* Bottled Water Reporter. April/May 2009.

713. Doss, J. K. 2008. Written testimony of Joseph K. Doss, President and CEO, International Bottled Water Association before the Subcommittee on Transportation Safety, Infrastructure Security, and Water Quality of the Environment and Public Works Committee, United States Senate; Hearing on Quality and Environmental Impacts of Bottled Water. September 10, 2008.

714. EWG (Environmental Working Group). 2008. Bottled Water Quality Investigation: 10 Major Brands, 38 Pollutants. Accessed July 5, 2009. http://www.ewg.org/reports/bottledwater

715. NRDC (National Resources Defense Council). 1999. Bottled water. Pure drink or pure hype? Accessed July 5, 2009. http://www.nrdc.org/water/drinking/bw/exesum.asp

716. EWG (Environmental Working Group). 2005. National Tap Water Quality Database. Accessed July 5, 2009. http://www.ewg.org/sites/tapwater/

717. Gibson, S., J. Johnson. 1979. *U.S. EPA Public Docket AR-226-0455.* St Paul, MN: 3M Company, Riker Laboratories. Absorption of FC–143–^{14}C in Rats after a Single Oral Dose.

718. U.S. EPA. 2004. Report 822R04003. *Drinking Water Health Advisory for Manganese.* Washington, DC: U.S. EPA.

719. Ljung, K., M. Vahter. 2007. Time to re-evaluate the guideline value for manganese in drinking water? *Environ. Health Perspect.* 115:1533–1538.

720. Smith, D., Gwiazda, R., Bowler, R. et al. 2007. Biomarkers of Mn exposure in humans. *Am. J. Ind. Med.* 50:801–811.

721. On Scene Coordinator Report on Deepwater Horizon Oil Spill (PDF) (Report). September 2011. Retrieved February 22, 2013. http://www.uscg.mil/foia/docs/dwh/fosc_dwh_report.pdf

4 Evaluation of Food and Food Contaminants

INTRODUCTION

The prevalence of hypersensitivity-related diseases, food intolerance, and chemical sensitivities in both the pediatric and adult population has increased dramatically over the last few years. Randolph[1] and Dickey[2] described the problem. The accelerating rates associated with morbidity, hypersensitivity, food intolerance, chronic degenerative disease, and chemical sensitivity are frequently the result of the total environmental pollutant overload in response to a significant instituting of toxic electromagnetic frequency (EMF) exposure or a chronic unrelenting series of exposures such as teeth fillings, breast implants, and other metal and synthetic prosthesis of which there are 220.

Among sensitized individuals, exposed to assorted inciting stimuli, many precipitate diverse sensitivities with or without immune sequelae with pathology but usually with transient or permanent and altered physiology. These transient and immune-altered physiologic responses are evidenced by clinical food sensitivity as well as varied lymphocyte, complements antibody (gamma globulin), vanilloid receptors, and/or oxidative cytokine responses which often results in inflammation. Recently, chemical and EMF exposures are recognized as the mechanism of disease development, and the resultant sensitivity-related illnesses (SRIs) may involve any major organ system, including the CNS, MS, GI, and GU or cardiovascular system. The majority of these have been observed to have food sensitivity as part of their problem. These illnesses may involve major neuropsychological manifestations from pollutant and food injury with accelerating rates of chemical exposure and bioaccumulation of these substances in the general population (GP) even though they do not always perceive them. An environmental proportion of chronic illness is overwhelmingly due to this food and chemical phenomenon.

The incidence and prevalence of allergy-related diseases, including asthma,[3] atopic dermatitis,[4] hay fever,[5] food allergy,[6–8] atopic conjunctivitis,[9] and eosinophilic esophagitis[10] have escalated considerably in the last two decades as has vascular inflammation as shown in the previous chapters. There has been increasing recognition, however, that not all sensitivities, including many types of food intolerance and chemical hypersensitivity reactions, are related to the classically understood concept of allergic phenomenon involving immunoglobulin (Ig)-E antibody-mediated allergic responses.[11–13] Food intolerance, for example, can precipitate a variety of outcomes, including headache, eczema, rhinosinusitis, vascular spasm, and cardiac arrhythmia that are unrelated to atopic disease.[14] To others working in the field, this increase in sensitivity is due to pollutant overload in our air, food, and water triggering the intracellular mechanisms making Ca^{2+} combining with protein kinase A and C and then being phosphorylated. Many of the other clinical phenomena include multiple neurovascular syndromes such as small vessel vasculopathy colitis, enteritis myotoxicity, neuritis, neuropathy, encephalopathy, and so on. For all of these, food sensitivity is part of the problem.

SRI, such as chemical sensitivity, therefore, refers to adverse clinical states elicited by exposure to low-dose diverse environmental triggers, including inhalants (such as pollens, molds, and terpenes), chemicals (such as natural gas, pesticides, herbicides, formaldehydes, synthetic perfumes, etc.), foodstuffs (such as gluten, casein, but more often specific food sensitivities, i.e., wheat, milk, and soy), and other various intolerances, biological compounds (such as molds, bacteria, virus, foods, and synthetic implants), or electrical stimuli[15] (such as electromagnetic radiation, smart meters, cell phones). Among individuals with SRI, there may be marked variation in the nature of the clinical or immune response, and sensitivity reactions may be apparent from early life, or may present as acquired problems where no preexisting difficulty was apparently evident.

Origins of SRI

Several determinants and mechanisms have been implicated in the escalating prevalence of SRI since Randolph[1] and Dickey[2] described and defined the problem. Etiological variables discussed in the literature as contributing to sensitivity states include microbial deprivation as described in the hygiene hypothesis,[16,17] nutritional transition and other factors resulting in arginine deficiency states,[18,19] environmental pollution with exposure to gaseous and particulate components of air contamination,[20] dissemination and widespread consumption of genetically modified foods,[21] climate change and meteorological and electromagnetic features,[22] and genetic factors.[23] It is unlikely, however, that the rise in SRI is primarily related to new genetic determinants as it is improbable that a sudden deterioration has occurred in the gene pool causing a ubiquitous propensity to sensitivity states. Furthermore, the marked disparity in geographic distribution of sensitivity-related health problems, including diseases such as asthma, points to environmental variables other than genomic variance.[24] However, it has been reported that environmental overload can alter genetics. This may be an overwhelming way that SRI occurs.

Several scientists and clinicians throughout the world have observed and studied specific events which appear to suggest a credible explanation for the emergence and rapid escalation in SRI. The 9/11 tragedy and recent warfare as occurred in the Gulf War and all the other acute disasters, such as the Gulf of Mexico oil spill, have shown that a significant percentage of previously well individuals working in theaters with toxicant exposures were noted to subsequently develop sensitivity conditions, hypersensitive states, and undiagnosed illnesses that were nonexistent prior to the exposures.[25–29] Severe health problems and previously nonexistent sensitivities were also documented in various survivors of the 1984 Bhopal industrial catastrophe in India where about a half million people were exposed to various toxins released by a pesticide plant.[30] Several case series and reports in the scientific literature have described a similar phenomenon of individuals developing previously nonexistent sensitivities following exposure to toxic insults.[31–34] It has also been noted that toxicant-exposed persons are considerably more likely to develop sensitivity-related health problems such as asthma.[35] In a recent book, Pall cites two dozen separate studies illustrating toxicant exposure as a prelude to the development of SRI.[36] In all probability, the disturbance of the cell membrane which allows Ca^{2+} to enter the cell may be the problem. When Ca^{2+} enters the cell, it can combine with protein kinase A and C. Then, when this complex is phosphorylated, it can increase the sensitivity 1000 times.[37] This can then disturb the food handling mechanism and propagate the illness by just eating the sensitive foods.[1,2,6]

Studies on workers occupationally exposed to various toxicants, for example, have revealed an increased prevalence of SRI[38,39] with significant differences between exposed versus nonexposed employees within the same occupation.[38] Dental employees exposed to mercury during amalgam removal, for instance, were noted to develop higher rates of symptoms suggestive of SRI.[40] Many other papers also report on sensitivity issues.[6]

Any major exposure or toxicant insult that is foreign to the body has the potential alone or in combination with other toxic stressors to induce or initiate a hypersensitivity state especially for foods. The primary toxicant insult or combination of insults may originate from various sources: (1) adverse chemical exposure—single major exposure or chronic low-dose chemical exposure, (2) insertion of foreign material into the body such as an implant,[41–44] (3) biological exposure such as an infection with mold or associated mycotoxins,[45] (4) major electrical or nuclear exposure,[46] (5) previous viral infection, that is, polio or recurrent neurovascular disease, that is, mononucleosis or bee sting, repetition,[6] (6) vast immunizations[6] given at once, and (7) head trauma, isolated but usually repeated.[6]

All of these can trigger the food handling mechanism leading to a constant triggering of illness by dust and daily living.

Although SRI can result from a single toxic insult, it appears that the path to SRI is determined by the total body pollutant load or the total body pollutant burden of accumulated exposures; the greater the total burden of accumulated exposures, the greater the total body burden of pollutants, the more likely a state of diminished tolerance and hypersensitivity ensues. Exposures contributing to the initiation of SRI may commence at any time during the life cycle, including the gestational phase through vertical transmission.[47] Prior to death, this total body pollutant overload can trigger the adverse food handling ability creating constant illness.

Exposure to primary toxicants may occur through ingestion, inhalation, dermal exposure, olfactory intake, vertical transmission as well as through injection or implantation as typically occurs with dental work, and surgical devices implantation. Adverse chemical exposures and mold exposure through the nose and respiratory tract appear to be the most common routes commencing after exposure to contaminated air in building settings[32,33,47–50] although EMF exposure is rapidly vying with the previously mentioned. Furthermore, the epidemiological escalation of SRI in the GP appears to have mirrored the rising prevalence of exposure by the population at large to multiple adverse agents in the environment such as pesticides, natural gas, and EMF transmitters. Finally, it has also been observed that SRI can be induced in animals by exposure to toxic insults (Figure 4.1).[51–53]

Rather than one specific type of chemical exposure, many different kinds of chemical agents have been implicated of which there are a myriad, such as natural gas, pesticides, herbicides, formaldehydes, volatile organic chemicals, and particulates. Also, molds and their mycotoxin metabolites whose total load can cause food sensitivities,[54–57] various types of pesticides, food additives, and gas, toxic foods,[58] solvents,[39] hydrogen sulfide,[59] and some toxic metals such as mercury[60,61] have been noted to instigate SRI. Initiation may develop after a single high-level exposure or insidiously after months or years of low-level exposure.[62] Initiating events, for example, may include exposures in situations such as a pesticide exposure, a natural gas leak in an apartment, employment in an auto body shop, close proximity to a gas well blowout or fracking, indoor air contamination following renovation, clerical work, off gassing from new office equipment, and so on. Medication used during gestation such as maternal antibiotic use can also act as an initiating agent for subsequent postnatal SRI.[63] All of these can trigger food sensitivity which then propagates the problem.

In response to an accumulated toxicant threshold, a state of impaired tolerance is initiated, which may develop within days of a serious primary exposure.[12] The degree of impaired tolerance or hypersensitivity often parallels the intensity of the total burden of bioaccumulated toxicants. Furthermore, the level of hypersensitivity is not fixed: If the body burden of toxicants is diminished, the hypersensitivity slowly begins to wane and individuals react to lesser degrees; if the body burden continues to accumulate, the hypersensitivity response worsens with more pronounced symptoms and sensitivity to an increasingly wider array of inciting compounds.[63] A clinical outcome ensues whereby minute exposures to assorted triggers evoke diverse signs and symptoms.[64] Minute exposures to foods can then propagate the sensitivity, causing chronic fatigue and brain dysfunction.

Triggering of SRI

Following the initiation phase, the exposed individual becomes hyperreactive to low levels of a wide spectrum of chemical, inhalant, food, or even electrical exposures that are not bothersome to healthy people. Specific incitants are not necessarily chemically related to the primary initiating exposure[65]—for example, a soldier initially exposed to chemical weapons which initiated the toxicant induced loss of tolerance (TILT) state may subsequently become sensitive to specific perfumes or cleaning agents and foods absent from the war theater. Between individuals, there will be variance in specific triggers—the exact nature of which presumably depends on various determinants, including the nature of the total load of exposures and the unique genomic background of that individual. Almost always, these patients become sensitive to specific foods which helps continue the problem and often deters healing. This food sensitivity is often masked until overdose for 4–7 days occurs or intradermal prevention is carried out.

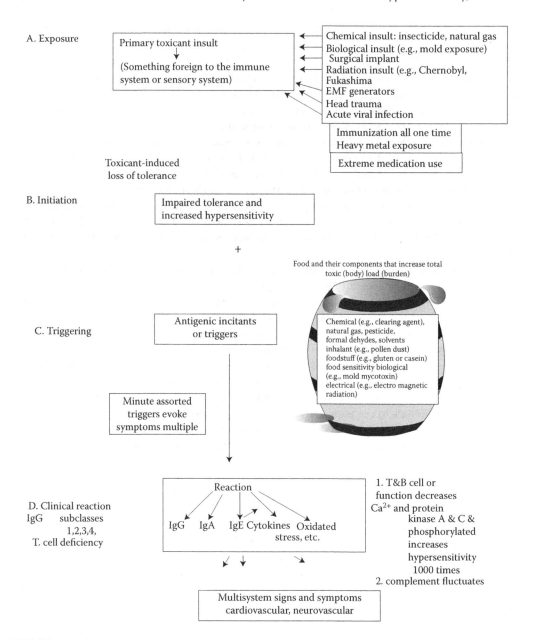

FIGURE 4.1 Sensory-related illness. (Adapted from Rea, W. J. 1992. *Chemical Sensitivity*, Vol. 1, p. 47. Boca Raton, FL: Lewis Publishers.)

Possible incitants include a wide array of chemicals such as automobile exhaust, flavoring agents in foods, assorted perfumes, petrochemicals, air fresheners, off-gassed household materials from carpets or paint, newsprint odors, synthetic chemicals from clothing, fillers in medications, and many more.[1,2,6] Incitants also include an array of foods as well as the additives within the foodstuffs. Germs such as bacteria, viruses, parasites, or molds in the environment can evoke reactions, as can inhalants such as pollens and terpenes. Some types of electromagnetic radiation as found with certain types of artificial lighting, smart meters, Wi-Fi, computers, and TV may also induce cytokine disturbances and trigger SRI.[66]

Although the assorted triggers evoking symptoms may vary considerably between individuals, it has repeatedly been demonstrated that certain triggers such as wheat, corn, milk, soy, monosodium glutamate (MSG), genetically modified organisms (GMOs), and pesticide-polluted foods, perfumes, and cleaners are common inciting stimuli especially for producing food sensitivities. In any one individual, it is often proportionate to the body burden of toxicants in that person; individuals with a heavy underlying total pollutant load will invariably have multiple triggers. Various publications are available which provide lists and tables of common triggers.[67]

Triggering responses can occur at incitant levels below olfactory threshold concentration levels, where the individual might not smell or sense the trigger.[12] The specific incitants triggering the reactions usually include compounds that the individual is frequently exposed to within their life—sensitivity tends to develop to agents that the body frequently encounters such as foods. Accordingly, the circle of intolerance[12] can change if individuals stay away from some compounds for a while or are exposed to new ones, and the circle will expand and contract depending on the ongoing severity of the initiating underlying burden of toxicants. The end result is that there are common compounds that most sensitive people react to which appears to be based on the frequency of previous exposure to these given antigens in their environment, that is, sensitized individuals usually become sensitive to antigens that are ubiquitous in their environment such as pollens, or compounds that they are frequently exposed to in their diet such as food, MSG, wheat, milk, soy, sugar, and casein.

Some toxic compounds act to initiate TILT, but these same compounds may also subsequently act as triggers for reactions. For example, cleaning solutions or biological compounds such as molds or foods can intensify the underlying toxicant load as well as provoking sensitivity reactions. Pharmaceutical products, compounds that are inherently foreign to the human body, can also add to the total burden of foreign compounds. Some drugs and fillers or excipients have within their preparations substances such as corn starch, lactose, or wheat which frequently act as incitants in susceptible hosts. As many chronically ill people are on several pharmaceuticals, these agents are often a source of ongoing stimulus,[68] including food sensitivity which will propagate the illness.

It has also been observed that some SRI patients with recurrent psychiatric manifestations appear to experience exacerbation of illness during seasons of high inhalant exposure from common environmental incitants such as mold, pollens, and weeds.[69] A recent study, for example, confirmed a significant positive association between allergy scores and anxiety scores.[70] Some mental health providers have casually referred to seasons of high inhalant exposure as the "bipolar season" because of anecdotal observation of increased admission rates to psychiatric facilities in such time periods. Foods and food intolerance are frequently overlooked in these seasons even though they may have a concurrent situation with some pollens and molds.

Food can influence the health of the chemically sensitive patient and patient with chronic degenerative disease in many ways. Depending on its nutritive quality, the natural toxic effects of food itself, and/or the additives and preservatives used to grow and treat it along with an individual's sensitivity to a particular food can affect either positively or negatively an individual's total pollutant load (burden), and thus his health. It cannot be emphasized enough that food and its contaminants are an important factor in both the development and treatment of chemical sensitivity and chronic degenerative disease. Also, because pollutant injury can cause excess or deficient nutrients intracellularly in the chemically sensitive patient and patient with chronic degenerative disease, adequate intake of less toxic nutrients is essential for good health. This intake which can occur for many years gradually shapes the susceptibility of the chemically sensitive patient and patient with chronic degenerative disease for poor health and wellness.

FOOD GROWN IN CONTAMINATED WATERS

Acidification of the world's oceans is already damaging coral reefs and could produce other unexpected chemical and biological consequences. Researchers now report that at low pH, phytoplankton take up less iron, a key nutrient needed for photosynthesis and growth. The results suggest ocean acidification could have a profound impact on these tiny one-celled plants which reside at the bottom of the food web and support commercially important fisheries.[71]

Seawater becomes more acidic when atmospheric carbon dioxide (CO_2) absorbed by the water is converted into carbonic acid. The acidity of oceans is changing very rapidly. The hydrogen ion concentration of surface ocean water (a reflection of pH) is now about 30% higher than it was 200 years ago, while atmospheric concentrations of CO_2 have risen by about 38%. Most of the research focus has been on how ocean acidification negatively impacts marine creatures, such as mollusks and corals that form shells or exoskeletons from calcium carbonate. Little attention has been paid to how increasing acidity changes the chemistry and biological availability of essential nutrients.

Shi et al.[72] measured the uptake of iron in *Thalassiosira weissflogii*, *Thalassiosira oceanica*, *Phaeodactylum tricornutum*, and *Emiliania huxleyi*. As the pH was lowered of model laboratory culture media from 8.6 to 7.7, they observed a significant decrease in the rate of iron uptake by all species. A similar trend occurred when laboratory phytoplankton were placed in natural seawater collected off the New Jersey coast and the open ocean near Bermuda. The average iron uptake rate decreased by 10%–20% between the highest and lowest pH conditions in natural seawater. "The average pH of ocean water today is 8.08."[71]

Much of the iron in ocean water is strongly bound to natural organic chelators, such as siderophores, which bind and release iron in different ways.[71] The team examined the effect on iron uptake of three chemically different model chelators, the synthetic chelator ethylenediaminetetraacetic acid (EDTA) and two siderophores, desferriferrioxamine B (DFB) and azotochelin. As the pH dropped, iron availability was dramatically reduced by EDTA and moderately reduced by DFB, but was unchanged by azotochelin.[71]

One conceivable consequence of limited iron due to ocean acidification could be a decline in phytoplankton populations, resulting in reduced fish harvests for human consumption. The thing they documented is a decrease in the bioavailability of dissolved iron in four laboratory organisms.

Phytoplankton species perform almost all marine photosynthesis, from air into organic matter and oxygen. Some of this organic matter sinks, carrying carbon into the deep oceans.[71] Calculations estimate this "carbon pump" has absorbed about a quarter of the CO_2 emitted by human activities. A decrease in iron availability through ocean acidification could restrict this carbon pump, resulting in an increase in atmospheric CO_2.[71]

On the other hand, marine organisms may evolve their own nutritional coping strategies. For instance, Sunda and colleagues[73] recently discovered that members of the bacterial genus *Marinobacter*, which live in close contact with phytoplankton that cause harmful algal blooms, produce a novel siderophore that tightly binds iron in the dark.[71] But when exposed to sunlight, the siderophore breaks down and releases an unbound form of iron that the phytoplankton readily takes up to drive photosynthesis. The relationship is mutually beneficial; when the *Marinobacter* and phytoplankton species are grown separately, both grow poorly compared with when they grow together.

Fish and shellfish are important and desirable sources of nutrition for many people. However, chemical and biological (bacteria, pathogens, metals such as mercury) contaminants can accumulate in fish and shellfish, making it unhealthy to consume them, especially in large quantities as shown earlier in this book.

Most states sample fish in their waters and then issue fish consumption advisories as a way of informing the public of risks associated with eating certain types and sizes of fish from certain bodies of contaminated water. Advisories are based on fish tissue monitoring data collected by states and tribes and are largely focused on areas of known or suspected contamination.

As one can observe, from 2009, the catfish which are bottom fish are still loaded with pesticide. Even DDT and DDE products are still present in the modern-day catfish. This makes them undesirable to eat. The bigger fish that eat them will also be contaminated.

PESTICIDE IN CATFISH

Overwhelmingly, the DDT toxics were still seen in catfish in 2009. The predominant one was DDE_{ppb} in 65% of the catfish and DDD_{ppb} in 29.8% of the fish. This was followed by *o,p*-DDD in

8.3%, dioxin in 7%, toxaphene in 6.4%, and endosulfan sulfate in 5.9%. These were followed by cypermethrins, endosulfans, esfenvalerates, hexachlorobenzenes, lindane, MGR-264, nonochlors, oxadiazon, piperonal, butexines, 4 varies other in fractions. It is clear that the old, long degradatory pesticides are still contaminating the catfish which are bottom feeders. Other lake fish had levels of Hg in them.

Mercury

Mercury is now found in all ocean fish due to the massive amount of Hg rained down from melting of the polar ice caps every year. The amount is established to be about 200 tons which then is eventually in the food chain of the sea.[71]

In the United States, 14% of the river miles, 28% of lake acreage, and 100% of the Great Lakes and their connecting waters are under fish consumption advisories meaning that the fish are contaminated with toxics. They have the potential of affecting health adversely. Those percentages have increased in recent years (Figure 4.2). The majority of chemically sensitive cannot eat fish for this reason.

Due to severe water contamination, fish advisories that limit or restrict consumption, especially of top-level predators (e.g., walleye and lake trout), are widespread across the United States. Advisories are issued for various contaminants. Mercury, dioxin, and polychlorinated biphenyls

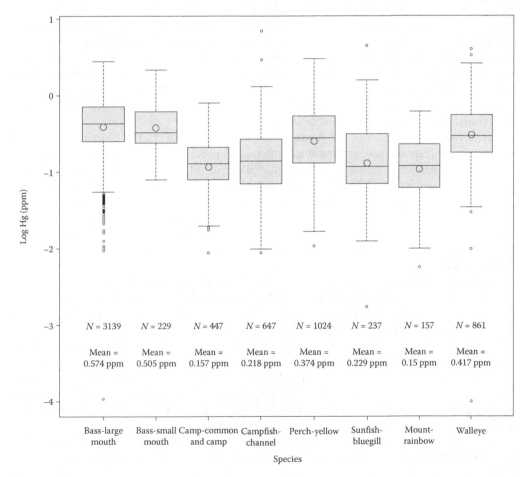

FIGURE 4.2 Log mercury level in the fish. (Adapted from EPA's Draft Report on the Environment 2003. Purer Water. Chapter 2, pp. 2–10.)

(PCBs) are responsible for many of the advisories throughout the United States. In January 2001, EPA and the U.S. Food and Drug Administration issued a nationwide advisory for women who are pregnant or may become pregnant. Combinations of these toxics are not looked into; therefore, the problems of multiple toxicity and sensitivities are not even looked into. The combination can make these problems much more severe.

Toxic chemicals enter the water of the Great Lakes (and therefore fish) from the atmosphere, industry effluents to tributaries, and sediments. They contain toxic substances from all the farms and ranches, and chemicals due to contamination of land from both farming and industry in the Midwest and the rest of the United States. These chemicals can be retained by plants and animals and increase in concentration through the food chain (bioaccumulation). Environmental data and modeling were used to estimate the relative contributions from each pathway to Lake Michigan. Total contaminant loads have decreased since the 1970s, and atmospheric deposition has increased in importance over time because of decreases in direct discharges to the lake and levels in sediments (Figure 4.2).

HYPERSENSITIVITY AND SENSITIZATION DURING CHILDHOOD ASSOCIATED WITH PRENATAL AND LACTATIONAL EXPOSURE TO MARINE POLLUTANTS

As shown in the Chippewa studies, exposures to marine contaminants are of much concern to populations that rely on seafood for their livelihood. Among the main contaminants resulting in increased exposures, methylmercury and PCBs share immunotoxic potentials.[74-76] Immunotoxicity is of particular concern when the exposures happen during the development of the neurovascular and immune system. Important windows of vulnerability are the intrauterine and the early postnatal periods, when unique immune maturational events take place.[77] Breast-feeding is thought to play an important role for the infant's immune system development, but the evidence is equivocal in regard to the extent of possible protection against allergic disease,[78-81] because of the toxic substances that pass through the placenta and the mother's milk.

As illustrated by studies on 2, 3, 7, 8-tetrachlorodibenzo-p-dioxin (TCDD),[82] an immunotoxicant may disrupt different immune maturational processes, depending upon the specific developmental timing of exposure.[77] Because the development of T-helper cell type 2 (Th2) functions is favored prenatally, and acquisition of Th1 functional capacities happens postnatal, the effects may depend on the age at peak exposure. For substances such as methylmercury, the peak exposure occurs during prenatal development, when the fetus shares the contaminant from the mother's diet; human milk is not an important exposure pathway for this substance.[83] However, lipophilic contaminants, such as PCBs, accumulate postnatally, so longer breast-feeding periods will result in higher body burdens in the child.[84,85]

Exposures to PCBs, methylmercury, and related substances are increased in the Arctic region,[74-76] especially where marine mammals are part of the traditional diet. The prevalence of allergy in the Arctic has generally been assumed to be low,[86] although the degree of sensitization has been dramatically increasing toward the end of the last millennium.[87]

Grandjean et al.[88] carried out a prospective study of a birth cohort in the Faroe Islands, a North Atlantic fishing community with increased average dietary exposures to methylmercury and PCBs from pilot whale meat and blubber.[89] Extended breast-feeding was common in this community.[90] Outcome parameters were total level of immunoglobulin E (IgE), grass-specific IgE, and occurrence of allergic disease. These studies did not look into each chemically sensitive and other hypersensitive mechanisms which might have given a more dismal picture.

According to Grandjean et al.[88] the strength of this study is that a population-based birth cohort was followed prospectively with repeated assessment of exposures to marine contaminants for comparison with the allergy and sensitization status up to 7 years of age. Compared with other populations, average exposures to both PCBs and methylmercury were high and ranges of exposures were wide, thereby adding statistical power to the study. Almost 90% of the children participated in the examinations at 5 and/or 7 years of age, and Grandjean et al. obtained IgE data at age 7 years from 71% of the children.

As a main finding, serum PCB concentrations at 7 years of age were positively associated with total IgE concentrations. Grandjean et al.[88] observed a similar tendency for the prenatal methylmercury exposure, although this correlation could be due to chance. Longer duration of breast-feeding also appeared to predict a higher IgE concentration at 7 years of age, but adjustment for the effect of PCB exposure reduced this association so that a chance finding could not be ruled out. For the grass-specific IgE concentration, the duration of breast-feeding again showed a positive correlation, now without a concomitant association with PCB. In addition, they observed an inverse association between grass-specific IgE levels and prenatal methylmercury exposure. Regarding clinical diagnoses, prenatal PCB exposures were inversely associated with a history of atopic dermatitis but showed a weak positive association with asthma. These diverse findings suggest that mechanisms for immunotoxicant effects for total and grass-specific IgE differ from those for asthma and atopic dermatitis. Indeed, we see this discrepancy all the time as the IgE is usually normal in the chemically sensitive patient. Since Grandjean's study group was the one who ate a lot of seafood, the toxics may have attacked cell walls causing the Ca^{2+} protein kinase A and C mechanism when phosphorylated increasing hypersensitivity. This mechanism could have triggered the asthma and other poorly correlated IgE mechanisms resulting in another type of hypersensitivity.

Because they based the clinical assessment of atopic disease only on examinations at ages 5 and 7 years and on maternal interview, the study cannot elucidate the possible role of immunotoxicants in the complex pathophysiological origins of these conditions. However, IgE concentrations have become routine clinical parameters in allergological diagnostics.[91] They chose total IgE as a marker of general IgE synthesis, and IgE specific to grass (*Phleum pratense*) as an important marker of sensitization, because grass pollen is ubiquitous and has previously been demonstrated to be the most common allergen in other North Atlantic environments.[86,92] Of course this is not necessarily true anymore. For grass pollen, they found 39 positives, corresponding to a sensitization rate of 8.3%, which is slightly lower than found in Western Greenland at 5–18 years of age; this difference is consistent with the lower age of their study population.

Markers of allergic reactions have previously been reported to be associated with a variety of environmental factors.[93–95] Sensitization reflected by a specific IgE is not necessarily governed by the same mechanisms as the ones determining total IgE level, as suggested by studies of parental smoking that showed associations in different directions for total IgE and skin test positivity.[96] Among indications of immune dysfunction associated with increased exposures to PCBs and dioxins, mononuclear cells from cord blood showed decreased *in vitro* secretion of tumor necrosis factor-α after mutagenic stimulation; this cytokine is an important proinflammatory stimulant.[75] Other exposure-related associations include differences in lymphocyte population ratios in peripheral blood from populations exposed to PCBs and related substances.[93,95,97] Laboratory animal studies suggest that mercury compounds may induce autoimmune disease and increases in interleukin-4 (IL4) production and IgE levels in certain rodent strains.[98] In human peripheral blood mononuclear cells *in vitro*, methylmercury concentrations of 100 µg/L were capable of inducing Th2 cytokine production, whereas γ-interferon production suppression occurred at 400 µg/L; in this model, mercury chloride stimulated increases in IL4 only at 1000 µg/L.[99]

In the present Grandjean[88] study, mutual correlations between PCB and methylmercury concentrations were weak and did not prevent characterization of their differing associations with the immunology parameters. In contrast, individual PCB congeners and ΣPCB concentrations in serum correlated very closely with one another. Close correlation also occurs with other persistent organic pollutants, such as *p,p'*-dichlorodiphenyldichloroethene (*p,p'*-DDE).[76,100] Although they focused on the ΣPCB concentration as a reliable overall marker of lipophilic contaminant exposure, they were unable to assess possible immunotoxic effects of individual PCB congeners or associated pollutants, which commonly occur in seafood together with PCBs.

Regarding other seafood constituents, maternal n-3 fatty acid intake from fatty fish is thought to affect the development of a child's immune system.[101] In the Faroes fishing community, positive correlations occur between serum concentrations of n-3 fatty acids and PCBs, although the latter mainly originates from pilot whale blubber.[89] Although n-3 fatty acids were not measured in the present study, the absence of any association between maternal fish intake during pregnancy and the immune parameters examined would argue against any important confounding due to maternal n-3 fatty acid intake during pregnancy. In a wider sense, confounding from other risk factors would likely be limited in this Nordic population with relatively uniform living circumstances, also taking into account the increased average level and wide range of exposures to the seafood contaminants.[102] Thus, the Grandjean[88] study considered a substantial number of social and obstetric variables as cofactors, none of which affected their findings. Their results therefore suggest that recommendations on marine food during pregnancy should take into consideration the possible immunotoxic impact of the contaminants.

The observed associations with developmental exposures to suspected immunotoxicants must be evaluated in light of the increased vulnerability of the developing immune system.[103] Because of the semiallogeneic pregnancy state, where graft rejection is suppressed, certain types of effects are more likely to be results of immunotoxicant exposures during the intrauterine developmental phase. During the early postnatal period, both immunosuppression and an increased risk of allergic disease can occur. The last-trimester fetus and the neonate usually exhibit comparatively depressed Th1-dependent functions, and current epidemiologic and experimental evidence on increased total IgE levels after exposure to various forms of stresses suggests that the postnatal acquisition of needed Th1 capacity could be a highly vulnerable target.[94,103] Accordingly, both dysfunction and misregulation are possible effects of developmental immunotoxicity.[103]

Although breast-feeding appeared to be positively associated with the total IgE concentration, the adjustment for PCB exposure attenuated this association to a nonsignificant level. The possible impact of lactational immunotoxicant exposure, as reflected by the postnatal serum PCB concentrations in the present study, would suggest that associations between breast-feeding and serum IgE concentrations in children could, at least in part, be due to immunotoxic food contaminants transferred via human milk. This is suggested by our two patients who had hyper IgE from birth.

Current evidence is equivocal concerning the effect of breast-feeding on the child's total serum IgE concentration. A prospective study in the United States found lower IgE concentrations at 8 years of age in breast-fed children, but only if the mother did not have an increased IgE level herself.[104] Further, in 258 Pakistani children 6 months to 12 years of age, a total IgE concentration above a reference level occurred in about 80% of bottle-fed children and only in half as many of those that were breast-fed.[105] However, in 215 Polish children 8 months to 18 years of age, the duration of breast-feeding was not associated with the total IgE concentration.[106]

Breast-feeding has often been considered a preventive factor in regard to allergy development, although some studies have suggested that breast-feeding may instead cause an increased risk.[78,79,81] Also, another Nordic study recently reported that longer breast-feeding was associated with a higher risk of atopic dermatitis but a lower risk of asthma.[107] The conundrums of statistically significant associations in opposite directions in different populations may be attributable to the effects of one or more independent risk factors that differ between the populations studied. However, data on immunotoxicant exposures are not available from the studies on breast-feeding regarding allergy development or serum IgE concentrations. The present study indicates that an effect of breast-feeding per se is likely to be small and may be negligible. Adjustment for lactational exposures to the immunotoxicants would seem necessary to assess the true magnitude of an independent effect of breast-feeding on allergy risks.

The associations of PCB and methylmercury exposures with indicators of allergy and allergic disease may involve both stimulation and inhibition of immune system functions. Based on the exposure assessments at three or four occasions, prenatal and postnatal exposures seem to have different effects. For methylmercury, they observed exposure-associated effects only in relation to prenatal exposures, and the much lower postnatal exposures did not reveal any clear associations. However, PCB and methylmercury may well target different components of the immune system, and their effects would also depend on the stage of development. Ideally, immune system dysfunction should therefore neither be assessed by means of a single or a few parameters nor at one stage of development only. We have found this to be true at the EHC-Dallas and EHC-Buffalo. Other types of immune factors such as T and B cells, complement and IgG subsets are often involved and immobilize contaminators. Deficiencies in these immune parameters clearly show an increase in contamination by toxics often producing chemical sensitivity and chronic degenerative disease.

Grandjean et al.[88] results may not necessarily be at odds with the "hygiene" hypothesis, which has been expressed in different terms regarding allergy and other diseases.[108] Rather, their data emphasize the need not to limit the focus only to gene–microbiome interactions but also to include environmental factors, such as immunotoxicants. Because their study provides evidence from a unique population with a well-characterized exposure to environmental chemicals from traditional food, the results provide insight into the potential effects of methylmercury and PCB exposures and their possible interaction with beneficial effects from breast-feeding. Even though the exposure in the Faroes may be less complex than elsewhere, the picture remains multifaceted.

Developmental immunotoxicity may predispose children to common diseases of increasing prevalence, such as childhood asthma and allergic diseases, and is therefore important from a public health perspective. Thus, their findings support the need for screening studies to identify immunotoxicants.[103] In this regard, immunosuppression should not be considered as the only relevant outcome, and effects associated with developmental exposures need to be considered independently from effects in mature organisms. Because of uncertainty regarding interpretation of results from different animal models, human studies remain crucial, and prospective studies must incorporate delayed adverse outcomes of developmental exposures.

PCBs AND FOODS

PCBs are persistent environmental toxicants associated with numerous adverse health effects. The widespread commercial use of PCBs, which peaked in the 1970s, contributed to the pervasive bioaccumulation of these toxicants in the environment.[102] Environmental exposure to PCBs is ongoing as a result of continued use and disposal of products containing these toxicants,[109] widespread bioaccumulation of PCBs in the biosphere, and bioconcentration in the food chain.[110] Meat and fish remain the primary source of PCB exposure for most of the adult human population and account for consistent PCB accumulation within human tissues.[111]

Several studies have evaluated associations of PCBs with human health effects and have demonstrated adverse reproductive,[112] developmental,[113] immunologic,[114] and neurologic[109] effects. The influence of PCBs on cancer risk is well established in animal studies[115,116]; however, human epidemiology studies are less consistent. Several epidemiologic studies derived from retrospective mortality analysis have linked occupational PCB exposure with an increased risk of developing malignant melanoma and brain cancer.[109,117–121] Interestingly, the risk of developing brain cancer has been shown to be independent of cumulative PCB exposure.[119,121] The risk of chemical sensitivity is high in PCB-exposed patients who do not get concerned. Therefore, their exposure must be considered for multiple reasons.

The ability of PCBs to accumulate in brain tissue[122–124] is likely related to their neurotoxicity. However, less is known about the effects of PCBs on brain endothelium. Previous research from Seelbach et al.[125] laboratory has demonstrated that PCBs can modulate properties of brain endothelial cells *in vitro* and enhance adhesion and transendothelial migration of tumor cells.[126–128] However, the interactions of PCBs with brain endothelium and the blood–brain barrier (BBB) *in vivo* are virtually unknown.

BLOOD–BRAIN BARRIER AND TOXICS

The BBB is anatomically situated at the level of the cerebral microvascular capillary endothelium and it regulates the blood–brain exchange. The tight junctions (TJs) limit passive paracellular movement of solutes, ions, and water across the BBB. They form the most apical element of the junctional complex and are composed of an intricate complex of transmembrane, accessory, and cytoplasmic proteins that connect the TJs to actin cytoskeleton and intracellular signaling systems.[129] The transmembrane proteins occludin and claudin-5 form the primary seal of the TJs. They bind to the intracellular proteins zonula occludens (ZO)-1, ZO-2, cingulin, and/or 7H6 that couple the TJs to the actin cytoskeleton of endothelial cells.[129] TJ proteins are also important in maintaining barrier polarity and are involved in cellular signaling. Disruption of the integrity of this system has been associated with several central nervous system pathologies.[130]

According to Seelbach et al.[125] a link between PCB exposure and pathology has been strongly established in the literature.[131,132] Both early childhood development and adult neurologic functions may be impaired by PCB exposure.[133–135] For example, a cohort analysis study performed on 7-year-old children showed that, in conjunction with mercury exposure, high umbilical cord PCB levels augmented neurobehavioral deficits later in life.[134] Further, epidemiologic studies support an association between PCB exposure and central nervous system disease, including Parkinson's disease, amyotrophic lateral sclerosis, non-Alzheimer-related dementia, and brain cancer in adults.[117,122,136] The BBB breakdown is a commonality in all of these central nervous system disease states[34]; however, the pathophysiologic influence of PCBs on the BBB function is not fully understood.

Research from Seelbach et al.[125] laboratory indicated that selected PCB congeners can stimulate proinflammatory properties.[128,137] These studies linked PCB exposure with prometastatic changes of cultured endothelial cells. Indeed, they demonstrated that exposure of endothelial cells to *ortho*-substituted PCBs can stimulate production of inflammatory mediators leading to adhesion and transmigration of THP-1 or breast cancer cells (MDA-MB-231).[126,128] It appears that activation of JAK3, EGFR, Src kinase, and MAP kinase signaling cascades may underlie these effects.[128,137] However, transendothelial migration of tumor cells may be further potentiated by disruption of endothelial cell junctions and hyperpermeability across the endothelial barrier. Therefore, in their study, they explored the influence of both coplanar and noncoplanar PCBs on molecular and functional properties of the BBB. They focused on three typical PCB congeners that maintain different structural properties, namely, PCB153, PCB126, and PCB118. Noncoplanar PCB153 accounts for the majority of PCBs found in environmental and in biological samples.[133] PCB126 belongs to the coplanar dioxin-like group of PCBs that act through an aryl hydrocarbon receptor (AhR) mechanism. In contrast, mono-*ortho*-substituted PCB118 is a weak AhR agonist.[138]

In their study, the molecular analysis of TJ proteins indicated that PCBs can differentially modulate TJ expression and/or localization. Exposure to PCB118 and PCB153 modulated expressional levels of claudin-5 and ZO-1, whereas PCB126 appeared to primarily influence the coassociation of occludin and ZO-1. These findings suggest that PCB congeners may be acting through different mechanisms to elicit the same functional effect (i.e., disrupted barrier integrity and increased permeability across the endothelial clefts). The precise mechanisms responsible for these events have yet to be elucidated; however, they are likely to involve redox-responsive reactions. Indeed, PCBs are potent generators of reactive oxygen species,[126,139,140] and the alterations of redox signaling contribute to the disruption of the BBB function.[141,142] The brain is highly sensitive to oxidative stress because of its high oxygen consumption, high iron and lipid content, and low activity for antioxidant defenses. Studies performed in their laboratory[143,144] and others[141,142] demonstrate that oxidative stress can alter the integrity of the BBB at the level of the TJs acting through Ras and Rho redox-responsive elements. The Ras GTPase pathway plays an important role in the regulation of claudin-5, ZO-1, and ZO-2,[144] and the Rho pathway is critical for TJ assembly.[142] Other redox-regulated candidate pathways that may be involved in PCB-induced alterations of TJ protein expression include MAP kinase[145] and PI3K.[146] Finally, these mechanisms may involve proteolysis of TJ proteins by matrix metalloproteinases (MMPs) and ubiquitination–proteasome systems.[127] Again with loosened TJ, Ca^{2+} can enter the cells, causing hypersensitivity and allowing chemical sensitivity to occur. However, a similar mechanism can occur to allow Ca^{2+} to enter, causing the triggering of hypersensitivity.

One of the major goals of Seelbach et al.'s[125] study was to develop a model to evaluate the effects of PCBs on the development of tumor metastases. They focused on brain metastases of melanoma cells, because metastatic brain tumors originating from malignant melanoma are seen frequently in clinical medicine.[147,148] Over the last 30 years, the mortality rate of malignant melanomas has increased by 50%.[149] Using a modification of previously published methods,[147,150,151] Seelbach et al.[125] introduced the highly metastatic melanoma cells into the internal carotid artery of fully immunocompetent mice. Because the internal carotid artery supplies the brain parenchyma with blood, tumor cell injection into brain vasculature mimics the metastatic process in humans in which circulating tumor cells adhere and invade capillary endothelium.[151] Their newly developed model resulted in the consistent development of metastatic nodules within brain parenchyma, an effect that was highly potentiated by preexposure to individual PCB congeners, especially PCB118. Several factors participate in the propensity of malignant melanoma to selectively target brain tissue[152,153]; however, tumor cell extravasation into the brain is dependent upon its interactions at the cerebral capillary endothelium. Thus, the leaky BBB due to PCB-induced alterations of TJ expression in brain microvessels may facilitate transcapillary transfer of tumor cells and other toxics to contribute to the development of brain metastasis or nonmalignant chemical sensitivity. In addition, those non-malignant directing of toxics and injury will give people cloudy brain function, short-term memory loss, weakness and fatigue, that is, a form imbalance found in the chemically sensitive patient. The peripheral chemicals absorbed through the skin, lung, and GI tract as well as the olfactory nerve can go to the brain, disturb the brain membranes in the frontal lobe and limbic system causing chemical hypersensitivity in SRI.

Seelbach et al.'s[125] study indicates that exposure to PCBs leads to disruption of the BBB integrity via modulation of TJ protein expression. Most important, they demonstrate for the first time that oral exposure to specific PCB congeners can enhance the rate of brain metastasis or chemical expansion. These results suggest that alteration of BBB integrity is the underlying mechanism of PCB-induced brain metastasis as well as chemical sensitivity and may also be involved in neuro-toxic and neurodevelopmental effects of these environmental toxicants even when carried by food.

The repeated exposure to other toxics or more PCB resulting in a leaky BBB will most likely cause the adverse cerebral response and the chemical sensitivity and chronic degenerative disease. It can then result in isolated to new total food sensitivity. These increased leaks will result in brain fog, lack of concentration, short-term memory loss, and so on.

The Integrated Atmospheric Deposition Network (IADN) and the Great Lakes Fish Monitoring Program (GLFMP) monitor persistent bioaccumulative toxic (PBT) pollutants in the air and fish, respectively, of the Great Lakes. Both programs show decreases in PBTs over time (Figures 4.2 through 4.5; Tables 4.1 and 4.2).

The total PCB loads at Fort Erie and NOTL for 2005 were calculated as the sum of the dissolved and particulate PCB loads (Table 4.2). The 2005 Niagara River load to Lake Ontario is represented by the NOTL load (147.22 kg/year). The largest source of uncertainty in this estimate is the dissolved PCB load.

OTHER TRIBUTARIES

For all of the other major tributaries to Lake Ontario, available PCB monitoring data were used to develop an annual loading regression for each tributary. PCB monitoring data from USEPA (2002 to 2008), NYSDEC (2007 to 2008), and USGS (Black River for 2004 to 2005)[154–156] for major U.S. tributaries to Lake Ontario were used to update and validate the loading regressions reported in

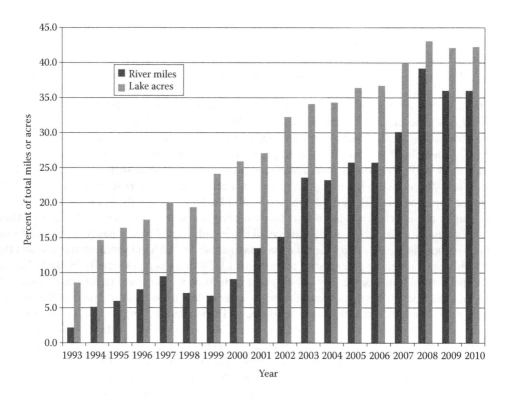

FIGURE 4.3 Trends in percentage of river miles and lake acres under fish consumption advisory, 1993–2010. (Adapted from EPA's Draft Report on the Environment 2003. Purer Water. Chapter 2:2-10.)

Atkinson et al.[157] A summary of the 2005 PCB load from Canadian and U.S. tributaries is shown in Table 4.3. Annual PCB loads from Canadian professional judgment were used to provide a reasonable estimate in instances where data were limited. A summary of the PCB sources to Lake Ontario in 2005 is presented in Table 4.3 and Figure 4.4. The NY direct point sources will be included in the wasteload allocation (WLA), while all other sources will be included in the load allocation (LA) for the total Maximum daily load (TMDL). An additional flux of PCBs to Lake Ontario is from the sediment; however, this flux was ignored because it is assumed to be at equilibrium under future TMDL condition (Figures 4.6 and 4.7).

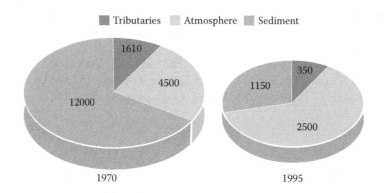

FIGURE 4.4 Bioaccumulative toxics in the Great Lakes. (Adapted from EPA's Draft Report on the Environment 2003. Purer Water. Chapter 2:2–11.)

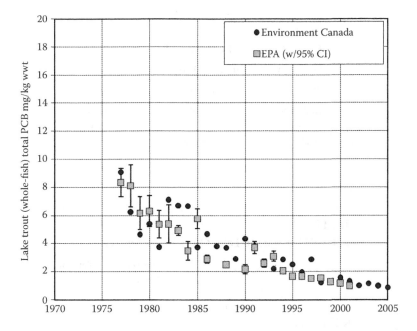

FIGURE 4.5 Average annual lake trout whole-fish total PCB concentration from 1977 to 2005 from USEPA. (Adapted from Elizabeth Murphy, USEPA, personal communication, November 7, 2006 and Environment Canada; Sean Backus, Environment Canada, personal communication, January 17, 2007.)

PCB has been shown to cause cancer and a number of serious noncancer health effects in animals and humans, including effects on the immune system, reproductive system, nervous system, and endocrine system. Studies in humans provide supportive evidence for the potential carcinogenicity and noncarcinogenic effects of PCB.[158] Of the various PCB congeners, several are considered to be similar to dioxin because of their structure and toxicity. The research results summarized in this report did not distinguish between these dioxin-like PCB congeners and other congeners. The scientific results described in this survey report typically are the sum of a subset of PCB congeners; the congeners included in the subset varied among researchers and can be found in the original references.

TABLE 4.1
Serum Polychlorinated Biphenyls in 30 Chemically Sensitive Patients

Patient	Compound	Above No.	Detection %	Limit Range	(0.3 mg/ppm) Mean Level (ppm)
F = 17	23'44' TETRA	0	0		
M = 13	23'44'5 PENTA	5	17	0.4–46.3	13.7
Age = 21–77 years	22'44'55 HEXA	11	37	0.3–90.5	12.4
Mean 52 years	233'44' PENTA	2	7	0.3–0.4	0.4
	22'344'5 HEXA	2	7	1.4–24.1	12.8
	22'344'5' HEXA	9	30	6.3–69.8	9.8
	22'344'5'6 HEPTA	0	0		
	22'344'55' HEPTA	0	0		
	22'344'55' HEPTA	16	53	0.3–31.8	4
	22'3'44'5 HEPTA	7	23	0.3–13.4	4.2

Source: Adapted from Environmental Health Center-Dallas.

TABLE 4.2
Estimated 2005 PCB Load (kg/year) at
Fort Erie and Niagara-On-The-Lake

Phase	Fort Erie	NOTL
Particulate	31.41	81.74
Dissolved	65.49	65.49
Total	96.89	147.22

TABLE 4.3
2005 PCB Loads to Lake Ontario, by Source

Source	2005 Load (kg/year)	Percent (%)
Nonpoint Sources		
Niagara River	147.22	63.1
New York tributaries[a]	13.00	5.6
Canadian tributaries[a]	22.00	9.4
Atmospheric deposition (wet and dry)	47.00	20.1
Point Sources		
NY direct point sources[b]	4.05	1.7
Total load	233.27	100[c]

[a] 2005 tributary loads are detailed in Table 4.3.
[b] 2005 NY direct point source loads are composed of facility loads and direct MS4 loads.
[c] Numbers may not add to 100% due to rounding.

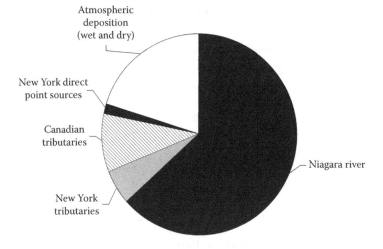

FIGURE 4.6 2005 PCB loads to Lake Ontario by source.

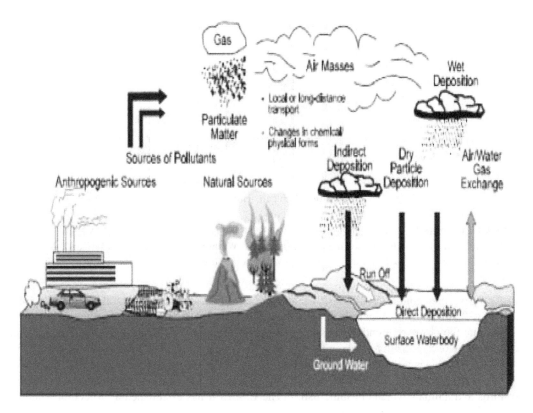

FIGURE 4.7 Atmospheric release, transport, and deposition processes. (Adapted from Aneja, V. P., P. A. Roelle, G. C. Murray et al. 2001. Atmospheric nitrogen compounds II: Emissions, transport, transformation, deposition and assessment. *Atmos. Environ.* 35:1903–1911.)

IMPROVEMENTS IN ECOSYSTEM HEALTH

Several examples of improved ecosystem health—as reflected in biomarkers—are reported in the Third Report to Congress. Newly published information is consistent with those findings.

Concentrations of PCB in fish generally have been declining in the Great Lakes since monitoring began in the 1970s and 1980s. Recent analytical results indicate that on average, total PCB concentrations in whole Great Lakes top predator fish have declined 5% annually between 1990 and 2003. This decline in PCB has been largely due to various remedial, mitigative, and pollution prevention efforts, such as the remediation of contaminated sediments and the reduction of PCB loadings to the Great Lakes.[159,160]

Figure 4.8 shows these trends for each of the lakes. In Lake Michigan, PCB concentrations in lake trout have declined consistently over the last two decades. PCB concentrations in lake trout of Lake Superior fluctuated through the early 1980s, with greater stabilization after that period. A slight increase was observed in 2000; however, this increase may have resulted from a change in collection sites, or the fact that the sample population was consuming more contaminated prey than the previous sample population collected from that site in 1998. In Lake Huron, an overall decline in PCB concentrations was observed with some periodic increases seen through 2000. As noted in Figure 4.9, walleye are collected in Lake Erie as the top predator fish instead of lake trout because they are more representative of conditions in that lake. PCB concentrations in Lake Erie increased in the late 1980s through the early 1990s, after which PCB concentrations suddenly declined. The period of increase corresponds with the introduction of zebra mussels into Lake Erie. Zebra mussels remove PCB contamination from open water and deposit it in the sediment making it available to bottom-feeding fish. Consequently, higher concentrations are observed in walleye since

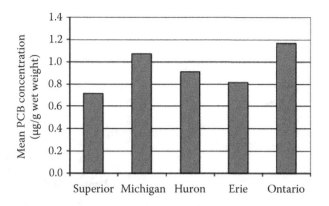

FIGURE 4.8   PCB fish contamination in Great Lakes top predator whole fish in 2002. (Adapted from U.S. EPA. 2006. Inventory Update Reporting [IUR]. IUR Data. Washington, DC: U.S. Environmental Protection Agency. Accessed July 8, 2009. http://www.epa.gov/oppt/iur/tools/data/.)

they prey on some bottom-feeding fish. Finally, in Lake Ontario, PCB concentrations have declined through 2000 with little observed fluctuation since the late 1990s.[160]

Despite the observed trends discussed above, concentrations in Great Lakes fish are still high enough to be of concern for consumption by wildlife and humans. The Great Lakes Water Quality Agreement includes a threshold concentration of total PCB in fish tissues (whole fish, calculated on a wet weight basis) of no more than 0.1 mg/g or parts per million (ppm) for the protection of birds and animals which consume fish.[161] The U.S. EPA has established a protection value for

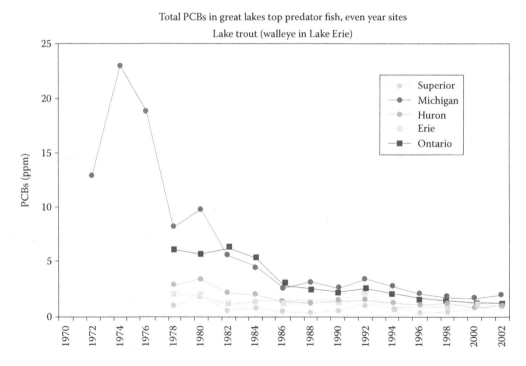

FIGURE 4.9   Bioaccumulative toxics in the Great Lakes. Atmospheric deposition of POCBs and DDT in the Great Lakes, 1992–1998. (Adapted from EPA's Draft Report on the Environment 2003. Purer Water. Chapter 2:2–13.)

fish-consuming wildlife and birds at 0.16 ppm in fish tissue.[162] Figures 4.8 and 4.9 demonstrate that PCB concentrations in all of the Great Lakes for top predator fish exceed these values. Furthermore, PCB levels in Great Lakes fish are high enough to warrant fish consumption advisories for humans for all five of the Great Lakes; these are discussed later in this section.

Reductions in PCB levels in herring gull eggs at Lakes Ontario and Erie occurred and were discussed in the Third Report to Congress. Current literature also reported reductions in PCB concentrations in gull eggs. For example, at sites on Lake Ontario, concentrations in herring gull eggs have decreased from approximately 70 mg/g (wet weight) in 1970–1974 to less than 10 mg/g in 1995–1999.[163] Levels of contamination vary spatially around the Great Lakes. Mean values of contaminants in herring gull eggs were calculated for the five-year period 1998–2002 around the Great Lakes. Across the 15 colonies examined, mean values ranged between 2 and 22 mg/g (wet weight) for total PCB; the highest concentration was in Saginaw Bay in Lake Huron.[164] Herring gull eggs provide a biomarker for colonial waterbirds, including other species such as terns and cormorants. Populations of most waterbird species in the Great Lakes have increased and become healthier than they were 30 years ago, as the majority of contaminant levels have decreased. However, more subtle health effects may still be found in these bird populations.[160]

In spite of these downward trends, levels of PCBs and other PBTs in certain types of fish still exceed health protection levels in all five lakes (Figure 4.9). Air data from Chicago showing elevated PCB levels suggest that cities still contain significant sources of PCBs. This would suggest that the water through the fish will be contaminated.

GLFMP samples are also being used to identify the presence of "new" bioaccumulating pollutants in the Great Lakes, such as certain brominated flame retardants.

Food grown in contaminated waters can cause severe illness. Pathogens associated with human or animal wastes can cause gastrointestinal illness, even death in people with compromised immune systems such as the chemically sensitive and chronic degenerated disease patients. Mollusks, mussels, and whelks are the main shellfish that can carry biotoxins causing common symptoms in humans, such as irritation of the eyes, nose, and throat as well as tingling lips and tongue, brain dysfunction, and cardiovascular dysfunction. Contaminated fish and shellfish are a particular concern to people in either of two high-risk categories: those with conditions that put them more at risk (e.g., pregnant women, nursing mothers, children, or people with compromised immune systems [i.e., chemical sensitivity, leukemia, etc.]); and people who consume fish as a primary food source (e.g., some tribes and ethnic groups). Because of their higher consumption rates, some communities have developed their own guidance to identify specific types of fish of concern (Minnesota Chippewa Tribe). Due to the widespread contamination of waters, we do not recommend fish for the chemically sensitive patient and patient with chronic degenerative disease.

The Minnesota Chippewa is an Indian tribal confederation with approximately 40,000 members. The tribe's six reservations occupy approximately 700,000 acres, 702 miles of streams, and 250,000 acres of wetlands. As water is an abundant natural resource for the tribe, its members rely heavily on fish caught in those waters as a source of food.

The major widespread contaminants in Minnesota Chippewa tribal waters are mercury, DDT, PCBs, plastics, dioxin, and furans. Fish consumption is the primary route of human exposure to these contaminants. Thus, the tribe chose as a primary environmental indicator the quantity of fish from its water that can be consumed safely by its most at-risk members: women of childbearing age, nursing mothers, and children. The tribally designated, treaty-protected quantity of preferred fish consumption is 224 grams (about 8 ounces) per day. The quantity of preferred fish that may be consumed safely by the most at-risk citizens are limited to 5% (about 0.4 ounces) or less. Lakes-specific guides for fish consumption are prepared for members of the tribe. The guides offer recommendations on the pounds per month of several fish species that is safe to consume. Unfortunately, these guidelines are arbitrary and not based on little human data. There is a large thrust (data on ocean fish) in the medical profession to eat more cold-water fish which we do not agree. Little is mentioned about the contamination of these fish causing the potential for more inflammation and, thus, heart

TABLE 4.4

35-Year-Old White Female with Mercury Toxicity

No. of Months	C	2	4	6
Hair	0	0	2+	4+ toxic
RBC	0	1+	3+	4+ toxic
Urine	0	1+	3+	4+ toxic

disease. We at the EHC-Dallas and EHC-Buffalo are to the point that we rarely recommend fish to our patients with chemical sensitivity and/or chronic degenerative disease due to the widespread chemical contamination. A case in point is shown in Table 4.4.

> This 35-year-old white woman had an extreme case of malnutrition, due to her food and chemical sensitivity. She was sensitive to foods that she could only tolerate 12 foods. She avoided fish for years and had subsequently lost her fish sensitivity. We recommended that she try various kinds of fish, no more than 3 ounces per week. We measured hair, RBC, and urine mercury levels. These were again measured every 2 months. The mercury was initially undetectable and as time went on the mercury levels became higher and higher. After 6 months, she had to stop eating fish because she was becoming toxic to mercury.

Other substances can come in the food chain. A new laboratory study demonstrating that poly-brominated diphenyl ethers (PBDEs) can alter human fetal brain cells may explain at least in part the neurotoxicity recently documented in epidemiologic studies of young children exposed to PBDEs (a brother FPCB) and previously shown in animal models.[165] The new study, the first to examine PBDE neurotoxicity in a human cell-based system, links the brain cell alterations to endocrine disruption. It is clear that the contamination of fish can be multifaceted. Therefore, all types of contamination can be found in fish such as plastics, pesticides, solvents, and many other chemicals which can result in chemical sensitivity, or exacerbate existing chemical sensitivity.

A wealth of data demonstrates that babies can be exposed to significant amounts of PBDE flame retardants both in the womb and through breast-feeding. Although all three PBDE formulations— penta, octa, and deca—are banned in Europe, and the penta and octa formulations were discontinued in the United States (deca also is banned in some states), PBDEs may still be used in some new U.S. products and in wares manufactured elsewhere. They also are found in a wide variety of older plastic consumer goods that remain in use in many homes, businesses, and automobiles. The PBDEs are known to migrate into indoor dust, posing a particularly high exposure risk to infants and toddlers because of their characteristic hand-to-mouth behavior.

To investigate how PBDEs may impact the developing fetal brain and thus sensitizing certain areas to develop abnormal functions, the team of scientists employed a method for evaluating human developmental neurotoxicity they had recently observed[166] as an alternative to animal testing. This method uses primary fetal human neural progenitor cells (hNPCs) cultured to produce complex three-dimensional cellular systems called neurospheres. Neurospheres undergo the same basic processes that occur during the early stages of normal human brain development: cell proliferation, differentiation, and migration. Tests conducted with neurospheres may help identify exogenous substances that disturb these basic processes *in vivo*.

The researchers focused on two of the PBDE compounds that accumulate the most in humans, BDE-47 and BDE-99. At concentrations below levels that cause cell death, they found these compounds could reduce the migration of the hNPCs, which suggests the possibility of adverse effects on brain development, and the effects increased with higher PBDE concentrations. At the highest tested concentration (10 μM), BDE-47 decreased the distance the cells migrated by more than 25% compared with unexposed cells, whereas the same concentration of BDE-99 decreased the distance by more than 30%. Additional testing established that both compounds also interfered with the differentiation of immature progenitor cells into neurons and oligodendrocytes.

Further tests suggested the PBDE compounds affected cell migration and differentiation by interfering with thyroid hormone signaling, an endocrine-disrupting effect that could be associated with additional impacts throughout a person's life. Follow-up work to determine whether PBDEs cause the same effects in rodent neurospheres would facilitate extrapolation from animals to humans. It is clear that thyroid dysfunction occurs in a multitude of people exposed to toxics. These can be from a multitude of toxic chemicals in food.

Other work has shown the tendency of PBDEs to accumulate in brain and neuronal cells, and the researchers used radiolabeled BDE-47 to measure an accumulation in test cells of approximately 60-fold. Considered with available human exposure data, these data suggest current PBDE exposure levels are likely to be of concern for human health, the authors write. Two recent studies have linked PBDEs with subtle changes in children's IQs and behavior.[167,168]

UNEP Offers Electronic Waste Predictions

The world's stockpile of e-waste—discarded computers, mobile phones, and other electronic devices—is growing by an estimated 40 million tons per year with little sign of stopping. UNEP estimates the number of discarded computers shipped to some developing countries could increase by as much as 500% by 2020. The informal recycling of electronics is a lucrative but highly hazardous cottage industry in many developing countries. The UNEP report therefore offers guidance for countries to build successful and safer e-waste management systems. Many environmental factors are present in the generation of disease but toxic overload can lead to food sensitivity and malnutrition.

Review of Environmental Factors in Malaria's Spread

A review by Chaves and Koenraadt[169] assesses the factors contributing to increases in malaria cases worldwide. They reported that climate change, human migration, and land-use changes all are causing malaria to spread into highland areas of East Africa, Indonesia, Afghanistan, and elsewhere. They systematically show how climate affects multiple biological components of malaria transmission and highlight the need for research to better understand the transmission dynamics of this disease and how to sustainably control or eliminate it. Certainly less pollution in air, food, and water would increase resistance to infectious diseases.

PAHs: Pathways to Waterways

Polycyclic aromatic hydrocarbons (PAHs), chemicals released during combustion of biomass and fossil fuels are ubiquitous in the environment. Rodenburg et al.[170] undertook a 4-year study to identify the primary routes by which PAHs end up in New York/New Jersey harbor. Their findings show stormwater runoff was the main pathway, contributing about half the harbors" PAH load, and atmospheric deposition was an important contributor of smaller PAH compounds. The results suggest that minimizing the flow of PAHs into waterways may require tweaking stormwater management plans to control runoff. These substances will get into seafood causing many fish to be contaminated. Again, Hg will bother the chemically sensitive patients.

Hyper IgE Syndrome

We at the EHC-Dallas and EHC-Buffalo have found a high incidence of contamination associated with hypersensitivity but only 10% triggered the IgE class. This hypersensitivity is rampant but through other mechanisms. However, we do have 17 patients with the hyper IgE syndrome (HIES) that is associated with chemical exposure.[6] These patients were universally sensitive to foods and

TABLE 4.5

Chemical Sensitivity Patients with HIES at EHC-Dallas, Measurement of IgE Levels and Eosinophils Levels >2000

Patient	Age	Race	Sex	IgE (<144)	Inhalant Test	Food Test	Chemical Test	Eosinophils (15–500 IU/mL)
1				57,000				78
2	20	W	F	48,653				1308
3	13	W	F	41,338	+	+	+	15
4				36,000	+			1010
5	51	W	M	17,900	+	75	75	1199
6				12,415	+			16
7				10,693	+			1018
8				9417	+			780
9	7	W	M	7094	+			600
10				6200	+			32
11	2	W	M	5607	+			720
12				5508	+			27
13	6	W	M	4289	+			48
14	45	W	F	4072	+			10
15	9	W	M	3343	+	171	71	1099
16	51	W	M	4289	+			
17	62	O	F		+	+	+	

2 from birth and 13 acquired as adults. Every one of the high IgE patients had multiple chemicals, including pesticides, solvents, and heavy metal associated with the HIES. Our series of hyper IgE patients is presented in Table 4.5.

HIES is a described illness with few reports in the literature. This series of chemically sensitive patients describes 17 cases aged 2–80 years, 3 males and 14 females of the HIES (IgE > 2000 U) exposed to chemicals (organochlorine, solvents, inorganic toxins [manganese, Hg, Cd]) before the symptoms started who developed immune dysfunction characterized by high levels of IgE, low T cells (81%), eosinophilia, recurrent upper respiratory infections, chronic eczema, recurrent candida, and food sensitivity. HIES represents an immunologically mediated response. The patients were studied in a less polluted environment, five times reduced by chemical analysis and particle counts. History, physical signs and symptoms, laboratory tests (RAST 100%), gamma globulins, T and B cells, and intradermal challenge (100%) proved that toxic chemicals were involved in the triggering of excess IgE. Short-term treatment responses were satisfactory to a regimen of massive avoidance of chemicals, food, and mold which were triggering agents, injection treatment of the neutralizing doses of these triggering agents, and specific nutrition supplementation were performed. Oxygen therapy and nutrient detoxification with sauna are good therapeutics for treatment in such cases. Hypersensitivity to chemical exposure should be ruled out or treated in patients with HIES. In conclusion, the HIES is uncommon but exists. It can be confused with parasites. The patients are very fragile. It is extremely difficult to treat and the patient is prone to anaphylaxis.

SOIL QUALITY AND NUTRITION: LESS CHEMICALLY CONTAMINATED FOODS

In order for the chemically sensitive patient and patient with chronic degenerative disease to receive sufficient nutrients, their foods should be grown in biodynamic composted nontoxic soil, which produces the highest nutritive quality possible. Attainment of food quality that is near that of foods grown on virgin soil is desirable. However, soil overuse and current factory farming methods make production of such food quality difficult. The development and adoption of newer, organic methods of food production are essential to future attainment of high-quality foods that are neither contaminated nor nutrient depleted by food preservation, storage, or preparation methods.

Recent studies on Kalahari Bushmen,[171] Hadza nomads in Tanzania,[172] Waorani Indians in the Amazon,[173] and the aborigines of Australia[174] show that these peoples had available a wide variety of food with high protein content as well as other nutritive qualities. Their fresh-eaten fish was uncontaminated with industrial toxics, by mycotoxins, or preservatives. Possibly one of the reasons these groups (especially the Waorani Indians) were virtually disease-free is because of their healthy diet. These data are now 20 years old and the facts have changed and chronic disease is creeping into these people's lives as time progresses and the nutrient environment becomes contaminated. Unfortunately, disease is now present in these people.

The soil of the hunter–gatherer societies had several advantages. It allowed nature to do the planting via the voluminous amount of seeds contained in the soil. This natural plant production assured plant variety and genetic divergence. Therefore, a diffuse number of plants were always present and available for soil restoration. This variety tended not to deplete the soil of specific nutrients such as minerals and humus and it also allowed for constant replenishment of soil nutrients. In addition, the hunter–gatherer societies allowed the soil to rest, at times, for years. Therefore, a less constant demand on the same soil nutrients occurred. These periods of rest further allowed for build-up of organic material in the soil thereby replenishing its nutritive value. Plant disease was less because of the balance of nature in the form of a varied number of plants and insects, as well as the strength of plant nutrient content.

The transition from hunter–gatherer societies to worldwide agricultural societies is now virtually complete as is the disease entities brought with toxic agriculture. With this transition has come a depletion of the nutrient value of the soil not only from centuries of overuse but also in an accelerated form from topsoil erosion as a result of mechanization and ill-advised farming techniques using pesticides and herbicides. Due to our explosion in technology, which allows more intensive farming on land that would previously have been rested, both overutilization of the land and thus nutrient depletion have resulted.

Due to the population of the earth being over 7 billion people, we will never be able to return to the type of food standard obtained by hunting and gathering food grown on virgin soils. As clinicians, we must now analyze each facet of food manufacturing and production to understand the positive and negative effects our present processes have on the quality of our food supply. We now have over 7 billion people to feed on a planet that should probably adequately support one half billion or less if nutritional value was taken into consideration.

In addition, commercial monocropping, which opposes nature's law of variety and rotation, contributes to the long-term depletion of soil nutrients. Finally, due to the demand for quantity, nutrient alteration with an increased demand for artificial fertilizers, pesticides, and herbicides has occurred. As marginal land that historically has not been as efficient for a particular crop being grown or animal being raised (e.g., raising tomatoes and corn on land to which cactus had adapted, or raising cattle on land on which buffalo and deer evolved, etc.) has been utilized, weakening of the nutrient content has occurred along with increased use of toxic substances to keep the land productive. This utilization of inappropriate land for the crops that nature has not intended to be grown as well as alteration of nutrient content continue to occur. Although food has become "inexpensive" as a result of this plentiful supply, the total cost of producing such lesser quality foods in terms of damage to both individual health and soil may be, in the final analysis, much higher than is immediately evident.

When an individual experiences nutrient depletion as a result of both an inadequate diet and excess exposure to pollutants, via his food and water supply as well as air environment, he may experience toxic overload with resultant chemical sensitivity or chronic degenerative disease.

The agricultural practices of the last 60 years now appear to pose a threat to man's optimum functioning as well as to the agricultural system because they have become increasingly dependent on sources and modalities that are not sustainable. These practices, including cultivation of limited genetic variant seed and crops and utilization of commercial farming methods that alter food quality (such as monocropping, mechanical disruption of the soil and application of synthetic fertilizers, herbicides, pesticides, and insecticides) have not always considered human health and nourishment as their primary goals.[175–178]

In contrast to the practices of hunter–gatherer societies, industrialized man has tampered with his natural food supply in order to produce a larger quantity of food with which to feed his ever-expanding population. However, the application of vast technological advances to food production in the twentieth century has not been the panacea it was once thought to be. While many benefits, such as easy availability of a large quantity, though often limited variety, of food, have been gotten from modern agricultural techniques and practices, many complications have also emerged. These complications include an ever-increasing depletion of soil nutrients with an increasing need for supplementation of synthetic nutrients and the increasing use of pesticides and herbicides to control plant disease. Also, our food-growing practices and our diet have been implicated in the onset of cancer and chronic diseases such as collagen disease and arteriosclerosis and they have also contributed to a rising susceptibility among the GP for chemical sensitivity and other chronic degenerative diseases such as neurovascular failure (multiple sclerosis, Alzheimer's, Parkinson's disease, and nonspecific neuropathy) and cancer and arteriosclerosis.

FACTORS CONTRIBUTING TO ALTERATION OF THE NUTRIENT VALUE OF FOODS

Factors that contribute to the alteration of the nutrient value of foods include cultivation of limited genetic variance of foods, monocropping and mechanical disruption of the soil, and the use of artificial fertilizers, herbicides, and pesticides. The chemical content of rain must also be considered because at times it is very contaminated and will contaminate the soil. The detrimental costs of this present food production practices in terms of human health and soil quality cannot be overestimated.

All the resistance factors, including plant strength and structural mechanics, will be similar in monocropping, in contrast to a field where plants are diversified and many, therefore, have variable levels of intrinsic resistance. The intrinsic resistance will often inhibit the spread of disease to additional plants since the disease is arrested by the ability of the strong plants to fend off insect or microbial infestations.

Mechanical farming of the soil using plows and discs tends to destroy earthworms, microbes, and other plants that seem to balance the nutrients in the soil. For example, nitrogen-fixing roots and bacteria may be destroyed, requiring artificial supplementation. In addition, these practices enhance erosion of high-quality topsoil, which then leaves lower-quality soils to supply nutrients to the plants. About 254 or more earthworms per cubic foot seem necessary for high-quality topsoil in order to ensure adequate aeration of soil and worm-derived fertilizer. Aeration into subsoil may be more difficult due to the absence of worms destroyed by mechanical disruption. Also, the moisture content of the subsoil may be depleted due to crusting of the topsoil and destruction of access channels by plows and discs. This decrease in the ability to hold moisture results in plant stress at the time of adverse weather conditions. Plants then become more prone to disease, and their nutrient quality diminishes. Beck has shown plants grown in organic soil with a minimum disruption have richer root system than commercial mechanical farm (Figure 4.10).

These mechanized methods sharply contrast with the "no till" techniques of sustainable agriculture that allow for a constant supply of nutrient-dense, high-quality foods for years. The commercial farming methods tend to destroy nutrient balance in the soil since, generally, they replace only nitrogen, phosphorus, and potassium. Therefore, soils prepared by commercial methods such as monocropping and limited supplementation may produce large crops of good-appearing foods that actually have decreasing nutrient value. Over time, the continuing use of these practices escalates nutrient depletion of the soil and plants. Because of the healthy appearance of these foods, neither

Commercial vs Organic Plant Growth

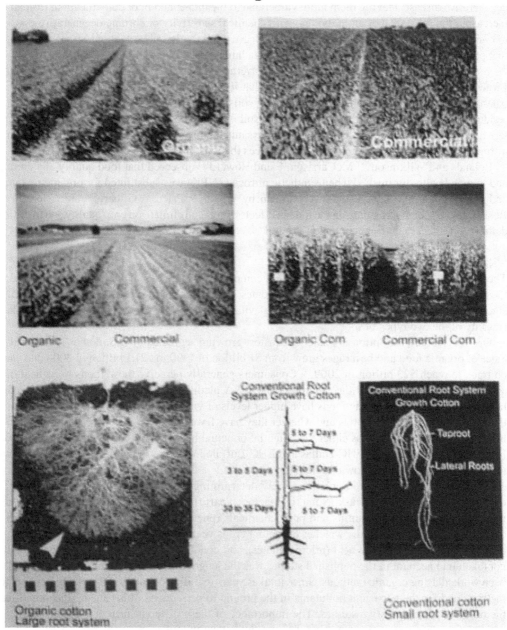

FIGURE 4.10 Malcolm Beck's commercial versus organic plants.

the farmer nor the consumer is aware of these insidious deficiencies. Unchecked, they magnify apparently continuing over each generation of foods with a resultant subtle decrease of natural quality of the foods as well as the soil in which they are raised. While falling short of providing the GP with an adequate nutrient supply, these foods have a significant impact on the person with chemical sensitivity and chronic degenerative disease. Usually, they aggravate the chemically sensitive patient and patient with chronic degenerative disease by exposing not detoxifying them to harmful chemicals, thus increasing their symptoms. Also, because the plants are nutrient-deficient, they fail to fuel the nutrient reserves of the chemically sensitive patients and patients with chronic degenerative disease, leaving them more vulnerable to the intake and poor detoxification. Instead of increasing the resistance of an individual with chemical sensitivity or chronic degenerative disease to contaminant exposures, this inadequate diet leaves them vulnerable. It should be kept in mind that plants can survive on fewer elements than can humans and other animals (usually 16).

Today, the content of organic matter in the average soil used for commercial growing in the United States has declined appreciably from what it was in its so-called "virgin state" (nature's balance) and is certainly much lower than that of soils fertilized with composted manures and crop residues. This reduction in organic matter in the soil is due to the lack of use of organic materials as fertilizers. Composted humus fertilization appears much more vital than fertilization with artificial nitrogen,[179] since it contains many more substances than just nitrogen (Table 4.6).[180]

Rolands and Wilkinson,[181] McCarrison,[182] and Howard[183] observed that food quality and animal and human health diminished when synthetic nitrogen (NPK) was substituted for organic manures and compost. Similar conclusions were drawn by Voisin,[184] Price,[185] Gilbert,[186] and Albrecht.[187] Bear[188] showed convincing data on the hidden effects of soil and climate on crop quality. Fertilization definitely influences nutrient content of foods.[189,190]

Organic Food

There are now over 1000 peer-reviewed studies comparing the nutritional quality of organic food to those commercially grown with artificial pesticides, herbicides, and fertilizers. Most of the studies since 2000 have emphasized the composure of vitamins, minerals, polyphenols, and antioxidant capacity of the two types of foods.

Organic food consumption is one of the fastest-growing segments of U.S. domestic foodstuffs. Sales of organic food and beverages grew from $1 billion in 1990 to $21.1 billion in 2008 and were on track to reach $23 billion in 2009.[191] Consumers generally perceive these foods to be healthier and safer for themselves and the environment.[192,193] A plethora of studies in the last two decades have assessed whether organic foods have higher levels of vitamins, minerals, and phytochemicals than conventionally raised foods and whether they have fewer pesticide residues. Far fewer studies have been conducted to assess either the potential or actual health benefits of eating organic foods. However, our studies at the EHC-Dallas and EHC-Buffalo in several thousand patients have shown this to be fine beyond a shadow of a doubt.

According to Crinnion and Benbrook et al.[194] determining the potential nutritional superiority of organic food is not a simple task. Numerous factors, apart from organic versus inorganic growing, influence the amount of vitamins and phytochemicals (phenols, flavonoids, carotenoids, etc.) in a crop. These factors include the weather (affecting crops year-to-year), specific environmental conditions from one farm to the next (microclimates), soil condition, and so on. Another major factor not taken into account in the published studies was the length of time the specific plots of land had been worked using organic methods. Since it takes years to build soil quality in a plot using organic methods and for the persistent pollutants in the ground to be reduced, this can significantly affect the outcome of comparative studies. The importance of these different factors is apparent from a review of the recent studies examining the nutrient content in tomatoes.

According to Crinnion,[194] differences between growers and soil quality of six recent studies of nutrient content of organic tomatoes, only one showed any significant differences between organic and conventional farms.[195] A California study of four different growers in one year found organically raised tomatoes have significantly higher levels of soluble solids and titratable acidity but lower red color, ascorbic acid, and total phenolics.[196] They also noted that differences among growers reached statistical significance. The authors did not note farm management skills as a possibility for the differences, suggesting it was due to differing soil conditions as well as the type of tomato used.

According to Crinnion et al.[194] in any well-designed study comparing organic versus conventional production systems, it is important that the total supply of nitrogen be equal. But one of the

TABLE 4.6
Effects of Fertilization Methods on Soil Properties[a]

Soil Parameter	Method of Fertilization		
	None	Normal NPK Treatment	Humus/Compost Treatment (One Form)[b]
Study A (4 years; $n^e = 20$)[c]			
pH	5.8 (fallow)	$6.0 \to 4.7$[c]	$6.8 \to 7.2$[d]
Study B (18 years; $n^e = 18$)[f]			
Humus (% dry wt)	2.3	2.8	2.4
Topsoil 0–4"	1.6	1.0	1.7[d]
Subsoil	(fallow)		
Subsoil density	1.5	1.53	1.36[d]
Phosphorus (ppm)			
Topsoil	70	130	120
Subsoil	50	40	70[d]
Biologic activity			
(CO_2 production)	85	81	112[d]
Earthworm holes			
(no./m^2)	25	25	92[d]
Study C (3 years; $n^e = 32$)[g]			
Nitrate runoff from fields (ppm)	–	40–59	7–11[d]

Source: Reprinted from *Nutritional Biochemistry and Metabolism with Clinical Applications*, 2nd ed., Linder, M. C., Ed., Food quality and its determinants, from field to table: Growing food its storage and preparation, p. 332, Copyright 1991, with permission from New York: Elsevier; W. J. Rea. 1994. *Chemical Sensitivity Vol II*. Page 585, Table 1. Reproduced by permission of Taylor and Francis Group, LLC, a division of Informa plc.

[a] Allocation of compost/humus increases the organic matter and phosphorus content of the lower layer of the soil, reduces nitrate runoff, reduces soil density (increases aeration), and enhances biologic activity.

[b] A sophisticated form of "organic" agriculture known as "biodynamics," practiced especially in Europe and Australia.

[c] Significant change ($p < 0.01$).

[d] Significant difference from NPK treatment ($p < 0.01$).

[e] Recalculated from Pfeiffer (1952) (Linder, 1973); n = number of samples/filed plots tested.

[f] Petterson and von Wistinghausen (1977).

[g] Koepf (1973).

major differences between organic and conventional farms is the forms in which nitrogen is present within the soil and cropping system.

On conventional farms, the majority of the nitrogen available to plants in the production season is applied as fertilizer in a synthetic form that is rapidly and readily available. On organic farms, on the other hand, nitrogen (N) is supplied in a complex matrix involving N stored in the soil, N affixed by legumes from nitrogen in the air, and N from composted manure, fish emulsion, and other soil amendments. These forms and sources of nitrogen are more slowly delivered and available to the plant.

The difference in forms of nitrogen on conventional and organic farms is important, as is the difference in how a person responds after eating a candy bar instead of an apple. Suppose the candy bar and apple has the same total amount of sugars, the rapidly available sugar in the candy bar triggers a spike in insulin (a problem for diabetics) causing a "sugar-high," followed by a "crash" in human stamina due to rapidly depleting energy (sugar) levels. With the apple though, the sugars are slowly released due to the prolonged breakdown of the apple tissue's complex matrix. There is no major spike in insulin, and instead a prolonged, steady period of available energy (sugar), with no sugar crash.

The rapidly available nitrogen in the conventional farming system diverts sugars from photosynthesis to produce more proteins and a spike in vegetative growth. And so the plant produces more leaves, and thus more chloroplasts, and then more carotenoids. Whereas in the organic system, the slower and prolonged supply of nitrogen does not trigger a spike in plant growth, allowing more photosynthetic sugars to be available for other metabolic functions such as producing more vitamin C and polyphenols.

There is also an environmental dimension to this story. Because N becomes available more gradually in organic systems, the N supply tends to more closely match plant needs. This results in more N winding up in the plant, and less running off the field after a heavy rain, leaching into the groundwater, or being lost to the atmosphere.

A 3-year study at the University of California (UC), Davis, found significant differences in phytochemical levels of tomatoes among varieties and from year-to-year.[197] Organically raised Burbank tomatoes were found to have significantly higher levels of ascorbic acid (26% higher) and the flavonoids quercetin (30% higher) and kaempferol (17%). But the other tomato cultivar (Ropreco), while showing 20% more kaempferol in the organic variety, had a less robust overall showing. This 3-year study also revealed significant differences in the nutrient content of the tomatoes from year-to-year within each plot. So, while the growing practices stayed the same, the weather conditions from year-to-year changed the outcome.

Science has made great progress in understanding the importance to human health of a range of secondary plant metabolites, many of which are essential vitamins and health-promoting antioxidants. According to Harborne,[198] secondary plant metabolites can be divided into four classes:

- Phenolic compounds (e.g., flavonoids and phenolic acids)
- Terpenoids (e.g., carotenoids and limonoids)
- Alkaloids (e.g., indoles)
- Sulfur-containing compounds (e.g., glucosinolates)

These phytochemicals play direct roles in plant responses to biotic (i.e., those caused by insects or plant disease) or abiotic (i.e., caused by weather extremes, or soil nutrient imbalances) sources of stress. They also account for and are the source of the color of foods and contribute to each food's unique flavor.

Climate has an enormous impact on nutrient levels from one year to the next, or when compared to others. Patterns of rainfall and temperatures, in particular, have a large impact on plant growth and development. For any given region, crop, and cultivar, there are weather patterns that will in most years clearly favor organic crop nutrient density, in contrast to conventionally grown crops, and vice versa. In addition, weather patterns and growing conditions may impact different nutrients in different ways.

According to Benbrook et al.[199] there were 236 valid matched pairs across 11 nutrients. The organic foods within these matched pairs were nutritionally superior in 145 or 61% of the cases while conventional foods were more nutrient dense in 87 matched pairs or 37%. Polyphenols and antioxidants were superior in three-fourths of the 59 matched pairs while contaminated foods were in potassium, phosphorus, and total protein levels in three-fourths of the 87 matched pairs. While a positive finding, these latter nutrients are clearly of lesser importance because they are greatly found in the American diet.

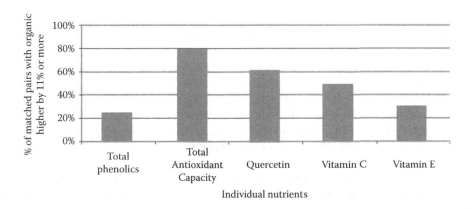

FIGURE 4.11 Percent of total matched pairs for a nutrient in which the organic sample nutrient levels exceed the conventional samples by more than 10%. (Adapted from Benbrook, C. et al. 2008. *Nutritional Superiority of Organic Food.*)

For five nutrients, Figure 4.11 shows the percent of total matched pairs for which the organic sample nutrient level exceeded the conventional sample level by 11% or more. Almost one-half of the 57 organic samples in these matched pairs exceeded the conventional sample nutrient level by 21% or more.

Another perspective reinforces the basic point. About 22% of the 145 matched pairs in which the organic samples were more nutrient dense fell within a difference of only 0%–10%, which can be regarded as minor. Almost two-thirds of the conventional matched pairs found to be more nutrient dense fell within the 0%–10% difference range.

Across all 236 matched pairs and 11 nutrients, the nutritional premium of the organic food averaged 25%. The differences documented in this study are sufficiently consistent and sizable to justify a new answer to the original question.

The magnitude of the significance of the differences in nutrient levels strongly favored the organic samples. One-fourth of the matched pairs in which the organic food contained higher levels of nutrients exceeded the level of conventional samples by 31% or more.

According to Benbrook et al.[199] our breadth of food choices, the quality and diversity of cuisine, and our increasing appreciation for fresh, local fruits, vegetables, and beverages are literally erupting across the landscape. But still, a significant and growing share of total meals is bought at fast food restaurants and in some families, more meals are consumed partially or fully in the car than at home.

The average American consumes less than half the recommended servings of fruits and vegetables, and so our intakes of essential vitamins and minerals can be grossly deficient despite years of public and private sector efforts to encourage fruit and vegetable consumption.

Intakes of added sugar, salt, and saturated fat clearly exceed recommended guidelines, and we consume and/or waste about 500 more calories per day than we did in 1970.

For millions of Americans, imbalanced and excessive consumption of food has displaced tobacco and smoking as the nation's number one, preventable cause of disease and premature death and disability.

Only one in two of Americans eat a healthy diet. Davis[200] found significant declines in the median concentrations of nutrients, protein, calcium, phosphorus, iron, riboflavin, and vitamin C in the average diet. It is clear from studies of 20,000 chemically sensitive patients with chronic degenerative disease that the use of organic food is far superior to conventional food.

Another UC-Davis study on flavonoid content of tomatoes (no ascorbic acid levels tested) was conducted using dried tomatoes that had been archived over a 10-year period.[201] The tomatoes were grown in experimental plots as part of the Long-Term Research on Agricultural Systems (LTRANS) project. Over the decade of crop production, it was found that organic tomatoes averaged 79% more quercetin and 97% more kaempferol than the conventionally grown tomatoes. Interestingly, while the flavonoid levels in tomatoes from conventional plots stayed relatively constant over 10 years, those from organic plots kept increasing each year. The increase in flavonoid levels corresponded with increasing levels of organic matter in the soil and the reduction of manure application after the plots became rich in organic matter. It is also interesting to note that, in the previously mentioned study,[197] the plots that provided Burbank and Ropreco tomatoes with higher flavonoid levels had been in organic-only care for 25 years prior to the beginning of the study, indicating the longer the soil has been worked using organic methods, the greater the nutritional difference from conventionally grown plot. Therefore, it appears that measuring produce from nonmature organic farms is not a valid method of comparison of the nutrient content of organic foods versus conventional foodstuffs.

Two other recent studies examined the difference between organically and conventionally grown tomatoes. The Italian study revealed that organic tomatoes have more salicylates than conventional tomatoes, but less ascorbic acid and lycopene.[202] The study specified that the tomatoes were grown in different parts of the same farm with sufficient distance between the organic and nonorganic plots to "prevent the drift of chemical treatments." How this was determined to be a safe distance was not revealed, and since chemicals have been shown to literally travel the globe, this is a questionable statement. The study also specified that the organic plots had been "organic" for only 3 years, which means they were not fully mature organic farms. This could account for the difference between these results and those of other tomato studies. The French study found results that were more consistent with the California studies, showing organic varieties had higher levels of ascorbic acid, carotenoids, and polyphenols than conventionally raised tomatoes.[203]

Understanding these factors puts studies of organic versus conventional growing practices into better perspective. Without an appreciation of these issues, the outcome of the study may not accurately reflect the true nutritional differences between agricultural methods.

Several reviews on nutritional differences between organic and nonorganic foods have been published in the last decade.[204–208] Earlier studies looked primarily at the mineral and vitamin content, while recent studies looked at phytochemicals (phenols, etc.) in the foods. Factors affecting variability discussed above must be kept in mind, something the earlier studies did not take into account. Factoring in these variables would presumably strengthen the findings reviewed below.

Lairon's review[204] reported that, regarding minerals, organic foods have 21% more iron and 29% more magnesium than nonorganic foods. When vitamins were studied, ascorbic acid was the most common vitamin found in higher quantities in many organic fruits and vegetables tested. Worthington[205] reached much the same conclusions stating that four nutrients were found in significantly higher levels in organic produce: ascorbic acid averaged 27% higher, iron 21% higher, magnesium 29% higher, and phosphorus 13.6% higher. Both Worthington and Lairon reported the studies they reviewed showed that conventional foods were typically higher in nitrates—15% higher in conventional foods according to Worthington. The systematic review by Dangour[206] that was published in the *American Journal of Clinical Nutrition* also reported significantly higher nitrate content in conventionally grown foods, although the authors changed the term from nitrate to "nitrogen compounds." They failed to find significant differences between organic and conventional foods for ascorbic acid, iron, or magnesium, but did report higher phosphorus levels in organic produce. Unfortunately, this widely publicized review did not include references for the 55 studies used for its conclusions, so validation of the findings is not possible.

Regarding nutrients the other reviews agree on, organic foods have more vitamin C, iron, phosphorus, and magnesium than conventional foods. While this is an important finding, it is cast in a brighter spotlight when it is recognized that during the last 50 years, vitamin C, phosphorus, iron, calcium, and riboflavin content has been declining in conventional foodstuffs grown in this country.[209]

Since quantities of some nutrients seem to be increasing in organic foods, organic foods appear to provide better nutrition.

In the last 20 years, the importance of the phytonutrient content of foods has been established. These compounds, including carotenoids, flavonoids, and other polyphenols, have been the focus of much study, and many are now provided as dietary supplements. Flavonoid molecules are potent antioxidants.[210–212] The carotenoid lycopene has been shown to help reduce cancer risk.[213] The anthocyanin compounds in berries have been shown to improve neuronal and cognitive brain functions and ocular health and protect genomic DNA integrity.[214] Because of the health benefits of phytonutrients, they have been the focus of much recent research on the nutritional value of organic foods (Table 4.7).

The nutrient density of many common foods has declined gradually over time in both the United States[209] and the United Kingdom.[232,233] The team led by Dr. Don Davis, University of Texas-Austin, examined changes between 1950 and 1999 in USDA food composition data for 43 garden crops. They found significant declines in median concentrations of six nutrients: protein (Pro), calcium (Ca), phosphorus (P), iron (Fe), riboflavin (Rib), and vitamin C (Vit C), as shown in Figure 4.9.

Declining average nutrient levels in the U.S. food supply have been brought about by what agronomists have labeled the "dilution effect," first coined in an important review article published in 1981.[234] The remarkable increases in per acre crop yields brought about over a half century through advances in plant breeding, the intensity of fertilizer and pesticide use, and irrigation are well known. However, few are aware that this achievement has come at a cost in terms of food nutritional quality.

A recent Critical Issue Report published by the Center in September 2007 describes in detail the evidence supporting the conclusion that there has been significant nutrient dilution across much of the U.S. food supply (including animal products). The report, "Still No Free Lunch: Nutrient Levels in U.S. Food Supply Eroded in Pursuit of Higher Yields," was written by Brian Halweil and is available from the Center's website (http://www.organic-center.org/science.nutriphp?action=view&report_id=115) (Figure 4.12).

NUTRIENT DECLINE IN CORN AND SOYBEANS

The steady decline of protein levels in U.S.-grown corn and soybeans has emerged as a major concern in the grain trade since, after all, livestock farmers buying corn and soybeans are basically paying for protein to fuel animal growth. These crops form the backbone of the animal-product portion of the food system, and so declines in average protein levels on the order of 20% in each crop are a cause of concern.

The declining protein content and quality of U.S. soybeans has, in all likelihood, been triggered in large part by the adoption of genetically modified, herbicide-tolerant varieties, especially Roundup Ready (RR) soybeans.

The nutritional inferiority of RR soybeans has been documented by a team of scientists at Midwestern land grant universities.[235] They compared the protein content and quality of soybeans grown in the 2000–2001 seasons in Argentina, Brazil, the United States, China, and India. Consistently, Argentinean soybean products contained the lowest level of crude protein, and at that time were about 95% RR.

Soybeans from Argentina contained 32.6% crude protein on a dry matter basis, compared with 39.3% in Brazil, 37.1% in U.S. beans, and 44.9% in Chinese soybeans, none of which were genetically altered. When this study was conducted, about one-half of U.S. soybeans were RR, explaining why the U.S. soybean protein levels were intermediate between the almost-all RR beans from Argentina, and conventional (i.e., no RR) soybeans from China.

Today, virtually all nonorganic soybeans planted in the United States are RR, and the depression in protein content, compared to conventional varieties, is likely comparable to the 25%-plus reduction reported in the Karr–Lilienthal study[235] between soybeans grown in Argentina and China.

TABLE 4.7
Nutrient Content of Foods: Organic versus Nonorganic

Food	Nutrients Tested	Results
Potatoes in Czechoslovakia	Ascorbic acid; chlorogenic acid (the polyphenol that is responsible for much of the antioxidant activity of coffee, and has been shown to protect paraoxonase activity)[215]	Organically grown potatoes had lower levels of nitrate and higher levels of ascorbic acid and chlorogenic acid[216]
Highbush blueberries[217] in New Jersey	Sugars, malic acid, total phenolics, total anthocyanins, and antioxidant activity	All nutrients tested were higher in organic than conventionally grown blueberries[219]
Strawberries, marionberries, and corn[218] from an organic farm in Oregon	Ascorbic acid and total polyphenols	All three foods had significantly higher amounts of ascorbic acid and total polyphenols than their conventionally grown counterparts[220]
Blackcurrants from five conventional and three organic farms in Finland	Total polyphenols	Significantly higher levels of total polyphenols and resveratrol in organic juice[223]
Syrah grapes from France	Anthocyanin content	Conventionally grown grapes had higher levels of anthocyanins, no information of history of the organic vineyards[222]
Grape juice from Brazil	Total polyphenols; resveratrol	Significantly higher levels of total polyphenols and resveratrol in organic juice[223]
Golden Delicious apples (3-year study)	Total antioxidant activity (total polyphenols provide 90% of the total antioxidant activity)[224]	Two of three years the antioxidant activity of organic apples was 15% higher than the conventional apples, no difference in the third year[225]
Plums	Ascorbic acid, α- and γ-tocopherol, β-carotene; total polyphenols	Organic orchards with soil left as natural meadow, ascorbate, tocopherols, and β-carotene were highest; in organic orchards with *Trifolium* groundcover, total polyphenols were highest, although highest levels of total polyphenols were in the conventional plums[226]
Peaches and pears (3-year study; 5-year-old orchard)	Total antioxidant activity, total polyphenols, ascorbic acid	Higher antioxidant, total polyphenols and ascorbic acid in organic fruit[227]
Red oranges from Italy	Total polyphenols, total anthocyanins, ascorbic acid, total antioxidant activity	Organic oranges had higher levels of total polyphenols, total anthocyanins, ascorbic acid, total antioxidant activity[228]
Varieties of wheat from India	Protein, starches, gluten	Higher protein, more easily digestible starch and gluten in the organic wheat; no information on history of the organic farms[229]
Oats from Sweden	Total polyphenols	No significant difference between organic and nonorganic; differences from year-to-year and among cultivars; no information on history of the organic farms[230]
Milk	Omega-3 fatty acids (α-linolenic [ALA] and eicosapentaenoic acid)	Organically raised dairy cattle yielded higher levels of omega3s,[231,232] no difference in vitamin A or E[233]
Grana Padano cheese from Italy	Conjugated linoleic acid (CLA), ALA	Higher levels of CLA and ALA in cheese samples from organic milk[234]

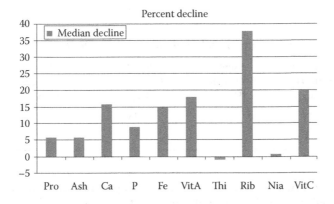

FIGURE 4.12   Trends in 43 garden crops; USDA data, 1950–1999.

In the case of corn, average protein levels have fallen about 20%, from around 9%–10% in the 1940s, to 7%–8% today, and sometimes fall below 6%.

The University of Illinois Long-Term Corn Experiment has been testing popular corn varieties for more than 100 years. Researchers report that: Among recent commercial corn hybrids, increased yields have further reduced total protein levels.[236]

A separate study found that protein in corn plants decreased about 0.3% every decade of the twentieth century, while starch increased by 0.3% each decade.[237]

They identified 191 matched pairs with valid comparisons of antioxidant, vitamin, and mineral levels. Of these, 119 organic samples within the matched pairs had higher nutrient levels, or 62% of the total matched pairs. The conventional samples contained higher levels of nutrients in 68 matched pairs, or 36%, as shown in Table 4.8. Nutrient levels were reported as equal in 2% of the matched pairs.

TABLE 4.8
Overview of Differences in the Nutrient Content in Organic and Conventional Foods in 191 Matched Pairs

Nutrient	Number of Matched Pairs	Number Organic Higher	Number Conventional Higher	Percent Organic Higher (%)	Percent Conventional Higher (%)
		Antioxidants			
Total phenolics	25	18	6	72	24
Total antioxidant capacity	8	7	1	88	13
Quercetin	15	13	1	87	7
Kaempferol	11	6	5	55	45
		Vitamins			
Vitamin C/ascorbic acid	46	29	17	63	37
β-Carotene	8	4	4	50	50
α-Tocopherol (vitamin E)	13	8	5	62	38
		Minerals			
Phosphorus	32	20	10	63	31
Potassium	33	14	19	42	58
Totals and averages	191	119	68	62	36

TABLE 4.9

Differences in Nitrate Levels in 18 Matched Pairs and Protein in 27 Matched Pairs

Nutrient	Number of Matched Pairs	Number Organic Higher	Number Conventional Higher	Percent Organic Higher(%)	Percent Conventional Higher (%)
Nitrates	18	3	15	16.7	83.3
Protein	27	4	23	14.8	85.2

They also analyzed two other nutrients—nitrates and protein. Across 18 matched pairs, nitrate levels in the conventional samples were higher in 83% of the pairs (undesirable), while protein levels were higher in 85% of the conventional samples in 27 matched pairs (desirable). These differences are shown in Table 4.9.

Magnitude of Differences

The magnitude of the differences in the nutrient levels in organic foods versus conventional foods is clearly greater in those pairs in which the organic food contained higher levels of nutrients. Table 4.10 displays the magnitude of differences in the 119 matched pairs in which the organic samples contained higher nutrient levels, while Table 4.9 reports the same information for matched pairs in which the conventional samples were found to contain higher levels of nutrients.

For the 119 matched pairs in which the organic food sample had higher nutrient levels, the magnitude of the difference was 21% or greater in 42% of the cases. The nutritional premium in favor of organic food was 31% or more in nearly one-quarter of the cases.

TABLE 4.10

Magnitude of Differences in 119 Matched Pairs Where the Organically Grown Food Contained Higher Levels of Nutrient

Nutrient	Number of Studies with Organic Greater than Conventional by				
	0%–10%	11%–20%	21%–30%	31%–50%	Over 50%
Antioxidants					
Total phenolics	9	4	1	4	
Total antioxidant capacity		3	2	1	1
Quercetin	2		3	1	7
Kaempferol	1	3	2	1	1
Vitamins					
Vitamin C/ascorbic acid	3	14	7	3	2
β-Carotene	1	1			2
α-Tocopherol (vitamin E)	3	2	1	1	1
Minerals					
Phosphorus	7	7	3	3	
Potassium	5	5	2	1	1
Totals	31	39	20	14	15

HERBICIDES, PESTICIDES, AND INSECTICIDES

It is obvious that the application of pesticides and herbicides to substances with high biological activity causes several disturbances in plant metabolism and commonly alters the nutritive values of plant products.[238–241]

According to Mohammodi,[242] a conventional wheat productivity utilizing follage, commercial fertilizers applied through pesticides can improve grain yield. However, this intensive production system also can degrade soil quality, enhance runoff to covering the soil with an improvision surface, and contribute to surface and imparting pollution and add to production cost.[242] See Chapter 2 on gastrointestinal section on glyphosate and atrazine complication for growing wheat, rye, soy, etc.

ANIMALS

In addition to the direct toxic contamination of plants, animals dependent on these plants for food are also contaminated. For example, an animal that eats plants sprayed with insecticide or contaminated with mycotoxins will incorporate this substance into its tissues.

Bald eagles were significantly affected by contaminants in the environment in the early 1960s and 1970s. Now monitoring them can provide a gross indication of general contaminant levels in the environment. In 1999, a consortium of the Michigan Department of Environmental Quality, the U.S. Fish and Wildlife Service, and researchers from Michigan State University and Clemson University initiated a bald eagle contaminant monitoring project. Ninety samples of blood and feathers were collected by nonlethal procedures from permanent inland nests, from nests in additional inland watersheds being assessed as part of the Michigan department's 5-year watershed assessment cycle, and from Great Lakes and connecting channel nests show changes in mean PCB levels and mean mercury levels, respectively, in bald eagles between the late 1980s and early 1990s, and in 1999. Specifically, PCB levels in the blood of bald eagles were dramatically lower in 1999 for inland nests and those in Lakes Superior, Michigan, and Huron. (Although Lake Erie did not show the same result, only one eagle was sampled there in 1999.) Similarly, mean mercury levels in bald eagle feathers declined in all geographic areas examined.

EFFECT OF DIFFERENT FERTILIZATION METHODS ON SOIL BIOLOGICAL INDEXES

Conventional wheat production utilizing tillage, commercial fertilizer applied through pesticides, and irrigation can improve the grain yield. However, this intensive production system also can degrade soil quality, enhance runoff by covering the soil with an impervious surface, contribute to surface and impurity pollution, and add to production cost.[243] Alternative systems have been developed that use renewable organic resources and minimize tillage to build soil organic matter and enhance soil quality. Fertilization is one of the soil and crop management practices, which exert a great influence on soil quality.[244] Farmyard manure (FYM) and compost are organic sources of nutrients that also have been shown to increase soil organic matter and enhance soil quality. It is well known that organic amendments, such as plant residues, FYM, and composts, have a number of benefits in soil physical and chemical properties. Many reports have also revealed different aspects of biology of soils amended with organic matters, including the number of general microorganisms,[245] biomass of bacteria and fungi,[246] enzyme activities,[247] and biochemical properties.[248] Microbial communities perform necessary ecosystem services, pathogen suppression, stabilization of soil aggregates, and degradation of xenobiotics.

Soil microbial biomass, activity, and community structure have been shown to respond to agricultural management practices. Alternation to no tillage or increased cropping intensity increases microbial biomass C (MBC) in response to increased nutrient reserves and improved soil structure and water retention.[249]

Enzyme activities have been indicated as soil properties suitable for use in the evaluation of the degree of alteration of soils in both natural and agroecosystems. Soil microbial properties have a strong correlation with soil health. Some research has already suggested the favorable effects of conservation, tillage practices, and organic fertilizers on soil enzyme activities.[247] The activity of dehydrogenase is considered an indicator of the oxidative metabolism in soils and thus of the microbiological activity, because it is exclusively intracellular and, theoretically, can function only within viable cells. Urease catalyzes the hydrolysis of urea to CO_2 and NH_3, which is of specific interest because urea is an important N fertilizer. Urease is released from living and disintegrated microbial cells, and in the soil it can exist as an extracellular enzyme absorbed on clay particles or encapsulated in humic complexes. Phosphatases catalyze the hydrolysis of both organic phosphate (P) esters and anhydrides of phosphoric acid into inorganic P. Phosphatase activity may originate from the plant roots (and associated mycorrhiza and other fungi), or from bacteria.[250]

Fertilization plays an important role in crop growth and soil improvement. This study was conducted to determine the best fertilization system for wheat production. Experiments were arranged in a complete block design with three replications in 2 years. Main plots consisted of six methods of fertilization including (N1): FYM; (N2): compost; (N3): chemical fertilizers; (N4): FYM + compost; (N5): FYM + compost + chemical fertilizers; and (N6): control. Main plots were arranged in subplots. The addition of compost or FYM significantly increased the soil MBC in comparison to the chemical fertilizer. The dehydrogenase, phosphatase, and urease activities in the N3 treatment were significantly lower than in the FYM and compost treatments.

The results indicated statistically significant ($p < 0.05$) differences in the level of MBC in the soil between various methods of fertilization. There were no significant differences between interaction effects of fertilization on MBC. The pattern of variation of MBC in the soil during the 2 years of study was similar. The addition of compost or FYM, significantly ($p < 0.05$) increased the soil MBC in comparison to the chemical fertilizer and the control. Higher levels of MBC in compost-treated soil could be due to greater amounts of biogenic materials such as mineralizable nitrogen, water-soluble carbon, and carbohydrates. Integrated use of chemical fertilizers and organic fertilizers (N5) brings in more MBC in soil compared to their single application. Similar observations were recorded by Leita et al.[251]. Fertilizers may meet up the demand of mineral nutrition required by the microbes but not that of carbon, which is a major component of microbial cells. Integrated application of organic and inorganic materials provides a balanced supply of mineral nutrients as well as carbon.

The activities of all enzymes varied significantly in different fertilization methods. The pattern of variation of enzyme activity in the soil during the 2 years of study was similar; however, urease activity was higher in the first year. The activities of all enzymes were generally higher in the N4 treatment than in the unfertilized and chemical fertilizer treatments (Table 4.11). There were no differences in phosphatase activity between the compost treatment and the FYM treatments. The dehydrogenase, phosphatase, and urease activities in the N3 treatment were significantly lower than in the FYM and compost treatments. As shown in Table 4.12, alkaline and acid phosphatase generally increased with compost application. Increased phosphatase activity could be responsible for hydrolysis of organically bound phosphate into free ions, which were taken up by plants. Tarafdar and Marschner[250] reported that plants can utilize organic P fractions from the soil by phosphatase activity enriched in the soil–root interface. The observed increase in enzymatic activities due to organic fertilizers amendments is in accordance with previous studies. Martens et al.[252] reported that addition of the organic matter maintained high levels of phosphatase activity in soil during a long-term study.

Giusquiani et al.[253] reported that phosphatase activities increased when compost was added at rates of up to 90 to 1 and the phosphatases continued to show a linear increase with compost rates of up to 270 to 1 in a field experiment. Application of nitrogen fertilizers significantly decreased urease activity while addition of organic manure increased its activity. The authors concluded that because

TABLE 4.11

Effects of Fertilization Methods on Dry Weight, Protein, and Vitamin Contents of Food Plants[a]

Vegetable	Regular NPK	Stable Manure	Manure and NPK	Composted Manure
			Methods of Fertilization	
Spinach				
Dry weight (7%)	6.9	9.4[b]	6.5	9.2[b]
Protein (% of control)	100	103	99	101
Nitrate-N (μg/g)	270	20[b]	280	10[b]
Ascorbate (μg/g)	340	560[b]	320	490[b]
β-Carotene (μg/g)	28	25	27	25
Sugar (% weight)	0.9	1.0	0.7	1.3[b]
Savoy cabbage				
Dry weight (%)	8.3	13.0[b]	8.7	14.2[b]
Protein (% of control)	100	133[b]	121[b]	135
Ascorbate (μg/g)	440	800[b]	430	780[b]
Celery				
Dry weight (%)	15.0	16.4[b]	15.3	15.9[b]
Protein (% of control)	100	142[b]	118	131[b]
Sugar (% of weight)	2.1	2.3	2.3	2.2

Source: Reprinted from *Nutritional Biochemistry and Metabolism with Clinical Applications*, 2nd ed., Linder, M. C., Ed., Food quality and its determinants, from field to table: Growing food its storage and preparation, p. 334, Copyright 1991, with permission from New York: Elsevier; W. J. Rea. 1994. *Chemical Sensitivity Vol II*. Page 589, Table 3. Reproduced by permission of Taylor and Francis Group, LLC, a division of Informa plc.

[a] Data from Schupan (1974). Crops were grown side by side in experimental pots containing a base of sand or "fen" soil plus the fertilizer indicated, all at the same level of nitrogen. Values shown are means for 4–6 average values (two types of pots planted 2 or 3 times = years). Protein values are given relative to the NPK-fertilized pots (controls).

[b] Indicates values significantly different from control (NPK-fertilized) ($p < 0.01$). (1) Fertilization has significant effects on plant dry weight (water content) as well as protein; mineral fertilizers tend to increase moisture content and decrease protein and dry matter. Differences in sugar and vitamin contents in favor of organic treatment may also occur. (2) Results vary with the particular food crop. (3) Spinach tends to absorb and accumulate nitrate when fertilized with inorganic nitrates.

the nitrogen fertilizers used in the experiments contained NH_4^+ and that the reaction products of urease being NH_4^+, microbial induction of urease activity had been inhibited. The effect of organic amendments on enzyme activities is probably a combined effect of a higher degree of stabilization of enzymes to humic substances and an increase in microbial biomass with increased soil carbon concentration.[252,254] This is also indicated by the strong correlation of protease, acid phosphatase, and urease with MBC concentrations. Only alkaline phosphatase activity showed statistically no significant correlations. Compost application increased dehydrogenase activity (Table 4.11). Stronger dehydrogenase activity in compost-applied plots may be due to higher organic matter content.[255]

Marinari et al.[256] reported that a higher level of dehydrogenase activity was observed in soil treated with compost and FYM compared to soil treated with mineral fertilizer. The enzyme activity in organic amendment soil increased by an average of twofold to fourfold compared with the unamended soil. Application of compost caused a significant increase in dehydrogenase activity.[252]

TABLE 4.12

Effect of Fertilization Methods on MBC and Soil Enzyme Activity

Treatment	MBC (µg)	Protease (µg)	Acid Phosphatase (µg)	Alkaline Phosphatase (µg)	Urease (µg)	Dehydrogenase (µg)
			Basal Fertilizer			
FYM (N1)	278.4c	86.5c	167.4b	2987.3b	49.6a	60.1b
Compost (N2)	312.6c	94.6bc	169.2b	3001.4b	44.4b	62.9ab
Chemical fertilizer (N3)	196.3d	87.1c	158.1c	2678.6c	28.8c	21.2d
FYM + Compost (N4)	409.5b	110.3a	226.6a	3314.4a	49.8a	63.8a
FYM + Compost + Chemical (N5)	691.2a	96.2b	169.2b	2879.1bc	29.4c	33.7c
Control (N6)	89.3c	73.1d	41.8d	2658.7c	27.9c	20.8d

Source: Reprinted from *Saudi Journal of Biological Sciences*, Vol. 19(3), Mohammadi, K., G. Heidari, M. T. K. Nezhad, S. Ghamari, Y. Sohrabi. Contrasting soil microbial responses to fertilization and tillage systems in canola rhizophere, pp. 377–383. Copright 2012 with permission from Elsevier.

Note: Mean values in each column with the same letter(s) are not significantly different using LSD tests at 5% of probability.

These results were similar to our finding that dehydrogenase in rhizosphere soil of N2 treatments was average three times higher than that of mineral fertilizer (N3) treatments. In addition, the higher organic matter levels in the compost treatments may provide a more favorable environment for the accumulation of enzymes in the soil matrix, since soil organic constituents are thought to be important in forming stable complexes with free enzymes.

Soil factors, including redox potential (Eh) and pH can affect the rate of enzyme-mediated reactions by influencing the redox status and ionization, respectively, as well as solubility of enzymes, substrates, and cofactors. In addition, some enzymes may predominate at specific pH levels. Application of compost and FYM caused a faster and higher reduction of soil, and at the same time increased the soil pH (Table 4.13).[257]

The Michigan Department of National Resources has also conducted an annual census of bald eagle nest in Michigan since 1961. The nests increased from 50 in 1961 to 366 in 2000. During that same period, bald eagle productivity, as measured by the number of young fledged per nest,

TABLE 4.13

Correlation Coefficients between Enzyme Activity and Microbial Biomass Carbon

	MBC	Protease	Acid Phosphatase	Alkaline Phosphatase	Urease	Dehydrogenase
MBC	1					
Protease	0.963*	1				
Acid phosphatase	0.982*	0.695*	1			
Alkaline phosphatase	0.219ns	0.682*	0.883*	1		
Urease	0.882*	0.133ns	0.598*	0.432ns	1	
Dehydrogenase	0.901*	0.913*	0.789*	0.712*		1

Source: Reprinted from *Saudi Journal of Biological Sciences*, Vol. 19(3), Mohammadi, G. Heidari, M. T. K. Nezhad, S. Ghamari, and Y. Sohrabi, Contrasting soil microbial responses to fertilization and tillage systems in canola rhizophere, pp. 377–383. Copyright 2012 with permission from Elsevier.

* $p < 0.01$; ns $p > 0.05$.

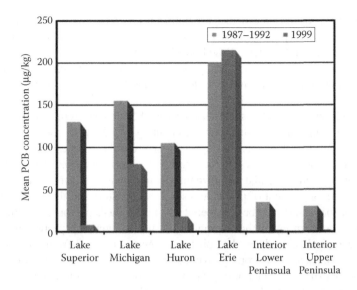

FIGURE 4.13 Mean polychlorinated biphenyls (PCB) concentration in nesting bald eagle feathers, 1987–1992 and 1999. (Adapted from Michigan Department of Environmental Quality, Office of Special Environmental Projects. *State of Michigan's Environment 2001: First Biennial Report.* 2001.)

increased more than 50%. The contaminant and population measures demonstrate that levels of key environmental contaminants in bald eagles within the Great Lakes Region have declined through the 1990s, and that population and productivity are increasing (Figures 4.13 and 4.14).

The largest use of pesticides is in agricultural production. That use fluctuates, depending on a number of factors such as weather or type of crop. According to the National Center for Food and Agricultural Policy (NCFAP), a private, nonprofit research organization, the use of agricultural pesticides increased between 1992 and 1997 from 892 million to 985 million pounds. The recent EPA report shows a similar increase in the use of all pesticides in this same time span, with leveling of use between 1997 and 1999.

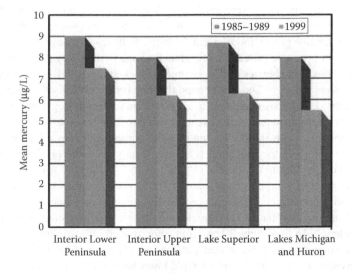

FIGURE 4.14 Mean mercury levels in nesting bald eagle feathers, 1985–1989 and 1999. (Adapted from Michigan Department of Environmental Quality, Office of Special Environmental Projects. *State of Michigan's Environment 2001: First Biennial Report.* 2001.)

Approximately half of those pesticides are herbicides used to control weeds that limit or inhibit the growth of a desired crop. Pesticides are also used in smaller quantities in rights-of-way, businesses, and home lawns and gardens. Based on EPA's national pesticide sales estimates, industrial, commercial, and governmental pesticide applications—many of which occur in urban environments—totaled 148 million pounds in 1999. Home and garden pesticide use was estimated to be 140 million pounds.

According to Crinnion, world pesticide use exceeded 5.0 billion pounds in both 2000 and 2001 (total cost, $64.5 billion) with the United States accounting for 1.2 billion pounds per year at an annual cost of $11 billion.[258] While the totals are staggering, so too is the infinitesimal amount of those 5 billion pounds a year that actually make it to the target pest—less than 0.1%.[259] No one has accounted for where the other 99.9% ends up, and it is known these compounds can travel thousands of miles around the globe.[180,260] Both the amount of pesticide residue on foodstuff and the amount released into the atmosphere are factors that should be considered when individuals purchase organically raised food.

Although organic farming methods prohibit the use of synthetic pesticides, the produce can be exposed to chemicals already in the soil from previous use and from compounds that percolate through the soil. Except for crops grown under cover, organic farms are also subject to exposure from pesticide drift from neighboring farms and global transport of chemicals. This exposure occurs from compounds that settle to the ground during both the growing season and the off season, and exposure can continue during transport and distribution. The level of various heavy metals in organically raised produce was higher in crops grown in open fields compared to the same crops grown in a greenhouse.[261] The researchers noted this was due to atmospheric contamination; root vegetables also absorbed toxins from the soil.

While no pesticides or herbicides can be used to grow crops that are certified organic, these crops are not free of insecticide residues, although significantly less so than the same foods grown by nonorganic methods (including integrated pest management systems).

Levels of pesticide residue on foods in the United States are monitored through the Pesticide Data Program (PDP) of the U.S. Department of Agriculture (USDA). A review that utilized the USDA data, along with data from Consumers Union and the Marketplace Surveillance Program of the California Department of Pesticide Regulation (CDPR), reported that organically raised foods had one-third the amount of chemical residues found in conventionally raised foods.[262] When compared to produce grown with integrated pest management techniques, the organic produce has 1% of the amount of residue. In addition, organic foods were much less likely than nonorganic product (by a factor of 10) to have two or more residues. Only 2.6% of organic foods had detectable multiple residues compared to 26% of conventionally grown foods. Data from the PDP reveal conventional produce with the highest percentages of positive (insecticide residue) findings were: celery (96%), pears (95%), apples (94%), peaches (93%), strawberries (91%), oranges (85%), spinach (84%), potatoes (81%), grapes (78%), and cucumbers (74%).[263] The study found that an average of 82% of conventional fruits were positive for insecticide residues compared to 23% of organic fruits. Regarding vegetables, 65% of conventionally grown produce tested positive, compared to 23% for organic vegetables.

Fruits and vegetables with the highest and lowest percentages of residues in the USDA study are similar to the listing of the most and least toxic foods available on the Internet through the Environmental Working Group (Table 4.14).[264] Table 4.15 lists the least toxic produce.

Not only have repeated studies shown that organic foods have lower levels of insecticides, clear evidence also indicates reduced pesticide exposure levels in consumers of organic foods. The reduced level of organophosphate (OP) pesticide on organic foods was demonstrated by a study of Seattle preschoolers.[265] In that study, 39 children were divided into two groups—those whose diets were at least 75% organic and those whose diets consisted predominately of conventionally grown foods. Children eating organic foods had a sixfold lower level of OP pesticide residues in their urine than those who ate more conventionally. The same research group tested preschoolers before and after changing their diets from conventionally grown to organic foods. When the shift was made to organic diets the urinary levels of malathion and chlorpyrifos became undetectable until their

TABLE 4.14
The Environmental Working Group's
12 Most Toxic Fruits and Vegetables
(in Order of Toxicity)

Peach	Nectarine	Lettuce
Apple	Strawberries	Grapes (imported)
Bell pepper	Cherries	Carrot
Celery	Kale	Pear

TABLE 4.15
The Environmental Working Group's Least
Toxic Produce

Onion	Asparagus	Papaya
Avocado	Sweet peas	Watermelon
Sweet corn	Kiwi	Broccoli
Pineapple	Cabbage	Tomato
Mango	Eggplant	Sweet potato

conventional diets were restored. Five different OP metabolites were measured with mean levels of 0.01, 0.2, 0.3, 4.6, and 5.1 μg/L while on conventional diets.[266]

Potential Health Benefits of Organic Foods

Since organically raised food typically has higher levels of health-promoting phytonutrients and certain vitamins and mineral and lower levels of insecticide residues, one could assume that they would provide health benefits. Unfortunately, studies looking at the potential health benefits of organic foods are scarce, and all but one are focused on implied health benefits. The majority of these studies look at antioxidant activity in humans, although some *in vitro* studies examined the anticancer potential of some organic food products.

Antioxidant Studies

Two studies examined whether drinking organic wine provides greater protection against LDL oxidation than conventional wine. Neither study (both by the same group of researchers in the same year) found a difference between organic and nonorganic wine; however, red wine of either agricultural method provided greater inhibition of LDL oxidation compared to white wine.[267,268] The chemically sensitive cannot tolerate either, therefore, the significance is moot.

A double-blind crossover trial of six Golden Delicious apple consumers was conducted to determine the difference in antioxidant activity between organic and nonorganic groups.[190] Golden Delicious apples have some of the lowest polyphenol content of any apple.[221] In this study, there was no difference noted in total polyphenol levels between organic and conventional apples, and thus no difference in antioxidant activity. Information on the maturity of the organic orchards was not available for review. As a follow-up study, fruits from mature organic orchards with higher polyphenol content, as noted above,[222] could be used with subsequent measurements to determine whether higher phenol levels would alter the antioxidant status in humans.

The use of nitrogen, phosphorus, and potash, the most prevalent fertilizer supplements in commercial farming, rose from 7.5 million nutrient tons (tons of a chemical nutrient in a fertilizer

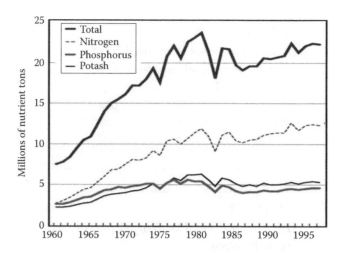

FIGURE 4.15   Use of fertilizer, 1960–1998. (Adapted from Daberkov, S. et al. *Agricultural Resources and Environmental Indicators: Nutrient Use and Management.* February 2003.)

mixture) in 1961 to nearly 24 million nutrient tons in 1981. Figure 4.15 displays trends in the use of fertilizer over the past 40 years.

EVIDENCE FOR INHIBITION OF CHOLINESTERASES IN INSECT AND MAMMALIAN NERVOUS SYSTEMS BY THE INSECT REPELLENT DEET

According to Corbel et al.[269] *N,N*-diethyl-3-methylbenzamide (deet) remains the gold standard for insect repellents. About 200 million people use it every year and over 8 billion doses have been applied over the past 50 years. Despite the widespread and increased interest in the use of deet in public health programs, controversies remain concerning both the identification of its target sites at the olfactory system and its mechanism of toxicity in insects, mammals, and humans. Here, they investigated the molecular target site for deet and the consequences of its interactions with carbamate insecticides on the cholinergic system. By using toxicological, biochemical, and electrophysiological techniques, Corbel et al.[269] showed that deet is not simply a behavior-modifying chemical but that it also inhibits cholinesterase activity, in both insect and mammalian neuronal preparations. Deet is commonly used in combination with insecticides and they show that deet has the capacity to strengthen the toxicity of carbamates, a class of insecticides known to block acetylcholinesterase (AChE). These findings question the safety of deet, particularly in combination with other chemicals, and they highlight the importance of a multidisciplinary approach to the development of safer insect repellents for use in public health.

Although aggregate use dipped in 1983, it increased most recently between 1996 and 1998 to more than 22 million nutrient tons. Use of most major fertilizers is concentrated on croplands in the Midwest. One can see the changes in fertilizers until 2020—some are lower and others much higher.

Chemicals and nutrients can move from their location of use or origin to a place in the environment where humans and other organisms can become exposed to them. People are exposed to chemicals in all aspects of their daily lives, through their clothing, use of everyday products, housing, automobiles, and buildings. The GP and the chemically sensitive patient and patient with chronic degenerative disease are at the mercy of the total environment pollutant load in air, food, and water.

One way people can be exposed to pesticides is through pesticide residue in food. The USDA's PDP measures pesticide residue levels in fruits, vegetables, grains, meat, and dairy products from across the country, sampling different combinations of commodities each year. In 2000, PDP collected and analyzed a total of 10,907 samples: 8912 fruits and vegetables, 178 rice, 716 peanut butter,

TABLE 4.16

U.S. Consumption of Selected Phosphate and Potash Fertilizers

Year Ending June 30	Grades 22% and Under	Grades over 22%	Phosphates Other Single Phosphates[a]	Superphosphates Diammonium Phosphate[b] (46-0)21	Monoammonium (18-Phosphate (11-Phosphate (51-55)-0)	Other Other Nitrogen-Phosphate Grades[c]	Potash Potassium Chloride	Other Single Nutrient[d]
1996	30,215	447,794	186,934	3,734,384	1,243,347	2,177,135	5,506,406	457,206
1997	47,292	385,015	263,078	3,720,928	1,319,346	2,536,936	5,651,965	632,309
1998	47,185	362,355	257,992	3,674,195	1,341,768	1,089,677	5,644,245	556,359
1999	63,696	357,937	298,969	3,170,287	1,275,382	2,889,072	5,197,078	555,813
2000	11,437	333,298	394,481	3,220,179	1,479,174	2,706,113	5,332,030	508,729
2001	16,268	328,555	362,989	3,202,905	1,520,808	2,484,279	5,316,632	535,018
2002	18,496	328,971	355,725	3,433,424	1,826,691	2,561,494	5,341,799	480,137
2003	21,164	250,038	201,126	3,186,701	1,830,901	2,442,941	5,454,374	669,143
2004	21,421	213,702	266,579	3,580,108	2,212,818	2,468,501	6,011,176	827,025
2005	15,635	191,061	262,045	3,392,521	2,234,194	2,634,712	5,577,417	804,916
2006	8993	173,939	230,781	2,999,062	2,327,598	2,598,068	4,889,824	800,355
2007	8621	142,133	286,356	2,853,687	2,682,723	2,771,531	5,790,888	810,272
2008	5194	120,821	280,330	2,608,738	2,773,322	2,537,635	5,514,846	763,255
2009	4963	72,419	267,610	1,820,559	2,012,258	2,147,515	3,338,415	625,827
2010	6721	78,185	368,670	2,320,718	2,652,038	2,905,750	5,197,711	760,566

Source: Adapted from ERS, TVA (Tennessee/Valley Authority), AAPFCO (Association of American Plant Food Control Officials), TFI (The Fertilizer Institute).

[a] All other single-phosphate materials excluding superphosphoric acid.
[b] 18-46-0 refers to the percentage of nitrogen, phosphate, and potash, respectively, contained in this fertilizer material.
[c] All nitrogen–phosphate materials other than diammonium phosphate and monoammonium phosphate.
[d] Other potash materials excluding potassium chloride and multiple-nutrient potash fertilizers.

and 1101 poultry which originated from 38 states and 21 foreign countries. In 2010, it increased more (Table 4.16).

Animals also become contaminated through production processes intended to enhance their marketability. Since some beef producers determined that fat interspersed through the muscle of beef improves its taste, methods intended to increase the fat content of beef, and hence its flavor and marketability, such as hormone supplementation, have been utilized. Also, commercial concerns about making available a large quantity of less expensive meats have led to more unfavorable production practices. Animals have been packed into feedlots and then to offset the effects of overcrowding and lack of exercise have been treated with pesticides, hormones, and antibiotics. As with chemically treated plants, the meat from these animals may appear nutritious, but the fact is that by the time this meat gets to market it may be heavily contaminated with residues from the treatments initially used to make it safe and enticing.

While these modern practices for beef production may be an economic boon for the middleman in a marketplace economy, they are not necessarily good for the health of the consumer or the profitability of the producer.

The alteration of our basic foods and their nutrient supply over the course of the twentieth and twenty-first century has had a long-term negative impact on our ability to maintain optimum human health and, certainly, in many instances, exacerbates chemical sensitivity and chronic degenerative disease. Often this impact has gone unnoticed because it initially manifests in subtle symptoms, such as loss of initiative, creativity, and overall vigor, rather than outright acute illness. Acute chemical sensitivity and chronic degenerative disease occur without recognition of the gradual loss of nutrient fuels for detoxification. Basic chronic nutrient depletion and overeating continue perhaps because the public has not been made aware of the inherent dangers of these new practices and because an abundance of easily accessible food keeps much of the industrialized world from starving. Further, the public does not protest current food production practices because the diseases produced by subtly inadequate or inappropriate nutrition are often chronic and common (e.g., cancer, atherosclerosis, arthritis) and lack cures. There is usually no recognizable (by casual observation) acute condition that is related to the nutrient quality of present-day commercial food, and, therefore, the public is, for the most part, unaware of its potential for effecting subtle, long-term nutrient alteration.

At the EHC-Dallas and EHC-Buffalo, we have observed a wide variety of adverse effects in chemically sensitive patients and patients with chronic degenerative disease who ate foods treated with artificial pesticides and fertilizers. These include symptoms involving the genitourinary, respiratory, dermal, neuromuscular, cardiovascular, and gastrointestinal systems.[241] Also, some cancers appear to be generated by contaminated diet. We have also observed thousands of chemically sensitive individuals who had no tolerance for foods treated with pesticides and chemical fertilizers. These patients have tolerated with impunity the same type of food that is less chemically contaminated, and most have even been restored to vigorous health.

The evidence is now strong that many researchers are developing strategies in favor of chemically less contaminated farming.[270–274] These strategies include crop rotation, companion planting, composted fertilization, and multianimal farms.

Another encouraging observation is that less polluted land and water can be restorative to contaminated animals and plants over a period of time. Plants become vigorous when nutrients in the soil are replenished. Animals and their offspring usually can clear harbored contaminants on less polluted land, as shown in a series of goats studied at the EHC-Dallas over a period of 4 years (Table 4.17) (CS, Vol. II, Table 6). All offspring were free of contaminants when their blood was measured by mass spectrometry and gas chromatography, as were most of the previously contaminated parents.

Chemical contamination of food, which will affect the chemically sensitive adversely, can result from various methods of transportation, preservation, and storage of foods. These methods can even contaminate organic food, making acquisition of pollutant-free food more difficult for the individual with chemical sensitivity and chronic degenerative disease. Each category of potential contamination of food, from its harvest to its preparation for consumption, is discussed separately. These methods of transportation, preservation, and storage of food involve the intentional and unintentional introduction of additives to food. Many chemical dump storage sites are being built and hopefully, at last, they will all be cleaned up (Figures 4.15 and 4.16).

Preservation and Storage

Our ability to preserve and store large quantities of foods has not entirely been a boon. With seasonal foods now available year round, individuals are able to consume large quantities of the same food repetitively. They, therefore, take in an increased volume of biological entities often from a monotonous diet. In so doing, their specific immune and enzyme detoxification systems, which would normally be able to rest during the time a food was "out of season" and unavailable, are continually taxed. Eventually, these systems can become overloaded and then weakened by this kind of constant demand, and an individual may then become a prime candidate for chemical sensitivity and chronic degenerative disease. For example, we have observed that some people who overeat watermelon during watermelon season and have a reaction usually recover by the next watermelon season if they cease eating the fruit. Once they eliminate the source of their exposure, their immune and enzyme detoxification systems specifically responsible for handling the biological entities of watermelon have time to recover. In contrast, an individual who continues to ingest too much corn,

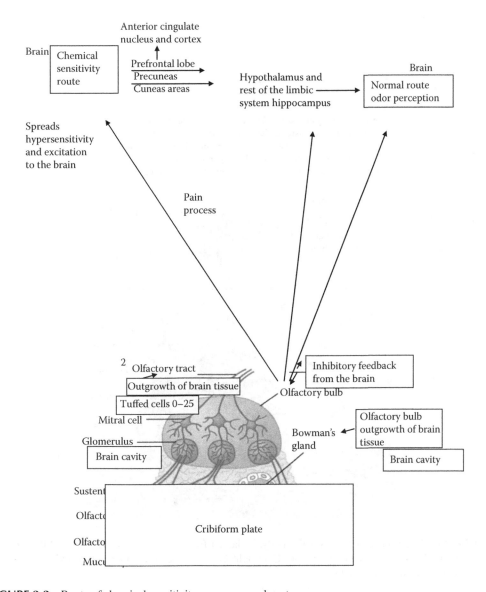

FIGURE 2.2 Route of chemical sensitivity versus normal route.

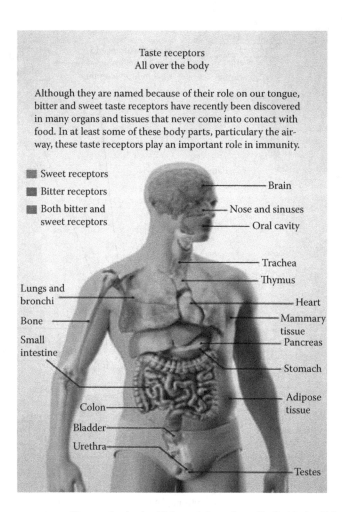

FIGURE 2.4 Taste receptors all over the body. (Adapted from Lee, R. J., N. A. Cohen. 2016. *Sci. Am.* 314(2):38–43; Reproduced with permission. Copyright © 2016 Scientific American, a division of Nature America, Inc. All rights reserved.)

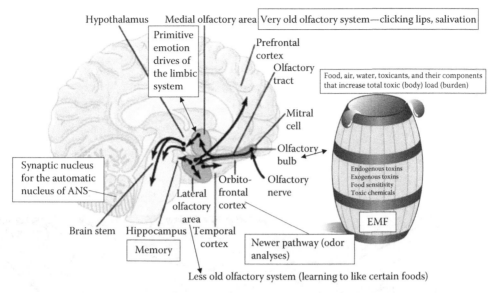

FIGURE 2.7 Neural connections of the olfactory system. (Modified from Guyton, A. C., J. E. Hall. 2002. In *Treaty of Medical Physiology*, 10th ed., A. C. Guyton, J. E. Hall, Eds., pp. 570–577. Rio de Janeiro: Guanabara Koogam SA; Rea, W. J., K. Patel. 2015. *Reversibility of Chronic Degenerative Disease and Hypersensitivity*, Vol. 2, page 58, Figure 2.3. Copyright 2009. Reproduced by permission of Taylor and Francis Group, LLC, a division of Informa plc.)

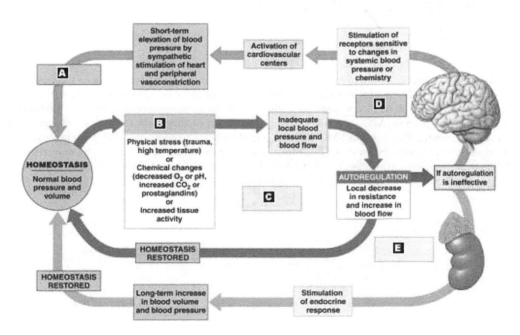

FIGURE 2.11 Cardiovascular regulation of hemodynamics occurs via local autoregulation, neural control, and hormones.

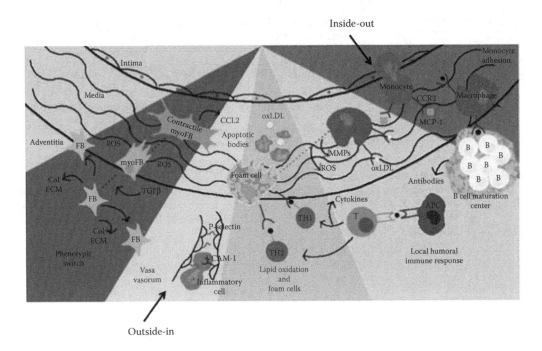

FIGURE 2.17 Theories of origin of vasa vasorum. Depiction of inside-out and outside-in theories of vascular inflammation. The outside-in theory assumes that inflammatory cells enter the vessel wall from the luminal side. The outside-in theory predicts that the inflammatory cells gain entry to the vessel wall via the adventitial vasa vasorum. APC, antigen-presenting cell; CCL2, chemokine ligand 2; Col, collagen; ECM, extracellular matrix; FB, fibroblast; MCP-1, monocyte chemoattractant protein 1; MMPS, matrix metalloproteinases; myoFB, myofibroblast; oxLDL, oxidized low-density lipoprotein; ROS, reactive oxygen species; TGFβ, transforming growth factor-β; Th1 and Th2, T helper cells 1 and 2; VCAM-1, vascular cell adhesion molecule 1. (Reprinted with permission from Maiellaro and Taylor.)

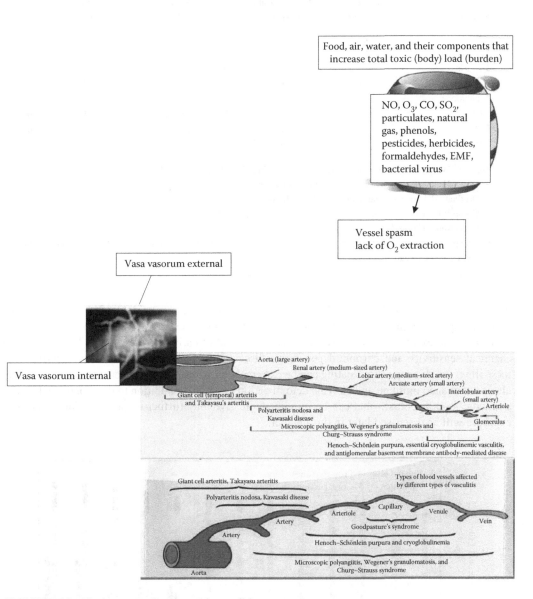

FIGURE 2.22 Environmentally triggered vasculitis.

TABLE 4.17

Goat Study: Clearing of Organochlorine Polluted Animals Grazing on Less Chemically Polluted Land

Substance	Group I[b]			Group II[c]		
	No. of Goats Tested[a]	No. of Goats Positive	%	No. of Goats Tested	No. of Goats Positive	%
DDT	10	1	10	13	0	0
Endo II	10	1	10	13	0	0
Dieldrin	10	1	10	13	0	0
Heptachlor epoxide	10	1	10	13	0	0
HCB	10	2	20	13	0	0
DDE	10	1	10	13	0	0
Total	10	3	30	13	0	0

Source: W. J. Rea. 1994. *Chemical Sensitivity Vol II*. Page 599, Table 6. Reproduced by permission of Taylor and Francis Group, LLC, a division of Informa plc.

[a] Original—10; second generation—13: The EHC-Dallas.

[b] Group I: Unselected commercial goats placed on a nonpesticided and nonherbicided pasture for 1 year. Then levels were measured.

[c] Group II: The second generation came from Group I. They were placed on the land without herbicides and pesticides for 1 year.

milk, apples, tomatoes, beef, or a host of any other foods that are available year round does not allow his specific handling system time to recover because these easily accessible foods can be frequently and excessively eaten. Not only can this kind of eating be the catalyst for the onset of chemical sensitivity and chronic degenerative disease, but also for those already suffering with these illnesses, this repetitious eating can be extremely harmful, since it appears to exacerbate their already-damaged immune and enzyme detoxification systems. In addition to the repetitive damage, a specific food mycotoxin that can be immunodepressive may further be present. This mycotoxin exposure will be discussed later in this chapter.

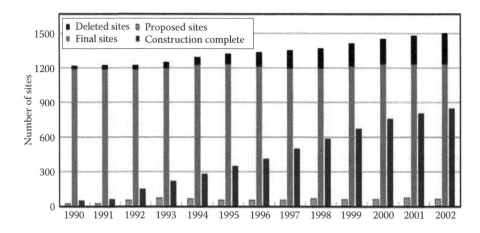

FIGURE 4.16 Superfund national priorities list (NPL) site totals by status and milestone, 1990–2002. (Adapted from EPA's Draft Report on the Environment 2003. Better Protected Land. Chapter 3:3–10.)

The negative results of eating a diet made of a diminished intake of fresh foods and repetitious intake of other foods have led to the development of the rotary diet, which is intended to combat these results.

Chemical Processing

Chemical processing effects can also create many pollutants. For example: New research suggest that the sweetener, high-fructose corn syrup could be tainted with mercury, putting millions of children at risk for developmental problems.

In 2004, Dufault,[275] an environmental health researcher at the Food and Drug Administration (FDA) stumbled upon an obscure Environmental Protection Agency report on chemical plants' mercury emissions. Some chemical companies make lye by pumping salt through large vats of mercury. Since lye is a key ingredient in making high fructose corn syrup (HFCS) (it is used to separate corn starch from the kernel). One sees vast contamination.

Dufault sent HFCS samples from three manufacturers that used lye to labs at the University of California-Davis and the National Institute of Standards and Technology. The labs found mercury in most of the samples.

In January, Dufault and her coauthors[275]—eight scientists from various universities and medical centers—published the findings in the peer-reviewed journal *Environmental Health*. People were ingesting 200 µg of the neurotoxin per week—three times more than the amount the FDA deems safe for children, pregnant women, women who plan to become pregnant, and nursing mothers.

But the FDA and the Corn Refiners Association, an industry trade group, claim there is nothing to worry about. Mercury poses different risks depending on its chemical form. In its unadulterated elemental state, mercury is relatively safe to ingest—the body absorbs only about a tenth of a percent of it. Inorganic forms of mercury, such as cinnabar, are more easily absorbed and therefore more dangerous than elemental. Organic forms, such as methylmercury, which originate from fossil fuel emissions and build up in the fatty tissue of tuna and other kinds of fish, are the worst; readily absorbed, they can cumulatively damage the brain and nervous system.

The corn syrup industry claims that no HFCS manufacturers currently use mercury grade lye, though it concedes some used to. (According to the EPA, four plants still use the technology.)

Hundreds of foreign plants still use mercury to make lye—which may then be used to make foods for export. Already, 11% of the sweeteners and candy on the U.S. market are imported.

A report issued by the Minnesota-based Institute for Agriculture and Trade Policy found low levels of mercury in 16 common food products, including certain brands of kid-favored foods, such as grape jelly and chocolate milk.

Preserving methods, such as canning harvested produce, diminish the nutrient content of food.[175] In the 1930s, Price showed that jaw malformation occurred almost exclusively in the offspring of native tribes who switched to a Western-type diet, the foods of which had been canned.[185] He further showed that cats fed a diet of food preserved by canning developed incapacitating physical degeneration by the third generation. For humans, this depletion of nutrients in food provides a basis for body dysfunction and the possible onset or exacerbation of chemical sensitivity.

In food storage, contamination can occur intentionally or inadvertently by chemical treatment for food shelf longevity, by insulation of containers having phenol or acrylic in cans, by treatment of grains and fruits with fungicides, by waxing vegetables, or by introducing gases such as ethylenes for ripening fruits (bananas). Fumigation elicits ethylene oxide, formaldehyde, or pesticide.[276,277] These pesticides are often found in the blood of the chemically sensitive, and these patients react adversely to them when they are used in a controlled challenge.

Containers may be oiled and treated with pesticides, phenolates, or acrylics, which may then leach off into the foods. Kalin and Brooks[278] have demonstrated human sensitivity to food contaminants emanating from plastic containers. At the EHC-Dallas, we have confirmed this observation on multiple occasions in the environmental control unit (Table 4.18) (CS, Vol II, p. 603, Table 8).

TABLE 4.18

Contaminants Found in Food Stored in Plastic versus Glass

Contaminant	Glass or Nonpetroleum Cellophane (Plant Derived)	Plastic Containers
Vinyl	Below detection limits	Present
Phthalates	Below detection limits	Present
Solvents	Below detection limits	Present
Chemically sensitive patients (500) challenged with previously tested food to which they showed no reaction	No reaction	450 with reactions

	Food in Glass Container	Food in Plastic Container
Reaction	0%	80%

Source: Adapted from Environmental Health Center-Dallas, 1984. Analysis performed by Dr. John Laseter; W. J. Rea. 1994. *Chemical Sensitivity Vol II.* Page 603, Table 8. Reproduced by permission of Taylor and Francis Group, LLC, a division of Informa plc.

Numerous other studies involving containerized foods have emphasized the migration of toxic substances from plastics into the foods they are storing.[279] Plastics particularly leach substances such as phthalates into stored oils and fats.

In addition, bleaching foods with sulfurs and chlorines may add to their contamination. Apples, asparagus, and french fried potatoes are examples of foods that are frequently bleached. Bleaching agents such as those used on asparagus and french fried potatoes give rise to methionine sulfox-amine.[1] We have seen many patients with chemical sensitivity who had no reactions to pure, organic food react to bleached food. Solvents used in extraction contain trichloroethylene[281] or hexane,[280] which are then found in the refined oils. Also, fried foods have chemical substances.

Other foods, for example, grains, are intentionally fungicided in order to inhibit mold growth. Foods treated with fungicides also adversely affect the chemically sensitive individual. Unfortunately, this intentional poisoning is used to prevent mold growth when an equally effective less toxic drying process could be used. In this latter process, grains are harvested and dried to a point of less than 10% moisture.[282]

The state of moisture that results from the application of water to foods in order to prevent wilting also determines whether microorganisms that cause rotting or poisoning of food can proliferate. Water treatment enhances mycotoxin formation.

To minimize nutrient losses during storage and transportation, foods must be kept cool. Therefore, environments controlled for temperature and moisture are used for apples, pears, oranges, grapefruit and other citrus, potatoes, sweet potatoes, carrots, and so on.

Preservatives, colorings, and flavorings, often aldehydes[283] and tartrazine dyes,[284] are intentionally added to commercially available food during its manufacturing and processing (Table 4.19) (CS, Vol. II, p. 601, Table 7). Some preservatives and dyes have long been known to aggravate chemical sensitivity. Many have now been banned for human use. Ninety-four of 100 tartrazine dyes, for example, have been banned, and the rest may be in the process of being eliminated (Lockey, S. D. 1978. Personal communication).

Foods may be further contaminated when pesticides and herbicides are often unintentionally added to them. For example, sulfur dioxide is added to some dry fruits as a preservative and FDC yellow dyes are added to some candies and other foods usually to enhance or level certain tastes. All of these additives have been reported to exacerbate symptoms of some people with chemical sensitivity.

TABLE 4.19

Sources of Synthetic Contamination of Food during Transportation, Storage, and Preparation

Transportation	Containers	Oiled burlap sacks, plastic sacks, solid containers,
Storage	Insecticides	fungicided cardboard boxes
	Fuel exhausts	Spraying en route to prevent infestation
	Heat	Animals breathing during transportation
	Gases for ripening	Pasteurization—milk—loss of nutrient
	Waxing	Ethylene—bananas, other fruits
	Fungicides	Cucumbers, turnips, green peppers
	Bleaching	Grains, peanuts, strawberries
	Containers	Chlorine, sulfuric acid—french fried potatoes, asparagus,
	Sweeteners	cut apples
	Colorings	Phenols, plastics, pesticides—cans, boxes, bottles
	Preservatives	Saccharin (sulfur), aspartame, refined sugar
	Emulsifiers	Tartrazines, other dyes—yellow, blue, green
	Thickeners and stabilizers	Antibiotics, BHA, BHT, propyl gallate, sulfurs, salt,
	Flavorings	formaldehyde, nitrates, nitrites—dried fruit, bacon, packed
	Extractors	goods, candies, other sweets, carrageenin
	Irradiation	Polysorbates
		Guar gums, other gums
		Aldehydes—fruit flavors
		Methylene chloride—decaffeinateds; hexanes—vegetable oils
		Fruit juice, milk, potatoes, onions, pork
Preparation	Smoking and barbecuing with synthetic fuel or natural woods—benzopyrenes, nitrosamines	
	Gas, oil roasting and broiling—hydrocarbons	
	Cookware—aluminum, plastic, cooper	
	Flavor enhancers—monosodium and monoammonium glutamate	
	Baking powder—aluminum	

Source: Adapted from Rea, W. J. 1992. *Chemical Sensitivity, Vol. II: Source of Total Body Load*, p. 601, Table 8. CRC Press: Boca Raton, FL.

Another source of food contamination is our nation's water supply. For example, many waters are contaminated by organochlorine pesticides, which have been found in freshwater fish. Usually, foods so contaminated are inedible for the person with chemical sensitivity. A study from Ontario[285] exemplifies the unintentional contamination of food by herbicides and pesticides.

Davies[285] calculated that a large part of the chemical load of humans in Canada comes from food sources in Ontario (Tables 4.20 and 4.21) (CS II, p. 606, Tables 9 and p. 608, Table 10).

In addition to Davies' finding, polybrominated biphenyls (PBBs) have been found in the milk of cattle fed contaminated feed in Michigan. Bekesi et al.[286] found suppressed immune systems in people who drank this milk, and we have seen several patients who emerged with chemical sensitivity as a result of drinking this milk. All commercially grown foods found at grocery stores in the United States have pesticides in them (Table 4.22) (CS II, pp. 593–596, Table 5),[287,288] and may far exceed the levels (which we believe are too high anyway) defined by government industry safety standards, according to a study by the Natural Resource Defense Council.[289] Many of our

TABLE 4.20

Pesticide Residue in Food in Lake Ontario Region

Chemical	Minimum Detection Limit	Root Vegetables Including Potatoes	Fruit	Leafy Vegetables	Milk	Eggs/Meat
Dibenzofurans	0.0000001	0.00013–0.000039	0.0066–0.000045	ND	0.00012–0.0.0000076	0.005–0.0000016
Dioxins	0.0000001	0.00001–0.0000012	0.0012–0.000005	0.000004	0.0000025–0.0000034	ND
Chlorobenzenes— di, tri, tetra	0.00001	0.0011	0.0044–0.00014	0.0004–0.00028	0.0012–0.00055	0.0016–0.0074
Pentachlorobenzene	0.00001	ND	ND	ND	ND	ND
Hexachlorobenzene	0.00001	0.00004	ND	0.00002	0.00016	0.00017
α-HCH	0.00001	ND	0.00002	ND	0.00013	0.00013
γ-HCH	0.00001	0.00005	0.0001	0.00007	ND	0.0021
Heptachlor	0.00001	ND	ND	ND	ND	ND
Aldrin	0.00001	ND	ND	ND	ND	ND
Oxychlordane	0.00001	ND	ND	0.00004	0.00008	0.00013
Heptachlor epoxide	0.00001	ND	ND	ND	0.00021	0.00012
α-Chlordane	0.00001	0.0001	0.00013	ND	0.0001	0.00012
γ-Chlordane	0.00001	0.00004	0.00006	0.00006	0.00002	ND
α-Endosulfan	0.00001	ND	0.0014	0.0038	ND	ND
p,p'-DDE	0.00001	0.00039	0.0046	0.00002	0.00027	0.0031
Dieldrin	0.00001	0.023	0.00011	0.0031	0.0019	0.0031
Endrin	0.00001	0.00037	0.00027	0.00032	0.00027	ND
β-Endosulfan	0.00001	0.00071	0.0057	0.017	0.0022	ND
p,p'-DDD	0.00001	0.00047	ND	0.00034	ND	0.00017
o,p'-DDT	0.00001	ND	ND	0.00002	ND	ND
p,p'-DDT	0.00001	0.065	0.00039	0.00042	0.0014	0.00031
Photomirex	0.00001	ND	ND	ND	ND	ND
Mirex	0.00001	ND	ND	ND	ND	ND
Methoxychlor	0.0001	ND	ND	ND	ND	ND
Total PCB	0.0001	ND	0.0007	ND	0.0001	0.0003

Source: Adapted from Davies, K. 1986. Human exposure routes to selected persistent toxic chemicals in the great lakes basin: A case study of Toronto and Southern Ontario region (Unpublished). Toronto: Department of Public Health; W. J. Rea. 1994. *Chemical Sensitivity Vol II.* Page 606–607 Table 9. Reproduced by permission of Taylor and Francis Group, LLC, a division of Informa plc.

Note: ND = not detected. Concentrations of selected persistent toxic organochlorines detected in food composition (1985) (μg/g).

chemically sensitive patients at the EHC-Dallas react severely to pesticide challenge, thus confirming both their presence and potential for adverse effects.

Consumers Union analyzed data collected by the USDA's PDP to compare the relative amounts and toxicity of pesticide residues in different foods. They obtained pesticide residue data on over 27,000 food samples tested by the PDP in 1994–1997. They weighted the amounts of residues present to account for differences in the toxicity of individual pesticide chemicals, and computed a toxicity index (TI) for each food. The TI integrates measures of the frequency of pesticide detection, the levels of residues present, and the relative toxicity of the detected

TABLE 4.21

Concentrations of Dioxin and Dibenzofurans, and Chlorobenzenes in Food in the Lake Ontario Region

Chemical	Minimum Detection Limit	Root Vegetables Including Potatoes	Fruit	Leafy Vegetables	Milk	Eggs/Meat
Dibenzofurans	0.0000001	0.00013– 0.000039	0.0066– 0.000045	ND	0.00012– 0.0000076	0.005– 0.000016
Dioxins	0.0000001	0.00001– 0.00000012	0.0012–0.000005	0.0000004	0.0000034– 0.0000025	ND
Chlorobenzenes- di, tri, tetra	0.00001	0.0011	0.0044–0.00014	0.0004– 0.00028	0.0012–0.00055	0.0016–0.0074

Source: Adapted from Davies, K. 1986. Human exposure routes to selected persistent toxic chemicals in the great lakes basin: A case study of Toronto and Southern Ontario region (Unpublished). Toronto: Department of Public Health; W. J. Rea. 1994. *Chemical Sensitivity Vol II*. Page 608, Table 10. Reproduced by permission of Taylor and Francis Group, LLC, a division of Informa plc.

residues, yielding an index of the relative toxicity loading of each food. The majority of foods have TI values between 10 and 300 and a few more have values between 300 and 600. That is the relative toxicity loading of the widely consumed foods tested by the PDP spans a range of at least 60-fold (Table 4.23).

Six foods had very low TIs (10 or less) each time they were tested: frozen/canned corn, mild, U.S. orange juice, U.S. broccoli, bananas, and canned peaches. Not quite as low were frozen/canned sweet peas, U.S. and imported apple juice, frozen winter squash from Mexico, tomatoes from Canada, Brazilian orange juice, and U.S. wheat (Table 4.24). Seven foods consistently had high or very high TIs each time tested: fresh peaches (both domestic and imported); frozen and fresh winter squash grown in the United States, domestic and imported apples, grapes, spinach and pears; and U.S.-grown green beans.

Some foods have residues of many more pesticides than others. Up to 37 different pesticide chemicals were detected in apples by the PDP, for example, and more than 20 are found in peaches, pears, and spinach, while 10 were found in broccoli and fewer than that in apple juice, orange juice, bananas, and corn. Individual food samples often have multiple residues on them. An apple grown in the United States typically contains four pesticides, and some have as many as 10 different residues. Peaches, winter squash, spinach, carrots, and grapes are more likely than not to have two or more residues in a sample. One sample of spinach had residues of 14 different pesticides on it.

Eleven of the 12 highest TI scores are for U.S.-grown foods. There are 39 cases with 10 or more samples of a food from a specific other country to compare with U.S. samples; in 26 cases (67%), U.S. samples had higher TIs. Some differences exist between importing countries, as well as between the United States and other countries. Cases where imports are worse include Chilean grapes, Canadian and Mexican carrots, Mexican broccoli and tomatoes, Argentine and Hungarian apple juice, and Brazilian orange juice. U.S. samples are worse than imports for fresh peaches, fresh and frozen winter squash, fresh green beans, apples, and pears. U.S. apple juice has a higher TI than apple juice from Germany or Mexico, and U.S. grapes have higher TIs than those from South Africa and Mexico. The size and differences vary from food to food. In two cases with the highest TIs of any foods, U.S. peaches have 10 times the TI of Chilean imports, and U.S. frozen winter squash has a TI 143 times as high as Mexican winter squash has. Only two imported foods, Mexican broccoli and Brazilian orange juice, have TIs more than 10-fold larger than those of U.S. samples, but in each case, the higher score is still comparatively low.

TABLE 4.22

Commercial Food[a] versus Less Chemically Contaminated Food[b]

Less Chemically Contaminated Food (Private Survey)[a]			Chemically Contaminated Commercial Foods (Private Survey) One Market[b]		Commercial Foods (EPA Survey) Multiple Markets	
Food	Pesticide	ppm	Pesticide	ppm	Pesticide	ppm
Beef	None	0	Trimethyl/parathion	Tr	Multiple	+[c]
Pork	Endrin	Tr	Dieldrin/endrin	0.8	Multiple	+
				0.15		
Broccoli	Aldrin	Tr	Lindane	1.13	Dacthal	0.01
Cabbage	None	0	Lindane	0.33	Lindane	+
Carrot	None	0	None	0	Botran	1.1
					Trifluralin	0.01–0.15
					DDE	0.03–0.12
					Endrin	0.01
					Dieldrin	0.01
					DDT	0.03
Watercress		0	Not studied	–	Thiodin	2.55
Cauliflower	None	0	None	0	Lindane	0.01
Celery	None	0	None	0	Pesticide	+
Corn	None	0	None	0	Herbicide	+
					Fumigant	+
					Fensulfothion	+
					Imidan	+
					Dieldrin	0.01
Cucumber	None	0	None	0	DDE	0.01–0.03
					Endosulfan	0.04
					Dioazinon	0.02
					Thiodan	4.1
					Aldicarb	0.05
					CIPC	0.01–0.17
					DDE	0.01–0.03
Lettuce	None	0	None	0	Endosulfan	0.04
					Dioazinon	0.02
					Thiodan	4.1
					Aldicarb	0.05
					CIPC	0.01–0.17
Potato	None	0	None	0	DDT	0.02
Spinach	None	0	Diazinon	0.48	DDE	0.02–0.04
					Dacthal	0.02
					Malathion	0.01–0.21
					Endosulfan	0.14
Strawberry	None				DDE	0.01–0.08
					Kelthane	0.07–3.7
					Mevinphos	0.02–0.28
String bean	None	0	Not done	Monitor 0.91		
Apple	None	0	Not done	Multiple +		
Avocado	None	0	Not done		Ethylene	+
Banana	None	0	Not done		Pesticide	+

(Continued)

TABLE 4.22 (*Continued*)
Commercial Food[a] versus Less Chemically Contaminated Food[b]

Less Chemically Contaminated Food (Private Survey)[a]			Chemically Contaminated Commercial Foods (Private Survey) One Market[b]		Commercial Foods (EPA Survey) Multiple Markets	
Food	Pesticide	ppm	Pesticide	ppm	Pesticide	ppm
Pear	None	0	Not done		Botran	0.77
Tomato	None	0	Not done		Fenvalerate	0.02
Beet (tops)	None	0			Dacthal	0.14
Orange	None	0			DDE	0.01
					Parathion	0.04
					Chlorpyrifos	0.01–0.12
					Ethion	0.19
					Kelthane	0.17–0.43
					Methidathion	0.05–0.53
Oatmeal	None	0			Fumigant	+
Rice	None	0			Fenthion	0.5
Radish	None	0			Fungicide	+
Bell pepper	None	0			Dactiral	1.43
Collard green	None	0	Not done		Monitor	1.78
			Not done		Diazinon	0.96
					Daconil	123
Daikon	None	0	Not done		Thiodan	0.69
Mushroom	None	0			Bravo/ Daconil	0.16
Parsley	None	0	Not done		Diazinon	2.16
Eggplant	None		Not done		Pesticide	+
Grape	None	0	Not done		Pesticide	+

Source: Adapted from Harris Hosen, MD, Port Arthur, Texas; W. J. Rea. 1994. *Chemical Sensitivity Vol II.* Page 593–596, Table 5. Reproduced by permission of Taylor and Francis Group, LLC, a division of Informa plc.
[a] Acquired through the EHC-Dallas less chemically contaminated network.
[b] Acquired at commercial grocery store.
[c] + = positive, ut: the number is unknown.

Generally, processed food has less pesticide than fresh. TI values for apple juice and orange juice are far lower than for the fresh fruits, and the TI for canned peaches is 1/1000 that of fresh peaches. Canned spinach has a TI about half as high as that for fresh spinach. Canned/frozen corn and canned/frozen peas also have among the lowest TI values, but no data on the fresh crops are available. Frozen and canned green beans and frozen winter squash each had TI scores higher than those for the corresponding fresh crops.

About 1% of the residues detected by the PDP in 1994, 4% in 1995 and 1996, and 5% in 1997 violated U.S. tolerances. Most violations are not excessive residues of legally registered pesticides, but rather, low levels of chemicals that are not registered for use on that food. Some violations are attributed to persistent residues in soils or to wind dispersal of pesticides applied legally to nearby fields, but we believe the PDP data show widespread illegal use of several insecticides on both U.S. and Mexican spinach.

TABLE 4.23
Foods with the Lowest Toxicity Index to the Highest Scores

Food	Score
Canned/frozen sweet corn (USA, 1995)	0.01
Canned/frozen sweet corn (USA, 1994)	0.02
Milk (USA, 1996)	1
Milk (USA, 1997)	1
Broccoli (USA, 1994)	2
Orange juice (USA, 1997)	2
Bananas (imports, 9 countries, 1994)	3
Bananas (imports, 7 countries, 1995)	4
Canned peaches (USA, 1997)	5
Canned/frozen peas (USA, 1994)	6
Grapes (Mexico, 1994)	10
Apple juice (USA, 1996)	11
Apple juice (Mexico, 1977)	12
Apple juice (Germany, 1997)	13
Apple juice (Argentina, 1996)	18
Apple juice (USA, 1997)	20

Note: The TI values for different foods shown in Table 4.24 range from 0.01 to 5376—a range of more than 500,000-fold. However, the majority of values fall between 10 and 300 on the TI scale. The scale is relative, and there is no firm dividing link between "acceptable" and "excessive" degrees of pesticide toxicity loading. Nevertheless, in our judgment, values of less than 10 can be considered very low toxicity loading, that is, the food is very "clean." Values above 00 indicate "high" toxicity loading, increasingly serious as scores get larger. TI values between 10 and 100 fall on a continuum rising from "low" through "moderate" toxicity loading.

Twenty-two different pesticides were detected in U.S. peaches in 1996, but one chemical—methyl parathion—accounts for more than 90% of the total toxicity load. Methyl parathion accounts for a large part of the TI values for apples, pears, green beans, and peas, as well as peaches. The high TIs for winter squash (fresh and frozen) from the United States are almost entirely due to residues of dieldrin, a very toxic, carcinogenic insecticide that was banned 25 years ago, but persists in some agricultural soils. A handful of other widely used insecticides and a few fungicides consistently account for the greatest fraction of toxicity loading in most crops.

The fact that a few very toxic pesticides account for most of the toxicity loading in PDP-tested crops has important policy implications. The risks associated with pesticides in foods can be sharply reduced by focusing risk management efforts on a few high-risk pesticide uses. Safer alternative exists to manage most pests against which these high-risk chemicals are used.[290]

Corn, bananas, and peas all have an inedible exterior husk, which tends to keep pesticide residues away from the edible portions of the foods. Processing typically further reduces residues. Only three of 1015 samples of corn tested in 2 years had any detectable residues. The very low score for U.S. broccoli reflects the rarity of residues in that food; the two most frequently detected insecticides were each found on less than 2% of 659 samples. Apple juice (imported and domestic) typically has only low residues of a few pesticides. The score for canned peaches, which is 1/1000 that for fresh peaches, reflects effects of processing, a longer time between harvest and consumption, and differences in pest management on peaches grown for processing as opposed to those grown for the fresh market.

A few other foods had scores nearly as low as those listed above: frozen/canned peas tested in 1995–1996 (TIs of 22 and 21); frozen winter squash from Mexico (1997, 21); orange juice from

TABLE 4.24
Highest Toxicity Indices (Those over 100 on the TI Scale)

Fresh peaches	United States, 1995	5376
Fresh peaches	United States, 1996	4848
Fresh peaches	United States, 1994	4390
Frozen winter squash	United States, 1997	3012
Fresh winter squash	United States, 1997	1706
Grapes	United States, 1994	1552
Fresh spinach	Mexico, 1996	623
Apples	United States, 1994	567
Fresh spinach	United States, 1995	554
Apples	United States, 1996	550
Frozen/canned green beans	United States, 1997	529
Apples	United States, 1995	521
Fresh spinach	United States, 1996	495
Fresh peaches	Chile, 1996	471
Pears	United States, 1997	435
Pears	Chile, 1997	415
Fresh peaches	Chile, 1994	381
Fresh peaches	Chile, 1995	366
Fresh spinach	United States, 1997	349
Grapes	Chile, 1996	339
Grapes	United States, 1995	329
Apples	New Zealand, 1994	298
Fresh green beans	United States, 1994	294
Apples	New Zealand, 1996	284
Apples	New Zealand, 1995	260
Fresh spinach	Mexico, 1997	256
Celery	United States, 1994	255
Grapes	Chile, 1995	241
Grapes	United States, 1996	228
Fresh green beans	United States, 1995	222
Frozen/canned green beans	United States, 1996	222
Canned spinach	United States, 1997	204
Pears	South Africa, 1997	201
Potatoes	United States, 1994	191
Grapes	Chile, 1994	181
Grapes	South Africa, 1996	169
Tomatoes	Mexico, 1997	159
Pears	Argentina, 1997	157
Oranges	United States, 1994	138
Carrots	Mexico, 1995	136
Tomatoes	Mexico, 1996	123
Lettuce	United States, 1994	122
Fresh spinach	Mexico, 1995	103

Note: The foods/origins/years are listed in descending order.

Brazil (1997, 23); fresh winter squash from Honduras (1997, 23); U.S. sweet potatoes (1997, 25); Canadian tomatoes (1997, 26); and wheat (1995–1997, 18, 29 and 32) (Table 4.19).

Seven crops (peaches, apples, pears, grapes, winter squash, spinach, and green beans) appear among the highest TI scores repeatedly, with scores above 200 essentially every time they were tested. For all but green beans and winter squash, imports and U.S. samples both have high (though often not equally high) TI scores. In most cases, the consistently high scores are attributable to the insect problems typically associated with growing these crops, and to the insecticides (mostly OPs) used on them.

NEURODEVELOPMENTAL DISORDERS AND PRENATAL RESIDENTIAL PROXIMITY TO AGRICULTURAL PESTICIDES

According to Shelton et al.[290] California is the top agriculture-producing state in the nation, grossing $38 billion in revenue from farm crops in 2010.[291] Each year, approximately 200 million pounds of active pesticide ingredients are applied throughout the state.[292] While pesticides are thought by some to be so critical for the modern agricultural industry, certain commonly used pesticides have been associated with abnormal and impaired neurodevelopment in children.[293–302] In addition, specific associations have been reported between agricultural pesticides and autism spectrum disorders (ASD)[303] and the broader diagnostic category under which autism falls, the pervasive developmental disorder.[304]

Developmental delay (DD) refers to young children who experience significant delays reaching milestones in relation to cognitive or adaptive development. Adaptive skills include communication, self-care, social relationships, and/or motor skills. In the United States, DD affects approximately 3.9% of all children 3–10 years of age, and is approximately 1.7 times more common among boys than girls.[305]

Autism is a developmental disorder with symptoms appearing by age 3. Specific deficits occur in domains of social interaction and language, and individuals show restricted and repetitive behaviors, activities, or movements (DSM-IV 2000) The ASDs represent lower severity, usually with regard to language ability. ASDs affect boys 4–5 times more than girls, and the Centers for Disease Control and Prevention (CDC) recently estimated a prevalence of 1.1% among children 8 years of age, a 78% increase since their 2007 estimate.[306] Available evidence suggests that causes of both ASD and DD are heterogeneous and that environmental factors can contribute strongly to risk.[307,308] Just lowering of IQ and creativity in a so-called normal group of children has been seen over the last 20 years, obviously that is due to gross environmental contamination.

The majority of pesticides sold in the United States are neurotoxic and operate through one of three primary mechanisms: (1) inhibition of AChE, (2) voltage-gated sodium channel disruption, and/or (3) inhibition of gamma-aminobutyric acid (GABA).[309] AChE primarily functions as an inhibitory neurotransmitter, but also has critical roles in the development of learning, cognition, and memory. GABA is also an inhibitory neurotransmitter, and is necessary for development and maintenance of neuronal transmission.

Though limited research has assessed *in utero* exposures to pesticides, animal models (rats) of early exposure to OPs showed more severe neurodevelopmental effects for males than for females.[310,311] According to Shelton et al.[290] based on previously published epidemiology or mechanistic considerations, they selected the following pesticide families to investigate for this analysis: OPs, carbamates, organochlorines, and pyrethroids. Potential mechanisms linking these select pesticide groups to autism pathophysiology were recently reviewed.[312]

According to Shelton et al.[290] the aim was to explore the relationship between agricultural pesticide applications and neurodevelopmental outcomes by (1) assessing the gestational exposure during pregnancy to Childhood Autism Risks from Genes and Environment (CHARGE) study mothers, (2) testing the hypothesis that children with ASD or DD had higher risk of exposure *in utero* than typically developing children, and (3) evaluating specific windows of vulnerability during gestation. Because of the well-defined case and control populations in the CHARGE study and the comprehensive availability of potential confounders, this analysis served as exploratory research to identify environmental risk factors for ASD and DD, and contributes to a broader understanding of the potential risks to neurodevelopment from agricultural pesticides in a diverse population of California residents.

According to Shelton et al.[290] the CHARGE study is an ongoing California population-based case–control study which aims to uncover a broad array of factors contributing to autism and DD.[313] Since 2003, the CHARGE study has enrolled over 1600 participants whose parents answer extensive questionnaires regarding environmental exposures including their place of residence during pregnancy. Here they report on ASD and DD in relation to gestational residential proximity to agricultural pesticide applications. The group of children with ASD includes approximately two-thirds with a diagnosis of full-syndrome autism or autistic disorder (68%) and one-third with a diagnosis of an ASD (32%). The DD group can also include children with short-term memory loss, lowered IgE, and various other developmental problems including other brain dysfunctions and ID (identification) loss.

Cases are recruited from children diagnosed with full-syndrome ASD or DD in one of the regional centers of the California Department of Developmental Services (DDS). Eligibility in the DDS system does not depend on citizenship or financial status, and is widely used across socio-economic levels and racial/ethnic groups. It is estimated that 75%–80% of the total population of children with an autism diagnosis are enrolled in the system.[314] In addition to recruitment through the regional centers, some CHARGE participants are also recruited through referrals from other clinics, self-referral, or general outreach. The referents are recruited from the GP identified through California birth records, and are frequently matched to the autism case population on sex, age, and the catchment area for the region they would have gone to, had they been a case. Children were eligible if they are 2–5 years of age, born in California, live with a biological parent who speaks either English or Spanish, and resides in the study catchment area. Currently, the catchment area for the CHARGE study participants consists of a 2-hour drive from the Sacramento area, but previously included participants from Southern California. Early in the study, recruitment in Southern California was terminated due to logistical difficulties that led to lower enrollment of GP controls.

Parents of children coming into the study with a previous diagnosis of ASD are administered the Autism Diagnostic Interview-Revised (ADI-R), surveyed regarding a wide range of environmental exposures, and asked to report all addresses where they lived from 3 months before conception to the time of the interview.

Participating children are administered the Autism Diagnostic Observation Schedule (ADOS), and combined with the ADI-R, is used to either confirm their diagnosis or reclassify them for purposes of our study. To rule out ASD, children who enter the study without an ASD diagnosis (from the DD or GP groups) are given the Social Communications Questionnaire (SCQ).[315]

Children with a previous diagnosis of DD are evaluated on both the Mullen Scales of Early Learning (MSEL) and Vineland Adaptive Behavioral Scale (VABS). DD is confirmed if they scored 15 on the SCQ and at or below 2 standard deviations lower than the mean (< 70) on the composite scores of MSEL and VABS. Those meeting criteria for one test, scoring < 77 on the other, and not qualifying for ASD, are classified as atypical and combined with the DD group (25 of the 168) for this analysis. For this sample, of those who entered the study as typically developing, 26 were reclassified with DD and 2 with ASD. Of those who entered as DD, 36 were reclassified with ASD. Only cases with completed diagnostic testing were included in the analysis presented here. Additional details on CHARGE study protocols have been published elsewhere.[313]

ESTIMATION OF PESTICIDE EXPOSURES

Since 1990, California has required commercial application of agricultural pesticides to be reported to the CDPR, which makes data publically available in the form of the annual Pesticide Use Report (PUR). As described by CDPR,[292] the PUR data include pesticide applications to parks, golf courses, cemeteries, rangeland, pastures, and along roadside and railroad rights-of-way. In addition, all postharvest pesticide treatments of agricultural commodities must be reported along with all pesticide treatments in poultry and fish production as well as some livestock applications. The primary exceptions to the reporting requirements are home and garden use and most industrial and institutional uses.[292]

The PUR database includes all commercial applications at the county level, requiring spatially explicit (latitude and longitude) reporting for commercial agricultural applications. The PUR database then compiles agricultural pesticide applications throughout the state by square mile areas (1.0 m^2 or 2.6 km^2) set by the U.S. Geological Survey, referred to as a meridian-township-range-section (MTRS). The amount of chemical applied is assigned to an MTRS by date, in pounds (each pound is 0.45 kg) of active ingredient only, excluding synergists and other compounds in the formulation. Mapping software (ArcGIS v10.0; ESRI, Redlands, CA) was used to create a geographic centroid (centermost point in the square mile) for each MTRS for use in this analysis.

Next, a spatial model was developed in ArcMap, which created three buffers of varying sizes around each residence with radii of 1.25 km, 1.5 km, and 1.75 km. Where the buffer intersected a centroid (or multiple centroids), the MTRS corresponding with that centroid was assigned to that residence; subsequently, pesticides applied in that MTRS (or multiple MTRSs) were considered exposures for that mother with the timing based on linking the date of application to the dates of her pregnancy. Each pregnancy therefore was assigned an exposure profile corresponding to applications made to the MTRS nearest the mother's home and days of her pregnancy on which those applications occurred (for a visual representation of the exposure model.

They classified chemicals in the PUR according to chemical structure as members of the OP, carbamate, pyrethroid, or organochlorine classes of pesticides. Subclasses of pyrethroids were categorized as type 1 and type 2 because they induce distinct behavioral effects in animal studies.[316,317] In addition, chlorpyrifos, an OP widely used in agriculture, was explored independently because previous research had associated higher levels of prenatal exposure with diminished psychomotor and mental development in children at 3 years of age.[299]

During model selection, they tested the joint versus independent effects of two classes of pesticides (e.g., pyrethroids and OPs) in models that contained each independent variable (dichotomous) for the two pesticides and an interaction variable of those two dichotomous variables. They also explored the possibility that another pesticide was responsible for the observed association due to correlation between pesticides (i.e., if one class is applied, another is more likely to be applied in that same buffer zone) by treating other classes of pesticides as potential confounders.

Final models were adjusted for paternal education (categorical), home ownership (binary), maternal place of birth (USA, Mexico, or outside the USA and Mexico), child race/ethnicity (white, Hispanic, other), maternal prenatal vitamin intake (binary; taken during the 3 months prior to pregnancy through the first month), and year of birth (continuous). Prenatal vitamin consumption in this time window was found in previous work to have an inverse association with ASD, meaning that early prenatal vitamin intake may confer a lower risk of ASD.[318] Other potential confounders explored but found not to satisfy criteria for confounding based on inclusion in the directed acyclic graph (DAG) or the change in estimate criterion were distance from a major freeway, maternal major metabolic disorders (diabetes, hypertension, and obesity), gestational age (days), latitude of residence, type of insurance used to pay for the delivery (public vs. private), maternal age, paternal age, and season of conception. Maternal age, though a known risk for ASD, does not differ significantly between cases and controls in the CHARGE study because the participating mothers of typical development (TD) children are older than the GP (Table 4.25).

During pregnancy, residences of the CHARGE study participants were distributed broadly throughout California, with the greatest concentrations in Sacramento Valley, followed by the San Francisco Bay area and Los Angeles. One-third lived within 1.5 km of an agricultural pesticide application from one of the four pesticide classes evaluated. ASD and TD groups had similar sociodemographic profiles, with some variation by regional center, prenatal vitamin intake, and maternal place of birth, and more ASD cases were recruited earlier in the study than DD or TD children. As described in "Methods," early in the study, challenges were encountered recruiting non-ASD participants in Southern California, resulting in a greater proportion

TABLE 4.25

Characteristics (*n*(%) or Mean ± SD) of CHARGE Study Population (*n* + 970)

Characteristic	ASD	Delayed	Typical	*p*-Value ASD vs. TD	*p*-Value DD vs. TD
Total	486	168	316		
Male	414 (85.2)	115 (68.5)	262 (82.9)	0.39	0.0003
Child's age at enrollment (months)	36.7 ± 9.7	38.3 ± 8.9	36.9 ± 8.9	0.73	0.11
Childs race/ethnicity				0.12	<0.0001
White	246 (50.6)	66 (39.3)	165 (52.2)		
Hispanic	130 (26.8)	60 (35.7)	73 (23.1)		
Other	110 (22.6)	41 (24.4)	78 (24.7)		
Mother's age (years)	31.3 ± 5.5	30.8 ± 6.6	31.1 ± 5.7	0.69	0.57
Father's age (years)	33.9 ± 6.4	33.1 ± 7.8	33.5 ± 7.0	0.49	0.52
Mother's education				0.12	<0.0001
High school or less	67 (13.8)	51 (30.4)	46 (14.6)		
Some college	197 (40.5)	68 (40.5)	100 (31.7)		
College or professional	222 (45.7)	49 (29.2)	170 (53.8)		
Father's education				0.58	<0.0001
High school or less	106 (21.8)	74 (44.1)	81 (25.6)		
Some college	153 (31.5)	47 (27.9)	91 (28.8)		
College or professional	225 (46.3)	44 (26.2)	144 (45.6)		
Regional center/region				<0.0001	0.01
Alta	174 (35.8)	82 (48.8)	131 (41.5)		
North Bay	64 (13.2)	19 (11.3)	53 (16.8)		
East Bay	81 (16.7)	17 (10.1)	65 (20.6)		
Valley Mountain	85 (17.5)	38 (22.6)	49 (15.5)		
Southern California	82 (16.9)	12 (7.1)	18 (5.7)		
Maternal birth place				0.07	0.0003
In the USA	367 (75.5)	127 (75.60)	259 (82.0)		
In Mexico	38 (7.8)	28 (16.7)	22 (7.0)		
Outside USA or Mexico	81 (16.7)	13 (7.7)	35 (11.1)		
Year of birth				0.0003	0.49
1999–2003	348 (71.6)	94 (56.0)	187 (59.2)		
2004–2008	138 (28.4)	74 (44.1)	129 (40.8)		
Homeowner	320 (65.8)	100 (59.5)	242 (76.6)	0.001	<0.0001
Private health insurance	402 (82.7)	118 (70.2)	270 (85.4)	0.31	<0.0001
Periconceptional prenatal vitamin	252 (52.0)	79 (53.0)	189 (59.8)	0.003	0.01
Known chromosomal abnormality	11 (2.3)	50 (32.7)	0 (0.0)	–	–

Source: Adapted from Shelton, J. F. et al. 2014. *Environ. Health Perspect.* 122 (10):A266.

of ASD participants relative to TD participants from that regional center. The DD case group, which was not matched, differed from the reference group on many characteristics, including sex, race/ethnicity, maternal birth place, regional center, maternal education, and paternal education and appears to be of substantially lower socioeconomic status than either the ASD or TD groups. Age of the child at enrollment was similar between the ASD and DD groups compared with the TD groups.

TABLE 4.26

Exposure to Pesticide Applications (Any vs. None) within 1.5 km of the Home during the 3 Months before Conception through Delivery According to Outcome (ASD *n* = 486, DD *n* = 168, TD *n* = 316)

	ASD			DD			TD		
Exposure	*n*	Unweighted %	Weighted %	*n*	Unweighted %	Weighted %	*n*	Unweighted %	Weighted %
No agriculturally applied pesticides	342	70.4	70.1	124	73.8	66.9	219	69.3	72.2
Any agriculturally applied pesticides	144	29.6	29.9	44	26.2	33.0	97	30.7	27.8
Organophosphates	125	25.7	26.6	32	19.1	25.2	84	26.6	24.9
Chlorpyrifos	61	12.6	14.4	20	11.9	18.4	45	14.2	12.4
Pyrethroids	106	21.8	22.5	36	21.4	28.3	67	21.2	20.1
Type 1 pyrethroids	49	10.1	10.4	17	10.1	16.3	29	9.2	7.9
Type 2 pyrethroids	100	20.6	20.9	34	20.2	26.9	63	19.9	19.1
Carbamates	54	11.1	11.0	13	7.7	11.1	30	9.5	7.3
Organochlorines	24	4.9	4.9	4	2.4	3.9	10	3.2	3.3

Source: Adapted from Shelton, J. F. et al. 2014. *Environ. Health Perspect.* 122 (10):A266.

Note: The development and use of CHARGE survey weights were designed to correct for the nonsociodemographically representative participation, that is, the differences in participants versus nonparticipants with regard to by sociodemographic factors such as maternal education, insurance payment type, birth regional center, birth place of mother, and child race. Survey weights are based on the probability of participation in the study.

In the CHARGE study population, of the pesticides evaluated, OPs were the most commonly applied agricultural pesticide near the home during pregnancy. In the group exposed to OPs within 1.5 km of the home, 21 unique compounds were identified, the most abundant of which was chlorpyrifos (20.7%), followed by acephate (15.4%), and diazinon (14.5%). The second most commonly applied class of pesticides was the pyrethroids, one-quarter of which was esfenvalerate (24%), followed by lambda-cyhalothrin (17.3%), permethrin (16.5%), cypermethrin (12.8%), and tau-fluvalinate (10.5%). Of the carbamates, approximately 80% were methomyl or carbaryl, and of the organochlorines, 60% of all applications were dienochlor. Among those exposed, only one-third were exposed to a single compound over the course of the pregnancy.

In the unweighted study population, little difference in exposure proportion was apparent, yet once the survey weights were applied, both case populations had higher exposure proportions than the TD controls, indicating that factors associated with exposure were also associated with study participation (Table 4.26). Because the study weights reflect the distributions of the three recruitment strata (ASD, DD, and TD controls) in the pool from which they were drawn, differences between case and control participation by regional center catchment area likely accounts for this effect. For example, DD cases proportionally underenrolled in the CHARGE study from the Valley Mountain regional center compared with the recruitment pool. Because the Valley region had the highest proportion of exposed participants, weights that accounted for the discrepancy between the proportions of DD cases enrolled from the Valley region would more accurately represent the population distribution of cases and controls.

By pounds applied, the amount of pyrethroids and OPs (continuous, unweighted) applied within 1.5 km of the home were strongly correlated with each other ($\rho = 0.74$, $p < 0.0001$) and to a lesser extent OPs with carbamates ($\rho = 0.45$, $p = 0.01$) and carbamates with pyrethroids ($\rho = 0.44$,

TABLE 4.27

Adjusted ORs[a] (95% CIs) for ASD and Residential Proximity to Agricultural Pesticide Applications (Any vs. None) within Prespecified Buffers, by Time Period[b]

Pesticide, Buffer Radius (km)	Pregnancy	Preconception	1st trimester	2nd trimester	3rd trimester
			Organophosphates		
1.25	1.60 (1.02, 2.51)	1.37 (0.76, 2.50)	1.53 (0.87, 2.68)	1.57 (0.87, 2.83)	1.99 (1.11, 3.56)
1.5	1.54 (1.00, 2.38)	1.38 (0.82, 2.31)	1.45 (0.88, 2.41)	1.85 (1.08, 3.15)	2.07 (1.23, 3.50)
1.75	1.26 (0.83, 1.92)	1.30 (0.80, 2.13)	1.02 (0.63, 1.65)	1.54 (0.93, 2.55)	1.99 (1.20, 3.30)
			Chlorpyrifos		
1.25	1.57 (0.82, 3.00)	1.07 (0.40, 2.89)	1.26 (0.52, 3.06)	2.55 (0.95, 6.84)	1.83 (0.72, 4.65)
1.5	1.66 (0.94, 2.93)	1.07 (0.46, 2.48)	1.32 (0.65, 2.70)	3.31 (1.48, 7.42)	1.78 (0.82, 3.87)
1.75	1.78 (1.05, 3.02)	1.25 (0.59, 2.65)	1.12 (0.58, 2.16)	2.63 (1.28, 5.41)	2.15 (1.04, 4.41)
			Pyrethroids		
1.25	1.34 (0.82, 2.20)	1.82 (0.92, 3.60)	1.59 (0.86, 2.96)	1.56 (0.83, 2.94)	1.64 (0.84, 3.19)
1.5	1.41 (0.89, 2.25)	1.82 (1.00, 3.31)	1.53 (0.88, 2.67)	1.69 (0.93, 3.06)	1.87 (1.02, 3.43)
1.75	1.27 (0.83, 1.96)	1.69 (0.97, 2.95)	1.14 (0.67, 1.91)	1.49 (0.87, 2.58)	1.83 (1.04, 3.23)
			Type 2		
1.25	1.40 (0.83, 2.34)	2.01 (0.97, 4.16)	1.64 (0.85, 3.17)	1.29 (0.65, 2.56)	1.51 (0.75, 3.05)
1.5	1.53 (0.94, 2.51)	1.98 (1.06, 3.71)	1.85 (1.01, 3.38)	1.45 (0.78, 2.73)	1.67 (0.87, 3.21)
1.75	1.30 (0.82, 2.05)	1.64 (0.92, 2.94)	1.32 (0.76, 2.29)	1.33 (0.75, 2.38)	1.56 (0.86, 2.84)
			Carbamates[c]		
1.25	1.37 (0.66, 2.84)	–	–	–	–
1.5	1.80 (0.81, 3.08)	–	–	–	–
1.75	1.43 (0.78, 2.62)	–	–	–	–

Source: Adapted from Shelton, J. F. et al. 2014. *Environ. Health Perspect.* 122 (10):A266.

[a] Multivariate multinomial conditional logistic regression with survey weights and strata variables far matching variables. All models were adjusted for paternal education, home ownership, maternal place of birth, child race/ethnicity, maternal prenatal vitamin intake (during the 3 months before pregnancy through the first month), and year of birth.

[b] Pregnancy: Conception (day 0) to the end of pregnancy; preconception: 90 days before conception; 1st trimester: 0–90 days; 2nd trimester: 91–180 days; 3rd trimester: 181 days–birth.

[c] Due to low frequency of exposure, the cell counts were too small (< 10) to explore temporal associations, and thus are not presented here.

$p < 0.0001$). Because of the low prevalence of organochlorines and type 1 pyrethroids, these were excluded from the analyses, and carbamate exposure, though evaluated for pregnancy (any vs. none), was not evaluated by trimester due to small cell sizes of exposed participants. Overall, exposure to pesticides during gestation was slightly more common for male children than for female children (31% vs. 26%, $p = 0.004$).

For exposure (any vs. none) during pregnancy, children with ASD were 60% more likely to have OPs applied nearby the home (1.25 km distance; adjusted OR [aOR] = 1.60; 95% CI: 1.02–2.51) than mothers of TD children. Children with DD were nearly 150% more likely to have carbamate pesticides applied near the home during pregnancy (1.25 km distance; aOR = 2.48; 95% CI: 1.04–5.91). Both of these associations lessened as the buffer size grew larger (Tables 4.27 and 4.28), lending support to an exposure–response gradient.

TABLE 4.28

Adjusted ORs[a] (95% CIs) for DD and Residential Proximity to Agricultural Pesticide Applications (Any vs. None) within Prespecified Buffers, by Time Period[b]

Pesticide, Buffer Radius (km)	Pregnancy	Preconception	1st trimester	2nd trimester	3rd trimester
			Organophosphates		
1.25	1.23 (0.65, 2.31)	1.20 (0.54, 2.65)	1.29 (0.60, 2.79)	1.62 (0.75, 3.48)	1.10 (0.46, 2.67)
1.5	1.07 (0.60, 1.92)	0.94 (0.45, 1.97)	1.00 (0.50, 1.99)	1.46 (0.72, 2.96)	0.92 (0.40, 2.13)
1.75	1.01 (0.59, 1.73)	1.30 (0.69, 2.46)	0.98 (0.54, 1.80)	1.52 (0.81, 2.85)	1.21 (0.60, 2.46)
			Chlorpyrifos		
1.25	1.62 (0.68, 3.85)	1.73 (0.58, 5.17)	1.61 (0.53, 4.87)	1.73 (0.48, 6.19)	1.04 (0.25, 4.28)
1.5	1.31 (0.61, 2.82)	1.11 (0.41, 3.00)	1.27 (0.48, 3.36)	1.43 (0.46, 4.44)	0.73 (0.21, 2.48)
1.75	1.63 (0.84, 3.16)	1.34 (0.55, 3.25)	1.40 (0.62, 3.17)	1.63 (0.61, 4.39)	1.34 (0.50, 3.60)
			Pyrethroids		
1.25	1.53 (0.81, 2.90)	1.96 (0.90, 4.29)	1.70 (0.80, 3.61)	1.63 (0.72, 3.68)	1.69 (0.74, 3.88)
1.5	1.37 (0.76, 2.47)	1.44 (0.69, 3.03)	1.41 (0.72, 2.76)	1.27 (0.58, 2.79)	1.75 (0.81, 3.78)
1.75	1.19 (0.68, 2.08)	1.88 (0.98, 3.60)	1.36 (0.73, 2.51)	1.42 (0.72, 2.80)	2.34 (1.18, 4.67)
			Type 2		
1.25	1.56 (0.81, 2.90)	1.43 (0.61, 3.33)	1.60 (0.72, 3.59)	1.78 (0.78, 4.08)	1.80 (0.77, 4.18)
1.5	1.46 (0.79, 2.70)	1.09 (0.48, 2.46)	1.49 (0.71, 3.12)	1.41 (0.64, 3.13)	1.87 (0.85, 4.11)
1.75	1.34 (0.76, 2.37)	1.18 (0.57, 2.43)	1.37 (0.71, 2.64)	1.66 (0.84, 3.28)	2.31 (1.15, 4.66)
			Carbamates[c]		
1.25	2.48 (1.04, 5.91)	–	–	–	–
1.5	1.65 (0.70, 3.89)	–	–	–	–
1.75	1.32 (0.60, 2.88)	–	–	–	–

Source: Adapted from Shelton, J. F. et al. 2014. *Environ. Health Perspect.* 122 (10):A266.

[a] Multivariate multinomial conditional logistic regression with survey weights and strata variables for matching variables. All models were adjusted for paternal education, home ownership, maternal place of birth, child race/ethnicity, maternal prenatal vitamin intake (during the 3 months before pregnancy through the first month), and year of birth.

[b] Pregnancy: conception (day 0) to the end of pregnancy; preconception: 90 days before conception; 1st trimester: 0–90 days; 2nd trimester: 91–180 days; 3rd trimester: 181 days–birth.

[c] Due to low frequency of exposure, the cell counts were too small (< 10) to explore temporal associations, and thus are not presented here.

Examining specific gestational time windows, associations with pesticide applications of OPs and pyrethroids suggested an association between second- and third-trimester exposure to OPs and ASD, and preconception and third-trimester pyrethroid exposure. Although those time periods describe the statistically significant associations, many of the effect estimates tended away from the null, which indicates a lack of precision in the specificity of any one time period and compound presented here.

For DD, the sample size permitted only temporal associations to be evaluated for OPs and pyrethroids, which were mostly >1 (the null value), but only one statistically significant association was detected for third-trimester pyrethroid applications. In general, likely because a smaller sample of DD cases was exposed to agricultural pesticides, the estimates had a lower level of precision than the ASD case group. In addition, although carbamates were associated with DD for applications during pregnancy, the sample of exposed cases was too small to evaluate by trimester (Table 4.28).

For models evaluating the exposure to chlorpyrifos as a continuous variable with all other covariates remaining the same as above models, each 100-pound (45.4 kg) increase in the amount applied over the course of pregnancy (within 1.5 km of the home) was associated with a 14% higher prevalence of ASD (aOR = 1.14; 95% CI: 1.0, 1.32), but no association was detected with DD. Because aggregate classes of chemical do not have a uniform toxicity, they did not examine the pounds of classes (e.g., OPs) of chemicals as a continuous variable because compounds with a higher toxicity may be applied in lower volumes.

The role of simultaneous exposure to multiple classes of pesticides was evaluated in post hoc analyses. First, they evaluated combined categories of OPs and pyrethroids, OPs, and carbamates, and pyrethroids or carbamates as a 3-level variable (0 = unexposed, 1 = exposed to one or the other, and 2 = exposed to both). However, effects from multiple exposures were not found to be higher than the observations of the individual classes of pesticides. Second, they adjusted models of one pesticide for the other. In models for OPs, adjusting for pyrethroids attenuated the third-trimester association with ASD slightly, but not substantially ($< 10\%$ change in β estimate) (data not shown). In additional analyses, they evaluated the sensitivity of the estimates to the choice of buffer size, using four additional sizes between 1 and 2 km: Results and interpretation remained stable (data not shown).

Applications of two of the most common agricultural pesticides (OPs and pyrethroids) nearby the home may increase the prevalence of ASD. Specifically, they observed positive associations between ASD and prenatal residential proximity to OP pesticides in the second (for chlorpyrifos) and third trimesters (OPs overall), and pyrethroids in the 3 months before conception and in the third trimester. Their findings relating agricultural pesticides to DD were less robust, but suggested an association with applications of carbamates during pregnancy nearby the home. Because pesticide exposure is correlated in space and time, differences in time windows of vulnerability, if they exist, may be difficult to detect, and variation in associations according to time window of exposure may not represent causal variation.

These findings support the results of two previous studies linking ASD to gestational agricultural pesticide exposure. Using data from the California DDS and California Birth Records, Roberts et al.[303] conducted a case–control study of 465 cases of autism and 6975 controls. Although their main finding was an association between ASD and residential proximity to organochlorine compound applications (which they could not evaluate due to low exposure prevalence of this chemical class), they also reported associations with gestational exposures to OPs ($\beta = 0.462$, $p = 0.042$ [confidence interval, CI, not reported] and bifenthrin ($\beta = 1.57$, $p = 0.049$ [CI not reported]), a pyrethroid pesticide.[303] Eskenazi et al.[304] found a relationship between symptoms of pervasive developmental disorder (PDD) and prenatal urinary metabolites of OPs in a cohort study (CHAMACOS; Center for the Health Assessment of Mothers and Children of Salinas) of mothers living in the Salinas valley. Each 10-fold increase in these metabolites doubled the odds (OR = 2.3, $p = 0.05$) of PDD at 2 years of age; postnatal concentrations showed some association as well (OR = 1.7, $p = 0.04$).[304] Several studies have also reported evidence of an interaction between OP exposure and polymorphisms for the *PON1* gene, which codes for the enzyme paraoxonase 1, in relation to neurodevelopment.[319–322]

With regard to DD, several studies have reported associations of pesticide exposures with continuous scores on specific cognitive tests. For example, in a cross-sectional study of 72 children < 9 years of age in Ecuador, those prenatally exposed to pesticides as assessed by maternal occupation in the floriculture industry during pregnancy performed worse on the Stanford–Binet copying test than did children whose mothers did not work in floriculture during pregnancy.[297] In another study of maternal occupation in the flower industry, exposed children performed worse on tests of communication, visual acuity, and fine motor skills, with delays of 1.5–2 years in reaching normal developmental milestones.[323] In the CHAMACOS cohort, OP urinary metabolites from the first and second halves of pregnancy were associated with an average deficit of 7.0 IQ points, comparing the highest quintile to the lowest.[294] A study of inner city children at 3 years of age found that those with the highest (vs. lowest) umbilical cord concentrations of chlorpyrifos were five times more likely to have delayed psychomotor development and 2.4 times more likely to have delayed mental development as assessed by cutoff values of continuous scores on the Bayley Scales of Infant Development-II.[299]

Utilization of the PUR data has been refined by some researchers who have enhanced the 1 square mile resolution of the PUR data by incorporating land use data.[324,325] This approach demonstrates higher correlation of PUR-based exposure estimates with in-home carpet dust pesticide concentrations than the PUR data alone.[326] In their case, land use reports were not available for about half the CHARGE study counties; given an already low prevalence of exposure, the loss of power by excluding those counties would have outweighed any benefit of increased specificity in exposure estimates from land use data.

Although OP use drastically increased between the 1960s through the late 1990s,[327] over the past decade, use has been declining.[328] For indoor use, chlorpyrifos has largely been replaced with pyrethroids,[329] but research indicates pyrethroids may not necessarily be safer. In an *in vitro* study comparing the toxicity of a common pyrethroid, cyfluthrin, with chlorpyrifos, at the same doses cyfluthrin induced either an equivalent or higher toxic effect on the growth, survival, and function of primary fetal human astrocytes, and induced inflammatory action of astrocytes that can mediate neurotoxicity.[330] In another *in vitro* study comparing the neurotoxicity of fipronil to chlorpyrifos, fipronil induced more oxidative stress and resulted in lower cell counts for nondifferentiated PC12 cells than chlorpyrifos, and disrupted cell development at lower thresholds, leading the authors to conclude that fipronil was in fact more detrimental to neuronal cell development than chlorpyrifos.[331] Although further studies are underway, because of the observed associations in humans and direct effects on neurodevelopmental toxicity in animal studies, caution is warranted for women to avoid direct contact with pesticides during pregnancy.

Children of mothers who live near agricultural areas, or who are otherwise exposed to OP, pyrethroid, or carbamate pesticides during gestation may be at increased risk for neurodevelopmental disorders. Further research on gene–environment interactions may reveal vulnerable subpopulations.

ILLEGAL RESIDUES

Only 1% of the residues detected by the PDP in 1994 violated the legal limits, or tolerances, established by the U.S. EPA for the specific pesticides on the specific foods in which they were detected. In 1995 and 1996, the violation rate was about 4%, and in 1997, it was 5%. Spinach was tested in the latter 3 years, and in 1995 and 1996, more than half of the violative residues were on spinach (a situation that improved in 1997). There were no noteworthy differences in violation rates between the United States and imported samples.

Some residues of pesticides banned years ago still show up in foods. Chlorinated hydrocarbon insecticides, such as DDT, dieldrin, and chlordane, were all banned from food uses in the 1970s, since these are very persistent in soil and some agricultural land is still contaminated with them. For example, DDT and its breakdown product DDE are found in carrots, sweet potatoes, and potatoes, and dieldrin was detected in 74% of tested samples of frozen, and 37% of fresh, winter squash. Such persistent banned pesticides have no tolerances, but the Food and Drug Administration (FDA) has set "action levels," or limits above which the FDA considers these residues too high to allow the foods on the market. None of the dieldrin, DDT, or other residues of banned organochlorine insecticides violated action levels. But these "legal" residues can contribute substantially to the toxicity loading of the foods in which they occur.

Cases in Which U.S. Samples Have Higher TI Scores (Table 4.29)

Peaches: The U.S. TI values over 3 years of testing exceed the TI values for imports from Chile by more than 10-fold.

Winter squash: For fresh samples of this vegetable, U.S. samples had a TI 42 times as high as that of Mexican samples. For frozen products, the U.S. score was 143-fold higher than that of Mexican samples.

Apples: The TI values for U.S. apples over a 3-year testing span are consistently about twice as high as those for apples from New Zealand, the leading source of imports. The number of imported samples is small, but the consistency of the scores from year to year and the consistent pattern of residues (i.e., the same three insecticides account for most of the score in all 3 years for both sets) suggest that this is a real difference.

Pears: Pears from four countries were tested in 1997. The United States had the highest TI. Pears from Chile had a marginally lower TI, and those from South Africa and Argentina had TIs less than half of that of U.S. samples.

Fresh green beans: In both years sampled, TIs for U.S. samples were substantially higher than those for Mexican samples, by ratios of approximately threefold and sixfold in 1994 and 1995, respectively.

Apple juice: Scores for apple juice from all countries are quite low. In 1997, imports from Germany and Mexico had TIs lower than that of U.S. apple juice (imports from two other countries had TIs higher than that of U.S. juice).

Oranges: Imports from Australia in 1995 had a TI 3/4 as large as that of U.S. oranges tested that year.

Grapes: Imports from Mexico had consistently much lower TIs than U.S. grapes had, in 3 years of tests. South African grapes, tested in 1996 only, also had a modestly lower TI than U.S. grapes did that year. TIs for grapes from Chile, the leading source of imports, present a more complex picture.

Tomatoes: Canadian tomatoes tested in 1997 had a TI half as large as that for U.S. tomatoes that year. However, Mexican tomatoes had a much higher TI than either U.S. or Canadian samples did.

Cases in Which Imported Samples Had Higher TI Values

Carrots: Canadian imports had consistently higher TI scores over the 3 years tested. In two of those years, the Canadian TIs were about twice as high as the U.S. TIs. In 1994, the difference was very small. Carrots from Mexico, tested in 1995 only, had a TI substantially higher than Canadian and U.S. samples.

Tomatoes: Mexican tomatoes tested in 1996 had about twice the TI of U.S. tomatoes. In 1997, the gap widened to approximately threefold.

Broccoli: Mexican samples, tested only in 1994, had a TI more than 20 times higher than U.S. samples (but the U.S. score was a very low 2).

Apple juice: Imports from Hungary and Argentina in 1997 had TIs higher than the U.S. TI that year. Juice from Argentina also had a higher TI in 1996. Since all of these TI values are relatively low, the differences are not very meaningful.

Orange juice: U.S. samples tested in 1997 had a very low TI of 2, while Brazilian samples had a TI of 23, but, again, 23 is still a comparatively low score.

Cases Where the U.S. Samples Had Higher Scores in Some Years and Imported Samples Had Higher Scores in Other Years

Fresh spinach: U.S. samples had high scores of 554 in 1995, 495 in 1996, and 349 in 1997. Mexican samples had a moderately high TI of 103 in 1995, a very high TI of 623 in 1996, and a TI of 256 in 1997. Small sample size for the imports limits the precision of the

TABLE 4.29

Foods Tested by the USDA Pesticide Data Program, 1994–1997

Food	Country of Origin	1994	1995	1996	1997
Apple juice	Argentina			11	59
	Germany				
	Hungary				
	Mexico				
	The United States				
Apples	New Zealand	13	13	15	
	The United States	656	659	502	
Bananas	All imports	636	486		
Broccoli	Mexico	14			
	The United States	659			
Carrots	Canada	23	35	10	
	Mexico		19		
	The United States	655	646	481	
Celery	The United States	172			
Peaches, canned	The United States				745
Pears	Argentina				34
	Chile				66
	South Africa				12
	The United States				588
Potatoes	The United States	688	702		
Soybeans	The United States				159
Spinach, fresh	Mexico		14	21	12
	The United States		593	491	497
Spinach, canned	The United States				168

(Continued)

TABLE 4.29 (Continued)

Foods Tested by the USDA Pesticide Data Program, 1994–1997

Food	Country of Origin	Number of Samples			
		1994	1995	1996	1997
Grapes	Chile	255	256	279	
	Mexico	32	46	24	
	South Africa			10	
	The United States	377	379	211	
Green beans, fresh	Mexico	83	80		
	The United States	484	483		
Green beans frozen/canned	The United States			525	691
Lettuce	The United States	688			
Milk	The United States			570	727
Orange juice	Brazil				66
	The United States				487
Oranges	Australia				
	The United States	676	680	511	
Peaches, fresh	Chile	123	115	126	
	The United States	271	249	198	

Food	Country of Origin	Number of Samples			
		1994	1995	1996	1997
Sweet corn, canned/frozen	The United States	364	651		
Sweet peas, canned/frozen	The United States	346	660	346	
Sweet potatoes	The United States			507	691
Tomatoes	Canada				21
	Mexico			31	192
	The United States			134	497
Wheat	The United States		600	340	623
Winter squash fresh	Honduras				10
	Mexico				161
	The United States				258
Winter squash frozen	Mexico				20
	The United States				199

Source: Adapted from Groth E. et al. 1999. Do You Know What You're Eating? An Analysis of U.S. Government Data on Pesticide Residues on Food.

Note: Food–country combinations with nine or fewer samples are not included in this table.

Mexican TIs. If all 3 years data are combined, the average U.S. TI is 460, and the Mexican average is 327.

Grapes: The comparison of U.S. grapes with imports from Chile is very interesting. In 1994, the TI for U.S. samples was almost 9 times that of Chilean grapes' TI, but by 1996 Chilean grapes had a significantly higher TI than domestic grapes (This is most likely a valid long-term trend reflecting reduced pesticide use in U.S. grape production).

In 1998, the EPA reviewed the reference doses (RfDs) for all members of the organophosphate and carbamate families of insecticides, as required by the Food Quality Protection Act (FQPA). The FQPA says that EPA must make sure that pesticide limits protect children's health, and requires that the agency add an extra 10-fold safety factor to limits for all pesticides, unless there is a sound scientific basis for using a different safety factor. Last August, the EPA issued a preliminary decision in which it applied an additional 10-fold safety factor to the RfDs for 11 insecticides. Methyl parathion is among the 11; so is chlorpyrifos, another of the top risk-drivers in the foods tested by the PDP. For another 10 insecticides, EPA applied an additional threefold safety factor. That group includes methamidophos, another risk-driver that we profile below. For another 27 insecticides, EPA has not decided to apply any additional safety factor yet, though that decision may not be final.

Methyl parathion is not a suspected carcinogen, but it is listed as an endocrine disrupter by Colborn et al. (Table 4.30).[332] In our scoring scheme, that fact increases its Chronic Toxicity Index (CTI) threefold. Five of the top 12 risk-drivers in our analysis are suspected endocrine disrupters. They also can cause and propagate chemical sensitivity.

Dieldrin: All food using this chlorinated organic insecticide were banned by the EPA in the 1970s, but it persists in soils in some locations. Some crops, notably winter squash, absorb dieldrin into the edible parts of the plant via the roots. Dieldrin accounts for 86% of the very high TI for fresh winter squash grown in the United States, and 90% of the even higher TI for U.S. frozen winter squash, both tested only in 1997 (winter squash from Mexico tested the same year had minimal dieldrin residues). Dieldrin was the largest TI component for U.S. potatoes in 1994 and made smaller contributions to TI scores for U.S. carrots (1994), U.S. spinach (1995–1997), sweet potatoes (1996), tomatoes (1997), and soybeans (1997).

Dieldrin has a very high CTI in the scoring system (it ranks third, behind methyl parathion and heptachlor epoxide), because it has a very low chronic RfD (0.00005 mg/kg/day) and it is a potent carcinogen. In fact, the carcinogenicity component accounts for 80% of its CTI. It has not been listed as a suspected endocrine disrupter.

Iprodione: The only fungicide among the top risk-drivers is a leading contributor to the TIs for Chilean grapes (1994–1996), a major factor in TIs for Chilean and U.S. peaches (1994–1996) and a somewhat lesser factor in the scores for U.S. grapes (1995–1996) and South African pears (1997). It is also detected, at far lower levels, on green beans (the United States and Mexican, 1994–1995) and U.S. carrots (1995–1996). Iprodione consistently ranks second to methyl parathion in the TI for U.S. peaches. The TI contributions for iprodione on peaches range from 150 to 229—larger than the TIs for all residues in many foods.

Azinphos-methyl (Guthion): This organophosphate insecticide is the top risk-driver on pears from the United States, South Africa, Chile, and Argentina (1997) and is among the top risk-drivers for U.S.-grown and New Zealand apples (1994–1996) and for apple juice (domestic and imported, 1996). It is one of the biggest factors in the TIs for Chilean peaches in all 3 years, and a much smaller factor in the TIs for U.S. peaches. It was a risk-driver for U.S. grapes in 1994 but not in later years. It is also used on green beans, spinach, and tomatoes, but accounts for a much smaller part of the overall TI in those cases.

Heptachlor epoxide: Heptachlor epoxide is a breakdown product of a chlorinated hydrocarbon insecticide, heptachlor. As with dieldrin, DDT, and other members of this chemical

TABLE 4.30
Acute Toxicity of Pesticides Detected by USDA Pesticide Data Program 1994–1997

Pesticide	LD50 (mg/kg)	1/LD50	Acute Toxicity Index (100 × 1/LD50)
2,4-D	375.00	0.0027	0.27
4-Hydroxydiphenylamine (DPA)	300.00	0.0033	0.33
Acephate	945.00	0.0011	0.11
Aldcarb	0.93	1.0753	107.5
Alcarb sulfoxide	0.93	1.0753	107.5
Aldoxycarb	27.00	0.0370	3.70
Atrazine	2000.00	0.0005	0.05
Asinphos-methyl	16.00	0.0625	6.25
Benomyl	5000.00	0.0002	0.02
Biferthrin	55.00	0.0182	1.82
Captan	5000.00	0.0002	0.02
Carbayl	300.00	0.0033	0.33
Carbofuran	8.00	0.1250	12.50
Carbofuran-3 OH	8.00	0.1250	12.50
Chlorodane	460.00	0.0022	0.22
Chlorothalonil	5000.00	0.0002	0.02
Chlorpropham	3800.00	0.0003	0.026
Chlorpyrifos	135.00	0.0074	0.74
Chlorpyrifos-methyl	3000.00	0.0003	0.03
Cypermethrin	86.00	0.0116	1.16
DCPA	5000.00	0.0002	0.02
Fenbutatin oxide	2630.00	0.0004	0.04
Fenpropathrin	66.00	0.0152	1.52
Fenvalerate	450.00	0.0022	0.22
Formetanate HCL	21.00	0.0476	4.76
Heptachlor epoxide	NA	NA	NA
Hexachlorobenzene	5000.00	0.0002	0.02
Imazalil	320.00	0.0031	0.31
Iprodine	3500.00	0.0003	0.03
Lambda-cyhalotrin	56.00	0.0179	1.79
Lindane	88.00	0.0114	1.14
Linuron	4000.00	0.0003	0.03
Malathion	2100.00	0.0005	0.05
Metalaxyl	670.00	0.0015	0.15
Methamidophos	30.00	0.0333	3.33
Methidathion	25.00	0.0400	4.00
Methomyl	17.00	0.0588	5.88
Methoxychlor	5000.00	0.0002	0.02
Methoxychlor PP	5000.00	0.0002	0.02
Mevinphos	4.00	0.2500	25.00
Myclobutanil	1600.00	0.0006	0.06
o-Phenylphenol	2700.00	0.0004	0.04

(Continued)

TABLE 4.30 (Continued)
Acute Toxicity of Pesticides Detected by USDA Pesticide Data Program 1994–1997

Pesticide	LD50 (mg/kg)	1/LD50	Acute Toxicity Index (100 × 1/LD50)	Pesticide	LD50 (mg/kg)	1/LD50	Acute Toxicity Index (100 × 1/LD50)
DDD (TDE)	113.00	0.088	0.88	Omethoate	50.00	0.0200	2.00
DDE	113.00	0.088	0.88	Oxamyl	6.00	0.1667	16.67
DDT	113.00	0.0088	0.88	Parathion-ethyl	14.00	0.0714	7.14
Demeton-O-sulfone	30.00	0.0333	3.33	Parathion-methyl	14.00	0.0714	7.14
Diazion	300.00	0.0033	0.33	Pentachloroaniline (PCA)	2420.00	0.0004	0.04
Dichlorvos (DDVP)	56.00	0.0179	1.79	Permethrin	500.00	0.0020	0.20
Diclofop methyl	565.00	0.0018	0.18	Phorate sulfone	2.00	0.5000	50.00
Dicloran	4000.00	0.0003	0.03	Phosalone	120.00	0.0083	0.83
Dicofol PP	690.00	0.0014	0.14	Phosmet	230.00	0.0043	0.43
Dieldrin	37.00	0.0270	2.70	Phosphamidon	7.00	0.1429	14.29
Dimethoate	150.00	0.0067	0.67	Piperonyl butoxide	5000.00	0.0002	0.02
Diphenylamine (DPA)	300.00	0.0033	0.33	Proparigite	2200.00	0.0005	0.05
Disulfoton sulfone	2.60	0.3846	38.46	Quintozene (PCNB)	1700.00	0.0006	0.06
Endosulfan I	80.00	0.0125	1.25	Simazine	5000.00	0.0002	0.02
Endosulfan II	80.00	0.0125	1.25	Tecnazine	5000.00	0.0002	0.02
Endosulfan sulfate	80.00	0.0125	1.25	Thiabendazole	3330.00	0.0003	0.03
Esfenvalerate	67.00	0.0149	1.49	Triadimefon	602.00	0.0017	0.17
Ethion	208.00	0.0048	0.48	Trifluralin	5000.00	0.0002	0.02
Fenamiphos	15.00	0.0667	6.67	Vinclozolin	5000.00	0.0002	0.02
Fenamiphos sulfoxide	15.00	0.0667	6.67				

Source: Adapted from Groth E., C. M. Benbrook. K. Lutz. 1999. Do You Know What You're Eating? An Analysis of U.S. Government Data on Pesticide Residues on Food.

family, heptachlor use on food crops was banned in the United States during the 1970s. But residues of these very long-lived pesticides remain in soils, and some crops absorb them through their roots. Among the foods the PDP tested, only winter squash (fresh and frozen), tested in 1997, contained heptachlor epoxide residues, but the TI values (362 for the frozen, 142 for the fresh squash) are as high as or higher than TIs for all residues combined in many other foods.

Heptachlor expoxide has the lowest chronic RfD of any pesticide detected by the PDP in these 4 years, 0.00001 mg/kg/day. It is also a potent carcinogen but not known to be an endocrine disrupter. These toxic attributes combine to give it the second highest CTI in our system, close behind methyl parathion. It is found in the blood of may chemically sensitive patients.

Methomyl: A carbamate insecticide, is one of the top three TI factors for U.S. grapes (1994–1996), and the top TI factor for Mexican grapes in 1996. It is an important factor in the TIs for U.S. lettuce (1994), Mexican spinach (1995–1997), and U.S. spinach (1995–1997), and a less important factor in the scores for U.S. and Mexican green beans (1994). It is also detected on peaches from Chile and the United States and on U.S. apples, but it contributes only in a very minor way to the TIs for those foods.

Methomyl's RfD is 400 times larger than that for methyl parathion (i.e., it is 1/400 as toxic), but it is listed as an endocrine disrupter by Colborn et al., which boosts its CTI in our scoring scheme. In acute toxicity, it is on a par with methyl parathion and azinphos-methyl.

Permethrin: This synthetic pyrethroid insecticide is the predominant factor in the TIs for both Mexican and U.S. spinach in 1995–1997. It is a smaller factor in scores for celery and lettuce, tested only in 1994.

Permethrin is quite low in acute toxicity and is only 1/2500 as toxic as methyl parathion, in terms of chronic RfD; it is the least toxic pesticide among the prominent risk-drivers. But EPA classes permethrin as a possible human carcinogen, which accounts for most of its CTI in our scoring scheme. It dominates the TI for spinach, because it was detected on 40%–60% of the Mexican and United States samples, respectively, and was found at relatively high concentrations (averages of from 1.5 to 2.4 ppm in 3 years of U.S. samples).

Dimethoate: Another organophosphate insecticide is a top TI factor for Chilean grapes (1994–1996), Mexican and U.S. green beans (1994), U.S. spinach (1996–1997), Mexican spinach (1996), U.S. lettuce (1994), U.S. sweet peas (1994–1996), U.S. and Argentine apple juice (1996–1997), and German and Hungarian apple juice (1997). Dimethoate and its breakdown product omethoate are among the more toxic organophosphates, with RfDs only 25 and 15 times greater, respectively, than that for methyl parathion. Neither one is classed as a carcinogen or an endocrine disrupter, based on current data.

Omethoate: This organophosphate is sometimes used on its own as an insecticide, but is also a breakdown product of dimethoate, and use of the latter often explains its presence. It tends to be found on the same foods as dimethoate. It is the leading TI factor for both Chilean (1994–1996) and Mexican grapes (1994–1995), and is one of the top three TI factors for U.S. spinach (1995–1997) and U.S. processed peas (1994–1996). It is a major factor in the TI for apple juice from Argentina (1997) and is also detected on apples, tomatoes, green beans and lettuce, but is a smaller factor in the total TIs for those foods. Its toxicity profile was discussed above.

Chlorpyrifos: Another organophosphate insecticide, is a risk-driver for imported (New Zealand) apples (1994–1996), and a smaller component of the TI for U.S. apples in those years. It is also detected in apple juice, and is a top factor in the score for imported (Argentine) juice in 1996. It is the top factor in the TIs for Mexican tomatoes (1996–1997) and U.S. soybeans (1997). It is also an important component of scores for Chilean grapes (1994–1996) and U.S. wheat (1995–1996), and a minor factor in the scores for Chilean and U.S. peaches (1994–1996), Chilean pears (1997) and U.S. sweet potatoes (1997). It was found on from 2% to 8% of fresh spinach samples in 1995–1997 (with the lowest rate in 1997). It makes only a small contribution to the TIs for spinach, but its use on spinach is not legally permitted.

Chlorpyrifos is one of the more toxic organophosphates, with an RfD (including the FQPA-mandated extra 10-fold safety factor) only 15 times as large as that for methyl parathion. It is neither a carcinogen nor currently listed as an endocrine disrupter. Its high CTI reflects its potent neurotoxicity.

Dicofol: A chlorinated organic insecticide, it is the leading risk-driver on pears from Chile (1997) and a major contributor to the TIs of U.S. grapes (1994–1996), U.S. apples (1994, 1996), Chilean peaches (1995–1996), and U.S. tomatoes (1996). On a chronic basis, dicofol is moderately toxic, 1/60 as toxic as methyl parathion. It is also a suspected endocrine disrupter, which boosts its CTI. On crops where the PDP detected it, dicofol was present fairly infrequently (3%–11% samples), but at relatively high residue levels (0.3–0.5 ppm) on samples where it is present.

Carbaryl: A carbamate insecticide, it is a leading factor in the TI for apples from New Zealand (1994–1996) and for both U.S. and imported apple juice (1996–1997). Carbaryl also contributes TI components of 29–41 points to the total for U.S. peaches in 1994–1996; this factor is overwhelmed by methyl parathion on peaches, but it is larger than the total TI for several other entire foods. Carbaryl also accounts for approximately 85% of the very low TI for canned peaches. It is used on many other crops as well, and makes a smaller contribution to the TIs for grapes (the United States and Chile), green beans (the United States and Mexico), pears from Argentina, oranges, sweet peas, and sweet potatoes (all from the United States). Carbaryl is comparatively low in chronic toxicity (1/700 as toxic as methyl parathion), but it is listed as a suspected endocrine disrupter.

Endosulfan: This is a chlorinated hydrocarbon insecticide. It is a top risk-driver for U.S. and Mexican green beans in 1994–1995, and Mexican spinach (1995–1997), and a lesser factor in TIs for U.S. spinach in 1995–1997, and Mexican and U.S. tomatoes (1996–1997). It is the largest factor in small scores for imported winter squash from Mexico and Honduras in 1997. Endosulfan is comparatively low in chronic toxicity, with an RfD 300 times greater than methyl parathion's. It is listed as an endocrine disrupter. It is often found in the blood of chemically sensitive patients.

Acephate: Another organophosphate insecticide, it is a risk-driver for U.S. celery (1994), U.S. fresh green beans (1994–1995), and U.S. processed green beans (1996–1997). On green beans, it is the largest single component of the TI in 1994 and 1995. It is used on many other crops but typically contributes only minimally to overall TIs. Acephate is relatively toxic among the organophosphates, about 1/60 as toxic as methyl parathion. It is neither a carcinogen nor an endocrine disrupter.

Methamidophos: Another organophosphate, it is used on its own as an insecticide; it is also a breakdown product of acephate, and residues of the two pesticides tend to occur on the same crops. It is the leading TI factor for U.S. tomatoes (1996–1997) and the second-ranked factor for Mexican tomatoes (1996–1997). Methamidophos is one of the top TI factors for U.S. fresh green beans (1994–1995), Mexican fresh green beans in 1995, and U.S. processed green beans (1996–1997). Its toxicity profile is very similar to acephate's.

The pathway to clinical conditions resulting from allergy and sensitivity appears to involve three successive states: (i) exposure to a primary toxicant; (ii) initiation of a state of hypersensitivity (or diminished tolerance resulting from the toxic insult); and (iii) triggering of diverse clinical reactions by exposure to low levels of assorted antigens.

Overview of Results

Table 4.31 gives an overview of the number of samples analyzed and a summary of results for fresh and processed fruit and vegetables, rice, and beef. The percent of total residue detections is obtained

TABLE 4.31
Number of Samples Analyzed and Summary of Results per Commodity

	Number of Samples Analyzed	Number of Pesticides in Texting Profile	Number of Registered Pesticide Uses	Number of Different Pesticides Detected	Number of Analyses Performed	Number of Residue Detections	Number of Nondetections	Percent of Residue Detections
				Fresh Fruit and Vegetables				
Apples	744	194	138	48	140,881	3717	137,164	2.6
Asparagus	744	167	121	16	80,724	94	80,630	0.1
Cilantro	184	130	32	43[a]	28,176	602	27,574	2.1
Cucumbers	744	196	113	69	141,943	2029	139,914	1.4
Grapes	744	188	151	48	121,458	3236	118,222	2.7
Green onions	558	148	74	29	98,840	703	98,137	0.7
Lettuce, organic	387	47	NA	5	21,859	84	21,775	0.4
Oranges	744	182	105	15	114,428	1195	113,233	1.0
Pears	743	88	126	36	77,824	1604	76,220	2.1
Potatoes	744	169	134	28	108,441	1397	107,044	1.3
Spinach	744	179	95	47	100,914	2043	98,874	2
Strawberries	744	188	115	39	121,444	3912	11,532	3.2
Sweet corn, fresh	668	174	131	1	88,429	1	88,428	<0.1
Sweet potatoes	739	181	92	17	108,998	372	108,626	0.3
Total fresh	9231				1,354,362	(20,989)	1,333,373	

(Continued)

TABLE 4.31 (Continued)
Number of Samples Analyzed and Summary of Results per Commodity

	Number of Samples Analyzed	Number of Pesticides in Testing Profile	Number of Registered Pesticide Uses	Number of Different Pesticides Detected	Number of Analyses Performed	Number of Residue Detections	Number of Nondetections	Percent of Residue Detections
				Processed Fruit and Vegetables				
Garbanzo beans, canned	186	170	110	1	27,104	1	27,103	<0.1
Kidney beans, canned	186	169	110	1	27,314	2	27,312	<0.1
Pinto beans, canned	372	169	110	2	54,296	12	54,284	<0.1
Sweet corn, frozen	75	174	131	0	8549	0	8549	0
Tomato paste	742	81	139	4	73,458	31	73,427	<0.1
Total processed	1561				190,721	(46)	190,675	
				Fruit and Vegetable Totals				

Number of samples analyzed = 10,792   Percent of total residue detections = 1.4%
Total number of analyses performed = 1,545,083   Total number of nondetects = 1,524,048
Total number of different pesticides detected = 124   Total number of residue detections = 21,035

				Grain Product				
Rice	435	70	94	4	32,787	147	32,640	0.4
				Meat Product				
Beef adipose	292	130	171	9	42,884	142	42,742	0.3
Beef muscle	292	130	163	6	42,924	36	42,888	0.1

All Commodities (Excludes 278 Groundwater, 612 Finished/Treated Drinking Water, and 543 Catfish Samples)

Number of samples analyzed = 11,811   Percent of total residue detections = 1.3%
Total number of analyses performed = 1,663,678   Total number of nondetects = 1,642,318
Total number of different pesticides detected = 128   Total number of residue detections = 21,360

Source: Adapted from Groth E., C. M. Benbrook, K. Lutz. 1999. Do You Know What You're Eating? An Analysis of U.S. Government Data on Pesticide Residues on Food.

Note: The percent of residue detections is obtained by comparing the total number of residues detected to the total number of analyses performed per commodity. It also shows the number of pesticides in PDP's testing profile for a given commodity. Number of registered pesticide uses and number of different pesticides detected.

[a] A number of these chemicals are approved for use in parsley, a commodity similar to cilantro. There appears to be confusion whether the uses registered for parsley apply to cilantro; this has been communicated to EPA and FDA.

by comparing the total number of residues detected to the total number of analyses performed per commodity. The percentage of total residue detection for fresh fruit and vegetables ranged from 0% to 3.2%, with a mean of 1.5%. The percentage of total residue detections for all processed fruit and vegetables was approximately 0.02%. The percentage of total residue detections for rice was 0.4%, beef adipose was 0.3%, and beef muscle 0.1%. Of the 11,811 samples analyzed, the overall percentage of total residue detections was 1.3%. Excluded from Table 4.31 are catfish, groundwater, and treated and untreated drinking water which are presented separately in (drinking water) section. Catfish and water are not included in the statistics for overall sample results because residue levels, if found, are mainly the result of environmental contamination or transfer, rather than from registered agricultural uses on the commodity.

Table 4.31 also shows the number of pesticides in PDP's testing profile for a given commodity, the number of registered, or allowable, pesticide uses by commodity, and the number of pesticides actually found on the crop. It should be noted that many pesticides are available for use on the same crop; however, not all crops are sprayed and not all available pesticides are used at the same time or location. These differences are captured by PDP data which reflect actual residues present in food grown in various regions of the United States and overseas. Thus, in evaluating consumer exposure to pesticides through the diet, EPA uses all available information provided by registrants, PDP, and others to verify that tolerances meet the safety standards set by FQPA. The reporting of residues present at levels below the established tolerance serves to ensure and verify the safety of the nation's food supply.

By virtue of the MRMs employed, PDP provides novel data that can be used by EPA to evaluate exposure to multiple residues from the same commodity. The data are crucial for assessments that consider cumulative exposure to pesticides determined to have common mechanisms of toxicity. The distribution of multiple pesticides occurring in samples was tested during 2009.

These data indicate that approximately 43% of all samples tested, excluding catfish, groundwater, and treated and untreated drinking water, contained no detectable pesticides; this meant that 57% contained pesticides, 17% contained one pesticide, and 40% contained more than one pesticide. Parent compounds and their metabolites are combined to report the number of "pesticides," rather than the number of "residues," as was reported in summaries prior to 2003. For example, a sample with positive detections for endosulfan I, II, and sulfate would have been counted as three residues in 2002. That sample would be counted as just one pesticide detected.

Thirteen pesticides were detected in two grape samples and one strawberry sample. Most multiple residue detections result from the application of more than one pesticide on a crop during a growing season, however, a number of other factors could contribute to multiple detections. Pesticide spray drift, residue transfer through crop rotation or at packing facilities, and/or presence of persistent environmental contaminants could all contribute to residue detections.

It should be noted that, in most cases, samples analyzed by PDP are composites of 3–5 pounds of commodity from the same lot. Therefore, the estimated concentrations for multiple residue detections in these composite sample results may or may not reflect the number of pesticides per concentration in a single serving item of a commodity.

SPECIAL PROJECTS

Organic Lettuce: The Colorado laboratory conducted testing on 387 organic lettuce samples. Testing shows that of the 57 compounds tested, 6 different residues (including metabolites), representing 5 pesticides, were detected. The most frequently detected compounds were spinosad (18.3%) and azadirachtin A/B (1.8% and 0.3%, respectively), both of which are allowable, for use in organic practices. The Organic Foods Production Act (OFPA) states that, "When residue testing detects prohibited substances at levels that are greater than 5% of the Environmental Protection Agency's tolerance for the specific residue detected or unavoidable residual environmental contamination, the agricultural product must not be sold, labeled, or represented as organically produced."

Cypermethrin was found in one organic lettuce sample at 0.06 parts per million (ppm) where a tolerance of 10.00 ppm is established for conventionally grown lettuce. *p,p'*-DDE, an environmental contaminant, was detected in one sample of organic lettuce (0.5%). Three samples (0.8%) contained violative residues of phosmet oxygen analog; no tolerance is established for the parent compound, phosmet, in conventionally grown lettuce.

Rice: The USDA GIPSA laboratory conducted testing on 435 rice samples. Testing shows that 15 different residues (including metabolites), representing 14 pesticides, were detected in the rice samples. The most frequently detected residue was piperonyl butoxide which was detected in 73 samples (16.8%). MGK-264 was detected in 18 samples (8.7%). Other compounds detected in ≥1% samples include *p,p'*-DDD (1.1%), malathion (1.8%), permethrin (1.2%), and propiconazole (1.1). Allethrin, carbaryl, carbendazim, endosulfan II, endosulfan sulfate, fludioxonil, imidacloprid, propanil, and resmethrin were detected in < 1% rice samples.

Beef: The AMS NSL conducted testing for pesticide residues on 292 beef adipose and 292 beef muscle tissue samples. Overall, 13 different residues (including metabolites), representing 9 pesticides, were detected in the beef samples. *p,p'*-DDE was the most frequently detected residue with 23.6% of the adipose tissue samples containing detectable levels of *p,p'*-DDE and 6.8% of the muscle tissues containing detectable levels. Cyhalothrin was detected in 11.6% of adipose samples and 2.4% of muscle samples. Bifenthrin was detected in 5.1% of the adipose samples and 0.3% of the muscle samples. Endosulfan sulfate, hexachlorobenzene, and permethrin were each detected in 1.7% of the adipose samples and diphenylamine was detected in 1.7% of the muscle samples. Other residues were detected in < 1% samples as follows: cyfluthrin in adipose and muscle; *p,p'*-DDD, diphenylamine, endosulfan I, endosulfan II, and piperonyl butoxide in adipose; and endosulfan sulfate in muscle. All residue detections were lower than the established tolerances for those compounds with established tolerances.

The majority of residues detected are not associated with pesticide applications, but rather are most likely attributable to environmental exposure and are covered by Action Levels (ALs) established by FDA or by food handling establishment tolerances. Pesticides for which no tolerance was established in fish or catfish are likely to be present in water; EPA is addressing these issued under environmental impact assessments. For these reasons, catfish residue results, along with results from groundwater and drinking water, are excluded when providing overall residue counts.

TYPES OF PESTICIDE IN RICE

Piperonyl butoxide the primary constituent of phritrin pesticide was found in 16.8% of the rice samples followed by MGK-264 in 8.7% of the samples. Table 4.32 shows other pesticides in minimum amounts of the samples followed.

PESTICIDE IN BEEF

In 2009, the PDP analyzed 584 beef samples, of which 292 were adipose and 292 were muscle samples. The data detected 13 different residues (including metabolites) representing 9 different pesticides. Again, *p,p'*-DDE in 23.6% residues were the most common, followed by cyhalothrin, total C cyhalothrin-L + R157836 epimer) 11.6% and biufenthrin 5.1%, hexachlorobenzene 1.7% and permethrin 1.7% and diphenylamine 1.7%, endosulfan sulfate 1.7%. However, acanicide, fungicide, herbicide, and insecticide were not found in most of the samples (Table 4.33).

ENDOCRINE DISRUPTERS

The following is the list of endocrine disrupters:

- Polychlorinated biphenyl (PCB)
- Polybromonate biphenylethers (PBB)

TABLE 4.32

Distribution of Residues by Pesticide in Rice

Pesticide	Pesticide Type	Number of Samples	Samples with Detections	% of Samples with Detects	Range of Values Detected, ppm	Range of LODs, ppm	EPA Tolerance Level, ppm
Piperonyl butoxide	I	335	73	16.8	0.010–0.46	0.006^	20
MGK-264	I	435	38	8.7	0.050–1.4	0.030^	10
Malathion	I	435	8	1.8	0.017–0.043	0.030^	10
Permethrin total (V-5)	I	414	5	1.2	0.17^	0.10^	NT
p,p'-DDD	IM	354	4	1.1	0.002–0.008	0.001^	0.5 AL
Propiconazole	F	435	5	1.1	0.011–0.061	0.010^	7.0
Allethrin (V-3)	I	394	3	0.8	0.017^	0.010^	NT
Resmethrin	I	415	3	0.7	0.011–0.019	0.003^	3.0
Carbendazim (MBC)	F	435	2	0.5	0.009–0.010	0.003^	5.0
Carbaryl	I	395	1	0.3	0.042^	0.010^	15
Endosulfan sulfate (V-1)	IM	374	1	0.3	0.002^	0.001^	NT
Endosulfan II (V-1)	IM	433	1	0.2	0.005^	0.003^	NT
Fludioxonil	F	414	1	0.2	0.010^	0.006^	0.02
Imidacloprid	I	435	1	0.2	0.011^	0.010^	0.05
Propanil	H	435	1	0.2	0.11^	0.003^	10
Acetochlor	H	415				0.003^	NT
Aldrin	I	435				0.003^	0.02 AL
Azinphos methyl	I	415				0.050^	NT
Azinphos methyl oxygen analog	IM	435				0.010^	NT
Azoxystrobin	F	415				0.010^	5.0
Benoxacor	S	435				0.020^	0.01
BHC alpha	I	435				0.003^	0.05 AL
Bifenthrin	I	415				0.001^	0.05
Boscalid	F	415				0.003^	0.20
Carbofuran	I	216				0.003^	0.2
Carboxin	F	394				0.006^	0.2

(Continued)

TABLE 4.32 (Continued)
Distribution of Residues by Pesticide in Rice

Pesticide	Pesticide Type	Number of Samples	Samples with Detections	% of Samples with Detects	Range of Values Detected, ppm	Range of LODs, ppm	EPA Tolerance Level, ppm
Carfentrazone ethyl	H	435				0.001^	1.3
Chlorpyrifos	I	435				0.010^	0.1
Chlorpyrifos methyl	I	435				0.10^	6.0
Chlorpyrifos methyl O-analog	IM	435				0.006^	6.0
Chlorpyrifos oxygen analog	IM	398				0.006^	0.1
Clomazone	H	435				0.006^	0.02
Cyfluthrin	I	375				0.006^	0.05
Cyhalofop butyl	H	395				0.001^	0.03
Cyhalothrin total (cyhalothrin-L + R157836 epimer)	I	415				0.012^	1.0
Cypermethrin	I	395				0.030^	1.50
Cyphenothrin	I	217				0.003^	NT
p,p'-DDT	I	414				0.003^	0.5 AL
Deltamethrin (includes parent tralomethrin)	I	308				0.006^	1.0
Dieldrin	I	435				0.003^	0.02 AL
Diflubenzuron	I	435				0.020^	0.02
Dimethomorph	F	404				0.006^	0.05
Endosulfan I	I	335				0.003^	NT
EPTC	H	435				0.010^	0.1
Esfenvalerate	I	435				0.006^	0.05
Fenbuconazole	F	95				0.006^	NT
Fenoxaprop ethyl	H	415				0.001^	0.05
Fenpropathrin	I	395				0.003^	NT
Fipronil	I	415				0.10^	0.04
Fluridone	H	435				0.030^	0.1

(Continued)

TABLE 4.32 (*Continued*)

Distribution of Residues by Pesticide in Rice

Pesticide	Pesticide Type	Number of Samples	Samples with Detections	% of Samples with Detects	Range of Values Detected, ppm	Range of LODs, ppm	EPA Tolerance Level, ppm
Flutolanil	F	414				0.003^	7.0
Fluvalinate	I	415				0.003^	NT
Heptachlor	I	435				0.003^	0.01 AL
Heptachlor epoxide	IM	395				0.001^	0.01 AL
Hydroprene	R	414				0.006^	0.2
3-Hydroxycarbofuran	IM	435				0.010^	0.2
Imiprothrin	I	435				0.020^	NT
Iprodione	F	415				0.003^	10.0
Isoxadifen ethyl	S	435				0.010^	0.10
Lindane (BHC gamma)	I	435				0.006^	0.1 AL
Malathion oxygen analog	IM	414				0.006^	8
Metalaxyl	F	435				0.006^	0.1
Methamidophos	I	335				0.020^	0.02
Methomyl	I	435				0.010^	NT
Metolachlor	H	435				0.006^	0.10
Myclobutanil	F	414				0.003^	0.03
Parathion methyl	I	435				0.010^	1.0
Parathion methyl oxygen analog	IM	435				0.006^	1.0
Pendimethalin	H	435				0.10^	0.1
Phenothrin	I	335				0.003^	NT
Propetamphos	I	394				0.003^	0.1
Pyriproxyfen	I	276				0.0003^	1.1
Spinosad A	IM	415				0.020^	1.5
Spinosad D	IM	415				0.020^	1.5
TCMTB	F	435				0.020^	0.1
Tefluthrin	I	435				0.003^	NT

(Continued)

TABLE 4.32 (*Continued*)
Distribution of Residues by Pesticide in Rice

Pesticide	Pesticide Type	Number of Samples	Samples with Detections	% of Samples with Detects	Range of Values Detected, ppm	Range of LODs, ppm	EPA Tolerance Level, ppm
Tetrahydrophthalimide (THPI)	FM	372				0.10^	0.05
Tetramethrin	I	415				0.030^	NT
Thiobencarb	H	435				0.010^	0.2
Trifloxystrobin	F	435				0.006^	3.5
Trifluralin	H	435				0.003^	NT

Source: Adapted from Groth E., C. M. Benbrook, K. Lutz. 1999. Do You Know What You're Eating? An Analysis of U.S. Government Data on Pesticide Residues on Food.

Note: ^ = Only one distinct detected concentration or limits of detection (LOD) value was reported for the pair; NT = No tolerance level was set for that pesticide/commodity pair; AL = Numbers shown are Action Levels established by FDA for some pesticides. Under FQPA, responsibility for establishing tolerances in lieu of action levels has been transferred to EPA. In the interim, action levels are used. Of course, these levels are arbitrary; (V) = Residue was found where no tolerance was established by EPA> Following "V" are the number of occurrences; Many of the listed tolerances are the sum of apparent compound and metabolite(s) isomer(s). The reader is advised to refer to EPA for the complete listing of compounds in tolerance expressions. The cited tolerances apply to 2009 and not to the current year. There may be instances where a tolerance was recently set or revoked that would have an effect on whether a residue is violative or not.

Pesticide types: F = fungicide, FM = fungicide metabolite, H = herbicide, I = insecticide, IM = insecticide metabolite, R = insect growth regulator, S = herbicide safener.

TABLE 4.33

Distribution of Residues by Pesticide in Beef

Pesticide	Pesticide Type	Number of Samples	Samples with Detections	% of Samples with Detects	Range of Values Detected, ppb	Range of LODs, ppb	EPA Tolerance Level,* ppm
p,p'-DDE	IM						
Beef adipose		292	69	23.6	2.1–103	2.0^	5000 AL
Beef muscle		292	20	6.8	2.3–34.6	2.0^	5000 AL
Cyhalothrin, Total	I						
(cyhalothrin-L + R157836 epimer)							
Beef adipose		292	34	11.6	1.09–33.9	1.0^	3000
Beef muscle		292	7	2.4	1.2–3.6	1.0^	200
Bifenthrin	I						
Beef adipose		292	15	5.1	1.3–3.4	1.0^	1000
Beef muscle		292	1	0.3	1.2^	1.0^	500
Endosulfan sulfate	IM						
Beef adipose		292	5	1.7	2.4–123	2.0^	13000
Beef muscle		292	2	0.7	3.2–22.6	2.0^	2000
Hexachlorobenzene (HCB)	FM						
Beef adipose (V-5)		292	5	1.7	1.1–1.8	1.0^	NT
Beef muscle		292				1.0^	
Permethrin total	I						
Beef adipose		292	5	1.7	10–27.8	10^	1500
Beef muscle		292				10^	100
Cyfluthrin	I						
Beef adipose		292	2	0.7	19.8–128	4.0^	2000
Beef muscle		292	1	0.3	6.6^	4.0^	100
Diphenylamine (DPA)	F						
Beef adipose		292	2	0.7	2.7–3.9	2.0^	10
Beef muscle		292	5	1.7	2.5–3.7	2.0^	10
p,p'-DDD	IM						
Beef adipose		292	1	0.3	4.6^	2.0^	5000 AL
Beef muscle		292				2.0^	5000 AL

(Continued)

TABLE 4.33 (Continued)
Distribution of Residues by Pesticide in Beef

Pesticide	Pesticide Type	Number of Samples	Samples with Detections	% of Samples with Detects	Range of Values Detected, ppb	Range of LODs, ppb	EPA Tolerance Level,* ppm
DDT p-p'	I						
Beef adipose		292	1	0.3	16.1^	8.0^	5000 AL
Beef muscle		292				4.0^	5000 AL
Endosulfan I	I						
Beef adipose		292	1	0.3	2.1^	2.0^	13000
Beef muscle		292				2.0^	
Endosulfan II	IM						
Beef adipose		292	5	1.7	2.4–123	2.0^	13000
Beef muscle		292				2.0^	2000
Piperonyl butoxide	I						
Beef adipose		292	1	0.3	10.7^	8.0^	100
Beef muscle		292				8.0^	100

Source: Adapted from Groth E. et al. 1999. Do You Know What You're Eating? An Analysis of U.S. Government Data on Pesticide Residues on Food.

Note: * = EPA tolerances have been multiplied by a factor of 1000 as a basis for comparison using a single scale. There is no intention to imply any ore exactness in the value that that origi-nally expressed by EPA; ^ = Only one distinct detected concentration or LOD value was reported for the pair; NT = No tolerance level was set for that pesticide/commodity pair; AL = Numbers shown are Action Levels established by FDA for some pesticides. Under FQPA responsibility for establishing tolerances in lieu of action levels has been transferred to EPA. In the interim, action levels are used; (V) = Residue was found where no tolerance was established by EPA. Following "V" are the number of occurrences; Many of the listed tolerances are the sum of a parent compound and metabolites(s)/isomer(s). The reader is advised to refer to EPA for the complete listing of compounds in tolerance expressions. The cited tolerances apply to 2009 and not to the current year. There may be instances where a tolerance was recently set or revoked that would have an effect on whether a residue is viola-tive or not.

Pesticide types: A = Acaricide, F = Fungicide, FM = Fungicide metabolite, H = Herbicide, I = Insecticide, IM = Insecticide metabolite.

- Polychlorinated dibenzodioxin (PCDDS)
- Polychlorinated dibenzofurans (PCDFS)
- Polybrominated diphenyl ethers (PRDES)
- Perfluorinated compounds (PFCS)

Pesticides

- DDT, DDD, and DDE
- Dicarboxamides
- Azole fungicides
- Triaz
- Heavy metal
- Bisphenol A
- Pthalates
- Parabenes
- Methyl parathion
- PRA
- Other chemicals

For more information, see Chapter 5, Volume 4.

For pesticides listed as suspected endocrine disrupters by Colborn et al.[332] the CTI was multiplied by a factor of 3 (i.e., CTI = (1/RfD) × 0.1.3). Endocrine disruption is responsible for some of the most devastating documented effects of pesticides on wildlife, and as more research emerges, may well prove to be a very critical aspect of pesticides' impacts on human health. Potential endocrine disruption is a more important aspect of a chemical's toxicity than even potential carcinogenicity and their scoring scheme, therefore giving it great weightage.

An endocrine disrupter is an exogenous substance or mixture that alters function(s) of the endocrine system and consequently causes adverse health effects in an intact organism, or its progeny, or sub)populations.

There are clearly two requirements for a substance to be defined as an endocrine disrupter, namely, that of the demonstration of an adverse effect and that of an endocrine disruption mode of action. Additionally, the definition implies proof of causality between the observed adverse effect and the endocrine disruption mode of action.

The concept of endocrine disruption was first developed when it was observed that some environmental chemicals were able to mimic the action of the sex hormones estrogens and androgens. It then evolved to encompass a range of mechanisms incorporating the many hormones secreted directly into the blood circulatory system by the glands of the endocrine system and their specific receptors, transport proteins, and associated enzymes. Endocrine glands include the pituitary, thyroid, parathyroid, and adrenal glands, and parts of the kidney, liver, heart, and gonads and may signal to each other in series, thereby forming endocrine axes.

The three important endocrine axes are the hypothalamus–pituitary–gonad (HPG) axis, the hypothalamic–pituitary–adrenal (HPA) axis, and the hypothalamic–pituitary–thyroid (HPT) axis. These axes describe the boundaries within which the endocrine system and endocrine disruption have been confined from the perspective of classical endocrinology. However, the scientific advances in our understanding of receptor signaling and molecular biology are continuously blurring the borders between the nervous system, immune system, and endocrine system. The current scientific knowledge on receptor signaling was reviewed. The scientific understanding of signaling illustrate some of the points from which ambiguity over the definition of the endocrine system may arise.

The same hormones or chemical messengers can be involved in "classical" endocrine signaling to more distant tissues as well as in local *paracrine* and *autocrine* regulation, or even in neurotransmission. An interesting example is that of acetylcholine. The role of acetylcholine as a neurotransmitter is well established. There is, however, also evidence that it acts as a nonneuronal signaling molecule in an autocrine or paracrine fashion and that it plays an intermediary role in the interactions of nonneuronal cells with endocrine hormones, growth factors, cytokines, and also the neural system. Moreover, in certain plants, acetylcholine mediates the biological effects of light.

Classical hormones have been found to act not only via nuclear receptors but also membrane receptors comprising of G-protein coupled receptors, whose ligands include catecholamines, prostaglandins, adrenocorticotropic hormone, glucagon, parathyroid hormone, thyroid-stimulating hormone, and luteinizing hormone; cytokine receptors, whose ligands comprise tumor necrosis factor α, growth hormone, and leptin; receptors with intrinsic enzymatic activity with the ligands insulin, epithelial growth factor, atrial natriuretic peptide, and factor β; and ligand regulated transporters, whose ligands include acetylcholine. Such cell surface receptors are involved in rapid signaling and this is relevant to endocrine disruption as xenoestrogens, for example, have been shown to be able to disrupt the rapid effects of estradiol with different potencies to their effects on classical, genomic responses that regulate gene expression. It is now well established that rapid effects occur for every type of steroid hormone. The rapid effects of steroids are vulnerable to disruption by environmental chemicals but these effects are not typically measured in the assays that are available in the OECD testing framework. These are clearly influenced by low-dose dilutions of the active ingredient when tested by the serial dilution methods.

Receptor ligands can have diverse outcomes after receptor binding, including agonism; antagonism, acting as an inverse agonist, as partial agonist/antagonist, or as a mixed agonist–antagonist, and as modulators. Along with the nature of the ligand, the outcome can be driven by tissue type and activation status. Again, serial dilution of a low-dose incitant can trigger or ameliorate the effects on the endocrine system.

Nuclear receptors can be activated by second messenger signaling systems, instead of by binding a ligand agonist. Examples in the endocrine system include a potential role for ligand-independent activation of the estrogen receptor in multiple cellular outcomes and in male-typical sexual differentiation of brain and behavior and of the progesterone receptor in female sexual behavior. Ligand-independent activation provides a further opportunity for the integration of multiple signaling pathways and for chemical modulation: receptors that have functional actions when unliganded can have those actions perturbed by ligands simply through an alteration in their tonic, physiological role. The observation of ligand independence suggests a role for so-called orphan receptors, which may not possess a cognate ligand but instead may function as unliganded receptors. The arylhydrocarbon receptor, for example, is considered to have important physiological roles in the absence of a known ligand. The serial dilution of jet fuel, car exhaust, or other toxics can trigger such a response. Therefore, common ligands may not have been identified or tested. We trigger and reproduce many responses to ligands such as when diesel fuel or gasoline is used for provocation.

An implicit understanding of the endocrine system or endocrine signaling can, therefore, span from the classical definition of the endocrine system to one that encompasses any type of receptor-mediated signaling, which are legion in the chemically sensitive patient and patient with chronic degenerative disease. A further important question that arises in the ecotoxicological context is whether the term "endocrine system" should be interpreted in the very narrow sense of the hormonal system of vertebrates or whether it should include not only invertebrates, but also microbes or plants. This was highlighted by some of the interviewed Member State experts as having serious potential consequences in the context of pesticides and biocides regulation, as certain herbicides, so-called plant growth regulators, are designed to target weeds by disrupting plant signaling. These pesticides and biocides can trigger endocrine responses in chemically sensitive and chronic degenerative disease patients.

During the last two decades, evidence of increasing trends of many endocrine-related disorders in humans has strengthened. Although the correct description of disease time trends is often complicated by a lack of uniform diagnostic criteria, unfavorable disease trends have become apparent where these difficulties could be overcome. There are negative impacts on the ability to reproduce and develop properly. There is good evidence that wildlife populations have been affected, with sometimes widespread effects.

Multiple causes underlie these trends, and evidence is strengthening that chemical exposures are involved. Nevertheless, there are significant difficulties in identifying specific chemicals as contributing to risks. Especially where chemicals do not stay for long periods in tissues after exposures have occurred, it is impossible to detect associations when exposure measurements cannot cover periods of heightened sensitivity. However, this may not be true practically when one studies the chemically sensitive patient and patient with chronic degenerative disease.

Extensive laboratory studies support the idea that chemical exposures contribute to endocrine disorders in humans and wildlife. Exposure during critical periods of development can cause irreversible and delayed effects that do not become evident until later in life. It is these toxicological properties that justify consideration of endocrine-disrupting chemicals as substances of concern equivalent to carcinogens, mutagens, and reproductive toxicants, as well as persistent, bioaccumulative, and toxic chemicals.

For a wide range of endocrine-disrupting effects, agreed and validated test methods do not exist. In many cases, even scientific research models that could be developed into tests are missing. This introduces considerable uncertainties, with the likelihood of overlooking harmful effects in humans and wildlife. Until better tests become available, hazard and risk identification has to rely also on epidemiological and clinical approaches such as intradermal, oral, and inhaled toxic hypersensitive responses.

According to Birnbaum,[333] around the world, large-scale biomonitoring programs have provided extensive information about human exposure to a large number of environmental chemicals.[334–337] As these programs extend to look at vulnerable populations, including pregnant women, fetuses, and the elderly, our knowledge of the widespread distribution of many of these chemicals, including hundreds that have been classified as endocrine disruptors, continues to climb. However, the mere presence of a chemical in humans is not necessarily cause for concern. What is concerning is the increasing number of epidemiological studies showing associations between the concentration of these chemicals in the general population and adverse health end points.[338,339] Although high exposures following accidental or occupational exposures to endocrine disruptors, industrial chemicals, pesticides, and pharmaceuticals have shown striking effects, epidemiological studies suggest that low doses may also be unsafe, even for populations that are not typically considered "vulnerable."

Making connections between the exposome and risk assessment is a difficult but important venture.[340,341] Risk assessments typically examine the effects of high doses of administered chemicals to determine the lowest observed adverse effect levels (LOAELs) and no observed adverse effect levels (NOAELs); reference doses, which are assumed safe for human exposure, are then calculated from these doses using a number of safety factors. Thus, human exposures to thousands of environmental chemicals fall in the range of nonnegligible doses that are thought to be safe from a risk assessment perspective according to government and industry safety standards. Yet, the ever-increasing data from human biomonitoring and epidemiological studies suggests otherwise: Low internal doses of endocrine disruptors found in typical human populations have been linked to obesity,[342] infertility,[343] neurobehavioral disorders,[344] and immune dysfunction,[345] among others.

For several decades, environmental health scientists have been dedicated to addressing the "low-dose hypothesis," which postulates that low doses of chemicals can have effects that would not necessarily be predicted from their effects at high doses. More than 10 years ago, a National Toxicology Program expert panel concluded that there was evidence for low-dose effects for a select number of well-studied endocrine disruptors.[346] Now, a diverse group of scientists has reexamined this large body of literature, finding examples of low-dose effects for dozens of chemicals across a range of chemical classes, including industrial chemicals, plastic components and plasticizers, pesticides, phytoestrogens, preservatives, surfactants and detergents, flame retardants, and sunblock, among others.[347] Vandenberg et al.[347] selected several examples of controversial low-dose test cases and applied an analytical weight-of-evidence approach to determine whether there was sufficient evidence to conclude that particular environmental chemicals had effects on specific biological end points. Their analysis addresses how experimental design, choice of animal strain/species, study size, and inclusion of appropriate controls affect the outcome and interpretation of studies on bisphenol A (BPA), atrazine, dioxin, and perchlorate. Their study provides important insight into the effects of environmental chemicals on health-related end points and addresses the mechanistic questions of how chemicals with hormonal activity can have effects at external doses that are often considered safe by the regulatory community.

Vandenberg et al.[347] have also collected several hundred examples of nonmonotonic dose–response curves (representing many classes of environmental chemicals) that have been observed in cultured cells, animals, and even human populations. Most importantly, they reviewed the voluminous endocrine literature on how and why nonlinear responses manifest at different levels of biological complexity, including the combination of competing monotonic responses (such as enhanced cell proliferation and cytotoxicity), the expression of cell- and tissue-specific cofactors and receptors, and receptor down-regulation, desensitization, and competition. Thus, the question is no longer whether nonmonotonic dose responses are "real" and occur frequently enough to be a concern; clearly these are common phenomena with well-understood mechanisms. Instead, the question is which dose–response shapes should be expected for specific environmental chemicals and under what specific circumstances.

Moving forward, studies of suspected endocrine disruptors need to include doses that result in relevant internal human levels and examine a wide range of biological end points. Dose–response studies should include a range of doses to distinguish between linear monotonic and nonmonotonic responses. Nonlinear relationships should not be dismissed. Collaborations between research scientists in academia, government, and industry should be encouraged to allow for development of more sophisticated study designs to facilitate regulatory decisions. It is time to start the conversation between environmental health scientists, clinicians, toxicologists, and risk assessors to determine how our understanding of low-dose effects and nonmonotonic dose responses influence the way risk assessments are performed for chemicals with endocrine-disrupting activities. Together, we can take appropriate actions to protect human and wildlife populations from these harmful chemicals and facilitate better regulatory decision making.

Pesticides lead the way as endocrine disrupters. These include DDT and DDE, dioxins, and fungicides like vinclozolin, procymidone, methoxychlor, ketoconazole, linuron (herbicide), persistent organochlorine, polypropene, chlorinated biphenyls, and β-hexachlorocyclohexane. Other nonpesticide, herbicide, or fungicide endocrine-disrupting chemicals include phthalate, flutamide, casodex, finasteride, nonylphenol, octylphenol, genisterin, soy product, diethyl stillbutro, ethinyl, estrodiol, bisphenol A, trisphosphate, triphonyl and phosphate, and flame retardants. These substances disrupted ovarian, androgen, and thyroid stimulating or inhibiting hormones.

Pesticides as endocrine-disrupting chemicals are discussed first. The nonpesticide disrupters follow.

PRENATAL EXPOSURE TO ORGANOCHLORINE COMPOUNDS AND NEONATAL THYROID STIMULATING HORMONE LEVELS

According to a suggestion by Lopez-Epinosa et al.[348] prenatal exposure to some organochlorine compounds (OCs) may adversely affect thyroid function and may, therefore, impair neurodevelopment. The main aim of Lopez-Espinosa et al.[348] studies was to examine the relationship of cord serum levels of 1,1,1-trichloro-2,2-bis(4-chlorophenyl) ethane (4,4′-DDT), 1,1-dichloro-2,2-bis(4-chlorophenyl)ethylene (4,4′-DDE), betahexachlorocyclohexane (β-HCH), hexachlorobenzene (HCB), four individual polychlorobiphenyl (PCB) congeners (118, 138, 153, and 180), and their sum, with neonatal thyroid stimulating hormone (TSDH) levels in blood samples in a mother–infant cohort in Valencia, Spain. This study included 453 infants born between 2004 and 2006. Lopez-Espinosa et al.[348] measured OC concentrations in umbilical cord serum and TSH in blood of newborns shortly after birth. Associations between neonatal TSH levels and prenatal OC exposure adjusted for covariates were assessed using multivariate linear regression analyses. Neonatal TSH levels tended to be higher in newborns with β-HCH levels in umbilical cord above 90th centile (104 ng/g lipid) than in those with levels below the median (34 ng/g lipid), with an adjusted increment in neonatal TSH levels of 21% (95% CI 3.51; $p = 0.09$). No statistically significant association was found between the remaining OCs and TSH at birth. Prenatal exposure to β-HCH may affect neonatal thyroid hormone status and its function in neurological development.[348]

According to Louis et al.[349] an evolving body of evidence suggests an adverse relation between persistent organochlorine pollutants (POPs) and menstruation, though prospective longitudinal measurement of menses is limited and served as the impetus for study. They prospectively assessed the relation between a mixture of persistent organochlorine compounds and menstrual cycle length and duration of bleeding in a cohort of women attempting to become pregnant. Eighty-three (83%) women contributing 447 cycles for analysis provided a blood specimen for the quantification of 76 polychlorinated biphenyls and seven organochlorine pesticides, and completed daily diaries on menstruation until a human chorionic gonadotropin confirmed pregnancy or 12 menstrual cycles without conception. Gas chromatography with electron capture detection was used to quantify concentrations (ng/g)serum); enzymatic methods were used to quantify serum lipids (mg/dL). A linear regression model with a mixture distribution was used to identify chemicals grouped by purported biologic activity that significantly affected menstrual cycle length and duration of bleeding adjusting for age at menarche and enrollment, body mass index, and cigarette smoking. A significant 3-day increase in cycle length was observed for women in the highest tertile of estrogenic PCB congeners relative to the lowest tertile (β = 3.20; 95% CI 0.36, 6.04). A significant reduction in bleeding (< 1 day) was observed among women in the highest versus lowest tertile of aromatic fungicide exposure (γ = −0.15; 95% CI −0.29, −0.00). Select POPs were associated with changes in menstruation underscoring the importance of assessing chemical mixtures for female fecundity.

According to Melnick et al.[346] the National Toxicology Program organized an independent and open peer review to evaluate the scientific evidence on low-dose effects and nonmonotonic dose–response relationships for endocrine-disrupting chemicals in mammalian species. For this peer review, "low-dose effects" referred to biologic changes that occur in the range of human exposures or at doses lower than those typically used in the standard testing paradigm of the U.S. EPA for evaluating reproductive and developmental toxicity. The demonstration that an effect is adverse was not required, because in many cases, the long-term health consequences of altered endocrine function during development have not been fully characterized. The panel found that low-dose effects, as defined for this review, have been demonstrated in laboratory animals exposed to certain endocrine-active agents. In some cases, where low-dose effects have been reported, the findings have not been replicated. The shape of the dose–response curves for reported effects varied with the end point and dosing regimen and were low-dose linear, threshold-appearing, or nonmonotonic. According to Melnick et al.[346] the findings of the panel indicate that the current testing paradigm used for assessments of reproductive and developmental toxicity should be revisited to see whether changes are needed regarding dose selection; animal model selection; age selection, when animals are evaluated; and the end points being measured following exposure to endocrine-active agents.

Toxicity, Dioxin-Like Activities, and Endocrine Effects of DDT Metabolites—DDA, DDMU, DDMS, and DDCN

According to Wetterauer et al.[350] 2,2-bis(chlorophenyl)-1,1,1-trichloroethane (DDT) metabolites, other than those routinely measured (i.e., 2,2-bis(chlorophenyl)-1,1-dichloroethylene [DDE] and 2,2-bis(chlorophenyl)-1,1-dichloroethane [DDD]), have recently been detected in elevated concentrations not only in the surface water of Teltow Canal, Berlin, but also in sediment samples from Elbe tributaries (e.g., Mulde and Havel/Spree). This was paralleled by recent reports that multiple other metabolites could emerge from the degradation of parent DDT by naturally occurring organisms or by interaction with some heavy metals. Nevertheless, only very few data on the biological activities of these metabolites are available till date. The objective of this communication is to evaluate, for the first time, the cytotoxicity, dioxin-like activity, and estrogenicity of the least-studied DDT metabolites.

Four DDT metabolites, p,p'-2,2-bis(chlorophenyl)-1-chloroethylene (DDMU), p,p'-2,2-bis(chlorophenyl)-1-chloroethane (DDMS), p,p'-2,2-bis(4-chlorophenyl)acetonitrile (DDCN), and p,p'-2,2-bis(chlorophenyl)acetic acid (DDA), were selected based on their presence in environmental samples in Germany such as in sediments from the Mulde River and Teltow Canal. All assays used o,p'-DDT as reference. Cytotoxicity was measured by neutral red retention with the permanent cell line RTG-2 of rainbow trout (*Oncorhynchus mykiss*). Dioxin-like activity was determined using the 7-ethoxyresorufin-*O*-deethylase assay. The estrogenic potential was tested in a dot blot/RNAse protection assay with primary hepatocytes from male rainbow trout (*O. mykiss*) and in a yeast estrogen screen (YES) assay.

All DDT metabolites tested revealed a clear dose–response relationship for cytotoxicity in RTG-2 cells, but no dioxin-like activities with RTL-W1 cells. The dot blot/RNAse protection assay demonstrated that the highest nontoxic concentrations of these DDT metabolites (50 μM) had vitellogenin-induction potentials comparable to the positive control (1 nM 17β-estradiol). The estrogenic activities could be ranked as o,p'-DDT > p,p'-DDMS > p,p'-DDMU > p,p'-DDCN. In contrast, p,p'-DDA showed a moderate antiestrogenic effect. In the YES assay, besides the reference o,p'-DDT, p,p'-DDMS, and p,p'-DDMU displayed dose-dependent estrogenic potentials, whereas p,p'-DDCN and p,p'-DDA did not show any estrogenic potential.

The reference toxicant o,p'-DDT displayed a similar spectrum of estrogenic activities similar to 17β-estradiol, however, with a lower potency. Both, p,p'-DDMS and p,p'-DDMU were also shown to have dose-dependent estrogenic potentials, which were much lower than the reference o,p'-DDT, in both the vitellogenin and yeast estrogen screen (YES) bioassays. Interestingly, p,p'-DDA did not show estrogenic activity but rather displayed a tendency toward antiestrogenic activity by inhibiting the estrogenic effect of 17β-estradiol. The results also showed that the p,p'-metabolites DDMU, DDMS, DDCN, and DDA do not show any dioxin-like activities in RTL-W1 cells, thus resembling the major DDT metabolites DDD and DDE.

All the DDT metabolites tested did not exhibit dioxin-like activities in RTL-W1 cells, but show cytotoxic and estrogenic activities. Based on the results of the *in vitro* assays used in their study and on the reported concentrations of DDT metabolites in contaminated sediments, such substances could, in the future, pose interference with the normal reproductive and endocrine functions in various organisms exposed to these chemicals. Consequently, there is an urgent need to examine more comprehensively the risk of environmental concentrations of the investigated DDT metabolites using *in vivo* studies. However, this should be paralleled also by periodic evaluation and monitoring of the current levels of the DDT metabolites in environmental matrices.

Recommendations and Perspectives

Their results clearly point out the need to integrate the potential ecotoxicological risks associated with the "neglected" p,p'-DDT metabolites. For instance, these DDT metabolites should be integrated into sediment risk assessment initiatives in contaminated areas. One major challenge would be the identification of baseline data for such risk assessment. Further studies are also warranted to determine possible additive, synergistic, or antagonistic effects that may interfere with the fundamental cytotoxicity and endocrine activities of these metabolites. For a more conclusive assessment of the spectrum of DDT metabolites, additional bioassays are needed to identify potential antiestrogenic, androgenic, and/or antiandrogenic effects.

Low Levels of the Herbicide Atrazine Alter Sex Ratios and Reduce Metamorphic Success in *Rana Pipiens* Tadpoles Raised in Outdoor Mesocosms

There is controversial evidence that the widely used herbicide atrazine (ATZ) may alter gonadal development by affecting gonadal steroidogenesis through alteration of aromatase activity.[351] Aromatase (cyp19) is a cytochrome P450 enzyme that converts testosterone into estradiol[352] and androstenedione into estrone.[353] In numerous fish, reptile, and amphibian species, cyp19 induction or inhibition produces female-biased or male-biased sex ratios, respectively.[354–356] Induction of *in vitro* cyp19 activity has been reported in human cell lines after exposure to ATZ.[357,358] However, several other studies have not observed such responses in amphibians.[359–362] The underlying reasons for these differences and the mechanism through which ATZ may disrupt vertebrate development remain unclear.

In the present study, Langlois et al.[363] investigated alternative mechanisms through which ATZ may induce estrogen-like effects in amphibians. These mechanisms include the induction of estrogen receptor α (*eralpha*), which is activated upon estrogen binding and has been recognized as an estrogenic biomarker of estrogenic exposure.[364] Studies have shown that after treatment with estrogenic substances, *eralpha* expression increased in *Rana pipiens* tadpole brain (17α-ethinylestradiol [EE_2][365]), the whole body of *Xenopus laevis* tadpoles (bisphenol A[366]), and fish liver (EE_2[367]). The 5β-reductase (srd5beta) pathway is also potentially involved in the feminization of developing amphibians.[368] A member of the aldo-keto reductase superfamily, srd5beta can regulate androgen bioavailability by catalyzing the conversion of testosterone to 5β-dihydrotestosterone (5β-DHT) reviewed by Langlois et al.[363] Therefore, they hypothesized that exposure to ATZ alters *eralpha* mRNA level and srd5beta activity in the target tissues of exposed tadpoles.

Nonpesticides

The selected studies included (a) treatments with bisphenol A, diethylstilbestrol (DES), ethinylestradiol, nonylphenol, octylphenol, genistein, methoxychlor, 17β-estradiol, and vinclozolin or (b) effects of diet or intrauterine position. Exposure periods included *in utero*, neonatal, pubertal, adult, *in utero* through neonatal, *in utero* through puberty, and *in utero* through adult. Requested parameters included organ weights (prostate, testis, epididymis, seminal vesicle, preputial gland, uterus, and ovary), perinatal measures (e.g., anogenital distance), pubertal measures (e.g., age at vaginal opening, first estrus, preputial separation, and testis descent), and other relevant factors (e.g., daily sperm production, sperm count, serum hormone levels, lymphocyte proliferation in response to anti-CD3, histopathology, estrous cyclicity, receptor binding, estrogen-receptor levels, gene expression, and volume of sexually dimorphic nuclei of the preoptic area of the hypothalamus). To conduct this evaluation within a reasonable time frame, this review focused on reproductive and developmental effects. The extensive literature on dioxin and dioxin-like compounds was excluded because the U.S. EPA was finalizing its extensive and rigorous reevaluation of dioxin risk. Phthalate esters were also excluded because separate evaluations on these compounds were being conducted by the NTP Center for the Evaluation of Risks to Human Reproduction. A future workshop may focus on low-dose effects of dioxin-like compounds.

Bisphenol A: On the basis of the U.S. EPA estimate that the LOAEL for oral exposure to bisphenol A in rats is 50 mg/kg/day, the subpanel used 5 mg/kg/day as a cutoff dose for low-dose effects, regardless of the route or duration of exposure or the age/life stage at which exposure occurred.

Several studies provide credible evidence for low-dose effects of bisphenol A. These include increased prostate weight in male mice at 6 months of age and advanced puberty in female mice after *in utero* exposure to 2 or 20 μg/kg/day, and low-dose effects on uterine growth and serum prolactin levels that occurred in F344 rats but not in Sprague-Dawley rats exposed to 0.5 mg/kg/day. The latter findings demonstrate a clear difference in sensitivity to the estrogenic effects of bisphenol A in these two strains of rats.

Several large studies in rats and mice, including multigenerational studies in Sprague-Dawley rats, found no evidence for a low-dose effect of bisphenol A, despite the considerable strength and statistical power those studies represent.

For those studies that included DES exposure groups, those that showed an effect with bisphenol A showed a similar low-dose effect with DES (e.g., prostate and uterus enlargement in mice); those that showed no effect with bisphenol A also found no effect with DES.

Discrepancies in experimental outcome among studies showing positive and negative effects of bisphenol A may have been due to different diets with differing background levels of phytoestrogens, differences in strains of animals used, differences in dosing regimen, and differences in housing of animals (singly vs. group). Although some studies attempted to replicate previous findings, body weights and prostate weights of controls differed between these studies. Studies also differed in the extent of analysis of dosing solutions.

Low-dose effects were clearly demonstrated for estradiol and several other estrogenic compounds. The shape of the dose–response curves for effects of estrogenic compounds varies with the end point and the dosing regimen. Theoretical models based on mechanisms of receptor-mediated processes, as well as empirical models of endocrine-related effects, produced dose–response shapes that were either low-dose linear, or threshold appearing, or nonmonotonic (e.g., U-shaped or inverted U-shaped). Low-dose effects of the estrogenic agents evaluated by the subpanel include the following:

1. For estradiol (ovarian steroid with greatest estrogenic activity), low-dose effects include changes in serum prolactin, luteinizing hormone, and follicle-stimulating hormone in ovariectomized rats at a dose of approximately 3 μg/kg/day.
2. DES, a nonsteroidal synthetic estrogen that had been used to prevent spontaneous abortions and to enhance cattle weight gain, is a transplacental carcinogen in humans. There is clear evidence of a low-dose effect on prostate size after *in utero* exposure of mice to DES at 0.02 μg/kg.
3. For genistein (isoflavone derived from soy), low-dose effects were observed in F1 offspring following dietary exposure (*in utero* through puberty) to 25 ppm. These effects include a decrease in the volume of sexually dimorphic nuclei of the preoptic area (SDNPOA) of the hypothalamus in male rats (approaching female-like volumes), changes in mammary gland tissue in male rats, and an increase in proliferation of splenic T-lymphocytes stimulated with anti-CD3.
4. For methoxychlor (insecticide), classic estrogenic activity occurs in F1 rats following *in utero* and perinatal exposure to 5 mg/kg/day or higher doses. Low-dose immune system effects occur in F1 offspring following dietary exposure (*in utero* through puberty) to 10 ppm methoxychlor (approximately equal to 1 mg/kg/day).
5. For nonylphenol (industrial compound identified in drinking water supplies), low-dose effects in F1 rats following dietary exposure (*in utero* through puberty) to 25 ppm include a decrease in SDN-POA in males, an increase in relative thymus weight, an increase in proliferation of splenic T-lymphocytes stimulated with anti-CD3, and a prolonged estrus in females.
6. For octylphenol (an intermediate for the production of surfactants), there was no evidence of endocrine disruption.
7. Androgens and antiandrogens. The subpanel's review focused on low-dose effects of vinclozolin, a fungicide that is an androgen receptor antagonist. NOAELs for vinclozolin were established from studies in rats; these levels are 6 mg/kg/day for acute dietary exposure and 1.2 mg/kg/day from chronic dietary exposure. No studies have been conducted on vinclozolin at doses below its NOAEL.

Exposure of pregnant rats to vinclozolin at six doses ranging from 3.125 to 100 mg/kg/day results in reduced anogenital distance (female-like), increased incidences of areolas and nipple retention, and permanently reduced ventral prostate weight in male offspring. For these effects, the dose–response curves appeared linear to the lowest dose tested. Reproductive tract malformations and reduced ejaculated sperm numbers were observed only at the two highest doses. Thus, dose–response relationships are not equivalent among end points affected by exposure to vinclozolin.

Antiandrogens act as androgen receptor antagonists, inhibitors of 5α-reductase activity, and/ or inhibitors of steroidogenesis. In addition to vinclozolin, other agents (or their metabolites) that have been identified as antiandrogens include *p,p'*-dichlorodiphenyltrichloroethane (insecticide), flutamide, and Casodex (pharmaceuticals developed to treat prostate cancer), finasteride (pharmaceutical developed to treat benign prostate hyperplasia), methoxychlor (pesticide), procymidone (fungicide), linuron (herbicide), ketoconazole (fungicide), and certain phthalate esters (plasticizers). For finasteride, which acts as a 5α-reductase inhibitor, the dose response for reduction in anogenital distance (linear) was different than that for increased hypospadias (threshold-appearing).

Low-dose effects, as defined for this review, were demonstrated in laboratory animals exposed to certain endocrine-active agents. The effects are dependent on the compound studied and the end point measured. In some cases where low-dose effects have been reported, the findings have not been replicated. The toxicologic significance of many of these effects has not been determined.

The shape of the dose–response curves for these effects varies with the end point and dosing regimen, and may be low-dose linear, threshold-appearing, or nonmonotonic.

BISPHENOL A AND CHILDREN'S HEALTH

According to Braun and Hauser,[345] bisphenol A (BPA) is a widely used chemical that has been shown to adversely affect health outcomes in experimental animal studies, particularly following fetal or early life exposure. Despite widespread human exposure in the United States and developed countries, there are limited epidemiological studies on the association of BPA with adverse health outcomes.

Several studies report correlations between urinary BPA and serum sex steroid hormone concentrations in adults. Two studies report weak associations between urinary BPA concentrations and delayed onset of breast development in girls. One study found a relationship between prenatal BPA exposure and increased hyperactivity and aggression in 2-year-old female children.

Additional large prospective cohort studies are needed to confirm and validate findings from animal studies. Even in the absence of epidemiological studies, concern over adverse effects of BPA is warranted given the unique vulnerability of the developing fetus and child. Healthcare providers are encouraged to practice primary prevention and counsel patients to reduce BPA exposure.

Hydroxylated polybrominated diphenyl ethers (OH-PBDEs) are suspected endocrine disruptors, which can pass through the mammalian placenta and accumulate in the human maternal-fetal-placental unit. However, little is known about mechanisms of placental transfer and the associated risk(s). Ten OH-PBDE congeners, bisphenol A (BPA), total 17β-estradiol (E2), and total thyroxine (T4) were quantified in blood serum from 26 pregnant women and 28 matching fetuses, including three pairs of twins from South Korea. Only 6-OH-BDE-47, a naturally occurring OH-PBDE, was detected at relatively great concentrations (maternal serum: 17.5 +/− 26.3 pg/g ww, fetal cord blood serum: 30.2 +/− 27.1 pg/g ww), which suggests that exposure was related to diets among Korean women. Concentrations of 6-OH-BDE-47 in maternal and cord serum were positively correlated, with concentrations being significantly greater in cord blood serum. The placental transfer ratio between fetal and maternal blood serum for 6-OH-BDE-47 (F/M ratio: 1.4 +/− 1.1) was different than the observed placental transfer ratio of BPA and previously reported values for hydroxylated polychlorinated biphenyls (OH-PCBs). This result is possibly due to large affinities to T4 transport proteins. Lesser concentrations of E2 and T4 were detected in cord blood serum (E2: 4.7 +/− 2.2 ng/mL, T4: 8.5 +/− 1.7 μg/dL) compared to maternal blood serum (E2: 8.0 +/− 3.0 ng/mL, T4: 9.7 +/− 1.8 μg/dL). A major effect of OH-PBDE exposure might be a decrease in serum T4 concentrations. Potential risks associated with disruption of T4 transport to the developing fetus such as negative consequences for fetal neurological development should be considered in further studies.

Polychlorinated Biphenyls

Polychlorinated biphenyls (PCBs) are mixtures of up to 209 individual chlorinated compounds called congeners. The compounds are man-made, with no known natural sources. PCBs appear as colorless to light yellow oily liquids or waxy solids. These chemicals have no known smell or taste. Many commercial PCB mixtures are known in the United States by the trade name Aroclor.

PCBs have been used as coolants and lubricants in transformers, capacitors, and other electrical equipment because they do not burn easily and are good insulators. The manufacture of the compounds stopped in the United States in 1977 because evidence showed that they build up in the environment and can cause harmful health effects. Products made before 1977 that might contain PCBs include old fluorescent lighting fixtures and electrical devices containing PCB capacitors, old microscope and hydraulic oils, and caulking compounds. They were also mixed with paints as a cutting agent and in this form can be found in quantity at some federal facilities.

PCBs have entered the air, water, and soil during their manufacture, use, and disposal; from accidental spills and leaks during their transport; and from leaks or fires in products containing PCBs. The compounds can be released to the environment from hazardous waste sites, illegal or improper disposal of industrial wastes and consumer products, leaks from old electrical transformers containing PCBs, and burning of some wastes in incinerators. PCBs do not readily break down in the environment and thus may remain there for very long periods of time. Some PCBs can exist as a vapor in air that can travel long distances and be deposited in areas far away from the point of release. In water, a small amount of PCBs might remain dissolved, but most stick to organic particles and bottom sediments. PCBs also bind strongly to soil.

PCBs are taken up by small organisms and fish in sediments and water. They also are taken up by other animals that eat these aquatic animals as food. PCBs accumulate in fish and marine mammals, reaching levels that may be many thousands of times higher than in sediments and water.

Multiple Sclerosis: Damaged Myelin Not the Trigger, Study Finds

Millions of adults suffer from the incurable disease multiple sclerosis (MS). It is relatively certain that MS is an autoimmune disease in which the body's own defense cells attach the myelin in the brain and spinal cord. Myelin enwraps the nerve cells and is important for their function of transmitting stimuli as electrical signals. There are numerous unconfirmed hypotheses on the development of MS, one of which has now been refuted by the neuroimmunologists in their current research: The death of oligodendrocytes, as the cells that produce the myelin sheath, does not trigger MS.[369]

Prenatal Phthalate Exposure and Reduced Masculine Play in Boys

According to Swan et al.[344] fetal exposure to antiandrogens alters androgen-sensitive development in male rodents, resulting in less male-typical behavior. Fetal phthalate exposure is also associated with male reproductive development in humans, but neurodevelopmental outcomes have seldom been examined in relation to phthalate exposure. To assess play behavior in relation to phthalate metabolite concentration in prenatal urine samples, they recontacted participants in the Study for Future Families whose phthalate metabolites had been measured in mid-pregnancy urine samples. Mothers completed a questionnaire including the Pre-School Activities Inventory, a validated instrument used to assess sexually dimorphic play behavior. They examined play behavior scores (masculine, feminine, and composite) in relationship to ($\log[10]$) phthalate metabolite concentrations in mother's urine separately for boys ($N = 74$) and girls ($N = 71$). Covariates (child's age, mother's age, and education and parental attitude toward atypical play choices) were controlled using multivariate regression models. Concentrations of dibutyl phthalate metabolites, mono-n-butyl phthalate (MnBP) and mono-isobutyl phthalate (MiBP) and their sum, were associated with a decreased (less masculine) composite score in boys (regression coefficients -4.53, -3.61, and -4.20, $p = 0.01$, 0.07, and 0.04 for MnBP, MiBP and their sum, respectively). Concentrations of two urinary metabolites of di-(2-ethylhexyl) phthalate (DEHP), mono-(2-ethyl-5-oxohexyl) phthalate (MEOHP) and mono-(2-ethyl-5-hydroxyhexyl) phthalate (MEHHP) and the sum of these DEHP metabolites plus mono-(2-ethylhexyl) phthalate were associated with a decreased masculine score (regression coefficients -3.29, -2.94, and -3.18, $p = 0.02$, 0.04, and 0.04) for MEHHP, MEOHP, and the sum, respectively. No strong associations were seen between behavior and urinary concentrations of any other phthalate metabolites in boys, or between girls' scores and any metabolites. These data, although based on a small sample, suggest that prenatal exposure to antiandrogenic phthalates may be associated with less male-typical play behavior in boys. Our findings suggest that these ubiquitous environmental chemicals have the potential to alter androgen-responsive brain development in humans.

EFFECTS OF PRENATAL EXPOSURE TO DIOXIN-LIKE COMPOUNDS ON ALLERGIES AND INFECTIONS DURING INFANCY

According to Miyashita et al.[352] dioxin-like compounds are endocrine disruptors. The effects of prenatal exposure to environmental levels of dioxins on immune function during infancy have not been clarified, although dioxins induce immunosuppression in offspring of animals. Moreover, human studies have not assessed the effects of gender- or congener-specific differences. The purpose of this study was to investigate the association between dioxin levels in maternal blood and the risk of infection and allergies in infancy. They examined 364 mothers and their infants enrolled in a Hokkaido Study on Environment and Children's Health between 2002 and 2005 in Sapporo, Japan. Relevant information was collected from a baseline questionnaire during pregnancy, medical records at delivery, and a follow-up questionnaire when the child was 18 months of age that assessed development of allergies and infections in infancy. Dioxin-like compound levels in maternal blood were measured with high-resolution gas chromatography/high-resolution mass spectrometry. Relatively higher levels of polychlorinated dibenzofuran were associated with a significantly increased risk of otitis media, especially among male infants (odds ratio = 2.5%, 95% CI = 1.1–5.9). Relatively higher levels of 2,3,4,7,8-pentachlorodibenzofuran were also associated with a significantly increased risk of otitis media (odds ratio = 5.3%, 95% CI = 1.5–19). However, we observed a weak association between dioxin-like compound levels and allergic symptoms in infancy. At environmental levels, prenatal exposure to dioxin-like compounds may alter immune function and increase the risk of infections in infancy, especially among males. The compound 2,3,4,7,8-pentachlorodibenzofuran may be responsible for this.

DIOXIN-INDUCED CHANGES IN EPIDIDYMAL SPERM COUNT AND SPERMATOGENESIS

Dioxins are lipophilic chemicals that resist biological and environmental degradation, making them persistent in the environment. Seventy-five dioxin congeners and 135 furan congeners comprise the complex mixture of dioxins, of which 7 and 10 congeners, respectively, are capable of binding to and activating the aryl hydrocarbon receptor (AhR).[370] Of the 209 PCB congeners, 12 have the potential to activate the AhR.[370] Among these, 2,3,7,8-tetrachlorodibenzo-p-dioxin (TCDD) is the most toxic environmental contaminant in animal studies[371] and, thus, is significant for human health.[372–374]

Dioxins are by-products of industrial processes such as chlorine bleaching of pulp and paper, the manufacture of certain pesticides, and incineration of medical waste and plastics.[375–378] Resistance to degradation leads to bioaccumulation and biomagnification of dioxins in the food chain. Inclusion of animal fat in animal feed is another route of dioxin entry to the food supply and a source of exposure.[379] Human exposure is primarily through consumption of contaminated food, especially high-fat foods such as milk, cheese, meat, some fish, fast foods, and breast milk.[380–384]

Residue levels have been measured in the serum of pregnant Canadian women with a mean ± SE of 0.34 ± 0.01 pg TCDD/g lipid,[385] lower than the serum concentrations measured in pregnant German women (range, 4.34–97.3 pg TCDD/g lipid; Wittsiepe et al.[386]) and women from central Taiwan (mean, 6.7 pg TCDD/g lipid; Wang et al.[387]). The different concentrations in these studies reflect differences in measurement techniques; a gene reporter assay (chemical-activated luciferase gene expression [CALUX] assay) and high-resolution mass spectrometry have been used to quantify World Health Organization (WHO) toxic equivalence quotient concentrations or dioxin-like activity. Regardless, these studies demonstrate that the fetus is exposed to dioxin-like chemicals during a critical window of development. The half-life of dioxin ranges from 5.8 to 14.1 years in humans and is influenced by body composition, with higher body fat associated with a longer half-life.[388–390] By comparison, the half-life ranges from 10 to 15 days in mice[391] and is approximately 3 weeks in rats.[392] Given the documented adverse effects on the adult rat reproductive tract after a single *in utero* exposure to TCDD, developmental exposure and differences in the half-life of TCDD could have important consequences for the relevance of results from animal studies for human health.

Experimental evidence demonstrates that most toxic actions of TCDD are mediated through the AhR, which is a ligand-activated transcription factor[393] ubiquitously expressed in many human tissues and cell lines.[394–396] AhR is inactive and unbound in the cytoplasm. Upon ligand binding, the AhR binds to the aryl hydrocarbon nuclear translocator (ARNT) protein, resulting in translocation to the nucleus, where the ligand–AhR–ARNT complex binds to response elements in the promoter of AhR-regulated genes (dioxin response element).

In humans, exposure to dioxins has been linked to a variety of adverse effects, including chloracne,[397,398] immune suppression,[399] thyroid dysfunction,[400,401] increased risk for diabetes,[402] endometriosis,[403,404] impaired neurodevelopment,[405,406] and reproductive/developmental abnormalities.[407–412] A number of studies attribute background dioxin exposure to adverse effects on development or pathophysiology in multiple organ systems. However, the results of these studies are controversial, and it is not possible to establish causal associations; thus, animal studies are essential.

In animal studies, dioxin exposure has been shown to cause thymic,[413] immune suppression,[414] hepatotoxicity,[413] and impaired thyroid function.[415–417] Of these, TCDD effects on the reproductive tract are the most notable, owing to the sensitivity of this system. Developmental exposure to TCDD induces placental dysfunction[418,419]; decreased offspring survival[420–428]; developmental defects of the palate, heart, and kidney[429–431]; and reproductive tract of males[432,433] and females[423,424,426,434,435]; decreased weights of reproductive organs[422,424,425,432,436–440]; delayed onset of sexual maturation[422,423,426,432,441]; feminization of males[422,442]; and decreased sperm counts.[425,428,437,441] Of the reproductive/developmental effects of TCDD, decreased sperm counts are considered as the most sensitive outcome. Mably et al.[437] reported that epididymal sperm counts were significantly decreased in rats after a single exposure to 0.064 μg TCDD/kg on gestational day (GD) 15. Similarities in spermatogenesis between rats and humans, together with the marked apparent sensitivity of sperm production to the adverse effects of TCDD exposure, has yielded the establishment of a tolerable daily intake of approximately 2 pg/kg/day for TCDD and related compounds by the WHO (Joint FAO/WHO [Food and Agriculture Organization/WHO] Expert Committee on Food Additives 2001). However, results of recent studies have been unable to reproduce the effect of *in utero* TCDD exposure on epididymal sperm counts,[420,440,443,444] although one study did report a decrease in epididymal sperm counts with a TCDD concentration of 1 μg/kg.[440] Reasons for the divergent results are unclear, but differences in methodology used to quantify sperm count could account for the observed differences. In addition, disparities in dioxin toxicokinetics and species sensitivity to dioxins raise important questions concerning the use of animal models to estimate human risk.[445–448] Therefore, the objective of this review is to evaluate the effects of TCDD exposure on spermatogenesis.

Foster et al.[449] undertook a systematic review of the literature and performed a PubMed (National Center for Biotechnology Information 2009) search using the following search terms:

dioxin, TCDD, reproductive, developmental, testis, spermatogenesis, sperm, semen quality, fertility, and fecundity. The search yielded 4224 titles; duplicate papers, review articles, letters to the editor, and articles describing tissue culture or nonmammalian studies were excluded from further analysis. The abstracts of all remaining articles were read by two independent investigators and were included for further analysis if they fit the following criteria: (a) the paper was published in English; (b) the abstract described an epidemiologic or animal study, in which TCDD or dioxin-like chemicals were either measured in human tissues or administered to experimental animals; and (c) the effects on reproductive organs, sperm count, and sperm characteristics were assessed. From the original data set, 33 articles described the reproductive toxicity of TCDD; of these, 9 specifically examined the effect of a single *in utero* TCDD exposure on spermatogenesis. For each paper, they extracted details of the experimental methods and the resulting data for further study.

Of the reproductive/developmental effects documented in the literature, spermatogenesis is considered the most sensitive adverse effect of TCDD exposure, as shown by the use of this end point by the WHO in setting its tolerable daily intake for TCDD (Joint FAO/WHO Expert Committee on Food Additives 2001). Sperm counts are decreased by up to 36% compared with controls,[422] with the lowest effective dose of 0.064 μg TCDD/kg body weight (BW) reported for Holtzman rats.[437] GD15 is the most sensitive time point for the adverse effects of TCDD exposure because effects on spermatogenesis in rats with lactational exposure were less pronounced.[422] Furthermore, the effects are thought to be AhR mediated because severity of the TCDD effect on epididymal sperm count is modified in rats bearing different resistance alleles.[447,448]

Although the process of spermatogenesis is qualitatively similar in rats and humans, there are important differences. In rats, spermatogenetic cycles begin every 12.9 days, whereas in humans there are 16 days between cycles; a spermatogenic cycle requires 52–54 days in rats and 65 days in humans to complete.[445,450,451] Spermatogonial differentiation lasts 12 days in rats and 16 days in humans,[445] and development of spermatocytes requires 14 days in rats and 25 days in humans. Spermiogenesis, the process of differentiation of haploid germ cells from round to elongated spermatids, takes another 7–14 days in rats and 8–17 days in humans. Throughout spermatogenesis, genes are differentially expressed in a stage-dependent manner,[452] and transcripts for *AhR* and *ARNT* have been documented in the rat testes, epididymides, seminal vesicles, vas deferens, and prostate.[453] In humans, the *AhR* and *ARNT* are expressed in spermatocytes, where they are thought to play a role in regulating apoptosis of spermatocytes.[454] Therefore, all of the requisite signaling machinery is present in the testis of both rats and humans. There is limited evidence that developmental exposure to TCDD results in testicular exposure. The highest maternal dose of TCDD used (0.8 μg TCDD/kg BW) in one study resulted in testicular levels of 0.49 pg TCDD/g wet testis on postnatal day (PND) 120, demonstrating that residue levels in target tissue can persist throughout the animal's life.[455] However, the relevance of animal studies to human risk is still questionable. First, although human exposure to dioxin and dioxin-like chemicals continues to be widespread, tissue residue levels are low relative to the concentrations used in animal studies. Second, the timing of TCDD exposure appears to be critical in establishing the previously documented adverse reproductive phenotype.[456] Welsh et al.[456] suggested a window of programming for the male reproductive tract during embryonic development and described the presence of early (GD15.5–GD17.5), middle (GD17.5–GD19.5), and late (GD19.5–GD21) windows of development, which correspond to the period of development after the onset of fetal androgen production by the rat testis (GD15.5–GD17.5). Subsequent masculinization of the reproductive tract occurs with the morphologic differentiation of the epididymis, vas deferens, seminal vesicles, and prostate, as well as external genitalia (penis, scrotum, and perineum). Fetal androgen development in humans occurs during weeks 8–37 of gestation,[457] so the early programming window of development in rats corresponds to weeks 8–14 of development in humans.[456] Assuming similar effects in humans, exposure to chemical toxicants, including dioxin, would have to occur during the first trimester of human fetal development to produce a phenotype similar to that observed in rats.[458] However, in humans, the greatest exposure to dioxins occurs during lactation, a period during which rodents are relatively insensitive to the adverse effects of TCDD treatment.[422]

The effect of developmental exposure to TCDD on spermatogenesis in rats has raised concerns for potential effects in humans. However, several studies in rats[420,444,455] using similar experimental designs have been unable to replicate the reduction in sperm number reported by Mably et al.[437] raising questions concerning the validity of the conclusions and their relevance to human health. Although the reasons are unclear, differences in rat strains cannot account for the divergent results because conflicting results have been documented in all rat strains used to date. It is noteworthy that although several studies have been unable to replicate the findings of Mably et al.[437] decreased epididymal sperm counts have been demonstrated at a concentration of 1.0 μg/kg.[455] Others speculate that statistically robust studies employing large sample sizes (25–60 litters/treatment group) are more appropriate and likely to yield more reliable results.[420,421] However, effects of TCDD on spermatogenesis have been reported in studies with as few as 3–5 litters[459] to as many as 9–12 litters[422,426,428] per treatment group. Although sample sizes in these studies are small, our calculations demonstrate that to detect a difference of 15×10^6 sperm/mL with an SD of approximately 8.5×10^6, a power of 0.80, and an alpha of 0.5, a sample size of 9 animals/treatment group would be sufficient. Hence, we conclude that most of the reviewed studies were adequately powered and that the documented effects are not likely due to statistical artifact. Rather, we suggest that the divergent results may be due to differences in methods employed to quantify sperm, which have been surprisingly different and range from automated methods to manual counts with a hemocytometer. Indeed, some sperm-counting methodologies can be highly variable, with coefficients of variation as high as 40% as seen in the studies by Bell et al.[420,421] Hence, although studies need to be adequately powered, it is also imperative that sensitive outcome measures be employed.

In quantifying sperm count in reproductive/developmental toxicity studies, they propose that there is a need to standardize the methods used, and they favor manual counts with a hemocytometer over automated methods. Furthermore, they found different methods of reporting sperm counts (daily sperm production [DSP]/whole testis,[459] DSP/g testis,[459] testicular spermatid head count,[424] and sperm counts from whole epididymis,[420,421] caput/corpus epididymis,[426,428,459] cauda epididymal sperm,[422,424,428,437,440,444,455,459] and ejaculated sperm,[424,428] thus making comparisons difficult. Only two studies[428,459] measured DSP, caput/corpus sperm, and caudal epididymal sperm counts, permitting assessment of potential target sites of TCDD. Interestingly, although both studies agree on the effect of TCDD on caudal epididymal sperm counts, they diverge on the measure of DSP. Furthermore, different time points have been employed to quantify sperm, ranging from PND49, representing puberty,[444,455] to 15 months of age,[424] with most studies quantifying sperm counts between PND63 and PND120, corresponding to postpubertal and adult stages, respectively. Because male rodents are not sexually mature before approximately PND50 and because a spermatogenic cycle takes 52–54 days to complete in the rat,[445,451] measurement of sperm counts in rats before PND70 is likely to produce ambiguous results. Nonetheless, six of eight studies reported a TCDD-induced decrease in cauda epididymal sperm counts,[422,426,428,437,440,459] whereas the evidence for changes in DSP are more variable, with only three of six studies finding a significant decrease.[422,428,437] The variable results for DSP are more difficult to interpret because sperm production can be affected by many factors, including nutrition, infection, and general health of the animal, as well as time from last ejaculation and toxicant effects on the hypothalamic–pituitary–testicular axis.

Prior studies have demonstrated treatment-related decreases in BW[422,428] and absolute testicular weight,[422,428,437] suggesting a potential effect of TCDD; however, relative testicular weights, when reported, were unchanged,[422,428,440] indicating that the testes were unaffected. Circulating levels of follicle-stimulating hormone (FSH), luteinizing hormone, and testosterone were unchanged,[422,437,455] suggesting that the hypothalamic–pituitary–testicular axis was also unaffected by TCDD. Morphologic assessment of the testes also failed to demonstrate evidence of treatment-related effects. In one study, testicular atrophy and separation of the caput and caudal regions with a loss of corpus epididymis was observed in two rats, which were excluded from the analysis.[455]

Other than abstinence, Sertoli cell number is a central determinant of sperm count.[460] In humans, Sertoli cell proliferation takes place during fetal, postnatal (0–8 months of age), and prepubertal development. Animal studies in mice and rats reveal that androgens primarily regulate Sertoli cell proliferation during the perinatal and prepubertal periods,[461–464] whereas FSH plays a more central role in the peripubertal period.[465] Direct effects of developmental exposure to TCDD on the spermatocyte to Sertoli cell ratios were measured in adult Holtzman rats exposed to TCDD on GD15.[437] TCDD did not affect the spermatocyte to Sertoli cell ratio at any age (PNDs 49, 63, or 120), leading to speculation of a defect in germ cell division or an increase in apoptosis of germ cells. Morphologic changes to the testis have been demonstrated in adult rats exposed to a single injection of either 3.0 or 5.0 µg TCDD/kg BW, whereas doses of 0.5 and 1.0 µg TCDD/kg BW had no effect on the testis.[466] In that study, the number of spermatids per testis was decreased by TCDD treatment, and the spaces between adjacent Sertoli cells were enlarged, indicating dissolution of the germinal epithelium. Similarly, contacts between Sertoli cells and spermatogonia were disrupted in a subchronic study in rats treated with an initial dose of 25 or 75 µg TCDD/kg BW followed by a once-weekly maintenance dose of either 5 or 15 µg/kg, respectively, for 10 weeks.[413] However, Sertoli cell changes were only seen at high doses, which are well beyond the concentrations reported to induce changes in DSP and epididymal sperm counts.[437] Thus, it is unlikely that TCDD-induced changes in sperm counts can be attributed to changes in Sertoli cell structure or function. Therefore, we propose that the primary effect of TCDD is not on the testes or on spermatogenesis. We postulate that adverse effects of TCDD are more likely related to developmental abnormalities of the reproductive tract and epididymal structure and/or function.

TCDD-induced changes in cauda epididymal sperm counts and decreased weights of androgen target tissues such as the seminal vesicle, epididymides, and prostate provide clear evidence of developmental toxicity. The mechanism(s) of action underlying these responses remains unclear. Modes and/or mechanisms of action of dioxin-induced changes in cauda epididymal sperm counts and reproductive tract structure and function of potential relevance to human health include dysregulation of androgen signaling and enhanced phagocytosis of germ cells (reviewed by Phillips and Tanphaichitr[712]) and enhanced epididymal sperm transit.

DEREGULATION OF ANDROGEN SIGNALING

Circulating levels of testosterone and dihydrotestosterone (DHT) were decreased in adult rats exposed to high concentrations of TCDD in both time-course (15 µg TCDD/kg BW) and dose–response (100 µg TCDD/kg BW) studies.[439] Similarly, serum testosterone concentrations were significantly reduced in adult male rats treated with 25.0 µg TCDD/kg BW and sacrificed 4 weeks later.[467] However, the concentration of TCDD needed to induce a change in circulating testosterone levels is very high relative to the doses that alter sperm counts and those documented in human exposure. Decreased seminal vesicle and epididymal weights corroborated the reduced circulating testosterone levels; however, DSP or testis weights were unaffected, suggesting that TCDD may have affected Leydig cell function, and morphologic assessment of the testes revealed a decrease in Leydig cell volume. In three different rat strains bred from TCDD-resistant and TCDD-sensitive strains, circulating levels of testosterone were decreased 17 days after treatment with a single oral dose of 1,000 µg TCDD/kg BW.[447] Similarly, *in utero* exposure to the highest dose of TCDD (an initial dose of 300 ng TCDD/kg BW followed by a maintenance dose of 60 ng TCDD/kg BW for the 2 weeks before mating) induced a 50% decrease in plasma testosterone levels.[441] Mably et al.[438] found a 60% decrease in plasma testosterone and a 41% reduction in DHT after *in utero* exposure to a single dose of TCDD, which although substantial, was not significant, whereas other investigators were unable to find treatment-induced changes in circulating androgen levels.[424,427,436] In contrast, 1 µg TCDD/kg BW administered on GD15 increased circulating levels of testosterone on PND70 in three different rat strains with different sensitivities to TCDD.[448] No differences in circulating levels of FSH or testosterone were documented in adult Holtzman rats exposed to TCDD on GD15.[437] Therefore, the reduction in sperm counts reported in animal studies is unlikely the consequence of TCDD-induced changes in serum androgen levels[447,448] or effects on Leydig cell structure or function.

Deregulation of testosterone signaling has been documented in several animal studies but not detected in others. TCDD treatment induced a decrease in androgen receptor (AR) gene expression in ventral prostate and decreased weight, both evidence of decreased androgen signaling.[455] Morrow et al.[468] reported that activation of the AhR in LnCAP prostate cells by TCDD could inhibit androgen-dependent proliferation, which was mediated by cross-talk between the AhR and the AR. Transcriptional regulation of AR signaling[469] by competition between the AR and the AhR for nuclear transcription factors is another possibility.[469] Competition between the AhR and AR for transcription factors has been documented in breast cancer cell lines[469]; however, although intriguing, its relevance to the testis and human cells *in vivo* and during development of the male reproductive tract remains unknown.

DEREGULATION OF EPIDIDYMAL FUNCTION

Reports that a single TCDD injection on GD15 results in decreased epididymal or cauda epididymal sperm counts without effect on testicular DSP are difficult to reconcile. We postulate that the adverse effects of TCDD are mediated via changes in epididymal function as opposed to effects on the testes. Changes in sperm transit through the excurrent duct system or increased removal of damaged sperm from the epididymis could provide reasonable alternative explanations to TCDD effects on spermatogenesis. Several laboratories have examined TCDD treatment on sperm transport through the epididymides with divergent results. High-dose *in utero* and lactational exposure to TCDD (an initial dose of 25–300 ng TCDD/kg followed by 5–60 ng TCDD/kg throughout premating, mating, pregnancy, and lactation) decreased the time for sperm to transit through the epididymis in Wistar rats.[441] In contrast, exposure to 1.0 μg TCDD/kg on GD15 had no effect on sperm transit in Holtzman rats, suggesting that phagocytosis of sperm in the epididymides is increased.[428] Exposure of C57BL/6 mice to TCDD (0.1–50 μg TCDD/kg) for 24 hours resulted in a decrease in spermatozoan mitochondrial membrane potential compared with vehicle-treated control mice.[470] The effect was not evident in AhR-knockout mice, demonstrating that the effect requires activation of the AhR. However, there was no increase in the number of apoptotic germ cells in the testis and no change in morphology of the testis and epididymis.

In general, phagocytosis of spermatozoa by the epithelial cells of the cauda epididymis is very low. It has previously been suggested that damaged spermatozoal cells can be phagocytosed,[471] but the interpretation of these data has been challenged.[472] Furthermore, if TCDD treatment did stimulate phagocytosis to the extent that sperm counts decreased by almost 40%, one would expect this to be obvious when examining the morphology of the epididymis. This does not appear to be the case, given the lack of reference of such an effect. A second possibility is that the blood–epididymal barrier is compromised, resulting in activation of the immune system, thus allowing macrophages to readily enter the lumen of the epididymis and attack maturing spermatozoa.[473] Although this may explain the loss of epididymal spermatozoa, we found no reports of large numbers of macrophages within the epididymal lumen. A more likely possibility is that spermatozoa transit time is altered, resulting in fewer spermatozoa stored in the cauda epididymis. The epididymis is a long, open-ended, and highly convoluted tubule.[474] Spermatozoa are stored in the cauda epididymis, but the retention of spermatozoa in this region is not well understood. Perhaps the best explanation is related to the length and high degree of convolution in this region of the epididymis. Changes in the convoluted nature of the cauda or the length of the cauda could directly affect the quantity of spermatozoa retained in the epididymis. Antiandrogenic compounds such as phthalates reportedly alter epididymal development and coiling of the epididymal tubule,[475] and flutamide significantly reduces the size of the cauda epididymis[476]; however, whether the length of the epididymal tubule is also reduced is unknown. Wilker et al.[459] reported that neonatal administration of TCDD resulted in a loss of epididymal segmentation, although they did not report whether this is associated with alterations in the cauda. Epididymal sperm transit time may also be affected by changes in the composition of epididymal fluid. Water is reabsorbed from the seminal fluid in the efferent ducts between the testis and epididymis,[477] a process regulated by estradiol and mediated by estrogen receptor-α (ERα).[478] TCDD is known to block estrogen action by activating the AhR, which has been shown to partly bind to the estrogen response element of estrogen-dependent genes.[479] In the epididymis, after treatment with antiestrogens, or in ERα-knockout mice, there is retention of water in the seminal fluid,[478] which is associated with a decrease in cauda epididymal sperm counts.[480] Less concentrated sperm would exhibit faster transit time, particularly in the cauda epididymis, because fluid pressure in the epididymal lumen would likely be increased. Thus, the effect of dioxin and dioxin-like chemicals on epididymal structure and function requires further study.

Semen quality and sperm counts have reportedly declined approximately 2% per year for about 50 years.[481] That provocative review[481] led to an explosion of studies, some of which reported a decline in semen quality[482–484] and some of which did not.[485] Although the reported decline in sperm counts remains controversial, there appears to be consensus for regional differences in semen quality.[486–488] Geographic differences in semen quality may also be accounted for by differences in race, genetic background, lifestyle, diet, and exposure to environmental toxicants.

Environmental contaminants have received growing attention, in part because animal studies have shown that some chemicals reduce sperm counts and because human exposure to environmental pollutants is potentially modifiable. Reduced sperm counts have been documented in studies of men occupationally exposed to different environmental contaminants,[489,490] but the relationship between dioxin exposure and semen quality remains ambiguous. No difference in semen quality was found in Taiwanese men exposed prenatally to rice oil contaminated with PCBs and polychlorinated dibenzofurans (Yu-Cheng accidental exposure), despite the occurrence of chloracne—clear evidence of AhR activation.[491] However, sperm concentration and sperm motility were decreased in dioxin-exposed young healthy men from Belgium, a region with high dioxin contamination,[492] and total sperm count was decreased in Belgium men from Flanders.[493] In 101 Flemish men, 5 months after exposure to PCB- and dioxin-contaminated food, Dhooge et al.[494] observed that semen volume was decreased but sperm concentration was increased with an increase in dioxin-like activity (CALUX assay). The increased sperm concentration can be explained by decreased semen volume in these men, whereas total and free testosterone levels were also decreased with increasing dioxin-like activity. In contrast, no relationship between dioxin-like activity and semen parameters was found in Inuit men and men from three European populations with tissue residue levels representative of background exposure.[495]

It is difficult to compare studies because of differences in reporting results, such as sperm count versus sperm concentration, methods of quantifying dioxin exposure, and differences in controlling for confounding factors such as age, smoking history, influence of mothers smoking during pregnancy, time from last ejaculation, use of medications known to affect semen quality, and health status of the study subjects. Another factor that may be important is the subject's age at the time of exposure, as shown in a recent study of semen quality in men acutely exposed to high levels of TCDD in Seveso, Italy.[412] In that study, men were stratified on the basis of their age at the time of exposure; men who were adults at the time of exposure showed no effects, while sperm counts were increased in men exposed during the peripubertal period. However, decreased sperm concentrations were observed in men who were between 1 and 9 years of age at the time of exposure (mean age, 6.2 years). Mocarelli et al.[412] also reported a decreased percentage of motile sperm and of progressively motile sperm, without any effect on circulating testosterone levels, suggesting a critical time window for dioxin exposure during which the developing reproductive tract is more sensitive; this is consistent with the animal literature. In contrast to the animal literature, these human exposures were associated with a decrease in semen characteristics, especially motility. Taken together, epidemiologic data suggest that dioxin exposure affects the function of sex glands with a decreased semen volume but with no change in sperm count; these data are, in part, consistent with the animal literature but contradictory to a definitive effect of dioxin on spermatogenesis. Moreover, although preliminary, the epidemiologic data also suggest that concentration and developmental stage at the time of exposure may be an important determinant of dioxin effects on semen quality in the human population.

PERSISTENT ORGANIC POLLUTANT EXPOSURE LEADS TO INSULIN RESISTANCE SYNDROME

Despite international agreements intended to limit the release of persistent organic pollutants (POPs) such as organochlorine pesticides, polychlorinated biphenyls (PCBs), polychlorinated dibenzo-*p*-dioxins (PCDDs), and polychlorinated dibenzofurans (PCDFs), POPs still persist in the environment and food chains.[486,496–500] Most human populations are exposed to POPs through consumption of fat-containing food such as fish, dairy products, and meat.[498] Humans bioaccumulate these lipophilic and hydrophobic pollutants in fatty tissues for many years because POPs are highly resistant to metabolic degradation.[498,501] The physiological impact associated with chronic exposure to low doses of different mixtures of POPs is poorly understood, but epidemiological studies have reported that Americans, Europeans, and Asian patients with type 2 diabetes accumulated greater body burdens of POPs, including 2,3,7,8-tetrachlorodibenzo-*p*-dioxin (TCDD), 2,2′,4,4′,5,5′-hexachlorobiphenyl (PCB153), coplanar PCBs (PCB congeners 77, 81, 126, and 169), *p,p′*-diphenyldichloroethene (DDE), oxychlordane, and *trans*-nonachlor.[502–507]

The incidences of type 2 diabetes and the insulin resistance syndrome have increased at a globally alarming rate, and >25% of adults in the United States have been estimated to be affected by metabolic abnormalities associated with insulin resistance.[508] Impaired insulin action is a central dysfunction of the insulin resistance syndrome characterized by abdominal obesity and defects in both lipid and glucose homeostasis, increasing the risk for developing type 2 diabetes, cardiovascular diseases, nonalcoholic fatty liver disease, polycystic ovarian disease, and certain types of cancer.[509,510] Although a sedentary lifestyle and consumption of high-fat food are considered major contributors to insulin resistance and obesity, these conventional risk factors can only partly explain the worldwide explosive prevalence of insulin resistance–associated metabolic diseases. They therefore sought to elucidate whether the exposure to POPs present in a food matrix could contribute to insulin resistance and metabolic disorders.

POPs accumulate in the lipid fraction of fish, and fish consumption represents a source of POP exposure to humans.[497,499,511] Therefore, certain European countries have dietary recommendations to limit the consumption of fatty fish per week.[512] On the other hand, n-3 polyunsaturated fatty acids present in fish oil have a wide range of beneficial effects,[513] including protection against high-fat (HF) diet–induced insulin resistance.[514] Accordingly, Ruzzin et al.[515] fed rats an HF diet containing either crude (HFC) or refined (HFR) fish oil obtained from farmed Atlantic salmon and investigated the metabolic impacts of POPs and their ability to interfere with n-3 polyunsaturated fatty acids.

In this study, Ruzzin et al.[515] demonstrate for the first time a causal relationship between POPs and insulin resistance in rats. *In vivo*, chronic exposure to low doses of POPs commonly found in food chains induced severe impairment of whole-body insulin action and contributed to the development of abdominal obesity and hepatosteatosis. Treatment *in vitro* of differentiated adipocytes with nanomolar concentrations of POP mixtures mimicking those found in crude salmon oil induced a significant inhibition of insulin-dependent glucose uptake. These data provide compelling evidence that exposure to POPs increases the risk of developing insulin resistance and metabolic disorders.

Despite intense investigations and establishment of both preventive and therapeutic strategies, insulin resistance–associated metabolic diseases such as type 2 diabetes, obesity, and nonalcoholic fatty liver disease have reached alarming proportions worldwide.[508,516,517] By 2015, the World Health Organization (WHO) estimates that >1.5 billion people will be overweight and that 338 million people will die from chronic diseases such as diabetes and heart disease.[518] Although physical inactivity and regular intake of high-energy diets are recognized contributors,[519,520] these lifestyle factors can only partially explain the explosive and uncontrolled global increase in metabolic diseases. Recently, the development of insulin resistance and inflammation was found to be exacerbated in humans and animals exposed to air pollution.[521,522] Furthermore, the widespread environmental contaminant bisphenol A was reported to impair pancreatic beta cells and trigger insulin resistance.[523] This data, together with the finding that type 2 diabetics accumulate significant body burdens of POPs,[504] provide additional evidence that global environmental pollution contributes to the epidemic of insulin resistance–associated metabolic diseases.

Although rats chronically fed the HFC diet for 28 days were exposed to a relatively high intake of organic pollutants, the concentrations of PCDDs/PCDFs and indicator PCBs in adipose tissue of these animals did not exceed those observed in Northern Europeans 40–50 years of age,[513] thereby indicating that doses of POP exposure sufficient to induce detrimental health effects were not excessive. Whether the exposure to lower levels of POPs would induce similar detrimental effects as those observed in the present study remains to be investigated.

Dietary interventions are current strategies to prevent or treat metabolic diseases, and nutritional guidelines are usually based on energy density and glycemic index of the diet; however, the levels of POPs present in food has received less attention. Given that POPs are ubiquitous in food chains,[498] such underestimation may interfere with the expected beneficial effects of some dietary recommendations and lead to poor outcomes. For instance, the presence of POPs in food products may, to some extent, explain the conflicting results regarding the protective effects of n-3 polyunsaturated fatty acids against the incidence of myocardial infarction.[524,525] Overall, better understanding of the interactions between POPs and nutrients will help improve nutritional education of patients with insulin resistance syndrome.

To protect consumer health, the presence of contaminants in food is internationally regulated. In the European Union legislation, certain POPs, including dioxins and dioxin-like PCBs, are regulated in foodstuffs.[526] Risk assessment of these organic pollutants is based on the ability of individual compounds to produce heterogeneous toxic and biological effects through the binding of the aryl hydrocarbon receptor. Interestingly, Ruzzin et al.[515] found that cultured adipocytes exposed to a PCDF or PCDD mixture have normal insulin action, even though the TEQ of these mixtures could be up to 3500 times higher than the TEQ of the non-*ortho*-substituted and mono-*ortho*-substituted PCB mixtures that impaired insulin action. These findings demonstrate that risk assessment based on WHO TEQs assigned to dioxins and dioxin-like PCBs is unlikely to reflect the risk of insulin resistance and the possible development of metabolic disorders.

Although the production of organochlorine pesticides has been restricted since the 1970s, the global production and use of pesticides are poorly controlled,[486,527] and the presence of these environmental chemicals in seafood still remains unregulated in European countries.[528] Of the POP mixtures tested *in vitro*, organochlorine pesticides were the most potent disruptors of insulin action. This powerful inhibitory effect of pesticides on insulin action likely explains the common finding emerging from several independent cross-sectional studies reporting an association between type 2 diabetes and the body burdens of *p,p'*-DDE, oxychlordane, or *trans*-nonachlor.[504–506] Therefore, widespread pesticide exposure to humans appears to be of particular global concern in relation to public health.

They draw two main conclusions from these observations. First, exposure to POPs present in the environment and food chains are capable of causing insulin resistance and impair both lipid and glucose metabolism, thus, supporting the notion that these chemicals are potential contributors to the rise in prevalence of insulin resistance and associated disorders. Second, although beneficial, the presence of n-3 polyunsaturated fatty acids in crude salmon oil (in the HFC diet) could not counteract the deleterious metabolic effects induced by POP exposure. Altogether, their data provide novel insights regarding the ability of POPs to mediate insulin resistance–associated metabolic abnormalities and provide solid evidence reinforcing the importance of international agreements to limit the release of POPs to minimize public health risks.

House Dust Concentrations of Organophosphate Flame Retardants in Relation to Hormone Levels and Semen Quality Parameters

According to Meeker et al.[529] organophosphate (OP) compounds, such as tris(1,3-dichloro-2-propyl) phosphate (TDCPP) and triphenyl phosphate (TPP), are commonly used as additive flame retardants and plasticizers in a wide range of materials. Although widespread human exposure to OP flame retardants is likely, there is a lack of human and animal data on potential health effects.

They explored relationships of TDCPP and TPP concentrations in house dust with hormone levels and semen quality parameters.

They analyzed house dust from 50 men recruited through a U.S. infertility clinic for TDCPP and TPP. Relationships with reproductive and thyroid hormone levels, as well as semen quality parameters, were assessed using crude and multivariable linear regression.

TDCPP and TPP were detected in 96% and 98% of samples, respectively, with widely varying concentrations up to 1.8 mg/g. In models adjusted for age and body mass index, an interquartile range (IQR) increase in TDCPP was associated with a 3% (95% CI, from −5% to −1%) decline in free thyroxine and a 17% (95% CI, 4%–32%) increase in prolactin. There was a suggestive inverse association between TDCPP and free androgen index that became less evident in adjusted models. In the adjusted models, an IQR increase in TPP was associated with a 10% (95% CI, 2%–19%) increase in prolactin and a 19% (95% CI, from −30% to −5%) decrease in sperm concentration.

OP flame retardants may be associated with altered hormone levels and decreased semen quality in men. More research on sources and levels of human exposure to OP flame retardants and associated health outcomes are needed.

Use of environmentally persistent polybrominated diphenyl ether (PBDE) flame retardants has been reduced because of concerns about health effects, but potential health effects of organophosphate (OP) flame retardants used as alternatives to PBDEs have not been extensively investigated, despite evidence of widespread human exposure. Meeker and Stapleton measured the OP flame retardants tris (1,3-dichloro-s-propyl) phosphate (TDCPP) and triphenyl phosphate (TPP) in house dust samples collected from 50 male infertility clinic patients and estimated associations with serum hormone concentrations (luteinizing hormone, follicle-stimulating hormone, estradiol, prolactin, free thyroxine, total triodothyronine, and thyrotropin) and semen quality parameters (concentration, motility, and morphology). The authors report that TDCPP and TPP were detected in 48 of 50 dust samples at widely varying concentrations. Models adjusted for potential confounders indicated that TDCPP and TPP were both positively associated with serum prolactin concentration, TDCPP was inversely associated with free thyroxine, and TPP was inversely associated with sperm concentration. The authors conclude that additional research to confirm these findings is warranted given evidence of potential effects and widespread exposure to these compounds.

Several chemicals commonly encountered in the environment have been associated with altered endocrine function in animals and humans, and exposure to some endocrine-disrupting chemicals may result in adverse effects on reproduction, fetal/child development, metabolism, neurologic function, and other vital processes.[530] Recent attention to the potential risks that environmental chemicals may pose to reproductive and developmental health has also been driven by reports of temporal downward trends in semen quality[481,531] and male testosterone levels[532,533]; increased rates of development anomalies of the reproductive tract, specifically hypospadias and cryptorchidism[534]; and increased rates of testicular cancer.[535–537] Public and scientific concern also stems from recent reports of inexplicable increases in the rates of thyroid cancer,[538,539] congenital hypothyroidism,[540] and neurologic development disorders such as autism.[541] Not only do these studies report temporal trends, but many also describe wide geographic variability in these measures and trends, which provides further evidence that environmental factors may play a role.

Flame retardants are used in construction materials, furniture, plastics, electronics equipment, textiles, and other materials. Until recently, polybrominated diphenyl ethers (PBDEs) accounted for a large proportion of flame retardants used in polyurethane foam and electronic applications.[542] However, in the past several years, common PBDE mixtures (i.e., pentaBDE and octaBDE) have been banned or voluntarily phased out in the United States and many parts of the world because of their persistence, bioaccumulation, and evidence for adverse health effects, including endocrine disruption and altered fetal development.[543,544] Thus, the use of alternate flame retardants has been on the rise,[545] as has scrutiny related to the potential environmental and human health consequences of alternate flame retardants. Compared with PBDEs and other brominated flame retardants (e.g., hexabromocyclododecane and tetrabromobisphenol A), organophosphorus (OP) flame retardants have received little attention with regard to human exposure and potential health effects. Trichloroalkyl phosphates, such as TDCPP, and triaryl phosphates, such as TPP, continue to be used as flame retardants and plasticizers in a wide variety of applications, resulting in widespread environmental dispersion.[546] Production and use of OP flame retardants has surpassed that of PBDEs in Europe,[546] and annual production of both TDCPP and TPP in the United States has been estimated to be between 10 and 50 million pounds per year.[547] As with PBDEs, OPs such as TDCPP and TPP are used as additive flame retardants that can be released into the surrounding environment over time.[548] Recent studies have reported that concentrations of OP flame retardants measured in house dust are on the same order of magnitude as PBDEs, and for some OPs, such as TPP, concentrations greatly exceed those of PBDEs.[546,549] Given that house dust is a primary source of exposure to PBDEs[550,551] and that PBDEs can be detected in the blood of nearly all individuals in the general population,[552] human exposures to OP flame retardants are also likely to be widespread.

The presence of TDCPP was reported in a significant proportion of human seminal plasma samples nearly three decades ago,[553] and high doses of OP flame retardants have been associated with adverse reproductive, neurologic, and other systemic effects (e.g., altered thyroid and liver weights) in laboratory animals.[542,548,554] To our knowledge, no studies exploring associations between nonoccupational exposure to OP flame retardants and human health end points have been conducted to date, although evidence exists for endocrine and reproductive effects in relation to other OP compounds. In the present study, we measured two OP flame retardants (TDCPP and TPP) in house dust and assessed relationships with hormone levels and semen quality parameters among men recruited from an infertility clinic as part of an ongoing study of environmental influences on reproductive health.

Semen Quality

Semen samples were analyzed for sperm concentration and motion parameters by a computer-aided semen analyzer (HTM-IVOS, version 10HTM-IVOS; Hamilton-Thorne Research, Beverly, Massachusetts). Setting parameters and the definition of measured sperm motion parameters for the computer-aided semen analyzer were established by manufacturer. To measure both sperm concentration and motility, 5 μL of semen from each sample was placed into a prewarmed (37°C) Makler counting chamber (Sefi Medical Instruments, Haifa, Israel). We analyzed a minimum of 200 sperm cells from at least four different fields from each specimen. Motile sperm was defined as World Health Organization (WHO) grade a sperm (rapidly progressive with a velocity ≥25 μm/s at 37°C) and grade b sperm (slow/sluggish progressive with a velocity ≥5 μm/s but < 25 μm/s) (WHO 1999). For sperm morphology, at least two slides were made for each fresh semen sample. The resulting thin smear was allowed to air dry for 1 hour before staining with a Diff-Quik staining kit (Dade Behring AG, Dudingen, Switzerland). They performed morphologic assessment with a Nikon microscope using an oil immersion 100 × objective (Nikon Company, Tokyo, Japan). They counted a minimum of 200 sperm cells from two slides for each specimen.

Results

Of the 50 dust samples collected, they detected TDCPP and TPP in 48 (96%) and 49 (98%) samples, respectively. The distribution of measured TDCPP and TPP concentrations. Concentrations of TDCPP and TPP were positively (right) skewed and varied widely, from < LOD (107 and 173 ng/g, respectively) to maximum values of 56 μg/g and 1800 μg/g, respectively. The distribution of age, BMI, serum hormone levels, and semen quality parameters among the men in the study are also presented.

Semen quality parameters were available for all 50 men with OP dust measures, and hormone levels were available for 38 of the men. In preliminary correlation analysis, TDCPP and TPP were moderately correlated (Pearson $r = 0.56$, $p = 0.0001$; Spearman $r = 0.33$, $p = 0.02$). TDCPP was inversely associated with free T_4 and positively associated with prolactin. They also found a suggestive inverse association between TDCPP and FAI, although the Spearman rank correlation for this relationship was stronger than the Pearson correlation (Spearman $r = -0.33$, $p = 0.04$). TPP was positively correlated with prolactin (not shown; Pearson $r = 0.37$; $p = 0.02$) and inversely associated with sperm concentration. The inverse association remained when the three men with a sperm concentration below the commonly used reference criteria of 20 million sperm/mL[555] were removed from the analysis (Pearson $r = -0.31$, $p = 0.03$).

In multivariable linear regression models adjusted for age and BMI, the inverse association between TDCPP and free T_4 and the positive association between TDCPP and prolactin remained. An IQR increase in dust TDCPP concentration was associated with a 2.8% (95% CI, −4.6% to −1.0%) decline in free T_4 relative to the population median. This relationship was robust to the exclusion of an outlying free T_4 value (0.88 ng/dL) from the model (not shown; $p = 0.01$). An IQR increase in TDCPP was also associated with a significant 17.3% (95% CI, 4.1%–32.2%) increase in serum prolactin. The suggestive inverse association between TDCPP and FAI was no longer evident in the multivariate models. The inconsistency between Pearson and Spearman correlations in the preliminary analysis led them to assess the potential for influential values in the results of parametric models. When excluding three subjects that had studentized residuals of >2 or < −2 in the original model, an IQR increase in TDCPP was associated with a suggestive 6.3% decline in FAI (95% CI, −13.8%–1.9%; $p = 0.13$).

In the present study, they found that OP flame retardants were detected in nearly 100% of house dust samples collected from 50 homes, and OP concentrations varied widely between homes. Meeker and Stapleton recently demonstrated that, in these samples, geometric mean TDCPP and TPP concentrations were on the same order of magnitude as the sum of 34 PBDE congeners.[549] TPP concentrations were considerably higher than PBDE concentrations and ranged up to maximum concentration of 1.8 mg/g compared with 0.04 mg/g for sum of PBDEs. Because of the ubiquity of these compounds in homes and other microenvironments,[556–558] their toxicity potential should be considered more fully, especially as replacements for recently banned or withdrawn PBDE formulations are sought.

They found an inverse association between TDCPP concentrations in house dust and serum free T_4 levels. Thyroid hormones are vital to a number of physiologic processes, including metabolism, reproduction, cardiovascular health, and neurodevelopment. Because thyroid hormone insufficiency can have serious adverse effects on a number of vital physiologic functions, even chemicals that cause only a subtle shift in thyroid hormone levels should be considered carefully in terms of societal impact at the population level.[559] They also found positive relationships between both TDCPP and TPP with prolactin. Prolactin is a protein hormone that serves a number of important functions involving reproduction, metabolism, maintenance of homeostasis in immune responses, osmotic balance, and angiogenesis[560,561] and is increasingly becoming used as a measure of neuroendocrine/dopaminergic function in environmental and occupational epidemiology studies.[562,563] Because dopamine is responsible for inhibiting prolactin secretion, increased circulating levels of prolactin may reflect deficiencies in dopamine release, transport, or uptake.[564] Finally, in these data, we also observed that an IQR increase in house dust TPP was associated with a substantial (19%) decline in sperm concentration. These findings may have substantial public health implications, given the likelihood of exposure to TPP among the general population, but more human and animal studies are needed to confirm our results.

Toxicology data relevant to the end points explored in the present study are limited.[542,548,554] TPP binds to the androgen receptor with moderate affinity[565] and activates enzymes involved in steroid hormone metabolism *in vitro.*[566] In addition, in rat studies, butylated TPP has been associated with endocrine effects, including reduced male fertility and altered female reproductive cycles.[567] Rats dosed with high levels of TDCPP had altered thyroid weights and an increased thyroid/body weight ratio compared with control animals, and high-dose males demonstrated a significant increase in testicular interstitial-cell tumors and had increased histopathologic abnormalities in the testis, epididymis, and seminal vesicle.[554]

Meeker and Stapleton[343] can also compare their findings with effects reported in association with other OP compounds. Consistent with the observation of an inverse association between TPP and sperm concentration, other OP flame retardants and plasticizers such as tricresyl phosphate (found in jet fuel exhausts that are piped into the cabin) are reproductive toxicants that have caused marked reductions in male fertility and semen quality measures in laboratory animals.[554] Their findings are also consistent with several reports on the more well-studied OP insecticides. For example, in their previous work among a larger and overlapping group of men from the ongoing study, urinary levels of 3,5,6-trichloro-2-pyridinol, a urinary metabolite of the OP insecticides chlorpyrifos and chlorpyrifos-methyl, were associated with increased prolactin[568] and reduced free T_4,[543] FAI,[544] and sperm motility.[569] A variety of OP pesticides have been linked to decreased semen quality in studies of occupationally exposed men.[570–573] Case studies of patients with acute OP pesticide poisoning have also reported decreased levels of circulating thyroid hormones and increased prolactin.[574,575] This is consistent with animal studies that reported inverse associations between chlorpyrifos and T_4 levels in mice and sheep,[576,577] and studies that reported increased prolactin levels, decreased dopamine and testosterone levels, and damaged male reproductive organs in rats exposed to the OP insecticide quinalphos.[578] Thus, the relationships observed in the present study may be consistent with those reported for OP insecticides. However, compared with OP triesters used as insecticides, OP flame retardants are more stable against hydrolysis, which makes them more persistent in the environment.[579] This potential for environmental persistence, combined with the widespread use and distribution of these compounds and the potential for adverse reproductive and neuroendocrine effects, serves as a further indication that more research is needed on the potential health effects resulting from exposure to OP flame retardants.

Meeker and Stapleton's study[343] has a number of limitations. First, the sample size was relatively small, which may have limited our ability to detect subtle associations between OP levels and hormone or semen quality markers. Second, because this represents the first study to assess the relationship between OP flame retardants and endocrine/reproductive outcomes in humans, a number of comparisons were made. Thus, the observation of a statistical relationship due to chance cannot be ruled out. Third, the study was cross-sectional in nature, so one cannot make conclusions regarding the temporality of the relationships observed. Fourth, one cannot rule out the presence of unmeasured confounders or coexposures that may explain our reported findings. However, they considered a number of potential confounding factors in the multivariable models. In addition, they previously reported that TDCPP and TPP were only moderately correlated with PBDE congeners and other brominated flame retardants (all correlation coefficients were ≤ 0.4).[549] Finally, they used house dust concentrations to estimate exposure to TDCPP and TPP. Because data on the prevalence, sources, and pathways of human exposure to TDCPP and TPP are lacking, this approach may be associated with exposure measurement error. However, if the measurement error were nondifferential, it would be expected to dilute exposure–outcome relationships toward the null.[580] Also, TDCPP and TPP are used (in a manner similar to that of PBDEs) as additive flame retardants in furniture foams, textiles, plastics, and electronics, which may result in exposure sources and pathways similar to those of PBDEs in the home and in other microenvironments where house dust plays a primary role in aggregate exposure.[550,551] Sensitive and specific biomarkers of exposure to these OP flame retardants are needed, as are studies comparing the contribution of OP concentrations in house dust and other environmental media (e.g., air and diet) to biomarker levels to determine important pathways of exposure and the most relevant media and time windows for the estimation of exposure in epidemiologic studies.

They found evidence that concentrations of OP flame retardants in house dust may be associated with altered hormone levels and decreased sperm concentration. More research is needed to determine the extent and sources of human exposure to OP flame retardants and associated effects on human health.

Zebrafish Seizure Model Identifies p,p'-DDE as the Dominant Contaminant of Fetal California Sea Lions That Accounts for Synergistic Activity with Domoic Acid

Another example of food contamination was shown by Tiedeken and Ramsdell.[581] They found California sea lions (CSLs; *Zalophus californianus*) are subject to multiple classes of environmental stressors, including exposure to persistent environmental contaminant burdens, infection by several pathogens, and episodic poisoning by toxins from harmful algal blooms.[582–584] It has been proposed that exposure to these different classes of stressors contributes to reproductive failure events in this species.[585,586] This and similar unusual mortality/morbidity trends or events provide leads toward identifying environmentally relevant stressor interactions in natural populations.[587] The last four decades of investigations into reproductive failure of the sea lion population in the California Channel Islands National Marine Sanctuary (CINMS) has revealed exposure to a mixture of stressors, including environmental contaminants (dichlorodiphenyltrichloroethanes [DDTs] and polychlorinated biphenyls [PCBs]) and disease (leptospirosis and San Miguel sea lion virus), along with the rising presence of the algal toxin domoic acid.[587] Research encompassing the complexity of potential stressors that converge by happenstance at a time or place of interest is referred to as "coincidental mixtures" and is considered among the most difficult areas for environmental health research.[588]

One component of these stressors, environmental chemical contaminants, has been documented in CINMS sea lion cows and found to be transferred to their fetuses through the placenta.[589] The most abundant of these compounds, 1,1-bis-(4-chlorophenyl)-2,2-dichloroethene(p,p'-DDE), has been described by food web bioaccumulation and physiologically based pharmacokinetic models to increase in the fetus during the course of development.[590,591] Another environmental stressor, the algal toxin domoic acid, causes abortion, premature parturition, or death of pregnant female sea lions and readily permeates the placenta to accumulate in amniotic fluid and poison the fetus.[585,592] The seasonality of massive algal blooms in the vicinity of the CINMS during the late spring upwelling periods places domoic acid exposure at the end of gestation for the CSL and at completion of neurodevelopment of the fetus.[593] This coincidence of two stressors, p,p'-DDE and domoic acid, in fetal sea lions—each known to promote neurodevelopmental toxicity—led to a testable exposure scenario for coincidental mixtures.

Tiedeken and Ramsdell[581] previously reported that p,p'-DDE exposure of zebrafish embryos increases the sensitivity and the manifestation of seizure behavior induced by domoic acid after brain maturation.[593] The body concentration of p,p'-DDE in zebrafish at the time of domoic acid exposure corresponded to the upper range found in fetal sea lions near term.[593] Given the complex body burden of persistent contaminants such as PCBs, polybrominated diphenyl ether (PBDEs), and persistent pesticides in addition to DDTs in fetal sea lions, a compelling question is whether other dominant contaminant components of these groups contribute to the p,p'-DDE effect to enhance domoic acid–induced toxicity.

Formulated mixture for fetal sea lion contaminants. Tiedeken and Ramsdell[581] previously reported that exposure to DDT or its metabolite DDE during zebrafish neurodevelopment enhances seizure behavior response to the algal toxin domoic acid after completion of brain maturation, a likely exposure scenario for the CSL population of the Channel Islands.[593] In the present study, they have expanded upon this finding to evaluate the influence of p,p'-DDE in the presence of co-occurring persistent contaminants. They formulated a mixture of organochlorine pesticides, PCBs, and PBDEs in defined proportion to the single component (p,p'-DDE) that they previously determined to enhance chemical-induced seizures after completion of brain development. Investigating the interaction of PCBs with p,p'-DDE is especially relevant to the CINMS sea lions whose increased body burdens of DDTs were correlated with prenatal mortality events,[582] but the co-occurrence of elevated burdens of PCBs and other stressors precluded firm conclusion of the adverse health effect of any contaminant.[586] To investigate this potential interaction, they formulated the contaminant mixtures to match levels determined in 14 premature CSL pups sampled during a domoic acid–associated mortality event in 2005 on San Miguel Island.[594]

The reconstituted mixture approach used here is based on the concentration in the fetal CSL that reflects transplacental transfer. Transplacental transfer of contaminants has been determined for both preterm and term CSLs and is best described by maternal load and fetal fat content.[589] Accordingly, they used levels measured in preterm CSL fetuses, a life stage in which domoic acid poisoning commonly occurs. Their experimental approach was twofold. In the first test, they used the most predominant contaminants—PCB-153 and PCB-138 (which represented up to 46% of total PCBs), β-HCH (100%), PBDE-47 (83%), and *trans*-nonachlor (80%)—formulated in proportion to levels reported for fetal CSL blubber. Finding no interactive effect with p,p'-DDE, they next increased the number of PCBs to a total of 20 congeners (to reach 95% of total PCBs) and PBDEs to a total of 4 congeners (to reach a total of 99% of the total measured content). Additionally, they administered this complex formulation by egg microinjection rather than bath exposure to assure consistent internal composition at the time of exposure to the chemical convulsant.

p,p'-DDE exposure of zebrafish embryos increases sensitivity of the fish to chemical convulsants. Their previous experiments indicated that this effect was apparent at bath exposure levels as low as 0.3 μM p,p'-DDE.[593] In the studies conducted here, they used both doses of 1.0 and 2.0 μM p,p'-DDE in the presence or absence of a contaminant formulation. The effects were determined in response to two chemical convulsants, PTZ and domoic acid. In addition to enhancing induced seizure behavior, p,p'-DDE also promotes a unique and readily observed head-shake behavior in response to the two chemical convulsants.[593] They observed no additional effects beyond those observed in p,p'-DDE–exposed embryos after coapplication of either the primary contaminant formulation or the complex contaminant formulation. This indicates that embryonic exposure to p,p'-DDE—and not exposure to co-occurring PCBs, β-HCH, PBDEs, and *trans*-nonachlor—is the primary contributor to greater sensitivity to domoic acid seizures at the completion of development.

Relevancy of dosage of formulated mixture to fetal sea lion exposure levels. The embryonic exposures they used for the zebrafish experiments are based on a previously determined observable effect level of p,p'-DDE to enhance domoic acid–induced seizures, with the effective dose calibrated to wet-weight body concentration at the time of completed neurodevelopment. This dose corresponds to modeled levels of whole-body p,p'-DDE in full-term CSL fetuses based on 1991 data of the mothers consuming fish contaminated with 1000 ng DDE/g wet weight.[590] When this dose is compared with actual wet-weight body concentrations of full-term CSLs, it corresponds to the highest levels of animals sampled in 2002, mid-range levels of animals sampled in 1996, and low exposure levels of animals sampled in 1972. The dosage of other organochlorines in their formulation is based on the ratio of individual congeners measured relative to mean p,p'-DDE values of 14 fetal sea lions. Hence, the total concentration of the complex contaminant mixture spans the range found in CINMS sea lions over a 30-year period and likely includes current concentrations found with the most susceptible population, that is, offspring of first-time pregnant animals, which are reported to have nearly a 10-fold higher concentration of DDTs and PCBs.[586]

Interaction of PCBs with p,p'-DDE. PCBs are the most abundant co-contaminant with DDE in the sea lions of the CINMS. Originally identified to occur in both pregnant females and fetuses, the higher concentrations of both PCBs and DDTs found in females with aborted fetuses during a 1970 mortality event suggested the potential for an interactive effect.[582] An experimental study of this sea lion population 2 years later showed the same trend, with eight times higher DDT concentrations and four times higher PCB concentrations in those females with aborted fetuses than in females with normal term deliveries.[586] However, the identification of two pathogens, one of which was associated with reproductive failure in livestock, added a confounding factor that precluded implicating a role for PCBs or DDTs in the reproductive poisoning of these sea lions.[586]

PCBs have been associated with developmental complications in children and experimental animals. Substantial epidemiologic and experimental research in animals using PCBs has demonstrated the adverse effects of PCBs during development, with a primary effect of diminishing thyroid hormone levels (reviewed by Ulbrich and Stahlmann[595]). Epidemiologic studies have shown interaction between DDE and the four primarily occurring PCB congeners (118, 138, 153, and 180) to be correlated with measures of attention in early infancy.[596] Developmental studies in rats comparing the commercial PCB mixture Arochlor 1254 with a formulation of PCBs, DDTs, and other persistent pesticides to match human blood composition lends insight to the interaction of these compounds.[597] Similarities between Arochlor 1254 and human blood formulation were best related to thyroid hormone–mediated actions, which are common for the PCB components of each mixture, whereas the presence of an organochloride/DDT component resulted in an overall increased toxicity and reproductive complications.[597] A differential action of DDT versus PCBs was noted in another study in which PCBs and HCH showed inverse correlation with thyroid hormone levels during pregnancy, whereas no correlation was found for DDT and thyroid hormone.[598] Hence, the different mode of action of PCBs may not affect seizure pathways modulated by developmental exposure to *p,p'*-DDE.

The lack of interaction Tiedeken and Ramsdell observed between PCBs and *p,p'*-DDE in increasing sensitivity to induced seizure behavior indicates that PCBs at the levels found in fetal sea lions do not contribute to this response. This response is similar to that found in a rodent study in which pregnant dams were given a PCB formulation to match human milk; the exposure did not alter *N*-methyl-D-aspartate receptors or long-term potentiation in the fetal hippocampus, but did reduce these end points in the occipital cortex.[599] The dominant PCB components of our complex contaminant formulation are similar to those in the human milk formulation. Accordingly, this PCB formulation lacks effect early in neurodevelopment (prior to synaptogenesis) on *N*-methyl-D-aspartate receptors, specifically their density, which mediate the excitotoxic effect of domoic acid in the region of the brain where domoic acid seizures originate.

Interaction of PBDEs with p,p'-DDE. In contrast to PCBs, PBDEs levels have been increasing in wildlife and humans over the last two decades and, like PCBs, are found in high levels in the blubber of CSLs.[600] Although PBDEs were not appreciably present at the time of the CSL mortality events of the 1970s, their presence over the last decade may play a role as other organochlorine contaminants are decreasing. Analysis of sea lion blubber from males stranded between 1993 and 2003 indicate that PBDEs probably reached their peak level (3900 ng/g lipid) during this period. The levels of PBDE measured in fetal sea lions of the CINMS are 10 times lower (320 ng/g lipid) than those reported in male sea lions.[594] The congener composition of both the male and fetal animals is very similar, with predominance of the penta-BDE congeners 47, 100, and 99. The 10-fold difference in concentrations between males and fetal sea lions is consistent with a similar magnitude of differences in PCBs and may be due to higher lifelong accumulation in males.[594,600,601] PBDEs transfer with a maternal–fetal coefficient near 1, with levels found in human maternal and fetal blood averaging 33 ng/g lipid,[602] about 10-times lower than those found in fetal sea lions.

PBDEs have neurotoxic effects comparable with those of PCBs in experimental animals, but supporting epidemiologic data are limited for the neurodevelopmental period (reviewed by Costa and Giordano[603]). PBDEs have shown adverse effects during neurodevelopment in mice, with a primary effect occurring during synaptogenesis, resulting in later-in-life changes in spontaneous behavior (hyperactivity) and impairments in learning and memory.[604] These effects have been described for PBDE-99 and PBDE-47, two major components found in our formulation. PBDE-99 has been reported to have an additive effect with PCB-52, a fact that is not surprising, given their similar effects on thyroid hormone levels and neurotoxicity.[604] An absence of chemical convulsant-enhanced seizure behavior in our zebrafish study indicates that PBDEs at the concentrations reported in fetal sea lions, in combination with PCBs, demonstrate no interaction on p,p'-DDE-induced developmental neurotoxicity.

Breast milk contaminated with chlorinated hydrocarbons is one of the most serious outcomes of the use of pesticides.[605] The discovery of DDT in mothers' milk in the United States was one of the main reasons for banning that chemical. In addition, dieldrin has been found in Australian beef, and lanolin used to coat the nipples of Australian mothers during breast-feeding was found to be contaminated with organophosphates, organochlorines, and carbophenothion insecticides.[605,606]

Food Preparation

Apart from food refining, several factors are responsible for the ultimate degree of nutrients lost in food preparation. These include the response of the food to temperature, light, oxygen, CO_2, pH, moisture, and microorganisms.

Toxins induced in foods through heat processing include carcinogens such as nitrosamines.[607] Therefore, preparation methods must be scrutinized when reactions to food occur.

Frandan and others have suggested that high-temperature cooking at 100°C causes toxins to be produced in food or after 110–120°C sugars caramelize, producing slightly mutagenic toxic substances. At 105–120°C, proteins start pyrolyzing into highly toxic or carcinogenic substances.[608-618]

Fats are damaged by heat, causing trans-fatty acids that may inhibit elongase and transferases. Heating fat also may produce polyaromatic hydrocarbons and other carcinogens. Most high-temperature cooking adversely affects the chemically sensitive person.[609,619-621] The combination of heating sugars and proteins produces a Maillard reaction, resulting in a yellow-golden color on bread. These toxic molecules have been shown to trigger congenital anomalies, hepatic toxicity, increased allergenicity, and increased aging.[609,621] Methods of food preparation can seriously affect the nutrient content of food. Low heat cooking using very little water, as done in steaming and pressure cooking, is the best method. Because the food does not come in contact with water when these methods are used, little or nonleaching of nutrients occurs. Also, broiling with an electric heat source has about the same degree of destruction as steaming and pressure cooking. Microwave cooking destroys nutrients to about the same degree as steaming, boiling, or broiling.

In contrast, open-flame cooking has deleterious effects on food nutrients. Benzo[a]pyrene are known carcinogens produced by open-flame cooking. Browning meat creates carcinogens such as polyaromatic hydrocarbons, which are enhanced with charcoal and liquid smoke. Gas flames also cause the formation of mutagens and carcinogens. Gas flames seem to be the most noxious for the chemically sensitive individual, as the gas actually penetrates the food it cooks. Also, boiling destroys heat-labile nutrients. Baking and reheating further destroy nutrients.

Genetically Engineered Foods

Genetically engineered crops are the result of technology developed in the 1970s that allow genes from one species to be forced into the DNA of an unrelated species. The inserted genes produce proteins that confer traits at a new plant, such as herbicide tolerance or pesticide production. The process of creating the GM crop can produce all sorts of side effects and the plants contain proteins that have never been in the food supply. In the United States, new types of food substances are normally classified as food additives, which must undergo extensive testing, including long-term animal feeding studies. If approved, the label of the food products containing the additive must list it as an ingredient.

There is an exception for substances that are deemed generally recognized as safe (GRAS). GRAS status allows a product to be commercialized without any additional testing. According to U.S. law, to be considered GRAS, the substance must be the subject of a substantial amount of peer-reviewed published studies (or equivalent) and there must be overwhelming consensus among the scientific community that the product is safe. GM foods had neither. Some experts contend that GM foods are illegal. In 1992, the FDA declared GMO crops are safe as long as the producers say they are. Such a lenient approach was largely the result of Monsanto's influence over the U.S. government.

There is much safety concern that the inserted gene has been found to transfer to the human gut bacteria and many even end up in human DNA.[613] Farmer and medical experts report that there are. many sick, sterile, and dead animals.[613]

According to Smith,[614] after feeding hamsters for 2 years over three generations, those on a GM soy diet lost their ability to procreate.

In India, animals that graze on Bt cotton have decreased by 71%. Some have shown problems with growth, organ development, and their immune systems. Smith,[614] says that 20%–55% of animals fed GM corn or soybean have spontaneous abortions. It also kills chicken embryo in 24–48 hours. With a GM gene present, you have decreased nutrient ability to take up nutrients. With the glyphosate it also decreases nutrient uptake.

Over 90% of the canola in the United States is GMO, antinutrients of soybean that are genetically engineered have as much as 7-times higher the amount of known allergen cold trypsin inhibiter when compared with non-GM soy in the cooked state.

A review of 19 mice and rat studies using GMO soy and corn showed significant disrupters to the gut and kidney with other organs affected. According to Smith[614] thousands of farm workers who harvest Bt cotton in India are complaining of skin rashes all over the body. Animals grazing on the Bt cotton plants after harvest have died.

Bt corn on mice gave rheumatoid arthritis, inflammatory bone disease, osteoporosis, arteriosclerosis, cancer, allergies, and ALS.

In the United States, 90%–95% of soy and corn of GMO contamination paths are at the farm level that include seeds, improperly cleaned equipment, cross-pollination, and coming of in grain handling and storage. GMO farmland has increased from 4 million acres to 30 million[614] over 93% of all U.S. soy production is GMO. The FDA neglected to regulate GMO animal sterility.

WAR ON WEEDS

Farmers, plant geneticists, chemists, and agronomists recently have been engaged in an arms race against weeds, particularly weeds that have evolved resistance to the common herbicide glyphosate. A second generation of herbicide-tolerant crops has been developed to battle resistant weeds, but they have sparked concerns about overreliance on chemical controls.

Introduced in the 1980s, glyphosate has been the best-selling herbicide since 2001. Monsanto, which markets glyphosate as Roundup, introduced crops engineered to be tolerant of glyphosate in the late 1990s, and farmers now plant Roundup Ready herbicide-tolerant corn, soybeans, and cotton on the majority of cultivated areas in the United States. Thanks to the popularity of the firm's Roundup Ready trait, last year, 94% of soybean acres were herbicide-tolerant, as was 73% of cotton acreage, and 72% of corn acreage, according to the Department of Agriculture.

Farmers liked glyphosate because it vastly simplified weed control. But it also led to the emergence of resistant weeds that are increasingly hard to kill.

Beginning in 2013, pending approval by USDA, farmers will be able to plant crops that have been genetically modified to also tolerate applications of the herbicides 2,4-dichlorophenoxyacetic acid (2,4-D) and 3,6-dichloro-2-methoxybenzoic acid (dicamba). Both herbicides have been in use for more than 40 years. The traits will be "stacked" to include tolerance to glyphosate as well as to 2,4-D or dicamba.

Dow AgroSciences' 2,4-D-tolerant corn, part of its Enlist Weed Control System, is the first of the new crops in line for USDA consideration and marketing to U.S. farmers. Monsanto plans to follow with its 2014 introduction of dicamba-tolerant soybeans, called Roundup Ready 2 Xtend. Both companies say that the emergence of weeds resistant to glyphosate will drive farmers' adoption of the new seeds (Figure 4.17).

Farmers would still be able to manage most weeds through applications of glyphosate, but for any resistant weeds that remain, they will have the option of adding 2,4-D or dicamba without worrying about damaging their crops. The firms are promoting the seeds as a way to control weeds, without having to resort to tilling or hand-weeding. So-called low-till or conservation tillage is a common soil conservation practice.

But in the long term, experts say, if farmers do not also use nonchemical methods for weed control, such as crop rotation, eventually weeds will emerge that are resistant to 2,4-D and dicamba as well as glyphosate.

The new crops will be a valuable tool to help diversify weed management programs.[615] However, if farmers depend too much on the new technology, "evolutionary nature is such that when you put enough selection pressure on a species, it will develop resistance." That pressure would create weeds that could survive 2,4-D or dicamba applications.

The specter of weeds brandishing multiple resistances has made the new crops a target for groups promoting sustainable agriculture. Others have raised alarms about risks associated with an increase in the use of 2,4-D and dicamba. For example, growers of crops that are susceptible to the herbicides are worried that more drift of 2,4-D and dicamba from treated fields will weaken or kill their crops.

For their part, Dow and Monsanto insist that the lessons learned from overreliance on glyphosate are changing farming practices. Never again, they say, will it be the norm to use the same herbicide,

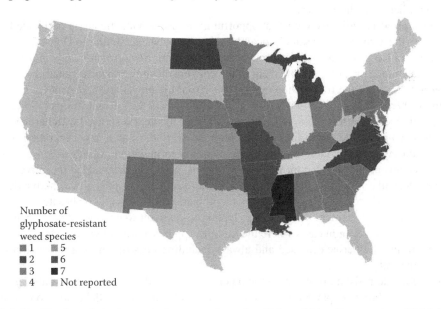

Number of
glyphosate-resistant
weed species
■ 1   ■ 5
■ 2   ■ 6
■ 3   ■ 7
▩ 4   ▩ Not reported

FIGURE 4.17 Number of glyphosate-resistant weed species. (Adapted from Bromgardner, M. M. War On Weeds. CEN RSS. 2012. Accessed April 15, 2016. http://cen.acs.org/articles/90/i21/War-Weeds.html.)

year after year, on the same crop in the same location. They dispute estimates that the use of 2,4-D or dicamba will greatly increase, and both firms have developed new, low-drift formulations of these herbicides that they say will minimize off-field migration.

At Dow, plant scientists began the search for a new herbicide-tolerance trait almost 10 years ago, with the emergence of weeds resistant to glyphosate. The company settled on 2,4-D as the target herbicide because it is already commonly used, kills a wide range of weeds, and has a mode of action that is different from glyphosate's. Both 2,4-D and dicamba are synthetic versions of the plant hormone auxin. Putting additional auxin on weeds triggers uncontrolled growth that leads to death.

To find genes that confer a tolerance to 2,4-D, scientists looked in bacteria that live in soils where 2,4-D has been used. One bacterium, *Ralstonia eutropha*, produces enzymes that break down the molecule into constituents that are not lethal to plants.

Dow's plant geneticists were able to insert the gene into corn, soy, and cotton. The resulting genotypes were tested for 2,4-D tolerance, and the successful plants were then tested for any impact on yield, grain quality, stress tolerance, or maturity. Well-behaved traits confer the desired advantage without also bringing along other metabolic changes that would weaken the crops.

While the Enlist crops were showing their stuff in field trials, Dow chemists worked on a new formulation of 2,4-D, called 2,4-D choline, to minimize volatility.[615] An application technology specialist at Dow AgroSciences explains that rather than traditional ester or amine forms of the molecule, which can volatilize in the environment, the new version is a more stable quaternary ammonium salt.

In addition, with less particle drift when application directions are followed. Dow recently reported that field tests of the formula showed a 92% reduction in volatility and a 90% reduction in drift.

Crops that contain the 2,4-D tolerance trait will also tolerate older versions of 2,4-D. However, Dow has developed a stewardship program that obligates farmers to use a premixed combination of 2,4-D choline and glyphosate. The program includes farmer education about using multiple herbicide modes of action, the requirement to use Dow's new herbicide mixture, and labeling instructions for proper application. State pesticide regulations generally require farmers to follow labeling guidelines when using herbicides.

Soybean growers will have their first opportunity to use a synthetic auxin herbicide beginning in 2014 with the arrival of Monsanto's dicamba-tolerant soybeans. Similar to Dow's 2,4-D trait, the dicamba-tolerance gene was isolated from a soil bacterium, *Stenotrophomonas maltophilia*. The bacteria metabolize dicamba with the help of the enzyme dicamba monooxygenase.

Monsanto licensed the trait technology in 2005 from the university, and Arnevik's team tested more than 100 resulting transformations. Years of field trials of the tolerant strains followed to make sure the trait does not affect yield, regardless of whether the field is sprayed with herbicide.

On the chemicals side, Monsanto worked with BASF to develop a new generation of dicamba that has reduced volatility compared with the common formulation available today. Current versions of dicamba are not labeled for use with soybeans, giving farmers added incentive to trade up to the new formula. Monsanto does not plan to require farmers to spray a dual-herbicide mixture; farmers in areas where resistant weeds are not a problem can stick with glyphosate.

On the other hand, farmers who do have glyphosate-resistant weeds should not depend just on a two-herbicide blend, even in cases where the mixture appears to kill all weeds. Monsanto and Dow promote varying the herbicides used and always including ones that have a residual effect when applied to the soil.

More herbicide-resistant traits are in the pipeline, which will increase the availability of diverse modes of action. For example, Syngenta and Bayer CropScience are collaborating on a *p*-hydroxyphenylpyruvate dioxygenase herbicide-tolerance trait for soybeans. And crops tolerant to three or more herbicides are not far behind.

Since the advent of Roundup Ready traits, however, farmers have not been in the habit of controlling for nonexistent weeds. To some extent, it is true that farmers might not change what they are doing until a resistant weed appears. Roundup Ready was so good that the farmers could forget what they knew in terms of weed management.

In addition to using a changing rotation of herbicides, farmers will need to change their agricultural practices to include crop rotation, cover cropping, and weed control after harvest. And in some areas, low-till practices will be more difficult to adhere to.

Monsanto promoted Roundup Ready as a weed system, and that is how Dow is promoting its crops.

Freese also points to research from Pennsylvania State University that projects a fourfold increase in the amount of 2,4-D used on corn after growers adopt the Enlist system. "It is postemergence use that causes most crop injury" and selects for resistant weeds.

For its part, Dow says that "rates of herbicide application per acre of corn will not increase with our new technology package." Without the new traits, farmers would still need to apply an ever-greater amount of herbicides to control weeds resistant to glyphosate. In addition, farmers would have to resort to cultivation practices that could increase soil erosion and pollution.

A group of U.S. growers organized as the Save Our Crops Coalition has asked USDA to take a close look at the problem of damage from 2,4-D drift. In a statement, the group, which includes fruit and vegetable growers, says "SOCC appreciates Dow's substantial efforts to develop a low-volatility formulation of 2,4-D."

For now, groups for and against the introduction of the new herbicide-tolerant crops are waiting on a ruling from USDA, which wrapped up its public comment period on the 2,4-D trait.

GMO—FOODS

GLYPHOSATE

The explosion of awareness about gluten sensitivity is hard to miss. Whether walking down supermarket aisles or ordering in restaurants, "gluten-free" proclamations call out in ever-increasing numbers. Pizza crust, hotdog buns, and cookies are offered with rice flour, corn meal, anything but wheat and its close relatives, like rye, barley, and spelt that contain gluten.

Technically, gluten refers to any of the more than 23,000 distinct proteins in wheat, and the term "gluten-related disorders" describes a wide spectrum of problems associated with its consumption.[617] Wheat is not the only grain of concern, as there are gluten-like proteins known as gliadins and glutenins found in most other cereal grains (Table 4.34). All of these are linked to reactions. The most well-known conditions linked to gluten sensitivity are celiac disease and wheat allergy, in part, because they are both specific immune responses that can be unequivocally confirmed. Those with celiac disease can experience adverse effects when exposed to gluten in the parts-per-million range levels and research shows that when it goes undiagnosed, it is associated with a nearly fourfold increased risk of death from all causes.[618]

Unfortunately, celiac disease and other forms of gluten-related disorders are often overlooked or misdiagnosed because the symptoms are so varied. They can affect cardiovascular, neurological, and skeletal systems, to name but a few[619]; in fact, there are over 300 health conditions and/or symptoms linked to gluten sensitivity.[620]

Celiac disease prevalence in Finland doubled in the last two decades, even when ruling out confounding factors such as better detection rates.[618] The growth in the United States is even worse. According to one 2009 study, celiac disease has increased more than fourfold in the United States during the past 50 years.[621] A 2010 study pushed that figure to a fivefold increase in celiac disease prevalence just since 1974.[622]

The same study found that the dramatic uptick was "due to an increasing number of subjects that lost the immunological tolerance to gluten in their adulthood."[623] Clearly, there is an environmental

TABLE 4.34

Gluten Like Proteins Found in Cereal Grains

Food	Total Protein	Gliadins (% of Total Protein)	Glutenins (% of Total Protein)
Wheat	10–15	40–50	30–40
Rye	9–14	30–50	30–50
Oats	8–14	10–15	−5
Corn	7–13	50–55	30–45
Rice	8–10	1–5	85–90
Sorghum	9–13	>60	
Millet	7–16	57	30
Buckwheat			High

Source: Adapted from Pizzorno J. E., Murray M. T., Eds. 1999. *Textbook of Natural Medicine.* 2nd ed. p. 1601. New York: Churchill Livingstone.

component to this trend. One theory popularized by the 2011 publication of Davis is that the increase in the incidence of celiac disease might be attributable to an increase in the gluten content of wheat resulting from wheat breeding. This view was echoed in a 2012 study published in the journal *BMC Medicine*[624]:

> One possible explanation is that the selection of wheat varieties with higher gluten content has been a continuous process during the last 10,000 years, with changes dictated more by technological rather than nutritional reasons.

A 2013 review of historical data commissioned by the U.S. Department of Agriculture, however, found no clear evidence of an increase in the gluten content of wheat in the United States during the twentieth century, and only a slight change in the twenty-first century. They did concede that an increase in the per capita consumption of wheat and gluten may play a role.[625] Additional environmental factors studied to play a role include: timing of gluten exposure,[626] breast feeding duration,[627] the composition of the intestinal microbiota,[628] herbicides and pesticides, and cesarean birth.[629,630] Also, the hypersensitivity phenomena resulting from more and large holes in GOMD membranes allowing Ca^{2+} to enter, when combined with protein kinase A and C and then phosphorylated, causes hypersensitivity to increase to 1000 times.

One of the most common explanations for the alarming increase in gluten-related health issues is both that detection of gluten problems has improved and that more practitioners are looking for it; hence, the greater numbers. While better detection and the new "popularity" of the disorder are certainly contributing, there is an accumulating body of research indicating a third factor is at play, namely, the exposure of the U.S. population to environmental toxins and other food allergens, whose combined influence is triggering the increase in the overall susceptibility to gluten. Support for this idea is found in the increased rates of gluten-related disorders over the past decade or two. These include autoimmune problems such as allergies and asthma, as well as gastrointestinal disorders such as Crohn's disease, irritable bowel syndrome (IBS), and acid reflux (GERD). Also, the increase in chemical sensitivity appears to be a major factor in our studies at the EHC-Dallas.

> There are over 300 health conditions and/or symptoms linked to gluten sensitivity, as confirmed by peer-reviewed studies.

Here, we will present evidence that strongly suggests that one significant addition to the American diet, genetically modified (GM) food, is a major contributor to gluten sensitivity reactions, and it also interferes with complete and rapid recovery. Also called GMOs, these are crops that have had foreign genes inserted into their DNA, usually from bacteria or viruses, to confer a particular trait. There are nine GM food crops currently being grown for commercial use; the six major ones are soy, corn, cotton (used for cooking oil production), canola (also used for cooking oil production), sugar beets (used for sugar production), and alfalfa (used as animal feed). All six are engineered to be herbicide tolerant, that is, to survive spray applications of weed killer. They, thus, contain high residue levels of these extremely toxic, endocrine-disrupting, and DNA-damaging agro chemicals. Some corn and cotton varieties are also equipped with genes that produce a toxic insecticide 1 Bt-toxin (from *Bacillus thuringiensis* soil bacteria). There are also zucchini, yellow squash, and papaya varieties that have viral genes designed to help them ward off certain viral infections.

Based on animal feeding research, case studies, and the properties of these crops, GMOs are linked with four types of disorders impact gluten reactions:

1. Leaky gut (aka "intestinal permeability")
2. Impaired digestive capacity (reduced enzymes, damage to microvilli)
3. Gut bacteria dysbiosis (overgrowth of pathogenic microbes)
4. Immune/allergenic response

It is well known that a significantly higher percentage of patients diagnosed with celiac disease have leaky gut,[631] whereby the junctures between the cells lining the intestinal wall (enterocytes) open up, allowing contents of the intestines to enter the bloodstream. (Technically, anyone who consumes gluten—whether a celiac sufferer or not—is susceptible to increased intestinal permeability. That is because the protein class in wheat known as α-gliadin can provoke the release of zonulin from our bodies, which can promote intestinal permeability to unhealthy levels.[632])

When the intestines are intact and functioning properly, usually only tiny by-products of digestion are ushered appropriately into the bloodstream for assimilation. Approximately 90% of proteins are fully broken down into smaller "peptides," with the remaining 10% capable of stimulating an antigenic response.[633] With gaps in the intestinal walls, however, a far larger percentage of undigested food particles (macromolecules), gut bacteria, and even consumed chemicals can all enter the bloodstream.

An example of the protective aspect of the immune system is that it can launch an attack on the undigested proteins, treating them as invaders. This will result in a number of inflammatory reactions and symptoms of a hypersensitized immune system. In addition, some of these proteins will exhibit the phenomenon of "molecular mimicry," where the person's immune system may attack a protein sequence in undigested wheat, for example, that resembles a sequence that also exists in the body's own tissue. This sets up the groundwork for a wide range of autoimmune conditions, whereby the immune system starts to attack parts of the body, losing "self-tolerance."

Celiac disease is one such example of this immune system "friendly fire," but in truth, there are literally hundreds of possible side effects and symptoms that can result from this process.

When considering the role of GMOs in "punching holes in the gut," the most obvious candidate is the GM corn *designed* to produce Bt-toxin. That is because the toxin is designed to create holes. It is not supposed to create holes in *human* cells. Rather, it is *supposed* to limit its destructive effects by targeting certain insect species, in which it breaks open small pores in the cells of their digestive tract and kills them.[634]

When Bt-corn was introduced into the diet in 1996, the biotech companies and their supporters in the U.S. EPA (which categorized these corn plants as *registered pesticides*) promised that the toxin was only dangerous to certain insects—it had no effect on humans or mammals. This assumption, however, was directly contradicted by several peer-reviewed published studies, and even by the statements of the EPA's Science Advisory Panel.[635]

The study most clearly related to the risk of leaky gut was published in February 2012.[636]

Researchers "documented that modified Bt toxins (from GM plants) are not inert on human cells, but can exert toxicity." In concentrations that are generally higher than that produced in average Bt corn, Bt-toxin disrupts the membrane in just 24 hours, causing fluid to leak. Thus, the main assumption used as the excuse to allow pesticide-producing corn into the diet appears to be totally false. Bt-toxin does interact with human cells boring small holes into intestinal walls.

The other primary assumption touted by regulators was that Bt-toxin would be fully broken down by the digestive processes in our stomach. But a 2011 Canadian study conducted disapproved that one as well. They discovered that 93% of the pregnant women tested had Bt-toxin from genetically engineered corn in their blood. And so too did 80% of their unborn fetuses.[637]

If the Bt-toxin had entered the bloodstream through holes that it created, it is likely that bacteria and food particles also got through and caused problems. Bt-toxin's presence in fetuses is of greater concern. The toxin may be disrupting cellular integrity throughout their system. Since fetuses do not have a fully developed blood–brain barrier, the hole-poking toxin may be active in their brains as well.

The authors of this Canadian study were faced with a question, "Why did so many of their subjects have Bt-toxin in their blood?" The toxin is expected to quickly wash out of the bloodstream. Therefore, the consumption of Bt-toxin must be quite frequent to explain why 9 of 10 subjects still have it in their blood. But this was Canada; and unlike Mexico, they do not eat corn chips and corn tortillas every day. They *do* eat lots of corn *derivatives* like corn sweeteners, but these highly processed foods no longer have the Bt-toxin present and, therefore, could not be the source.

But livestock in North America do eat Bt corn as a main component of their diets.

Canadians eat the meat and dairy products of these corn-fed animals every day. The authors of the study, therefore, speculated that the source of the Bt-toxin in the blood could have been the meat or dairy. This would mean that the Bt-toxin protein remains intact through the animals' entire digestive process and then again through the humans' digestive process. While this may be true, there is another possible explanation with very serious consequences for those who eat GMOs.

In spite of numerous claims by the biotech industry that it would never happen, research confirmed that part of the DNA "transgene" inserted into GMO crops can actually transfer into the DNA of our gut bacteria.[638] They found that part of the gene from the herbicide-tolerant Roundup Ready (RR glyphosate) soybean had integrated into the DNA of the intestinal flora of three out of seven subjects tested (Nature of Biotechnology 2004). The transfer of the RR gene had occurred before the subjects came to the research facility, apparently from consuming GM soy in some previous meal(s). The percentage of subjects with the integrated GM genes may have been higher if the study had been conducted in the United States. This was done in the United Kingdom, however, where the intake of GM soy is but a fraction of that eaten in North America (Figures 4.18 through 4.21).

The gut bacteria that contained part of the Roundup Ready gene were not killed when exposed to Roundup's active ingredient, glyphosate. In other words, the gut bacteria were herbicide-tolerant. This suggests that the transferred genes from GMOs continue to function after they have integrated into our gut bacteria. If so, we may have GM proteins continuously being produced inside the intestines long after eating of GMOs stops.

The funding for this research was cut off, so the researchers never did test whether the Bt gene in corn likewise transfers. But this might provide a far more plausible explanation why so many subjects tested positive for Bt-toxin. The Bt-toxin genes could have transferred from corn chips or corn tortillas into gut bacteria, where they produced the toxin on a continuous basis inside the intestinal tract. Then, it could have altered the permeability of the cell walls, entered the bloodstream, and then also traveled through the placenta into the unborn fetuses of pregnant test subjects.

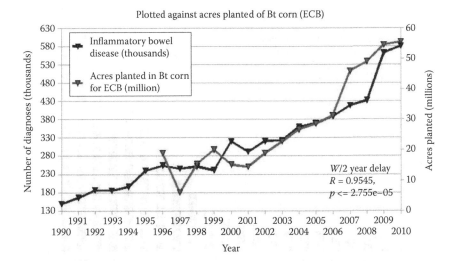

FIGURE 4.18 Hospital discharge diagnoses of inflammatory bowel disease. (Adapted from Smith, J. Can Genetically Engineered Foods Explain the Exploding Gluten Sensitivity? Gluten and GMOs. 2013. Accessed April 15, 2016. http://responsibletechnology.org/media/images/content/Exploding-Gluten-Sensitivity_. pdf?key=38810328.)

Bᴛ Cᴏʀɴ ᴀɴᴅ Gʟᴜᴛᴇɴ Sᴇɴsɪᴛɪᴠɪᴛʏ

If leaky gut is a precursor and a contributing factor to the many types of gluten sensitivity, then the introduction of Bt corn into the U.S. diet may be responsible for increasing the number of reactive eaters. It also may help explain why a range of gastrointestinal and inflammatory disorders have also risen sharply after GMOs were introduced (see Figure 4.21).

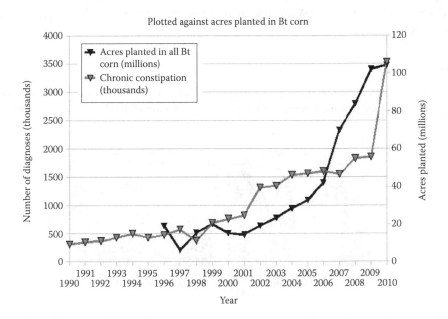

FIGURE 4.19 Hospital discharge diagnoses of chronic constipation. (Adapted from Smith, J. Can Genetically Engineered Foods Explain the Exploding Gluten Sensitivity? Gluten and GMOs. 2013. Accessed April 15, 2016. http://responsibletechnology.org/media/images/content/Exploding-Gluten-Sensitivity_.pdf?key=38810328.)

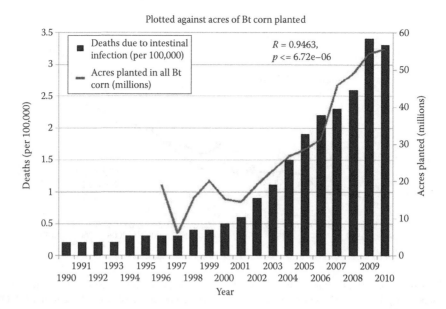

FIGURE 4.20 Deaths due to intestinal infection. (Adapted from Smith, J. Can Genetically Engineered Foods Explain the Exploding Gluten Sensitivity? Gluten and GMOs. 2013. Accessed April 15, 2016. http://responsibletechnology.org/media/images/content/Exploding-Gluten-Sensitivity_.pdf?key=38810328.)

On the other hand, if the leaky gut is being caused by conditions such as celiac disease, then Bt corn may be exacerbating the problems, possibly converting asymptomatic people into those who suffer acutely.

In either case, removing Bt corn from the diet would make sense in the treatment, and possibly prevention, of this debilitating disease. In addition, leaky gut is exacerbated by each of the other three disorders also linked to GMOs, impaired digestion, disrupted gut bacteria, and increased allergen exposure.

IMPAIRED DIGESTION

If the digestive system is not functioning properly, then food particles are not broken down as quickly or as completely. One obvious result is poor absorption of food. If a person is not gaining

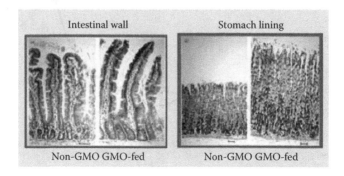

FIGURE 4.21 Rats fed genetically engineered potatoes suffered from potentially precancerous cell growth in their digestive tracts. (Adapted from Smith, J. Can Genetically Engineered Foods Explain the Exploding Gluten Sensitivity? Gluten and GMOs. 2013. Accessed April 15, 2016. http://responsibletechnology.org/media/images/content/Exploding-Gluten-Sensitivity_.pdf?key=38810328.)

sufficient nutrition from the foods they consume, their overall health, including their immune system, can suffer.

With poor digestion, proteins can remain intact for longer than normal periods in the gastrointestinal (GI) tract. This can result in the larger, undigested food particles becoming the "food" of pathogenic gut bacteria, leading to their overgrowth. This further compromises digestion and immunity. When protein putrefies, it can also release excess hydrogen sulfide (as toxic as cyanide gas) which irritates and inflames the mucous membranes. Undigested proteins also have a greater likelihood of provoking autoimmune reactions, in which the immune system attacks parts of the body, and which can contribute to upsetting the delicate balance between the innate (Th1) and adaptive (Th2) poles of immunity. Th2-dominance is a type of immune hypersensitization where formerly harmless foods provoke harmful immune responses.

If the leaky gut remains unchecked, the constant antigenic challenges presented by these larger food particles entering the bloodstream will continue to foment inappropriate antibody responses, inflammation, and the development of more serious autoimmune disease.

One of the debilitating side effects of celiac disease is the flattening of the microvilli along the intestinal walls. These cells are what absorbs broken-down food into the bloodstream for use by the whole body. Normally, they stick out like tiny fingers, dramatically increasing the surface area that can be used for digesting. (The total surface area of the intestinal villi of a healthy human being is equivalent to a tennis court.)

In celiac disease patients, the immune system adversely responds to gluten proteins causing destruction in the microvilli, and a filling in of the crypts between them, resulting in a flattened, highly dysfunctional surface. Because the surface area for nutrient absorption is drastically reduced and/or functionally disabled, celiac disease patients often suffer from a variety of disorders related to poor digestion and malnutrition.

When the wall of the intestines are irritated (in the case of celiac disease or in general), the body produces less of cholecystokinin (CCK). This, in turn, reduces the digestive enzymes produced by the pancreas, as well as the bile produced in the liver. Without sufficient levels, digestion is slowed down, particularly of proteins. Thus, gluten sensitivity carries a one-two punch: reducing digestion by damaging cell walls, and exacerbating nutrient malabsorption by reducing digestive enzymes and bile. This can become a vicious cycle if the larger food particles result in bacterial overgrowth, which in turn, can further irritate the lining of the intestines, further lowering digestive capability directly, and through reduced CCK levels.

As discussed above, Bt-toxin was found to poke holes in human cells. It is certainly possible that this can disrupt the digestive capability of the gut lining, as well as lower CCK levels. A study on mice also looked at the impact of Bt-toxin on the microvilli and discovered a real problem.

Using both natural Bt-toxin from bacteria, as well as that produced in an experimental GM crop (potato), the toxin damaged the microvilli of mouse intestines (ileum). Some microvilli were broken off and discontinuous; others were shortened.[636] This is very similar to the type of damage that gluten proteins cause to the intestines.

The high levels of glyphosate-based herbicides in Roundup Ready crops may also directly damage the structure and function of the gut wall. A study on glyphosate exposure in carnivorous fish revealed remarkable adverse effects throughout the digestive system,[639] including "disruption of mucosal folds and disarray of microvilli structure" in the intestinal wall, along with an exaggerated secretion of mucin throughout the alimentary tract.

Another study using GM potatoes also caused severe disruption of the cells lining the digestive tract of rats in just 10 days. Damage included potentially precancerous growth and abnormal cell architecture. The foreign gene inserted into the potato *did* produce a pesticide, but *not* the Bt-toxin. Instead, it was outfitted with a gene from a snowdrop plant that produced an insecticide GNA lectin. The big revelation from the study, however, was that the lectin itself was not the cause of the damage to the intestines and stomach. When other rats were fed the lectin itself, no such damage took place. This research lays the blame squarely on the unpredicted side effects of the process of genetically engineering a crop. In other words any GMO crop, irrespective of what gene is inserted, can theo-retically cause this type of profound damage to the digestive tract.[637,640]

According to U.S. hospital discharges and ambulatory admissions records data, inflammatory bowel syndrome skyrocketed since the introduction of GMOs.

Livestock Ulcers and Corroded Intestines

According to Collado et al., the GMO-fed stomachs of pigs were inflamed, discolored, and had multiple ulcers. The non-GMO stomachs were healthy.[641] Danish pig farmers reported that when they switched pigs from GM soy to non-GM soy feed in April 2012, deaths from ulcers and bloat disappeared entirely during the next year. Tursi et al.[642] by contrast, 36 animals were lost over the previous 2 years to these maladies. Animals also recovered from chronic diarrhea, increased con-ception rate and litter size, eliminated birth defects, and reduced their need for antibiotics by 2/3.

Some butchers in the United States also see a marked difference between the organs of cattle fed GM versus non-GM fed. Instead of the healthy, intact intestines that they see in the non-GMO animals, the GMO-fed ones are thin and corroded, and tear easily. The changes are not just in the intestines and not just in cattle. Collado et al.[641] confirms that based on autopsies, "There is a big difference in the liver and the intestinal tract on these animals on GMOs," including cows, pigs, sheep, horses, and even dogs on a corn-based diet.

This type of damage to the structural integrity of the intestinal wall might directly reduce its capability to digest nutrients. Furthermore, the unhealthy gut lining may also reduce the production of CCK, which will then lower bile and digestive enzyme production in the pancreas. Consumption of GMOs, however, might damage the pancreatic cells directly leading to lower digestive capability.

Roundup Ready Soybeans and Reduced Digestive Enzymes

Pregnant mice were fed GM soybeans, and their offspring continued on the diet for 8 months. Compared to controls fed non-GMO soybeans, the pancreas suffered a profound reduction in diges-tive enzyme production.[640] α-Amylase, a major enzyme that degrades carbohydrates, was 77% lower among 2-month-old mice pups, and remained 75% and 60% lower in months five and eight. Young mice (1 month) also had reduced amounts of a protein digesting enzyme precursor (zymo-gen), which is essential for healthy breakdown of the proteins in food.

Nearly all GMO soybeans are Roundup Ready, engineered to survive otherwise deadly doses of Roundup herbicide. As a result, Roundup Ready (RR) soybeans (as well as RR corn, cotton, canola, sugar beets, and alfalfa) end up with physiologically significant amounts of Roundup absorbed into the plant tissues and deposited into the food portion. When analyzing the dangerous impacts of RR soybeans, it is unclear whether the primary causative factor is the genetic engineering of the plant or the high Roundup content in the food, but their individual toxicities may work in concert and synergize.

An analysis of the properties and effects of glyphosate, the active ingredient in Roundup, shows how this toxin may contribute to many of the problems discussed. For example, carnivorous fish exposed to glyphosate showed decreased activity of protease, lipase, and amylase, important pro-teins involved with the digestion of proteins, fats, and carbohydrates, in the esophagus, stomach, and intestine.[642] Glyphosate also has profoundly harmful effects on the bacteria living inside the intestines.

Bacteria living inside the human plays a critical role in digestion, immunity, detoxification, and even the production of nutrients (e.g., the entire B group of vitamins is produced through their activ-ity). Together, they function like another essential organ. In fact, some researchers in the field have suggested we reclassify ourselves as "meta-organisms" as there are about 10 times the number of bacteria cells in the digestive tract as there are human cells in the entire body. The relationship with the internal bacteria plays an immensely important role in health.

A proper balance of bacteria supports not only many aspects of physical health, but also mental health. The "gut–brain axis" depends on the health of the flora residing in the gastrointestinal tract. As much as 95% of serotonin, for instance, is synthesized in the gut through the bacterial conversion of the essential amino acid L-tryptophan.

One of the hallmark features of gluten sensitivity is gastrointestinal symptoms such as gas, bloating, constipation, diarrhea, and cramping all of which indicate an imbalance in the gut flora.

In fact, gluten-sensitive individuals often have documented imbalances in their gut flora. This is especially true for those with celiac disease.[643–646] While we do not know whether the gut flora imbalance precedes the sensitization to gluten, or vice versa, it is likely that both processes play a role.

Glyphosate was patented as a broad-spectrum biocide which is a very powerful antibiotic. In tiny amounts, it can significantly reduce the population of the healthy bacterial varieties in the digestive tract and promote the overgrowth of dangerous pathogenic bacteria according to research with poultry[647] and cattle.[648]

Introduction of Roundup Ready Canola (and Use of Roundup on Canadian Farms) Appears to Correlate with Childhood Celiac Diagnoses in an Alberta Hospital

The implications for health may be quite profound and complex. In celiac patients, for example, the healthy *Bifidobacterium* strains can affect certain components of the immune system especially the cytokines. The cytokines that provoke inflammation are reduced by the *Bifidobacterium* bacteria, while the type that is anti-inflammatory (IL-10) is increased.[647] But *Bifidobacterium* is easily killed by glyphosate. The result could be a generalized increase in inflammation, which is now recognized as the basis for numerous diseases.

Highly pathogenic bacteria such as those that produce *Salmonella* or botulism poisoning are highly resistant to glyphosate. Furthermore, some of the healthy bacteria that are killed normally keep some of the pathogenic bacteria in check. Glyphosate use kills lactic-acid-producing bacteria in the gut of cattle, allowing the bacteria that produce deadly botulism to flourish. This might explain the increase in chronic botulism in cattle.[649,650] Cases of sudden infant death syndrome are also linked to the botulism toxin.[651]

In addition to the risk of producing acute toxins, such as the one that causes botulism poisoning, bacterial pathogens can activate the potent signaling molecule zonulin. Zonulin, as described above, can induce a breakdown of the tight junctions in cells lining the gut, leading to leaky gut.[652] Indeed, some of the same bacterial growth stimulated through glyphosate exposure, for example, *Clostridium botulinum*,[653] *Clostridium perfringens*,[40] and *Salmonella* infections,[654] have been found to increase intestinal permeability.

Collado et al.[641] specifically saw a huge increase in the overgrowth of *Clostridium perfringens* type A in livestock within a year of the introduction of RR soy and corn in 1996. This condition, which affects the liver, has resulted in sudden deaths of pigs and cows, as well as chronic conditions.

The bacterial overgrowth from glyphosate may be just one of the reasons why Collado, switched from a genetically modified grain to one that is not genetically modified, dramatic improvements in health has occurred. Both the immune and digestive systems are much healthier in animals on non-GMO feed.

Butchers have noted that livestock fed on GMOs have a different smell. According to Collado et al.[641] "the pigs fed GMOs have a very dramatic difference in their microflora. They have a terrible odor compared to the normal microflora because of that changed bio-environment." Similarly, the organs and tissues are discolored, possibly due to the proliferation of this different flora. A village in Andhra Pradesh, India lost all 13 buffaloes after they grazed on Bt cotton plants for a single day. Natural cotton plants did not have any negative effects over the previous 7 years.

While it is clear that roundup residues in GM crops can damage the gut microflora, there is preliminary evidence suggesting that Bt-toxin might be a similar culprit, especially in animals. In India, farmers allow sheep, goat, and buffalo to graze on cotton plants after harvest. When genetically engineered Bt cotton was introduced into the country, the results were tragic. Thousands of animals died; even more suffered from a variety of disorders.[655]

Sanchez et al.[643] suggests that the Bt-toxin produced in the cotton plant kills the cellulose-digesting bacteria normally found in the animals' rumen.

This would explain why autopsies of the dead sheep revealed shriveled intestines, and an autopsy of a dead buffalo showed undigested food in the rumen, at least three days after consumption. According to Sanchez et al.[643] since the cellulose was never broken down, the food never made it into the intestines.

U.S. agriculture consultant Nadal et al.[644] reports that when his client, who was raising miniature cattle (3 feet high), switched from non-GMO to GMO corn feed, he may have come across the same issue. The animals "were not able to process the food correctly, and they would bloat up and die." The farmer quickly lost about 90% of his herd, but was able to save the rest by switching back to non-GMO corn.

An unpublished study by the India-based Navdanya organization also found a significant reduction in soil bacteria over 3 years in fields where Bt cotton was planted, compared to natural cotton. This supports the theory that Bt-toxin, which is produced even by the roots of the plants, is a natural enemy of certain types of bacteria and therefore a "natural antibiotic."

If those types of bacteria were only found in rumens, it may not be a problem for humans; since we do not have rumens. On the other hand, the Bt-toxin may interact with other gut bacteria to cause harm. This appears to be the case in insects; a study showed that Bt-toxin only killed certain insects when gut bacteria were present.[654] When bacteria were first removed by administering antibiotics, the toxin was no longer lethal. The authors suggest that Bt-toxin can cause otherwise benign gut bacteria to exert pathogenic effects. The mechanics of how this happens, and whether it also impacts humans, is not known. It may be a direct impact on the bacteria; transfer of the Bt-toxin gene to the gut bacteria (which may dramatically increase the amount of toxin produced) or simply the transport of healthy bacteria through the "leaky gut" created by the Bt-toxin, where it then becomes toxic.

DIRECT EXPOSURE TO ALLERGENS

Sensitivity to gluten is just one of many immune reactions to food that is on the increase. According to the CDC statistics, hospital-confirmed extreme food allergies have been steadily increasing over the past 15 years. It is well known that if a person is experiencing an allergic reaction to one substance, they can become more vulnerable to reactions from other potential triggers. At low levels of stimulation, the immune system can remain quiet. But once the allergen load reaches a critical threshold, the person may react to many things that were tolerated before that point. This is the spreading phenomena seen in many food-sensitive patients who have chemical sensitivity.

GMOS AS ALLERGENS

If GMOs either provoke allergic responses or somehow damage the immune system (immunotoxic), their entrance into the food supply in large quantities could boost allergic reactions to other non-GMO foods which is often seen in the chemically sensitive. Determining whether a GMO is allergenic, however, can be very difficult. The foods contain genes and their proteins from bacteria and viruses that have never been part of the human food supply in the past. People are not usually allergic to a food until they have eaten it several times. It would, therefore, be difficult to know in advance if the new foreign protein was an allergen.

Bt-toxin protein matches an egg yolk allergen; and GM papaya protein also finds a match in the database.[656] This is why a rotation diet is necessary for many food-sensitive chemically sensitive patients.

The Bt protein also fails two other tests recommended by the WHO. The protein remains stable for too long when exposed to heat and to simulated stomach acid and digestive enzymes.[657]

Thus, it shares the characteristic with many allergens of not being quickly degraded during digestion.

If their foreign GM proteins trigger reactions, the danger is compounded by the fact that genes can transfer into the DNA of human gut bacteria and may continuously produce the protein from within the intestines. This could trigger reactions 24/7, permanently elevating the load on the immune system.[658] This is one reason why external lactobacillus is necessary for treating some food-intolerant chemically sensitive patients.

If the Roundup Ready soybean protein is an allergen, this might explain why soy allergies in the United Kingdom jumped by 50% just after GMOs were introduced in the late 1990s.[659]

Bt-Toxin as an Allergen, and Promoter of Reactions to Other Foods

In addition to failing the WHO allergy criteria, there are many other studies that implicate Bt-toxin as an allergen. In its natural state derived from soil bacteria, Bt-toxin has triggered immune responses in mice[657] and in farm workers,[635] and allergic- and flu-like symptoms in hundreds of exposed citizens.[660]

The Bt-toxin is produced in GM corn by inserting the toxin-creating gene from the natural soil bacteria. It is not the same, however, as the spray version. It is far worse. It is designed to be more toxic, and produced in concentrations that are thousands of times greater than the spray, and it does not wash off or biodegrade in sunlight, like the natural version does. It is no wonder that an Italian government study showed that mice fed Bt corn had dramatic immune responses.[659] Furthermore, thousands of Indian farm workers who harvest Bt cotton are also experiencing allergic- and flu-like symptoms.[661]

When scientists exposed mice to natural Bt-toxin, not only did they react to the toxin directly, afterwards, their immune systems were triggered by substances that formerly did not cause a response.[662] This illustrates how exposure to one GM food might cause an increase in allergies to many natural foods. One usually sees this phenomena in the chemically sensitive patients.

Genetic Engineering Produces Unexpected New or Increased Allergens

Irrespective of which foreign gene is inserted into a plant, the very process of insertion, followed by cloning that cell into a plant, causes massive collateral damage to the plants' natural DNA. There can be hundreds or thousands of mutations throughout the DNA, and these, in turn, can introduce new allergens or toxins, or elevate levels of existing harmful proteins. Neither GMO companies nor federal regulators screen for most of these types of unexpected side effects, and even if they did, the complexity of possible allergens and allergenic reactions produced would make a truly comprehensive and accurate assessment virtually impossible.

After Monsanto's Bt corn was on the market, independent scientists decided to take a look at the impacts of the insertion process on the expression of natural genes in the corn plant.[663] They found 43 proteins that had been inadvertently increased, decreased, newly introduced, or were completely missing. One of the newly introduced proteins that is not found in the natural corn variety is gamma zein, a known allergen. This means that the corn sold on the U.S. market has an unlabeled new allergen that might be provoking reactions in sensitive consumers.

In a 1996 study by Monsanto in the *Journal of Nutrition*, scientists acknowledge an increase by 27% of a known soy allergen trypsin inhibitor. Since trypsin is a major enzyme produced by the pancreas and used in the breakdown of food proteins, an inhibition of trypsin activity could result in greatly increasing the length of time that allergenic proteins from our diet remain undegraded in the digestive tract. This would allow more time to provoke allergic responses.

The 27% increase was found in raw soybeans. Trypsin inhibitor is usually degraded substantially by cooking. In Monsanto's study, they did cook soybeans and compare the composition of selective components. But for some reason, they chose not to include the results in the paper. The trypsin inhibitor was hardly broken down at all. As a result, it was as much as seven times higher in the cooked GM soy compared to the non-GM version of the identical variety of soybeans.[664]

Others discovered that GM soybeans contain a unique, unexpected protein that was able to bind with IgE antibodies, suggesting that it may provoke dangerous allergic reactions. The same study revealed that one human subject showed a skin prick immune response only to GM soy, but not to natural soy.[21] The results of this research, however, must be considered preliminary, as the non-GM soy control was a "wild" type and not easily comparable to the GM variety. The ideal control soy would have been the same *natural* soy variety as that which had been genetically engineered (isogenic).

HARMLESS PROTEINS CAN TURN HARMFUL IN GMOS

Australian scientists produced a genetically engineered pea with a gene from the kidney bean. The gene produces an antinutrient (α-amylase inhibitor) that interferes with the digestive system of the pea weevil larvae, causing them to starve to death. These bug-killing peas passed all the studies that are usually conducted on GMOs before regulators wave them onto the world market.

But the developers of the peas decided to do one more test that no GM food developer had done before or since. They supplemented mice diets with GM peas, non-GM peas, or kidney beans, then subjected the animals to a battery of tests. Only mice fed GM peas had an immune response to GM protein. In addition, the mice fed the GM peas started to react to egg albumin, while those fed non-GM peas or kidney beans did not.[659] This fact parallels the spreading phenomena that is seen in the severe chemically sensitive patient who continues to be sensitive to more foods the more the treatment is neglected with nonrotation in appropriate diet.

The findings suggest that GM peas might cause allergies in humans, as well as promote reactions to a wide range of other foods. According to Carman, if a GM food was introduced onto supermarket shelves and caused an immune reaction, it would be very difficult to find the culprit, particularly if it caused reactions to other, different foods, as this GM pea was found to do.

What is fascinating about this research is that the identical protein found in its original state, in the kidney bean did not provoke reactions. It was only after the gene was transferred into the peas and the protein was produced in that new environment that it became harmful and potentially deadly. The scientists later discovered that the sugar molecules that often attach to proteins had a subtle difference in their shape. Since sugar attachments are known to trigger reactions, they blamed the mice reaction on this unpredicted side effect of genetic engineering.

No other GM crop is evaluated for the presence or changes in sugar chains. Any of them might be provoking allergic responses, as well as enhancing reactions to other foods formerly considered harmless.

We have observed how gluten sensitivity and celiac disease involve a combination of inflammatory and other immune responses, altered gut bacteria, as well as destruction of intestinal integrity. We have further observed that genetically modified foods may trigger immune reactions, impair gut bacteria, and damage gut integrity and digestive capacity. While there is insufficient research to prove that GMO consumption *causes* gluten sensitivity, the evidence does show how it may, at least, exacerbate the symptoms, or contribute to the conditions that may lead to the development of sensitivity to gluten.

Although 64 countries either ban GMOs outright or require mandatory labeling, the United States is not one of them.

ASSOCIATIONS BETWEEN POLYCYCLIC AROMATIC HYDROCARBON-RELATED EXPOSURES AND *P53* MUTATIONS IN BREAST TUMORS

Breast cancer is the second leading cancer-related cause of death among women in the United States.[665] Previous epidemiologic and experimental investigations suggest that polycyclic aromatic hydrocarbons (PAHs) may be associated with breast cancer.[666–670] However, despite strongly positive associations in animal models and some evidence of a positive association in humans, the carcinogenicity of these chemical compounds on the human breast remains unclear.

PAHs are ubiquitous environmental pollutants formed by incomplete combustion of organic material.[671] These chemicals have estrogenic properties,[672] are known carcinogens in humans[671] and cause mammary tumors in laboratory animals.[667,673] Exposure to PAHs in the general population occurs primarily through charred, smoked, and broiled foods; leafy vegetables[674]; wood- and coal-burning stoves[675]; air pollution[676]; and tobacco smoke.[677] PAH–DNA adducts,[669] lifetime intake of grilled/smoked meat,[678] and long-term passive smoking, but not current or former active smoking,[679] have been associated with breast cancer in our study population. They cause chemical sensitivity even though at times it is not perceived.

Cigarette smoke is associated with PAH–DNA adducts in human lymphocytes,[680] and the PAH benzo[*a*]pyrene (B[*a*]P) from cigarette smoke induces neoplastic transformation of human breast epithelial cells.[681] However, smoking has been inconsistently linked to breast cancer but has in lung cancer and chemical sensitivity in epidemiologic research, with more consistently positive findings reported for long-term passive smoking and among genetically susceptible subgroups.[682–684]

PAHs are formed on the surface of "welldone" meat,[685] but epidemiologic studies examining meat intake or doneness have yielded inconclusive results.[686,687] These studies have primarily focused on recent dietary habits, whereas lifetime intake may be more relevant for carcinogenesis. Steck et al.[678] observed a positive association between lifetime intake of grilled and smoked meat and breast cancer among postmenopausal women (middle vs. lowest tertile of intake, odds ratio [OR] = 1.47; 95% CI, 1.11–1.95; highest vs. lowest tertile of intake, OR = 1.47; 95% CI, 1.12–1.92).

PAHs are metabolized through activation and detoxification pathways. When PAH exposure is high or detoxification is insufficient, PAH–DNA adducts form, including in breast tissue.[688,689] Adducts persist when repair mechanisms are inadequate.[690] Therefore, PAH–DNA adducts reflect both exposure to PAHs and host response—which differs because of variation in metabolism and/or DNA repair capacity between individuals—and are consistently associated with breast cancer in epidemiologic research.[688]

The p53 protein is a transcription factor that regulates cell proliferation, differentiation, apoptosis, and DNA repair and therefore plays an important role in normal cell function and neoplastic transformation.[691] Certain carcinogens may be associated with specific mutation patterns in the *p53* tumor suppressor gene, and these characteristic patterns of DNA damage may contribute information about disease etiology by lending biologic support to exposure–disease associations and by helping to evaluate potential mechanisms of carcinogenesis.[692] Smoking has been associated with breast tumor *p53* mutational spectra.[693] They hypothesized that associations between PAH-related exposures and breast cancer would differ according to tumor *p53* mutation status, effect, type, and number and we investigated this possibility using data from a population-based study.

RESULTS

Associations between PAH-related exposures and selected *p53* mutation types are presented. They were unable to statistically evaluate relations for all mutation types because of small numbers of certain mutations. They found consistently elevated associations between PAH-related exposures and G:C → A:T transitions at CpG sites as well as insertions/deletions. PAH-related exposures showed different directions of association with G:C → A:T transitions at non-CpG sites, A:T → G:C transitions, and G:C → T:A transversions (data not shown). PAH exposures were also inconsistently related to *p53* missense, nonsense, and silent mutations. Frameshift mutations were consistently associated with PAH-related exposures, and these associations were strongest for PAH–DNA adducts. Few effect estimates for mutation type or effect reached statistical significance.

They also examined associations of p53 mutation status with active smoking and lifetime intake of grilled and smoked meat using referent groups consisting of never smokers with low intake of grilled and smoked meat. The use of this approach strengthened associations between

PAH-related factors and p53 mutation–negative cancer, whereas associations with p53 mutation–positive cancer were essentially unchanged. In these analyses, p53 mutation–negative cancer was associated with smoking history (ever vs. never; OR = 1.31; 95% CI, 1.03–1.67), current smoking (OR = 1.43; 95% CI, 1.06–1.93), and lifetime intake of grilled and smoked meat (OR = 1.61; 95% CI, 1.27–2.05).

Relations between PAH-related exposures and G:C → A:T transitions at CpG sites, insertions/deletions, and frameshift mutations were also strengthened by using the alternative referent groups. For example, examining associations between current smoking and insertions/deletions and between grilled and smoked meat intake and G:C → A:T transitions at CpG sites yielded ORs of 3.06 (95% CI, 0.87–10.77) and 2.68 (95% CI, 0.89–8.09), respectively. They did not examine mutation number, A:T → G:C transitions, or :C → T:A transversions due to low numbers of subjects with these mutations. Results were not altered substantially for missense, nonsense, and silent mutations (data not shown). Comparing current smokers who had high lifetime intake of grilled and smoked meat with never smokers who had low intake of grilled and smoked meat yielded ORs of 1.53 (95% CI, 1.07–2.20) for *p53* mutation–negative cancer, 4.24 (95% CI, 1.00–17.94) for G:C → A:T transitions at CpG sites, 4.49 (95% CI, 1.05–19.25) for insertions/deletions, and 4.43 (95% CI, 1.04–18.98) for frameshift mutations.

In this population-based analysis, Mordukhovich et al.[694] found that participants with breast tumor *p53* mutations were less likely to be exposed to PAH-related sources than were participants with *p53* mutation–negative cancer. However, frameshift mutations and number of mutations were consistently elevated in exposed subjects, and tumors of women exposed to PAH-related sources showed a pattern of increased G:C → A:T transitions at CpG sites and insertions/deletions. Associations of PAH-related exposures with *p53* mutation status, type, and effect were strengthened by minimizing PAH exposure in referent groups.

This is the first study to examine associations of dietary PAH intake, PAH–DNA adducts, and passive smoking with breast tumor *p53* mutations. It is the third study to examine associations between active smoking and breast cancer *p53* mutations, and has a larger sample size than the previous investigations.[693,695] Few studies have looked at the relations between exogenous exposures and *p53* mutations in breast cancer, although such research has the potential to provide insights regarding breast cancer etiology.

They found a relatively low prevalence of *p53* mutations (15%) among their participants, which is consistent with the wide range reported in the literature (11%–35%).[695–697] This variation across studies may be due to differences between study populations, such as differences in distribution of age and race.[698,699] Methodologic errors in mutation detection may also have contributed to the modest mutation prevalence. However, they selected a method previously shown to have a high sensitivity[700] and that has been used successfully in various applications, including detection of *p53* mutations in hematologic malignancies.[701]

Immunohistochemical staining estimates p53 protein expression and is widely used as a proxy measure for detection of *p53* mutation status. However, the sensitivity of this method relative to mutation analysis is <75% for breast cancer,[702] and immunohistochemistry is subject to a number of methodologic limitations.[703,704]

Mordukhovich et al.[694] detected overexpression in 36% of tumor samples,[705] which is consistent with the range reported in the literature (30%–40%),[706,707] but they did not find evidence of heterogeneity in the ORs for the associations between PAH-related exposures and p53-positive cancer as defined by protein expression status and the corresponding PAH exposures and p53-negative breast cancer. This is consistent with the results of one study of smoking and p53 overexpression,[708] and inconsistent with two other studies that noted an association between smoking and p53-positive breast cancer among younger women.[709,710] Potential explanations for the discrepant findings across investigations include the inability to identify specific *p53* mutational subtypes when using immunohistochemistry as a proxy, differences in metabolic activation and detoxification of PAHs between study populations, and chance findings.

Conway et al.[693] found that current smokers were more likely and former smokers were less likely than never smokers to have p53 mutation, positive breast cancer. In contrast, they found that both current and former smokers were less likely than never smokers to have p53 mutation–positive cancer. Another epidemiologic study found positive, nonsignificant associations between smoking history and p53 mutation prevalence.[698] However, the number of p53 mutation–positive cases ($n = 34$, mutation prevalence $= 11\%$) was substantially smaller than in their study ($n = 128$, mutation prevalence $= 15\%$) or in the study by Conway et al. ($n = 108$, mutation prevalence $= 24\%$), and the results appeared to be unstable. Reasons potentially underlying inconsistent results between studies include differences in age and race distributions and in metabolism and detoxification of PAHs between study populations, varying definitions of current smoking status, methodologic differences in mutation analysis, and chance findings.[711]

REFERENCES

1. Randolph, T. G. 1962. *Human Ecology and Susceptibility to the Chemical Environment*, p. 71. Springfield, IL: Thomas.
2. Dickey, L. D. 1976. *Clinical Ecology*. Springfield, IL: Charles C. Thomas.
3. Lau, S., R. Nickel, B. Niggemann, C. Grüber, C. Sommerfeld, S. Illi, M. Kulig, J. Forster, U. Wahn. 2002. The development of childhood asthma: Lessons from the German Multicentre Allergy Study (MAS). *Paediatr. Respir. Rev.* 3 (3):265–272. doi: 10.1016/s1526-0542(02)00189-6.
4. Kiyohara, C., K. Tanaka, Y. Miyake. 2008. Genetic susceptibility to atopic dermatitis. *Allergol. Int.* 57 (1):39–56.
5. Sih, T., O. Mion. 2010. Allergic rhinitis in the child and associated comorbidities. *Pediatr. Allergy Immunol.* 21 (1 Pt 2):e107–e113.
6. Rea, W. J. 1992. *Chemical Sensitivity (Volume 1): Tools of Diagnosis and Methods of Treatment*. Boca Raton, FL: CRC Press.
7. Miller, C. S. 1996. Chemical sensitivity: Symptom, syndrome or mechanism for disease? *Toxicology* 111 (1–3):69–86.
8. Cochrane, S. et al. 2009. Factors influencing the incidence and prevalence of food allergy. *Allergy* 64 (9):1246–1255.
9. Isolauri, E., M. Kalliomaki, S. Rautava, S. Salminen, K. Laitinen. 2009. Obesity—extending the hygiene hypothesis. *Nestle Nutr. Workshop* 64:75–89.
10. Nantes Castillejo, O., J. Zozaya, F. Jimenez-Perez, J. Martinez-Penuela, F. Borda. 2009. Incidence and characteristics of eosinophilic esophagitis in adults. *An. Sist. Sanit. Navar.* 32 (2):227–234.
11. Gelincik, A. et al. 2008. Confirmed prevalence of food allergy and non-allergic food hypersensitivity in a Mediterranean population. *Clin. Exp. Allergy* 38 (8):1333–1341.
12. Miller, C. S., N. A. Ashford. 2000. Multiple chemical intolerance and indoor air quality. Chapter 27. In *Indoor Air Quality Handbook*, J. D. Spengler, J. M. Samet, J. F. McCarthy, Eds. New York: McGraw-Hill.
13. Sicherer, S. H., H. A. Sampson. 2010. Food allergy. *J. Allergy Clin. Immunol.* 125 (Suppl 2): S116–S125.
14. Millichap, J. G., M. M. Yee. 2003. The diet factor in pediatric and adolescent migraine. *Pediatr. Neurol.* 28 (1):9–15.
15. Rea, W. J., Y. Pan, E. J. Fenyves, I. Sujisawa, N. Suyama, G. H. Ross. 1991. Electromagnetic field sensitivity. *J. Bioelectr.* 10:241–256.
16. Bjorksten, B. 2009. The hygiene hypothesis: Do we still believe in it? *Nestle Nutr. Workshop Ser.* 64:11–22.
17. Kalliomaki, M., E. Isolauri. 2002. Pandemic of atopic diseases—A lack of microbial exposure in early infancy? *Curr. Drug Targets* 2 (3):193–199.
18. Maarsingh, H., J. Zaagsma, H. Meurs. 2008. Arginine homeostasis in allergic asthma. *Eur. J. Pharmacol.* 585 (2–3):375–384.
19. Meurs, H., H. Maarsingh, J. Zaagsma. 2003. Arginase and asthma: Novel insights into nitric oxide homeostasis and airway hyperresponsiveness. *Trends Pharmacol. Sci.* 24 (9):450–455.
20. D'Amato, G., G. Liccardi, M. D'Amato, S. Holgate. 2005. Environmental risk factors and allergic bronchial asthma. *Clin. Exp. Allergy* 35 (9):1113–1124.
21. Yum, H. Y., S. Y. Lee, K. E. Lee, M. H. Sohn, K. E. Kim. 2005. Genetically modified and wild soybeans: An immunologic comparison. *Allergy Asthma Proc.* 26 (3):210–216.

22. D'Amato, G., L. Cecchi. 2008. Effects of climate change on environmental factors in respiratory allergic diseases. *Clin. Exp. Allergy* 38 (8):1264–1274.

23. van den Oord, R. A., A. Sheikh. 2009. Filaggrin gene defects and risk of developing allergic sensitisation and allergic disorders: Systematic review and meta-analysis. *BMJ* 339:b2433.

24. Gold, D. R., R. Wright. 2005. Population disparities in asthma. *Annu. Rev. Public Health* 26:89–113.

25. Bell, I. R., M. Walsh, A. Gross, J. Gersmeyer, G. Schwartz, P. Kanof. 1997. Cognitive dysfunction and disability in geriatric veterans with self-reported intolerance to environmental chemicals. *J. Chron. Fatigue Syndr.* 3 (3):15–42.

26. Fukuda, K. et al. 1998. Chronic multisymptom illness affecting Air Force veterans of the Gulf War. *JAMA* 280 (11):981–988.

27. Fiedler, N., H. Kipen, B. Natelson, J. Ottenweller. 1996. Chemical sensitivities and the Gulf War: Department of Veterans Affairs Research Center in basic and clinical science studies of environmental hazards. *Regul. Toxicol. Pharmacol.* 24 (1 Pt 2):S129–S138.

28. Fiedler, N., N. Giardino, B. Natelson, J. E. Ottenweller, C. Weisel, P. Lioy, P. Lehrer, P. Ohman-Strickland, K. Kelly-Mcneil, H. Kipen. 2004. Responses to controlled diesel vapor exposure among chemically sensitive Gulf War veterans. *Psychosom. Med.* 66 (4):588–598.

29. Reid, S., M. Hotopf, L. Hull, K. Ismail, C. Unwin, S. Wessely. 2002. Reported chemical sensitivities in a health survey of United Kingdom military personnel. *Occup. Environ. Med.* 59 (3):196–198.

30. Nemery, B. 1996. Late consequences of accidental exposure to inhaled irritants: RADS and the Bhopal disaster. *Eur. Respir. J.* 9 (10):1973–1976.

31. Cone, J. E., T. A. Sult. 1992. Acquired intolerance to solvents following pesticide/solvent exposure in a building: A new group of workers at risk for multiple chemical sensitivities? *Toxicol. Ind. Health* 8 (4):29–39.

32. Welch, L. S., R. Sokas. 1992. Development of multiple chemical sensitivity after an outbreak of sick-building syndrome. *Toxicol. Ind. Health* 8 (4):47–50.

33. Simon, G. E., W. J. Katon, P. J. Sparks. 1990. Allergic to life: Psychological factors in environmental illness. *Am. J. Psychiatry* 147 (7):901–906.

34. Tabershaw, I. R., W. C. Cooper. 1966. Sequelae of acute organic phosphate poisoning. *J. Occup. Med.* 8 (1):5–20.

35. Gauderman, W. J., E. Avol, F. Lurmann, N. Kuenzli, F. Gilliland, J. Peters, R. Mcconnell. 2005. Childhood asthma and exposure to traffic and nitrogen dioxide. *Epidemiology* 16 (6):737–743.

36. Pall, M. L. 2007. *Explaining 'Unexplained Illness': Disease Paradigm for Chronic Fatigue Syndrome, Multiple Chemical Sensitivity, Fibromyalgia; Post-Traumatic Stress Disorder, Gulf War Syndrome and Others.* New York: Harrington Park Press.

37. Hennies, K., H.-P. Neitzke, H. Voigt. 2000. Mobile telecommunications and health.

38. Zibrowski, E. M., J. M. Robertson. 2006. Olfactory sensitivity in medical laboratory workers occupationally exposed to organic solvent mixtures. *Occup. Med.* 56 (1):51–54.

39. Yu, I. T., N. L. Lee, X. H. Zhang, W. Q. Chen, Y. T. Lam, T. W. Wong. 2004. Occupational exposure to mixtures of organic solvents increases the risk of neurological symptoms among printing workers in Hong Kong. *J. Occup. Environ. Med.* 46 (4):323–330.

40. Moen, B., B. Hollund, T. Riise. 2008. Neurological symptoms among dental assistants: A crosssectional study. *J. Occup. Med. Toxicol.* 3:10.

41. Rea, W. J., J. R. Butler, J. L. Laseter, I. R. DeLeon. 1984. Pesticides and brain function changes in a controlled environment. *Clin. Ecol.* 2 (3):145–150.

42. Rea, W. J. 1976. Environmentally triggered thrombophlebitis. *Ann. Allergy* 37 (2):101–109.

43. Brautbar, N., A. Campbell, A. Vojdani. 1995. Silicone breast implants and autoimmunity: Causation, association, or myth? *J. Biomater. Sci.* 7 (2):133–145.

44. Miller, C. S., T. J. Prihoda. 1999. A controlled comparison of symptoms and chemical intolerances reported by Gulf War veterans, implant recipients and persons with multiple chemical sensitivity. *Toxicol. Ind. Health* 15 (3–4):386–397.

45. Steyn, P. S., W. C. Gelderblom, G. S. Shephard, F. R. van Heerden. 2009. Mycotoxins with a special focus on aflatoxins, ochratoxins and fumonisins (Part 14, Chapter 146). In *General and Applied Toxicology*, 3rd ed., B. Ballantyne, T. C. Marrs, T. Syversen, Eds. New Jersey: Wiley.

46. Barnes, J. G. 2001. "Sensitivity syndromes" related to radiation exposures. *Med Hypotheses* 57 (4):453–458.

47. Gordon, M. 1987. Reactions to chemical fumes in radiology departments. *Radiography* 53 (608):85–89.

48. Ashford, N., C. Miller. 1998. *Chemical Exposures: Low Levels and High Stakes*, 2nd ed. New York: John Wiley and Sons.

49. Lax, M. B., P. K. Henneberger. 1995. Patients with multiple chemical sensitivities in an occupational health clinic: Presentation and follow-up. *Arch. Environ. Health* 50 (6):425–431.

50. Miller, C. S., H. C. Mitzel. 1995. Chemical sensitivity attributed to pesticide exposure versus remodeling. *Arch. Environ. Health* 50 (2):119–129.

51. Rogers, W. R., C. S. Miller, L. Bunegin. 1999. A rat model of neurobehavioral sensitization to toluene. *Toxicol. Ind. Health* 15 (3–4):356–369.

52. Overstreet, D. H., C. S. Miller, D. S. Janowsky, R. W. Russell. 1996. Potential animal model of multiple chemical sensitivity with cholinergic supersensitivity. *Toxicology* 111 (1–3): 119–134.

53. Sorg, B. A., T. Hochstatter. 1999. Behavioral sensitization after repeated formaldehyde exposure in rats. *Toxicol. Ind. Health* 15 (3–4):346–355.

54. Lee, T. G. 2003. Health symptoms caused by molds in a courthouse. *Arch. Environ. Health* 58 (7):442–446.

55. Pestka, J. J., I. Yike, D. G. Dearborn, M. D. Ward, J. R. Harkema. 2008. Stachybotrys chartarum, trichothecene mycotoxins, and damp building-related illness: New insights into a public health enigma. *Toxicol. Sci.* 104 (1):4–26.

56. Mahmoudi, M., M. E. Gershwin. 2000. Sick building syndrome. III. Stachybotrys chartarum. *J. Asthma* 37 (2):191–198.

57. Hintikka, E. L. 2004. The role of stachybotrys in the phenomenon known as sick building syndrome. *Adv. Appl. Microbiol.* 55:155–173.

58. Ziem, G., J. McTamney. 1997. Profile of patients with chemical injury and sensitivity. *Environ. Health Perspect.* 105 (Suppl 2):417–436.

59. Kilburn, K. H. 2003. Effects of hydrogen sulfide on neurobehavioral function. *South Med. J.* 96 (7):639–646.

60. Stejskal, V., J. Stejskal. 2006. Toxic metals as a key factor in disease. *Forword. Neuro. Endocrinol. Lett.* 27 (Suppl 1):3–4.

61. Stejskal, V. D., A. Danersund, A. Lindvall, R. Hudecek, V. Nordman, A. Yaqob, W. Mayer, W. Bieger, U. Lindh. 1999. Metalspecific lymphocytes: Biomarkers of sensitivity in man. *Neuro. Endocrinol. Lett.* 20 (5):289–298.

62. Miller, C. S. 1999. Are we on the threshold of a new theory of disease? Toxicant-induced loss of tolerance and its relationship to addiction and abdiction. *Toxicol. Ind. Health* 15 (3–4):284–294.

63. Rea, W. J. 1997. *Chemical Sensitivity (Volume 4): Tools of Diagnosis and Methods of Treatment.* Boca Raton, FL: Lewis Publishers.

64. Miller, C. S. 1997. Toxicant-induced loss of tolerance—An emerging theory of disease? *Environ. Health Perspect.* 105 (Suppl 2):445–453.

65. Sorg, B. A., J. R. Willis, R. E. See, B. Hopkins, H. H. Westberg. 1998. Repeated low-level formaldehyde exposure produces cross-sensitization to cocaine: Possible relevance to chemical sensitivity in humans. *Neuropsychopharmacology* 18 (5):385–394.

66. Kalinina, N. H., I. D. Nikiforova, K. A. Syssoev, V. A. Sidorenko. 1999. Immunological aspects of osteoporosis in Chernobyl cleanup workers. Conference proceedings. *International Conference on the Effects of Low and Very Low Doses of Ionizing Radiation on Human Health.* June 16–18.

67. Sears, M. 2007. The medical perspective on environmental sensitivities. Government of Canada: Canadian Human Rights Commission (available at http://www.chrc-ccdp.ca/research_program_recherche/esensitivities_hypersensibilitee/toc_tdm-en.asp] Accessed Oct 11, 2009.)

68. Miller, C. S., T. J. Prihoda. 1999. The Environmental Exposure and Sensitivity Inventory (EESI): A standardized approach for measuring chemical intolerances for research and clinical applications. *Toxicol. Ind. Health* 15:370–385.

69. Randolph, T. G., R. Moss. 1980. *An Alternative Approach to Allergies.* New York: Lippincott & Crowell.

70. Postolache, T. T., S. Zimmerman, M. Lapidus, J. Cabassa, D. D'agostino, P. Langenberg, L. Tonelli. 2009. Changes in severity of allergy and anxiety symptoms are positively correlated in patients with recurrent mood disorders who are exposed to seasonal peaks of aeroallergens. *J. Allergy Clin. Immunol.* 123 (2):313–322.

71. Potera, C. 2010. Will ocean acidification erode the base of the food web? *Environ. Health Perspect.* 118 (4):118a–157.

72. Shi, D. L., Y. Xu, B. M. Hopkinson, F. M. M. Morel. 2010. Effect of ocean acidification on iron availability to marine phytoplankton. *Science* 327:676–679.

73. Sunda, W. G., S. A. Huntsman. 1992. Feedback interactions between zinc and phytoplankton in seawater. *Limnol. Oceanogr.* 37:25–40.

74. Belles-Isles, M., P. Ayotte, E. Dewailly, J. P. Weber, R. Roy. 2002. Cord blood lymphocyte functions in newborns from a remote maritime population exposed to organochlorines and methylmercury. *J. Toxicol. Environ. Health A* 65 (2):165–182.

75. Bilrha, H., R. Roy, B. Moreau, M. Belles-Isles, E. Dewailly, P. Ayotte. 2003. In vitro activation of cord blood mononuclear cells and cytokine production in a remote coastal population exposed to organochlorines and methyl mercury. *Environ. Health Perspect.* 111:1952–1957.

76. Heilmann, C., P. Grandjean, P. Weihe, F. Nielsen, E. BudtzJorgensen. 2006. Reduced antibody responses to vaccinations in children exposed to polychlorinated biphenyls. *PLoS Med.* 3 (8):e311.

77. Dietert, R. R. 2008. Developmental immunotoxicology (DIT): Windows of vulnerability, immune dysfunction and safety assessment. *J. Immunotoxicol.* 5 (4):401–412.

78. Bergmann, R. L., T. L. Diepgen, O. Kuss, K. E. Bergmann, J. Kujat, J. W. Dudenhausen, U. Wahn. 2002. Breastfeeding duration is a risk factor for atopic eczema. *Clin. Exp. Allergy* 32 (2):205–209.

79. Kirsten, G. F. 2009. Does breastfeeding prevent atopic disorders? *Curr. Allergy Clin. Immunol.* 22 (1):24–26.

80. Kramer, M. S., L. Matush, I. Vanilovich, R. Platt, N. Bogdanovich, Z. Sevkovskaya, et al. 2007. Effect of prolonged and exclusive breast feeding on risk of allergy and asthma: Cluster randomised trial. *BMJ* 335 (7624):815.

81. van Odijk, J., I. Kull, M. P. Borres, P. Brandtzaeg, U. Edberg, L. A. Hanson, A. Høst, M. Kuitunen, S. F. Olsen, S. Skerfving, J. Sundell, S. Wille. 2003. Breastfeeding and allergic disease: A multidisciplinary review of the literature (1966–2001) on the mode of early feeding in infancy and its impact on later atopic manifestations. *Allergy* 58 (9):833–843.

82. Kerkvliet, N. I. 2009. AHR-mediated immunomodulation: The role of altered gene transcription. *Biochem. Pharmacol.* 77 (4):746–760.

83. Grandjean, P., P. Weihe, L. Needham, V. Burse, D. Patterson, E. Sampson, P. Jorgensen, M. Vahter. 1995. Relation of a seafood diet to mercury, selenium, arsenic, and polychlorinated biphenyl and other organochlorine concentrations in human milk. *Environ. Res.* 71 (1):29–38.

84. Barr, D. B., P. Weihe, M. D. Davis, L. L. Needham, P. Grandjean. 2006. Serum polychlorinated biphenyl and organochlorine insecticide concentrations in a Faroese birth cohort. *Chemosphere* 62 (7):1167–1182.

85. Patandin, S., N. Weisglas-Kuperus, M. A. de Ridder, C. Koopman-Esseboom, W. A. van Staveren, C. G. van der Paauw, P. J. Sauer. 1997. Plasma polychlorinated biphenyl levels in Dutch preschool children either breast-fed or formula-fed during infancy. *Am. J. Public Health* 87 (10):1711–1714.

86. Krause, T. G., A. Koch, L. K. Poulsen, B. Kristensen, O. R. Olsen, M. Melbye. 2002. Atopic sensitization among children in an arctic environment. *Clin. Exp. Allergy* 32 (3):367–372.

87. Krause, T., A. Koch, J. Friborg, L. K. Poulsen, B. Kristensen, M. Melbye. 2002. Frequency of atopy in the Arctic in 1987 and 1998. *Lancet* 360 (9334):691–692.

88. Grandjean, P., L. K. Poulsen, C. Heilmann, U. Steuerwald, P. Weihe. 2010. Allergy and sensitization during childhood associated with prenatal and lactational exposure to marine pollutants. *Environ. Health Perspect.* 118 (10):1429–1433.

89. Steuerwald, U., P. Weihe, P. J. Jorgensen, K. Bjerve, J. Brock, B. Heinzow, E. Budtz-Jørgensen, P. Grandjean. 2000. Methylmercury exposure and health effects in humans: A worldwide concern. *J. Pediatr.* 136 (5):599–605.

90. Grandjean, P., P. J. Jorgensen, P. Weihe. 1994. Human milk as a source of methylmercury exposure in infants. *Environ. Health Perspect.* 102:74–77.

91. Weinmayr, G. et al. 2009. International variations in associations of allergic markers and diseases in children: ISAAC phase two. *Allergy* 65 (6):766–775.

92. Clausen, M., S. Kristjansson, A. Haraldsson, B. Bjorksten. 2008. High prevalence of allergic diseases and sensitization in a low allergen country. *Acta Paediatr.* 97 (9):1216–1220.

93. Nagayama, J., H. Tsuji, T. Iida, R. Nakagawa, T. Matsueda, H. Hirakawa, T. Yanagawa, J. Fukushige, T. Watanabe. 2007. Immunologic effects of perinatal exposure to dioxins, pcbs and organochlorine pesticides in Japanese infants. *Chemosphere* 67 (9):S393–S398.

94. Poulsen, L. K., L. Hummelshoj. 2007. Triggers of IgE class switching and allergy development. *Ann. Med.* 39 (6):440–456.

95. Tusscher, G., W. Ten, P. A. Steerenberg, H. Van Loveren, J. G. Vos, A. Egk Von Dem Borne, M. Westra, J. W. Van Der Slikke, K. Olie, H. J. Pluim, J. G. Koppe. 2003. Persistent hematologic and immunologic disturbances in 8-year-old dutch children associated with perinatal dioxin exposure. *Environ. Health Perspect.* 111 (12):1519–1523.

96. Strachan, D. P., D. G. Cook. 1998. Health effects of passive smoking. 5. Parental smoking and allergic sensitisation in children. *Thorax* 53 (2):117–123.

97. van Den Heuvel, R. L., G. Koppen, J. A. Staessen, E. D. Hond, G. Verheyen, T. S. Nawrot, H. A. Roels, R. Vlietinck, G. Schoeters. 2002. Immunologic biomarkers in relation to exposure markers of pcbs and dioxins in Flemish adolescents (Belgium). *Environ. Health Perspect.* 110 (6):595–600.

98. Nielsen, J. B., P. Hultman. 2002. Mercury-induced autoimmunity in mice. *Environ. Health Perspect.* 110 (suppl 5):877–881.

99. de Vos G., S. Abotaga, Z. Liao, E. Jerschow, D. Rosenstreich. 2007. Selective effect of mercury on Th2-type cytokine production in humans. *Immunopharmacol. Immunotoxicol.* 29 (3–4):537–548.

100. Heilmann, C., E. Budtz-Jorgensen, F. Nielsen, B. Heinzow, P. Weihe, P. Grandjean. 2010. Serum concentrations of antibodies against vaccine toxoids in children exposed perinatally to immunotoxicants. *Environ. Health Perspect.* 118:1434–1438.

101. Furuhjelm, C., K. Warstedt, J. Larsson, M. Fredriksson, M. Fagerås Böttcher, K. Fälth-Magnusson, K. Duchén. 2009. Fish oil supplementation in pregnancy and lactation may decrease the risk of infant allergy. *Acta Paediatr.* 98 (9):1461–1467.

102. Longnecker, M. P. et al. 2002. Comparison of polychlorinated biphenyl levels across studies of human neurodevelopment. *Environ. Health Perspect.* 111 (1):65–70.

103. Dietert, R. R. 2008. Developmental immunotoxicology (DIT): Windows of vulnerability, immune dysfunction and safety assessment. *J. Immunotoxicol.* 5 (4):401–412.

104. Wright, A. L., D. Sherrill, C. J. Holberg, M. Halonen, F. D. Martinez. 1999. Breast-feeding, maternal IgE, and total serum IgE in childhood. *J. Allergy Clin. Immunol.* 104 (3 pt 1):589–594.

105. Satwani, H., A. Rehman, S. Ashraf, A. Hassan. 2009. Is serum total IgE levels a good predictor of allergies in children? *J. Pak. Med. Assoc.* 59 (10):698–702.

106. Daniluk, U., M. Kaczmarski, K. Sidor. 2008. Chosen factors and high total concentration of immunoglobulin E (IgE) in children. *Pol. J. Environ. Stud.* 17 (4):473–478.

107. Giwercman, C., L. B. Halkjaer, S. M. Jensen, K. Bonnelykke, L. Lauritzen, H. Bisgaard. 2010. Increased risk of eczema but reduced risk of early wheezy disorder from exclusive breast-feeding in high-risk infants. *J. Allergy Clin. Immunol.* 125 (4):866–871.

108. Bach, J. F. 2002. The effect of infections on susceptibility to autoimmune and allergic diseases. *N. Engl. J. Med.* 347 (12):911–920.

109. Prince, M. M., A. M. Ruder, M. J. Hein, M. A. Waters, E. A. Whelan, N. Nilsen, E. M. Ward, T. M. Schnorr, P. A. Laber, K. E. Davis-King. 2006. Mortality and exposure response among 14,458 electrical capacitor manufacturing workers exposed to polychlorinated biphenyls (PCBs). *Environ. Health Perspect.* 114 (10):1508–1514.

110. Norstrom, K., G. Czub, M. S. McLachlan, D. Hu, P. S. Thorne, K. C. Hornbuckle. 2009. External exposure and bioaccumulation of PCBs in humans living in a contaminated urban environment. *Environ. Int.* doi: 10.1016/j.envint.2009.03.005 (Online 24 April 2009).

111. Schneider, A. R., E. T. Porter, J. E. Baker. 2007. Polychlorinated biphenyl release from resuspended Hudson River sediment. *Environ. Sci. Technol.* 41:1097–1103.

112. Leoni, V. et al. 1989. PCB and other organochlorine compounds in blood of women with or without miscarriage: A hypothesis of correlation. *Ecotoxicol. Environ. Safety* 17 (1):1–11.

113. Jorissen, J. 2007. Literature review. Outcomes associated with postnatal exposure to polychlorinated biphenyls (PCBs) via breast milk. *Adv. Neonatal Care* 7:230–237.

114. Glynn, A., A. Thuvander, M. Aune, A. Johannisson, P. Darnerud, G. Ronquist, S. Cnattingius. 2008. Immune cell counts and risks of respiratory infections among infants exposed pre- and postnatally to organochlorine compounds: A prospective study. *Environ. Health* 7 (1):62.

115. Glauert, H. P., J. C. Tharappel, S. Banerjee, N. L. Chan, I. Kania-Korwel, H. Lehmler, E. Y. Lee, L. W. Robertson, B. T. Spear. 2008. Inhibition of the promotion of hepatocarcinogenesis by 2,2′,4,4′,5,5′-hexachlorobiphenyl (PCB-153) by the deletion of the p50 subunit of NF-κb in mice. *Toxicol. Appl. Pharmacol.* 232 (2):302–308.

116. Lehmann, L., H. L. Esch, P. A. Kirby, L. W. Robertson, G. Ludewig. 2007. 4-Monochlorobiphenyl (PCB3) induces mutations in the livers of transgenic Fisher 344 rats. *Carcinogenesis* 28:471–478.

117. Hopf, N. B., M. A. Waters, A. M. Ruder. 2009. Cumulative exposure estimates for polychlorinated biphenyls using a job-exposure matrix. *Chemosphere* 76:185–193.

118. Knerr, S., D. Schrenk. 2006. Carcinogenicity of "nondioxin-like" polychlorinated biphenyls. *Crit. Rev. Toxicol.* 36:663–694.

119. Loomis, D., S. R. Browning, A. P. Schenck, E. Gregory, D. A. Savitz. 1997. Cancer mortality among electric utility workers exposed to polychlorinated biphenyls. *Occup. Environ. Med.* 54:720–728.

120. Robinson, C. F., M. Petersen, S. Palu. 1999. Mortality patterns among electrical workers employed in the U.S. construction industry, 1982–1987. *Am. J. Ind. Med.* 36:630–637.

121. Sinks, T., G. Steele, A. B. Smith, K. Watkins, R. A. Shults. 1992. Mortality among workers exposed to polychlorinated biphenyls. *Am. J. Epidemiol.* 136:389–398.

122. Caudle, W. M., J. R. Richardson, K. C. Delea, T. S. Guillot, M. Wang, K. D. Pennell, G. W. Miller. 2006. Polychlorinated biphenyl-induced reduction of dopamine transporter expression as a precursor to Parkinson's disease-associated dopamine toxicity. *Toxicol. Sci.* 92:490–499.

123. Saghir, S. A., L. G. Hansen, K. R. Holmes, P. R. Kodavanti. 2000. Differential and non-uniform tissue and brain distribution of two distinct 14C-hexachlorobiphenyls in weanling rats. *Toxicol. Sci.* 54:60–70.

124. Sipka, S., S. Eum, K. W. Son, S. Xu, V. G. Gavalas, B. Hennig, M. Toborek. 2008. Oral administration of pcbs induces proinflammatory and prometastatic responses. *Environ. Toxicol. Pharmacol.* 25 (2):251–259.

125. Seelbach, M., L. Chen, A. Powell, Y. Jung Choi, B. Zhang, B. Hennig, M. Toborek. 2009. Polychlorinated biphenyls disrupt blood–brain barrier integrity and promote brain metastasis formation. *Environ. Health Perspect.* 118 (4):479–484.

126. Choi, W., S. Y. Eum, Y. W. Lee, B. Hennig, L. W. Robertson, M. Toborek. 2003. PCB 104-induced proinflammatory reactions in human vascular endothelial cells: Relationship to cancer metastasis and atherogenesis. *Toxicol. Sci.* 75:47–56.

127. Eum, S. Y., I. E. András, P. O. Couraud, B. Hennig, M. Toborek. 2008. PCBs and tight junction expression. *Environ. Toxicol. Pharmacol.* 25:234–240.

128. Eum, S. Y., Y. W. Lee, B. Hennig, M. Toborek. 2004. VEGF regulates PCB 104-mediated stimulation of permeability and transmigration of breast cancer cells in human microvascular endothelial cells. *Exp. Cell Res.* 296:231–244.

129. Abbott, N. J., L. Ronnback, E. Hansson. 2006. Astrocyte-endothelial interactions at the blood-brain barrier. *Nat. Rev. Neurosci.* 7:41–53.

130. Weiss, N., F. Miller, S. Cazaubon, P. O. Couraud. 2009. The blood–brain barrier in brain homeostasis and neurological diseases. *Biochim. Biophys. Acta* 1788:842–857.

131. Hennig, B., G. Reiterer, Z. Majkova, E. Oesterling, P. Meerarani, M. Toborek. 2005. Modification of environmental toxicity by nutrients: Implications in atherosclerosis. *Cardiovasc. Toxicol.* 5:153–160.

132. Safe, S. 1989. Polychlorinated biphenyls (PCBs): Mutagenicity and carcinogenicity. *Mutat. Res.* 220:31–47.

133. Faroon, O., D. Jones, C. de Rosa. 2001. Effects of polychlorinated biphenyls on the nervous system. *Toxicol. Ind. Health* 16:305–333.

134. Grandjean, P. et al. 2001. Neurobehavioral deficits associated with PCB in 7-year-old children prenatally exposed to seafood neurotoxicants. *Neurotoxicol. Teratol.* 23 (4):305–317.

135. Petersen, M. S., J. Halling, S. Bech, L. Wermuth, P. Weihe, F. Nielsen, P. J. Jørgensen, E. Budtz-Jørgensen, P. Grandjean. 2008. Impact of dietary exposure to food contaminants on the risk of Parkinson's disease. *Neurotoxicology* 29 (4):584–590.

136. Steenland, K., M. J. Hein, R. T. Cassinelli, M. M. Prince, N. B. Nilsen, E. A. Whelan, M. A. Waters, A. M. Ruder, T. M. Schnorr. 2006. Polychlorinated biphenyls and neurodegenerative disease mortality in an occupational cohort. *Epidemiology* 17 (1):8–13.

137. Eum, S. Y., Y. W. Lee, B. Hennig, M. Toborck. 2006. Interplay between epidermal growth factor receptor and Janus kinase 3 regulates polychlorinated biphenyl-induced matrix metalloproteinase-3 expression and transendothelial migration of tumor cells. *Mol. Cancer Res.* 4:361–370.

138. Hestermann, E. V., J. J. Stegeman, M. E. Hahn. 2000. Relative contributions of affinity and intrinsic efficacy to aryl hydrocarbon receptor ligand potency. *Toxicol. Appl. Pharmacol.* 168:160–172.

139. Hassoun, E. A., H. Wang, A. Abushaban, S. J. Stohs. 2002. Induction of oxidative stress in the tissues of rats after chronic exposure to TCDD, 2,3,4,7,8-pentachlorodibenzofuran, and 3,3′,4,4′,5-pentachlorobiphenyl. *J. Toxicol. Environ. Health A* 65:825–842.

140. Hennig, B., P. Meerarani, R. Slim, M. Toborek, A. Daugherty, A. E. Silverstone, L. W. Robertson. 2002. Proinflammatory properties of coplanar PCBs: In vitro and *in vivo* evidence. *Toxicol. Appl. Pharmacol.* 181 (3):174–183.

141. Haorah, J., S. H. Ramirez, K. Schall, D. Smith, R. Pandya, Y. Persidsky. 2007. Oxidative stress activates protein tyrosine kinase and matrix metalloproteinases leading to blood-brain barrier dysfunction. *J. Neurochem.* 101:566–576.

142. Persidsky, Y., D. Heilman, J. Haorah, M. Zelivyanskaya, R. Persidsky, G. A. Weber, H. Shimokawa, K. Kaibuchi, T. Ikezu. 2006. Rho-mediated regulation of tight junctions during monocyte migration across the blood–brain barrier in HIV-1 encephalitis (HIVE). *Blood* 107:4770–4780.

143. András, I. E., H. Pu, J. Tian, M. A. Deli, A. Nath, B. Hennig, M. Toborek. 2005. Signaling mechanisms of hiv-1 tat-induced alterations of claudin-5 expression in brain endothelial cells. *J. Cereb. Blood Flow Metab.* 25 (9):1159–1170.

144. Zhong, Y., E. J. Smart, B. Weksler, P. O. Couraud, B. Hennig, M. Toborek. 2008. Caveolin-1 regulates human immunodeficiency virus-1 Tat-induced alterations of tight junction protein expression via modulation of the Ras signaling. *J. Neurosci.* 28:7788–7796.

145. Krizbai, I. A., H. Bauer, N. Bresgen, P. M. Eckl, A. Farkas, E. Szatmári, A. Traweger, K. Wejksza, H. Bauer. 2005. Effect of oxidative stress on the junctional proteins of cultured cerebral endothelial cells. *Cell Mol. Neurobiol.* 25 (1):129–139.

146. Schreibelt, G. et al. 2007. Reactive oxygen species alter brain endothelial tight junction dynamics via RhoA, PI3 kinase, and PKB signaling. *FASEB J.* 21 (13):3666–3676.

147. Fidler, I. J., G. Schackert, R. D. Zhang, R. Radinsky, T. Fujimaki. 1999. The biology of melanoma brain metastasis. *Cancer Metastasis Rev.* 18:387–400.

148. Gonzalez-Martinez, J., L. Hernandez, L. Zamorano, A. Sloan, K. Levin, S. Lo, Q. Li, F. Diaz. 2002. Gamma knife radiosurgery for intracranial metastatic melanoma: A 6-year experience. *J. Neurosurg.* 97:494–498.

149. Geller, A. C., D. R. Miller, G. D. Annas, M. F. Demierre, B. A. Gilchrest, H. K. Koh. 2002. Melanoma incidence and mortality among US whites, 1969–1999. *JAMA* 288:1719–1720.

150. Chen, L., K. R. Swartz, M. Toborek. 2009. Vessel microport technique for applications in cerebrovascular research. *J. Neurosci. Res.* 87:1718–1727.

151. Zhang, Z., T. Hatori, H. Nonaka. 2008. An experimental model of brain metastasis of lung carcinoma. *Neuropathology* 28:24–28.

152. Palmieri, D., A. F. Chambers, B. Felding-Habermann, S. Huang, P. S. Steeg. 2007. The biology of metastasis to a sanctuary site. *Clin. Cancer Res.* 13:1656–1662.

153. Rolland, Y., M. Demeule, L. Fenart, R. Béliveau. 2009. Inhibition of melanoma brain metastasis by targeting melanotransferrin at the cell surface. *Pigment Cell Melanoma Res.* 22:86–98.

154. Litten, S. 2009. Toxics Chemicals in NYS Tributaries to Lake Ontario: A Report on Sampling Undertaken in 2007 and 2008 with Special Emphasis on the Polychlorinated Dibenzodioxins and Furans. Report to the U.S. Environmental Protection Agency. March 2009.

155. Coleates, R., S. Hale. 2009. Field Data Report: Lake Ontario Tributaries 2007–2008. USEPA.

156. Richards, R. P., D. V. Eckhardt. 2006. *Tributary Loadings of Priority Pollutants to Lake Ontario: A Prototype Approach Employing Surrogate Parameters.* USEPA Grant #GL982840-03-0. Prepared for USEPA, Region 2.

157. Atkinson, J. F., J. V. DePinto, K. Beljan, E. Verhamme, W. M. Larson. 2008. *TMDL Development for PCBs in Lake Ontario.* Final Report Submitted to USEPA-Region 2, New York, New York, in Partial Fulfillment of Project No. 92768806 (97 pp).

158. U.S. EPA. 1998. Integrated Risk Information System: Polychlorinated Biphenyls (PCBs). Last Revised on 01/02/1998. Accessed April 05, 2016. http://www.epa.gov/iris/subst/0294.htm.

159. U.S. Environmental Protection Agency (U.S. EPA). 2007. Contaminants in Top Predator Fish. *Great Lakes National Program Office.* Accessed April 05, 2016. http://www.epa.gov/glnpo/glindicators/fish-toxics/topfishb.html#Contaminant%20Concent rations%20in%20Top%20Predator%20Fish.

160. Environment Canada (EC) and U.S. Environmental Protection Agency (U.S. EPA). 2005. *State of the Great Lakes 2005.* Environment Canada (En161-3/0-2005E) and the United States Environmental Protection Agency (EPA 905-R-06-001). Accessed April 05, 2016. http://binational.net/solec/English/SOLEC%202004/Tagged%20PDFs/SOGL%202005%20Report/English%20Version/Complete%20Report.pdf.

161. United States and Canada. 1987. Great Lakes Water Quality Agreement of 1978, as amended by Protocol signed November 18, 1987. Ottawa and Washington. Accessed April 05, 2016. http://www.epa.gov/glnpo/glwqa/1978/index.html.

162. U.S. EPA. 2005. National Coastal Condition Report II. Office of Research and Development/ Office of Water. EPA-620/R-03/002. December 2004. Accessed April 05, 2016. http://www.epa.gov/owow/oceans/nccr/2005/index.html.

163. Environment Canada and the United States Environmental Protection Agency. State of the Great Lakes. 2003. Accessed April 05, 2016. http://www.epa.gov/glnpo/solec/solec_2002/State_of_the_Great_Lakes_2003_Summary_ Report.pdf.

164. Weseloh, D., V. Chip, C. Pekarik, S. R. De Solla. 2006. Spatial patterns and rankings of contaminant concentrations in herring gull eggs, from 15 sites in the Great Lakes and connecting channels, 1998–2002. *Environ. Monit. Assess.* 113:265–284.

165. Schreiber, T., K. Gassmann, C. Götz, U. Hübenthal, M. Moors, G. Krause, H. F. Merk, N. Nguyen, T. S. Scanlan, J. Abel, C. R. Rose, E. Fritsche. 2009. Polybrominated diphenyl ethers induce developmental neurotoxicity in a human *in vitro* model: Evidence for endocrine disruption. *Environ. Health Perspect.* 118 (4):572–578.

166. Moors, M., T. Dino Rockel, J. Abel, J. E. Cline, K. Gassmann, T. Schreiber, J. Schuwald, N. Weinmann, E. Fritsche. 2009. Human neurospheres as three-dimensional cellular systems for developmental neurotoxicity testing. *Environ. Health Perspect.* 117 (7):1131–1138.

167. Roze, E., L. Meijer, A. Bakker, K. N. Van Braeckel, P. J. Sauer, A. F. Bos. 2009. Prenatal exposure to organohalogens, including brominated flame retardants, influences motor, cognitive, and behavioral performance at school age. *Environ. Health Perspect.* 117:1953–1958.

168. Herbstman, J., A. Sjödin, M. Kurzon, S. Lederman, R. Jones, V. Rauh, L. Needham, D. Tang, M. Niedzwiecki, R. Wang, F. Perera. 2010. Prenatal exposure to PBDEs and neurodevelopment. *Environ. Health Perspect.* 118 (5):712–719.

169. Chaves, L., C. Koenraadt. 2010. Climate change and highland malaria: Fresh air for a hot debate. *Q. Rev. Biol.* 85 (1):27–55.

170. Rodenburg, L. A., S. N. Valle, M. A. Panero, G. R. Munoz, L. M. Shor. 2010. Mass balances on selected polycyclic aromatic hydrocarbons (PAHs) in the New York/New Jersey harbor. *J. Environ. Qual.* 39:642–653.

171. Diamond, J. 1987. The worst mistake in the history of the human race. *Discover* May:64–66.

172. Woodburn, J. 1968. An introduction to Hadza ecology. In *Man the Hunter*, R. B. Lee, I. DeVore, Eds., pp. 49–55. Chicago: Aldine.

173. Davis, E. W., J. A. Yost. 1983. The ethnobotany of Waorani of eastern Ecuador. *Bot. Mus. Leafl.* 3:159–217.

174. McArthur, M. 1960. Food consumption and dietary levels of groups of Aborigines living on naturally occurring foods. In *Records of the American-Australian Scientific Expedition to Arnhem Land*, Vol. 2, C. P. Mountford, Ed., pp. 90–135. Melbourne: Melbourne University Press.

175. Hill, S. B., J. A. Ramsay. 1977. Limitations of the energy approach in defining priorities in agriculture. In *Agriculture and Energy*, W. Lockeretz, Ed., pp. 713–731. New York: Academic Press.

176. Pelletier, K. R., Ed. 1979. *Holistic Medicine: From Pathology to Optimum Health*. New York: Delacorte (Dell).

177. Hill, S. B. 1977. *Energy and the Canadian Food System with Particular Reference to New Brunswick*. Report to New Brunswick Government's Agricultural Resources Study Group. Fredericton, N. B.

178. Hill, S. B. 1979. Eco-agriculture: The way ahead. *Agrologist* 8 (4):9–11.

179. Linder, M. C., Ed. 1991. Food quality and its determinants, from field to table: Growing food, its storage, and preparation. In *Nutritional Biochemistry and Metabolism with Clinical Applications*, 2nd ed., p. 332. New York: Elsevier.

180. Li, J., T. Zhu, F. Wang, X. Qiu, W. Lin. 2006. Observation of organochlorine pesticides in the air of the Mt. Everest region. *Ecotoxicol. Environ. Safety* 63 (1):33–41.

181. Rolands, M. J., B. Wilkinson. 1930. The vitamin B content of grass seeds in relationship to manures. *Biochem. J.* 24 (1):199–204.

182. McCarrison, S. R. 1926. The effect of manorial conditions on nutritional value of millet and wheat. *J. Med. Res.* 14:351.

183. Howard, S. A. 1945. *Farming and Gardening for Health or Disease*. London: Faber and Faber.

184. Voisin, A. 1965. *Fertilizer Application*. London: Crosby Lockwood.

185. Price, W. A. 1945. *Nutrition and Physical Degeneration*, 4th ed. Los Angeles: Paul B. Hoeber.

186. Gilbert, F. A. 1957. *Mineral Nutrition and the Balance of Life*. Norman: University of Oklahoma Press.

187. Albrecht, W. A. 1975. *The Albrecht Papers*, Charles Walters, Jr., Ed., p. 515. Raytown, MI: Acres.

188. Bear, F. E., S. J. Toth, A. L. Prince. 1948. Variation in mineral composition of vegetables. *Soil Sci. Soc. Am. Proc.* 13:380–384.

189. Linder, M. C., Ed. 1991. Food quality and its determinants, from field to table: Growing food, its storage, and preparation. In *Nutritional Biochemistry and Metabolism with Clinical Applications*, 2nd ed., p. 335. New York: Elsevier.

190. Briviba, K., B. A. Stracke, C. E. Rüfer, B. Watzl, F. P. Weibel, A. Bub. 2007. Effect of consumption of organically and conventionally produced apples on antioxidant activity and DNA damage in humans. *J. Agric. Food Chem.* 55 (19):7716–7721.

191. U.S. Department of Agriculture. Accessed January 20, 2010. http://www.ers.usda.gov/briefing/organic/demand.htm.

192. Magnusson, M. K., A. Arvola, U. K. Hursti, L. Åberg, P. Sjödén. 2003. Choice of organic foods is related to perceived consequences for human health and to environmentally friendly behaviour. *Appetite* 40 (2):109–117.

193. Lockie, S., K. Lyons, G. Lawrence, J. Grise. 2004. Choosing organics: A path analysis of factors underlying the selection of organic food among Australian consumers. *Appetite* 43:135–146.

194. Crinnion, W. J. 2010. Organic foods contain higher levels of certain nutrients, lower levels of pesticides, and may provide health benefits for the consumer. *Altern. Med. Rev.* 15 (1):4–12.

195. Juroszek, P., H. M. Lumpkin, R. Yang, D. R. Ledesma, C. Ma. 2009. Fruit quality and bioactive compounds with antioxidant activity of tomatoes grown on-farm: Comparison of organic and conventional management systems. *J. Agric. Food Chem.* 57 (4):1188–1194.

196. Barrett, D. M., C. Weakley, J. V. Diaz, M. Watnik. 2007. Qualitative and nutritional differences in processing tomatoes grown under commercial organic and conventional production systems. *J. Food Sci.* 72:C441–C451.

197. Chassy, A. W., L. Bui, E. N. C. Renaud, M. Van Horn, A. E. Mitchell. 2006. Three-year comparison of the content of antioxidant microconstituents and several quality characteristics in organic and conventionally managed tomatoes and bell peppers. *J. Agric. Food Chem.* 54 (21):8244–8252.

198. Harborne, J. B. 1999. Classes and Functions Of Secondary Products from Plants. *Chemicals from Plants Perspectives on Plant Secondary Products*, 1–25.

199. Benbrook, C., X. Zhao, J. Yanez, N. Davies, P. Andrews. 2008. New Evidence Confirms the Nutritional Superiority of Plant-Based Organic Foods. *Nutritional Superiority of Organic Food.*.

200. Davis, D. R., M. D. Epp, H. D. Riordan. 2004. Changes in USDA food composition data for 43 garden crops, 1950 to 1999. *J. Am. Coll. Nutr.* 23 (6):669–682.

201. Mitchell, A. E., Y. Hong, E. Koh, D. M. Barrett, D. E. Bryant, R. Ford Denison, S. Kaffka. 2007. Ten-year comparison of the influence of organic and conventional crop management practices on the content of flavonoids in tomatoes. *J. Agric. Food Chem.* 55 (15):6154–6159.

202. Rossi, F., F. Godani, T. Bertuzzi, M. Trevisan, F. Ferrari, S. Gatti. 2009. Health-promoting substances and heavy metal content in tomatoes grown with different farming techniques. *Eur. J. Nutr.* 48 (4):259–250.

203. Caris-Veyrat, C., M. Amiot, V. Tyssandier, D. Grasselly, M. Buret, M. Mikolajczak, J. Guilland, C. Bouteloup-Demange, P. Borel. 2004. Influence of organic versus conventional agricultural practice on the antioxidant microconstituent content of tomatoes and derived purees; consequences on antioxidant plasma status in humans. *J. Agric. Food Chem.* 52 (21):6503–6509.

204. Lairon, D. 2009. Nutritional quality and safety of organic food. A review. Agron. Sustain. Dev. Accessed April 07, 2016. http://www.agronomy-journal.org/index.pbp?option=articleS[access=standard&Itemid=129&url=/articles/agro/abs/first/a8202/a8202.html.

205. Worthington, V. 2001. Nutritional quality of organic versus conventional fruits, vegetables, and grains. *J. Altern. Complement Med.* 7:161–173.

206. Dangour, A. D., S. K. Dodhia, A. Hayter, E. Allen, K. Lock, R. Uauy. 2009. Nutritional quality of organic foods: A systematic review. *Am. J. Clin. Nutr.* 90 (3):680–685.

207. Magkos, F., F. Arvaniti, A. Zámpelas. 2006. Organic food: Buying more safety or just peace of mind? A critical review of the literature. *Crit. Rev. Food Sci. Nutr.* 46:23–56.

208. Dangour, A., A. Aikenhead, A. Hayter, E. Allen, K. Lock, R. Uauy. 2009. Comparison of putative health effects of organically and conventionally produced foodstuffs: A systematic review. Accessed April 07, 2016. http://www.nutriwatch.org/04Foods/fsa/health.pdf.

209. Davis, D. R., M. D. Epp, H. D. Riordan. 2004. Changes in USDA food composition data for 43 garden crops, 1950 to 1999. *J. Am. CoU. Nutr.* 23:669–682.

210. Vanacker, S., M. Tromp, G. Haenen, W. Vandervijgh, A. Bast. 1995. Flavonoids as scavengers of nitric oxide radical. *Biochem. Biophys. Res. Commun.* 214 (3):755–759.

211. Duthie, G., A. Crozier. 2000. Plant-derived phenolic antioxidants. *Curr. Opin. Lipidol.* 11:43–47.

212. Pietta, P. G. 2000. Flavonoids as antioxidants. *J. Nat. Prod.* 63:1035–1042.

213. Karppi, J., S. Kurl, T. Nurmi, T. H. Rissanen, E. Pukkala, K. Nyyssönen. 2009. Serum lycopene and the risk of cancer: The Kuopio Ischaemic Heart Disease Risk Factor (KIHD) Study. *Ann. Epidemiol.* 19 (7):512–518.

214. Zafra-Stone, S., T. Yasmin, M. Bagchi, A. Chatterjee, J. A. Vinson, D. Bagchi. 2007. Berry anthocyanins as novel antioxidants in human health and disease prevention. *Mol. Nutr. Food Res.* 51 (6):675–683.

215. Gugliucci, A., D. H. Bastos. 2009. Chlorogenic acid protects paraoxonase 1 activity in high density lipoprotein from inactivation caused by physiological concentrations of hypochlorite. *Fitoterapia* 80:138–142.

216. Hajšlová, J., V. Schulzová, P. Slanina, K. Janné, K. E. Hellenäs, C. Andersson. 2005. Quality of organically and conventionally grown potatoes: Four-year study of micronutrients, metals, secondary metabolites, enzymic browning and organoleptic properties. *Food Addit. Contam.* 22 (6):514–534.

217. Wang, S. Y., C. Chen, W. Sciarappa, C. Y. Wang, M. J. Camp. 2008. Fruit quality, antioxidant capacity, and flavonoid content of organically and conventionally grown blueberries. *J. Agric. Food Chem.* 56 (14):5788–5794.

218. Asami, D. K., Y. J. Hong, D. M. Barrett, A. E. Mitchell. 2003. Comparison of the total phenolic and ascorbic acid content of freeze-dried and air-dried marionberry, strawberry, and corn grown using conventional, organic, and sustainable agricultural practices. *J. Agric. Food. Chem.* 51:1237–1241.

219. Dani, C., L. S. Oliboni, R. Vanderlinde, D. Bonatto, M. Salvador, J. A. Henriques. 2007. Phenolic content and antioxidant activities of white and purple juices manufactured with organically- or conventionally-produced grapes. *Food Chem. Toxicol.* 45 (12): 2574–2580.

220. Vian, M. A., V. Tomao, P. O. Coulomb, J. M. Lacombe, O. Dangles. 2006. Comparison of the anthocyanin composition during ripening of syrah grapes grown using organic or conventional agricultural practices. *J. Agric. Food Chem.* 54 (15):5230–5235.

221. Lamperi, L., U. Chiuminatto, A. Cincinelli, P. Galvan, E. Giordani, L. Lepri, M. Del Bubba. 2008. Polyphenol levels and free radical scavenging activities of four apple cultivars from integrated and organic farming in different Italian areas. *J. Agric. Food Chem.* 56 (15):6536–6546.

222. Stracke, B. A., C. E. Rüfer, F. P. Weibel, A. Bub, B. Watzl. 2009. Three-year comparison of the polyphenol contents and antioxidant capacities in organically and conventionally produced apples (*Malus domestica* Bork. cultivar 'Golden Delicious'). *J. Agric. Food Chem.* 57 (11):4598–4605.

223. Lombardi-Boccia, G., M. Lucarini, S. Lanzi, A. Aguzzi, M. Cappelloni. 2006. Nutrients and antioxidant molecules in yellow plums (*Prunus domestica* L.) from conventional and organic productions: A comparative study. *J. Agric. Food Chem.* 54 (10):3764.

224. Carbonaro, M., M. Mattera, S. Nicoli, P. Bergamo, M. Cappelloni. 2002. Modulation of antioxidant compounds in organic vs conventional fruit (peach, *Prunus persica* L., and pear, *Pyrus communis* L.). *J. Agric. Food Chem.* 50 (19):5458–5462.

225. Tarozzi, A., S. Hrelia, C. Angeloni, F. Morroni, P. Biagi, M. Guardigli, G. Cantelli-Forti, P. Hrelia. 2005. Antioxidant effectiveness of organically and non-organically grown red oranges in cell culture systems. *Eur. J. Nutr.* 45 (3):152–158.

226. Punia, N. D., N. Khetarpaul. 2008. Physicochemical characteristics, nutrient composition and consumer acceptability of wheat varieties grown under organic and inorganic fanning conditions. *Int. J. Food Sci. Nutr.* 59:224–245.

227. Dimberg, L. H., C. Gissen, J. Nilsson. 2005. Phenolic compounds in oat grains (*Avena sativa* L.) grown in conventional and organic systems. *Amhio* 34:331–337.

228. Ellis, K. A., G. Innocent, D. Grove-White, P. Cripps, W. G. Mclean, C. V. Howard, M. Mihm. 2006. Comparing the fatty acid composition of organic and conventional milk. *J. Dairy Sci.* 89 (6):1938–1950.

229. Molkentin, J., A. Giesemann. 2007. Differentiation of organically and conventionally produced milk by stable isotope and fatty acid analysis. *Anal. Bioanal. Chem.* 388:297–305.

230. Ellis, K. A., A. Monteiro, G. T. Innocent, D. Grove-White, P. Cripps, W. G. Mclean, C. V. Howard, M. Mihm. 2007. Investigation of the vitamins A and E and β-carotene content in milk from UK organic and conventional dairy farms. *J. Dairy Res.* 74 (4):484–491.

231. Prandini, A., S. Sigolo, G. Piva. 2009. Conjugated linoleic acid (CLA) and fatty acid composition of milk, curd and Grana Padano cheese in conventional and organic farming systems. *J. Dairy Res.* 76:278–282.

232. Mayer, A-M. 1997. Historical changes in the mineral content of fruits and vegetables. *Br. Food J.* 99 (6):207–211.

233. White, P. J., M. R. Broadley. 2005. Historical variation in the mineral composition of edible horticultural products. *J. Hortic. Sci. Biotechnol.* 80 (6):660–667.

234. Jarrell, W. M., R. B. Beverly. 1981. The dilution effect in plant nutrition studies. In *Advances in Agronomy*, Vol. 34, N. C. Brady, Ed., pp. 197–224.

235. Karr-Lilienthal, L. K., M. R. Merchen, C. M. Grieshop, M. A. Flahaven, D. C. Mahan, N. D. Fastinger, M. Watts, G. C. Fahey. 2004. Ileal amino acid digestibilities by pigs fed soybean meals from five major soybean-producing countries. *J. Anim. Sci.* 82 (11):3198–3209.

236. Uribelarrea, M., F. E. Below, S. P. Moose. 2004. Grain composition and productivity of maize hybrids derived from the Illinois protein strains in response to variable nitrogen fertilizer. *Crop Sci.* 44:1593–1600.

237. Pollak, L. M., M. P. Scott. 2005. Breeding for Grain Quality Traits, Maydica. 50:247–257; Paul Scott, Research Geneticist, USDA-ARS, Ames, Iowa, discussion with author, Accessed April 07, 2016, pscott@iastate.edu.

238. Mott, L., M. Broad. 1984. *Pesticides in Food: What the Public Needs to Know*, pp. 86–87. San Francisco: Natural Resources Defense Council, Inc.

239. Calabrese, E. J. 1980. *Nutrition and Environmental Health, Vol. 1, The Vitamins*, p. 63. New York: John Wiley and Sons.

240. Westley, J. 1980. Rhodanese and the sulfane pool. In *Enzymatic Basis of Detoxication*, W. B. Jakoby, Ed., pp. 256–257. New York: Academic Press.

241. Rea, W. J. 1992. *Chemical Sensitivity*, Vol. 1, p. 47. Boca Raton, FL: Lewis Publishers.

242. Mohammadi, K. 2011. Effect of different fertilization methods on soil biological indexes. *Int. J. Biol. Biomol. Agric. Food Biotechnol. Eng.* 5 (6):329–332.

243. Rice, P. J., L. L. McConnell, L. P. Heighton, A. M. Sadeghi, A. R. Isensee, J. R. Teasdale, A. A. Abdul-Baki, J. A. Harman-Fetcho, C. J. Hapeman. 2001. Runoff loss of pesticides and soil: A comparison between vegetative mulch and plastic mulch in vegetable production systems. *J. Environ. Qual.* 30:1808–1821.

244. Chander, K., S. Goyal, D. P. Nandal, K. K. Kapoor. 1998. Soil organic matter, microbial biomass and enzyme activities in a tropical agroforestry system. *Biol. Fertil. Soils* 27:168–172.

245. Nishio, M., S. Kusano. 1980. Fluctuation patterns of microbial numbers in soil applied with compost. *Soil Sci. Plant Nutr.* 26:581–593.

246. Lundquist, E. J., L. E. Jackson, K. M. Scow, C. Hsu. 1999. Changes in microbial biomass and community composition and soil carbon and nitrogen pools after incorporation of rye into three California agricultural soils. *Soil Biol. Biochem.* 31:221–236.

247. Kandeler, E., D. Tscherko, H. Spiegel. 1999. Long-term monitoring of microbial biomass, N mineralisation and enzyme activities of a Chernozem under different tillage management. *Biol. Fertil. Soils* 28:343–351.

248. Lynch, J. M. 1983. *Soil Biotechnology*, p. 191. Oxford: Blackwell.

249. Biederbeck, V. O., R. P. Zentner, C. A. Campbell. 2005. Soil microbial populations and activities as influenced by legume green fallow in a semiarid climate. *Soil Biol. Biochem.* 37:1775–1784.

250. Tarafdar, J. C., H. Marschner. 1994. Phosphatase activity in the rhizosphere and hyphosphere of VA mycorrhizal wheat supplied with inorganic and organic phosphorus. *Soil Biol. Biochem.* 26:387–395.

251. Leita, L., M. De Nobilli, C. Mondini, G. Muhlbacova, L. Marchiol, G. Bragato, M. Contin. 1999. Influence of inorganic and organic fertilization on soil microbial biomass, metabolic quotient and heavy metal bioavailability. *Biol. Fertil. Soils* 4:371–376.

252. Martens, D. A., J. B. Johanson, J. W. T. Frankenberger. 1992. Production and persistence of soil enzymes with repeated addition of organic residues. *Soil Sci.* 153:53–61.

253. Giusquiani, P. L., G. Gigliotti, D. Businelli. 1994. Long-term effects of heavy metals from composted municipal waste on some enzyme activities in a cultivated soil. *Biol. Fertil. Soils* 17:257–262.

254. Crecchio, C., M. Curci, R. Mininni, P. Ricciuti, P. Ruggiero. 2001. Short term effects of municipal solid waste compost amendments on soil carbon and nitrogen content, some enzyme activities and genetic diversity. *Biol. Fertil. Soils* 34:311–318.

255. Wlodarczyk, T., W. Stepniewski, M. Brzezinska. 2002. Dehydrogenase activity, redox potential, and emissions of carbon dioxide and nitrous oxide from Cambisols under flooding conditions. *Biol. Fertil. Soils* 36:200–206.

256. Marinari, S., G. Masciandaro, B. Ceccanti, S. Grego. 2000. Influence of organic and mineral fertilizers on soil biological and physical properties. *Bioresor. Technol.* 72:9–17.

257. Nayak, D. R., Y. J. Babe, T. K. Adhya. 2007. Long-term application of compost influences microbial biomass and enzyme activities in a tropical Aric Endoaquept planted to rice under flooded condition. *Soil Biol. Biochem.* 39:1897–1906.

258. Pesticides industry sales and usage. 2000 and 2001 market estimates. Accessed April 08, 2016. http://www.epa.gov/oppbead1/pestsales/01pestsales/market_estimates2001.pdf.

259. Pimentel, D. 1995. Amounts of pesticides reaching target pests: Environmental impacts and ethics. *J. Agric. Environ. Ethics* 8:17–29.

260. Harner, T., K. Pozo, T. Gouin, A. M. Macdonald, H. Hung, J. Cainey, A. Peters. 2006. Global pilot study for persistent organic pollutants (POPs) using PUF disk passive air samplers. *Environ. Pollut.* 144:445–452.

261. Pandey, J., U. Pandey. 2009. Accumulation of heavy metals in dietary vegetables and cultivated soil horizon in organic farming system in relation to atmospheric deposition in a seasonally dry tropical region of India. *Environ. Monit. Assess.* 148:61–74.

262. Baker, B. P., C. M. Benbrook, E. Groth, K. Lutz Benbrock. 2002. Pesticide residues in conventional, integrated pest management (IPM)-grown and organic foods: Insights from three US data sets. *Food Addit. Contam.* 19:427–446.

263. U.S. Food and Drug Administration. Pesticide residue monitoring program 2000. Accessed April 08, 2016. http://www.fda.gov/Food/FoodSafety/FoodContaminantsAdulteration/Pesticides/ Residue MonitoringReports/ucml25171.htm.

264. Crinnion, W. J. 2010. Organic foods contain higher levels of certain nutrients, lower levels of pesticides, and may provide health benefits for the consumer. *Altern. Med. Rev.* 15 (1):4–12.

265. Curl, C. L., R. A. Fenske, K. Elgethun. 2003. Organophosphorus pesticide exposure of urban and suburban preschool children with organic and conventional diets. *Environ. Health Perspect.* 111:377–382.

266. Lu, C., K. Toepel, R. Irish, R. A. Fenske, D. B. Barr, R. Bravo. 2006. Organic diets significantly lower children's dietary exposure to organophosphorus pesticides. *Environ. Health Perspect.* 114 (2):260–263.

267. Kalkan Yildirim, H., Y. Delen Akcay, U. Guvenc, E. Yildirim Sozmen. 2004. Protection capacity against low-density lipoprotein oxidation and antioxidant potential of some organic and nonorganic wines. *Int. J. Food Sci. Nutr.* 55:351–362.

268. Delen Akcay, Y., H. Kalkan Yildirim, U. Guvenc, E. Yildirim Sozmen. 2004. The effects of consumption of organic and nonorganic red wine on low-density lipoprotein oxidation and antioxidant capacity in humans. *Nutr. Res.* 24:541–554.

269. Corbel, V., M. Stankiewicz, C. Pennetier, D. Fournier, J. Stojan, E. Girard, M. Dimitrov, J. Molgó, J. Hougard, B. Lapied. 2009. Evidence for inhibition of cholinesterases in insect and mammalian nervous systems by the insect repellent deet. *BMC Biol.* 7 (1):47.

270. Besson, J.-M., H. Vostmann. 1978. *Towards a Sustainable Agriculture*, p. 243. Aatau, Switzerland: Verlag Wirz.

271. Oelhalf, R. C. 1978. *Organic Agriculture: Economic and Ecological Comparisions with Conventional Methods*, p. 271. Montclair, NJ: Allanheld, Osmun.

272. Youngberd, G. 1978. The alternative agriculture movement. *Policy Stud. J.* 6 (4):524–530.

273. Buesching, D. 1979. The alternative agriculture movement: Origins, development and current composition. *Agric. World* 5 (7):1–8.

274. Peters, S. 1980. The land in trust: A social history of the organic farming movement. Ph.D. thesis. Montreal: Department of Sociology, McGill University (unpublished).

275. Dufault, R., Z. Berg, R. Crider, R. Schnoll, L. Wetsit, S. G. Gilbert, H. M. Kingston, M. M. Wolle, G. M. Mizanur Rahman, D. R. Lak. 2015. Blood inorganic mercury is directly associated with glucose levels in the human population and may be linked to processed food intake. *Integr. Mol. Med.* 2 (3):181–194.

276. Murphy, S. D. 1986. Toxic effects of pesticides. In *Cassarett and Doull's Toxicology: The Basic Science of Poisons*, 4th ed., M. O. Amdur, J. Doull, C. D. Klaassen, Eds., pp. 610–611. New York: Pergamon Press.

277. Ecobichon, D. J. 1991. Toxic effects of pesticides. In *Cassarett and Doull's Toxicology: The Basic Science of Poisons*, 4th ed., M. O. Amdur, J. Doull, C. D. Klaassen, Eds., pp. 610–611. New York: Pergamon Press.

278. Kalin, E. W., C. R. Brooks. 1963. Systemic toxic reactions to soft plastic food containers. *Med. Ann. D. C.* 32 (1):1–8.

279. Till, D. E., P. S. Scwartz, K. R. Sidman, J. R. Valentine, R. H. Whelan. 1982. Plasticizer migration from polyvinyl chloride film to solvent and foods. *Food Chem. Toxic* 20:95–104.

280. Baselt, R. C. 1982. *Disposition of Toxic Drugs and Chemical in Man*, 2nd ed., p. 375. Davis, CA: Biomedical Publications.

281. Baselt, R. C. 1982. *Disposition of Toxic Drugs and Chemical in Man*, 2nd ed., p. 753. Davis, CA: Biomedical Publications.

282. Tainsh, A. R. 1917–1947. The role of fungi in peace and war, p. 403. Copyright A. R. Tainsh, Stockholm, Oct. 28, 1987. Unpublished papers.

283. Committee on Aldehydes, Board on Toxicology and Environmental Health Hazards, Assembly on Life Sciences, National Research Council. 1981. *Formaldehyde and Other Aldehydes*, p. 28. Washington, DC: National Academy Press.

284. Taylor, S. 1987. Allergic and sensitivity reactions to food component. In *Nutritional Toxicology*, Vol. II, J. N. Hathcock, Ed., p. 173. Orlando: Academic Press.

285. Davies, K. 1986. Human exposure routes to selected persistent toxic chemical in the great lakes basin: A case study of Toronto and Southern Ontario region (Unpublished). Toronto: Department of Public Health.

286. Bekesi, J. G., H. A. Anderson, J. P. Roboz, J. Roboz, A. Fischbein, I. J. Selikoff, J. F. Holland. 1979. Immunologic dysfunction among PBB-exposed Michigan dairy farmer. *Ann. N. Y. Acad. Sci.* 230:717–729.

287. U. S. Food and Drug Administration. 1987. Food and drug administration pesticide program: Residues in foods. Washington, DC: U.S. Food and Drug Administration.

288. Saifer, P., M. Zellerbach. 1984. *Detox.* Los Angeles, CA: Jeremy P. Tarcher.

289. Natural Resources Defence Council. 1984. *Pesticides in Food: What the Public Needs to Know.* San Francisco, CA: Natural Resources Defense Council.

290. Shelton, J. F., E. M. Geraghty, D. J. Tancredi, L. D. Delwiche, R. J. Schmidt, B. Ritz, R. L. Hansen, I. Hertz-Picciotto. 2014. Neurodevelopmental disorders and prenatal residential proximity to agricultural pesticides: The CHARGE study. *Environ. Health Perspect.* 122 (10):A266.

291. California Department of Food and Agriculture. 2010. California Agricultural Production Statistics. Accessed April 08, 2016. http://www. cdfa.ca.gov/statistics/.

292. CDPR (California Department of Pesticide Regulation). 2014. *Pesticide Use Reporting (PUR).* Accessed April 08, 2016. http://www.cdpr. ca.gov/docs/pur/purmain.htm.

293. Bouchard, M. F., D. C. Bellinger, R. O. Wright, M. G. Weisskopf. 2010. Attention-deficit/hyperactivity disorder and urinary metabolites of organophosphate pesticides. *Pediatrics* 125 (6):e1270–e1277.

294. Bouchard, M. F. et al. 2011. Prenatal exposure to organophosphate pesticides and IQ in 7-year-old children. *Environ. Health Perspect.* 119 (8):1189–1195.

295. Engel, S. M., G. S. Berkowitz, D. B. Barr, S. L. Teitelbaum, J. Siskind, S. J. Meisel, J. G. Wetmur, M. S. Wolff. 2007. Prenatal organophosphate metabolite and organochlorine levels and performance on the brazelton neonatal behavioral assessment scale in a multiethnic pregnancy cohort. *Am. J. Epidemiol.* 165 (12):1397–1404.

296. Eskenazi, B., A. R. Marks, A. Bradman, L. Fenster, C. Johnson, D. B. Barr, N. P. Jewell. 2006. In utero exposure to dichlorodiphenyltrichloroethane (DDT) and dichlorodiphenyldichloroethylene (DDE) and neurodevelopment among young Mexican American children. *Pediatrics* 118 (1):233–241.

297. Grandjean, P., R. Harari, D. B. Barr, F. Debes. 2006. Pesticide exposure and stunting as independent predictors of neurobehavioral deficits in Ecuadorian school children. *Pediatrics* 117 (3):e546–e556.

298. Guillette, E. A., M. M. Meza, M. G. Aquilar, A. D. Soto, I. E. Garcia. 1998. An anthropological approach to the evaluation of preschool children exposed to pesticides in Mexico. *Environ. Health Perspect.* 106:347–353.

299. Rauh, V. A., R. Garfinkel, F. P. Perera, H. F. Andrews, L. Hoepner, D. B. Barr, R. Whitehead, D. Tang, R. W. Whyatt. 2006. Impact of prenatal chlorpyrifos exposure on neurodevelopment in the first 3 years of life among inner-city children. *Pediatrics* 118 (6):e1845–e1859.

300. Ribas-Fito, N., M. Torrent, D. Carrizo, L. Munoz-Ortiz, J. Julvez, J. O. Grimalt, J. Sunyer. 2006. In utero exposure to background concentrations of DDT and cognitive functioning among preschoolers. *Am. J. Epidemiol.* 164 (10):955–962.

301. Torres-Sánchez, L., S. J. Rothenberg, L. Schnaas, M. E. Cebrián, E. Osorio, M. Del Carmen Hernández, R. M. García-Hernández, C. Del Rio-Garcia, M. S. Wolff, L. López-Carrillo. 2007. In utero P,p'-DDE exposure and infant neurodevelopment: A perinatal cohort in Mexico. *Environ. Health Perspect.* 115 (3):435–439.

302. Young, J. G., B. Eskenazi, E. A. Gladstone, A. Bradman, L. Pedersen, C. Johnson, D. B. Barr, C. E. Furlong, N. T. Holland. 2005. Association between in utero organophosphate pesticide exposure and abnormal reflexes in neonates. *Neurotoxicology* 26 (2):199–209.

303. Roberts, E. M., P. B. English, J. K. Grether, G. C. Windham, L. Somberg, C. Wolff. 2007. Maternal residence near agricultural pesticide applications and autism spectrum disorders among children in the California Central Valley. *Environ. Health Perspect.* 115:1482–1489. doi: 10.1289/ehp.10168.

304. Eskenazi, B., A. R. Marks, A. Bradman, K. Harley, D. B. Barr, C. Johnson, N. Morga, N. P. Jewell. 2007. Organophosphate pesticide exposure and neurodevelopment in young Mexican-American children. *Environ. Health Perspect.* 115 (5):792–798.

305. Boyle, C. A., S. Boulet, L. A. Schieve, R. A. Cohen, S. J. Blumberg, M. Yeargin-Allsopp, S. Visser, M. D. Kogan. 2011. Trends in the prevalence of developmental disabilities in US children, 1997–2008. *Pediatrics* 127 (6):1034–1042.

306. Centers for Disease Control and Prevention. 2012. Prevalence of Autism Spectrum Disorders—Autism and Developmental Disabilities Monitoring Network, 14 Sites, United States, 2008. Accessed May 27, 2014. http://www.cdc.gov/mmwr/preview/ mmwrhtml/ss6103a1.htm.

307. Hallmayer, J. et al. 2011. Genetic heritability and shared environmental factors among twin pairs with autism. *Arch. Gen. Psychiatry* 68 (11):1095–1102.

308. Mendola, P., S. G. Selevan, S. Gutter, D. Rice. 2002. Environmental factors associated with a spectrum of neurodevelopmental deficits. *Ment. Retard. Dev. Disabil. Res. Rev.* 8 (3):188–197.

309. Casida, J. E. 2009. Pest toxicology: The primary mechanisms of pesticide action. *Chem. Res. Toxicol.* 22 (4):609–619.

310. Levin, E. D., N. Addy, A. Nakajima, N. C. Christopher, F. J. Seidler, T. A. Slotkin. 2001. Persistent behavioral consequences of neonatal chlorpyrifos exposure in rats. *Brain Res. Dev.* 130 (1):83–89.

311. Levin, E. D., O. A. Timofeeva, L. Yang, A. Petro, I. T. Ryde, N. Wrench, F. J. Seidler, T. A. Slotkin. 2010. Early postnatal parathion exposure in rats causes sex-selective cognitive impairment and neurotransmitter defects which emerge in aging. *Behav. Brain Res.* 208 (2):319–327.

312. Shelton, J. F., I. Hertz-Picciotto, I. N. Pessah. 2012. Tipping the balance of autism risk: Potential mechanisms linking pesticides and autism. *Environ. Health Perspect.* 120:944–951.

313. Hertz-Picciotto, I., L. A. Croen, R. Hansen, C. R. Jones, J. van de Water, I. N. Pessah. 2006. The CHARGE study: An epidemiologic investigation of genetic and environmental factors contributing to autism. *Environ. Health Perspect.* 114:1119–1125.

314. Croen, L. A., J. K. Grether, J. Hoogstrate, S. Selvin. 2002. The changing prevalence of autism in California. *J. Autism Dev. Disord.* 32 (3):207–215.

315. Rutter, M., A. Bailey, S. K. Berument, C. Lord, A. Pickles. 2003. *Social Communication Questionnaire (SCQ).* Los Angeles: Western Psychological Services.

316. Agency for Toxic Substances and Disease Registry. 2003. Toxicological Profile for Pyrethrins and Pyrethroids. Accessed February 22, 2014. http://www.atsdr.cdc.gov/toxprofiles/tp155.pdf.

317. Breckenridge, C. B., L. Holden, N. Sturgess, M. Weiner, L. Sheets, D. Sargent, D. M. Soderlund, J. S. Choi, S. Symington, J. M. Clark, S. Burr, D. Ray. 2009. Evidence for a separate mechanism of toxicity for the Type I and the Type II pyrethroid insecticides. *Neurotoxicology* 30 (suppl 1):S17–S31.

318. Schmidt, R. J., R. L. Hansen, J. Hartiala, H. Allayee, L. C. Schmidt, D. J. Tancredi, F. Tassone, I. Hertz-Picciotto. 2011. Prenatal vitamins, one-carbon metabolism gene variants, and risk for autism. *Epidemiology* 22 (4):476–485.

319. Costa, L. G., T. B. Cole, A. Vitalone, C. E. Furlong. 2005. Measurement of paraoxonase (PON1) status as a potential biomarker of susceptibility to organophosphate toxicity. *Clin. Chim Acta* 352 (1–2):37–47.

320. D'Amelio, M. et al. 2005. Paraoxonase gene variants are associated with autism in North America, but not in Italy: Possible regional specificity in gene–environment interactions. *Mol. Psychiatry* 10 (11):1006–1016.

321. Furlong, C. E., T. B. Cole, G. P. Jarvik, C. Pettan-Brewer, G. K. Geiss, R. J. Richter, D. M. Shih, A. D. Tward, A. J. Lusis, L. G. Costa. 2005. Role of paraoxonase (PON1) status in pesticide sensitivity: Genetic and temporal determinants. *Neurotoxicology* 26 (4):651–659.

322. Lee, P. C., S. L. Rhodes, J. S. Sinsheimer, J. Bronstein, B. Ritz. 2013. Functional paraoxonase 1 variants modify the risk of Parkinson's disease due to organophosphate exposure. *Environ. Int.* 56:42–47.

323. Handal, A. J., S. D. Harlow, J. Breilh, B. Lozoff. 2008. Occupational exposure to pesticides during pregnancy and neurobehavioral development of infants and toddlers. *Epidemiology* 19 (6):851–859.

324. Nuckols, J. R., R. B. Gunier, P. Riggs, R. Miller, P. Reynolds, M. H. Ward. 2007. Linkage of the California Pesticide Use Reporting Database with spatial land use data for exposure assessment. *Environ. Health Perspect.* 115:684–689.

325. Rull, R. P., B. Ritz. 2003. Historical pesticide exposure in California using pesticide use reports and land-use surveys: An assessment of misclassification error and bias. *Environ. Health Perspect.* 111:1582–1589. doi: 10.1289/ehp.6118.

326. Gunier, R. B. et al. 2011. Determinants of agricultural pesticide concentrations in carpet dust. *Environ. Health Perspect.* 119:970–976.

327. U.S. Department of Agriculture. 2006. Pest Management Practices. Accessed June 2, 2014. http://www.ers.usda.gov/ersDownloadHandler.ashx?file=/media/873656/pestmgt.pdf.

328. U.S. Environmental Protection Agency. 2011. Pesticide Industry Sales and Usage: 2006 and 2007 Market Estimates. Accessed May 27, 2014. http://www.epa.gov/opp00001/pestsales/07pestsales/market_estimates2007.pdf.

329. Williams, M. K., A. Rundle, D. Holmes, M. Reyes, L. A. Hoepner, D. B. Barr, D. E. Camann, F. P. Perera, R. M. Whyatt. 2008. Changes in pest infestation levels, self-reported pesticide use, and permethrin exposure during pregnancy after the 2000–2001 U.S. Environmental Protection Agency restriction of organophosphates. *Environ. Health Perspect.* 116:1681–1688.

330. Mense, S. M., A. Sengupta, C. Lan, M. Zhou, G. Bentsman, D. J. Volsky, R. M. Whyatt, F. P. Perera, L. Zhang. 2006. The common insecticides cyfluthrin and chlorpyrifos alter the expression of a subset of genes with diverse functions in primary human astrocytes. *Toxicol. Sci.* 93 (1):125–135.

331. Lassiter, T. L., E. A. MacKillop, I. T. Ryde, F. J. Seidler, T. A. Slotkin. 2009. Is fipronil safer than chlorpyrifos? Comparative developmental neurotoxicity modeled in PC12 cells. *Brain Res. Bull.* 78 (6):313–322.

332. Colborn, T., D. Dumanoski, J. Peterson Meyers. 1996. *Our Stolen Future.* New York: Dutton.

333. Birnbaum, L. S. 2012. Environmental chemicals: Evaluating low-dose effects. *Environ. Health Perspect.* 120 (4):A143–A144.

334. Barr, D. B., A. O. Olsson, L. Wong, S. Udunka, S. E. Baker, R. D. Whitehead, M. S. Magsumbol, B. L. Williams, L. L. Needham. 2010. Urinary concentrations of metabolites of pyrethroid insecticides in the general U.S. population: National Health and Nutrition Examination Survey 1999–2002. *Environ. Health Perspect.* 118 (6):742–748.

335. Bilau, M. et al. 2008. Dietary exposure to dioxin-like compounds in three age groups: Results from the Flemish environment and health study. *Chemosphere* 70 (4):584–592.

336. Churchill, J. E., D. L. Ashley, W. E. Kaye. 2001. Recent chemical exposures and blood volatile organic compound levels in a large population-based sample. *Arch. Environ. Health* 56 (2):157–166.

337. Woodruff, T. J., A. R. Zota, J. M. Schwartz. 2011. Environmental chemicals in pregnant women in the United States: NHANES 2003–2004. *Environ. Health Perspect.* 119:878–885.

338. Braun, J. M., R. Hauser. 2011. Bisphenol A and children's health. *Curr. Opin. Pediatr.* 23 (2):233–239.

339. Crain, D. A. et al. 2008. Female reproductive disorders: The roles of endocrine-disrupting compounds and developmental timing. *Fertil. Steril.* 90 (4):911–940.

340. Paustenbach, D., D. Galbraith. 2006. Biomonitoring: Is body burden relevant to public health? *Regul. Toxicol. Pharmacol.* 44 (3):249–261.

341. Rappaport, S. M., M. T. Smith. 2010. Environment and disease risks. *Science* 330 (6003):460–461.

342. Carwile, J. L., K. B. Michels. 2011. Urinary bisphenol A and obesity: NHANES 2003–2006. *Environ. Res.* 111 (6):825–830.

343. Meeker, J. D., H. M. Stapleton. 2010. House dust concentrations of organophosphate flame retardants in relation to hormone levels and semen quality parameters. *Environ. Health Perspect.* 118:318–323.

344. Swan, S. H., F. Liu, M. Hines, R. L. Kruse, C. Wang, J. B. Redmon, A. Sparks, B. Weiss. 2010. Prenatal phthalate exposure and reduced masculine play in boys. *Int. J. Androl.* 33 (2):259–269.

345. Miyashita, C., S. Sasaki, Y. Saijo, N. Washino, E. Okada, S. Kobayashi, K. Konishi, J. Kajiwara, T. Todaka, R. Kishi. 2011. Effects of prenatal exposure to dioxin-like compounds on allergies and infections during infancy. *Environ. Res.* 111 (4):551–558.

346. Melnick, R. et al. 2002. Summary of the National Toxicology Program's Report of the Endocrine Disruptors Low-Dose Peer Review. *Environ. Health Perspect.* 110 (4):427–431.

347. Vandenberg, L. N. et al. 2012. Hormones and endocrine-disrupting chemicals: Low-dose effects and nonmonotonic dose responses. *Endocr. Rev.* 33 (3):378–455.

348. Lopez-Espinosa, M. A.-J., E. Vizcaino, M. Murcia, V. Fuentes, A. Garcia, M. Rebagliato, J. O. Grimalt, F. Ballester. 2009. Prenatal exposure to organochlorine compounds and neonatal thyroid stimulating hormone levels. *J. Expos. Sci. Environ. Epidemiol.* 20 (7):579–588.

349. Louis, G. M. B., L. I. Rios, A. Mclain, M. A. Cooney, P. J. Kostyniak, R. Sundaram. 2011. Persistent organochlorine pollutants and menstrual cycle characteristics. *Chemosphere* 85 (11):1742–1748.

350. Wetterauer, B., M. Ricking, J. C. Otte, A. V. Hallare, A. Rastall, L. Erdinger, J. Schwarzbauer, T. Braunbeck, H. Hollert. 2011. Toxicity, dioxin-like activities, and endocrine effects of DDT metabolites—DDA, DDMU, DDMS, and DDCN. *Environ. Sci. Pollut. Res.* 19 (2):403–415.

351. Hayes, T., K. Haston, M. Tsui, A. Hoang, C. Haeffele, A. Vonk. 2002. Herbicides: feminization of male frogs in the wild. *Nature* 419:895–896.

352. Lephart, E. D. 1996. A review of brain aromatase cytochrome P450. *Brain Res. Brain Res. Rev.* 22:1–26.

353. Simpson, E. R., M. S. Mahendroo, G. D. Means, M. W. Kilgore, M. M. Hinshelwood, S. Graham-Lorence, B. Amarneh, Y. Ito, C. R. Fisher, M. D. Michael. 1994. Aromatase cytochrome P450, the enzyme responsible for estrogen biosynthesis. *Endocr. Rev.* 15:342–355.

354. Chardard, D., C. Dournon. 1999. Sex reversal by aromatase inhibitor treatment in the newt Pleurodeles waltl. *J. Exp. Zool.* 283:43–50.

355. Navarro-Martin, L., M. Blazquez, F. Piferrer. 2009. Masculinization of the European sea bass (*Dicentrarchus labrax*) by treatment with an androgen or aromatase inhibitor involves different gene expression and has distinct lasting effects on maturation. *Gen. Comp. Endocrinol.* 160:3–11.

356. Richard-Mercier, N., M. Dorizzi, G. Desvages, M. Girondot, C. Pieau. 1995. Endocrine sex reversal of gonads by the aromatase inhibitor letrozole (CGS 20267) in *Emys orbicularis*, a turtle with temperature-dependent sex determination. *Gen. Comp. Endocrinol.* 100:314–326.

357. Heneweer, M., M. van den Berg, J. T. Sanderson. 2004. A comparison of human H295R and rat R2C cell lines as *in vitro* screening tools for effects on aromatase. *Toxicol. Lett.* 146:183–194.

358. Holloway, A. C., D. A. Anger, D. J. Crankshaw, M. Wu, W. G. Foster. 2008. Atrazine-induced changes in aromatase activity in estrogen sensitive target tissues. *J. Appl. Toxicol.* 28:260–270.

359. Coady, K. K. et al. 2005. Effects of atrazine on metamorphosis, growth, laryngeal and gonadal development, aromatase activity, and sex steroid concentrations in *Xenopus laevis*. *Ecotoxicol. Environ. Saf.* 62:160–173.

360. Hecker, M. et al. 2005. Effects of atrazine on CYP19 gene expression and aromatase activity in testes and on plasma sex steroid concentrations of male African clawed frogs (*Xenopus laevis*). *Toxicol. Sci.* 86:273–280.

361. Hecker, M. et al. 2005. Plasma concentrations of estradiol and testosterone, gonadal aromatase activity and ultrastructure of the testis in Xenopus laevis exposed to estradiol or atrazine. *Aquat. Toxicol.* 72:383–396.

362. Oka, T., O. Tooi, N. Mitsui, M. Miyahara, Y. Ohnishi, M. Takase, A. Kashiwagi, T. Shinkai, N. Santo, T. Iguchi. 2008. Effect of atrazine on metamorphosis and sexual differentiation in *Xenopus laevis*. *Aquat. Toxicol.* 87:215–226.

363. Langlois, V. S., A. C. Carew, B. D. Pauli, M. G. Wade, G. M. Cooke, V. L. Trudeau. 2009. Low levels of the herbicide atrazine alter sex ratios and reduce metamorphic success in *Rana pipiens* tadpoles raised in outdoor mesocosms. *Environ. Health Perspect.* 118 (4):552–557.

364. Lutz, I., S. Blodt, W. Kloas. 2005. Regulation of estrogen receptors in primary cultured hepatocytes of the amphibian *Xenopus laevis* as estrogenic biomarker and its application in environmental monitoring. *Comp. Biochem. Physiol. C Toxicol. Pharmacol.* 141:384–392.

365. Duarte, P., N. S. Hogan, D. Lean, V. L. Trudeau. 2006. Regulation and endocrine disruption of aromatase in the brain of developing Rana pipiens [Abstract]. In *27th Annual Meeting of the Society of Environmental Toxicology and Chemistry of North America*, 5–9 November 2006, Montreal, Québec, Canada. Abstract 559. Accessed March 3, 2010. http://montreal.setac.org/montreal/pdf/SETAC_abstractbook_2006.pdf.

366. Levy, G., I. Lutz, A. Kruger, W. Kloas. 2004. Bisphenol-A induces feminization in *Xenopus laevis* tadpoles. *Environ. Res.* 94:102–111.

367. Filby, A. L., K. L. Thorpe, G. Maack, C. R. Tyler. 2007. Gene expression profiles revealing the mechanisms of anti-androgen and estrogen-induced feminization in fish. *Aquat. Toxicol.* 81:219–231.

368. Duarte-Guterman, P., V. S. Langlois, K. Hodgkinson, B. D. Pauli, G. M. Cooke, M. G. Wade, V. L. Trudeau. 2010. The aromatase inhibitor fadrozole and the 5-reductase inhibitor finasteride affect gonadal differentiation and gene expression in the frog *Silurana tropicalis*. *Sex Dev.* 3:333–341.

369. Locatelli G. et al. 2012. Primary oligodendrocyte death does not elicit anti-CNS immunity. *Nat. Neurosci.* 15 (4):543–550.

370. Van den Berg, M. et al. 2006. The 2005 World Health Organization reevaluation of human and mammalian toxic equivalency factors for dioxins and dioxin-like compounds. *Toxicol. Sci.* 93:223–241.

371. Denison, M. S., S. R. Nagy. 2003. Activation of the aryl hydrocarbon receptor by structurally diverse exogenous and endogenous chemicals. *Annu. Rev. Pharmacol. Toxicol.* 43:309–334.

372. Birnbaum, L. S. 1994. Endocrine effects of prenatal exposure to PCBs, doxins, and other xenobiotics: Implications for policy and future research. *Environ. Health Perspect.* 102:676–679.

373. Larsen, J. C. 2006. Risk assessments of polychlorinated dibenzo-pdioxins, polychlorinated dibenzofurans, and dioxin-like polychlorinated biphenyls in food. *Mol. Nutr. Food Res.* 50:885–896.

374. Schecter, A., L. Birnbaum, J. J. Ryan, J. D. Constable. 2006. Dioxins: An overview. *Environ. Res.* 101:419–428.

375. Anderson, D. R., R. Fisher. 2002. Sources of dioxins in the United Kingdom: The steel industry and other sources. *Chemosphere* 46:371–381.

376. Hewitt, L. M., J. L. Parrott, M. E. McMaster. 2006. A decade of research on the environmental impacts of pulp and paper mill effluents in Canada: Sources and characteristics of bioactive substances. *J. Toxicol. Environ. Health B Crit. Rev.* 9:341–356.

377. Lin, L. F., W. J. Lee, G. P. Chang-Chien. 2006. Emissions of polychlorinated dibenzo-*p*-dioxins and dibenzofurans from various industrial sources. *J. Air Waste Manag. Assoc.* 56:1707–1715.

378. Thornton, J., M. McCally, P. Orris, J. Weinberg. 1996. Hospitals and plastics. Dioxin prevention and medical waste incinerators. *Public. Health Rep.* 111:298–313.

379. Hoogenboom, L. A., J. C. Van Eijkeren, M. J. Zeilmaker, M. J. Mengelers, R. Herbes, J. Immerzeel, W. A. Traag. 2007. A novel source for dioxins present in recycled fat from gelatin production. *Chemosphere* 68:814–823.

380. Schecter, A., L. Li. 1997. Dioxins, dibenzofurans, dioxin-like PCBs, and DDE in U.S. fast food, 1995. *Chemosphere* 34:1449–1457.

381. Schecter, A., P. Cramer, K. Boggess, J. Stanley, J. R. Olson. 1997. Levels of dioxins, dibenzofurans, PCB, and DDE congeners in pooled food samples collected in 1995 at supermarkets across the United States. *Chemosphere* 34:1437–1447.

382. Schecter, A., M. Dellarco, O. Papke, J. Olson. 1998. A comparison of dioxins, dibenzofurans and coplanar PCBs in uncooked and broiled ground beef, catfish and bacon. *Chemosphere* 37:1723–1730.

383. Schecter, A., J. J. Ryan, O. Papke. 1998. Decrease in levels and body burden of dioxins, dibenzofurans, PCBS, DDE, and HCB in blood and milk in a mother nursing twins over a thirty-eight month period. *Chemosphere* 37:1807–1816.

384. Schecter, A., P. Cramer, K. Boggess, J. Stanley, O. Papke, J. Olson, A. Silver, M. Schmitz. 2001. Intake of dioxins and related compounds from food in the U.S. population. *J. Toxicol. Environ. Health A* 63:1–18.

385. Foster, W. G., A. C. Holloway, C. L. Hughes Jr. 2005. Dioxin-like activity and maternal thyroid hormone levels in second trimester maternal serum. *Am. J. Obstet. Gynecol.* 193:1900–1907.

386. Wittsiepe, J., P. Furst, P. Schrey, F. Lemm, M. Kraft, G. Eberwein, G. Winneke, M. Wilhelm. 2007. PCDD/F and dioxin-like PCB in human blood and milk from German mothers. *Chemosphere* 67:S286–S294.

387. Wang, S. L., C. Y. Lin, Y. L. Guo, L. Y. Lin, W. L. Chou, L. W. Chang. 2004. Infant exposure to polychlorinated dibenzo-p-dioxins, dibenzofurans and biphenyls (PCDD/Fs, PCBs)—correlation between prenatal and postnatal exposure. *Chemosphere* 54:1459–1473.

388. Michalek, J. E., R. C. Tripathi, S. P. Caudill, J. L. Pirkle. 1992. Investigation of TCDD half-life heterogeneity in veterans of Operation Ranch Hand. *J. Toxicol. Environ. Health* 35:29–38.

389. Michalek, J. E., J. L. Pirkle, S. P. Caudill, R. C. Tripathi, D. G. Patterson Jr, L. L. Needham. 1996. Pharmacokinetics of TCDD in veterans of Operation Ranch Hand: 10-year follow-up. *J. Toxicol. Environ. Health* 47:209–220.

390. Michalek, J. E., J. L. Pirkle, L. L. Needham, D. G. Patterson Jr, S. P. Caudill, R. C. Tripathi, P. Mocarelli. 2002. Pharmacokinetics of 2,3,7,8-tetrachlorodibenzo-p-dioxin in Seveso adults and veterans of operation Ranch Hand. *J. Expo. Anal. Environ. Epidemiol* 12:44–53.

391. Grassman, J. A., S. A. Masten, N. J. Walker, G. W. Lucier. 1998. Animal models of human response to dioxins. *Environ. Health Perspect.* 106 (Suppl. 2):761–775.

392. Rose, J. Q., J. C. Ramsey, T. H. Wentzler, R. A. Hummel, P. J. Gehring. 1976. The fate of 2,3,7,8-tetrachlorodibenzo-p-dioxin following single and repeated oral doses to the rat. *Toxicol. Appl. Pharmacol.* 36:209–226.

393. Robles, R., Y. Morita, K. K. Mann, G. I. Perez, S. Yang, T. Matikainen, D. H. Sherr, J. L. Tilly. 2000. The aryl hydrocarbon receptor, a basic helixloop-helix transcription factor of the *PAS* gene family, is required for normal ovarian germ cell dynamics in the mouse. *Endocrinology* 141:450–453.

394. Dolwick, K. M., J. V. Schmidt, L. A. Carver, H. I. Swanson, C. A. Bradfield. 1993. Cloning and expression of a human Ah receptor cDNA. *Mol. Pharmacol.* 44:911–917.

395. Harper, P. A., R. D. Prokipcak, L. E. Bush, Golas C. L., Okey A. B. 1991. Detection and characterization of the Ah receptor for 2,3,7,8-tetrachlorodibenzo-p-dioxin in the human colon adenocarcinoma cell line LS180. *Arch. Biochem. Biophys.* 290:27–36.

396. Li, W., P. A. Harper, B. K. Tang, A. B. Okey. 1998. Regulation of cytochrome P450 enzymes by aryl hydrocarbon receptor in human cells: CYP1A2 expression in the LS180 colon carcinoma cell line after treatment with 2,3,7,8-tetrachlorodibenzo-p-dioxin or 3-methylcholanthrene. *Biochem. Pharmacol.* 56:599–612.

397. Baccarelli, A., A. C. Pesatori, D. Consonni, P. Mocarelli, D. G. Patterson Jr., N. E. Caporaso, P. A. Bertazzi, M. T. Landi. 2005. Health status and plasma dioxin levels in chloracne cases 20 years after the Seveso, Italy accident. *Br. J. Dermatol.* 152:459–465.

398. Baccarelli, A., R. Pfeiffer, D. Consonni, A. C. Pesatori, M. Bonzini, D. G. Patterson Jr., P. A. Bertazzi, M. T. Landi. 2005. Handling of dioxin measurement data in the presence of non-detectable values: Overview of available methods and their application in the Seveso chloracne study. *Chemosphere* 60:898–906.

399. Weisglas-Kuperus, N., S. Patandin, G. M. Berbers, T. J. Sas, P. H. Mulder, P. J. Sauer, H. Hooijkaas. 2000. Immunologic effects of background exposure to polychlorinated biphenyls and dioxins in Dutch preschool children. *Environ. Health Perspect.* 108:1203–1207.

400. Koopman-Esseboom, C., D. C. Morse, N. Weisglas-Kuperus, I. J. Lutkeschipholt, C. G. Van der Paauw, L. G. Tuinstra, A. Brouwer, P. J. Sauer. 1994. Effects of dioxins and polychlorinated biphenyls on thyroid hormone status of pregnant women and their infants. *Pediatr. Res.* 36:468–473.

401. Pavuk, M., A. J. Schecter, F. Z. Akhtar, J. E. Michalek. 2003. Serum 2,3,7,8-tetrachlorodibenzo-p-dioxin (TCDD) levels and thyroid function in Air Force veterans of the Vietnam War. *Ann. Epidemiol.* 13:335–343.

402. Longnecker, M. P., J. E. Michalek. 2000. Serum dioxin level in relation to diabetes mellitus among Air Force veterans with background levels of exposure. *Epidemiology* 11:44–48.

403. Eskenazi, B., P. Mocarelli, M. Warner, S. Samuels, P. Vercellini, D. Olive, L. Needham, D. Patterson, P. Brambilla. 2000. Seveso Women's Health Study: A study of the effects of 2,3,7,8-tetrachlorodibenzo-p-dioxin on reproductive health. *Chemosphere* 40:1247–1253.

404. Heilier, J. F., J. Donnez, F. Nackers, R. Rousseau, V. Verougstraete, K. Rosenkranz, O. Donnez, F. Grandjean, D. Lison, R. Tonglet. 2007. Environmental and host-associated risk factors in endometriosis and deep endometriotic nodules: A matched case-control study. *Environ. Res.* 103:121–129.

405. Koopman-Esseboom, C., N. Weisglas-Kuperus, M. A. de Ridder, C. G. Van der Paauw, L. G. Tuinstra, P. J. Sauer. 1996. Effects of polychlorinated biphenyl/dioxin exposure and feeding type on infants' mental and psychomotor development. *Pediatrics* 97:700–706.

406. Vreugdenhil, H. J., C. I. Lanting, P. G. Mulder, E. R. Boersma, N. WeisglasKuperus. 2002. Effects of prenatal PCB and dioxin background exposure on cognitive and motor abilities in Dutch children at school age. *J. Pediatr.* 140:48–56.

407. Dimich-Ward, H., C. Hertzman, K. Teschke, R. Hershler, S. A. Marion, A. Ostry, S. Kelly. 1996. Reproductive effects of paternal exposure to chlorophenate wood preservatives in the sawmill industry. *Scand. J. Work Environ. Health* 22:267–273.

408. Halldorsson, T. I., I. Thorsdottir, H. M. Meltzer, M. Strom, S. F. Olsen. 2009. Dioxin-like activity in plasma among Danish pregnant women: Dietary predictors, birth weight and infant development. *Environ. Res.* 109:22–28.

409. Leijs, M. M., J. G. Koppe, K. Olie, W. M. van Aalderen, P. Voogt, T. Vulsma, M. Westra, G. W. ten Tusscher. 2008. Delayed initiation of breast development in girls with higher prenatal dioxin exposure; a longitudinal cohort study. *Chemosphere* 73:999–1004.

410. Mocarelli, P., P. Brambilla, P. M. Gerthoux, D. G. Patterson Jr., L. L. Needham. 1996. Change in sex ratio with exposure to dioxin [Letter]. *Lancet* 348:409.

411. Mocarelli, P. et al. 2000. Paternal concentrations of dioxin and sex ratio of offspring. *Lancet* 355:1858–1863.

412. Mocarelli, P. et al. 2008. Dioxin exposure, from infancy through puberty, produces endocrine disruption and affects human semen quality. *Environ. Health Perspect.* 116:70–77.

413. Chahoud, I., R. Krowke, A. Schimmel, H. J. Merker, D. Neubert. 1989. Reproductive toxicity and pharmacokinetics of 2,3,7,8-tetrachlorodibenzo-p-dioxin. 1. Effects of high doses on the fertility of male rats. *Arch. Toxicol.* 63:432–439.

414. Hogaboam, J. P., A. J. Moore, B. P. Lawrence. 2008. The aryl hydrocarbon receptor affects distinct tissue compartments during ontogeny of the immune system. *Toxicol. Sci.* 102:160–170.

415. Fan, F., K. K. Rozman. 1995. Short- and long-term biochemical effects of 2,3,7,8-tetrachlorodibenzo-p-dioxin in female Long-Evans rats. *Toxicol. Lett.* 75:209–216.

416. Henry, E. C., T. A. Gasiewicz. 1987. Changes in thyroid hormones and thyroxine glucuronidation in hamsters compared with rats following treatment with 2,3,7,8-tetrachlorodibenzo-pdioxin. *Toxicol. Appl. Pharmacol.* 89:165–174.

417. Kohn, M. C. 2000. Effects of TCDD on thyroid hormone homeostasis in the rat. *Drug Chem. Toxicol.* 23:259–277.

418. Ishimura, R., T. Kawakami, S. Ohsako, K. Nohara, C. Tohyama. 2006. Suppressive effect of 2,3,7,8-tetrachlorodibenzop-dioxin on vascular remodeling that takes place in the normal labyrinth zone of rat placenta during late gestation. *Toxicol. Sci.* 91:265–274.

419. Kawakami, T., R. Ishimura, K. Nohara, K. Takeda, C. Tohyama, S. Ohsako. 2006. Differential susceptibilities of Holtzman and Sprague-Dawley rats to fetal death and placental dysfunction induced by 2,3,7,8-teterachlorodibenzo-p-dioxin (TCDD) despite the identical primary structure of the aryl hydrocarbon receptor. *Toxicol. Appl. Pharmacol.* 212:224–236.

420. Bell, D. R. et al. 2007. Toxicity of 2,3,7,8-tetrachlorodibenzo-p-dioxin in the developing male Wistar(Han) rat. I: No decrease in epididymal sperm count after a single acute dose. *Toxicol. Sci.* 99:214–223.

421. Bell, D. R. et al. 2007. Toxicity of 2,3,7,8-tetrachlorodibenzo-p-dioxin in the developing male Wistar(Han) rat. II: Chronic dosing causes developmental delay. *Toxicol. Sci.* 99:224–233.

422. Bjerke, D. L., R. E. Peterson. 1994. Reproductive toxicity of 2,3,7,8- tetrachlorodibenzo-p-dioxin in male rats: Different effects of in utero versus lactational exposure. *Toxicol. Appl. Pharmacol.* 127:241–249.

423. Flaws, J. A., R. J. Sommer, E. K. Silbergeld, R. E. Peterson, A. N. Hirshfield. 1997. In utero and lactational exposure to 2,3,7,8-tetrachlorodibenzo-p-dioxin (TCDD) induces genital dysmorphogenesis in the female rat. *Toxicol. Appl. Pharmacol.* 147:351–362.

424. Gray, L. E. Jr., J. S. Ostby. 1995. In utero 2,3,7,8-tetrachlorodibenzo-p-dioxin (TCDD) alters reproductive morphology and function in female rat offspring. *Toxicol. Appl. Pharmacol.* 133:285–294.

425. Gray, L. E. Jr., W. R. Kelce, E. Monosson, J. S. Ostby, L. S. Birnbaum. 1995. Exposure to TCDD during development permanently alters reproductive function in male Long Evans rats and hamsters: Reduced ejaculated and epididymal sperm numbers and sex accessory gland weights in offspring with normal androgenic status. *Toxicol. Appl. Pharmacol.* 131:108–118.

426. Gray, L. E., C. Wolf, P. Mann, J. S. Ostby. 1997. In utero exposure to low doses of 2,3,7,8-tetrachlorod-ibenzo-p-dioxin alters reproductive development of female Long Evans hooded rat offspring. *Toxicol. Appl. Pharmacol.* 146:237–244.

427. Roman, B. L., R. J. Sommer, K. Shinomiya, R. E. Peterson. 1995. In utero and lactational exposure of the male rat to 2,3,7,8- tetrachlorodibenzo-p-dioxin: Impaired prostate growth and development without inhibited androgen production. *Toxicol. Appl. Pharmacol.* 134:241–250.

428. Sommer, R. J., D. L. Ippolito, R. E. Peterson. 1996. In utero and lactational exposure of the male Holtzman rat to 2,3,7,8- tetrachlorodibenzo-p-dioxin: Decreased epididymal and ejaculated sperm numbers without alterations in sperm transit rate. *Toxicol. Appl. Pharmacol.* 140:146–153.

429. Aragon, A. C., P. G. Kopf, M. J. Campen, J. K. Huwe, M. K. Walker. 2008. In utero and lactational 2,3,7,8-tetrachlorodibenzo-p-dioxin exposure: Effects on fetal and adult cardiac gene expression and adult cardiac and renal morphology. *Toxicol. Sci.* 101:321–330.

430. Birnbaum, L. S., M. W. Harris, L. M. Stocking, A. M. Clark, R. E. Morrissey. 1989. Retinoic acid and 2,3,7,8-tetrachlorodibenzo-p-dioxin selectively enhance teratogenesis in C57BL/6N mice. *Toxicol. Appl. Pharmacol.* 98:487–500.

431. Theobald, H. M., R. E. Peterson. 1997. In utero and lactational exposure to 2,3,7,8-tetrachlorodibenzo-rho-dioxin: Effects on development of the male and female reproductive system of the mouse. *Toxicol. Appl. Pharmacol.* 145:124–135.

432. Gray, L. E., J. S. Ostby, W. R. Kelce. 1997. A dose-response analysis of the reproductive effects of a single gestational dose of 2,3,7,8-tetrachlorodibenzo-p-dioxin in male Long Evans Hooded rat offspring. *Toxicol. Appl. Pharmacol.* 146:11–20.

433. Vezina, C. M., S. H. Allgeier, R. W. Moore, T. M. Lin, J. C. Bemis, H. A. Hardin, T. A. Gasiewicz, R. E. Peterson. 2008. Dioxin causes ventral prostate agenesis by disrupting dorsoventral patterning in developing mouse prostate. *Toxicol. Sci.* 106:488–496.

434. Heimler, I., A. L. Trewin, C. L. Chaffin, R. G. Rawlins, R. J. Hutz. 1998. Modulation of ovarian follicle maturation and effects on apoptotic cell death in Holtzman rats exposed to 2,3,7,8- tetrachlorodibenzo-p-dioxin (TCDD) in utero and lactationally. *Reprod. Toxicol.* 12:69–73.

435. Wolf, C. J., J. S. Ostby, L. E. Gray Jr. 1999. Gestational exposure to 2,3,7,8-tetrachlorodibenzo-p-dioxin (TCDD) severely alters reproductive function of female hamster offspring. *Toxicol. Sci.* 51:259–264.

436. Loeffler, I. K., R. E. Peterson. 1999. Interactive effects of TCDD and p,p'-DDE on male reproductive tract development in in utero and lactationally exposed rats. *Toxicol. Appl. Pharmacol.* 154:28–39.

437. Mably, T. A., D. L. Bjerke, R. W. Moore, A. Gendron-Fitzpatrick, R. E. Peterson. 1992. In utero and lactational exposure of male rats to 2,3,7,8-tetrachlorodibenzo-p-dioxin. 3. Effects on spermatogenesis and reproductive capability. *Toxicol. Appl. Pharmacol.* 114:118–126.

438. Mably, T. A., R. W. Moore, R. E. Peterson. 1992. In utero and lactational exposure of male rats to 2,3,7,8-tetrachlorodibenzop-dioxin. Effects on androgenic status. *Toxicol. Appl. Pharmacol.* 114:97–107.

439. Moore, R. W., C. L. Potter, H. M. Theobald, J. A. Robinson, R. E. Peterson. 1985. Androgenic deficiency in male rats treated with 2,3,7,8-tetrachlorodibenzo-p-dioxin. *Toxicol. Appl. Pharmacol.* 79:99–111.

440. Ohsako, S., Y. Miyabara, M. Sakaue, R. Ishimura, M. Kakeyama, H. Izumi, J. Yonemoto, C. Tohyama. 2002. Developmental stage-specific effects of perinatal 2,3,7,8-tetrachlorodibenzo-p-dioxin exposure on reproductive organs of male rat offspring. *Toxicol. Sci.* 66:283–292.

441. Faqi, A. S., I. Chahoud. 1998. Antiestrogenic effects of low doses of 2,3,7,8-TCDD in offspring of female rats exposed throughout pregnancy and lactation. *Bull. Environ. Contam. Toxicol.* 61:462–469.

442. Mably, T. A., R. W. Moore, R. W. Goy, R. E. Peterson. 1992. In utero and lactational exposure of male rats to 2,3,7,8-tetrachlorodibenzo-p-dioxin. 2. Effects on sexual behavior and the regulation of luteinizing hormone secretion in adulthood. *Toxicol. Appl. Pharmacol.* 114:108–117.

443. Bell, D. R. et al. 2007. Relationships between tissue levels of 2,3,7,8- tetrachlorodibenzo-p-dioxin (TCDD), mRNAs, and toxicity in the developing male Wistar(Han) rat. *Toxicol. Sci.* 99:591–604.

444. Yonemoto, J., T. Ichiki, T. Takei, C. Tohyama. 2005. Maternal exposure to 2,3,7,8-tetrachlorodibenzo-p-dioxin and the body burden in offspring of Long-Evans rats. *Environ. Health Prev. Med.* 10:21–32.

445. Adler, I. D. 1996. Comparison of the duration of spermatogenesis between male rodents and humans. *Mutat. Res.* 352:169–172.

446. Aylward, L. L., J. C. Lamb, S. C. Lewis. 2005. Issues in risk assessment for developmental effects of 2,3,7,8-tetrachlorodibenzo-pdioxin and related compounds. *Toxicol. Sci.* 87:3–10.

447. Simanainen, U., A. Adamsson, J. T. Tuomisto, H. M. Miettinen, J. Toppari, J. Tuomisto, H. M. Miettinen, J. Toppari, J. Tuomisto, M. Viluksela. 2004. Adult 2,3,7,8-tetrachlorodibenzo-p-dioxin (TCDD) exposure and effects on male reproductive organs in three differentially TCDD-susceptible rat lines. *Toxicol. Sci.* 81:401–407.

448. Simanainen, U., T. Haavisto, J. T. Tuomisto, J. Paranko, J. Toppari, J. Tuomisto, R. E. Peterson, M. Viluksela. 2004. Pattern of male reproductive system effects after in utero and lactational 2,3,7,8-tetrachlorodibenzo-p-dioxin (TCDD) exposure in three differentially TCDD-sensitive rat lines 2. *Toxicol. Sci.* 80:101–108.

449. Foster, W. G., S. Maharaj-Briceño, D. G. Cyr. 2009. Dioxin-induced changes in epididymal sperm count and spermatogenesis. *Environ. Health. Perspect.* 118 (4):458–464.

450. Hess, R. A., D. J. Schaeffer, V. P. Eroschenko, J. E. Keen. 1990. Frequency of the stages in the cycle of the seminiferous epithelium in the rat. *Biol. Reprod.* 43:517–524.

451. Robb, G. W., R. P. Amann, G. J. Killian. 1978. Daily sperm production and epididymal sperm reserves of pubertal and adult rats. *J. Reprod. Fertil.* 54:103–107.

452. Pang, A. L., W. Johnson, N. Ravindranath, M. Dym, O. M. Rennert, W. Y. Chan. 2006. Expression profiling of purified male germ cells: Stage-specific expression patterns related to meiosis and postmeiotic development. *Physiol. Genomics.* 24:75–85.

453. Roman, B. L., R. S. Pollenz, R. E. Peterson. 1998. Responsiveness of the adult male rat reproductive tract to 2,3,7,8-tetrachlorodibenzo-p-dioxin exposure: Ah receptor and ARNT expression, CYP1A1 induction, and Ah receptor down-regulation. *Toxicol. Appl. Pharmacol.* 150:228–239.

454. Schultz, R., J. Suominen, T. Varre, H. Hakovirta, M. Parvinen, J. Toppari, M. Pelto-Huikko. 2003. Expression of aryl hydrocarbon receptor and aryl hydrocarbon receptor nuclear translocator messenger ribonucleic acids and proteins in rat and human testis. *Endocrinology* 144:767–776.

455. Ohsako, S. et al. 2001. Maternal exposure to a low dose of 2,3,7,8-tetrachlorodibenzo-p-dioxin (TCDD) suppressed the development of reproductive organs of male rats: Dose-dependent increase of mRNA levels of 5alpha-reductase type 2 in contrast to decrease of androgen receptor in the pubertal ventral prostate. *Toxicol. Sci.* 60:132–143.

456. Welsh, M., T. K. Saunders, M. Fisken, H. M. Scott, G. R. Hutchison, L. B. Smith, R. M. Sharpe. 2008. Identification of a programming window for reproductive tract masculinization, disruption of which leads to hypospadias and cryptorchidism. *J. Clin. Invest.* 118:1479–1490.

457. Siiteri, P. K., J. D. Wilson. 1974. Testosterone formation and metabolism during male sexual differentiation in the human embryo. *J. Clin. Endocrinol. Metab.* 38:113–125.

458. Sharpe, R. M. 2009. *Male Reproductive Health Disorders and the Potential Role of Exposure to Environmental Chemicals.* London: CHEM Trust. Accessed February 17, 2010. http://www.chemtrust. org. uk/documents/ProfRSHARPE-MaleReproductiveHealthCHEMTrust09.pdf.

459. Wilker, C., L. Johnson, S. Safe. 1996. Effects of developmental exposure to indole-3-carbinol or 2,3,7,8-tetrachlorodibenzop-dioxin on reproductive potential of male rat offspring. *Toxicol. Appl. Pharmacol.* 141:68–75.

460. Sharpe, R. M., C. McKinnell, C. Kivlin, J. S. Fisher. 2003. Proliferation and functional maturation of Sertoli cells, and their relevance to disorders of testis function in adulthood. *Reproduction* 125:769–784.

461. Atanassova, N. N., M. Walker, C. McKinnell, J. S. Fisher, R. M. Sharpe. 2005. Evidence that androgens and oestrogens, as well as follicle-stimulating hormone, can alter Sertoli cell number in the neonatal rat. *J. Endocrinol.* 184:107–117.

462. De Gendt, K. et al. 2004. A Sertoli cell-selective knockout of the androgen receptor causes spermatogenic arrest in meiosis. *Proc. Natl. Acad. Sci. U. S. A.* 101:1327–1332.

463. Tan, K. A., K. De Gendt, N. Atanassova, M. Walker, R. M. Sharpe, P. T. Saunders, E. Denolet, G. Verhoeven. 2005. The role of androgens in Sertoli cell proliferation and functional maturation: Studies in mice with total or Sertoli cell-selective ablation of the androgen receptor. *Endocrinology* 146:2674–2683.

464. Tan, K. A., K. J. Turner, P. T. Saunders, G. Verhoeven, K. De Gendt, N. Atanassova, R. M. Sharpe. 2005. Androgen regulation of stagedependent cyclin D2 expression in Sertoli cells suggests a role in modulating androgen action on spermatogenesis. *Biol. Reprod.* 72:1151–1160.

465. Johnston, H., P. J. Baker, M. Abel, H. M. Charlton, G. Jackson, L. Fleming, T. R. Kumar, P. J. O'Shaughnessy. 2004. Regulation of Sertoli cell number and activity by follicle-stimulating hormone and androgen during postnatal development in the mouse. *Endocrinology* 145:318–329.

466. Chahoud, I., J. Hartmann, G. M. Rune, D. Neubert. 1992. Reproductive toxicity and toxicokinetics of 2,3,7,8-tetrachlorodibenzo-pdioxin. 3. Effects of single doses on the testis of male rats. *Arch. Toxicol.* 66:567–572.

467. Johnson, L., R. Dickerson, S. H. Safe, C. L. Nyberg, R. P. Lewis, T. H. Welsh Jr. 1992. Reduced Leydig cell volume and function in adult rats exposed to 2,3,7,8-tetrachlorodibenzop-dioxin without a significant effect on spermatogenesis. *Toxicology* 76:103–118.

468. Morrow, D., C. Qin, R. Smith, S. Safe. 2004. Aryl hydrocarbon receptor inhibition of LNCaP prostate cancer cell growth and hormone-induced transactivation. *J. Steroid Biochem. Mol. Biol.* 88:27–36.

469. Kollara, A., T. J. Brown. 2006. Functional interaction of nuclear receptor coactivator 4 with aryl hydrocarbon receptor. *Biochem. Biophys. Res. Commun.* 346:526–534.

470. Fisher, M. T., M. Nagarkatti, P. S. Nagarkatti. 2005. Aryl hydrocarbon receptor-dependent induction of loss of mitochondrial membrane potential in epididydimal spermatozoa by 2,3,7,8- tetrachlorodibenzo-p-dioxin (TCDD). *Toxicol. Lett.* 157:99–107.

471. Sutovsky, P., R. Moreno, J. Ramalho-Santos, T. Dominiko, W. E. Thompson, G. Schatten. 2001. A putative, ubiquitin-dependent mechanism for the recognition and elimination of defective spermatozoa in the mammalian epididymis. *J. Cell Sci.* 114:1665–1675.

472. Cooper, T. G., C. H. Teung, R. Jones, M. C. Orgebin-Crist, B. Robaire. 2002. Rebuttal of a role for the epididymis in sperm quality control by phagocytosis of defective sperm. *J. Cell Sci.* 115:5–7.

473. Cyr, D. G., M. Gregory, E. Dufresnes, E. Dube, P. T. K. Chan, L. Hermo. 2007. The orchestration of occludin, claudins, catenins and cadherins as players involved in maintenance of the blood-epididymal barrier in animals and humans. *Asian J. Androl.* 9:463–475.

474. Robaire, B., B. Hinton, M. C. Orgebin-Crist. 2006. The epididymis. In *Physiology of Reproduction*, 3rd ed., E. Knobil, J. Neil, Eds., pp. 1071–1148. New York: Elsevier.

475. Barlow, N., P. M. D. Foster. 2003. Pathogenesis of male reproductive tract lesions from gestation through adulthood following in utero exposure to di(n-butyl) phthalate. *Toxicol. Pathol.* 31:397–410.

476. McKinnell, C., N. Atanassova, K. Williams, J. S. Fisher, M. Walker, K. J. Turner, T. K. Saunders, R. M. Sharpe. 2000. Suppression of androgen action and the induction of gross abnormalities of the reproductive tract in male rats treated neonatally with diethylstilbesterol. *J. Androl.* 22:323–338.

477. Hess, R. A. 2002. The efferent ductules: Structure and functions. In *The Epididymis: From Molecules to Clinical Practice*, B. Robaire, B. T. Hinton, Eds., pp. 49–80. New York: Plenum.

478. Zhou, Q. et al. 2001. Estrogen action and male fertility: Roles of the sodium/hydrogen exchanger-3 and fluid reabsorption in reproduction tract function. *Proc. Natl. Acad. Sci. U. S. A.* 98:14132–14137.

479. Safe, S., F. Wang, W. Porter, R. Duan, A. McDougal. 1998. Ah receptor agonist as endocrine disruptors: Antiestrogenic activity and mechanisms. *Toxicol. Lett.* 102:343–347.

480. Ruz, R., M. Gregory, C. E. Smith, D. G. Cyr, R. A. Hess, D. B. Lubahn, R. A. Hess, L. Hermo. 2006. Expression of aquaporins in the efferent ducts, sperm counts, and sperm motility in estrogen receptor-α deficient mice fed lab chow versus casein. *Mol. Reprod. Dev.* 73:226–237.

481. Carlsen, E., A. Giwercman, N. Keiding, N. E. Skakkebaek. 1992. Evidence for decreasing quality of semen during past 50 years. *BMJ* 305:609–613.

482. Auger, J., J. M. Kunstmann, F. Czyglik, P. Jouannet. 1995. Decline in semen quality among fertile men in Paris during the past 20 years. *N. Engl. J. Med.* 332:281–285.

483. Irvine, S., E. Cawood, D. Richardson, E. MacDonald, J. Aitken. 1996. Evidence of deteriorating semen quality in the United Kingdom: Birth cohort study in 577 men in Scotland over 11 years. *BMJ* 312:467–471.

484. Younglai, E. V., J. A. Collins, W. G. Foster. 1998. Canadian semen quality: An analysis of sperm density among eleven academic fertility centers. *Fertil. Steril.* 70:76–80.

485. Pal, P. C., M. Rajalakshmi, M. Manocha, R. S. Sharma, S. Mittal, D. N. Rao. 2006. Semen quality and sperm functional parameters in fertile Indian men. *Andrologia* 38:20–25.

486. Jorgensen, N. et al. 2001. Regional differences in semen quality in *Eur. Hum. Reprod.* 16:1012–1019.
487. Jorgensen, N. et al. 2002. East-west gradient in semen quality in the Nordic-Baltic area: A study of men from the general population in Denmark, Norway, Estonia and Finland. *Hum. Reprod.* 17:2199–2208.
488. Jorgensen, N., C. Asklund, E. Carlsen, N. E. Skakkebaek. 2006. Coordinated European investigations of semen quality: Results from studies of Scandinavian young men is a matter of concern. *Int. J. Androl.* 29:54–61.
489. De Celis, R., A. Feria-Velasco, M. Gonzalez-Unzaga, J. Torres-Calleja, N. Pedron-Nuevo. 2000. Semen quality of workers occupationally exposed to hydrocarbons. *Fertil. Steril.* 73:221–228.
490. Eskenazi, B., A. Wyrobek, L. Fenster, D. Katz, M. Sadler, J. Lee, M. Hudes, D. M. Rempel. 1991. A study of the effect of perchloroethylene exposure on semen quality in dry cleaning workers. *Am. J. Ind. Med.* 20:575–591.
491. Guo, Y. L., P. C. Hsu, C. C. Hsu, G. H. Lambert. 2000. Semen quality after prenatal exposure to poly-chlorinated biphenyls and dibenzofurans. *Lancet* 356:1240–1241.
492. Van Waeleghem, K., N. De Clercq, L. Vermeulen, F. Schoonjans, F. Comhaire. 1996. Deterioration of sperm quality in young healthy Belgian men. *Hum. Reprod.* 11:325–329.
493. Comhaire, F. H., A. M. Mahmoud, F. Schoonjans. 2007. Sperm quality, birth rates and the environment in Flanders (Belgium). *Reprod. Toxicol.* 23:133–137.
494. Dhooge, W., N. van Larebeke, G. Koppen, V. Nelen, G. Schoeters, R. Vlietinck, J. M. Kaufman, F. Comhaire. 2006. Serum dioxin-like activity is associated with reproductive parameters in young men from the general Flemish population. *Environ. Health Perspect.* 114:1670–1676.
495. Toft, G. et al. 2007. Semen quality in relation to xenohormone and dioxin-like serum activity among Inuits and three European populations. *Environ. Health Perspect.* 115 (Suppl. 1):15–20.
496. Atlas, E., C. S. Giam. 1981. Global transport of organic pollutants: Ambient concentrations in the remote marine atmosphere. *Science* 211 (4478):163–165.
497. Dougherty, C. P., S. H. Holtz, J. C. Reinert, L. Panyacosit, D. A. Axelrad, T. J. Woodruff. 2000. Dietary exposures to food contaminants across the United States. *Environ. Res.* 84 (2):170–185.
498. Fisher, B. E. 1999. Most unwanted. *Environ. Health Perspect.* 107:A18–A23.
499. Schafer, K. S., S. E. Kegley. 2002. Persistent toxic chemicals in the US food supply. *J. Epidemiol Community Health* 56 (11):813–817.
500. Van den Berg, H. 2009. Global status of DDT and its alternatives for use in vector control to prevent disease. *Environ. Health Perspect.* 17:1656–1663.
501. Kiviranta, H., J. T. Tuomisto, J. Tuomisto, E. Tukiainen, T. Vartiainen. 2005. Polychlorinated dibenzo-p-dioxins, dibenzofurans, and biphenyls in the general population in Finland. *Chemosphere* 60 (7):854–869.
502. Fierens, S., H. Mairesse, J. F. Heilier, C. De Burbure, J. F. Focant, G. Eppe, E. De Pauw, A. Bernard. 2003. Dioxin/polychlorinated biphenyl body burden, diabetes and endometriosis: Findings in a population-based study in Belgium. *Biomarkers* 8 (6):529–534.
503. Henriksen, G. L., N. S. Ketchum, J. E. Michalek, J. A. Swaby. 1997. Serum dioxin and diabetes mellitus in veterans of Operation Ranch Hand. *Epidemiology* 8 (3):252–258.
504. Lee, D. H., I. K. Lee, K. Song, M. Steffes, W. Toscano, B. A. Baker, D. R. Jacobs Jr. 2006. A strong dose-response relation between serum concentrations of persistent organic pollutants and diabetes: Results from the National Health and Examination Survey 1999–2002. *Diabetes Care* 29 (7):1638–1644.
505. Rignell-Hydbom, A., L. Rylander, L. Hagmar. 2007. Exposure to persistent organochlorine pollutants and type 2 diabetes mellitus. *Hum. Exp. Toxicol.* 26 (5):447–452.
506. Turyk, M., H. A. Anderson, L. Knobeloch, P. Imm, V. W. Persky. 2009. Prevalence of diabetes and body burdens of polychlorinated biphenyls, polybrominated diphenyl ethers, and p,p′-diphenyldichloroethene in Great Lakes sport fish consumers. *Chemosphere* 75 (5):674–679.
507. Wang, S. L., P. C. Tsai, C. Y. Yang, Y. L. Guo. 2008. Increased risk of diabetes and polychlorinated biphe-nyls and dioxins—A 24-year follow-up study of the Yucheng cohort. *Diabetes Care* 31 (8):1574–1579.
508. Ford, E. S., W. H. Giles, A. H. Mokdad. 2004. Increasing prevalence of the metabolic syndrome among U.S adults. *Diabetes Care* 27 (10):2444–2449.
509. Biddinger, S. B., C. R. Kahn. 2006. From mice to men: Insights into the insulin resistance syndromes. *Annu. Rev. Physiol.* 68:123–158.
510. Reaven, G. M. 2005. Why Syndrome X? From Harold Himsworth to the insulin resistance syndrome. *Cell Metab.* 1 (1):9–14.
511. Hites, R. A., J. A. Foran, D. O. Carpenter, M. C. Hamilton, B. A. Knuth, S. J. Schwager. 2004. Global assessment of organic contaminants in farmed salmon. *Science* 303 (5655):226–229.

512. Scientific Advisory Committee on Nutrition. 2004. Advice on Fish Consumption: Benefits and Risks. Accessed February 19, 2010. http://cot.food.gov.uk/pdfs/fishreport2004full.pdf.

513. Jump, D. B. 2002. The biochemistry of n-3 polyunsaturated fatty acids. *J. Biol. Chem.* 277 (11):8755–8758.

514. Storlien, L. H., E. W. Kraegen, D. J. Chisholm, G. L. Ford, D. G. Bruce, W. S. Pascoe. 1987. Fish oil prevents insulin resistance induced by high-fat feeding in rats. *Science* 237 (4817):885–888.

515. Ruzzin, J. et al. 2009. Persistent organic pollutant exposure leads to insulin resistance syndrome. *Environ. Health Perspect.* 118 (4): 465–471.

516. Angulo, P. 2002. Nonalcoholic fatty liver disease. *N. Engl. J. Med.* 346 (16):1221–1231.

517. Zimmet, P., K. G. Alberti, J. Shaw. 2001. Global and societal implications of the diabetes epidemic. *Nature* 414 (6865):782–787.

518. WHO. 2005. Chronic Diseases: A Vital Investment. Geneva: World Health Organization. Accessed February 19, 2010. http://www.who.int/chp/chronic_disease_report/contents/en/index.html.

519. Hill, J. O., J. C. Peters. 1998. Environmental contributions to the obesity epidemic. *Science* 280 (5368):1371–1374.

520. Roberts, C. K., B. J. Barnard. 2005. Effects of exercise and diet on chronic disease. *J. Appl. Physiol.* 98 (1):3–30.

521. Kelishadi, R., N. Mirghaffari, P. Poursafa, S. S. Gidding. 2009. Lifestyle and environmental factors associated with inflammation, oxidative stress and insulin resistance in children. *Atherosclerosis* 203 (1):311–319.

522. Sun, Q. et al. 2009. Ambient air pollution exaggerates adipose inflammation and insulin resistance in a mouse model of diet-induced obesity. *Circulation* 119 (4):538–546.

523. Alonso-Magdalena, P., S. Morimoto, C. Ripoll, E. Fuentes, A. Nadal. 2006. The estrogenic effect of bisphenol A disrupts pancreatic β-cell function *in vivo* and induces insulin resistance. *Environ. Health Perspect.* 114:106–112.

524. Guallar, E. et al. 1999. Omega-3 fatty acids in adipose tissue and risk of myocardial infarction—The EURAMIC study. *Arterioscler. Thromb.* 19 (4):1111–1118.

525. Rissanen, T., S. Voutilainen, K. Nyyssonen, T. A. Lakka, J. T. Salonen. 2000. Fish oil-derived fatty acids, docosahexaenoic acid and docosapentaenoic acid, and the risk of acute coronary events—The Kuopio Ischaemic Heart Disease Risk Factor Study. *Circulation* 102 (22):2677–2679.

526. European Union. 2006. Amending regulation (EC) No 466/2001 setting maximum levels for certain contaminants in foodstuffs as regards dioxins and dioxin-like PCBs. Commission Regulation (EC) No 199/2006. *Official Journal of the European Union* L32:34–38. Accessed February 19, 2010. http://www.health.gov.mt/fsc/fsc_euleg_files/RegEC199_2006e.pdf.

527. Nweke, O. C., W. H. Sanders III. 2009. Modern environmental health hazards: A public health issue of increasing significance in Africa. *Environ. Health Perspect.* 117:863–870.

528. European Union. 2008. Amending regulation (EC) No 396/2005 on maximum residue levels of pesticides in or on food and feed of plant and animal origin, as regards the implementing powers conferred on the Commission. Regulation (EC) No 299/2008. *Official Journal of the European Union* L97:37–71. Accessed February 19, 2010. http://eur-lex.europa.eu/LexUriServ/LexUriServ.do?uri=OJ:L:2008:097:0 067:0071:EN:PDF.

529. Meeker, J. D., H. M. Stapleton. 2009. House dust concentrations of organophosphate flame retardants in relation to hormone levels and semen quality parameters. *Environ. Health Perspect.* 118 (3): 318–323.

530. Diamanti-Kandarakis, E., J. P. Bourguignon, L. C. Giudice, R. Hauser, G. S. Prins, A. M. Soto, R. T. Zoeller, A. C. Gore. 2009. Endocrine-disrupting chemicals: An Endocrine Society scientific statement. *Endocr. Rev.* 30:293–342.

531. Swan, S. H., E. P. Elkin, L. Fenster. 2000. The question of declining sperm density revisited: An analysis of 101 studies published 1934–1996. *Environ. Health Perspect.* 108:961–966.

532. Andersson, A. M., T. K. Jensen, A. Juul, J. H. Petersen, T. Jørgensen, N. E. Skakkebaek. 2007. Secular decline in male testosterone and sex hormone binding globulin serum levels in Danish population surveys. *J. Clin. Endocrinol. Metab.* 92:4696–4705.

533. Travison, T. G., A. B. Araujo, A. B. O'Donnell, V. Kupelian, J. B. McKinlay. 2007. A population-level decline in serum testosterone levels in American men. *J. Clin. Endocrinol. Metab.* 92:196–202.

534. Paulozzi, L. J. 1999. International trends in rates of hypospadias and cryptorchidism. *Environ. Health Perspect.* 107:297–302.

535. Adami, H. O., R. Bergström, M. Möhner, W. Zatonski, H. Storm, A. Ekbom, S. Tretli, L. Teppo, H. Ziegler, M. Rahu. 1994. *Int. J. Cancer.* 59:33–38.

536. Bergström, R., H. O. Adami, M. Möhner, W. Zatonski, H. Storm, A. Ekbom, S. Tretli, L. Teppo, O. Akre, T. Hakulinen. 1996. Increase in testicular cancer incidence in six European countries: A birth cohort phenomenon. *J. Natl. Cancer Inst.* 88:727–733.
537. Huyghe, E., T. Matsuda, P. Thonneau. 2003. Increasing incidence of testicular cancer worldwide: A review. *J. Urol.* 170:5–11.
538. Davies, L., H. G. Welch. 2006. Increasing incidence of thyroid cancer in the United States, 1973–2002. *JAMA* 295:2164–2167.
539. Enewold, L., K. Zhu, E. Ron, A. J. Marrogi, A. Stojadinovic, G. E. Peoples, S. S. Devesa. 2009. Rising thyroid cancer incidence in the United States by demographic and tumor characteristics, 1980–2005. *Cancer Epidemiol. Biomarkers Prev.* 18:784–791.
540. Harris, K. B., K. A. Pass. 2007. Increase in congenital hypothyroidism in New York State and in the United States. *Mol. Genet. Metab.* 91:268–277.
541. Hertz-Picciotto, I., L. Delwiche. 2009. The rise in autism and the role of age at diagnosis. *Epidemiology* 20:84–90.
542. Babich, J. A. 2006. *CPSC Staff Preliminary Risk Assessment of Flame Retardant (FR) Chemicals in Upholstered Furniture Foam.* Bethesda, MD: Consumer Product Safety Commission. Accessed January 27, 2010. http://www.cpsc.gov/library/foia/foia07/brief/ufurn2.pdf.
543. Meeker, J. D., D. B. Barr, R. Hauser. 2006. Thyroid hormones in relation to urinary metabolites of non-persistent insecticides in men of reproductive age. *Reprod. Toxicol.* 22:437–442.
544. Meeker, J. D., L. Ryan, D. B. Barr, R. Hauser. 2006. Exposure to nonpersistent insecticides and male reproductive hormones. *Epidemiology.* 17:61–68.
545. Stapleton, H. M., J. G. Allen, S. M. Kelly, A. Konstantinov, S. Klosterhaus, D. Watkins, M. D. McClean, T. F. Webster. 2008. Alternate and new brominated flame retardants detected in U.S. house dust. *Environ. Sci. Technol.* 42:6910–6916.
546. Reemtsma, T., J. B. Quintana, R. Rodil, M. Garcia-Lopez, I. Rodriguez. 2008. Organophosphorus flame retardants and plasticizers in water and air I. Occurrence and fate. *Trends. Anal. Chem.* 27:727–737.
547. U.S. EPA. 2006. *Inventory Update Reporting (IUR).* IUR Data. Washington, DC: U.S. Environmental Protection Agency. Accessed July 8, 2009. http://www.epa.gov/oppt/iur/tools/data/.
548. U.S. EPA. 2005. Furniture Flame Retardancy Partnership: Environmental Profiles of Chemical Flame-Retardant Alternative for Low-Density Polyurethane Foam. EPA 742- R-05-002. Washington, DC: U.S. Environmental Protection Agency. Accessed January 27, 2010. http://www.epa.gov/dfe/pubs/flameret/ffr-alt.htm.
549. Stapleton, H. M., S. Klosterhaus, S. Eagle, J. Fuh, J. D. Meeker, A. Blum, T. F. Webster. 2009. Detection of organophosphate flame retardants in furniture foam and U.S. house dust. *Environ. Sci. Technol.* 43:7490–7495.
550. Johnson-Restrepo, B., K. Kannan. 2009. An assessment of sources and pathways of human exposure to polybrominated diphenyl ethers in the United States. *Chemosphere* 76:542–548.
551. Lorber, M. 2008. Exposure of Americans to polybrominated diphenyl ethers. *J. Expo. Sci. Environ. Epidemiol.* 18:2–19.
552. Sjodin, A., L. Y. Wong, R. S. Jones, A. Park, Y. Zhang, C. Hodge, E. Dipietro, C. McClure, W. Turner, L. L. Needham, D. G. Patterson Jr. 2008. Serum concentrations of polybrominated diphenyl ethers (PBDEs) and polybrominated biphenyl (PBB) in the United States population: 2003–2004. *Environ. Sci. Technol.* 42:1377–1384.
553. Hudec, T., J. Thean, D. Kuehl, R. C. Dougherty. 1981. Tris(dichloropropyl) phosphate, a mutagenic flame retardant: Frequent cocurrence in human seminal plasma. *Science* 211:951–952.
554. National Research Council (NRC). 2000. *Toxicological Risks of Selected Flame-Retardant Chemicals.* Washington, DC: National Research Council, National Academies Press. https://doi.org/10.17226/9841.
555. WHO. 1999. *WHO Laboratory Manual for Examination of Human Semen and Semen–Cervical Mucus Interaction.* Cambridge, UK: Cambridge University Press. https://www.slideshare.net/netopenscienart/who-laboratory-manual-for-the-examination-of-human-semen-and-spermcervical-mucus-interaction.
556. Marklund, A., B. Andersson, P. Haglund. 2003. Screening of organophosphorus compounds and their distribution in various indoor environments. *Chemosphere* 53:1137–1146.
557. Marklund, A., B. Andersson, P. Haglund. 2005. Organophosphorus flame retardants and plasticizers in air from various indoor environments. *J. Environ. Monit.* 7:814–819.
558. Takigami, H., G. Suzuki, Y. Hirai, Y. Ishikawa, M. Sunami, S. Sakai. 2009. Flame retardants in indoor dust and air of a hotel in Japan. *Environ. Int.* 35:688–693.
559. Miller, M. D., K. M. Crofton, D. C. Rice, R. T. Zoeller. 2009. Thyroiddisrupting chemicals: Interpreting upstream biomarkers of adverse outcomes. *Environ. Health Perspect.* 117:1033–1041.

560. Ben-Jonathan, N., C. R. LaPensee, E. W. LaPensee. 2008. What can we learn from rodents about prolactin in humans? *Endocr. Rev.* 29:1–41.

561. Freeman, M. E., B. Kanyicska, A. Lerant, G. Nagy. 2000. Prolactin: Structure, function, and regulation of secretion. *Physiol. Rev.* 80:1523–1631.

562. de Burbure, C. et al. 2006. Renal and neurologic effects of cadmium, lead, mercury, and arsenic in children: Evidence of early effects and multiple interactions at environmental exposure levels. *Environ. Health Perspect.* 114:584–590.

563. Meeker, J. D., M. G. Rossano, B. Protas, M. P. Diamond, E. Puscheck, D. Daly, N. Paneth, J. J. Wirth. 2009. Multiple metals predict prolactin and thyrotropin (TSH) levels in men. *Environ. Res.* 109:869–873.

564. Felt, B., E. Jimenez, J. Smith, A. Calatroni, N. Kaciroti, G. Wheatcroft, B. Lozoff. 2006. Iron deficiency in infancy predicts altered serum prolactin response 10 years later. *Pediatr. Res.* 60:513–517.

565. Fang, H., W. Tong, W. S. Branham, C. L. Moland, S. L. Dial, H. Hong, Q. Xie, R. Perkins, W. Owens, D. M. Sheehan. 2003. Study of 202 natural, synthetic, and environmental chemicals for binding to the androgen receptor. *Chem. Res. Toxicol.* 16:1338–1358.

566. Honkakoski, P., J. J. Palvimo, L. Penttila, J. Vepsalainen, S. Auriola. 2004. Effects of triaryl phosphates on mouse and human nuclear receptors. *Biochem. Pharmacol.* 67:97–106.

567. Latendresse, J. R., C. L. Brooks, C. D. Flemming, C. C. Capen. 1994. Reproductive toxicity of butylated triphenyl phosphate and tricresyl phosphate fluids in F344 rats. *Fundam. Appl. Toxicol.* 22:392–399.

568. Meeker, J. D., S. R. Ravi, D. B. Barr, R. Hauser. 2008. Circulating estradiol in men is inversely related to urinary metabolites of nonpersistent insecticides. *Reprod. Toxicol.* 25:184–191.

569. Meeker, J. D., L. Ryan, D. B. Barr, R. F. Herrick, D. H. Bennett, R. Bravo, R. Hauser. 2004. The relationship of urinary metabolites of carbaryl/naphthalene and chlorpyrifos with human semen quality. *Environ. Health Perspect.* 112:1665–1670.

570. Padungtod, C., D. A. Savitz, J. W. Overstreet, D. C. Christiani, L. M. Ryan, X. Xu. 2000. Occupational pesticide exposure and semen quality among Chinese workers. *J. Occup. Environ. Med.* 42:982–992.

571. Recio-Vega, R., G. Ocampo-Gomez, V. H. Borja-Aburto, J. MoranMartinez, M. E. Cebrian-Garcia. 2008. Organophosphorus pesticide exposure decreases sperm quality: Association between sperm parameters and urinary pesticide levels. *J. Appl. Toxicol.* 28:674–680.

572. Yucra, S., J. Rubio, M. Gasco, C. Gonzales, K. Steenland, G. F. Gonzales. 2006. Semen quality and reproductive sex hormone levels in Peruvian pesticide sprayers. *Int. J. Occup. Environ. Health* 12:355–361.

573. Yucra, S., M. Gasco, J. Rubio, G. F. Gonzales. 2008. Semen quality in Peruvian pesticide applicators: Association between urinary organophosphate metabolites and semen parameters. *Environ. Health* 7:59. doi: 10.1186/1476-069X-7-59 [Online November 17, 2008].

574. Guven, M., F. Bayram, K. Unluhizarci, F. Kelestimur. 1999. Endocrine changes in patients with acute organophosphate poisoning. *Hum. Exp. Toxicol.* 18:598–601.

575. Satar, S., D. Satar, S. Kirim, H. Leventerler. 2005. Effects of acute organophosphate poisoning on thyroid hormones in rats. *Am. J. Ther.* 12:238–242.

576. De Angelis, S., R. Tassinari, F. Maranghi, A. Eusepi, A. Di Virgilio, F. Chiarotti, L. Ricceri, A. Venerosi Pesciolini, E. Gilardi, G. Moracci, G. Calamandrei, A. Olivieri, A. Mantovani. 2009. Developmental exposure to chlorpyrifos induces alterations in thyroid and thyroid hormone levels without other toxicity signs in CD-1 mice. *Toxicol. Sci.* 108:311–319.

577. Rawlings, N. C., S. J. Cook, D. Waldbillig. 1998. Effects of the pesticides carbofuran, chlorpyrifos, dimethoate, lindane, triallate, trifluralin, 2,4-D, and pentachlorophenol on the metabolic endocrine and reproductive endocrine system in ewes. *J. Toxicol. Environ. Health A* 54:21–36.

578. Sarkar, R., K. P. Mohanakumar, M. Chowdhury. 2000. Effects of an organophosphate pesticide, quinalphos, on the hypothalamo-pituitary-gonadal axis in adult male rats. *J. Reprod. Fertil.* 118:29–38.

579. Reemtsma, T., J. B. Quintana, R. Rodil, M. Garcia-Lopez, I. Rodriguez. 2008. Organophosphorus flame retardants and plasticizers in water and air I. Occurrence and fate. *Trends Anal. Chem.* 27:727–737.

580. Armstrong, B. 2004. Exposure measurement error: Consequences and design issues. In *Exposure Assessment in Occupational and Environmental Epidemiology*, M. J. Nieuwenhuijsen, Ed., pp. 181–200. New York: Oxford University Press.

581. Tiedeken, J. A., J. S. Ramsdell. 2009. Zebrafish seizure model identifies p,p'-DDE as the dominant contaminant of fetal California sea lions that accounts for synergistic activity with domoic acid. *Environ. Health Perspect.* 118 (4):545–551.

582. DeLong, R. L., W. G. Gilmartin, J. G. Simpson. 1973. Premature births in California sea lions: Association with high organochlorine pollutant residue levels. *Science* 181:1168–1170.

583. Gerber, J. A., J. Roletto, L. E. Morgan, D. M. Smith, L. J. Gage. 1993. Findings in pinnipeds stranded along the central and northern California coast, 1984–1990. *J. Wildl. Dis.* 29 (3):423–433.

584. Scholin, C. A. et al. 2000. Mortality of sea lions along the central California coast linked to a toxic diatom bloom. *Nature* 403 (6765):80–84.

585. Brodie, E. C., F. M. D Gulland, D. J. Greig, M. Hunter, J. Jaakola, J. S. Leger, T. A. Leighfield, F. M. Van Dolah. 2006. Domoic acid causes reproductive failure in California sea lions (*Zalophus californianus*). *Mar. Mamm. Sci.* 22 (3):700–707.

586. Gilmartin, W. G., R. L. DeLong, A. W. Smith, J. C. Sweeny, B. W. De Lappe, R. W. Risebrough, L. A. Griner, M. D. Dailey, D. B. Peakall. 1976. Premature parturition in the California sea lion. *J. Wildl. Dis.* 12:104–114.

587. Greig, D. L., F. M. D Gulland, C. Kreuder. 2005. A decade of live California sea lion (*Zalophus californianus*) strandings along the central California coast: Causes and trends, 1991–2000. *Aquat. Mamm.* 31 (1):11–22.

588. Sexton, K., D. Hattis. 2007. Assessing cumulative health risks from exposure to environmental mixtures—Three fundamental questions. *Environ. Health Perspect.* 115:825–832.

589. Greig, D. J., G. M. Ylitalo, A. J. Hall, D. A. Fauquier, F. Gulland. 2007. Transplacental transfer of organochlorines in California sea lions (*Zalophus californianus*). *Environ. Toxicol. Chem.* 26 (1):37–44.

590. Connolly, J. P., D. Glaser. 2002. p,p'-DDE bioaccumulation in female sea lions of the California Channel Islands. *Continental Shelf Res.* 22 (6–7):1059–1078.

591. You, L., E. Gazi, S. Archibeque-Engle, M. Casanova, R. B. Conolly, H. D. Heck. 1999. Transplacental and lactational transfer of p,p'-DDE in Sprague-Dawley rats. *Toxicol. Appl. Pharmacol.* 157 (2):134–144.

592. Maucher, J. M., J. S. Ramsdell. 2007. Maternal–fetal transfer of domoic acid in rats at two gestational time points. *Environ. Health Perspect.* 115:1743–1746.

593. Tiedeken, J. A., J. S. Ramsdell. 2009. DDT exposure of zebrafish embryos enhances seizure susceptibility: Relationship to fetal p,p'-DDE burden and domoic acid exposure of California sea lions. *Environ. Health Perspect.* 117:68–73.

594. Goldstein, T., T. S. Zabka, R. L. Delong, E. A. Wheeler, G. Ylitalo, S. Bargu, M. Silver, T. Leighfield, F. Van Dolah, G. Langlois, I. Sidor, J. L. Dunn, F. M. Gulland. 2009. The role of domoic acid in abortion and premature parturition of California sea lions (*Zalophus californianus*) on San Miguel Island, California. *J. Wildl. Dis.* 45 (1):91–108.

595. Ulbrich, B., R. Stahlmann. 2004. Developmental toxicity of polychlorinated biphenyls (PCBs): A systematic review of experimental data. *Arch. Toxicol.* 78 (5):252–268.

596. Sagiv, S. K., J. K. Nugent, T. B. Brazelton, A. L. Choi, P. E. Tolbert, L. M. Altshul, S. A. Korrick. 2008. Prenatal organochlorine exposure and measures of behavior in infancy using the Neonatal Behavioral Assessment Scale (NBAS). *Environ. Health Perspect.* 116:666–673.

597. Bowers, W. J., J. S. Nakai, I. Chu, M. G. Wade, D. Moir, A. Yagminas, S. Gill, O. Pulido, R. Meuller. 2004. Early developmental neurotoxicity of a PCB/organochlorine mixture in rodents after gestational and lactational exposure. *Toxicol. Sci.* 77 (1):51–62.

598. Chevrier, J., B. Eskenazi, N. Holland, A. Bradman, D. B. Barr. 2008. Effects of exposure to polychlorinated biphenyls and organochlorine pesticides on thyroid function during pregnancy. *Am. J. Epidemiol.* 168 (3):298–310.

599. Altmann, L., W. R. Mundy, T. R. Ward, A. Fastabend, H. Lilienthal. 2001. Developmental exposure of rats to a reconstituted PCB mixture or Aroclor 1254: Effects on long-term potentiation and [3H]MK-801 binding in occipital cortex and hippocampus. *Toxicol. Sci.* 61 (2):321–330.

600. Stapleton, H. M., N. G. Dodder, J. R. Kucklick, C. M. Reddy, M. M. Schantz, P. R. Becker, F. Gulland, B. J. Porter, S. A. Wise. 2006. Determination of HBCD, PBDEs and MeO-BDEs in California sea lions (*Zalophus californianus*) stranded between 1993 and 2003. *Mar. Pollut. Bull.* 52 (5):522–531.

601. Le Boeuf, B. J., J. P. Giesy, K. Kannan, N. Kajiwara, S. Tanabe, C. Debier. 2002. Organochloride pesticides in California sea lions revisited. *BMC Ecol.* 2 (1):11. doi: 10.1186/1472-6785- 2-11 [Online December 12, 2002].

602. Mazdai, A., N. G. Dodder, M. P. Abernathy, R. A. Hites, R. M. Bigsby. 2003. Polybrominated diphenyl ethers in maternal and fetal blood samples. *Environ. Health Perspect.* 111:1249–1252.

603. Costa, L. G., G. Giordano. 2007. Developmental neurotoxicity of polybrominated diphenyl ether (PBDE) flame retardants. *Neurotoxicology* 28 (6):1047–1067.

604. Dencker, L., P. Eriksson. 1998. Susceptibility in utero and upon neonatal exposure. *Food Addit. Contam.* 15 (Suppl.):37–43.

605. Luke, B. G. 1988. Pesticides in human food: Breast milk. *Paper presented at the Symposium of the Australian Society for Environmental Medicine.* Melbourne: Australia, March 1988.

606. News release. 1987. Lanolin products cleared. *Natl. Health Med. Res. Council* 41:1–2.

607. Preussmann, R. 1975. Chemische carcinogene in der menchlichen umwelt. In *Handbuch der allgemeinene Pathologie,* Vol. 6, Part 6, pp. 421–594. Berlin: Springer-Verlag.

608. Steinberg, D., S. Tarthasarthy, T. E. Carew, J. C. K. Khoo, J. L. Witztum. 1989. Beyond cholesterol: Modifications of low density lipoproteins that increase its atherogenicity. *N. Engl. J. Med.* 320:915–924.

609. Fradin, J., R. Dumas, L. Leforestier. 1992. *Toxicity of Heated Food in Relation to the Reached Temperatures.* Paris: Institut de Medecine Environmentale 4.

610. Bruce, W. R. 1987. Recent hypotheses for the origin of colon cancer. *Cancer Res.* 47:4237–4242.

611. Wargovitch, M. J., A. Medline, W. R. Bruce. 1983. Early histopathologic events to evolution of colon cancer in C57BL/6 and CF1 mice treated with 1.2-dimethylhydrazine. *J. Natl. Cancer Inst.* 71:125–131.

612. Kaneda, T., M. Masaki, S. Tane, M. Ueta. 1977. *Abst. 6th Annual Meeting of the Environmental Mutagen Society of Japan,* p. 42.

613. *European Communities submission to World Trade Organization dispute panel, January 28, 2005.*

614. Smith, J. 2010. *Genetically Modified Soy Linked to Sterility, Infant Mortality in Hamsters.* The Huffington Post. Accessed April 12, 2016. http://www.huffingtonpost.com/jeffrey-smith/genetically-modified-soy_b_544575.html.

615. Shaw, D., S. Culpepper, M. Owen, A. Price, R. Wilson. 2012. Herbicide-resistant weeds threaten soil conservation gains: finding a balance for soil and farm sustainability. CAST Issue Paper 49.

616. Hillger, D., K. Qin, D. M. Simpson, P. Havens. 2010. Reduction in drift and voltality of enlist duo with colex-D technology. *2010 North Central Weed Science Society Conference Proceedings* 65:38.

617. Ji, S. 2012. Wheat Contains Not One, but 23K Potentially Harmful Proteins. *GreenMedInfo.com.* Accessed October 24, 2013. http://www.greenmedinfo.com/blog/wheat-contains-not-one-23k-potentiallyharmful-proteins.

618. Rubio-Tapia, A. et al. 2009. Increased prevalence and mortality in undiagnosed celiac disease. *Gastroenterology* 137 (1):88–93.

619. Helms, S. 2005. Celiac disease and gluten-associated diseases. *Altern. Med. Rev.* 10 (3): 172–193.

620. Gluten Research on 300+ Adverse Health Effects. October 2, 2013. www.GreenMedInfo.com.

621. Catassi, C., D. Kryszak, B. Bhatti, C. Sturgeon, K. Helzlsouer, S. L. Clipp, D. Gelfond, E. Puppa, A. Sferruzza, A. Fasano. 2010. Natural history of celiac disease autoimmunity in a USA cohort followed since 1974. *Ann. Med.* 42 (7):530–538.

622. Sapone, A. et al. 2012. Spectrum of gluten-related disorders: Consensus on new nomenclature and classification. *BMC Med.* https://doi.org/10.1186/1741-7015-10-13.

623. Kasarda, D. D. 2013. Can an increase in celiac disease be attributed to an increase in the gluten content of wheat as a consequence of wheat breeding? *J. Agric. Food Chem.* 61 (6):1155–1159.

624. Sellitto, M. et al. 2012. Proof of concept of microbiome-metabolome analysis and delayed gluten exposure on celiac disease autoimmunity in genetically at-risk infants. *PLoS One* 7 (3):e33387.

625. Henriksson, C., A. M. Bostrom, I. E. Wiklund. 2013. What effect does breastfeeding have on coeliac disease? A systematic review update. *Evid. Based. Med.* 18 (3):98–103.

626. Cinova J., G. De Palma, R. Stepankova, O. Kofronova, M. Kverka, Y. Sanz, L. Tuckova. 2011. Role of intestinal bacteria in gliadin-induced changes in intestinal mucosa: Study in germ-free rats. *PLoS One* 6 (1):e16169.

627. Decker, E., M. Hornef, S. Stockinger. 2011. Cesarean delivery is associated with celiac disease but not inflammatory bowel disease in children. *Gut Microbes* 2 (2):91–98.

628. Arranz, E., J. Bode, K. Kingstone, A. Ferguson. 1994. Intestinal antibody pattern of coeliac disease: Association with gamma/delta T cell receptor expression by intraepithelial lymphocytes, and other indices of potential coeliac disease. *Gut* 35 (4):476–482.

629. Drago, S. et al. 2006. Gliadin, zonulin and gut permeability: Effects on celiac and non-celiac intestinal mucosa and intestinal cell lines. *Scand. J. Gastroenterol.* 41 (4):408–419.

630. Visser, J., J. Rozing, A. Sapone, K. Lammers, A. Fasano. 2009. Tight junctions, intestinal permeability, and autoimmunity: Celiac disease and type 1 diabetes paradigms. *Ann. N. Y. Acad. Sci.* 1165:195–205.

631. How Does Bt Work? University of California San Diego. Accessed October 14, 2013. http://www.bt.ucsd. edu/how_bt_work.html.

632. Bt Plant-Pesticides Risk and Benefits Assessment. EPA Scientific Advisory Panel. 2001. https://www. epa.gov/regulation-biotechnology-under-tsca-and-fifra/fifra-scientific-advisory-panel-meetings-related.

633. Mesnage, R., E. Clair, S. Gress, C. Then, A. Szekacs, G. E. Seralini. 2013. Cytotoxicity on human cells of Cry1Ab and Cry1Ac Bt insecticidal toxins alone or with a glyphosate-based herbicide. *J. Appl. Toxicol.* 33 (7):695–699.

634. Aris, A., S. Leblanc. 2011. Maternal and fetal exposure to pesticides associated to genetically modified foods in Eastern Townships of Quebec, Canada. *Reprod. Toxicol.* 31 (4):528–533.

635. Netherwood, T., S. M. Martin-Orue, A. G. O'Donnell, S. Gockling, J. Graham, J. C. Mathers, H. J. Gilbert. 2004. Assessing the survival of transgenic plant DNA in the human gastrointestinal tract. *Nat. Biotechnol.* 22 (2):204–209.

636. Fares, N. H., A. K. El-Sayed. 1998. Fine structural changes in the ileum of mice fed on delta-endotoxin-treated potatoes and transgenic potatoes. *Nat. Toxins* 6 (6):219–233.

637. Senapati, T., A. Mukerjee, A. Ghosh. 2009. Observations on the effect of glyphosate based herbicide on ultra structure (SEM) and enzymatic activity in different regions of alimentary canal and gill of *Channa punctatus*. *J. Crop Weed* 5 (1):236–245.

638. Ewen, S. W., A. Pusztai. 1999. Effect of diets containing genetically modified potatoes expressing *Galanthus nivalis* lectin on rat small intestine. *Lancet* 354 (9187):1353–1354.

639. Carmen, J., H. Vlieger, L. Ver Steeg, V. Sneller, G. Robinson, C. Clinch-Jones, J. Haynes, J. Edwards. 2013. A Long-term study on pigs fed a combined genetically modified (GM) soy and GM maize diet. *Organic Systems.* 8 (1):38–54.

640. Malatesta, M., C. Caporaloni, L. Rossi, S. Battistelli, M. Rocchi, F. Tonucci, G. Gazzanelli. 2002. Ultrastructural analysis of pancreatic acinar cells from mice fed on genetically modified soybean. *J. Anat.* 201 (5):409–415.

641. Collado, M. C., E. Donat, C. Ribes-Koninckx, M. Calabuig, Y. Sanz. 2009. Specific duodenal and faecal bacterial groups associated with paediatric coeliac disease. *J. Clin. Pathol.* 62 (3):264–269.

642. Tursi, A., G. Brandimarte, G. Giorgetti. 2003. High prevalence of small intestinal bacterial overgrowth in celiac patients with persistence of gastrointestinal symptoms after gluten withdrawal. *Am. J. Gastroenterol.* 98 (4):839–843.

643. Sanchez, E, I Nadal, E Donat, C Ribes-Koninckx, M Calabuig, Y Sanz. 2008. Reduced diversity and increased virulence-gene carriage in intestinal enterobacteria of coeliac children. *BMC Gastroenterol.* 8:50.

644. Nadal, I., E. Donat, C. Ribes-Koninckx, M. Calabuig, Y. Sanz. 2007. Imbalance in the composition of the duodenal microbiota of children with coeliac disease. *J. Med. Microbiol.* 56 (12):1669–1674.

645. Shehata, A. A., W. Schrodl, A. A. Aldin, H. M. Hafez, M. Kruger. 2013. The effect of glyphosate on potential pathogens and beneficial members of poultry microbiota *in vitro*. *Curr. Microbiol.* 66 (4):350–358.

646. Kruger, M., A. A. Shehata, W. Schrodl, A. Rodloff. 2013. Glyphosate suppresses the antagonistic effect of *Enterococcus spp.* on Clostridium botulinum. *Anaerobe* 20:74–78.

647. Laparra, J. M., M. Olivares, O. Gallina, Y. Sanz. 2012. Bifidobacterium longum CECT 7347 Modulates Immune Responses in a Gliadin-Induced Enteropathy Animal Model. *PLoS One* 7 (2):e30744.

648. Kruger, M., A. Grosse-Herrenthey, W. Schrodl, A. Gerlach, A. Rodloff. 2012. Visceral botulism at dairy farms in Schleswig Holstein, Germany: Prevalence of *Clostridium botulinum* in feces of cows, in animal feeds, in feces of the farmers, and in house dust. *Anaerobe* 18 (2):221–223.

649. Fasano, A. 2011. Zonulin and its regulation of intestinal barrier function: The biological door to inflammation, autoimmunity, and cancer. *Physiol Rev.* 91 (1):151–175.

650. Miyashita, S. I., Y. Sagane, K. Inui, S. Hayashi, K. Miyata, T. Suzuki, T. Ohyama, T. Watanabe, K. Niwa. 2013. Botulinum toxin complex increases paracellular permeability in intestinal epithelial cells via activation of p38 mitogen-activated protein kinase. *J. Vet. Med. Sci.* 75 (12):1637–1642.

651. Goldstein, J., W. E. Morris, C. F. Loidl, C. Tironi-Farinati, B. A. McClane, F. A. Uzal, M. E. Fernandez Miyakawa. 2009. Clostridium perfringens epsilon toxin increases the small intestinal permeability in mice and rats. *PLoS One* 4 (9):e7065.

652. Zhang, Y. G., S. Wu, Y. Xia, J. Sun. 2013. Salmonella infection upregulates the leaky protein claudin-2 in intestinal epithelial cells. *PLoS One* 8 (3):e58606.

653. *Mortality in sheep flocks after grazing on Bt cotton fields—Warangal District.* Report of the Preliminary Assessment. 2006.

654. Broderick, N. A., K. F. Raffa, J. Handelsman. 2006. Midgut bacteria required for *Bacillus thuringiensis* insecticidal activity. *Proc. Natl. Acad. Sci. U. S. A.* 103 (41):15196–15199.

655. Paganelli, A., V. Gnazzo, H. Acosta, S. L. Lopez, A. E. Carrasco. 2010. Glyphosate-based herbicides produce teratogenic effects on vertebrates by impairing retinoic acid signaling. *Chem. Res. Toxicol.* 23 (10):1586–1595.

656. Evaluation of Allergenicity of Genetically Modified Foods. Report of a Joint FAO/WHO Expert Consultation on Allergenicity of Foods Derived from Biotechnology. 2001. Accessed October 24, 2013. http://www.fao.org/fileadmin/templates/agns/pdf/topics/ec_jan2001.pdf.

657. Freese, W., D. Schubert. 2004. Safety testing and regulation of genetically engineered foods. *Biotechnology and Genetic Engineering Reviews*; 21. Accessed October 24, 2013. http://www.center-forfoodsafety.org/files/freese_safetytestingandregulationofgeneticallyebgineeredfoods_nov212004_62269.pdf.

658. Kleter, G. A., A. A. Peijnenburg. 2002. Screening of transgenic proteins expressed in transgenic food crops for the presence of short amino acid sequences identical to potential, IgE - binding linear epitopes of allergens. *BMC Struct. Biol.* 2:8.

659. Vazquez, R. I., L. Moreno-Fierros, L. Neri-Bazan, G. A. De La Riva, R. Lopez-Revilla. 1999. Bacillus thuringiensis CrylAc protoxin is a potent systemic and mucosal adjuvant. *Scand. J. Immunol.* 49 (6):578–584.

660. Townsend, M. 1999. Why soya is a hidden destroyer. *Daily Express*.

661. Bernstein, I. L., J. A. Bernstein, M. Miller, S. Tierzieva, D. I. Bernstein, Z. Lummus, M. K. Selgrade, D. L. Doerfler, V. L. Seligy. 1999. Immune responses in farm workers after exposure to *Bacillus thuringiensis* pesticides. *Environ. Health Perspect.* 107 (7):575–582.

662. Green, M., M. Heumann, R. Sokolow, L. R. Foster, R. Bryant, M. Skeels. 1990. Public health implications of the microbial pesticide *Bacillus thuringiensis*: An epidemiological study, Oregon, 1985–86. *Am J Public Health* 80 (7):848–852.

663. Zolla, L., S. Rinalducci, P. Antonioli, P. G. Righetti. 2008. Proteomics as a complementary tool for identifying unintended side effects occurring in transgenic maize seeds as a result of genetic modifications. *J. Proteome. Res.* 7 (5):1850–1861.

664. Finamore, A., M. Roselli, S. Britti, G. Monastra, R. Ambra, A. Turrini, E. Mengheri. 2008. Intestinal and peripheral immune response to MON810 maize ingestion in weaning and old mice. *J. Agric. Food Chem.* 56 (23):11533–11539.

665. American Cancer Society. 2008. *Cancer Facts and Figures.* Atlanta, GA: American Cancer Society.

666. Bonner, M. R., D. Han, J. Nie, P. Rogerson, J. E. Vena, P. Muti, M. Trevisan, S. B. Edge, J. L. Freudenheim. 2005. Breast cancer risk and exposure in early life to polycyclic aromatic hydrocarbons using total suspended particulates as a proxy measure. *Cancer Epidemiol. Biomarkers Prev.* 14:53–60.

667. el-Bayoumy, K., Y. H. Chae, P. Upadhyaya, A. Rivenson, C. Kurtzke, B. Reddy, S. S. Hecht. 1995. Comparative tumorigenicity of benzo[a]pyrene, 1-nitropyrene and 2-amino-1-methyl-6-phenylimidazo[4,5-b]pyridine administered by gavage to female CD rats. *Carcinogenesis* 16:431–434.

668. Gammon, M. D. et al. 2002. Environmental toxins and breast cancer on Long Island. I. Polycyclic aromatic hydrocarbon DNA adducts. *Cancer Epidemiol. Biomarkers Prev.* 11:677–685.

669. Gammon, M. D. et al. 2004. Polycyclic aromatic hydrocarbon-DNA adducts and breast cancer: A pooled analysis. *Arch. Environ. Health* 59:640–649.

670. Rundle, A., D. Tang, H. Hibshoosh, A. Estabrook, F. Schnabel, W. Cao, S. Grumet, F. P. Perera. 2000. The relationship between genetic damage from polycyclic aromatic hydrocarbons in breast tissue and breast cancer. *Carcinogenesis* 21:1281–1289.

671. Samanta, S. K., O. V. Singh, R. K. Jain. 2002. Polycyclic aromatic hydrocarbons: Environmental pollution and bioremediation. *Trends Biotechnol.* 20:243–248.

672. Santodonato, J. 1997. Review of the estrogenic and antiestrogenic activity of polycyclic aromatic hydrocarbons: Relationship to carcinogenicity. *Chemosphere* 34:835–848.

673. Hecht, S. S. 2002. Tobacco smoke carcinogens and breast cancer. *Environ. Mol. Mutagen* 39:119–126.

674. Phillips, D. H. 1999. Polycyclic aromatic hydrocarbons in the diet. *Mutat. Res.* 443:139–147.

675. Lewis, R. G., C. R. Fortune, R. D. Willis, D. E. Camann, J. T. Antley. 1999. Distribution of pesticides and polycyclic aromatic hydrocarbons in house dust as a function of particle size. *Environ. Health Perspect.* 107:721–726.

676. Lioy, P. J., A. Greenberg. 1990. Factors associated with human exposures to polycyclic aromatic hydrocarbons. *Toxicol. Ind. Health* 6:209–223.

677. Besaratinia, A., J. C. Kleinjans, F. J. Van Schooten. 2002. Biomonitoring of tobacco smoke carcinogenicity by dosimetry of DNA adducts and genotyping and phenotyping of biotransformational enzymes: A review on polycyclic aromatic hydrocarbons. *Biomarkers* 7:209–229.

678. Steck, S. E., M. M. Gaudet, S. M. Eng, J. A. Britton, S. L. Teitelbaum, A. I. Neugut, R. M. Santella, M. D. Gammon. 2007. Cooked meat and risk of breast cancer—Lifetime versus recent dietary intake. *Epidemiology* 18:373–382.

679. Gammon, M. D., S. M. Eng, S. L. Teitelbaum, J. A. Britton, G. C. Kabat, M. Hatch, A. B. Paykin, A. I. Neugut, R. M. Santella. 2004. Environmental tobacco smoke and breast cancer incidence. *Environ. Res.* 96:176–185.

680. Shantakumar, S. et al. 2005. Residential environmental exposures and other characteristics associated with detectable PAH-DNA adducts in peripheral mononuclear cells in a population-based sample of adult females. *J. Expo. Anal. Environ. Epidemiol.* 15:482–490.

681. Russo, J., Q. Tahin, M. H. Lareef, Y. F. Hu, I. H. Russo. 2002. Neoplastic transformation of human breast epithelial cells by estrogens and chemical carcinogens. *Environ. Mol. Mutagen.* 39:254–263.

682. Ambrosone, C. B., S. Kropp, J. Yang, S. Yao, P. G. Shields, J. ChangClaude. 2008. Cigarette smoking, N-acetyltransferase 2 genotypes, and breast cancer risk: Pooled analysis and meta-analysis. *Cancer Epidemiol. Biomarkers Prev.* 17:15–26.

683. Terry, P. D., M. Goodman. 2006. Is the association between cigarette smoking and breast cancer modified by genotype? A review of epidemiologic studies and meta-analysis. *Cancer Epidemiol. Biomarkers Prev.* 15:602–611.

684. Terry, P. D., T. E. Rohan. 2002. Cigarette smoking and the risk of breast cancer in women: A review of the literature. *Cancer Epidemiol. Biomarkers Prev.* 11:953–971.

685. Kazerouni, N., R. Sinha, C. H. Hsu, A. Greenberg, N. Rothman. 2001. Analysis of 200 food items for benzo[a]pyrene and estimation of its intake in an epidemiologic study. *Food Chem. Toxicol.* 39:423–436.

686. Holmes, M. D., G. A. Colditz, D. J. Hunter, S. E. Hankinson, B. Rosner, F. E. Speizer, W. C. Willett. 2003. Meat, fish and egg intake and risk of breast cancer. *Int. J. Cancer* 104:221–227.

687. Zheng, W., D. R. Gustafson, R. Sinha, J. R. Cerhan, D. Moore, C. P. Hong, K. E. Anderson, L. H. Kushi, T. A. Sellers, A. R. Folsom. 1998. Well-done meat intake and the risk of breast cancer. *J. Natl. Cancer Inst.* 90:1724–1729.

688. Gammon, M. D., R. M. Santella. 2008. PAH, genetic susceptibility and breast cancer risk: An update from the Long Island Breast Cancer Study Project. *Eur. J. Cancer* 44:636–640.

689. Santella, R. M. 1999. Immunological methods for detection of carcinogen-DNA damage in humans. *Cancer Epidemiol. Biomarkers Prev.* 8:733–739.

690. Braithwaite, E., X. Wu, Z. Wang. 1999. Repair of DNA lesions: Mechanisms and relative repair efficiencies. *Mutat. Res.* 424:207–219.

691. Levine, A. J. 1997. p53, the cellular gatekeeper for growth and division. *Cell* 88:323–331.

692. Greenblatt, M. S., W. P. Bennett, M. Hollstein, C. C. Harris. 1994. Mutations in the p53 tumor suppressor gene: Clues to cancer etiology and molecular pathogenesis. *Cancer Res.* 54:4855–4878.

693. Conway, K. et al. 2002. Prevalence and spectrum of p53 mutations associated with smoking in breast cancer. *Cancer Res.* 62:1987–1995.

694. Mordukhovich, I. et al. 2009. Associations between polycyclic aromatic hydrocarbon–related exposures and P53 mutations in breast tumors. *Environ. Health Perspect.* 118 (4):511–518.

695. Van Emburgh, B. O. et al. 2008. Polymorphisms in drug metabolism genes, smoking, and p53 mutations in breast cancer. *Mol. Carcinog.* 47:88–99.

696. Goldman, R., P. G. Shields. 1998. Molecular epidemiology of breast cancer. *In Vivo* 12:43–48.

697. Tennis, M. et al. 2006. p53 Mutation analysis in breast tumors by a DNA microarray method. *Cancer Epidemiol. Biomarkers Prev.* 15:80–85.

698. Bowen, R. L., J. Stebbing, L. J. Jones. 2006. A review of the ethnic differences in breast cancer. *Pharmacogenomics* 7:935–942.

699. Klauber-Demore, N. 2005. Tumor biology of breast cancer in young women. *Breast Dis.* 23:9–15.

700. Qiu, P., H. Shandilya, J. D'Alessio, K. O'Connor, J. Durocher, G. Gerard. 2004. Mutation detection using Surveyor nuclease. *Biotechniques* 36:702–707.

701. Mitani, N., Y. Niwa, Y. Okamoto. 2007. Surveyor nuclease-based detection of p53 gene mutations in haematological malignancy. *Ann. Clin. Biochem.* 44:557–559.

702. Lacroix, M., R. A. Toillon, G. Leclercq. 2006. p53 and breast cancer, an update. *Endocr. Relat. Cancer* 13:293–325.

703. Hall, P. A., W. G. McCluggage. 2006. Assessing p53 in clinical contexts: Unlearned lessons and new perspectives. *J. Pathol.* 208:1–6.

704. McCabe, A., M. Dolled-Filhart, R. L. Camp, D. L. Rimm. 2005. Automated quantitative analysis (AQUA) of *in situ* protein expression, antibody concentration, and prognosis. *J. Natl. Cancer Inst.* 97:1808–1815.

705. Rossner, P. et al. 2008. Mutations in p53, p53 protein overexpression and breast cancer survival. *J. Cell Mol. Med.* doi: 10.1111/j.158 [Online October 16, 2008].
706. Erdem, O., A. Dursun, U. Coskun, N. Gunel. 2005. The prognostic value of p53 and cerB2 expression, proliferative activity and angiogenesis in node-negative breast carcinoma. *Tumori* 91:46–52.
707. Iwase, H., Y. Ando, S. Ichihara, S. Toyoshima, T. Nakamura, S. Karamatsu, Y. Ito, H. Yamashita, T. Toyama, Y. Omoto, Y. Fujii, S. Mitsuyama, S. Kobayashi. 2001. Immunohistochemical analysis on biological markers in ductal carcinoma *in situ* of the breast. *Breast Cancer* 8:98–104.
708. Furberg, H., R. C. Millikan, J. Geradts, M. D. Gammon, L. G. Dressler, C. B. Ambrosone, B. Newman. 2002. Environmental factors in relation to breast cancer characterized by p53 protein expression. *Cancer Epidemiol. Biomarkers Prev.* 11:829–835.
709. Gammon, M. D., H. Hibshoosh, M. B. Terry, S. Bose, J. B. Schoenberg, L. A. Brinton, J. L. Bernstein, W. D. Thompson. 1999. Cigarette smoking and other risk factors in relation to p53 expression in breast cancer among young women. *Cancer Epidemiol. Biomarkers Prev.* 8:255–263.
710. van der Kooy, K., M. A. Rookus, H. L. Peterse, F. E. Van Leeuwen. 1996. p 53 protein overexpression in relation to risk factors for breast cancer. *Am. J. Epidemiol* 144:924–933.
711. Anttonen, M. J., R. O. Karjalainen. 2006. Highperformance liquid chromatography analysis of black currant (*Rives nigrurri* L.) fruit phenolics grown either conventionally or organically. *J. Agric. Food Chem.* 54:7530–7538.
712. Phillips, K. P., N. Tanphaichitr. 2008. Human exposure to endocrine disrupters and semen quality. *J. Toxicol. Environ. Health B Crit. Rev.* 11:188–220.

5 Microbiological, West Nile Virus, and Lyme Disease

VIRAL

MOSQUITO-BORNE DISEASE

Mosquitoes are important vectors (agents) in the transmission of animal diseases. Mosquito-borne diseases involve the transmission of viruses and parasites from animal to animal, animal to person, or person to person, without afflicting the insect vectors with symptoms of disease.

ACTION IN MOSQUITOES

Mosquitoes carrying such arboviruses stay healthy because their immune systems recognize the virions as foreign particles and "chop off" the virus's genetic coding, rendering it inert. Human infection with a mosquito-borne virus occurs when a female mosquito bites someone while its immune system is still in the process of destroying the virus's harmful coding.[1] It is not completely known how mosquitoes handle eukaryotic parasites so they can carry them without being harmed. Data have shown that the malaria parasite *Plasmodium falciparum* alters the mosquito vector's feeding behavior by increasing the frequency of biting in infected mosquitoes, thus increasing the chance of transmitting the parasite.[2]

CONTROL

When a mosquito bites, it also injects saliva and anticoagulants into the blood which may also contain disease-causing viruses or other parasites. This cycle can be interrupted by killing the mosquitoes, isolating infected people from all mosquitoes while they are infectious, or vaccinating the exposed population. All three techniques have been used, often in combination, to control mosquito-transmitted diseases. Window screens, introduced in the 1880s, were called "the most humane contribution the 19th century made to the preservation of sanity and good temper."[3]

EPIDEMIOLOGY

Mosquitoes are estimated to transmit diseases to more than 700 million people annually in Africa, South America, Central America, Mexico, and much of Asia with millions of resulting deaths. In Europe, Russia, Greenland, Canada, the United States, Australia, New Zealand, Japan, and other temperate and developed countries, mosquito bites are now mostly an irritating nuisance; but still cause some deaths each year.[4]

Historically, before mosquito-transmitted diseases were brought under control, they caused tens of thousands of deaths in these countries and hundreds of thousands of infections.[5] Mosquitoes were shown to be the method by which yellow fever and malaria were transmitted from person to person by Walter Reed, William C. Gorgas, and associates in the U.S. Army Medical Corps first in Cuba and then around the Panama Canal in the early 1900s.[6,7] Since then other diseases have been shown to be transmitted the same way.

Mosquitoes are a perfect example of one of the many organisms that can house diseases. Of the known 14,000 infectious microorganisms, 600 are shared between animals and humans. Mosquitoes are known to carry many infectious diseases from several different classes of microorganisms, including viruses and parasites. Mosquito-borne illnesses include malaria, West Nile virus (WNV), elephantiasis, dengue fever, yellow fever, and so on. These infections are normally rare to certain geographic areas. For instance, dengue hemorrhagic fever (DHF) is a viral mosquito-borne illness usually regarded only as a risk in the tropics. However, cases of dengue fever have been popping up in the United States along the Texas–Mexico border where it has never been seen before.

TYPES

Protozoa

The mosquito genus *Anopheles* carries the malaria parasite (*Plasmodium*). Worldwide, malaria is the leading cause of premature mortality, particularly in children under the age of 5, with around 2 million deaths annually, according to the Centers for Disease Control (CDC).

Helminthiasis

Some species of mosquito can carry the filariasis worm, a parasite that causes a disfiguring condition (often referred to as elephantiasis) characterized by a great swelling of several parts of the body; worldwide, around 10 million people are living with a filariasis disability.

Virus

The viral diseases yellow fever, dengue fever, and chikungunya are transmitted mostly by *Aedes aegypti* mosquitoes.

Other viral diseases such as epidemic polyarthritis, Rift Valley fever, Ross River fever, St. Louis encephalitis (SLE), WNV, Japanese encephalitis (JE), La Crosse (LAC) encephalitis, and several other encephalitis-type diseases are carried by several different mosquitoes. Eastern equine encephalitis (EEE) and western equine encephalitis (WEE) occur in the United States where they cause disease in humans, horses, and some bird species. Because of the high mortality rate, EEE and WEE are regarded as two of the most serious mosquito-borne diseases in the United States. Symptoms range from mild flu-like illness to encephalitis, coma, and death.[8]

Viruses carried by arthropods such as mosquitoes or ticks are known collectively as arboviruses. WNV was accidentally introduced in the United States in 1999 and by 2003 had spread to almost every state with over 3000 cases in 2006.

Culex and *Culiseta* are also involved in the transmission of disease.

TRANSMISSION

A mosquito's period of feeding is often undetected; the bite only becomes apparent because of the immune reaction it provokes. When a mosquito bites a human, it injects saliva and anticoagulants. For any given individual, with the initial bite there is no reaction but with subsequent bites the body's immune system develops antibodies and a bite becomes inflamed and itchy within 24 hours. This is the usual reaction in young children. With more bites, the sensitivity of the human immune system increases, and an itchy red hive appears in minutes where the immune response has broken capillary blood vessels and fluid is collected under the skin. This type of reaction is common in older children and adults. Some adults can become desensitized to mosquitoes and have little or no reaction to their bites, while others can become hypersensitive with bites causing blistering, bruising, and large inflammatory reactions, a response known as Skeeter syndrome.

MOSQUITO-BORNE DISEASES

Mosquitoes cause more human suffering than any other organism—over 1 million people worldwide die from mosquito-borne diseases every year. Not only can mosquitoes carry diseases that afflict humans but also transmit several diseases and parasites that dogs and horses are very susceptible to. These include dog heartworm, WNV, and EEE. In addition, mosquito bites can cause severe skin irritation through an allergic reaction to the mosquito's saliva—this is what causes the red bump and itching. Mosquito-vectored diseases include protozoan diseases, that is, malaria, filarial diseases such as dog heartworm, and viruses such as dengue, encephalitis, and yellow fever: CDC Travelers' Health provides information on travel to destinations where human-borne diseases might be a problem.

Malaria, Dog Heartworm, Dengue, Yellow Fever, Eastern Equine Encephalitis, St. Louis Encephalitis, La Crosse Encephalitis, Western Equine Encephalitis, West Nile Virus

Malaria

Malaria is an ancient disease probably originating in Africa. The malaria parasite (*Plasmodium*) is transmitted by female *Anopheles* mosquitoes. The term malaria is derived from the Italian "malaria" or "bad air" because it was thought to come on the wind from swamps and rivers. Scientists conducted extensive research on the disease during the 1880s and early 1900s. Approximately 40% of the world's population is susceptible to malaria, mostly in the tropical and subtropical areas of the world. It was by and large eradicated in the temperate area of the world during the twentieth century with the advent of DDT and other organochlorine and organophosphate mosquito control insecticides. However, more than 1 million deaths and 300–500 million cases are still reported annually in the world. It is reported that malaria kills one child every 40 seconds. In the United States, malaria affected colonization along the eastern shore and was not effectively controlled until the 1940s when the *Anopheles* mosquitoes were controlled. Resurgence occurred during the 1960s and early 1970s in the United States due to returning military personnel from Vietnam. *Anopheles quadrimaculatus* was the primary vector of the *Plasmodium vivax* (Protozoa) in the United States. Antimalarial drugs have been available for more than 50 years and recently scientists in Britain and the United States have cracked the code of the malaria parasite genome, a step that may help boost the campaign against the disease.

Dog Heartworm (*Dirofilaria immitis*)

Dog heartworm (*Dirofilaria immitis*) can be a life-threatening disease for canines. The disease is caused by a roundworm. Dogs and sometimes other animals such as cats, foxes, and raccoons are infected with the worm through the bite of a mosquito carrying the larvae of the worm. It is dependent on both the mammal and the mosquito to complete its lifecycle. The young worms (called microfilaria) circulate in the blood stream of the dog. These worms must infect a dog. Once inside the mosquito, the microfilariae leave the gut of the mosquito and live in the body of the insect where they develop for 2–3 weeks. After transforming twice in one mosquito, the third stage infective larvae move to the mosquito's mouthparts, whey they will be able to infect an animal. When the mosquito blood feeds, the infective larvae are deposited on the surface of the victim's skin. The larvae enter the skin through the wound caused by the mosquito bite. The worms burrow into the skin where they remain for 3–4 months. If the worms have infected an unsuitable host such as a human, the worms usually die. The disease in dogs and cats cannot be eliminated but it can be controlled or prevented with pills and/or injections. Some risk is present when treating dogs infected with heartworms but death is rare, still prevention is the best practice. Of course, good residual mosquito control practices reduce the rate of mosquito transmission. Until the late 1960s, the disease was restricted to southern and eastern coastal regions of the United States. Now, however, cases have been reported in all 50 states and in several provinces of Canada.

Arthropod-borne viruses (arboviruses) are the most diverse, numerous, and serious diseases transmitted to susceptible vertebrate hosts by mosquitoes and other blood-feeding arthropods. Humans and domestic animals can develop clinical illness but usually are "dead-end" hosts because they do not produce significant viremia, and do not contribute to the transmission cycle. There are several virus agents of encephalitis in the United States. WNV, EEE, WEE, SLE, LAC encephalitis, dengue, and yellow fever all of which are transmitted by mosquitoes. Another virus, Powassan, is a minor cause of encephalitis in the northern United States, and is transmitted by ticks. A new Powassan-like virus has recently been isolated from deer ticks. Encephalitis is global, in Asia, for example, about 50,000 cases of JE are reported annually.

Dengue

Dengue is a serious arboviral disease of the Americas, Asia, and Africa. Although it has a low mortality, dengue has very severe symptoms and has become more serious both in frequency and mortality, in recent years. *A. aegypti* and *Aedes albopictus* are the vectors of dengue. The spread of dengue throughout the world can be directly attributed to the proliferation and adaptation of these mosquitoes. Over the last 16 years, dengue has become more common, for example; in south Texas five cases were reported in causing one death. More recently, Hawaii recorded 85 cases of dengue during 2001 and the Florida Keys reported over 20 cases in 2010. In 2004, Venezuela has reported more than 11,600 cases of classic dengue fever and over 700 cases of DHF. Indonesia dengue outbreak has caused over 600 deaths and more than 54,000 cases. In 1999, Laredo and Nuevo Laredo had an outbreak of almost 100 cases.

Yellow Fever

Yellow fever, which has a 400-year history, occurs only in tropical areas of Africa and the Americas. It has both an urban and jungle cycle. It is a rare illness of travelers anymore because most countries have regulations and requirements for yellow fever vaccination that must be met prior to entering the country. Every year about 2,300,000 cases occur with 30,000 deaths in 33 countries. It does not occur in Asia. Over the past decade, it has become more prevalent. In 2002, one fatal yellow fever death occurred in the United States in an unvaccinated traveler returning from a fishing trip to the Amazon. In May 2003, 178 cases and 27 deaths caused by yellow fever were reported in south Sudan. In the Americas, 226 cases of jungle yellow fever have been reported with 99 deaths.

Eastern Equine Encephalitis

Eastern Equine Encephalitis (EEE) is spread to horses and humans by infected mosquitoes. It is among the most serious of a group of mosquito-borne arboviruses that can affect the central nervous system (CNS) and cause severe complications and even death. EEE is found in North America, Central and South America, and the Caribbean. It has a complex life cycle involving birds and a specific type of mosquito including several *Culex* species and *Culiseta melanura*. These mosquitoes feed on infected birds and become carriers of the disease and then feed on humans, horses, and other mammals. Symptoms may range from none at all to a mild flu-like illness with fever, headache, and sore throat. More serious infections of the CNS lead to a sudden fever and severe headache followed quickly by seizures and coma. About half of these patients die from the disease. Of those who survive, many suffer permanent brain damage and require lifetime institutional care. There is no specific treatment. A vaccine is available for horses, but not for humans.

St. Louis Encephalitis

St. Louis Encephalitis (SLE) is transmitted from birds to man and other mammals by infected mosquitoes (mainly some *Culex* species). SLE is found throughout the United States, but most often along the Gulf of Mexico, especially Florida. Major SLE epidemics occurred in Florida in 1959, 1961, 1962, 1977, and 1990. The elderly and very young are more susceptible than those between 20 and 50 years of age. During the period 1964–1998 (35 years), a total of 4478 confirmed cases of SLE were recorded in the United States. Symptoms are similar to those seen in EEE and like SEE, there is no vaccine. Mississippi's first case of SLE since 1994 was confirmed in June 2003. Previously the last outbreak of SLE in Mississippi was in 1975 with over 300 reported cases.

La Crosse Encephalitis

La Crosse encephalitis (LAC) is much less common than EEE or SLE, but occurs in all 13 states east of the Mississippi, particularly in the Appalachian region. It was reported first in 1963 in La Crosse, Wisconsin, and the vector is thought to be a specific type of woodland mosquito (*Aedes triseriatus*) called the tree-hole mosquito, with small mammals the usual warm-blooded host. It occurs in children younger than 16 and once again there is no vaccine for LAC encephalitis.

Western Equine Encephalitis

Western equine encephalitis (WEE) was first recognized in 1930 in a horse in California. It is found west of the Mississippi including parts of Canada and Mexico. The primary vector is *Culex tarsalis* and birds are the most important vertebrate hosts with small mammals playing a minor role. Unlike LAC encephalitis, it is nonspecific in humans and since 1964 fewer than 1000 cases have been reported. As with EEE, a vaccine is available for horses against WEE but not for humans. In Arizona, infected chicken flocks were found in three counties.

West Nile Virus

West Nile virus (WNV) emerged from its origin in 1937 in Africa (Uganda) into Europe, the Middle East, west and central Asia, and associated islands. It is a *Flavivirus* (family Flaviviridae) with more than 70 identified viruses. Serologically, it is a JE virus antigenic complex similar to SLE, JE, and Murray Valley encephalitis viruses. Similar to other encephalitides, it is cycled between birds and mosquitoes and transmitted to mammals (including horses) and man by infected mosquitoes. WNV might be described in one of four illnesses: West Nile fever (WNF) might be the least severe and is characterized by fever, headache, tiredness, and aches or a rash; like the "flu." This might last a few days or several weeks. At least 63% of patients report symptoms lasting over 30 days, with the median being 60 days. The other types are grouped as "neuroinvasive disease" which affects the nervous system. West Nile encephalitis affects the brain and West Nile meningitis (WNM, meningoencephalitis) causes an inflammation of the brain and membrane around it (CDC).

It first appeared in North America in 1999 in New York (Cornell Environmental Risk Analysis Program) with 62 confirmed cases and seven human deaths. Nine horses died in New York in 1999. In 2001, 66 human cases (10 deaths) were reported in 10 states. It occurred in birds or horses in 27 states and Washington, D.C., Canada, and the Caribbean. There were 733 horse cases in 2001 with Florida reporting 66% of the cases, approximately 33% were fatal. In 2001, more than 1.4 million mosquitoes were tested for WNV in the United States (2004) and over 43 species of mosquitoes have tested positive for WNV transmission, the *Culex pipiens* group seems to be the most common species associated with infecting people and horses. Currently, 65 mosquito and 300 bird species have tested positive in the United States for this virus.

During 2002, the number of areas reporting WNV grew to 44 states and five Canadian provinces. The only states not reporting WNV were Alaska, Arizona, Hawaii, Nevada, Oregon, and Utah that year. Intrauterine transmission (CDC MMWR [Morbidity and Mortality Weekly Report]) and laboratory infections (CDC MMWR) were reported for the first time. In all, over 3800 human cases with 232 fatalities in 39 states and Washington, D.C. were recorded. More than 24,350 horse cases of WNV were confirmed or reported in 2002. There is a vaccine for horses. Even alligators (CDC-EID [Emergency Infectious Disease]) were found infected in Georgia.

As of 2010, there have been 30,491 cases of WNV reported to CDC. Of these, 12,650 have resulted in meningitis/encephalitis and 119 were fatal. CDC estimates that there have been at least 1.5 million infections (82% are asymptomatic) and 341,000 cases of WNF, but the disease is grossly underreported due to its similarity to other viral infections.

Canada's first dead bird (a blue jay) from WNV in 2004 was confirmed in Ontario in May 2004. WNV was confirmed in two birds in Puerto Rico near the former U.S. Roosevelt Roads Navy Base (southeastern Puerto Rico).

Britain's Health Protection Agency has started its annual surveillance program for possible human cases of WNV infection. The program which has been used for the last 3 years operates during the summer, when there is WNV activity in other countries. The UK has not reported WNV, but is developing a West Nile Virus Contingency Plan.

WNV is a mosquito-borne zoonotic arbovirus belonging to the genus *Flavivirus* in the family Flaviviridae. This *Flavivirus* is found in the temperate and tropical regions of the world. It was first identified in the West Nile subregion in the East African nation of Uganda in 1937. Prior to the mid-1990s, WNV disease occurred only sporadically and was considered a minor risk for humans, until an outbreak in Algeria in 1994, with cases of WNV-caused encephalitis, and the first large outbreak in Romania in 1996, with a high number of cases with neuroinvasive disease. WNV has now spread globally, with the first case in the Western Hemisphere being identified in New York City in 1999,[9] over the next 5 years, the virus spread across the continental United States, north into Canada, and southward into the Caribbean Islands and Latin America.

The main mode of WNV transmission is via various species of mosquitoes, which are the prime vectors, with birds being the most commonly infected animal and serving as the prime reservoir host—especially passerines, which are of the largest order of birds, Passeriformes. WNV has been found in various species of ticks, but current research suggests they are not important vectors of the virus. WNV also infects various mammal species, including humans, and has been identified in reptilian species, including alligators and crocodiles, and also in amphibians. Not all animal species that are susceptible to WNV infection, including humans, and not all bird species develop sufficient viral levels to transmit the disease to uninfected mosquitoes, and are thus not considered major factors in WNV transmission.[10,11]

Approximately 80% of WNV infections in humans are subclinical, which cause no symptoms.[12]

In the event of being bitten by an infected mosquito, familiarity of the symptoms of WNV on the part of laypersons, physicians, and allied health professionals affords the best chance of receiving timely medical treatment, which may aid in reducing associated possible complications and also appropriate palliative care.

Signs and Symptoms

The incubation period for WNV—the amount of time from infection to symptom onset—is typically from 2 to 15 days. Headache can be a prominent symptom of WNV fever, meningitis, encephalitis, meningoencephalitis, and it may or may not be present in poliomyelitis-like syndrome. Thus, headache is not a useful indicator of neuroinvasive disease (CDC).

WNF, which occurs in 20% of cases, is a febrile syndrome that causes flu-like symptoms.[13] Most characterizations of WNF generally describe it as a mild, acute syndrome lasting 3–6 days after symptom onset. Systematic follow-up studies of patients with WNF have not been done, so this information is largely anecdotal. In addition to a high fever, headache, chills, excessive sweating, weakness, fatigue, swollen lymph nodes, drowsiness, pain in the joints, and flu-like symptoms are also observed. Gastrointestinal symptoms that may occur include nausea, vomiting, loss of appetite, and diarrhea. Less than one-third of patients develop a rash.

West Nile neuroinvasive disease (WNND), which occurs in <1% of cases, is when the virus infects the CNS resulting in meningitis, encephalitis, meningoencephalitis, or a poliomyelitis-like syndrome.[14] Many patients with WNND have normal neuroimaging studies, although abnormalities may be present in various cerebral areas including the basal ganglia, thalamus, cerebellum, and brainstem.[14]

West Nile virus encephalitis (WNE) is the most common neuroinvasive manifestation of WNND. WNE presents with similar symptoms to other viral encephalitis with fever, headaches, and altered mental status. A prominent finding in WNE is muscular weakness (30%–50% of patients with encephalitis), often with lower motor neuron symptoms, flaccid paralysis, and hyporeflexia with no sensory abnormalities.[15] "WNV is now the most common cause of epidemic viral encephalitis in the United States, and it will likely remain an important cause of neurological disease for the foreseeable future."[16]

WNM usually involves fever, headache, and stiff neck. Pleocytosis, an increase of white blood cells in cerebrospinal fluid (CSF), is also present. Changes in consciousness are not usually seen and are mild when present.

West Nile meningoencephalitis is inflammation of both the brain (encephalitis) and meninges (meningitis).

West Nile poliomyelitis (WNP), an acute flaccid paralysis syndrome associated with WNV infection, is less common than WNM or WNE. This syndrome is generally characterized by the acute onset of asymmetric limb weakness or paralysis in the absence of sensory loss. Pain sometimes precedes the paralysis. Paralysis can occur in the absence of fever, headache, or other common symptoms associated with WNV infection. Involvement of respiratory muscles, leading to acute respiratory failure, can sometimes occur.

Nonneurologic complications of WNV infection that may rarely occur include fulminant hepatitis, pancreatitis,[17] myocarditis, rhabdomyolysis,[18] orchitis,[19] nephritis, optic neuritis[20] and cardiac dysrhythmias, and hemorrhagic fever with coagulopathy.[21] Chorioretinitis may also be more common than previously thought.[22]

Cutaneous manifestations, specifically rashes, are not uncommon in WNV-infected patients; however, there is a paucity of detailed descriptions in case reports and there are few clinical images widely available. Punctate erythematous macular and popular eruptions, most pronounced on the extremities, have been observed in WNV cases and in some cases, histopathologic findings have shown a sparse superficial perivascular lymphocytic infiltrate, a manifestation commonly seen in viral exanthems. A literature review provides support that this punctuate rash is a common cutaneous presentation of WNV infection.[23]

Virology

WNV is one of the JE antigenic serocomplex of viruses.

Transmission

WNV is transmitted through female mosquitoes, which are the prime vectors of the virus. Only females feed on blood, and different species have evolved to take a blood meal on preferred types of vertebrate hosts. The infected mosquito species vary according to geographical area; in the United States, *Culex pipiens* (Eastern United States), *Culex tarsalis* (Midwest and West), and *Culex quinquefasciatus* (Southeast) are the main sources.[24]

Diagnosis

Diagnosis of WNV infections is generally accomplished by serologic testing of blood serum or CSF, which is obtained via a lumbar puncture. Typical findings of WNV infection include lymphocytic pleocytosis, elevated protein level, reference glucose and lactic acid levels, and no erythrocytes.

Definitive diagnosis of WNV is obtained through detection of virus-specific antibody immunoglobulin M (IgM) and neutralizing antibodies.

Prevention

Personal protective measures can be taken to greatly reduce the risk of being bitten by an infected mosquito.

Using insect repellent on exposed skin to repel mosquitoes. EPA-registered repellents include products containing DEET (*N,N*-diethyl-meta-toluamide) and picaridin (KBR 3023). DEET concentrations of 30%–50% are effective for several hours. Picaridin, available at 7% and 15% concentrations, needs more frequent application. DEET formulations as high as 50% are recommended for both adults and children over 2 months of age. Protect infants <2 months of age by using a carrier draped with mosquito netting with an elastic edge for a tight fit. DEET is toxic and should not be used.

When using sunscreen, apply sunscreen first and then repellent. Repellent should be washed off at the end of the day before going to bed.

Wear long-sleeve shirts, which should be tucked in, long pants, and hats to cover exposed skin. Apply permethrin-containing (e.g., Permanone) or other insect repellents to clothing, shoes, tents, mosquito nets, and other gear for greater protection. Permethrin is not labeled for use directly on skin. Most repellent is generally removed from clothing and gear by a single washing, but permethrin-treated clothing is effective for up to five washings. Of course, permethrin is toxic and should not be used either on skin or clothes.

Be aware that most mosquitoes that transmit disease are most active during twilight periods (dawn and dusk or in the evening). A notable exception is the Asian Tiger mosquito, which is a daytime feeder and is more apt to be found in, or on the periphery of, shaded areas with heavy vegetation. They are now widespread in the United States and in states such as Florida they have been found in 67 counties.[25]

Staying in air-conditioned or well-screened housing, and/or sleeping under an insecticide-treated bed net. Bed nets should be tucked under mattresses and can be sprayed with a repellent if not already treated with an insecticide.

Monitoring and Control

WNV can be sampled from the environment by the pooling of trapped mosquitoes via carbon dioxide-baited light traps and gravid traps, testing blood samples drawn from wild birds, dogs and sentinel monkeys, as well as testing brains of dead birds found by various animal control agencies and the public.

Dead birds, after necropsy, have their various tissues tested for virus by either RT-PCR or IHC, where virus shows up as brown-stained tissue because of a substrate–enzyme reaction.

West Nile control is achieved through mosquito control, by elimination of mosquito breeding sites such as abandoned pools, applying larvacide to active breeding areas and targeting the adult population via aerial spraying of pesticides which we do not recommend.

Treatment

No specific treatment is available for WNV infection. In severe cases, treatment consists of supportive care that often involves hospitalization, intravenous fluids, respiratory support, and prevention of secondary infections.

Prognosis

While the general prognosis is favorable, current studies indicate that WNF can often be more severe than previously recognized, with studies of various recent outbreaks indicating that it may take as long as 60–90 days to recover.[16,26] Patients with milder WNF are just as likely as those with more severe manifestations of neuroinvasive disease to experience multiple long-term (>1 + years) somatic complaints such as tremor, and dysfunction in motor skills and executive functions. Patients with milder illness are just as likely as patients with more severe illness to experience adverse outcomes.[27] Recovery is marked by a long convalescence with fatigue. One study found that neuroinvasive WNV infection was associated with an increased risk for subsequent kidney disease.[28,29] Many virus and bacteria are triggered by outdoor air conditions including such entities as WNV and Lyme disease. Each will be discussed.

WEST NILE VIRUS

According to Petersen et al.,[30] WNV has become endemic in all 48 contiguous states as well as all Canadian provinces since its discovery in North America in New York City in 1999.[19] It has produced the three largest arboviral neuroinvasive disease (encephalitis, meningitis, or acute flaccid paralysis) outbreaks ever recorded in the United States, with nearly 3000 cases of neuroinvasive disease recorded each year in 2002, 2003, and 2012.

WNV is maintained in a bird–mosquito–bird transmission cycle. Although WNV has been detected in 65 different mosquito species and 326 bird species in the United States, only a few

Culex mosquito species derive transmission of the virus in nature and subsequent spread to humans. Increased ambient temperature shortens the incubation time from infection to infectiousness in mosquitoes and increases viral transmission efficiency to birds, both critical factors for arboviral amplification.[31,32] At smaller scales, urban and agricultural land convers,[33] rural irrigated landscapes,[34] increased temperature,[35] increased rainfall,[36] and several socioeconomic factors such as housing age and community drainage patterns,[37] per capita income,[34] and density of poorly maintained swimming pools[38] relate to higher incidence in some locations. Nevertheless, considerable challenges remain in predicting how, when, and where these factors will combine to produce the focal, intense outbreaks that now characterize WNV ecology in the United States (Figure 5.1).

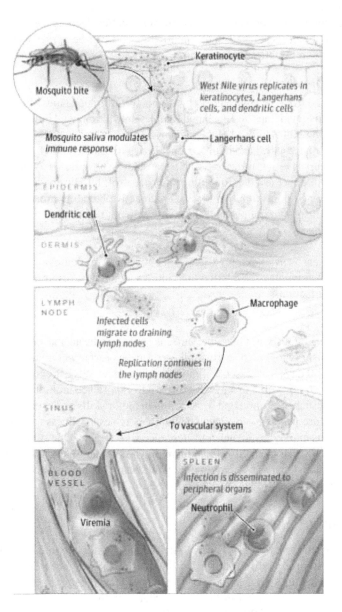

FIGURE 5.1 Schematic of pathogenesis of West Nile virus infection. (Reproduced with permission from Petersen, L. R., A. C. Brault, R. S. Nasci. West Nile virus: Review of the literature. 2013. *JAMA*, Vol. 310(3):308–315. Copyright 2013. American Medical Association. All rights reserved.)

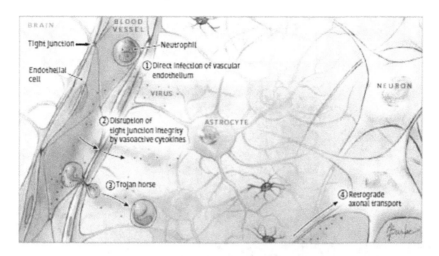

FIGURE 5.2 West Nile virus neuroinvasive mechanisms. (Reproduced with permission from Petersen, L. R., A. C. Brault, R. S. Nasci. West Nile virus: Review of the literature. 2013. *JAMA*, Vol. 310(3):308–315. Copyright 2013. American Medical Association. All rights reserved.)

WNV is capable of replicating and eliciting pathology in the brain (i.e., neurovirulence); however, a critical prerequisite to generating neuroinvasive disease in humans is the virus' capacity to gain access to the CNS (i.e., neuroinvasiveness).

WNV neuroinvasive mechanisms include: (1) direct viral crossing of the blood–brain barrier due to cytokine-mediated increased vascular permeability, (2) passage through the endothelium of the blood–brain barrier, (3) a Trojan horse mechanism in which infected tissue macrophages are trafficked across the blood–brain barrier, and (4) retrograde axonal transport of the virus to the CNS via infection of olfactory or peripheral neurons.[39] Regardless of how the virus enters the CNS, murine models of infection have shown persistent viral replication in various tissues, including the CNS, suggesting a potential etiology for long-term neurological sequelae observed in patients with neuroinvasive disease (Figure 5.2).[39]

Although the number of patients with neuroinvasive disease fluctuates annually, some regions experience persistently higher incidence. Ninety-four percent of patients with WNV infection have symptom onsets in July through September.[40] Extrapolations from neuroinvasive disease case reporting in the United States suggest that through 2010 approximately 3 million persons were infected, of whom 780,000 developed WNF.[41] In Canada, WNV was first detected in southern Ontario in 2001 and by 2009 the virus distribution had extended westward to British Columbia. Through October 2012, 975 patients with neuroinvasive disease have been reported in Canada (Figures 5.3 and 5.4).

TRANSMISSION TO HUMANS

According to Petersen et al.,[30] mosquito bites account for nearly all human infections. WNV can also be transmitted via transfused platelets, red blood cells, and fresh frozen plasma[42] as well as through heart, liver, lung, and kidney transplants.[43] Transmission via organ transplant has occurred from donors with detectable viremia, suggesting viral sequestration in organs shortly after viremia has cleared.

One possible transplacental transmission following a second trimester infection resulted in an infant with chorioretinitis, lissencephaly, and cerebral white matter loss. Fortunately, fetal abnormalities due to intrauterine infection are uncommon: none of 72 live infants born to 71 women infected during pregnancy had malformations linked to WNV infection or had conclusive laboratory evidence of congenital infection.[44] Nevertheless, three neonates born to women infected within 3 weeks pre partum developed symptomatic WNV disease at or shortly after birth, indicating the possibility of

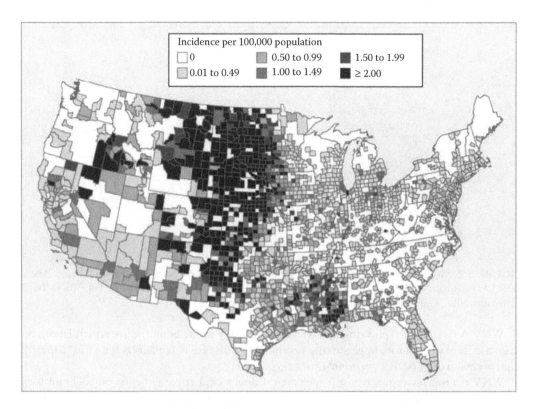

FIGURE 5.3 Map average annual human neuroinvasive disease incidence in the United States, 1999–2012. (Reproduced with permission from Petersen, L. R., A. C. Brault, R. S. Nasci. West Nile virus: Review of the literature. 2013. *JAMA*, Vol. 310(3):308–315. Copyright 2013. American Medical Association. All rights reserved.)

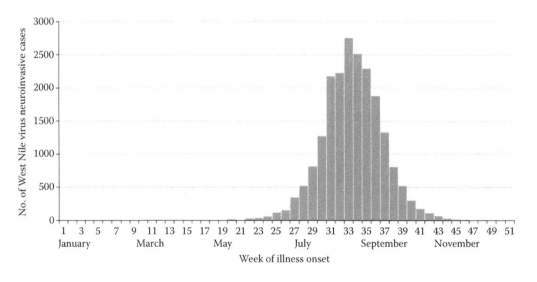

FIGURE 5.4 Cumulative number of human West Nile virus neuroinvasive disease cases by week of onset, 1999–2012. (Reproduced with permission from Petersen, L. R., A. C. Brault, R. S. Nasci. West Nile virus: Review of the literature. 2013. *JAMA*, Vol. 310(3):308–315. Copyright 2013. American Medical Association. All rights reserved.)

intrauterine infection or infection at the time of delivery. Other rare or suspected modes of transmission include breast milk transmission, percutaneous or conjunctival exposure to laboratory workers and by unknown means in patients undergoing dialysis and workers at a turkey breeder farm.[45]

INFECTION AND ILLNESS

According to Petersen et al.,[30] it is not known what proportion of persons develop WNV infection following an infected mosquito bite. Persons with a genetic defect in the OAS1 gene (HGNC8086), which modulates host response to exogenous viral RNA, are more likely to have anti-WNV antibodies than persons without this defect, suggesting that immune response function determines who becomes infected after exposure.[46] Among persons who become infected, approximately 25% develop WNF[47] and 1 in 150–250 develops neuroinvasive disease.[41,48] Risk factors for developing WNF following infection are poorly defined. A follow-up study of asymptomatic, viremic blood donors indicated that increasing viral load and female sex, but not age, subsequently increased the risk of developing WNF.[47] A smaller follow-up study of viremic blood donors suggested that younger persons were more likely to develop WNF.[49] In contrast, *advancing age profoundly* increases the risk of neuroinvasive disease, particularly encephalitis.[40,50] The risk may approach 1 in 50 among persons aged at least 65 years, a rate 16 times higher than that for persons aged 16–24 years.[50] In addition, a history of cancer, diabetes, hypertension, alcohol abuse, renal disease, and chemokine receptor CCR5 deficiency as well as male sex may increase the risk of neuroinvasive disease.[39,40,50–53] Persons infected through transplant of infected organs are at extreme risk of developing neuroinvasive disease[43]; however, conflicting data exist regarding risk among previous organ recipients infected via mosquito bite.[54,55]

Case fatality rates among patients with neuroinvasive disease generally approximate 10%.[40] Advanced age is the most important risk factor for death, ranging from 0.8% among those aged less than 40 years to 17% among those aged at least 70 years.[40] Encephalitis with severe muscle weakness, changes in the level of consciousness, diabetes, cardiovascular disease, hepatitis C virus infection, and immunosuppression are possible risk factors for death.[9,40,52] Patients discharged from the hospital following acute WNV illness experience a twofold to threefold increase in long-term, all-cause mortality compared with age-adjusted population norms, although not all of this increase may be attributable to WNV.[56]

According to Petersen et al.,[30] detection of IgM antibody in serum or CSF using the IgM antibody-capture enzyme-linked immunosorbent assay (MAC-ELISA) forms the cornerstone of WNV diagnosis in most clinical settings. Because IgM antibody does not cross the blood–brain barrier, its presence in CSF indicates CNS infection. At least 90% of patients with encephalitis or meningitis have demonstrable IgM antibodies in CSF within 8 days of symptom onset. The WNV-specific IgM antibody may not be detected initially in serum or plasma. One study showed that only 58% of patients with WNF had a positive MAC-ELISA result at clinical presentation.[57] Nevertheless, MAC-ELISA testing of acute- and convalescent-phase sera will provide definitive diagnosis. Testing for IgG antibodies has no utility in the acute clinical diagnostic setting.

How easy it has been to forget that WNV was the last major emerging infection of the twentieth century. This virus mysteriously appeared in Queens, New York, late in the summer of 1999, after an apparent single-chance introduction by unknown means.[58] This mosquito-transmitted virus was new to the Western Hemisphere. Infected crows were literally dropping from the sky, and severe, sometimes fatal, human disease occurred with no warning. Complacency regarding the risk of mosquito-borne illness had led to major reductions in New York City's vector control program years earlier.[59] Controversy accompanied the decision to use wide-scale aerial pesticide applications to reduce exposure to disease-carrying mosquitoes. These measures had not been used in New York City in many years and raised concerns about human toxicity and environmental damage. Similar concerns were expressed when spraying was performed in other urban centers in subsequent years.

When studies conducted in 1999 found that WNV had spread well beyond Queens,[47] experts in vector-borne diseases correctly predicted that the virus would have a permanent presence in North America. As noted by Petersen and colleagues[42] in their review, the virus swept across North America to the Pacific coast in only 5 years and is now found throughout the Western Hemisphere from Canada to Argentina. Petersen et al. also indicate that WNV has caused an estimated 3 million human infections just through 2010 with more than 16,000 reported neuroinvasive cases and almost 1600 deaths in the United States.

Last year's WNV outbreak, the deadliest since the virus first emerged, with 286 deaths touched all 48 contiguous states, although Texas (and Dallas County in particular) had the heaviest disease burden.

From May 30 to December 30, there were 173 cases of neuroinvasive disease related to WNV, 225 cases of the less-severe WNF, and 19 deaths reported through the National Electronic Disease Surveillance System also identified 17 virus-positive blood donors.

Of the patients with neuroinvasive disease, nearly all (96%) required hospitalization, 35% received intensive care, and 18% underwent assisted ventilation. The case fatality rate was 10%.

The rate of neuroinvasive disease was 7.3 per 100,000 residents, substantially higher than the rate during 2006 (2.91 per 100,000), which saw the largest WNV outbreak in Dallas County before last year.

A rapid rise in human disease cases followed shortly behind increased infection detected among mosquitoes in the area, primarily the southern house mosquito *(Culex quinquefasciatus)*.

The number of days in winter with a hard freeze (low temperature <28°F) was the strongest predictor of disease; fewer such days corresponded to more disease (p < 0.001).

Officials in Dallas County resorted to aerial spraying of insecticides to suppress mosquito levels during the outbreak, sparking some concern about health problems. But the researchers found that the spraying was not associated with more emergency department visits for respiratory symptoms, including asthma exacerbations, or skin rash. However, hypersensitivity, cardiovascular and neurological diseases were not reported.

Such measures remain important because "West Nile virus has become and will remain a formidable clinical and public health problem for years to come."

"Thus, sustainable, community-based surveillance and vector management programs are critical, particularly in metropolitan areas with a history of West Nile virus and large human populations at risk. Community response plans must include provisions for rapidly implementing large-scale adult mosquito control interventions when surveillance indicates such measures as necessary." However, aerial spraying was not used in Dallas County in the summer of 2013 and only six fatalities were reported.

"Effective West Nile virus prevention and control require an integrated vector management approach that includes source reduction by minimizing breeding sites; using larvacides where breeding sites cannot be eliminated; and monitoring for the presence of virus in adult mosquitoes, coupled with targeted pesticide use, when virus is found."

The U.S. Centers for Disease Control and Prevention (CDC) is currently engaged in a massive fear mongering campaign that would have everyone in America believe that the so-called WNV is spreading uncontrollably like wildfire. Though the CDC admits that only a miniscule percentage of people have even a remote chance of contracting the virus, the agency is still pushing for the mass spraying of cities with toxic pesticides, and actively encouraging people to coat themselves in toxic DEET chemicals to deter mosquitoes.

REAL TYPHOID CULPRIT

Molecular Biology: Lone protein toxin now a drug target brings on dramatic disease state, researchers say.

Most human infections of *Salmonella* bacteria cause stomach upset, diarrhea, and vomiting. But the Typhi strain of *Salmonella* is much worse. It causes typhoid, which each year kills more than 200,000 people worldwide. Most deaths occur in developing countries where people do not receive antibiotics in time to cure the illness.

Now mouse studies found that a toxic protein complex produced by the bacterium even in the absence of the microbe itself causes most typhoid symptoms such as lethargy, stupor, and weight loss, and leads to death.[60] The one major symptom not linked solely to this toxin is typhoid's characteristic high fever.

They also determined the complex's atomic-resolution crystal structure for the first time. The study could lead to new antibiotics and vaccines to fight typhoid. The *Salmonella* strain that produces the toxin has developed resistance to some existing antibiotics, and vaccines against typhoid have limited efficacy.

Typhoid toxin is a protein complex produced by *Salmonella typhi* when it infects animals and people. The complex was discovered in 2004 Galan's group. When the toxin enters cells, it damages the host DNA and halts cell growth and replication, thus producing many of the disease symptoms.

The toxin's structure has an exceptional feature: Two of its three subunits, CdtB and PltA, are connected by only a single disulfide linkage. This tenuous link is "striking department from other known toxin structures." The CdtB-PltA subunits nestle into the toxin's third component, the bowl-shaped PltB subunit.

Galán et al.[61] found that the toxin's disease effects are activated primarily by CdtB and that PltB aids the toxin's entry into cells by interacting with cell surface glycoproteins. PltA's function remains unclear; also used were carbohydrate arrays to identify specific types of cell surface glycoproteins the toxin is able to latch onto, gaining entry into host cells.

With most of typhoid's symptoms pegged to CdtB, that means the fever associated with typhoid is almost certainly caused by lipopolysaccharides on the bacterial surface. So the bacterium's CdtB and lipopolysaccharide components together may "account for the full spectrum of pathology."

This report is "the first time the virulence of an organism has been directly linked to the ability of bacteria to induce cellular DNA damage in a host."

LYME DISEASE

Lyme disease is a rapidly growing disease throughout the United States. It was first thought to be only in the southeastern United States. However, it now has been shown to grow in the entire North American continent causing a lot of chronic disease wherever it is found.

The causative spirochete of Lyme disease, *Borrelia burgdorferi* and *Babesia*, are the most common human tick-borne pathogen in the Northern Hemisphere. They are also probably the most complex bacteria known, as they have over 132 genes and 21 plasmids, with 90% of this genetic material unrelated to any known bacterium.

These genes facilitate adaptation of the organism in different forms and in different hosts with multiple mechanisms to evade and weaken host defenses. By comparison, the spirochete *Treponema pallidum pallidum* (the organism that causes syphilis) is a comparatively simple organism with only 22 genes and much less adaptive capability.

Lyme disease is currently viewed as being a mostly zoonotic tick-borne disease. The human mouth contains 400 different species of bacteria, as well as viruses and parasites. By contrast, ticks live in filth and feed on the blood of rodents and a variety of other animals, meaning that there are likely numerous other human pathogens besides *B. burgdorferi* potentially transmitted by tick bites. These other known and unknown pathogens may result in interactive coinfections. In addition, several opportunistic infections (mostly viral) are associated with *B. burgdorferi* infections.

Adding to the complexity and confusion is that here is no consensus regarding the definition of Lyme disease. Some define it with very narrow criteria, whereas others define it with broader clinical and laboratory criteria. No good laboratory test exists.

Some believe chronic persistent infection does not exist and speculate that persistent symptoms are associated with a self-perpetuating immune process that continues after the infection has cleared. However, no self-perpetuating immune process without persistent infection has ever been scientifically proven. However, we constantly referred patients who have had antibiotic treatment for 1–2 years who have not improved. When we treat the abnormal T-cells with the known autogenous lymphocytic factor (ALF) and gamma globulin deficiency with gamma globulin and mold and chemical sensitivity deficiency with gamma globulin and a variety of antigens they improve.

In contrast, those who consider a broader disease definition view the aberrant immune process as being associated with a persistent infectious process. Although multiple controversies surround Lyme disease, most agree that many of the symptoms associated with Lyme Disease/Tick borne disease (LYD/TBD) are mediated by immune processes.

LYD/TBD is associated with multisystemic symptoms, including psychiatric symptoms. Currently, there are 240 peer-reviewed articles demonstrating the association between LYD/TBD and psychiatric symptoms.

The most common mental symptoms include fatigue; nonrestorative sleep; impairments of executive functioning, attention, memory, and processing speed; sensory hyperacusis; and low frustration tolerance, irritability, depression, and anxiety.

Psychiatric symptoms are more significant with *Babesia* and *Bartonella* coinfections. A combination of our current limitations in understanding this disease, misinformation regarding this disease, and the failure to diagnose and treat it in the early stages results in a significant burden of psychiatric illness associated with LYD/TBD.[62]

IMMUNE EFFECTS OF LYME DISEASE

Recent attention has focused on the association between LYD/TBD and immune-mediated psychiatric symptoms.[63,64] Acute infections are usually associated with an early inflammatory reaction followed by adaptive immunity and a resolution of symptoms, but in Lyme disease this progression does not always occur. Instead, inflammation can persist without adaptive immunity, autoimmune symptoms may occur, and reinfections are common.

The complex genetic sophistication of *B. burgdorferi* allows it to adapt to multiple environments and disseminate and evade the host's immune system.[65] In a compromised environment, *B. burgdorferi* can survive by converting from a spirochetal form to granular and cystic forms. After entry, *B. burgdorferi* activates local inflammation yet evades host defenses and facilitates dissemination by potentially masquerading with host components such as plasmin and complement.[66]

B. burgdorferi is recognized by immune cells and attacked by complement and antibodies. *B. burgdorferi* responds by downregulating its surface proteins and hiding in the extracellular matrix.[67]

Some of the psychiatric sequelae may be associated with direct effects, such as possible toxin release, cell penetration, and lysis. In other infections, most symptoms are instead associated with immune effects. These immune effects include persistent inflammation with cytokine effects, the release of proinflammatory lipoproteins from the outer coat of *B. burgdorferi* and autoimmunity.

There are most likely other immune effects from the other coinfections and opportunistic infections seen with tick-borne diseases. For example, coinfections with *Anaplasma phagocytophilum* results in impairment in the ability to mount strong early inflammatory Th1-responses as demonstrated by a reduction of interleukin (IL)-12.[68]

There is a time progression of immune processes and a resulting progression of immune-mediated symptoms seen with LYD/TBD. Initial stages may include an erythema migrans ("bull's eye") rash, a flu-like illness, cranial nerve and other early neurologic symptoms, and musculoskeletal symptoms. Next, fatigue and cognitive impairments may occur. Subsequently, depression and other psychiatric symptoms are common, and in some cases late-stage disease is associated with dementia.

Autoimmune effects may also parallel these changes and may increase with peaks in anti-neuronal antibody production. The disease progression is associated with a progressive sequence of immune effects. Fatigue and cognitive impairments are associated with the action of proinflammatory cytokines, depression is associated with inflammation-induced changes in tryptophan catabolism, and dementia is associated with CNS *gliosis*. All of these symptoms may be temporarily exacerbated in response to a Jarisch–Herxheimer immune reaction provoked by antibiotic treatment.[64]

CNS PENETRATION

B. burgdorferi may reach the CNS either through peripheral nerves or through the blood stream. Although CNS penetration is well documented, it is still not clear how *B. burgdorferi* passes the blood–brain barrier. Two possible explanations include penetration between endothelial cells or transcellular passage.[67] When early CNS penetration occurs, the more common early CNS symptoms include painful meningoradiculitis with inflammation of the nerve roots and lancinating radical pain, lymphocytic meningitis, and various forms of cranial or peripheral neuritis.[69]

EARLY IMMUNE EFFECTS

According to Bransfield,[70] the erythema migrans rash is associated with polymorphonuclear cells replaced by a few infiltrating macrophages that are then replaced by a lymphocytic infiltrate.[71] Associated with these cellular changes are a humoral inflammatory reaction that includes tumor necrosis factor-alpha (TNF-alpha), IL-6, chemokines (CXCL1 and IL-8), NF-kappa B factors, metalloproteinases-1, -3, and -12, superoxide dismutase and C3a and C4a complement increases.[72,73]

High levels of proinflammatory cytokines (TNF-alpha), transforming growth factor-beta, and IL-6 early in the disease correlate with recovery, whereas low levels of proinflammatory cytokines correlate with chronicity.[74]

SYMPTOMS OF INFECTION

According to Bransfield,[70] it is important to recognize that infection without CNS penetration can have immune effects in the brain. Infections provoke proinflammatory cytokines that can cross the blood–brain barrier and affect neural and mental functioning. Like many infections, LYD/TBD has been associated with the proinflammatory cascade, which initially manifests as "sickness syndrome" symptoms.

Interferon treatment is a useful model to understand the earlier and later effects of inflammation upon mental functioning. Early interferon treatment symptoms include fatigue and cognitive impairments, whereas later symptoms are more emotional and behavioral in nature and include depression, anxiety, mania, irritability, impulsiveness, hostility, apathy, and relapse of substance abuse.[75]

The symptoms associated with the proinflammatory cascade in LYD/TBD have been associated with the proinflammatory cytokines IL-6, IL-8, IL-12, IL-17, IL-18, interferon-gamma, neopterin, and the chemokines CXCL12 and CXCL13. In addition, the outer coat of *B. burgdorferi* consists of lipoproteins that are proinflammatory, including the VlsE lipoprotein. Pathophysiologic changes are associated with oxidative stress, excitotoxicity, changes in homocysteine metabolism, and altered tryptophan catabolism.

B. burgdorferi reproduces in a cyclic manner, similar to relapsing fever and malaria. This cyclic reproduction is also associated with a cyclic provocation of proinflammatory cytokines and a cyclic appearance of symptoms associated with inflammation, such as fatigue, apathy, and the multiple cognitive and mood impairments associated with Lyme encephalopathy.[62,64]

BEHAVIORAL SYMPTOMS

According to Bransfield,[70] elevations of proinflammatory cytokines are associated with suicide attempts, self-destructive behavior, aggressive behavior, and fatigue, and the severity of suicidal tendencies correlates with the level of IL-6 in the CSF.[76] Similar to what is seen with interferon treatment, when inflammation persists with Lyme disease, mood and behavioral symptoms become apparent.

Persistent immune stimulation of the brain is associated with changes in tryptophan catabolism that include an increase of the enzyme indoleamine 2,3-dioxygenase. This enzyme reduces the conversion of tryptophan into serotonin, melatonin, and kynurenic acid (a neuroprotective N-methyl-D-aspartate [NMDA] antagonist) and instead converts tryptophan into kynurenine, which results in an increase in the production of quinolinic acid, an excitotoxin and NMDA agonist that can cause excitotoxicity and contribute to the cognitive, mood, and behavioral symptoms seen in many LYD/TBD patients.[64,77]

Quinolinic acid levels in the cerebral spinal fluid of Lyme disease patients is higher in patients with CNS infections and correlates with the severity of CNS symptoms, including depression.[77,78] Violent behavior is sometimes seen associated with LYD/TBD; it appears to be immune mediated and is often bizarre, senseless, and unpredictable.[79]

The stress of chronic infections causes a vicious cycle of chronic stress and nonrestorative sleep that contributes to perpetuating the disease process and is associated with decreased regenerative functioning, compromised immunity, oxidative stress, decreased resistance to infectious disease.[62,80]

AUTOIMMUNE EFFECTS

According to Bransfield,[70] autoimmune mechanisms provoked by *B. burgdorferi* in chronic Lyme disease have been implicated in the pathogenesis of psychotic symptoms[81] and neurologic symptoms of the central and peripheral nervous systems.[82]

In addition, *B. burgdorferi* outside the brain can release outer coat lipoproteins and flagella that may provoke antineuronal antibody production (molecular mimicry) that can disseminate to the brain; then multiple mechanisms can evoke autoimmune symptoms in the brain, including intrusive symptoms, obsessiveness, movement, disorders, paranoia, and other symptoms.[79,83–85]

LATE-STAGE IMMUNE CNS EFFECTS

According to Bransfield,[70] the three principal mechanisms leading to the injury of neuronal cells are: (1) the secretion of cytotoxic substances by leukocytes and glial cells, (2) direct cytotoxicity, and (3) autoimmune-triggered processes via molecular mimicry. An interaction between *B. burgdorferi* and the neural cells can cause dysfunction by adherence, invasion, and cytotoxicity of neural cells. In addition, *B. burgdorferi* outer surface protein A induces apoptosis and astrogliosis. *B. burgdorferi* spirochetes interacting with Schwann and glial cells also appear to produce nitric oxide, and the spirochetes can induce cytokines such as IL-6 or TNF-alpha in glial cells, both of which are neurotoxic and might provoke autoimmune reactions.[64]

When there is inflammation within the CNS, the chemokine CXCL134, which is produced by monocytes and dendritic cells in response to the spirochetal encounter, is found in high concentrations in the CSF.[67] Also, the inflammatory response elicited by *B. burgdorferi* in glial cells contributes to damage of oligodendrocytes that are vital for the function and survival of neurons.[86]

There are multiple known and unknown mechanisms through which *B. burgdorferi* can induce the neuronal dysfunction that leads to late-stage clinical symptoms.

Dementia

According to Bransfield,[70] multiple studies and a meta-analysis of 86 studies have demonstrated that dementia is accompanied by a significant inflammatory response. Because CNS *B. burgdorferi* infections are associated with CNS inflammation and systemic LYD/TBD are also associated with low-grade inflammatory processes, it supports clinical observations that rapidly progressive dementia can be associated with CNS infection and that slowly progressive dementia can be associated with systemic LYD/TBD.[87]

Autism

Autism spectrum disorders have been associated with a number of infections, including LYD/TBD. Both inflammatory and autoimmune processes that adversely affect developing fetal neural tissue appear to be involved in the pathophysiology. Effects upon the developing fetus from the mother's immune system and infection of the infant that adversely alters developing neural tissue are both possible pathophysiologic processes.[88–90]

The blood–brain barrier is permeable during fetal development and can be compromised by infections and environmental exposures throughout life. The absence of a complete barrier allows immune components access to the brain. Individuals with autism show increased proinflammatory cytokines in the brain as well as activation of microglia.[89]

Additionally, antibodies that target brain tissues have been described in both children with autism and their mothers, and antineuronal antibodies can be present in LYD/TBD patients. These immunologic phenomena may interfere with normal brain development and function, potentially contributing to developmental impairments and/or autistic spectrum symptoms.[89,91] When autism spectrum disorder is associated with chronic *B. burgdorferi* infection, effective treatment with antibiotics can reduce the infection, thereby reducing the immune provocation and in turn, reducing the symptoms.[92]

Most symptoms associated with Lyme disease and other tick-borne diseases are immune mediated. A progressive sequence of immune effects is associated with a progressive development of cognitive, psychiatric, neurologic, and somatic symptoms. These progressive immune effects include persistent inflammation with cytokine effects, the release of proinflammatory lipoproteins from the outer coat of *B. burgdorferi*, and autoimmunity.

Prolonged inflammation, particularly the type associated with chronic infection within the CNS, is associated with further cognitive impairments, more severe psychiatric symptoms, gliosis, and dementia. Autoimmune effects also can be present at the same time and can include antineuronal antibodies and *B. burgdorferi* lipoproteins that can disseminate from the periphery to inflame the brain.

These immune reactions can result in psychiatric symptoms such as obsessiveness, movement disorders, paranoia, and others. Autism spectrum disorders associated with Lyme disease and other tick-borne diseases appear mediated by a combination of inflammatory and autoimmune mechanisms from the mother's and/or infant's immune system. Understanding this pathophysiology will help physicians create new treatment options.

Functional Brain Imaging and Neuropsychological Testing in Lyme Disease

Differentiating neuropsychiatric Lyme disease from a primary psychiatric disorder can be a daunting task. Functional brain imaging and neuropsychological testing can be particularly valuable in helping to make diagnostic distinctions. In addition to a review of the relevance of functional imaging to neuropsychiatry in general, recent findings are presented regarding the use of single photon emission computed tomographic (SPECT) imaging in Lyme disease.

According to Fallon et al.,[91] primary care physicians and medical specialists are increasingly being asked to evaluate patients whose primary diagnosis may be either Lyme disease or a psychiatric disorder. Differentiating the two can be difficult at times, particularly because the manifestations of Lyme disease include secondary neuropsychiatric disorders.[1] Patients with Lyme disease may experience short-term memory loss, severe depression, panic attacks, unrelenting anxiety, impulsivity, paranoia, obsessive compulsive disorder, personality changes marked by irritability and mood swings, and rarely, manic episodes or psychotic states. Depression of at least 2 weeks' duration, by far the most common concomitant second psychiatric disorder, may occur in as many as 70% of patients with chronic Lyme disease at some point during their illness.[92]

The suggestion that these states are related to the Lyme infection is based on three findings: the frequency of psychiatric disorders is greater among patients with Lyme disease than among those with other medical conditions[92]; patient's psychiatric disorders may improve with antibiotic treatment alone[93]; and many patients who developed these neuropsychiatric conditions reported being psychiatrically healthy prior to the onset of Lyme disease.[94]

Lyme disease is not the only medical illness that can have psychiatric manifestations. Others include syphilis, AIDS, viral pneumonia, carcinoma of the brain or pancreas, hypoxia, endocrinopathies, vitamin B_{12} or folate deficiencies, temporal-lobe epilepsy, Wilson's disease, and collagen vascular diseases such as systemic lupus erythematosus. Failure to recognize the medical abnormality underlying what appears to be a "classic" psychiatric disorder is not uncommon. Koranyi[95] reported that nearly one-fifth of a sample of psychiatric outpatients had a medical condition as the cause of their psychiatric disorder and that this physical condition had been missed by the referring physician in about one-third of the cases.[96]

Patients with irritable bowel syndrome, chronic fatigue syndrome, and chronic Lyme disease may be mislabeled as having hypochondriasis or somatization disorder.[97,98] Such mislabeling may have particularly detrimental effects on the patient with Lyme disease as a delay in diagnosis and treatment may result in a curable acute infection becoming a chronic treatment-refractory illness.

While mislabeling Lyme disease as a primary psychiatric disorder can be damaging, so too can incorrectly labeling a primary psychiatric disorder as Lyme disease. Patients may then be exposed to unnecessary antibiotic treatment and possible secondary superinfection. Of equal concern is that comprehensive psychiatric care may be delayed because patients fear that seeking mental health care will result in their being stigmatized as a "crock" or a mentally ill patient. Tragic consequences may result. Major depression, for example, results in completed suicide in 15% of cases.[99]

To aid the clinician in the task of differentiating Lyme disease from primary psychiatric disorder, the Fallon et al.,[92] article focuses on four aspects of the evaluation that can be particularly helpful: clinical presentation, laboratory testing, neuropsychological testing, and functional brain imaging.

CLINICAL PRESENTATION

Differentiation between the emotional and cognitive abnormalities due to Lyme disease and those of a primarily psychological etiology may be aided by the following considerations. First, does the patient have markers of a nonpsychiatric disease such as an erythema migrans rash, migrating polyarthralgia or arthritis, myalgia, severe headaches, increased sound or light sensitivity, paresthesia, diffuse fasciculation, cardiac conduction delay, word-finding problems, short-term memory loss, cranial neuropathies, and/or radicular or shooting pains?[100]

Second, is the psychiatric disorder itself unusual? For example, in the case of depression, is it characterized by marked mood liability, in which the patient bursts into tears for no apparent reason or in which moods fluctuate from normal to extreme irritability over short periods? In the case of panic disorder, does the acute anxiety last longer than the usual 10-minute interval characteristic of most primary panic attacks?

Third, does the patient show a poor response to medications that typically would be helpful or that previously had helped that same patient? Fourth, is the psychiatric disorder of new onset in a person with no new identifiable stressors or secondary gain? Lack of a psychological precipitant for a psychiatric disorder of a new onset should raise the possibility of an underlying medical illness.

Fifth, is there a history of a psychiatric disorder or a strong family history of psychiatric disturbances, such that the patient's current condition may be unrelated to Lyme disease, exacerbated by Lyme disease, or triggered but not perpetuated by Lyme disease? As a rule, whenever a patient older than the age of 40 years develops a psychiatric disorder for the first time without apparent cause, an organic etiology must be suspected.

LABORATORY TESTS

According to Fallon et al.,[92] laboratory testing is an essential component of the diagnostic assessment both to provide evidence of exposure to *B. burgdorferi* and to exclude other diseases that might have neuropsychiatric presentations, such as systemic lupus erythematosus, multiple sclerosis, vitamin deficiencies, and endocrinopathies. The ELISA and the Western blot are the most commonly employed indirect serological tests. Although these tests are extremely helpful in confirming Lyme disease when both tests give evidence of reactivity, these tests can be misleading when equivocal results are obtained or are negative.

For example, some patients with Lyme disease may have Western blot results that indicate the presence of only a few of the bands that the CDC considers specific for Lyme disease, that is, the results are suggestive of Lyme disease but do not meet the standard of five bands required by the CDC for a positive Western blot and are therefore interpreted as "nonreactive." For some such patients, additional bands may become evident after treatment.[101]

Others may have meaningful evidence of exposure to *B. burgdorferi*, such as reactivity at the highly specific 31 kDa (OspA) and 34 kDa (OspB) sites. Unfortunately, according to Fallon et al.,[92] bands are not included in the CDC's top 10 list of diagnostic bands, many laboratories will not report them and therefore fail to provide the clinician with all of the important data. In the absence of definitive indirect diagnostic tests, additional testing that more directly detects the presence of the spirochete may be helpful.

The PCR assay for *B. burgdorferi,* if done at a reputable laboratory with good quality-control standards, may detect the presence of the DNA and therefore suggest active infection.[102] The Lyme urine antigen test, in the absence of a concurrent urinary tract infection, may be helpful in detecting the presence of *B. burgdorferi* protein shedding.[103] However, more research needs to be conducted regarding both the sensitivity and specificity of this test. Critical to proper interpretation of serological testing is that the tests be done at laboratories that have excellent quality control and high levels of sensitivity and specificity.

Tests of other involved areas, such as the CSF and joint cavities, are also essential components of a thorough evaluation. In chronic neuropsychiatric Lyme disease, Lyme ELISA of the serum may not always be sufficiently sensitive to detect disease, as suggested by a recent study in which 22% of patients had a negative whole sonicated *B. burgdorferi* ELISAs despite having culture or PCR-proven disease.[104]

Although CSF studies in early neurological Lyme disease are often abnormal, with evidence of intrathecal antibody production in 70%–90% of cases of Lyme meningitis, routine CSF antibody studies in chronic Lyme encephalopathy may be misleadingly normal. In a study of 35 patients with late neurological Lyme disease who had *B. burgdorferi* spA antigen in the CSF on experimental testing, 43% had normal CSF antibody study results and 20% had no evidence of either Lyme antibodies or other typical CSF abnormalities.[105] Normal CSF results therefore cannot be used to rule out neuroborreliosis.

NEUROPSYCHOLOGICAL TESTING

Patients with Lyme encephalopathy present with recent memory, word-finding, and spatial disorientation problems, make dyslexic-like number reversals or letter reversals when writing and are markedly distractible, such that they have trouble staying focused and completing projects. Often accompanied by a family member who sets as a surrogate memory source, such patients easily get confused, may forget key experiences, or may go off on a tangent and be unable to recall the initial question.

On neuropsychological tests, 50%–60% of patients with chronic neurological Lyme disease have evidence of objective impairment.[106,107] The impairment may involve memory, attention and concentration, verbal fluency, perceptual motor functioning, and/or conceptual ability. Often, objective cognitive deficits on neuropsychological testing can be demonstrated despite normal findings from a neurological examination and of electroencephalographic, CSF, and MRI studies.[107,108]

According to Fallon et al.,[92] while a patient may not appear to have memory problems on a routine clinical evaluation, clinically significant abnormalities may be evident on formal neuropsychological testing. Such tests, then, are valuable both as a means of confirming the presence of objective impairment and as a baseline from which to measure subsequent response to treatment. Tests that are particularly helpful include the Wechsler Memory Scale, the Busenke Selective Reminding test, and the Controlled Oral Word Association test. Patients with Lyme encephalopathy have significantly more memory problems than patients with other disorders that share certain features with Lyme disease, such as fibromyalgia or mild depression.[109]

Fatigue, anxiety, and depression, however, can cause a patient to perform poorly on neuropsychological tests. The psychiatric disorder itself may be primary, that is, unrelated to the biology of Lyme disease or secondary to the pathophysiological processes induced by *B. burgdorferi*. Regardless of whether the psychiatric disorder is primary or secondary, it behooves the physician to treat the concomitant psychiatric disorder aggressively in order to optimize the patient's functioning and more clearly evaluate the need for additional antibiotic treatment.

In the presence of active infection, however, psychiatric disorders related to CNS Lyme disease may be resistant to psychopharmacological treatment but may respond to such treatment following adequate antibiotic therapy.

Typically, mildly depressed patients will show few if any objective memory deficits on neuropsychological testing, while patients with Lyme encephalopathy will show mild-to-severe levels of impairment, particularly in verbal fluency and verbal short-term memory.

When neuropsychological tests do reveal deficits among depressed patients, the deficits may occur because of lack of effort and poor concentration rather than actual deficits in storage or retrieval. Depressed patients tend to give up easily when tested, responding "I don't know." Whereas patients with primary memory disorders, such as in Alzheimer's disease, more commonly make a determined effort but give incorrect answers.[110] Depressed patients tend to have good automatic or incidental learning (e.g., recalling what they had for breakfast or recalling the day of the week), whereas encephalopathic patients more typically have poor automatic learning.

In a study of 15 patients with chronic Lyme disease and memory complaints, nine had abnormal neuropsychological test results, while six had normal scores[107]; five of the six cognitively normal patients had the highest depression scores of the entire group of 15, confirming that moderate depression causes the perception of memory problems in some patients who do not have evidence of objective impairment. These moderately depressed patients, if treated for their psychiatric problem would likely experience an improvement of both mood and cognition.

As depression becomes more severe, however, neuropsychological tests may show impairment in many cognitive areas. The deficits in moderately to severely depressed patients typically involve spatial and holistic tasks, as well as tasks that require speed or sustained motor effort.[111] In addition, deficits may be seen on intelligence tests and in verbal learning and free recall.[112] Therefore, to get the most information from a set of neuropsychological tests, the clinician would be wise to treat a patient's concomitant mood disorder prior to initiation of the testing, thereby removing a confounding variable in test interpretation.

FUNCTIONAL BRAIN IMAGING

Functional brain imaging techniques, such as SPECT and positron emission tomography (PET), provide a dynamic picture of the brain's functioning: metabolism, blood flow, and chemistry. While structural imaging techniques are very helpful in identifying gross changes in brain structure, functional imaging techniques allow us to appreciate the working physiology of the brain.

PET studies have confirmed that regional cerebral blood flow changes are generally coupled with changes in regional brain metabolism. Decreased metabolic activity results in hypoperfusion, whereas increased metabolic activity results in hyperperfusion. Although hypoperfusion may occur as a result of vascular changes, functional brain imaging is particularly valuable to neuropsychiatrists for its ability to detect changes in perfusion that are secondary to metabolic changes. In comparison to PET scanning, SPECT scanning is about 3–4 times less expensive, is more widely available, and with the more recent SPECT scanners, is able to provide spatial resolution images of 6–9 mm, closely approaching the 406 mm resolution of PET studies. We at the EHC-Dallas have used the triple camera SPECT scan for years with good success.

SPECT scanners typically use a rotating gamma camera with one to three detector heads. The image data are subsequently reconstructed and reoriented in three orthogonal (coronal, sagittal, and transaxial) image planes. Although PET imaging can be used to provide a quantitative assessment of regional perfusion or metabolic abnormalities, the technique is invasive, requiring arterial sampling; to void the necessity of arterial sampling, the analysis of PET and SPECT scans is best done in a semiquantitative fashion.

MRI scans of patients with neurological Lyme disease may demonstrate punctate white matter lesions on T2-weighted images, similar to those seen in demyelinating disorders, such as multiple sclerosis.[108] This is most often seen among patients with evidence of meningitis or encephalitis. The white matter lesions may resolve after antibiotic treatment. In the later stage neurological Lyme disease, however, brain MRI scans are generally normal even though the patient may continue to have debilitating neuropsychiatric problems.[113]

Functional brain imaging by means of SPECT has recently emerged as a new and very useful tool in the evaluation of patients with Lyme disease. In patients with Lyme disease, SPECT scans typically show multifocal areas of decreased perfusion in both the cortex and the subcortical white matter.[114–118] In a review of 35 patients consecutively referred to Columbia Presbyterian Medical Center (New York) for technetium-99 m SPECT imaging who were suspected of having neurological sequelae to Lyme disease, 18 (51.4%) had significant perfusion abnormalities.[116]

Of these 18 patients, 17 had regional cortical abnormalities, 15 had a heterogeneous pattern of uptake, 14 had reduced tracer uptake in the periventricular white matter, and 11 had a global reduction of cortical perfusion. Most commonly involved were the frontal, temporal, and parietal lobes. Among the 18 patients whose SPECT scans were abnormal, 13 had normal brain MRI studies. A significant limitation of this study[116] is that patients were not prospectively categorized according to the diagnostic certainty of Lyme disease. Because all patients, including those with probable but not definite Lyme disease, were grouped together, the findings from this report must be considered tentative.

In a more recent report from investigators at Columbia,[118] 20 patients with seropositive chronic Lyme disease who had been previously treated with antibiotics were evaluated by techmetium-99 m-HMPAO (hexamethylpropyleneamine oxime) SPECT before and after repeated antibiotic treatment. The two scans of each patient with Lyme disease were read in random order by radiologists blind to the treatment received and to the temporal order of scans. The scans of 14 patients with non-Lyme neurological or systemic disease were interspersed so that radiologists would be blind to diagnosis as well.

In 800 patients with a positive triple camera SPECT scan at the EHC-Dallas, we found the majority to be associated with chemical sensitivity-induced vasculitis though some were Lyme induced. Ninety-six percent (27 of the 28 abnormal Lyme SPECT images showed a heterogeneous pattern, but this pattern was nonspecific, as it was also seen in the control patients with Creutzfeldt–Jakob disease, cerebral vasculitis, and chronic fatigue syndrome. Forty-one percent of the Lyme scans showed improved perfusion on the second scan, with the suggestion of more improvement among patients treated with intravenous antibiotics (5 of 10) than among patients given other forms of treatment (2 of 7).

In an abstract consistent with the above findings of a heterogeneous pattern of uptake, Logigian et al.[114] reported on eight patients with seropositive Lyme disease who were studied with use of the more objective quantitative SPECT method. All had reduced perfusion in a multifocal distribution, especially in the white matter. Only one of the eight had MRI white matter abnormalities. Six of the eight had abnormal spinal fluid, of whom three had intrathecal antibody production. All had neuropsychological deficits of verbal and visual memory. Six months following intravenous antibiotic treatment, quantitative SPECT scans of five of the patients revealed a pattern of improved flow.

In a more recent report, Logigian[115] contrasted the brain perfusion patterns of 13 patients with definite Lyme encephalopathy (as defined by the presence of objective deficits on neuropsychological testing), 9 patients with possible Lyme encephalopathy (no objective deficits), and 26 normal controls. Patients with definite Lyme encephalopathy had significantly more deficits than patients with possible encephalopathy, who in turn had significantly more deficits than normal controls.

When the 13 patients with definite Lyme encephalopathy were given intravenous ceftriaxone, a partial reversal in brain perfusion deficits was observed 6 months later. These results suggest that SPECT perfusion deficits are greater with more severe disease, that SPECT deficits may be seen even in the absence of objective neuropsychological deficits, and that the perfusion deficits are at least partially reversible. However, a simple clinical observation is found. These patients cannot stand on their toes with their eyes closed or walk a straight line. This clinical correlation is almost always (99%) correlated with a positive triple camera SPECT scan. It denotes cerebral vasculitis usually with chemical exposure etiology but can also be Lyme as the cause.

Hypoperfusion defects visualized on SPECT scans in Lyme disease may result from any process that alters the radiotracer distribution, including vascular delivery to neurons, transport of the tracer into the cells, and retention of the radioactive tracer in the cells. Problems may arise secondary to direct infection of neurons, from cellular dysfunction due to the indirect effects of neurotoxic immunomodulators such as cytokines, or from decreased perfusion through arterioles secondary to vasculitis. In other words, areas of hypoperfusion may result from a cellular, metabolic, and/or vascular problem.

In what ways, then, are SPECT scans helpful in the diagnostic assessment? First, SPECT scan with diffuse abnormalities may help to confirm that an objective abnormality is present in a patient suspected or having a purely factitious or psychogenic disorder. Second, a normal SPECT scan of a patient with prominent neuropsychiatric symptoms may suggest that a psychiatric disorder is the primary cause of the patient's cognitive or emotional distress and therefore lead the clinician to recommend reevaluation of the patient's psychiatric treatment. Third, an improvement in SPECT perfusion after treatment provides evidence that the brain has not been permanently damaged and that the treatments are resulting in physiological change.

Consider the following case: A 27-year-old previously healthy man who lived in an area of hyperendemicity for Lyme disease developed intense fatigue and intermittent paranoid delusions that he was being followed. Over the subsequent months, headaches, memory lapses, mental "cloudiness," and episodic inability to perform routine activities emerged. Cognitive deterioration advanced such that he no longer recognized members of his own family.

After admission to an intensive care unit and a full battery of tests, the diagnosis of CNS Lyme disease was made on the basis of positive ELISAs of the serum and CSF (0.267 and 0.265 optical density, respectively; cutoff, 0.112 optical density) and mild pleocytosis (6 WBCs/mm^3). Results of MRI and electroencephalography were normal. After treatment for 3 weeks with intravenous ceftriaxone, he was able to identify his family and friends and wished to return to work. However, over the subsequent few weeks after further intravenous antibiotic therapy had been discontinued, his confusion and memory problems returned (he would get lost in his own house), and new symptoms appeared: swollen knees, arthralgia in his toes and hands, and numbness on his right side.

Upon return to the infectious disease specialist, the patient and his family were told that his symptoms were probably not due to Lyme disease because he had already received the recommended course of treatment. A second spinal tap again showed pleocytosis (6 WBCs/mm^3), but the Lyme serologies, performed at a different laboratory, were now negative. Nevertheless, in response to pressure from the family and differing opinions from other specialists, the patient was retreated for 2 more weeks with intravenous antibiotics. This time his condition did not improve.

A team of psychiatrists evaluated the patient and concluded that he had a "dissociative disorder" rather than Lyme disease and should be transferred to a psychiatric inpatient facility. At this point, unable to feed himself or to speak coherently, he was removed from the care of the hospital by his family, who had arranged for him to be treated privately. Four months after discharge, a brain SPECT scan was done. Although clinically able to feed himself, he still had severe cognitive deficits; he did not know his name or any details of the prior year.

Was this a dissociative disorder? When his SPECT scan was compared to the scan of a patient with no abnormalities, findings were as follows. The SPECT scan of the patient with Lyme disease revealed marked hypoperfusion throughout the cortex as well as the appearance of dilated ventricles. As this patient had a normal MRI scan with no evidence of structural abnormalities such as dilated ventricles, it was concluded that the SPECT image indicated gray matter perfusion deficits as well as prominent white matter deficits, which gave the appearance of a dilated ventricle because the radiotracer deposition was so markedly reduced in the periventricular area. The SPECT scan findings were more consistent with a medical disease diffusely affecting brain function rather than a primary dissociative disorder, as the latter does not typically cause profound perfusion deficits.

It should be emphasized that the absence of perfusion abnormalities on a SPECT or PET scan does not prove absence of a disease process. As has been shown in studies of Alzheimer's disease, during the early stages of the illness, 45% of patients will not have perfusion abnormalities.[119] In Lyme disease, therefore a normal SPECT scan may indicate that either the brain is not involved or the brain involvement is in its early states or resolving.

In order to better appreciate the utility of SPECT imaging, a brief review of patterns of perfusion seen in other areas of clinical neuropsychiatry is required. Familiarity with these patients may enable one to more clearly state that a patient's neuropsychiatric disorder is primarily psychiatric or secondary to another illness. For example, the pattern of primary depression is different from the pattern of Alzheimer's dementia and from that of CNS Lyme disease. Although clinical judgment must still take precedence in the evaluation of the patient, these functional imaging techniques can substantially improve diagnostic confidence.

In primary depression, one most commonly sees decreased uptake in the left anterolateral prefrontal cortex and less commonly, decreased flow in the temporal lobes.[120] Left frontal-lobe normalization of flow may occur after successful treatment of depression.[121,122] This pattern of decreased frontal blood flow commonly seen in primary depression is also typical of depression secondary to other illnesses such as Parkinson's disease, Huntington's chorea, epilepsy, HIV dementia, and presumably, Lyme disease. Nevertheless, in Lyme disease accompanied by depression, as in most medical conditions with secondary depression, one would expect to see abnormal perfusion extending beyond the frontal-lobe areas as well.

In early Alzheimer's disease, one typically sees decreased flow in the temporal and posterior parietal areas, with sparing of the sensorimotor strip and occipital cortex, while in later Alzheimer's disease the frontal lobe may also be involved.[123,124] Temporoparietal abnormalities may be evident on functional imaging before atrophy is seen on CT or MRI scans.

This pattern of temporoparietal hypoperfusion distinguishes Alzheimer's disease from several other dementing illnesses, such as AIDS–dementia complex which shows a more diffusely heterogeneous pattern, and depressive pseudodementia, which tends to localize to the frontal lobes.[125] A parietal hypoperfusion pattern, however, overlaps with Parkinson's disease, dementia and as seems to be true from our xenon[94,124] SPECT studies (Fallon, 1996; unpublished data), with Lyme disease-related memory problems.

In early Huntington's disease, one may see decreased flow in the caudate nucleus, putamen, and cingulated gyrus by means of PET scanning.[126] Similarly, SPECT imaging has revealed markedly decreased flow in the caudate.[127]

Psychiatric disorders other than depression may also have characteristic functional imaging patterns. In obsessive–compulsive disorder, functional imaging studies may show increased flow in the frontal cortex and the caudate.[128] In schizophrenia, patients with positive symptoms (delusions, hallucinations) may have temporal-lobe hypoperfusion, while patients with negative symptoms (amotivation, flat affect) may have frontal-lobe hypoperfusion.[129,130]

Therefore, in evaluation of a depressed patient who presents with equivocal Lyme serologies but a clinical picture suggestive of Lyme disease, a SPECT scan may be very helpful. If the SPECT scan shows either a global reduction in flow or diffuse areas of heterogeneous tracer uptake, then this scan indicates another physiological process, in addition to or instead of that which causes depression is involved. Assuming that other medical causes of globally or heterogeneously reduced tracer uptake have been ruled out, then the diagnosis of Lyme disease is further supported but not necessarily confirmed.

One cannot conclude from a SPECT scan that a patient has Lyme disease, as similar SPECT scan patterns may be seen with other diseases as well. However, the diffusely abnormal SPECT scan does alert the clinician to the presence of an organic etiology other than that which causes primary depression.

Other disease processes that may cause a brain SPECT scan to show patchy, heterogeneous tracer uptake include vascular dementia,[131,132] chronic fatigue syndrome,[133] CNS lupus,[134] HIV encephalopathy,[135,136] and chronic or acute stimulant abuse.[137] Studies have shown, for example, that the SPECT scans of patients with AIDS–dementia complex could not be differentiated from the SPECT scans of patients who were chronic cocaine abusers.[137] Therefore, in the interpretation of a SPECT scan that has revealed heterogeneous uptake, the above disorders certainly need to be considered.

Although there are important correlations between abnormalities in the clinical presentation and abnormal SPECT findings, it is not clear how closely improvements in clinical functioning are paralleled by improvements in brain perfusion. For example, it is known that metabolic or flow defects may persist after a stroke or trauma, despite normal neurological examination findings.[123] Our clinical experience with Lyme disease patients indicates that improvement in SPECT perfusion abnormalities may occur rapidly or lag behind clinical improvement by many months.[117]

CONCLUSION

Physicians challenged with difficult differential neuropsychiatric diagnoses will benefit from employing an approach in which the clinical presentation and history are primary and other modalities are used to test the clinical impression. These additional modalities include laboratory testing of the serum and CSF, neuropsychological testing, and neuroimaging procedures.

SPECT scans, in their ability to detect diffuse cerebral abnormalities in the absence of other objective findings, such as an abnormal CSF, MRI, or focal neurological signs may be particularly helpful in the process of differentiating neuropsychiatric Lyme disease from primary psychiatric disorders. Intradermal provocation and the Lyme antigen under environmentally controlled conditions could reproduce the symptoms and was the most efficacious in the diagnosis of Lyme disease. However, they took the Lyme antigen off the market.

REFERENCES

1. Locke, S. F. 2008. *Bug vs Bug: How do Mosquitoes Survive Deadly Viruses Unscathed?* Scientific American.
2. Koella, J. C, F. L. Sorensen, R. A. Anderson. 1998. The malaria parasite, *Plasmodium falciparum*, increases the frequency of multiple feeding of its mosquito vector, *Anopheles gambiae*. *Proc. Royal Soc. B* 265(1398): 763–768. doi: 10.1098/rspb.1998.0358. Retrieved April 15, 2016.
3. History/reason of Mosquito Control in New Jersey. 2000. Accessed October 12, 2017. https://www.bing.com/search?q=History%2Freason+of+Mosquito+Control+in+New+Jersey.+2000&src=IE-SearchBox&FORM=IENTTR&conversationid=
4. Fradin, M. S. 1998. Mosquitoes and mosquito repellents: A clinician's guide. *Ann. Intern. Med.* 128: 931–940. Retrieved April 15, 2016.
5. Caldwell Crosby, M. 2005. *The American Plague.* p. 12, New York: Berkley Books. ISBN 0-425-21202-5.

6. McCullough, D. 1977. *The Path Between the Seas: The Creation of the Panama Canal 1870-1914.* Simon & Schuster, ISBN 0-671-24409-4.
7. Caldwell Crosby, M. 2005. *The American Plague*, pp. 100–202. New York: Berkley Books. ISBN 0-425-21202-5.
8. Mosquito-Borne Disease. Centers for Disease Control and Prevention. 2015. Accessed April 15, 2016. http://www.cdc.gov/ncidod/diseases/list_mosquitoborne.htm.
9. Nash, D. et al. 2001. The outbreak of West Nile virus infection in the New York City area in 1999. *N. Engl. J. Med.* 344(24):1807–1814.
10. Steinman, A., C. Banet-Noach, S. Tal, O. Levi, L. Simanov, S. Perk, M. Malkinson, N. Shpigel. 2003. West Nile virus infection in crocodiles. *Emer. Infect. Dis.* 9(7):887–889.
11. Klenk, K. et al. 2004. Alligators as West Nile virus amplifiers. *Emerg. Infect. Dis.* 10(12):2150–2155.
12. Centers for Disease Control and Prevention. 2015. Accessed April 18, 2016. http://www.cdc.gov/west-nile/index.html.
13. Olejnik, E. 1952. Infectious adenitis transmitted by *Culex molestus. Bull. Res. Counc. Isr.* 2:210–211.
14. Davis, L. E., R. DeBiasi, D. E. Goade, K. Y. Haaland, J. A. Harrington, J. B. Harnar, S. A. Pergam, M. K. King, B. K. DeMasters, K. L. Tyler. 2006. West Nile virus neuroinvasive disease. *Ann. Neurol.* 60(3): 286–300.
15. Flores Anticona, E. M., H. Zainah, D. R. Ouellette, L. E. Johnson. 2012. Two case reports of neuroinvasive west Nile virus infection in the critical care unit. *Case Rep. Infect. Dis.* 2012:839458.
16. Carson, P. J., P. Konewko, K. S. Wold, P. Mariani, S. Goli, P. Bergloff, R. D. Crosby. 2006. Long-term clinical and neuropsychological outcomes of West Nile virus infection. *Clin. Infect. Dis.* 43(6): 723–730.
17. Asnis, D. S., R. Conetta, A. A. Teixeira, G. Waldman, B. A. Sampson. 2000. The West Nile Virus outbreak of 1999 in New York: The Flushing Hospital experience. *Clin. Infect. Dis.* 30(3):413–8.
18. Montgomery, S. P., C. C. Chow, S. W. Smith, A. A. Marfin, D. R. O'Leary, G. L. Campbell. 2005. Rhabdomyolysis in patients with west Nile encephalitis and meningitis. *Vector-Borne Zoonotic Dis.* 5(3):252–257.
19. Smith, R. D., S. Konoplev, G. DeCourten-Myers, T. Brown. 2004. West Nile virus encephalitis with myositis and orchitis. *Hum. Pathol.* 35(2):254–258.
20. Anninger, W. V., M. D. Lomeo, J. Dingle, A. D. Epstein, M. Lubow. 2003. West Nile virus-associated optic neuritis and chorioretinitis. *Am. J. Ophthalmol.* 136(6):1183–1185.
21. Paddock, C. D. et al. 2006. Fatal hemorrhagic fever caused by West Nile virus in the United States. *Clin. Infect. Dis.* 42(11):1527–1535.
22. Shaikh, S. and M. T. Trese. 2004. West Nile virus chorioretinitis. *Br. J. Ophthalmol.* 88(12):1599–1560.
23. Anderson, R. C., K. B. Horn, M. P. Hoang, E. Gottlieb, B. Bennin. 2004. Punctate exanthem of West Nile Virus infection: Report of 3 cases. *J. Am. Acad. Dermatol.* 51(5) 820–823.
24. Hayes, E. B., N. Komar, R. S. Nasci, S. P. Montgomery, D. R. O'Leary, G. L. Campbell 2005. Epidemiology and transmission dynamics of West Nile virus disease. *Emerg. Infect. Dis.* 11(8):1167–1173.
25. Rios, L., J. E. Maruniak. 2011. Asian tiger mosquito, *Aedes albopictus* (Skuse) (Insecta: Diptera: Culicidae). *Department of Entomology and Nematology, University of Florida.* EENY-319.
26. Watson, J. T., P. E. Pertel, R. C. Jones, A. M. Siston, W. S. Paul, C. C. Austin, S. I. Gerber. 2004. Clinical characteristics and functional outcomes of West Nile fever. *Ann. Intern. Med.* 141(5):360–365.
27. Klee, A. L., B. Maidin, B. Edwin, I. Poshni, F. Mostashari, A. D. Fine, A. Layton, D. Nash. 2004. Long-term prognosis for clinical West Nile virus infection. *Emerg. Infect. Dis.* 10(8):1405–1411.
28. Nolan, M. S., A. S. Podoll, A. M. Hause, K. M. Akers, K. W. Finkel, K. O. Murray. 2012. Prevalence of chronic kidney disease and progression of disease over time among patients enrolled in the Houston West Nile virus cohort. *PLoS ONE* 7(7):e40374.
29. New Study Reveals: West Nile virus is far more menacing & harms far more people. 2012. *The Guardian Express.* Retrieved April 18, 2016.
30. Petersen, L. R., A. C. Brault, R. S. Nasci. 2013. West Nile virus: Review of the literature. *JAMA* 310(3):308–315.
31. Kilpatrick, A. M., M. A. Meola, R. M. Moudy, L. D. Kramer. 2008. Temperature, viral genetics, and the transmission of West Nile virus by *Culex pipiens* mosquitoes. *PLoS Pathog.* 4(6):e1000092.
32. Reisen, W. K., Y. Fang, V. M. Martinez. 2006. Effects of temperature on the transmission of West Nile virus by *Culex tarsalis* (Diptera: Culicidae). *J. Med. Entomol.* 43(2):309–317.
33. Bowden, S. E., K. Magori, J. M. Drake. 2011. Regional differences in the association between land cover and West Nile virus disease incidence in humans in the United States. *Am J. Trop. Med. Hyg.* 84(2):234–238.

34. DeGroote, J. P., R. Sugumaran. 2012. National and regional associations between human West Nile virus incidence and demographic, landscape, and land use conditions in the coterminous United States. *Vector Borne Zoonotic Dis.* 12(8):657–665.

35. Hartley, D. M., C. M. Barker, A. Le Menach, T. Niu, H. D. Gaff, W. K. Reisen. 2012. Effects of temperature on emergence and seasonality of West Nile virus in California. *Am. J. Trop. Med. Hyg.* 86(5):884–894.

36. Landesman, W. J., B. F. Allan, R. B. Langerhans, T. M. Knight, J. M. Chase. 2007. Inter-annual associations between precipitation and human incidence of West Nile virus in the United States. *Vector Borne Zoonotic Dis.* 7(3):337–343.

37. Ruiz, M. O., E. D. Walker, E. S. Foster, L. D. Haramis, U. D. Kitron. 2007. Association of West Nile virus illness and urban landscapes in Chicago and Detroit. *Int. J. Health. Geogr.* 6:10.

38. Reisen, W. K., R. M. Takahashi, B. D. Carroll, R. Quiring. 2008. Delinquent mortgages, neglected swimming pools, and West Nile virus, California. *Emerg. Infect. Dis.* 14(11):1747–1749.

39. Cho, H., M. S. Diamond. 2012. Immune responses to West Nile virus infection in the central nervous system. *Viruses.* 4(12):3812–3830.

40. Lindsey, N. P., J. E. Staples, J. A. Lehman, M. Fischer. 2010. Surveillance for human West Nile virus disease. *MMWR Surveill. Summ.* 59(2):1–17.

41. Petersen, L. R., P. J. Carson, B. J. Biggerstaff, B. Custer, S. M. Borchardt, M. P. Busch. 2012. Estimated cumulative incidence of West Nile virus infection in US adults, 1999–2010. *Epidemiol. Infect.* 310:1–5, published online ahead of print May 2012.

42. Pealer, L. N. et al. 2003. Transmission of West Nile virus through blood transfusion in the United States in 2002. *N. Engl. J. Med.* 349(13):1236–1245.

43. Nett, R. J., M. J. Kuehnert, M. G. Ison, J. P. Orlowski, M. Fischer, J. E. Staples. 2012. Current practices and evaluation of screening solid organ donors for West Nile virus. *Transpl. Infect. Dis.* 14(3):268–277.

44. O'Leary, D. R. et al. 2006. Birth outcomes following West Nile Virus infection of pregnant women in the United States, 2003–2004. *Pediatrics.* 117(3):e537–e545.

45. Petersen, L. R., E. B. Hayes. 2008. West Nile virus in the Americas. *Med. Clin. North. Am.* 92(6): 1307–1322. ix.

46. Lim, J. K. et al. 2009. Genetic variation in OAS1 is a risk factor for initial infection with West Nile virus in man. *PLoS Pathog.* 5(2):e1000321.

47. Zou, S., G. A. Foster, R. Y. Dodd, L. R. Petersen, S. L. Strame. 2010. West Nile fever characteristics among viremic persons identified through blood donor screening. *J. Infect. Dis.* 202(9):1354–1361.

48. Mostashari, F. et al. 2001. Epidemic West Nile encephalitis, 1999, New York. *Lancet* 358(9278):261–264.

49. Brown, J. A., D. L. Factor, N. Tkachenko, S. M. Templeton, N. D. Crall, W. J. Pape, M. J. Bauer, D. R. Ambruso, W. C. Dickey, A. A. Marfin. 2007. West Nile viremic blood donors and risk factors for subsequent West Nile fever. *Vector Borne Zoonotic Dis.* 7(4):479–488.

50. Carson, P. J. et al. 2012. Neuroinvasive disease and West Nile virus infection, North Dakota, USA, 1999–2008. *Emerg. Infect. Dis.* 18(4):684–686.

51. Lindsey, N. P., J. E. Staples, J. A. Lehman, M. Fischer. 2012. Medical risk factors for severe West Nile Virus disease, United States, 2008–2010. *Am. J. Trop. Med. Hyg.* 87(1):179–184.

52. Murray, K. et al. 2006. Risk factors for encephalitis and death from West Nile virus infection. *Epidemiol. Infect.* 134(6):1325–1332.

53. Bode, A. V., J. J. Sejvar, W. J. Pape, G. L. Campbell, A. A. Marfin. 2006. West Nile virus disease: A descriptive study of 228 patients hospitalized in a 4-county region of Colorado in 2003. *Clin. Infect. Dis.* 42(9):1234–1240.

54. Freifeld, A. G., J. Meza, B. Schweitzer, L. Shafer, A. C. Kalil, A. R. Sambol. 2010. Seroprevalence of West Nile virus infection in solid organ transplant recipients. *Transpl. Infect. Dis.* 12(2):120–126.

55. Kumar, D., M. A. Drebot, S. J. Wong, G. Lim, H. Artsob, P. Buck, A. Humar. 2004. A seroprevalence study of West Nile virus infection in solid organ transplant recipients. *Am. J. Transplant.* 4(11):1883–1888.

56. Lindsey, N. P., J. J. Sejvar, A. V. Bode, G. L. Campbell. 2012. Delayed mortality in a cohort of persons hospitalized with West Nile virus disease in Colorado in 2003. *Vector Borne Zoonotic Dis.* 12(3):230–235.

57. Tilley, P. A., J. D. Fox, G. C. Jayaraman, J. K. Preiksaitis. 2006. Nucleic acid testing for West Nile virus RNA in plasma enhances rapid diagnosis of acute infection in symptomatic patients. *J. Infect. Dis.* 193(10):1361–1364.

58. Komar, N., S. Langevin, S. Hinten, N. M. Nemeth, E. Edwards, D. L. Hettler, B. S. Davis, R. A. Bowen, M. L. Bunning. 2003. Experimental infection of North American birds with the New York 1999 strain of West Nile virus. *Emerg. Infect. Dis.* 9(3):311–322.

59. Kilpatrick, A. M., P. Daszak, M. J. Jones, P. P. Marra, L. D. Kramer. 2006. Host heterogeneity dominates West Nile virus transmission. *Proc. Biol. Sci.* 273(1599):2327–2333.

60. Song, J., X. Gao, J. E. Galán. 2013. Structure and function of the *Salmonella Typhi* Chimaeric A2B5 typhoid toxin. *Nature* 499 (7458):350–354.

61. Galán, J. E., M. Lara-Tejero, T. C. Marlovits, S. Wagner. 2014. Bacterial type III secretion systems: Specialized nanomachines for protein delivery into target cells. *Annu. Rev. Microbiol.* 68(1):415–438.

62. Bransfield, R. 2011. Neuropsychiatric Lyme disease: Pathophysiology, assessment & treatment. Paper presented at *2nd ILADS European Meeting*; May 28, 2011; Augsburg, Germany.

63. Fallon, B. A., E. S. Levin, P. J. Schweitzer, D. Hardesty. 2010. Inflammation and central nervous system Lyme disease. *Neurobiol. Dis.* 37:534–541.

64. Bransfield, R. 2012. The psychoimmunology of Lyme/tick-borne diseases and its association with neuropsychiatric symptoms. *Open Neurol. J.* 6:88–93.

65. Coburn, J., J. R. Fischer, J. M. Leong. 2005. Solving a sticky problem: New genetic approaches to host cell adhesion by the Lyme disease spirochete. *Mol. Microbiol.* 57(5):1182–1195.

66. Auwaerter, P. G., J. Aucott, J. S. Dumler. 2004. Lyme borreliosis (Lyme disease): Molecular and cellular pathobiology and prospects for prevention, diagnosis and treatment. *Expert. Rev. Mol. Med.* 6(2):1–22.

67. Rupprecht, T. A., U. Koedel, V. Fingerle, H. W. Pfister. 2008. The pathogenesis of Lyme neuroborreliosis: From infection to inflammation. *Mol. Med.* 14(3–4):205–212.

68. Jarefors, S., M. Karlsson, P. Forsberg, I. Eliasson, J. Ernerudh, C. Ekerfelt. 2006. Reduced number of interleukin-12 secreting cells in patients with Lyme borreliosis previously exposed to *Anaplasma phagocytophilum*. *Clin. Exp. Immunol.* 143(2):322–328.

69. Pfister, H. W., T. A. Rupprecht 2006. Clinical aspects of neuroborreliosis and post-Lyme disease syndrome in adult patients. *Int. J. Med. Microbiol.* 296(Suppl 40):11–16.

70. Bransfield, R. C. 2012. Relationship of inflammation and autoimmunity to psychiatric sequelae in Lyme disease. *Psychiatr. Ann.* 42(9):337–341.

71. Chong-Cerrillo, C., E. S. Shang, D. R. Blanco, M. A. Lovett, J. N. Miller. 2001. Immunohistochemical analysis of Lyme disease in the skin of naive and infection-immune rabbits following challenge. *Infect Immun.* 69(6):4094–4102.

72. Schramm, F., A. Kern, C. Barthel, S. Nadaud, N. Meyer, B. Jaulhac, N. Boulanger. 2012. Microarray analyses of inflammation response of human dermal fibroblasts to different strains of *Borrelia burgdorferi Sensu stricto*. *PLoS One.* 7(6):e40046.

73. Shoemaker, R. C., P. C. Giclas, C. Crowder, D. House, M. M. Glovsky. 2008. Complement split products C3a and C4a are early markers of acute Lyme disease in tick bite patients in the United States. *Int. Arch. Allergy Immunol.* 146(3):255–261.

74. Widhe, M., M. Grusell, C. Ekerfelt, M. Vrethem, P. Forsberg, J. Ernerudh. 2002. Cytokines in Lyme borreliosis: Lack of early tumour necrosis factor-alpha and transforming growth factor-beta1 responses are associated with chronic neuroborreliosis. *Immunology* 107(1):46–55.

75. Constant, A., L. Castera, R. Dantzer, P. Couzigou, V. de Ledinghen, J. Demotes-Mainard, C. Henry. 2005. Mood alterations during interferon-alpha therapy in patients with chronic hepatitis C: Evidence for an overlap between manic/hypomanic and depressive symptoms. *J. Clin. Psychiatry* 66(8):1050–1057.

76. Lindqvist, D., S. Janelidze, P. Hagell, S. Erhardt, M. Samuelsson, L. Minthon, O. Hansson, M. Björkqvist, L. Träskman-Bendz, L. Brundin. 2009. Interleukin-6 is elevated in the cerebrospinal fluid of suicide attempters and related to symptom severity. *Biol. Psychiatry* 66:287–292.

77. Halperin, J. J. and M. P. Heyes. 1992. Neuroactive kynurenines in Lyme borreliosis. *Neurology* 42(1):43–50.

78. Wichers, M. C., G. H. Koek, G. Robaeys, R. Verkerk, S. Scharpé, M. Maes. 2005. IDO and interferon-induced depressive symptoms: A shift in hypothesis from tryptophan depletion to neurotoxicity. *Mol. Psychiatry* 10:538–544.

79. Bransfield, R. 2012. Can infections and immune reactions to them cause violent behavior? *Neurol Psychiatry Brain Res.* 18(3):42.

80. Greenberg, H. E., G. Ney, S. M. Scharf, L. Ravdin, E. Hilton. 1995. Sleep quality in Lyme disease. *Sleep* 18(10):912–916.

81. Carter, C. J. 2011. Schizophrenia: A pathogenetic autoimmune disease caused by viruses and pathogens and dependent on genes. *J. Pathog..* doi:10.4061/2011/128318.

82. Schluesener, H. J., R. Martin, V. Sticht-Groh. 1989. Autoimmunity in Lyme disease: Molecular cloning of antigens recognized by antibodies in the cerebrospinal fluid. *Autoimmunity* 2(4):323–330.

83. Alaedini, A., N. Latov. 2005. Antibodies against OspA epitopes of *Borrelia burgdorferi* crossreact with neural tissue. *J. Neuroimmunol.* 159:192–195.

84. Sigal, L. G., A. H. Tatum. 1988. Lyme disease patients' serum contains IgM antibodies to *Borrelia burgdorferi* that cross-react with neuronal antigens. *Neurology* 38:1439–1442.

85. Sigal, L. H. 1993. Cross-reactivity between *Borrelia burgdorferi* Flagellin and a human axonal 64.000 molecular weight protein. *J. Infect. Dis.* 167:1372–1378.

86. Ramesh, G., S. Benge, B. Pahar, M. T. Philipp. 2012. A possible role for inflammation in mediating apoptosis of oligodendrocytes as induced by the Lyme disease spirochete *Borrelia burgdorferi*. *J. Neuroinflam.* 9(1):72.

87. Miklossy, J. 2011. Alzheimer's disease—A neurospirochetosis analysis of the evidence following Koch's and Hill's criteria. *J. Neuroinflam.* 8:90.

88. Bransfield, R. C., J. S. Wulfman, W. T. Harvey, A. I. Usman. 2008. The association between tickborne infections, Lyme borreliosis and autism spectrum disorders. *Med. Hypotheses.* 70:967–974.

89. Bransfield, R. C. 2009. Preventable cases of autism: Relationship between chronic infectious diseases and neurological outcome. *Pediatr. Health.* 3:125–140.

90. Nicholson, G. 2008. Chronic bacterial and viral infections in neurodegenerative and neurobehavioral diseases. *Lab Med.* 39:291–299.

91. Fallon, B. A., S. Das, J. J. Plutchok, F. Tager, K. Liegner, R. V. Heertum. 1997. Functional brain imaging and neuropsychological testing in Lyme disease. *Clin. Infect. Dis.* 25:S57–S63.

92. Fallon, B. A., J. A. Nields, J. J. Burrascano, K. Liegner, D. DelBene, M. R. Liebowitz. 1992. The neuropsychiatric manifestations of Lyme borreliosis. *Psychiatr. Q.* 63(1):95–117.

93. Pachner, A. R., P. Duray, A. C. Steere. 1989. Central nervous system manifestations cause of Lyme disease. *Arch. Neurol.* 46:790–795.

94. Fallon, B. A., J. A. Nields. 1994. Lyme disease: A neuropsychiatric illness. *Am. J. Psychiatry.* 151:1571–1583.

95. Koranyi, E. K. 1980. Somatic illness in psychiatric patients. *Psychosomatics.* 21:887–891.

96. Barsky, A. J., G. Wyshak, K. S. Latham, G. L. Klerman. 1991. Hypochondriacal patients, their physicians, and their medical care. *J. Gen. Intern. Med.* 6(5):413–419.

97. Johnson, S. K., J. DeLuca, B. H. Natelson. 1996. Assessing somatization disorder in Lyme disease, as similar SPECT scan patterns may be seen with the chronic fatigue syndrome. *Psychosom. Med.* 58:50–57.

98. Noyes, R., R. G. Kathol, M. M. Fisher, B. M. Phillips, M. T. Suelzer, C. S. Holt. 1993. The validity of DSM-III-R hypochondriasis. *Arch. Gen. Psychiatry.* 50:961–970.

99. Wilner, A., L. Wilner, R. Fishman. 1979. Psychiatric adolescent inpatients: 8–10 year follow-up. *Arch. Gen. Psychiatry.* 36:698–700.

100. Fallon, B. A., J. A. Nields, J. J. Burrascano, K. Liegner, D. DelBene, M. R. Liebowitz. 1992. The neuropsychiatric manifestations of Lyme borreliosis. *Psychiatr. Q.* 63:95–117.

101. Fein, L. A. 1996. Multivariate analysis of 160 patients with Lyme disease [abstract]. In: *Program and abstracts of the 9th Annual International Conference on Lyme Borreliosis and Other Tick-Borne Disorders.* Boston: Lyme Disease Foundation.

102. Keller, T. L., J. J. Halperin, M. Whitman. 1992. PCR detection of *Borrelia burgdorferi* DNA in cerebrospinal fluid of Lyme neuroborreliosis patients. *Neurology.* 42:32–42.

103. Harris, N. S., B. G. Stephens. 1995. Detection of *Borrelia burgdorferi* antigen in urine from patients with Lyme borreliosis. *J. Spirochetal. Tick-Borne Dis.* 2.37–41.

104. Oksi, J., J. Uksila, A. M. Marjam, J. Nikoskelainen, M. K. Viljanen. 1995. Antibodies against whole sonicated *Borrelia burgdorferi* spirochetes, 41-kilodalton flagellin and P39 protein in patients with PCR- or culture-proven late Lyme borreliosis. *J. Clin. Microbiol.* 33:2260–2264.

105. Coyle, P. K., S. E. Schutzer, Z. Deng, L. B. Krupp, A. L. Belman, J. L. Benach, B. J. Luft. 1995. Detection of *Borrelia burgdorferi*–specific antigen in antibody-negative cerebrospinal fluid in neurologic Lyme disease. *Neurology.* 45:2010–2015.

106. Logigian, E. L., R. F. Kaplan, A. C. Steere. 1990. Chronic neurologic manifestations of Lyme disease. *N. Engl. J. Med.* 323:1438–1444.

107. Krupp, L. B., D. Masur, J. Schwartz, P. K. Coyle, L. J. Langenbach, S. K. Fernquist, L. Jandorf, J. J. Halperin. 1991. Cognitive functioning in late Lyme borreliosis. *Arch. Neurol.* 48:1125–1129.

108. Halperin, J. J., H. L. Pass, A. K. Anand, B. J. Luft, D. J. Volkman, R. J. Dattwyler. 1988. Nervous system abnormalities in Lyme disease. *Ann. N.Y. Acad. Sci.* 539:24–34.

109. Kaplan, R. F., M. E. Meadows, L. C. Vincent, E. L. Logigian, A. C. Steere. 1992. Memory impairment and depression in patients with Lyme encephalopathy: Comparison with fibromyalgia and nonpsychotically depressed patients. *Neurology.* 42:1263–1267.

110. McGlynn, S. M., A. N. Kaszniak. 1991. When metacognition fails: Impaired awareness of deficit in Alzheimer's disease. *J. Cog. Neuroscience.* 3:183–189.

111. Weingartner, H., E. Silberman. 1982. Models of cognitive impairment: Cognitive changes in depression. *Psychopharmacol. Bull.* 18:27–42.

112. Miller, W. R. 1975. Psychologic deficits in depression. *Psychol. Bull.* 82:238–260.

113. Coyle, P. K. 1992. Neurologic Lyme disease. *Semin. Neurol.* 12:200–208.

114. Logigian, E. L., K. A. Johnson, M. F. Kijewski, R. F. Kaplan, B. L. Holman, A. C. Steere. 1997. Cerebral hypoperfusion in Lyme encephalopathy: A quantitative SPECT study. *Neurology.* 49(6):1661–1670.

115. Logigian, E. L., K. A. Johnson, M. F. Kijewski R. F. Kaplan, J. A. Becker, K. J. Jones, B. M. Garada, B. L. Holman, A. C. Steere. 1996. Reversible cerebral hypoperfusion in Lyme encephalopathy as demonstrated by quantitative single photon emission computed tomography (SPECT) [abstract no D612]. In: *Program and abstracts of the 7th International Congress on Lyme Borreliosis* (San Francisco):134.

116. Das, S., J. Plutchok, K. B. Liegner, B. A. Fallon, R. A. Fawwaz, R. L. Van Heertum. 1996. TC-99m HMPAO brain SPECT detection of perfusion abnormalities in Lyme disease patients with clinical encephalopathy. In: *Program and abstracts of the 43rd Annual Meeting of the Society of Nuclear Medicine* (Denver).

117. Liegner, K. B., M. D. Agricola, B. A. Fallon, S. Das. 1996. Serial brain SPECT scanning with TC-99 m HMPAO in patients with chronic Lyme encephalitis and encephalopathy undergoing prolonged intravenous antibiotic treatment. In: *Program and abstracts of the 7th International Congress on Lyme Borreliosis* (San Francisco):149.

118. Plutchok, J. J., R. S. Tikofsky, K. B. Liegner. 1997. Serial brain SPECT imaging in chronic Lyme encephalopathy. In: *Program and abstracts of the 44th Annual Meeting of the Society of Nuclear Medicine* (San Antonio).

119. Jagus, W. J. 1994. Functional imaging in dementia: An overview. *J. Clin. Psychiatry.* 55(11, suppl):5–11.

120. Mayberg, H. S., P. J. Jeffery, H. N. Wagner, S. G. Simpson. 1991. Regional cerebral blood flow in patients with refractory unipolar depression measured with TC-99 m HMPAO SPECT. *J. Nucl. Med.* 32:951.

121. Baxter, L. R., J. M. Schwartz, M. E. Phelps, J. C. Mazziotta, B. H. Guze, C. E. Selin, R. H. Gerner, R. M. Sumida. 1989. Reduction of prefrontal cortex glucose metabolism common to three types of depression. *Arch. Gen. Psychiatry* 46:243–250.

122. Dube, S., J. A. Dobkin, K. A. Bowler. 1993. Cerebral perfusion changes with antidepressant response in major depression. *Biol. Psychiatry* 33:47A–40.

123. Mayberg, H. S. 1994. Clincal correlates of PET- and SPECT- indentified defects in dementia. *J. Clin. Psychiatry* 55(Suppl 11):12–21.

124. Eberling, J. L., W. J. Jagust, B. R. Reed, M. G. Baker. 1992. Reduced temporal lobe blood flow in Alzheimer's disease. *Neurobiol. Aging* 13:483–491.

125. Friedland, R. P., W. J. Jagust. 1990. Positron and single photon emission tomography in the differential diagnosis of dementia. In: *Positron Emission Tomography in Dementia: Frontiers of Clinical Neuroscience Series.* Vol. 10. Duara R, Ed. pp. 161–77. New York: Wiley-Liss.

126. Mayberg, H. S., S. E. Starkstein, C. E. Peyser, J. Brandt, R. F. Dannals, S. E. Folstein. 1992. Paralimbic frontal lobe hypometabolism in depression associated with Huntington's disease. *Neurology* 42:1791–1797.

127. Cummings, J. L. 1993. The neuroanatomy of depression. *J. Clin. Psychiatry* 54(Suppl 11):14–20.

128. Baxter, L. R., M. J. Schwartz, K. S. Bergman, M. P. Szuba, B. H. Guze, J. C. Mazziotta, A. Alazraki, C. E. Selin, H. K. Ferng, P. Munford. 1992. Caudate glucose metabolic rate changes with both drug and behavior therapy for obsessive-compulsive disorder. *Arch. Gen. Psychiatry* 49:681–689.

129. Tamminga, C. A., G. K. Thaker, R. Buchanan, B. Kirkpatrick, L. D. Alphs, T. N. Chase, W. T. Carpenter. 1992. Limbic system abnormalities identified in schizophrenia using PET with fluorodeoxyglucose and neocortical alterations with deficit syndrome. *Arch. Gen. Psychiatry* 49:522–530.

130. Liddle, P. F., K. J. Friston, C. D. Frith, S. R. Hirsch, T. Jones, R. S. Frackowiak. 1992. Patterns of cerebral blood flow in schizophrenia. *Br. J. Psychiatry* 160:179–186.

131. Deisenhammer, E., F. Reisecker, F. Leblhuber, H. Markut, K. Hoell, J. Trenkler, H. Steinhaeusel. 1989. Single photon emission computed tomography (SPECT) and X-ray CT in patients with dementia. *Psychiatry Res.* 29:443–445.

132. Komatani, A., K. Yamaguchi, Y. Sugai, T. Takanashi, M. Kera, M. Shinohara, S. Kawakatsu. 1988. Assessment of demented patients by dynamic SPECT of inhaled xenon-133. *J. Nucl. Med.* 29:1621–1626.

133. Schwartz, R. B., A. L. Komaroff, B. M. Garada, M. Gleit, T. H. Doolittle, D. W. Bates, R. G. Vasile, B. L. Holman. 1994. SPECT imaging of the brain: Comparison of findings in patients with chronic fatigue syndrome, AIDS dementia complex, and major unipolar depression. *Am. J. Roentgenol.* 162:943–951.

134. Rubbert, A., J. Marienhagen, K. Pirnier, B. Manger, J. Grebmeier, A. Engelhardt, F. Wolf, J. R. Kalden. 1993. Single-photon emission computed tomography analysis of cerebral blood flow in the evaluation of central nervous system involvement in patients with systemic lupus erythematosus. *Arthritis Rheum.* 36:1253–1262.

135. Rubbert, A., E. Bock, J. Schwab, J. Marienhagen, H. Nüsslein, F. Wolf, J. R. Kalden. 1994. Anticardiolipin antibodies in HIV infection: Association with cerebral perfusion defects as detected by Tc 99m-HMPAO SPECT. *Clin. Exp. Immunol.* 98:361–368.

136. Tran Dinh, Y. R., H. Mamo, J. Cervoni, C. Caulin, A. C. Saimot. 1990. Disturbances in the cerebral perfusion of human immune deficiency virus-1 seropositive asymptomatic subjects: A quantitative tomography study of 18 cases. *J. Nucl. Med.* 31:1601–1607.

137. Holman, G. L., B. Garada, K. A. Johnson, J. Mendelson, E. Hallgring, S. K. Teoh, J. Worth, B. Navia. 1992. A comparison of brain perfusion SPECT in cocaine abuse and AIDS dementia complex. *J. Nucl. Med.* 33:1312–1315.

6 Treatment Options for Chemical Sensitivity

INTRODUCTION TO INTEGRATED PHYSIOLOGY FOR TREATMENT

AVOIDANCE OF INCITANTS (1) MECHANISMS

As stated throughout this book, the dynamics of homeostasis are regulated locally by the cellular homeostatic mechanism. Generally, this is the ground regulation system,[1,2] which functions through the skin, mucous membranes, sensory nerves, and connective tissue matrix with the end blood vessels, the end autonomic nerves, the fibroblasts, and macrophages. This function is in conjunction with the peripheral sensory, dorsal root, local spinal, regional, and central nervous system. The brain also helps regulate this physiology by the principal of allostasis (an additional process of maintaining homeostasis by variability). The immune, endocrine, and neurological systems also perform as the amplification systems. The vascular system distributes the oxygen and nutrients and removes the wastes. This ground regulation system and its allostatic principle not only regulates the dynamics of homeostasis but also is responsible for all vital functions and is a part of every inflammatory and defense process throughout the body. Therefore, manipulation of the ground regulation system is of paramount importance to achieve, obtain, and maintain wellness in chemically and electrically sensitive patients and patients with episodic chronic degenerative disease.

In our experience, to avoid triggering agents and maintain health in chemically and electrically sensitive patients and patients with episodic chronic degenerative disease, these patients must stay in the alarm stage of Selye.[3] Usually, these patients are in the masked stage causing unknown disease processes. This alarm stage dictates that the nonspecific and total body load is continually reduced resulting in the patient being constantly in the deadapted state. In this state, the patient immediately perceives incoming incitants and acts upon and neutralizes them usually by eliminating the offending substances, specifically sensory and motor dermal negation neutralizations; nutrient supplementation; oxygen administration, or sauna, or immune boosters, or modulations; and avoidance of pollutants in air, food, and water. This process, thus, regulates the dynamics of homeostasis more efficiently by obtaining and maintaining the basal steady state, which is the key to treatment of chemical, electrically sensitive, and chronic degenerative disease.

We like to picture the body as a barrel, which over the long term has a sponge effect, parking pollutants in each layer of fat or CT matrix like an onion and/or in the cells of the sponge. Subject to therapy, the body's barrel will be drained by clearing contaminants layer by layer akin to the peeling of an onion. This process is very laborious in the severely damaged chemical and electrically sensitive patients because they have to undergo reactions before each stage of clearing occurs. Since the environmental receptor system of the matrix and peripheral sensory nerves, such as vanilloids, GABA, NMDA, nitric oxide, and peroxynitrite receptors, touches and measures every cell, organ, and system in the body. The ground regulation system (of which connective tissue, autonomic nervous system [ANS], and end capillaries are a part) feeds and receives information to and from every cell in the body. Hence, therapy can be instituted from any area of this system.[2]

The secondary amplification systems (gamma globulin, complements, and T and B cells) as well as the local areas such as the autonomic–somatic nervous system, endocrine system, and immune and nonimmune detoxification systems are easy to access (i.e., vanilloid, dorsal root ganglion, etc.) (Figure 6.1).

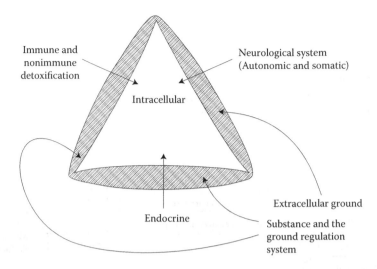

FIGURE 6.1 The environmental receptors of the ground regulation system feed information to every cell in the body, including the secondary amplification systems such as the autonomic–somatic nervous system, endocrine system, and the immune and nonimmune detoxification systems. (Adapted from Rea, W. J. 1994. *Chemical Sensitivity*, Vol. 4. Boca Raton, FL: CRC Press.)

It must be emphasized that since the peripheral sensory and spinal sensory nerves, as well as the autonomic afferent nerves are involved in the ground regulation system, nerve injury involves (by the law of nerve injury) an increase in sensitivity of all nerve channels distal to the injury. This sensitivity occurs when the incitant is combined with protein kinase 1 and 3 and is phosphorylated, increasing the sensitivity up to 1000 times. Therefore, the hypersensitivity stage to the nerve distal to the chemical or electromagnetic injury occurs (even with the immune system being invaded), thus, making the individual chemically and/or electrically sensitive.

When triggered, they make therapy difficult at times but easy at others. Because of the connective tissue and the receptors, that is, the muscarinic, GABA, vanilloid, NMDA, nitric oxide, and peroxynitrite, its collection and dissemination of information is ubiquitous. Thus, the glucocorticoid receptors (GRs) will allow many types and avenues of therapy. Because of this vastness and organization for maintaining the dynamics of homeostasis and allostasis, noxious stimuli can enter the surface or endothelium and the system modulation by sensory, peripheral, and dorsal root ganglion nerves anywhere in the body and trigger the dynamics of the homeostatic response. Therefore, accessing, obtaining, or enhancing therapy can occur almost anywhere in the body. For example, nutritional therapy used as an intervention at the gut level may affect the skeletal muscle by relieving muscle aches and spasm or in the bladder to relieve spasm (vanilloid and other receptors). Similarly, the precise and specific treatment dose of the injection of antigens at the intradermal or subcutaneous level in the arm may change cardiac or brain functions in a positive way as we have observed thousands of times at our center. Manipulation of this ground regulation system toward efficient dynamics of homeostasis and allostasis is most important since the spread of dysfunction into secondary amplifiers, such as the immune, nonimmune neural ganglion, or endocrine system, which often occurs, is much more energy draining and difficult to treat without medication. The strategy of environmental therapy is to eliminate the pollutant entry in air, food, and water. If possible, to contain the pollutant or other noxious stimuli within the local or regional area of the connective tissue or receptors of the fat or end organ, where it has been introduced, and to stop distal chronic triggering of these secondary homeostatic amplification systems. This goal can be accomplished if the total local defense system is strong, the pollutant exposure is not chronic or overwhelming, the nutrition is correct, and the pollutant load is not too toxic or in excess (Figure 6.2).

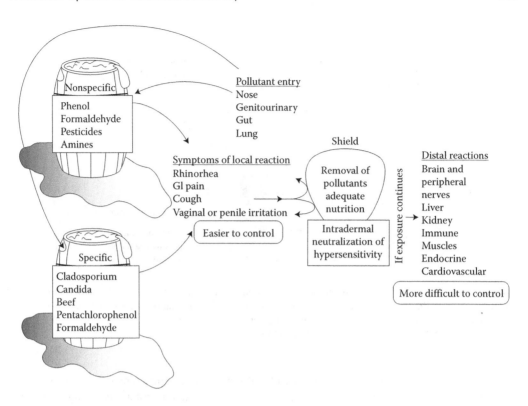

FIGURE 6.2 Therapy for chemical sensitivity and chronic degenerative disease is directed at containing the triggering of the ground regulation system to the local level of pollutant entry. The system reacts totally but not uniformly. (Adapted from Rea, W. J. 1994. *Chemical Sensitivity*, Vol. 4. Boca Raton, FL: CRC Press.)

When a patient with chronic degenerative disease or chemically sensitive patient is chronically triggered by noxious stimuli (bacteria, protozoan, virus, toxic chemical exposure), reactions usually occur locally (e.g., rhinorrhea) and distally (e.g., arrhythmia or memory loss), depending upon the body's ability to contain a local injury and response. Once triggered by noxious stimuli, the ground regulation system reacts totally, but not uniformly, accounting for some of the variability in quantity and variety of responses observed in different patients with chronic degenerative disease and chemically sensitive patients who may be exposed to the same or different pollutant incitants. The homeostatic and dyshomeostatic reactions depend upon sites, duration, and specific types of stresses (bacterial, fungal, electrical magnetic frequency [EMF], or chemical) as well as the total body pollutant load. These stresses can disrupt the local connective tissue matrix.[4]

The dynamics of homeostatic responses depend upon the integrity and resistance at the local entry point of the ground regulation system, as well as the degree of the ground regulation system peripheral autonomy that remains after repeated chronic exposures. The ground regulation system has significant peripheral autonomy not usually under the control of the central nervous system. However, with sensory nerve involvement it can rapidly change. This autonomy can be lost as local inflammation persists. This potential loss of local autonomy is one reason that our treatment is designed to stop local noxious stimuli-induced reactions, since distal, secondary responses are much more difficult to control and are less efficient in clearing. These distal homeostatic responses are less energy efficient and reduce endurance, which may cause weakness and pain in the individual.

Since the ground regulation system initially reacts in a completely nonspecific way, a great variety of stressors and noxious stimuli (total body load increase) can accumulate in the body and derail energy efficient dynamics of homeostatic functions. Therefore, reduction of total body load of as many pollutants as possible by avoidance of noxious stimuli, supplementation with nutrition,

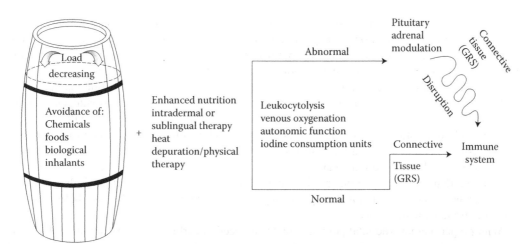

FIGURE 6.3 Effects of treatment between the ground regulation system and the immune system in chemically sensitive patients. (Adapted from Rea, W. J. *Chemical Sensitivity*, Vol. 4. Boca Raton, FL: CRC Press.)

injection, or sublingual neutralization of specific incitants to the patient who is hypersensitive is necessary. Heat depuration/physical therapy techniques will help to correct this system, allowing it to move toward the stable dynamics of homeostasis and allostasis. As shown throughout this book, the ground regulation system reacts in accordance with Selye's alarm reaction.[3] The dynamics of homeostatic disturbances are defined from its principles, that is, 3–4-hour finite reactions with changes in WBC (leukocytolysis), peripheral venous oxygenation with variable oxygen extraction, changes in autonomic nerve and electrical function, and the ability to tolerate 500,000 injected dead bacterial stimuli, as well as end tissue and organ temperature and electrical tone changes (Figure 6.3).

Therefore, massive avoidance of both primary, that is, xenobiotics, fungi, viruses, bacteria, and secondary stressors (e.g., foods and previously damaged foci) will stop the reaction, eliminating changes in WBCs (leukocytolysis), arterial and venous oxygenation, autonomic function, and others. Finally, with chronic pollutant overload, there eventually develops a disassociation of the normal integrated function of the ground regulation system with the immune system.

This disruption is always combined with exhaustion of the pituitary–adrenal function that cannot always be restored to normal with the nondrug or surgical means available till date. Thus, most of our therapies are directed toward preventing this disassociation, since up to this point the body has a great propensity to heal itself. At times, drugs, avoidance, nutrition, or surgery prevent the disassociation results and allow nonmedication treatment again.

The techniques described in this volume when activated, including the numerous receptors such as the muscarinic, vanilloids, GABA, sodium channel, NMDA, nitric oxide, and peroxynitrate receptors, will reduce the specific and nonspecific total body pollutant load on the ground regulation system and the immune system, even in some fixed-named diseases (such as early lupus erythematosus, early rheumatoid arthritis, colitis, vasculitis, etc.). But with excess and prolonged chronic overload, there is a dissolution of normal interphase between the ground regulation system with the peripheral sensory nerves and their receptors, which are vanilloid and others, and the immune system, which occurs in late-stage, fixed-named disease and the disease becomes autonomous.[5,6] Early changes in complement, T and B lymphocytes, gamma globulins, blastogenic receptors, and cell-mediated immunity abnormalities can be corrected utilizing our programs. As we have observed several times, even early production of mild-to-moderate auto-antibodies can be helpful to return to normal by our therapy if the total body pollutant load is reduced. However, sometimes our treatment modalities will only work partially, and the use of immune suppressants or modulators (i.e., autogenous lymphoystic factor) may be necessary in advanced cases of autoimmune and suppressed immune disease. In our opinion regarding patient treatment, the techniques of massive avoidance of pollutants in air, food, and water; specific antigen neutralization injection therapy for biological inhalants, foods, some chemicals, terpenes, some bacteria and viruses; nutrition therapy; heat depuration/physical therapy; oxygen therapy; acupuncture type modalities and specific point dose phototherapy; neural therapy, especially cold laser and directed infrared therapy for certain patients; homeopathy; osteopathic manipulation; and the administration of immune and nonimmune neural modulators such as autogenous lymphocytic factor (ALF), gamma globulin, and autogenous vaccines will usually allow efficient dynamics of homeostasis and allostasis to be returned and wellness to be restored to the patient. We are constantly astounded at how much reversibility is still present in early fixed-named diseases such as asthma, cardiomyopathy, chronic sinuitisis, colitis, enteritis, arrhythmia, genealogical disturbance, fibromyalgia, arthritis, and so on. At times, even surgery for inflamed target organs or removal of an inflammation producing prosthesis should always be tried before institution of chronic toxic drug therapy.

With proper therapy, the total pollutant load is reduced in earlier stages of fixed-named disease and most nonfixed-named chronic degenerative diseases (metabolic syndrome, fibromyalgia) and chemical sensitivities can be reversed. Once the body is in the reversal process, then energy released by the mitochondria in auto-oxidative enzymatic processes can be taken up by the interstitial water, complexed with proteoglycans (PG) and glycosaminoglycans (GAG) of the extracellular matrix (ECM). The matrix is capable of absorbing and cooling the heat-generating redox reactions, but, at the same time, it makes available the energy that is generated by these reactions to be used for maintaining the dynamics of homeostasis (Figure 6.4).

Because the energy generated is the energy resulting from the restored dynamics of homeostasis and allostasis, the defense mechanism of the body is restored. Thus, the efficient use of energy by the avoidance of triggering agent therapies for treatment in early fixed-named and nonfixed-named disease is the key to achieving the patient's health. To a significant extent, the behavior of high-energy electrons originates from the oxidative breakdown of carbon–hydrogen bonding, for example, in glucose breakdown.[7] By pollutant avoidance techniques and positive nutrition, the pollutant stress on mitochondria and the ECM is unloaded, which improves health in chemically or electrically sensitive patients and/or patients with episodic chronic degenerative disease.

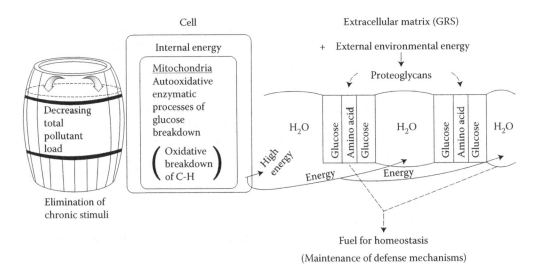

FIGURE 6.4 Proper therapy for chemically sensitive patients allows high energy to be released from the mitochondria, which is to be taken up to water and complexed with proteoglycans of the extracellular matrix to supply the fuel need for homeostasis and, thus, maintenance of the defense mechanisms. (Adapted from Rea, W. J. *Chemical Sensitivity*, Vol. 4. Boca Raton, FL: CRC Press.)

Lowering the total body pollutant load allows important intracellular and extracellular antioxidant systems (i.e., intracellular and extracellular superoxide dismutase, catalase, and glutathione peroxidase), the extracellular space, and the sensitized peripheral sensory nerves and their receptors (i.e., vanilloid receptors [VRs] and vitamins C, A, E, and many others) to reach their functional base efficiently, usually resulting in the normal dynamics of homeostasis.[4,8] The electron and proton displacements that appear in enzymatic oxygen metabolism mainly lead to the formation of multiple free radicals (OH, H_2O_2, and O_2), which, if in excess, will disturb the function of the tissue and cause inflammation and even destroy tissue. This factor is the reason for keeping the total pollutant load decreased on a daily basis in chemically or electrically sensitive patients and those with chronic degenerative disease, because even a healthy person has limits of how much free radical stress he can tolerate. Failure to do so leads to fixed-named, irreversible autonomous disease.

Furthermore, external as well as internal energy is taken into a physiological redox potential of the organism via the environmental receptor system of the extracellular ground substance. If the enzymatic stages responsible for electron and proton transfer are disturbed, which can occur locally (e.g., through chronic noxious stimuli overload, resulting in inadequate blood supply, which results in local tissue hypoxia), resulting in an accumulation of free radicals or more possibly an accumulation of local free radical induced injury.[4] This injury predisposes the local tissue to further injury by less noxious incitants (secondary homeostatic foci). If this process of free radical production is prolonged, the resulting nonphysiological alteration of the redox potential of the basic ground substance, cells, and vascular tree leads to the development of chronic inflammatory processes,[2,9] which are observed in patients with chronic degenerative disease and those who are chemically sensitive.

Hence, the therapy for episodic chronic degenerative disease and chemical sensitivity is based on the avoidance of pollutants in air, food, and water (which create free radicals ready to cause inflammation), as well as the replacement of nutrient fuels in the form of vitamins, minerals, amino acids, and lipids, thus decreasing the tendency toward inflammation.

Intradermal injection neutralization of biological inhalants, foods, bacteria, viruses, and chemicals, as well as tolerance modulator administration, such as ALF, autogenous vaccines, and mycotic immune modulators, are directed at correcting the dynamics of the hypersensitivity portion of homeostasis through basic cellular and connective tissue modulation due to the rapid information dissemination capabilities of the ground regulation system.

The hypersensitivity part of the homeostatic mechanism is often missed. Because of ignoring the hypersensitivity, often the therapy is less than satisfactory or even fails in some patients. Avoidance of pollutants also certainly eliminates the hypersensitivity phase in many environmentally wounded patients. However, others have to be administered precise neutralizing injections in order to regain their health.

The sugar polymers of the ECM provide biological information transmission and storage due to high water binding and ion exchange capacity, resulting in a rapid regulation of homeostasis. Thus, avoidance and interdermal neutralization are effective treatments. Due to the redox system, the connective tissue matrix takes up and gives off electrons.[7] Therefore, every situation, such as pollutant exposure in patients with chronic degenerative disease or who are chemically sensitive, that alters electrical tone can then be encoded in the connective tissue matrix, especially in ordered water.

The information is continued on and reciprocally (feedback) spread to processes throughout the organism, resulting in an adverse systemic reaction(s) that clinically leads to fatigue, headaches, brain fog, and so on. At the same time, excess extracellular electrons and protons in the form of oxygen and hydroxyl radicals, which appear in every enzyme-guided transformation, can be intercepted by water and sugar polymers, with the resulting heat used for further stimulation of biological processes and the generation of pyroelectricity throughout the area. This process brings about more efficient neutralization of the entering pollutants.

When the physiological conditions deteriorate with excess chemical or noxious stimuli overload, metabolic change such as vascular spasm, dying of the cells of the microcirculation, shunting, and hypoxia results, which further enhances the illness. The nonspecific mesenchyme reaction is triggered with fibroblasts being activated and the extracellular sol turns to gel or gel to sol, depending on the area of the body involved, thus changing the ECM structure as well as the electrical charges. Structural changes then alter the metabolic response adversely, causing symptom production.

Preventing this physical conversion phenomenon in the ECM and vascular tree are very important for optimum function since autonomy changes, when the conversion of gel to sol or vice versa occurs. An example of this change occurs when endothelial cells change to mesenchymal cells after long-term peritoneal dialysis. The fibrocytes proliferate until the peritoneum undergoes fibrosis and is no longer capable of dialysis. Another example would be the chronic degenerative state of the individual who develops the metabolic syndrome, where homeostasis and allostasis is altered. This patient is characterized by obesity, insulin resistance, microalbuminuria and impaired fibrinolysis, elevated triglycerides, low HDL cholesterol, and high blood pressure. Often a reactive problem is present indicating inflammation.[10] This condition is a precursor to arteriosclerotic coronary disease, where the nonspecific mesenchyme reaction leads to coronary thrombosis (Figure 6.5).

By using modalities such as subcutaneous injections of the appropriate neutralizing doses of biological inhalants, foods, bacteria, viruses, and some chemicals and avoiding chemical, EMF, mycotoxins, or volatile organs exposures, the episodic chronic degenerative diseased and periodic chemically sensitive individual can be helped to prevent disease by avoiding this conversion of gel to sol form or sol to gel. These proceedings maintain the autonomy of the dynamics of homeostasis and allostasis. Once this physical conversion of both the tissue architecture and physiology occurs and autonomy of homeostasis is lost, all therapies will be much more difficult and, perhaps, impossible to use. Once autonomy of the dynamics of homeostasis and allostasis changes, it has a tendency to remain fixed, that is, arteriosclerosis in coronary thrombosis, because if severe anatomical architecture changes, emphysema and lung failure may occur. At this stage, here, fixed-named disease occurs with its own autonomous triggering of dyshomeostatic responses, that is, myocardial infarction, spondylolisthesis, and so on. This homeostatic and allostatic regulatory capacity of the ECM, thus, has major implications in the treatment of the periodic chemically sensitive patients and those with episodic chronic degenerative disease, before fixed-named disease occurs. It is possible to influence positively, both the structure and function of the whole body.[1,2,9] Because of its vastness, the ECM system can be altered by input at almost any area of the body, with resultant positive trends toward or negative trends away from homeostasis and allostasis. The great advantage of the vastness of the ground regulation system is that many types of therapy will aid in the recovery from chemical sensitivity or chronic degenerative disease. Pollutant avoidance treatment also will often aid in rejuvenating the secondary amplification systems such as the immune and nonimmune

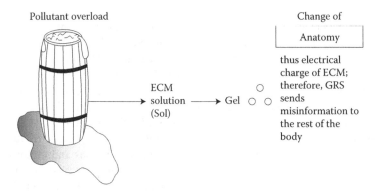

FIGURE 6.5 Environmental therapy helps prevent the changes in the regulatory capacity of the extracellular matrix and its ground regulation system in chemically sensitive patients, since it is possible to positively influence both structure and function of the whole body. (Adapted from Rea, W. J. *Chemical Sensitivity*, Vol. 4. Boca Raton, FL: CRC Press.)

enzyme detoxification systems, the endocrine, vascular, and ANS, as well as the central nervous system (CNS) and any other damaged system in the body.[11]

To really understand system-based therapy in the episodic chemically sensitive patients and the ones with episodic chronic degenerative disease, one must realize that the modern Newtonian concepts of classical physics and Virchow's classic cellular pathology, both linear in reasoning (that A causes B, i.e., *Mycobacteria tuberculosis* bacilli cause pulmonary tuberculosis or a streptococcal bacteria cause pharyngitis), have some use in the treatment of chemical sensitivity and chronic degenerative disease, but, overall, they are somewhat outdated. Therapy for chemical sensitivity and chronic degenerative disease, although incorporating some of Virchow's and Newton's concepts, is mostly based on multidimensional functional association centered on the fact that biological systems do not always show linearity. They frequently show hormesis, as illustrated in the varied responses. They may show low dose structure and high dose inhibition or vice versa. Even though these systems are multifactoral, nonlinear, and open, they are also highly integrated and are subject to a vital biological flow, equilibrium of dynamic homeostasis, and allostasis (Figure 6.6).

The biological systems exchange energy and material with their surrounding environments and are, thus, open systems. The failure of many people to understand this fact explains why the clinicians also apparently misunderstand the diagnosis and treatment of chemical sensitivity (periodic homeostatic disturbance) and episodic chronic degenerative disease (aperiodic homeostatic disturbance). In contrast to the classical closed system (mechanical, Newtonian), open systems show that when there is an influx of nonchaotic energy, information about the presence of this energy (i.e., food, pesticides, natural gas, and formaldehyde) can spread through the entire system and eventually the whole body. Thus, introduction of xenobiotic chemicals, as seen in chemically sensitive patients and those with chronic degenerative disease, disturbs this information-transmission process, and removal of these pollutants (avoidance of pollutants and/or injections neutralization or air pollutants, food, and water pollutants) allows the body to restore the dynamics of homeostasis and allostasis.

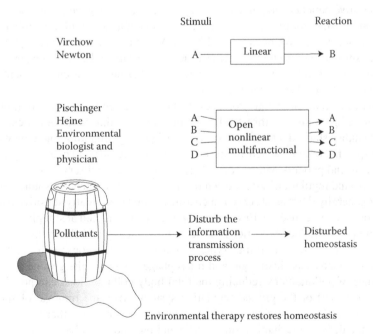

FIGURE 6.6 The causes of and therapy for chemically sensitive patients are based on multi-dimensional function association. Biological systems do not show linearity but are highly integrated and are subject to biological flow equilibrium. (Adapted from Rea, W. J. *Chemical Sensitivity*, Vol. 4. Boca Raton, FL: CRC Press.)

The information dissemination capabilities of the ground regulation system, the system that was reported by Heine and Draczynski[12] and originally defined, described, and worked out by Pischinger in 1975,[13] appear to be present in any area of the body that is manipulated in the treatment of chemical sensitivity and chronic degenerative disease. Even the sensory nerve sensitization and the vanilloid to their receptor systems, avoidance appears to also be involved in the treatment of chemical sensitivity and chronic degenerative disease. The ease of therapeutic manipulation in this ground regulation system area is because of easy access through the environmental receptor system of the sensory nerves and the connective tissue matrix. The initial ground regulation system detoxification is then followed by detoxification and restoration of the orderly function of the amplification systems (the immune and nonimmune enzyme detoxification systems and the neurovascular and endocrine systems).

The entire field of activity of the ground regulation system is the extracellular ground substance and sensory nerves. This activity is coupled with cells in relationship to the central homeostatic mechanism in the brain. The origins of where both homeostasis and allostasis occurs. However, since the connective tissue matrix engulfs cells, there is communication set up between the two by PG, GAG, and hyaluronic acid calyx's integrins attached to and penetrating the cell membrane to intracellular connections.

The lymphatic's and lymphatic organs are also connected with the ECM and the ground regulation system. Again emphasizing why environmental manipulation coupled with lymphatic's often improves the message dynamics of homeostasis and allostasis in chemically sensitive patients or patients with chronic degenerative disease.

All organ cells depend on the intact function of the ground regulation system for their existence. It appears as if organic diseases, including chemical or electrical sensitivity and chronic degenerative disease, initially originate as a dysfunction of this ground regulation system and its connections throughout the organism. If homeostatic deregulating noxious substances such as heavy metals, solvents, or pesticides are removed from the body, the system tends to re-regulate, returning the dynamics of homeostasis and allostasis to normal, as observed in most of the properly treated chemically sensitive patients and patients with episodic chronic degenerative disease studied at the EHC-Dallas and Buffalo for the last 25 years. The effects of a variety of noxious substances on the ground regulation system have been studied by the Vienna group for 40 years.[14–16] These noxious substances are similar to those that trigger chemical sensitivity and chronic degenerative disease at the EHC-Dallas and Buffalo, for the last 40 years, as well as numerous environmental and complementary medicine clinics throughout the world.

The dynamics of the functional processes of the ground regulation system (normal, dysfunction, and changes in stimulation threshold) were measured on thousands of patients by the Vienna group. These studies showed a two-layer system of triggering inflammation. One was specific and the other nonspecific, both of which we have observed in over 40,000 chemically and electrically sensitive patients and patients with chronic degenerative disease observed at the EHC-Dallas and Buffalo. The ground regulation system often reacting at the near speed of sound can react locally, regionally, or generally,[13,17,18] as observed in chemically and electrically sensitive patient or patient with chronic degenerative disease. Environmental therapy is directed at stopping or modulating all of the environmentally induced reactions. As seen in chemically and electrically sensitive patients, a variety of stimuli can set off similar types of reactions in the nonspecific part of the defense mechanism for homeostasis (histiocyte and microphage stages) in the ground regulation system. Thus, avoidance of pollutants by reducing the total body pollutant load can positively affect this local and regional part of the ground regulation system. Also, the removal of specific incitants (i.e., staphylococcus, lead, pesticides, and EMF waves) can affect the other functions triggered by specific parts the defense mechanism (monocytic and lymphocytic phase) and the ground regulation system.

Perger,[16] working at the University of Vienna, showed tremendous cost savings by manipulating the ground regulation system of chemically triggered chronic diseases. Some diagnoses included disseminated sclerosis, ulcerative colitis, rheumatic diseases, autonomic dysfunction, and even some cancers. We have found, as did Perger with his patients,[16] cost-reducing procedures such as avoidance, injection therapy, and nutritional therapy in the treatment of chemically sensitive patients and patients with chronic diseases are very efficacious.

Heine and Draczynski[12] showed that the mesh structure of the ECM produced by the connective tissue cells (macrophages, fibroblasts, and mast cells) was the basis of both information encoding and information dissemination, with reciprocal feedback effects occurring between these cells. This finding allows for environmental manipulation of one area of the body that will positively influence the rest of the generalized condition of chemically sensitive patients or patients with chronic degenerative disease.

GROUND REGULATION SYSTEM

To better understand environmental therapy for chemically sensitive patients and/or patients with chronic degenerative disease, one should understand the principles and facts of chemical and electrical sensitivity[4] and episodic chronic degenerative disease, as well as the physiology of the ground regulation system. Therefore, a detailed description of the ground regulation system and its physiology related to treatment follows.

The structure and function of the ground substance (ECM) and the ground regulation system for obtaining and maintaining homeostasis and allostasis is complicated but very understandable in chemically and electrically sensitive patients and patients with episodic chronic degenerative disease. (Several facts about this substance and its information disseminating system will be discussed.)

According to Heine et al.[10] cells have a reciprocal (feedback) relationship to their environment with seawater being the primary homeostatic regulation system of a single cell. The ion composition of the structured extracellular space of multicellular organisms corresponds to this seawater environment. The milieu surrounding a cell forms a structured basic substance in multistructured organisms, the ECM (Figure 6.7), which has a significant effect on determining the genetic as well as environmental expressivity of a cell.[10]

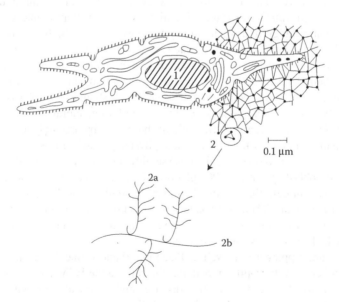

FIGURE 6.7 (1) Fibroblast synthesizing extracellular matrix. The proteoglycan network pattern (2) is enlarged (arrow). Proteoglycans (2a) are bound to hyaluronic acid (2b) in the ground substance. (From Heine, H. 1991. *Matrix and Matrix Regulation: Basis for a Holistic Theory in Medicine*, A. Pischinger, Ed., H. Heine, Eng. Trans. N. Mac Lean, p. 23. Brussels, Belgium: Editions Haug International. With permission.)

Three-dimensional architecture of the matrix can actually radically halt metabolism and aberrancy such as malignancy, as shown by Bissel.[19] Homeostasis and allostasis are paramount in running and correcting the system.

For example, we have observed some chemically sensitive and chronic degenerative disease patients with acquired or genetic sulfonation, methylation, and acetylation defects who respond favorably to reduction of their total body load of chemicals, which require sulfonation, methylation, or acetylation for detoxification. This reduction would decrease the triggering of the ground regulation system and eventually cellular function, allowing chemically sensitive patient or patient with chronic disease to regulate toward homeostasis and allostasis and allowing the condition to become quiescent and for the inflammation to subside.

The molecular biology of this connective tissue matrix involves sugar polymers, either in free form or bound to a variety of proteins, lipids, and water. These sugar polymers form the extracellular ground substance communication matrix and the individual sugar surface film, the glycocalyx of a cell. One of the cardinal injuries of the homeostasis and allostasis mechanism with pollutant or other noxious stimuli exposure is the alteration of sugar metabolism, which may increase two to threefold before nutritional depletion occurs. Thus, these sugar surfaces and structures may be injured by pollutant overload in chemically sensitive patients or patients with chronic degenerative disease, but possibly, in any given patient, they can be restored with chronic pollutant avoidance and positive nutritional and injection therapy.

These proven modalities send chemically sensitive patients and patients with chronic degenerative disease toward stabilizing the dynamics of homeostasis. Since connective tissue engulfs or underlays all cells, organs, and lobules, it should be emphasized that connective tissue has more than mechanical binding and space-filling properties, though these are important physiologically.

Because connective tissue is the only organ in the body that has direct contact with all of the body parts, it is a vital medium for transmission of end, peripheral, and spinal sensory or of afferent autonomic nerve function, as well as nutrient and oxygen flow from end vessels. Here, basement membrane characteristics and dynamics are important, both to deliver and remove the appropriate substance(s) for effective intracellular function. Molecular sieve effect reciprocal (feedback) effects pass through the ground regulation system everywhere in the body, resulting in the connective tissue acting as both an information medium with all cells[20–22] as well as a molecular sieve.

Since one can enter the ground regulation system anywhere in the body, the understanding of this transmitter function of the connective tissue is essential in treating chemically sensitive patients and patients with chronic degenerative disease, since specific neutralization dose injection therapy and specific total body load reduction will have a significant impact on the patient's physiology, at times changing even tissue architecture in a positive way. It should be emphasized that everything that comes from the blood vessels passes through the capillary membrane sieve via the extracellular network of ground substance transport cannuliculi that works by assembly–disassembly processes always being dynamic change by the structure and physiology. Substances such as serine proteases, hydrolases, lysozymes, and so on cause the disassembly process of the cannuliculi and connective tissue, while the fibroblasts producing PG, glucosamine, and collagen can cause the assembly and reassembly of the cannuliculi, thus, again changing the architecture. The process is very dynamic, occurring many times a day. There are concentration fields (i.e., electrolytes and metabolites) that direct the formation of the cannuliculi, which directs the nutrient and wastes to and from the cell and the capillary bed where the sieve effect occurs.[23]

Reicker et al.[24] and Eppinger,[25] as well as Pischinger[13] and Heine,[26] feel strongly that the functional connection between the capillary bed and the cell via the ECM and its disturbances are the starting point of many chronic degenerative diseases and chemical sensitivity. We would agree. When one integrates these scientists' opinions with the stepwise progression of pollutant injury,[4] one can see a complete version of the genesis of periodic dyshomeostatic chemical sensitivity and aperiodic dyshomeostatic episodic chronic degenerative disease and, therefore, the rationale of avoidance and specific neutralization dose injection treatment.

It appears that the ground regulation system is primarily affected in all diseases.[10] Chemical sensitivity (periodic homeostatic disturbance) and chronic degenerative diseases (aperiodic episodic homeostatic disturbance) are clearly the two types of degenerative responses that initially occur before fixed-name disease. Furthermore, due to its homeostatic orientation, the ground regulation system plays a significant role in healing when it is unloaded through pollutant or noxious stimuli avoidance. Once the chemically sensitive patients or patients with chronic degenerative disease learns how to keep his pollutant load down, thus maintaining a deadaptive state, complete healing will often occur, resulting in excellent energy and total health.

The intra- and extracellular principle used in treating these homeostatic disturbances of chemically sensitive patients and patients with chronic degenerative disease is that the human physiology and matrix autonomy is geared toward homeostasis and allostasis intact. Given a chance, the individual's own healing powers will come into play and restore health in chemically sensitive patients or patients with chronic degenerative disease. Thus, decreasing the total body pollutant load, restoring nutrition, and implementing specific antigen neutralization injection therapy for the hypersensitivity to biological inhalants, foods, bacteria, viruses, and some chemicals will aid the body in clearing the chemical sensitivity and often also chronic degenerative disease.

PHYSIOLOGY OF AVOIDANCE AND OTHER TREATMENT MODALITIES

Heine examined Pischinger's model[27] of the ECM and its homeostatic and allostatic regulatory mechanisms; sensory nerve paradigm is important in understanding the treatment of the homeostatic disturbances of chemical sensitivity and chronic degenerative disease. EMF, mycotoxin, solvent, and a detailed analysis of the connective tissue matrix and its ground regulation system physiology follows.

First: The total environmental pollutants load is significant because it will be difficult to reduce the ambient intake of pollutants if the environmental pollutant load is too high. Controlled less polluted internal environments for work and home will be necessary.

Second: The sensory afferent nerves from the periphery, the dorsal sensory spinal ganglion, the autonomic afferent and the trigeminal afferent nerves and the brain receptors must remain or revert to rising desensitization in order to easily assess the incoming pollutants in an orderly fashion. This needs to occur so that chaos does not occur in the internal detoxifying and adjustment mechanisms.

Third: The ECM permeates the extracellular space and always reacts totally and rapidly but not necessarily uniformly. Due to this fact, the reciprocal information network allows therapy to be instituted anywhere in the body to restore local, regional, or central homeostasis.

Fourth: The ECM forms a meshwork of high polymer sugar protein complexes, which engulf and order water, with the negatively charged PG predominating. This configuration of tissue with the charges allows excellent rapid communication with the cell and rapid reciprocal (feedback) information. This interchange often occurs at the near speed of light. These changes can be activated by injection therapy whether in a specific dose of an antigen or a solitary acupuncture needle, or a local anesthetic. Avoidance of pollutants and decreasing of the local or total body pollutant load works over a period of time.

These areas and processes are followed by structural glycoproteins (collagen, elastin, fibronectin, immunomodulin, laminin, etc.) and GAG, which form a molecular sieve that must be penetrated (transit route) by the entire metabolic products and eminating from the capillaries including the toxics that are trapped in the matrix going to and from the cell. Actually the body is a series of sieves from the point of noxious stimuli entry to their exit. The size of the filter pores of the molecular sieve is determined by the concentration of PG/GAG and their negative charge and is ever changing. It is dynamic with multiple changes in the pore size occurring during the day depending upon the need for proper filtration.

Local and central reciprocal (feedback) information will influence the size of the filter pores, thus allowing appropriate substances to flow through but often stopping inappropriate substances, depending on whether or not the information is correct for the particular situation of pollutant exposure versus nonexposure. Of course, this molecular sieve will help isolate noxious stimuli so the macrophages can clear them when avoidance therapy is used and autophagia is triggered. Fasting usually clears proteinacious slag from the connective tissue matrix and mesh filtration system.

Fifth: The negative charge of PG/GAG makes them capable of water binding and ion exchange which is extremely important in righting a pollutant exposure and preventing a pollutant injury. Since PG/GAGs are guarantors of isotonic, isosmia, and isotonia, the basic electrostatic tone reacts to every change in the ECM with deviations in the electropotential which if strained can cause fatigue[28] but if normalized produces energy. An example of pollutants entering the ECM and causing disturbance of the ground regulation system is the onset of odor sensitivity in the periodically homeostatically disturbed chemically sensitive patients—which if allowed deterioration, can cause illness and incapacity in certain patients. Here, the dynamics of homeostasis and allostasis are disturbed, allowing for the increase in odor perception and triggers of the fatigue mechanism. Often the odor hypersensitivity is masked and not perceived thus allowing more pollutants to enter the body. This fact of electropotential deviation allows the clinician great latitude in treating the homeostatically and allostatically compromised patient by using techniques of massive avoidance of pollutants, specific antigen neutralization injection, acupuncture, particularly laser acupuncture, neuro therapy and homeopathy as well as nutrients for detoxification of pollutants which usually restores the patient to health.

Sixth: The information encoded in the ECM can inform the cell membrane as a potential of the glycocalyx leading to cell reaction via depolarization of the cellular membrane (e.g., muscle and nerve cells) or via activation of secondary messengers on the membrane (cyclic adenosine monophosphate, inosite triphosphate, and so on, which transmit coded information to cytoplasmic enzymes (Figure 6.8).

This information lands in the cell nucleus where it comes into contact with the epigenetic and genetic material. If the epigenetic material is triggered, the environmental pollutant can then alter the nongenetic and genetic response favorably to the patient to improve health or nonfavorably to yield fatigue with brain or body dysfunction. Information is followed by transcription of the epigenetic mechanism to DNA parts by the various types of RNA. After transfer into the cytoplasm, the various RNA types in the endoplasmic reticulum start translation of the information into protein products individual to the cell (e.g., pollutant exposure results in increased activity of the rough endoplasmic reticulum, increasing the glucuronic conjugation mechanisms and thus allowing for increased pollutant detoxification, and (if the system is overloaded, not allowing significant detoxification to occur).[29] Also, the smooth endoplasmic reticulum produces its products which are usually structural proteins or enzymes, and so on.

Seventh: The mesh-type macromolecular superstructure of PG/GAG also plays an important role in the mechanical coherence of tissue.[30] For example, through this coherence, the terminal axons for the ANS fibers are subject to specific mechanical and electrical tension, which can react with the release of the neurotransmitters and neuropeptides, as well as electrical impulses. As often observed in chemically sensitive patients, excess release or clearing through detoxification or neurotransmitters may cause multiple symptoms. Often symptoms of released neurotransmitters can be neutralized by specific intradermal injection therapies. Noxious stimuli avoidance therapy does help change the electrical tension and helps prevent the release of noxious neurotransmitters and neuropeptides.

Eighth: The highly malleable PG/GAG forms a shock-absorbing system that works like a lubricating substance that changes by a high-energy consuming step to a visco-elastic substance (gel to sol or sol to gel) when severed and repeated mechanical demands occur. The piezoelectric effect occurs, generating electrical charges that are fed into the energy gathering system, thus sending signals locally and distally. These rheological changes also belong to the encoding of information in the ground substance,[29] especially in ordered water. Many chemically sensitive patients and patients with chronic degenerative disease have been observed to exacerbate with exercise,

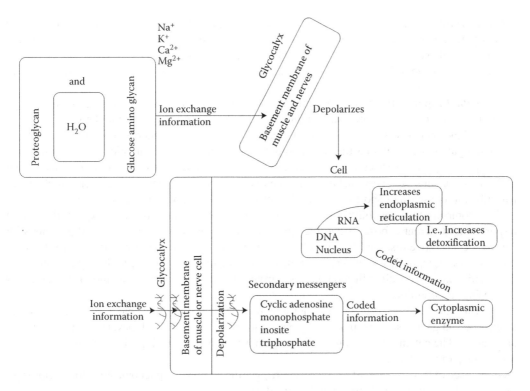

FIGURE 6.8 Therapy in chemically sensitive patients can be varied and more effective, since blockage or damage of individual components enables other subsystems to take over function completely or partially, for long-term or short-term periods, until defective components can be repaired. (Adapted from Rea, W. J. *Chemical Sensitivity*, Vol. 4. Boca Raton, FL: CRC Press.)

massage, or lesser mechanical traumas, presumably as a result of this conversion process. The patients become labile due to chemical or other noxious incitant overload. However, with proper oxygen therapy, alkalinization by bicarbonates (tri-salts of Na^+, Ca^{2+}, and K^+), laser and specific directed acupuncture, provocative intradermal neutralization of incitant, and gentle massage, the chronic fatigue caused by the acidosis can often be overcome and the patient can get back to exercising again.

Ninth: The ECM is connected to the endocrine system by the capillaries and by the CNS via the peripheral autonomic nerve endings. Both systems are connected to the brain, and therefore superior regulatory centers can be influenced by manipulating this ECM. Often, each of these anatomical areas is seen to be involved in some cases of the homeostatic and allostatic disturbances of chemical sensitivity[31] and chronic degenerative disease. Pituitary, hypothalamic, thyroid, adrenal, pancreatic are often involved in pollutant injury causing a series of endocrine malfunctions including fatigue, sleep disorders, insulin swings, or diabetes.

Tenth: Once the pollutant load is decreased, allostasis can become helpful in that occasionally biofeedback or psychological therapy will help correct homeostatic malfunction in those dyshomeostatic and dysallostatic patients who have experienced psychological trauma. Since capillaries, autonomic nerve fibers and connective tissue cells, which wander through connective tissue and regulate the ECM (macrophages, leukocytes, and mast cells) are all mutually informative through released cell products prostaglandins, lymphokines, cytokines, protease inhibitors, etc), this entire anatomical arrangement results in a vast, intermeshed, communication system that has a significant adjustment and performance capacity for the body's homeostasis.[32] Local and/or general dysfunction of any of these substances in this ECM will cause the homeostatic disturbances that exacerbate chemical sensitivity (periodic) or chronic degenerative (aperiodic) disease. Therapy is directed at a homeostatic and allostatic regulation of these substances so that harmonic resonance of information can be restored. Reduction of total body load has often been noted to decrease release of cell products and maintain equilibrium of chemically sensitive patients or patients with chronic degenerative disease.

Eleventh: In spite of the higher specialization of subsystems such as the immune and neurological systems and their associated susceptibility,[33] and the nonimmune enzyme detoxification systems[34] and the endocrine systems,[35] the overabundance of this highly intermeshed biological system (ground regulation system) aids the body in rapid compensation. This anatomical and informational make-up has a great therapeutic advantage in that it can compensate for the failure of individual components or subsystems by enabling other components or subsystems to take over completely or partially, for long-term or short-term periods, until defective components can be repaired.[36,37]

This compensatory capability of the ground regulation system appears to explain the varied responses to different exposures and therapies by chemically sensitive patients and patients with chronic degenerative disease. Because of this phenomenon, avoidance of pollutants will decrease this system's susceptibility to being triggered, and specific injection therapy for biological inhalants, food, and some chemicals will modulate the ground regulation system in a similar manner, thus decreasing susceptibility.

Twelfth: The ECM is a protein and caloric regulator because PGs are able to store carbohydrate as glucose and galactose, protein as NH groups, fat as carbohydrate with oxygen ester (fatty acids) and water.[37] The patient may become obese or gain weight around the hips. Fasting and rotary diets usually help this problem.

Avoidance of food for at least 12 hours will trigger the autophagic phenomenon which helps right physiology by clearing out debris including dead cells.

If the ground regulation system becomes too deregulated, as seen in some advanced chemically sensitive patients and some chronic degenerative diseased individuals, protein malnutrition will occur. Conversely obesity or weakness with dysfunction may also result from ground regulation system deregulation and in other patients.

The need for oral or intravenous hyperalimentation in the malnourished chemically sensitive patient or patient with chronic degenerative disease will be presented later along with various nutrient regimens for those patients with different ratios of sugar to protein to fat. Sometimes low-calorie diets will be needed for the obese chemically sensitive patients and patients with chronic degenerative disease.

Since collagen fibrils need polysaccharides for side-to-side polymerization,[37] protein can be stored in the body in the form of collagen and PG. Therefore, the entire ground substance of the organism has the capacity to be a protein store. This fact emphasizes why it takes a long period of time to restore nutrition completely in malnourished chemically sensitive patients and patients with episodic chronic degenerative disease, and subsequently, to complete function of all systems since each protein, sugar, and fat will need to be replaced. Though a normal ratio of collagen to polysaccharide in stored protein is 5%–95%, pathological states such as chemical sensitivity or chronic degenerative disease can yield different ratios. For example, from 42% collagen to 58% of polysaccharide has been found in some pathological conditions, such as amyloid or protein storage disease.[38] Stored protein in differing quantities and combinations can bind many of the molecules, such as immunoglobulins, lipoprotein, fibrinogen, complement, albumin, amino acids, glycoproteins, and foreign antigen proteins, sialic acid, cholesterol, xenobiotics, and carboxyhemoglobin.[38]

If the stored substances exceed the various individual storage area's capacity for breakdown (usually basement membranes and EC matrix), there is an increased shift of these substances to the transient routes, resulting in inflammatory micro to macro angiopathies. This type of inflammation is seen as are the more advanced homeostatic disturbances in chemical sensitivity (vasculitis) and chronic degenerative disease (i.e., diabetes mellitus).

Heine[38] showed one example of this altered collagen polysaccharide deposition in that carboxy-hemoglobin deposits were found on vessel walls in smokers who eventually developed endarteritis obliterans. Both Heine[38] and Pischinger[39] believe that these deposits of metabolic waste ("slag") can be worked on by protein fasting. Our findings are in agreement with these scientists, and we have utilized this procedure of total fast in over 10,000 patients with chemical sensitivity and chronic degenerative disease. Fasting appears to eliminate the metabolic waste that causes the vasculitis seen in the homeostatic disturbances of patients with chemical sensitivity and chronic degenerative disease.

The reason some chemically sensitive patients repair more slowly than others after fasting is that different individuals have different regeneration capacities.[38] This repair process is dependent not only on the completion of a successful fast (which mobilizes lipophilic xenobiotics from fat stores and lipid membranes) but also nonlipophilics such as heavy metals including mercury (Hg), cadmium (Cd), and lead (Pb) from the matrix trap which will reduce total body pollutant load while restoring homeostasis. Also, this regeneration capacity is dependent on the availability of nutrients, the lipophilicity of chemicals, and the extent of the pollutant damage to the individual. At the EHC-Dallas and Buffalo, we have fasted more than 10,000 chemically sensitive patients and patients with chronic degenerative disease over the last 30 years under various stages of environmental control. It has been one of our most effective tools in relieving vasculitis and autonomic nervous system dysfunction neuropathy and brain dysfunction, gastrointestinal and genitourinary upset; and olfactory, chronic pulmonary diseases and muscular-skeletal dysfunction and other chronic dyshomeostatic maladies that have vessel involvement.

Thirteenth: Fasting and rotary diets aid in improving the homeostatic function of chemically and electrically sensitive patient and patient with chronic degenerative disease, because by a reduction of the constant shedding of vesicular elements from connective tissue cells and defense cells in the ECM[39] are eliminated by autophagy. These vesicles are eliminated by the release of a large number of biologically active substances such as lysosomes.

These substances, then, release local proteolytic and hydrolytic enzymes, cytokines, prostaglandins, thromboxanes, and leukotrienes, which then place a constant strain on the dynamics of homeostasis and repair mechanisms of chemically sensitive patients and patients with chronic degenerative disease. Fasting decreases the number of vesicles and cytokines released, and so on, and relieves the stress in chemically sensitive patient and patient with chronic degenerative disease.

The release of the enormous quantities of tissue hormones from the lysis of leukocytes also occurs in chemical sensitivity and chronic degenerative disease, and these toxic waste elements may alter the pH downward and alter autocrine and paracrine regulation to the regulators of homeostasis and allostasis.[2,39–41] If this breakdown occurs in excess (most chemically sensitive patients and some patients with chronic degenerative disease have low WBC counts and/or low pH after a reaction), then the slowing of this process by fasting and other avoidance techniques with the inherent decrease in xenobiotic load, alkalinization by trisalts, plus better tissue oxygenation by oxygen administration enhances the homeostatic functions of self-healing powers in chemically sensitive patients and patients with chronic degenerative disease. The ground regulation system returns to normal homeostatic function and the chemical sensitivity or chronic degenerative disease decrease is eliminated (Table 6.1).

Recent findings suggest that folic acid deficiency (and a consequent increase in the levels of homocysteine) may increase the risk of Alzheimer's disease and Parkinson's disease, stroke, and psychiatric disorder.[42–44] Folate plays a critical role in one carbon metabolism by facilitating the remethylation by methione from homocysteine.[45] By increasing homocysteine levels and impairing DNA synthesis, methylation and repair of folate deficiency can damage cells including neurons.[43,46] Improved brain function can be found with antioxidants such as vitamin E,[47] *Gingko biloba* extract,[48] and creatine.[49]

While dietary supplements help brain function it has become more evident that underfeeding with caloric restriction and the time interval between feeding are highly significant in brain

TABLE 6.1

Benefits of Fasting, Rotary Diets, and Alkalinization on the Ground Regulation System of Chemically Sensitive Patients

1. Eliminates the vesicular elements in the connective tissue
2. Decreases the release of biologically active substances such as
   a. Proteolytic and hydrolytic enzymes
   b. Cytokines
      i. Prostaglandins
      ii. Thromboxanes
      iii. Leukotrienes
3. Decreases the release of tissue hormones from leukocytolysis
4. Increases pH
5. Alters the autocrine and paracrine regulation to the regulators of homeostasis
6. Decreases xenobiotic overload

Source: Adapted from Environmental Health Center-Dallas, 2002.

longevity and sharpness. The dietary restriction regimes (McAison) used in animal studies involve a reduction in overall calories by 30%–50% and on an increase in intermeal interval (i.e., eating every other day) with maintenance of the composition of the diet in terms of vitamins, minerals, protein, and so on. This type of regime in animals can extend the brain function one third of a life time and longer. Life spans for round worms, rodents, and monkeys can be increased up to 50% by reducing calorie intake.[50–52] Caloric restriction reduces the incidence of age-related cancer, cardiovascular diseases, and immune defects in rodents.[50] We have observed this improvement of gastrointestinal functions and the immune defects in our chemically sensitive patients and patients with chronic degenerative disease. Although biochemical energy production is required to sustain cell viability and functions excessive energy production may cause cells to become damaged and then by being more susceptible to disease.

By adapting to food availability, the individual stores energy by forming glycogen and lipids. When food supplies are scarce the energetic stress induces changes in gene expression that result in changes in cellular metabolism mobilizing the lipids and glycogen to be utilized. When dietary restriction (30%–50% less calories) and every other day fasting is utilized there is a decrease in body temperature, blood pressure, glucose, and insulin levels. In chemically sensitive humans the body temperature decreases just the opposite of normal rate. Dietary restrictions retards age-related increases in the levels of glial fibrillar acidic protein and oxidative damage to proteins and DNA.[53,54] The retardation of many age-related gene expression, are also found with dietary restriction and fasting. These genes involved were those of oxidative-stress responses, innate immunity, and energy metabolism.

Mice maintained a 40% reduction of an added carbohydrate, the diet did not show deficits in learning and memory motor control and avoidance learning.[53]

The rats feeding with alternate day fasting improved glucose transport and mitochondrial function of the brain synaptosomes when challenged with oxidative stress.[55]

Dietary restriction prevented age-related alterations of the levels of serotonin and dopamine in the cerebral cortex of rats.[56] Preservation of neurotransmitters signaling is likely to be critical for the ability of dietary restrictions to maintain the function of the nervous system. We have found that fasting for 1–4 days in chemically sensitive patients and patients with chronic degenerative disease improved their brain functions sharply.

Lee et al.[57–59] reported that periodic fasting in adult rats and mice increases neurogenesis in their brains. These occurred especially among the neural stem cells of the hippocampus, which correlated with improved learning[55] showed that with fasting gluconeogenesis also occurred.

Rats maintained on dietary restriction for 2–4 months exhibited increased resistance to epilepsy and Alzheimer's disease.[60–63] Some studies show an increase in vulnerability of hippocampal and cortical neurons to excitotoxicity and apoptosis by a mechanism involving enhanced release of calcium from the endoplasmic reticulum.[64] Dietary restrictions also protect against oxidative stress. We find that fasting, clean water, and less polluted air also decreased oxidative stress in our chemically sensitive patients and patients with chronic degenerative disease. The vulnerability of nigro-striatal dopaminergic neuron to MPTP toxicity was decreased in mice maintained on dietary restriction. Therefore, more dopaminergic neurons survived exposure and deficients in motor function were markedly decreased.[65]

Fourteenth: Ordered water is the most important element of the ECM because when its quantity is reduced, the brush shape of the PGs folds in and there is an adverse functional effect of the transit routes on the EC matrix, thus hindering total body communication.[66] This adverse effect causes disequilibrium and inappropriate function of the ground regulation system occurs. Clinically, hydration with a less-polluted spring, distilled, or filtered water keeps this aspect of the ground regulation system functioning.

Fifteenth: The degree of leukocyte resistance in chemically and electrically sensitive patients and patients with chronic degenerative disease to environmental factors, such as physical, chemical, and pharmacological stimuli, appears to be much less than the normal individual. Therefore, large degrees of cellular and matrix swelling occur and can be positively influenced by environmental therapy. One great benefit of environmental therapy is the loss of edema seen in treated chemically sensitive patients and patients with chronic degenerative disease, which restores homeostasis and allostasis. Another benefit is the mobilization of toxics by avoidance, heat therapy, and proper nutrition which will strengthen the leukocytes and replenish macrophages.

The data derived from the treatment techniques discussed in this volume show that there are many types of therapy to aid chemically sensitive patients and patients with chronic degenerative disease in recovery of orderly homeostasis. These treatment techniques have a sound natural physiological basis.

Heine[67] emphasizes that the physiological lysis of numbers of leukocytes is more than the number of leukocytes present in the total quantity of blood in a 24-hour period by a factor of about 6 without any numerical change in the figures in the differential blood count. Studies at the EHC-Dallas have shown a similar phenomenon. Heine[67] has shown an increase in lysis of the leukocytes in pathological states such as autonomic dystonia, headache, and allergic phenomena. For example, penicillin sensitivity and most other sensitivity would be a homeostatic regulation disturbance—specifically, an inhibition of homeostatic regulation. Other chemical exposures increase lysis resulting in an increase in sensitivity and deterioration of the body physiology. The breakdown of leukocytes is a nonspecific reaction. The absence of cytolytic capacity has been shown to damage the reticular endothelial system (RES). Stern and Willhelm[68] have shown that loading the (RES) reticular endothelial system with a specific chemical, that is, x-ray dye, causes a loss of lytic function of the serum with damage to the RES. Leukolysis appears to be dependent upon physical chemical factors such as pH, rH, and border surface activity. Since most chemically sensitive patients have low WBC counts, one sees an increase in leukocytolysis with pollutant exposure and reactions that produce a low pH. Stern and Willhelm[68] have demonstrated various stages of intracellular degeneration on his darkfield microscopic studies. These studies emphasize the destruction of damaged cells, and they emphasize the pro-inflammatory effect as well as the tendency toward homeostasis and allostasis. When reducing the total body pollutant load and treating with alkalinization, reactivity decreases, less local tissue reaction occurs and results in pH increases, as the leukocytolysis lessens.

There appears to be an increased sensitivity in the periodic homeostatically and allostatically disturbed chemically sensitive patients which, when xenobiotic exposure occurs, allows for increased leukocytolysis out of proportion with physiological parameters. This increased reactivity, with an increased leukocytolytic pool is an estimate of the reactivity of the ECM, and thus, the ground regulation system[69] and explains the hypersensitivity stage of chemical sensitivity. Thus, if an individual

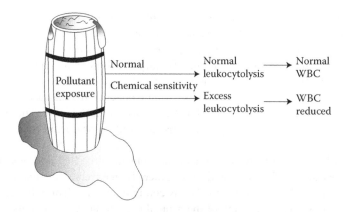

FIGURE 6.9 Leukocytolysis as a guide to successful therapy in chemically sensitive patients. (Adapted from Rea, W. J. *Chemical Sensitivity*, Vol. 4. Boca Raton, FL: CRC Press.)

has increased leukocytolysis with a decrease in WBC, as seen in many chemically sensitive and some chronic degenerative diseased individuals with the same amount of xenobiotic exposure as a nonsensitive individual, this individual would predictably have an extrasensitive ground regulation system which would result in dyshomeostasis and dysallostasis. This condition would telegraph its sensitivity throughout the body resulting in distal homeostatic reaction (e.g., more sensitivity to odors of chemicals, foods, mold, pollen, etc.) followed by dyshomeostatic reactions. Also, when incitants combines with protein kinase 1 and 3 it is then phosphorylated and increases the hypersensitivity by 1000 times.[69] The untreated chemically sensitive patient fits this scenario exactly (Figure 6.9).

The one thing that is not addressed in correcting the physiology of the ground regulation system is the microcirculation and its ability to deliver oxygen to all cells and tissue of the body. (See section on Oxygen Therapy.)

Circadian Clock

Fifteenth, the Circadian Clock on a molecular level, has open-ended systems such as the ground regulation system, are compelled to oscillation and fluctuation due to their instability, which corresponds to their principle of activation and inhibition and their spring effect. Due to their anatomical structure and physiological response including their electrical (sugar), insulation (amino acids) and conduction (water) properties, their rhythms at a molecular level are subject to external rhythms such as day and night or seasonally induced rhythms.

The homeostatic responses in chemically sensitive and episodic chronic degenerative diseased individuals have been observed to be extremely sensitive to these seasonal (winter versus summer) and daily variations[70] (particularly cloud cover versus sunny days) and therefore will have a wider variation of molecular responses.

The circadian clock in mammals is expressed within pacemaker neurons of the suprachiasmatic nucleus (SCN) that in turn maintain proper phase alignment of peripheral tissue clocks present in nearly all cells. Thus, the brain SCN clock provides "standard time" for all peripheral tissue clocks. In experimental models, clock disruption leads to disorders in glucose metabolism, confirming the role for these genes as key regulators of metabolism and supporting the hypothesis originally proposed by McKnight and colleagues that circadian cycles are intimately interconnected with metabolic cycles.[71] Accumulating evidence has revealed that multiple clock genes participate in metabolic homeostasis, suggesting that these proteins have evolved overlapping (or convergent) functions, both as intrinsic "hands" of the clock and as regulators of metabolism. While still at an early stage, emerging studies in humans suggest parallels in the role of circadian genes and metabolic homeostasis. At the epidemiological level, it has been suggested that increased activity during what was 'rest' time in the premodern world, together with sleep disruption, have been associated with increased prevalence of obesity, diabetes, and cardiovascular disease, in addition to certain cancers and inflammatory disorders. This review highlights advances in understanding the molecular coupling between metabolic and clock networks, and its relevance to gene–environment and brain–behavioral systems important in energy balance and metabolic disease.

Features of the circadian clock in all organisms include its persistence under constant conditions, a periodicity that is temperature compensated, and its entrainment to light from the sun. In mammals, cell autonomous circadian clocks are generated by a transcriptional autoregulatory feedback loop composed of the transcriptional activators, CLOCK and BMAL1, and their target genes, *Period* and *Cryptochrome*, which rhythmically accumulate and form a repressor complex that interacts with CLOCK-BMAL1, to inhibit their own transcription.[72] This autoregulatory loop is posttranscriptionally regulated by casein kinases (CK1ε and CK1δ), which target the PER proteins for degradation via the SCF/β-TrCP–ubiquitin ligase complex, and by AMP kinase, which targets the CRY proteins for degradation via the SCF/FBXL3–ubiquitin ligase complex by the 26S proteosome (Figure 6.10).

The prevailing model of the circadian clock involves the transcription–translation feedback loop, but less is known concerning nontranscriptional mechanisms that may generate circadian oscillations. In cyanobacteria, cycles of protein phosphorylation are sufficient to generate biological rhythms in the absence of transcription.[73] In the mammalian SCN, changes in cyclic AMP levels alter period length, an additional example of posttranslational signaling as a mechanism controlling circadian cycles,[74] and recent work has shown that the SCN neuronal coupling network itself

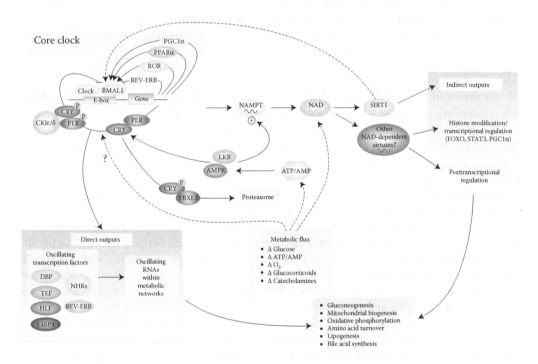

FIGURE 6.10 Direct and indirect outputs of the core clock mechanism. The core clock consists of a series of transcription/translation feedback loops that synchronize diverse metabolic processes through both direct and indirect outputs, including gluconeogenesis and oxidative metabolism. The clock also receives reciprocal input from nutrient signaling pathways (including SIRT1 and AMPK), which function as rheostats to couple circadian cycles to metabolic flux, especially in peripheral tissues. (Adapted from Takahashi, J. S., J. Bass. 2010. *Science* 330 (6009):1349–1354; The American Association for the Advancement of Science. Circadian Integration of Metabolism and Energetics. Reprinted with permission from AAAS.)

has intrinsic oscillatory function that can emerge in the absence of cell autonomous oscillators.[75] RNAi screening of mammalian cells also indicates coupling of the peripheral clock to PI-3 kinase signaling.[76]

Fibroblast cell lines display approximately 24 hours oscillation of core clock genes, demonstrating that the clock is not only expressed in neurons but also in peripheral tissues.[77] Intrinsic oscillation of clocks in liver cells can be entrained by food, whereas oscillation of the brain clock is resilient and entrained primarily by light.[78] A recurring theme in understanding the coupling between circadian and metabolic systems is the recognition that the two systems are reciprocally regulated; food entrains the liver clock, whereas light acts through the brain clock to control feeding time.

Crosstalk between the Clock and Metabolic Transcription Networks Involves

Nuclear hormone receptors and the phase alignment of metabolic gene expression cycles

These findings raise the possibility that disruption of nuclear hormone receptor (NHR) cycles may perturb the clock, and conversely, that delay, advance or reduced amplitude of circadian oscillations may impair NHR function. Knock-in mice of the NHR co-repressor NCor display increased energy expenditure, and a shift in the oscillation in the abundance of RNAs encoding oxidative, glycolytic, and respiratory genes, indicating that disruption of the phase of expression of NHRs contributes to metabolic deregulation.[79] Mistiming of gene expression rhythms as a cause of metabolic deregulation has also been suggested by studies in *Rev-erbα* mutant animals, in which a phase shift in oscillating rhythms of metabolic gene transcription, rather than changes in total abundance of RNA, correspond with altered energy balance.[80] Misalignment between gene transcription cycles within metabolic tissues and the behavioral cycle (of fasting and feeding) may be sufficient to alter energy homeostasis. For instance, high fat feeding provided at the incorrect circadian time leads to greater weight gain in mice than isocaloric feeding at the normal circadian time.[81]

Direct versus Indirect Role of Clock Transcription Factors in Metabolic Gene Regulation

It is possible that disruption within the core clock may be transmitted to metabolic outputs through alterations in NHRs or directly by actions of clock activators or repressors. For example, PER2 directly occupies promoters of certain metabolic genes.[82] Alternatively, the clock activator loop drives D-element-binding-protein expression, providing indirect regulation of gluconeogenic genes.[83] This raises the question as to whether the effects of clock gene disruption relate to direct alterations in "timing" per se, or to indirect effects arising due to independent activity of the clock factors on metabolic networks. The dichotomy between circadian versus noncircadian actions of clock proteins may not be fully valid, since the rhythmic abundance in the expression level of these proteins in turn may produce rhythmic changes in metabolism. For example, CRY, a rhythmically expressed clock repressor, modulates gluconeogenesis through interference with glucagon and inhibition of cyclic AMP signaling.[84] Conceptually, the question of timing versus expression as a cause of metabolic disorders following disruption of clock genes is akin to the difference between a musical performer playing the wrong notes or playing the right notes at the wrong time. One experimental approach to tease apart the role of circadian timing per se in physiology would be to test whether physiological defects could be corrected by alignment of the internal period with the external light cycle (i.e., a test of "resonance"). In plants, various period-length mutants have improved photosynthesis and growth when exposed to external light cycles that matched the endogenous circadian period.[85]

An intriguing question remains the extent to which NHRs modulate circadian systems according to changing environmental conditions, such as humoral or nutritional factors. For example, variation in the concentration of glucocorticoid hormone, retinoic acid, heme, and fatty acids affect GRs, retinoic acid receptor (RAR), REV-ERBα, neuronal Per-Arnt-Sim (PAS) doman protein 2 (NPAS2), and PPARs. Therefore, variation in cellular concentrations of any one of these ligands may influence Bmal1 transcription, and thereby modulate local cellular circadian rhythms. Within the brain, heme and carbon monoxide may modulate NPAS2 activity,[86] whereas within the vascular cells, retinoic acid influences circadian oscillations through activation of RARα and RXRα.[87] Similarly, rhythmic variation in NHR ligands may exert distinct effects on local tissue clock function at different times in the day–night cycle.

Sleep and Forced Circadian Misalignment: Genetic Models and Human Studies

Ties between circadian disruption and metabolic disturbance have garnered attention, including large cross-sectional sampling of populations subjected to shift work. Extensive studies also indicate a correlation between sleep time and body mass index (BMI). Disruption in specific phases of sleep may be connected to metabolic function. Subtle tones sufficient to selectively deprive subjects of slow wave sleep without producing conscious wakefulness were sufficient to impair glucose tolerance.[88] Neuroanatomic studies also indicate interconnections between regions of hypothalamus important in circadian signaling, energetics, and sleep.[89,90] At the molecular level, *orexin* (hypocretin), originally discovered as a neuropeptide produced in the feeding-stimulatory neurons of lateral hypothalamus, is positioned at the intersection of neuronal systems controlling sleep, circadian output, and metabolism.[90] Analysis of orexin receptor 2 knockout mice indicates that lack of orexin signaling increases susceptibility to obesity (rather than the original expectation that orexin, a potent wakefulness-inducing peptide, would induce adiposity).[91] Orexin receptor 2 mutations also account for canine narcolepsy, and orexin deficiency is a hallmark of the disease in humans.[92] Activity of the orexin neuron is modulated by glucose and integrates signals downstream of leptin-responsive neurons within the arcuate nucleus. Leptin also impacts sleep, possibly independently of effects on body weight, raising the need to further define leptin actions in this process.[93] Manipulation of orexin signaling, an integrator of energetic and circadian signals, may, thus, provide opportunities to intervene not only in disorders of sleep but also related metabolic complications.

In humans exposed to a light–dark cycle lengthened to 28 hours, out of synchrony with the endogenous clock, the sleep–wake cycle is driven at 28 hours, whereas the melatonin and body temperature rhythm free-runs with approximately 24-hour period.[94] Such "forced desynchrony," a manipulation that is intended to simulate deleterious effects of jet-lag or shift work, caused impaired glucose tolerance and hypoleptinemia. Whether circadian disruption might also effect endocrine pancreas insulin secretion, hepatic gluconeogenesis, and glucose disposal in skeletal muscle in humans awaits further study; however, these results emphasize the clinical linkages between circadian function and metabolic homeostasis.

Coupling and Outputs: How Do Clocks Sense and Respond to Nutrient Signals?

Under homeostatic conditions, the clock acts as a driver of metabolic physiology (Figure 6.11). However, with perturbations in either circadian or metabolic systems, such as forced behavioral misalignment with shift work, or conversely, high-fat feeding, a vicious cycle ensues in which disruption of metabolic pathways damp and lengthen circadian oscillations.[95] The identity of metabolic sensors that may act as intermediates in coupling circadian cycles with physiologic systems remains to be identified. For instance, do changes in cell nutrient signaling in turn produce changes in circadian clock function? Does metabolic disease lead to altered amplitude or phase of circadian cycles within brain or peripheral organs? Two lines of research have begun to address these questions: first, involving the cellular pathway of adenosine monophosphate concentrations, and second, involving NAD+ metabolism. Using phosphopeptide mapping, Lamia et al. identified a consensus motif for phosphorylation by adenosine monophosphate-activated protein kinase (AMP-K), a sensor of AMP/ATP ratio, within the CRY protein.[96] AMP kinase activator 5-aminoimidazole-4-carboxamide-1-β-D-ribofuranoside (AICAR) promoted degradation of CRY, which was abrogated by mutation of the AMP-K consensus motif. AMP-K knockout mouse embryonic fibroblasts (MEFs) also displayed altered rhythmicity, leading to the proposal that AMP concentration directly couples circadian rhythms to nutrient state in peripheral cells.

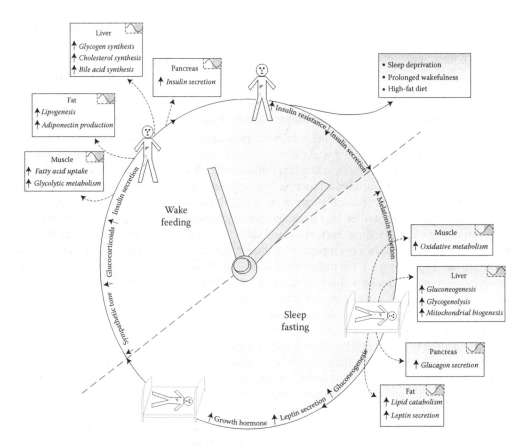

FIGURE 6.11 The clock partitions behavioral and metabolic processes according to time of day. The clock coordinates appropriate metabolic responses within peripheral tissues with the light/dark cycle. For example, the liver clock promotes gluconeogenesis and glycogenolysis during the sleep/fasting period, whereas it promotes glycogen and cholesterol synthesis during the wake/feeding period. Proper functioning of peripheral clocks keeps metabolic processes in synchrony with the environment, which is critical for maintaining health of the organism. Different tissues exhibit distinct clock-controlled properties; thus, ablation of the clock in certain tissues will cause opposing effects on metabolic function as uncovered through dynamic challenges at different times in the cycle under different nutrient conditions. Aging, diet, and environmental disruption such as shift work may also affect integration of circadian and metabolic systems. (Adapted from Takahashi, J. S., J. Bass. 2010. *Science* 330 (6009):1349–1354; From Rabinowitz, J. D. and White, E. 2010. The American Association for the advancement of science. *Autophagy and Metabolism.* 330 (6009):1344–1348. Reprinted with permission from AAAS.)

A second example in metabolic coupling with the core clock originated with the finding that the mammalian ortholog of the yeast sirtuin deacetylases (for silent information regulator), proteins that activate or silence chromatin according to availability of fuel, comprises part of an additional feedback loop with the core clock.[97,98] Sirtuins are present in transcription complexes with the clock, and in turn modulate activity of clock transcription factors. CLOCK-BMAL1 activates the major pathway for mammalian NAD^+ synthesis, involving its regeneration from nicotinamide mediated by nicotinamide phosphoribosyltransferase (NAMPT).[99,100] NAD^+ concentration in cells varies across the light–dark cycle, consistent with a role for NAD^+ as an oscillating metabolite linking metabolic cycles with the clock. Both NAMPT and SIRT1, similar to the NHRs and AMPK, are regulated not only by the clock but also by the nutritional status of the organism. For example, fasting increases NAMPT expression in an AMPK-dependent manner in skeletal muscle, whereas fasting and caloric restriction increase SIRT1 activity across multiple tissues. Thus, regulation of the clock by NAD^+ and SIRT1 allows for fine-tuning and synchronization of the core molecular clock with the environment. Because NAD^+-dependent deacetylases regulate gluconeogenesis and many other pathways,[101] it will be important to further delineate the role of clock in NAD^+-driven metabolism. A second NAD^+-regulated pathway has recently been linked to circadian feeding cycles: PARP-1 activity is circadian in the liver and interacts with the CLOCK protein to poly-ADP-ribosylate it. Since PARP-1 is regulated by NAD^+, this provides yet another pathway for metabolic signals to regulate the core clock pathway.[102] Collectively, these findings identify incoming (AMPK and PARP-1) and outgoing (NAD^+/Sirtuin) sensors that couple nutrient availability, metabolism, and the clock.

In recent past 20 years, the mystery of biological timing has been transformed through genetic discovery. As a consequence, availability of molecular clock genes has now provided tools to understand the physiological functions of the circadian system in unprecedented detail. As we experimentally dismantle the clock, the interdependence of timing and energetics seems inextricable. Major gaps in our understanding include: (i) the connection between brain and peripheral tissue clocks in metabolic homeostasis; (ii) the interplay between circadian and sleep disruption in energetics; (iii) the relationship between nutrient state and circadian homeostasis; and (iv) the impact of circadian clock systems on human physiology. Ultimately, such studies will yield deeper insight into the interconnections between genes, behavior, and metabolic disease.

Many patients are worse in the winter than in the summer. Others are sensitive to the ion and pressure changes of the sunspots (solar storms), and some are sensitive to weather fronts. The most important intracellular pacer is the rhythmic synthesis of ATP by the cell mitochondria[103] bound to the cell membrane. It is the circadian rhythm of "secondary messengers," such as the ANS and the sympathetic associated cyclic adenosine monophosphate,[103] that causes some symptoms in chemically sensitive patients and patients with chronic degenerative disease.[35] In the ECM, the most important pacer is the rhythm of the relationship of sugar biopolymers to the molecule swarms of fluid-crystal water and ions. For example, Heine[103] observed the control of circadian rhythm over urine flow, where illness would increase polyuria at night. This phenomenon in chemically sensitive and chronic degenerative ill patients appears to be one of increased water retention during their 24-hour low spots of circadian rhythm with edema resulting, which often is mobilized as the day goes on. Patients who have avoided pollutants while being treated in the environmentally controlled unit have shown massive mobilization of edema followed by diuresis.

Circadian temperature variations are also important indicators of molecular rhythms in the relationship between the extracellular rhythms in the ECM and the cells. These relationships are accentuated in the homeostatic physiology of chemically sensitive and episodic chronic degenerative diseased individual due to the person's subnormal temperatures. Many circadian rhythms are dependent upon the endocrine system, while many xenoestrogens or estrogen mimics such as DDT, kepone, toxaphene, dieldrin, endosulfans, trazine herbicides, aromatic hydrocarbon, heptachlor epoxide, trans-nonachlor, and methychlor are found in chemically sensitive patients, which potentially disrupt the rhythm.[47] Thus, one can see why the reduction or elimination of these substances by avoidance, nutrition supplementation, and heat depuration therapy would restore circadian rhythms, enabling the ground regulation system to move toward stabilizing the dynamics of homeostasis and restore health in chemically sensitive patients.

Defense Mechanism

Sixteenth, the unloading of the cellular phases of the defense mechanism must also be addressed when one is designing therapy for chemically sensitive patients and patients with episodic chronic degenerative disease. The goal of therapy is to keep the dynamics of the homeostatic regulatory physiology in chemically sensitive patient in phase I and II of the defense reaction so that easy reversibility of the damage following an exposure can be obtained. Most often, chemically or electrically sensitive patient and patient with episodic chronic degenerative disease presents in stage IV, making therapy more difficult.

Initially, when a pollutant or microbe enters the body, there is an abrupt drop in pH from cleavage of acetate, sulfates, and so on by proteases released from macrophages, so that the mononuclear

TABLE 6.2
Therapy in Chemically Sensitive Patient is Directed at the Correction of the Cellular Phases of the Defense Mechanism of Homeostasis

Incitant Enters the Body

a. Acute exposure
1. Decrease in pH, mononuclear histiocytes released from local binding to surround incitant. Release of tissue hormones (leukotriene, interferon, prostaglandin, etc.) occur. Cell membrane changes.
2. Microphage phase: Changes in microcapillary permeability with edema and delivery of immunoglobulin; leukocytes migrate; ATPase is activated by calcium increase and magnesium decrease. Severe local and mild passive generalized reaction occurs.
3. Macrophage phase: Humoral, autonomic, shock phase, monocytosis with macrophage increase and activation of the entire defense mechanism. Monocyte factor is released, giving an increase in monocytes and, macrophages, and in leukocytolysis with a decrease in venous oxygenation, and activation of serum B and G globulin.

b. Chronic exposure
1. Lymphocytic phase: Lymphocytes surrounding vessels and areas of inflammation.

Source: Adapted from Environmental Health Center-Dallas, 2002.

---

histocytes (phase I) are released from local binding (Table 6.2). Once released, these tissue macrophages attempt to wall off the foreign compound or noxious invasion. With the release of tissue hormones (i.e., prostaglandin, leukotrienes, interferon, etc.), noxious substances initiate an abrupt drop in pH and a change in cell membranes, which in turn starts the rapid emergency reaction that is initially biophysical with the slower biochemical properties being than set off as part of the response chain. Treatment with bicarbonates of sodium (Na), potassium (K), and calcium (Ca^{2+}) may often stop or reverse the process, if it is chronic causing the patient to be acutely and chronically ill. Often a tablespoonful is given orally; it may also be given intravenously.

Changes in permeability of the microcapillary wall occur. Not only do these changes in permeability result in the local microphage phase (phase II) with a very localized response but also a more passive generalized response occurs. There is a leak in the vascular wall resulting in edema for dilution of the noxious substance and delivery of immunoglobulin, which can be effective immediately, if the immunoglobulin has a memory for a previous similar noxious exposure.[35,104] These can immediately counteract the incitant giving energy; however, if the incitant is chronic specific, gamma globulins 1, 2, 3, and 4 will often become depleted, resulting in recurrent infection, fatigue, weakness, muscle and joint ache, as well as an increase of chemical sensitivity.

In addition, there is a migration of leukocytes to the noxious area. ATPase is activated by increase in calcium levels and magnesium level decreases since much energy is needed to combat and overcome the invasion. Chemically sensitive patients and patients with episodic chronic degenerative disease often become weak and fatigued at this stage. If pollutant overload is chronic or in excess, this homeostatic process will be hampered, and chronic chemical sensitivity and/or chronic degenerative disease initiates.

Clearly, avoidance techniques and good nutrition will aid in recovery and help the individual to recover normal homeostatic physiology at this stage of injury. All efforts at reduction of exposure should take place to keep chemically sensitive patients and patients with chronic degenerative disease in the first two stages of injury. At the EHC-Dallas, we have observed once that chemically sensitive patients or patients with episodic chronic degenerative disease was treated and functioning in the alarm stage, dealing with noxious stimuli exposure immediately, the individual rapidly resumed the normal dynamics of physiologic homeostatic health without damaging the defense mechanism. Some patients are aided by injection of gamma globulin. Gamma globulin is now one of our routine measurements, especially subsets 1, 2, 3, and 4, which are deficient in about 20% of the severe chemically sensitive patients. Treatments by injection and avoiding pollutants are deemed necessary and appropriate for hypersensitive patients. Nutritional and oxygen therapy, as well as autogenous lymphocytic factor (ALF) also helps. If noxious stimuli continue, the ATPase is weakened followed by homeostatic dysfunction and spreading disease. Chemically or electrically sensitive patients and patients with episodic chronic degenerative disease exhibit more weakness accompanied by somatic symptoms such as headache, myalgia, rhinitis, fatigue, and so on. Although initially low to begin this phase, magnesium elevates as the reaction continues, stopping the production of ATPase. The macrophage phase (phase III) then occurs with humoral autonomic, antishock, monocytic phase with activation of the organism's entire defense mechanisms (change to the humoral antishock phase of Selye[3]). Monocytic factor is needed in this phase which depends upon an increase in calcium and a decrease in magnesium in tissue fluid. The results are an increase in monocytes and thus, macrophages, and decrease in lymphocytes, an increase in leukocytolysis, a decrease in venous oxygenation, and activation of serum B and G globulin. Administration of magnesium and alkali salts and institution of pollutant avoidance often arrest these processes, thus allowing chemically sensitive individual's homeostatic physiology to revert to the alarm stage. The defense mechanism is restored. Finally, if the pollutant load is not eliminated, the defense mechanism deteriorates in response to the chronic pollutant exposure keeping the homeostatic physiology of chemically sensitive patients and patients with chronic degenerative disease in this stage (the lymphocytic phase V). This is the stage of the defense mechanism which is seen in most untreated chemically sensitive and many chronic degenerative diseased (chronically ill) patients presenting for their first consultation.

Seventeenth, loose soft connective tissue, which still corresponds to the embryonic mesenchyme, is distributed all over the body. It is particularly rich in the ECM, and thus particularly reactive to any noxious or disturbing substance. Even the connection between hard substances (i.e., tendons, fascia, and scars) penetrated by soft connective tissue accompanied by vessels and nerves[105] is a clear illustration of the importance of loose connective tissue bearing the ECM. The loose connective tissue's purpose includes maintaining the functional capacity of these hard substances. Closely circumscribed perforations in the superficial body fascia (diameter 3–7 μm) have been shown to be particularly significant, since only at these places is the penetration of vessel–nerve bundles of the dermis invested in loose connective tissue penetrating deeply. These peripheral and spinal nerves and afferent autonomic nerves can become sensitized. According to Heine,[106] these penetration points correlate morphologically with the acupuncture points, which when sensitized can become very fragile causing more hypersensitivity. Even the bone, vessel, and nerve exit points correspond to acupuncture points.[106] Obviously, these acupuncture points can be diseased or distorted, which can also create homeostatic disturbances and in some at certain ages can prevent the ability to hold normalizing physiology. However, in particular, chemically sensitive patients and patients with episodic chronic degenerative disease often has peripheral neuropathy or tender trigger points that are relieved by specific antigen injection therapy, acupuncture, neural therapy, avoidance, and nutritional programs, which will restore information and energy flow.

The dysfunction of the homeostatic physiology of the chemical or electrical sensitivity and episodic chronic degenerative disease is initially based on histochemical and biochemical disturbances of function. The point of initiation of this function or dysfunction appears to be the ground regulation system, followed by amplification by the immune and/or nonimmune enzyme detoxification systems, autonomic and somatic nervous systems, endocrine system, and vascular trees. The function of the ground regulation system can be altered by every functional disturbance of the tissues anywhere in the body since there are multiple feedback mechanisms. These facts allow for many of the aforementioned treatments of the disturbed homeostatic physiology in chemical sensitivity and chronic degenerative disease to be entered at different parts of the body. For example, treatment with cranial fascial manipulation can enter the system at the head and neck, while intradermal injection therapy can enter it via the arms or legs. Testosterone, estrogen, and progesterone administration will often dampen the pollutant triggered responses and allow improvement in the patient with chemical sensitivity or episodic chronic degenerative disease.

The homeostatic regulatory systems and their pathways may be stressed by chemical or any noxious substance overload. Minimal chronic inflammation results if the stimuli are not removed. Due to their lack of specific symptoms—usually muscle and fascial pain and fatigue—that can be related clinically to cause and effect, these minimal inflammations can only be detected with difficulty and scientific precision. These secondary homeostatic foci if not eliminated or minimized will continue to trigger dyshomeostasis, resulting in severe to irreversible fixed-named disease. Here, massage and acupuncture help. At this stage, early symptoms, which appear to be diffused and not related to etiology, may occur. However, if the patient is deadapted by total load reduction, the patient reverts back to Selye's alarm state,[3] where cause/effect can be proven by challenge. We have housed patients in the environmentally controlled unit and deadapted literally thousands of them by reducing their total body load during this stay. Inhaled, oral, or intradermal challenge was then used to reproduce the reaction with the prodrome of inflammation. If the exposure is repeated constantly, the chronic mild inflammation will reoccur.

Since the chronic inflammation of early chemical sensitivity or chronic degenerative disease may be so mild that there may be a clinical subliminal response of the regulatory systems as adaptation manifests. Each maladaptation results in symptoms, but clinically, they are not covertly related to cause. Thus, mild responses often allow the inflammation to go on for years, chronically stimulating the dynamics of the homeostatic mechanism making it more vulnerable to lesser and lesser noxious stimuli until nontoxic stimuli such as food triggers it. However, since the chemical load continues or increases, the regulatory systems (cellular, tissue, humoral, and neural) are under preliminary stress. The result is periodic metabolic deterioration that results in lability of the molecular oscillating and fluctuating processes.[107] The result of this lability is an excessive response to all additional stimuli. However, there may be some areas that are more responsive than others, that is, some patients have extreme sound or light sensitivity and only moderate sensitivity to chemicals. Some chemically sensitive patients may have severe sensitivity to the odor of formaldehyde or phenol, yet have very little sensitivity to light or sound. This molecular metabolic response is classic for chemically sensitive patients who are ambient dose, odor sensitive, and extremely liable to most stimuli.

Eventually, tolerance is lost and supersensitivity to chemical odors manifests. Pollutant reduction through avoidance of toxic substances in air, food, and water and through mobilization and elimination of toxic chemicals by heat depuration/physical therapy will help to quell the inflammation, thereby allowing for a movement toward homeostasis and decreased chemical sensitivity.

We have observed this process in nearly 40,000 chemically or electrically sensitive patients and/or patients with episodic chronic degenerative disease who were studied at the EHC-Dallas and Buffalo. Nutrient supplementation will often give the ground regulation system enough fuel to stop the inflammation and let the ground regulation system heal. Nutrient supplementation can also alter the degenerative metabolism of homeostasis, but this prescription should be looked at like giving antibiotics without cleaning the dirty wound. Therefore, fasting a patient both in the environmentally controlled unit and on an outpatient basis clears the "slag" PG from the cannulicula of the ground regulation system and removes the stimulus prohibiting the return of the homeostasis, thus allowing the nutrient therapy to work better.

Specific antigen injection neutralization also directly interferes with the switch and spreading mechanisms, thus regulating the dynamics of homeostasis and decreasing the lability of the matrix. Autogenous modulators appear to do the same again, allowing nutrient replacement to work.

Primarily, this metabolic and molecular oscillating and fluctuating structural lability concerns the segmental homeostatic regulatory complex to which the xenobiotic stimulating or inhibiting focus is connected.[35] This is the point where avoidance therapy is most efficacious. Eventually, with continued chronic external stimuli (i.e., initially triggered by phenol but then by total chemical overload), there are adverse effects to the metabolism of all organs, which result in homeostatic deregulation and inflammation.[107] Further consequences of chronic pollutant overload are an extension of this homeostatic regulatory change, leading to the appearance of homeostatic regulatory degeneration with both informational and tissue changes. In early homeostatic disturbances observed in chemical sensitivity and chronic disease, one frequently observes segmental reactions involving one region of the body. It is much easier to stop the process with appropriate environmental therapy at the early stage. As the sensitivity increases and spreading occurs, it is more difficult to successfully deliver an appropriate therapy.

The crossing over of the homeostatic regulatory symptoms to the contralateral side of the body shows the secondary involvement of the area/organ, which trumpets the onset of severe homeostatic dysfunction, where local and perhaps regional containment of the incitant is lost. The "sidedness" of chemically sensitive patient is usually observed during the course of illness. Some cases of chemical sensitivity are graphic.[35,108] Almost all chemically sensitive patients have one side of the body that is more affected than the other, usually correlating with an unbalanced ANS.

If this labilized system is affected by a second noxious stimuli (e.g., pesticide) or even a common nontoxic stimuli (e.g., food), this "secondary stress" homeostatic disturbance foci is responded to inadequately and excessively, and a remote homeostatic disturbance is set off by the ground regulation system, whose points of localization are determined by the dyshomeostatic focal point area where the secondary injury occurred. We have repeatedly observed this phenomenon in the disturbed dynamics of homeostatic physiology of the untreated chemically sensitive patients. Eighty percent of chemically sensitive patients have secondary food and biological inhalant sensitivity as the spreading phenomenon has already occurred. If these secondary sensitivities are not treated with reduction of the total load, specific injection therapy, massage, cranial manipulation, sauna, nutrition, and laser therapy, these sensitivities alone will keep the patients ill.

As seen in early normal hormonal homeostasis and chemical sensitivity and described by Heine[2] in his work, a short-lasting stimulus leads to partial depolarization of PG, which is corrected and terminated through charge replacement at once if the system is open and functionally healthy. Chronic minimal duration stimuli (i.e., constant intermittent noxious incitant intake) form localized inflammatory foci, which when observed in the more advanced cases of chemical sensitivity and chronic degenerative disease are the cause of lasting depolarization processes, which eventually lead to structural changes in the entire ground regulation system. At the end of this degeneration process, the transformation of the sol is in the direction of the gel or gel to sol, depending on what is the condition of the normal anatomy and physiology of that particular organ or area. Once the transformation occurs, there is an alteration in the direction of the biological activity of the ordered water field lying in between the molecular filaments. Water alters PG/GAG by losing its polarization, structure, and order and thus its charge. Then, when triggered, it gives misinformation to the system.[107] Trincher[107] has shown that crystalline water decreases with warming, and this process occurs with destabilization.

According to Pischinger[1] and Heine,[2] the cell whose metabolism and biological activity is regulated by the extracellular ground regulation system, is a generator of electromagnetic information.[107] Calculated field strengths and showed that the results from the relationship between speed of sound and membrane thickness is a resonating oscillation in the microwave field (~1 Tera H_2). Popp[109] and Bergsmann[110] showed that the electromagnetic oscillation of coherent light presented an information system in all living organisms, where the transition of oxygen from the stimulated singlet state to the molecular triplet state was recognized as a laser source with a wavelength of 634 nm. This system appears to be highly significant in the field of cell regeneration. Bergsmann[110] showed that cells are capable of releasing resonance and dampen phenomena in low frequencies.

It is clear that the basic physics of chemical sensitivity and episodic chronic degenerative diseases are electromagnetic and that there are some severely affected chemically sensitive patients who have electromagnetic sensitivity.[70] Fifty percent of these patients can be triggered by external electromagnetic waves generated by a frequency generator as we have done at the EHC-Dallas. For example, a 35-year-old white female was exposed to EMF from constantly using a computer and from being exposed with insecticide sprayed in her home and at work. She developed a short-term memory loss, confusion, and brain fog, as well as atrial flutter. She was refractory to medication and entered the ECU. Her signs and symptoms cleared within five days after fasting and with breathing clean air. Once she was stabilized with a rotary diet of organic food and glass bottled spring water, she was challenged in a screened room by using a standard frequency generator with different frequencies and blanks in a double-blind manner. Signs and symptoms were recorded and computerized pupillography was used to measure the ANS changes. Her EMF sensitivity was triggered at frequencies 60–180 Hz and 240 Hz, while 50 Hz, 190 Hz, and 200 Hz did not trigger the sensitivity. None of the blanks triggered autonomic changes.

Apparently, the ground regulation system is entered, triggering diffuse and specific responses that are extremely difficult to deal with therapeutically. However, reduction of the total electromagnetic and chemical load, as well as positive nutrition, acupuncture, specific antigen injection therapy, and simple grounding will reverse some responses of these patients. Some specific laser therapy appears to help with some of these situations in individual cases.

These colloidal (sol to gel and gel to sol) structural changes and then electrical changes have their primary effect on the immediate environment, where the initial chemical or noxious stimulus overload occurs, resulting in electrolability, incoherence of the ground regulation system, followed by the distal dynamics of dyshomeostasis. This overload always affects the whole system, when the overload is of chronic duration, thus altering the dynamics of the homeostatic regulatory quality. Again, it must be emphasized that every denatured homeostatic regulatory process creates preconditions for further worsening of the homeostatic regulatory basis. Thus, worsening of the periodically disturbed chemically sensitive patient and aperiodically disturbed patient with episodic chronic degenerative diseased patient occurs. Therefore, one wants to keep the total body load decreased by safe diet, less polluted food, and less polluted air in the home and work place. Not only the neural processes but also the local tissue and humoral regulatory systems are affected, and the interaction of a variety of regulatory systems is affected in the sense of the macro-organic network.

The spreading of the dysfunction of the ground regulation system takes place to and from feedback with neural and humoral systems.[109] The spreading phenomenon of chemical sensitivity[3,7] correlates well with Heine[106] and Perger's[111] concepts. Spreading of noxious triggers to other organs always signals a worsening of chemically sensitive patient or patient with chronic episodic degenerative disease, making therapy more difficult. Initially, safe exposure limits are set and exceeded to the isolation properties of serous membranes, septa and fascia spreading may occur. Often physical therapy, exercise, osteopathic manipulation, neurotherapy, or laser acupuncture will temporarily arrest the symptoms of chemical sensitivity and chronic degenerative disease.

However, if the total body load is not decreased by avoidance therapy alone, those therapeutic processes will not hold their positive and therapeutic results. It should emphasized, however, that the use of these other modalities in place of load reduction over the short- and long-term often leads to an exacerbation of the deterioration of the homeostatic disturbance in the patient with chemical sensitivity or chronic degenerative with the disease getting worse. According to Bergsmann,[110] these local and regional barriers can be crossed by building up biological connections in the loose areolar connective tissues via lymphatics, arteries, and veins in the sense of biologically closed electric circuits. Therefore, excess load as seen in chemical sensitivity and chronic degenerative disease would allow crossing of the local and regional, barriers stimulating the connections and, thus, spreading of the chemical sensitivity to other organs. Environmental therapy stops the spreading, often reverses, localizes, or regionalizes the response, thus allowing chemically and electrically sensitive patients and patients with episodic chronic degenerative disease to return to the deadapted state, thus improving the defense mechanism. If the overload can be reduced chronically, total repair may occur.

The electrolability and oscillation capacity of the ground regulation system structures also require their sensitivity to electrostatic and electromagnetic environmental influences such as static fields, air electricity charges, and electromagnetic impulse fields (spherics). This lability to electromagnetism is often observed in chemically sensitive patients and patients with chronic disease who does poorly with weather changes, such as is seen in pre-storms and storms,[70] exposure to fluorescent lights, televisions, cell phones, smart meter, WiFi, and other electrical generators.[70] These areas of disturbances are very difficult to counteract since there are few defenses for them. However, fasting and good environmental control, which results in total body pollutant load reduction, appears to be the best defense if the nutrition is corrected.

As described earlier, the Heine¹and Pischinger cylinder is the connective tissue ground system, which is stretched out against the surface of the body in form of cylinders that surround the nerve–vessel bundles piercing the superficial fascia in a membrane-like structure. This cylinder has little conductivity but is capable of oscillation and is an organ of perception for electromagnetic and magnetic dimensions. Therefore, the resulting intrinsic organic homeostatic regulatory processes can be altered effectively by a variety of completely different techniques, such as reduction of total body pollutant load, heat depuration/physical therapy, massages, electromagnetic field administration, needle pricks with acupuncture, specific antigen intradermal neutralization, local anesthesia, laser beams, grounding, and even removal of affected organs and synthetic parts. Thus, the dynamics of homeostasis are restored in chemically sensitive patients or patients with chronic degenerative disease and economy of function once again occurs, resulting in a healthy individual. This economy of function appears to be the last function to be healed after the defense mechanism is stabilized. The successfully treated chemically sensitive patients or patients with chronic degenerative disease has excellent resistance to infections and chronic disease because he has learned to keep his total body load decreased and, hence, stays in the alarm stage at all times. Since he usually uses slight symptom onset (i.e., slight brain fog or dullness or muscle aches) as an early warning, he always stays in the Selye deadapted alarm stage, immediately acting to eliminate and neutralize the noxious stimuli. If the energy decreases, he immediately fasts, gets better air and nutrition, and then is restored to full energy and health. He lives a medication-free, creative life.

Each modality of treatment will be discussed in detail. These include avoidance therapy in air, food, water, EMF, chemicals, specific injection therapy for biological inhalant, food, chemicals, bacteria, virus, nutritional supplementation and replacement, tolerance modulators, surgery acupuncture, neural therapy, and the combination of the two using laser acupuncture, homeopathy, cranial sacral manipulation, osteopathic manipulation, energy balancing, and physical therapy.

AVOIDANCE THERAPY: DETAILS OF HOW TO ELIMINATE SPECIFIC INCITANTS

Avoidance of pollutants and potential noxious stimuli in air, food, and water is the most important therapy for patients with chemical and electrical sensitivity or chronic degenerative disease. This type of therapy reduces, both, the total body pollutant and other noxious stimuli load, thus allowing the body to return to normal dynamic homeostatic function. If one follows and uses the principle and facts gathered in the environmental control unit the lowering of this total body load can take from one to seven days in the mild-to-moderately sensitive patient, and up to several months or even years in a few severe chronically ill patients with an aperiodic or chronic periodic homeostatic disturbance (Table 6.3).

TABLE 6.3

Treatment of Pollutants by Avoidance Decreasing Total Body Pollutant Load

1. Water contaminants	7. Pollens, dust, other particulates
2. Food and food pollutants and pollutants sensitivity	8. Neuro transmitters
3. Chemicals—Toxicity and sensitivity	9. Air pollution—outside, indoors
4. Molds and mycotoxins—pollutants and sensitivity	10. Virus
5. Terpenes	11. Bacteria
6. Algae	

Source: Adapted from Environmental Health Center-Dallas and Buffalo, 2016.

While studying pollutants and eliminating them under environmentally controlled unit conditions, one will usually be able to restore the dynamics of homeostasis. These pollutants, such as natural gas, insecticides, chemical solvents, formaldehyde, mycotoxins, particulates, and EMF, should be reduced indoors so that the total pollutant load is at least five times of that of a regular building.

OUTDOOR AIR POLLUTION

Outdoor air pollution is somewhat variable, depending upon the air and water emitters. Each city and country area has its own pollutants. However, depending on size and location some have more pollutants than the others. Large cities have car and truck pollutants as the big generators. Some are in narrow valleys or at the bottom of canyons. Others have giant generators such as oil refineries or electrical generating plants. Some have pesticide factories, others have metal generator factors, computer and metal, plants, and so on. Rural area in farm lands are exposed to pesticides, herbicides, and fertilizers; other natural sulfur generating areas like volcanoes; pine and cedar terpenes, forests, and others; mold and mycotoxin; algae areas; and methane gas leaks from the earth.

Although some air pollutants are ingested or absorbed through the skin, they usually enter the body by way of inhalation or directly from the nose to the brain. All routes are particularly hazardous for chemically sensitive patients and patients with chronic degenerative disease. The volume of air that passes through the lungs is considerable at 4.3 L/minute, which translates into approximately 2.7 metric tons for 2260 m^3/year. When an individual inhales an air contaminant at the rate of 1 mg/m^3 in one year, he/she has inhaled about 2.3 g of pollutants. The seriousness of this situation becomes readily apparent when the numerous pollutants available for inhalation are acknowledged. This seriousness is especially true for particulate matter 2.5 μm or less in diameter, which has been shown to cross the alveolar-vascular membrane causing damage to the local and distal cardiovascular tree. In addition, many gases, such as carbon monoxide, ozone, nitrous oxides, sulfur dioxides, and methane gas, can cause inflammation resulting in chronic vascular and neural inflammation. These pollutants are stored in the body at varying rates and lengths of time, depending on many factors including the quantity and quality of immune and enzyme detoxification available, the status of the nutrient pool, as well as the type of toxins involved. Chemically sensitive patients and patients with chronic degenerative disease appear to experience greater absorption, slower detoxification, and more inappropriate handling of inhaled environmental toxic chemicals than is seen in the normal population. However, the total and specific environmental pollutant load can also damage the normal population when occurring over a long period of time.

Outdoor air pollution has long been thought to enhance, or at times even cause disease processes. The history of awareness of the environmental aspects of this dates back to Hippocrates, who mentions it in his work "Air, Waters and Places."

Prior to the fourteenth century, outdoor air pollution as we know it today was virtually unknown, with the possible exception of that produced by volcanoes, pine forests (29% of the total natural pollutants), forest fires, swamps emitting methane gas (70% of total natural pollutants), high mold areas, some sulfur spring areas, sunspot influences, sandstorms, and positive ion winds. From these sources, the pollutants of nature such as methane, terpenes, and sulfur compounds emanate.

Manmade pollution became severe around the time of the industrial revolution. This pollution increased gradually as industrialization spread over the earth (Figure 6.12 and Table 6.2). As European forests were decimated and the burning of soft coal introduced, manmade pollution evolved on a greater scale.

Increased industrialization and mechanization on the earth, circa 1850, brought a dramatic increase in manmade pollution. Generally, the levels of both inorganic and organic pollutants increased. Evidence suggests that while chemical sensitivity and chronic degenerative disease has existed for at least 2000 years. The incidence has increased since the industrial revolution and has

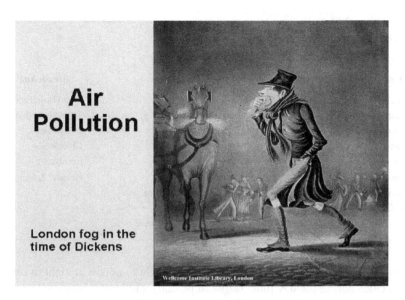

FIGURE 6.12   London fog in the time of Dickens.

since increased in the last 30 years. Today, large amounts and kinds of pollutants occur all over the United States (Table 6.4) apparently causing chemical sensitivity and chronic degenerative disease.

Air pollution is also a global problem, as we have learned from many incidents (Table 6.5). The nuclear explosion at Chernobyl in Russia in 1986 and Fukashima in Japan, for example, showed that each part of the earth is at the mercy of the other. Radioactive material from those explosions fell around the circumference of the earth. Other instances of global deposition of pollutants have been observed. Pesticide used to spray for grasshopper epidemics in West Africa for instance, ended up in Florida 5 days after spraying.

Ozone occurs from the photolysis of nitrogen oxides and when hydrocarbons, aldehydes, and other gases are converted by photochemical processes to peroxy radicals. Anthropogenetically derived ozone may peak as high as 0.60 ppm, with an average of hourly concentrations of 0.20– 0.30 ppm. This phenomenon is commonly seen in Southern California and 0.05–1.5 ppm is found in eastern urban areas. The average concentration of ozone in the atmosphere is 0.27 ppm. Background concentrations in cities are 0.5–1 ppb with levels reaching 1–2 ppm at peak hours. Ozone concentrations in the rural areas east of the Mississippi River range from 0.03 to 0.10 ppm. Ozone background

---

TABLE 6.4

Pollutants Occurring All Over the United States

Particulates

Ozone (O_3)

Carbon monoxide (CO)

Sulfur oxides (SO_2 and SO_3), hydrogen sulfide (H_2S), and acid gases (HF, HCl)

Nitrogen oxides (NO_2 and others)

Lead (Pb) and other metals

Volatile organics (VOCs), solvents, pesticides, and methane (CH_4)

Bioaersols: molds, bacteria, pollen, and others

Radiation

Standards for air pollutant concentrations

WiFi, smart meters

TABLE 6.5
Some Air Pollutants

Outdoor Air	Indoor Air	Breath Analysis
Perchloroethylene	Crotenaldehyde	Methyl ethyl acetylene
Trichloroethylene	Benzaldehyde	Tetrachloroethylene
D-Limonene	Formaldehyde	D-Limonene
1-Ethyl-4-methylbenzene	Camphor	Glycidor
α-Pinene	Hexaldehyde	Eucalyptor
Benzaldehyde	Linalool	Hexane, 2, 3-dimethyl
Formaldehyde	1-Ethyl-4-methylbenzene	
Hexaldehyde	4-Methyl heptanes	
	2,2,5-Trimethyl pentane	

in these areas is less than 0.03 ppm. Urban ozone is thought to persist at night in rural areas but it dissipates in cities during the day time. Ozone apparently can be transported long distances, as is evidenced by these elevated levels in rural areas east of the Mississippi. The concentration of ozone is cumulative; therefore, most of the safety standards (0.12 ppm at peak hour) are inadequate for protecting optimal human health (Figure 6.13). Concentrations of ozone in major cities, such as Chicago (0.2 ppm), Los Angeles (0.36 ppm), Washington, D.C. (0.17 ppm), and Dallas-Fort Worth (0.12 ppm) (Figures 6.14 and 6.15), have constantly exceeded this stand (Figure 6.16).

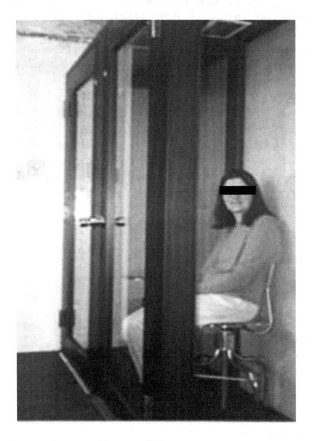

FIGURE 6.13 Booth in an environmentally controlled room.

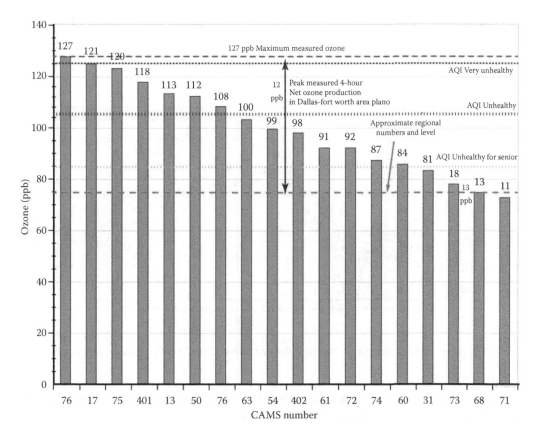

FIGURE 6.14   Dallas-fort worth daily maximum ozone running 8-hour average by site for August 9, 2002. (Adapted from www.tnrcc.state.Tx.US/updated/air/monops/airpollevents/2002/020809dfw-c.gif.)

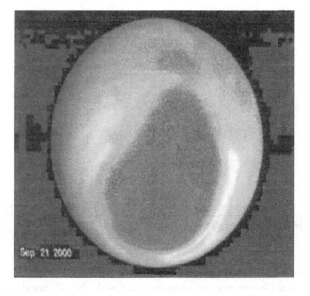

FIGURE 6.15   The hole in the earth's ozone layer as seen from space NASA. (Adapted from http://www.gsfg. nasa.gov/topstory/20020103greenhouse.html.)

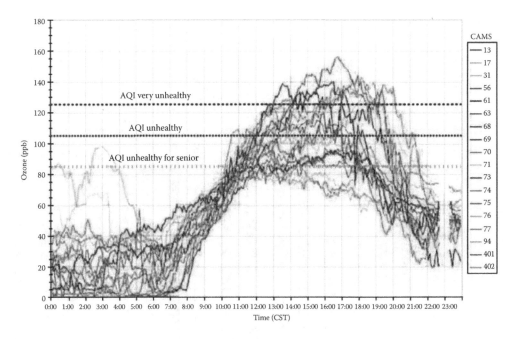

FIGURE 6.16 Dallas-fort worth high noncompliant ozone levels from 18 EPA monitoring sites on September 8, 2002.

Chemically sensitive patient reacts adversely to high ozone exposure, which may create increased free radicals and, thus, stress the antipollutant enzymes.

Lead

Lead is a significant component of outdoor air pollution. It results mainly from leaded fuel emitted from motor vehicles and battery factories. Lead levels from the beginning of time are shown in Figure 6.17.

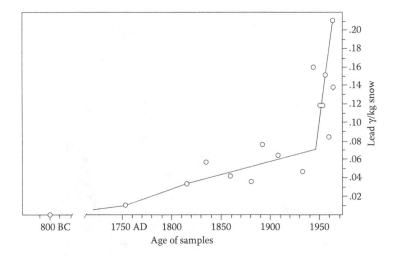

FIGURE 6.17 Industrial lead pollution at Camp Century, Greenland since 800 BC μg/kg (micrograms per kilogram). (Reprinted from *Geochimica et Cosmochimica. Col.* 33(10). Chemical concentrations of pollutant lead aerosols, terrestrial dusts and sea salts in Greenland and Antartica snow strata. Copyright 1969. With permission from Elsevier.)

The Romans were the first to build lead smelters, and in doing so, they became the first to contaminate the earth with lead. The industrial revolution of the eighteenth century then spurred the onset of large-scale lead contamination. Finally, the mechanization of the earth in the 1950s brought about the grossest increase in air, food, and water pollution. This increase in lead over time, probably, has contributed to increased chemical sensitivity and chronic degenerative disease.

Outdoor air pollution plays a critical role in human health and especially that of the chemically sensitive and chronic degenerative disease patients. Moderate levels of outdoor air pollutants, such as $PM_{2.5}$ or PM_{10}, CO, O_3, NO_2, and SO_2, have been linked to significantly higher rates of asthma,[112-114] heart attacks,[115,116] stroke,[117,118] and many other health problems. In many of these studies, adverse health effects are seen even though air pollutant levels are well below US EPA standards. In addition, a large percentage of indoor air pollutants come from the outdoors.[119,120] Outdoor pollutants affect our patients with chemical sensitivity and chronic degenerative diseases.[121]

The outdoor air pollutants analyzed were: particulates (<2.5 μm, $PM_{2.5}$), ozone (O_3: 1 hour averages), carbon monoxide (CO), Sulfur oxide (SO_2), and nitrogen oxides (NO and NO_2). Patients were monitored and results were recorded for change in symptoms and signs.

First, the monthly variations of the pollutants were studied by taking the maximum readings for every day and calculating their average value for the whole month. Figures 6.3 through 6.6 show the monthly variations of the above pollutants combined for the 4 years studies.

$PM_{2.5}$ showed a significant maximum in July and a minimum around December (Figure 6.1), indicating a definite yearly periodicity.

In conclusion, $PM_{2.5}$, O_3, CO, and NO show strong yearly periodicity, whereas SO_2 and NO_2 have weaker indication for a year periodicity.

A comparison of the annual average of the above six pollutants during the 4 year measurements show no significant improvements, only some fluctuations (Figure 6.7). Again, more research and data are needed to understand these fluctuations. Patient responses were also recorded. Winter months (from the second week of December to the first week of March) had longer stays and treatment periods from 1 week to 10 days. People generally were worse at these times (Figure 6.8—length of stay) (p. 2248, Table, 31.27, CS, Vol. 4).

A number of previous studies have examined relationships between the months of the year and levels of pollutants such as $PM_{2.5}$, CO, O_3, and SO_2. Many studies have found that $PM_{2.5}$ levels are higher in the winter months.[122,123] Some studies (in Los Angeles and California, United States; Seoul, South Korea; Athens, Greece; and New Delhi, India) have found that CO is highest in winter months,[124-127] although other studies (in Milan, Italy and New Jersey) have found higher levels in summer months.[128,129] The higher levels of $PM_{2.5}$ and CO seen in winter months may be related to the higher rates of burning fossil and biomass fuels in the colder winter months; however, in the southern part of the United States, particulate count of <2.5 μm is recorded from May through September due to the influx of African dust in the environment. Our patients' health is always worse on high particulate days, probably, because they have vasculitis throughout the year. Apparently, since both seasons (winter and summer) are high for pollutants, it suggests why patients have so much more trouble. For patients, the winter is when cold air is denser. This would cause a jamming of air pollutants into a smaller area causing more concentrated points of respirable substances.

Ozone is invariably higher in the warmer weather summer months.[125,126,130] Most ozone is produced by complex reactions with hydrocarbons, nitrogen oxides, and sunlight; these reactions are more efficient in warmer weather. The higher levels of ozone, due to prolonged and hotter sunshine as well as more cars being on the road, give acute reactions to our patients.

Sulfur dioxide has been reported to be higher in the winter.[125,127,130] Since we do not have levels that exceed EPA standards, we do not see adverse patient response from sulfur dioxide. Nitrogen dioxide has also been reported to be somewhat higher in the winter as compared to summer.[125-127,130] This may be due to coal or gas-fired apparatus for heating or some other unknown mechanism. We are not sure why these substances of CO, nitrous oxides, and sulfur dioxides are higher in the winter, but they certainly can cause changes in the health of the hypersensitive patient and those with chronic degenerative disease.

One salient point that we have noticed in our patients is that if the total load of the environmental pollutants (particularly nitrous oxides, sulfur dioxides, carbon monoxides, and ozone) are combined and high levels persist, the patients have more adverse health effects; therefore, no specific pollutant of the aforementioned would have to be extremely high in order to have adverse health effects. They all could be a little high and have the affect of increasing the total body load, thus rendering it vulnerable to dysfunction. Another finding that has become obvious during the course of over 30 years of unit study is that the severely chemically sensitive patient has a much slower clearing response in the winter months of December, January, and February. Even though the pollutant loads are the same in the ECU as in the summer, these inpatients are slow to clear as are the outpatients. These months always yield longer stays (28 vs. 17 days for summer) in the ECU. Patients have many more unexplained chronic symptoms with slower clearing at this time than at other times during the year. The etiology of this slow clearing of symptoms is at present uncertain, but probably it has something to do with how the sun hits the earth in the Northern Hemisphere in the winter versus the summer, the length of time the Sun is out (more pollution tends to occur in the winter because the nights are longer), and perhaps different electrical phenomena. The density of the air increases during these months and is thought to account for many of the problems. Winter days, at times, may be clearer, but then the high pressure presses pollutants to the earth's surface.

Wind seemed to be another factor in dispersing of pollutants and causing or relieving health effects. If the wind was below 5 miles an hour, pollutants seemed to back up and the patients got worse. If the wind was above 5 miles an hour, pollutants tended to disperse and patients improved their symptoms.[130] In conclusion, pollutant levels though varied over the four years had a similar pattern and overall were elevated but not increasing. Adverse effects of high outdoor air pollution were observed in patients with chemical sensitivity and chronic degenerative disease and were found in all seasons. The more prolonged chronic effects occurred in the winter months, but more acute affects were observed on high ozone and particulate days during the summer months.[130]

Air: Less Polluted Indoor

The essentials for creating a less polluted home environment are determined by whether one builds a new home or refurbishes an old one. Each will be discussed separately.

The purpose of the environmentally controlled unit is to maximize the control of outdoor and indoor pollutants. In doing so, the environmentally controlled unit has an ultimate goal to create an oasis for patients with chemical sensitivity (periodic homeostatic disturbance) and with chronic degenerative disease (aperiodic homeostatic disturbance) in order to restore and maintain normal homeostasis throughout a lifetime.

Of course, location of the home under ideal circumstances would be away from all noxious stimuli generators, including cities with a population of over 50,000 rural farm area, where there are insecticides, herbicides, and areas where there is a lot of electromagnetic generation. These areas would include seashores, ranch areas, and areas where there are national parks, and so on. The least polluted area as shown in Volume III is in the Big Bend National Park in Texas followed by park areas in Arkansas, New Mexico, Northeastern Arizona, Wyoming, Montana, Idaho, Extreme Northern California, and Oregon. Some areas in South Padre Island in Texas toward the southern end are still less polluted as are the outer banks of North Carolina.

Most of the time the ideal home location is not possible; therefore, the creation of an environmentally controlled unit type environment for the home and, if possible, in the workplace is extremely important and essential in order to obtain and maintain normal homeostatic function. Less polluted homes are temporary until the population is diminished and the WiFi is controlled.

New Home

The construction of a new home will cost a little more than a converted home; however, the mainte-nance will be less. If the patient is electrically sensitive the house is extensively shielded.

Ideally, if the patient is not electrically sensitive and the house is well grounded, steel studs (usu-ally a problem for the EMF sensitive patient) can be used. If the patient is EMF sensitive then no smart meter or WiFi or no metal can be used and the house will have to be built with all wood and/or stone.

Brick, cement block (some are toxic so care must be taken in selection), and stone can be used as an alternative to steel or aluminum studs. Concrete is very efficient. It appears to be better than steel and sheetrock. However, caution should be used unless there is give to grounding or it can be hazardous (Figures 6.18 and 6.19).

Pine studs can be used if sealed with foil (Figure 6.20). Metal lathe can be used on the exterior with stucco, brick, or hard wood. However, caution in the use of any metal must be used for the electromagnetically sensitive patient. A minimum use of metal is desired to be used in house con-structed for these patients because of the possibility of electric and magnetic attraction for entrances and earth forces.

Magnesium oxide blown in foam can be used for insulation (Figure 6.21).

Metal lathe will then be used for the inside walls followed by nontoxic plaster. Glazed ceramic tile and nontoxic grout can be used for the walls and floors (Figure 6.22).

Safe substitutes for the walls, ceiling, and floors can be hard wood (Figure 6.23), glass (Figure 6.24), ceramic tile (Figure 6.25), stone (Figure 6.26), Adobe brick (Figure 6.27), or porcelain (Figure 6.28).

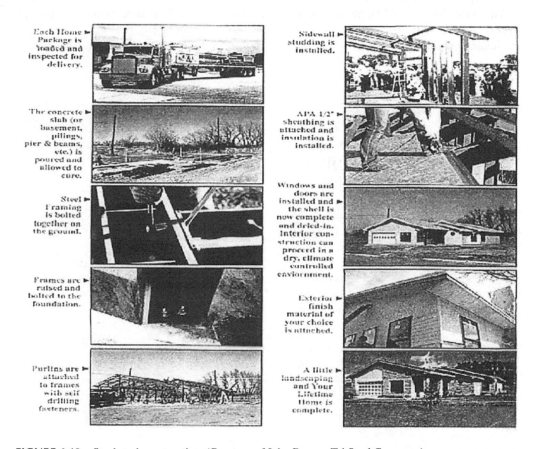

FIGURE 6.18   Steel stud construction. (Courtesy of John Brown, Tri Steel Company.)

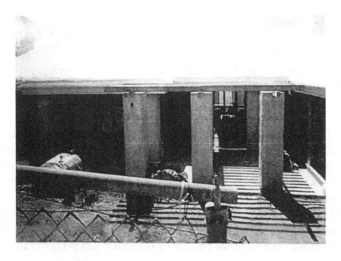

FIGURE 6.19 Concrete beam and studs.

Hardwood or aluminum windows can be used. No carpets are recommended. Pitched roofs of tile, sheet metal, or aluminum shingles can be used.

Heating and cooling by hot water are best illustrated in Figure 6.24.[131] The sources for heating the water should be outside and may then be electric, gas, oil, coal, or wood. If inside, only electric heat pumps should be used.

Air return ducts should be galvanized with multiple filters of aluminum, charcoal, paper, and glass beads (Figure 6.29).[131]

Plumbing should be of copper or porcelain pipes.

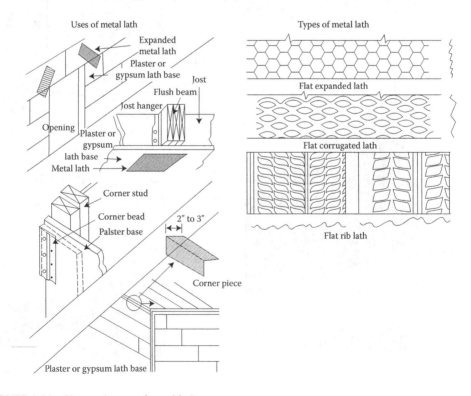

FIGURE 6.20 Uses and types of metal lathes.

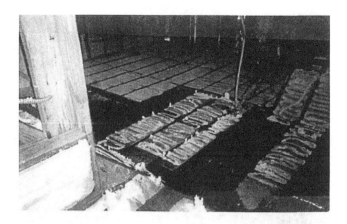

FIGURE 6.21   Insulation: magnesium oxide.

Sealants for areas that may leak should be pure silicone and used outside, not inside, the home.[132,131,131]

Old Houses

One must be careful when renovating old houses because some unknown contaminants may be present like old termite proofing with DDT (half-life—50 years) or chlorodane (half-life—20 years)

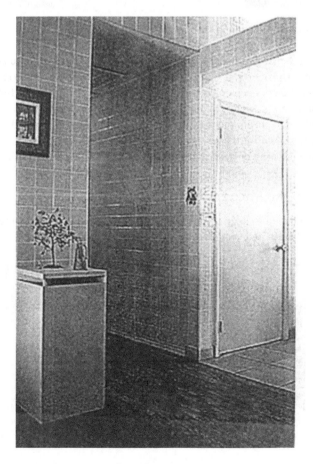

FIGURE 6.22   Glazed ceramic tile on walls and floor.

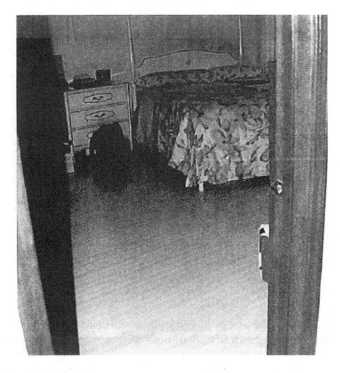

FIGURE 6.23 Painted hardwood floor.

compounds. If an old house has had a lot of internal insecticide use or these substances have been tested and found on the property, it will be very dangerous to one's health to renovate. In addition, house interiors that have not been contaminated with creosote, heating oils, fungicides, lead paints, and particularly molds are difficult to find.

Once these details have been attended to and evaluated, one can proceed with renovation using the materials already shown for the new house construction (Figure 6.30). Local air handling units should also be used consisting of steel housing, metal, charcoal, paper (accordion, no glue) and glass.

AVOIDANCE OF MOLD AND MYCOTOXINS: REMEDIES

Dehumidifier(s) are needed to keep the relative humidity (ambient air moisture) between 30°—and 50° Rh during remediation and sometimes after remediation.

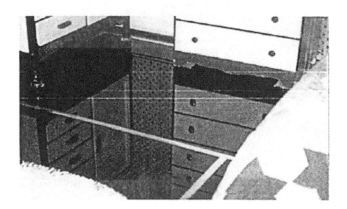

FIGURE 6.24 Glass floor.

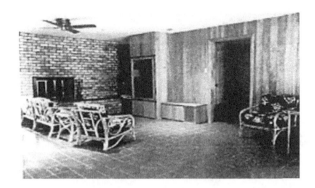

FIGURE 6.25   Ceramic floor, brick and hardwood walls.

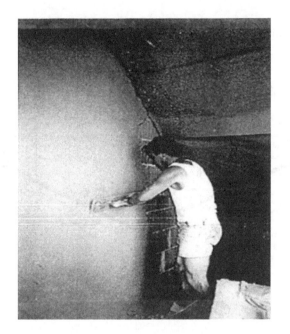

FIGURE 6.26   Plaster on stone wall.

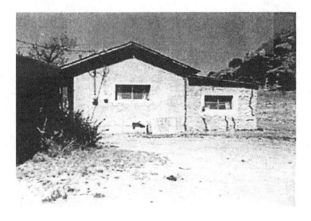

FIGURE 6.27   Adobe walls—adobe home.

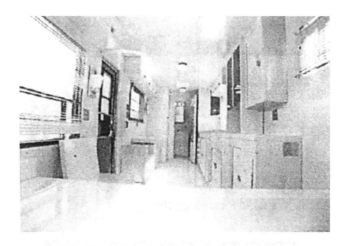

FIGURE 6.28 Trailer with porcelain ceiling, walls and floors.

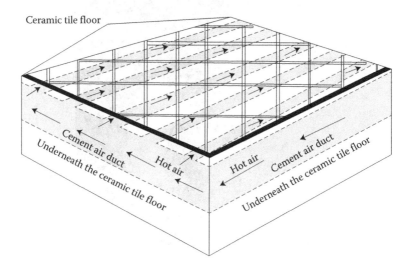

FIGURE 6.29 Heating from cement air duct beneath ceramic tile flooring.

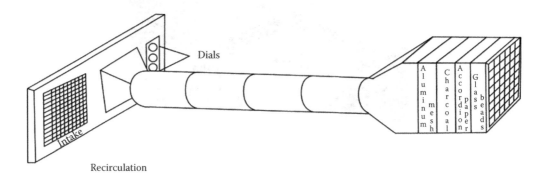

FIGURE 6.30 Filtration through air conditioning.

Before effective remediation can begin, the cause of the water intrusion or damage must be repaired or corrected. Cracks or breaches in the foundation walls, leaks in the roof, leaky windows, plumbing leaks or drips, or heavy condensation from unwrapped piping. Any source of excess moisture or dampness needs to be corrected.

Deconstruction

The next critical step in effective mold remediation is the removal of all nonsalvageable wet or contaminated building materials—and all means all. All materials must be removed, even those inside tight spaces and crevices. This includes damaged wallboards, paneling, decorative wood boards, wallpaper, and fiberboards. Insulation in ceilings, walls or floors, must also be removed. Nonsalvageable carpeting, floor boards, vinyl flooring, hardwood flooring, sub-flooring, and so on must be removed too, and these must preferably be double-bagged and then discarded. No contaminated materials must remain. Any remaining mold can grow back inside the ceiling, wall, or floor cavities after reconstruction. Often padded furniture such as couches, love seats padded chairs, box springs, mattresses, and so on, must also be discarded. Books and other paper items often transport mold spores and mold toxins and may need to be discarded as well. Remember, it is critical that all work be done with negative air pressure.

Containment

Heavy duty plastic sheeting, usually at least 6 millimeters thick, must be installed over entries or openings in walls or ceilings, separating work areas from nonaffected areas prior to beginning work. Remember, no one should be inside the containment area except those performing the remediation, and the flaps should be kept taut at all times.

After removal of contaminated materials, the next stage is cleaning exposed framing and surfaces. First, there is the rough or initial cleaning. Second, the detailed surface cleaning and sanitizing. Rough or initial cleaning may involve media blasting, such as baking soda or dry ice blasting, which removes viable mold. With smaller jobs, wire brushing or power brushing and light sanding may be used instead of media blasting. After the initial removal of heavy visible mold, all of exposed remaining surfaces must be thoroughly wet-wiped, sanitized, and Hepa-vacuumed. That is everything must be meticulously wet-wiped (not dry-wiped) and Hepa-vacuumed: furniture, contents such as books, knick knacks, walls, ceiling, windows and floors; utilities, plumbing pipes— everything! And they must be cleaned (wet-wiped) to as near dust-free as possible. Clothes have to be wet or damp with a cleaning agent or biocide—a product that can kill mold. Washing of materials must be done at least six times.

Chemicals

There is a plethora of chemical agents that can be used. Many of these products, while quite effective, can be mild to very caustic and require extensive ventilation (supplied air). Bleach is not recommended but many people use it. There are a number of noncaustic and nonallergenic products on the market, such as commercial grade hydrogen peroxide (37%) vinegar, and enzyme-based cleaners, which are effective and safer for occupants and technicians, releasing little or no VOCs (volatile organic compounds).

After treating surfaces with a biocide, a good soap or cleaner is needed to remove heavy debris and staining. This can range from a household soap to a commercial low-VOC degreaser.

Encapsulation

Encapsulation is the sealing of cleaned or treated surfaces with a kind of paint—a primer of sorts— often with antimicrobial properties that help to protect the substrate such as porous material like wood from subsequent fungal growth. Encapsulation may not be needed after media blasting, since it thoroughly cleans the wood and removes the roots (fungus mycelia). But encapsulation is most definitely needed if the surfaces were cleaned by hand or by other chemicals, since these methods are not as thorough as cleaning with a blasting media.

Ammonia

A final wipe should include an ammonia solution (3%–20% ammonia) to neutralize the mold trichothecenes. Although a single agent cannot neutralize all mold toxins, ammonia has been proven to be the most effective single agent against the mycotoxins produced by mold. Trichothecenes are very toxic (poisonous to humans and other animals) and difficult to destroy. So, spraying, fogging, or wet-wiping with ammonia in the middle or final cleaning stages is important to abate this very harmful chemical. Ammonia is also an effective biocide (mold killer); however, some contractors prefer to use it only at the final stages of the cleaning process because of its pungent nature.

Ozone

Ozone (O_3) is a natural occurring gas. However, there are generators that can produce ozone. Ozone is great for destroying bacteria, viruses, VOCs, MVOCs, odors, and molds. In short, it purifies the air. Ozonation at the very end of the remediation process is a very good idea. Ozonation should be performed by a contractor experienced in ozone generation to assure no one is in the home when the ozone is applied, and that ozone levels have returned to a safe level before anyone re-enters the home.

Post-Remediation Testing and Assessment

Post-remediation air and surface sampling, along with a visual inspection, are highly recommended to insure the remediation was successful. Measurement for high humidity, mold spores, and residual mold toxins should be made. This post clean up assessment is usually performed by a hygienist or mold inspector—preferably by a different person than the one performing the remediation. We like mold plates because the spore counts are erratic. Any plate that grows less than five of mold colonies means the room is decontaminated. Many buildings are still contaminated after mycotoxins clean up and cannot be lived in by the mold-sensitive patient.

To insure that mold contamination is remediated appropriately, do not take it lightly. Follow the professional protocols, and you could prevent years of suffering and spending thousands of dollars on ineffective remediations and medical treatment.

EVALUATION OF FIVE ANTIFUNGAL AGENTS USED IN REMEDIATION PRACTICES AGAINST SIX COMMON INDOOR FUNGAL SPECIES

Chakravarty and Kovar[133] investigated the effect of five antifungal agents (Sanimaster, hydrogen peroxide, isopropyl alcohol, bleach, and Sporicidin) used in fungal remediation practices on the growth and spore germination of six commonly occurring indoor fungal species (*Alternaria alternata, Aspergillus niger, Chaetomium globosum, Cladosporium herbarum, Penicillium chrysogenum,* and *Stachybotrys chartarum*). These antifungal agents significantly inhibited the growth and spore germination within 12 hours of treatment. When the antifungal agents were washed off with distilled water, no significant differences were observed in spore germination after 24 hours of incubation period. Two weeks after treatment, in vitro fungal growth was not inhibited compared with nontreated control. In the treated wood blocks, colony forming units of these fungi were viable after 2 weeks of treatment.

Recently, fungi (both mold and yeast) have become one of the leading causes of indoor air quality (IAQ) complaints.[134–141] Fungi become a problem within a built environment, where excessive humidity or moisture is present for an extended period of time.[135–149] The problem can originate from sudden water releases, such as a ruptured pipe or large spill that goes untreated, or from a chronic condition, such as a leaking roof or plumbing failure. Even high humidity or warm, moist air condensing on cool surfaces can cause fungal problems. Studies have shown that fungal occurrence in indoor environments was high during fall and summer seasons.[150] Environmental factors such as high temperature and relative humidity are among the factors contributing to the high occurrence of indoor fungi.

Fungi can grow almost anywhere in a building if conditions are favorable (moisture, temperature, and substrate) for their growth and activities.[151–153] If there is visible fungal growth on painted wall surfaces, it is possible that fungi may also be growing inside the wall cavity. The environment inside the walls of a structure often differs drastically from the outside and could create perfect conditions for fungal growth. If the wall remains wet for a prolonged period, fungal growth on the back side of gypsum board will likely be worse than that on the front. A noninvasive but limited approach for observing fungal growth within the interstitial space (e.g., wall or ceiling cavity) can be performed using a borescope. Air sampling for the presence of fungal spores within the interstitial space can be performed using an inner wall sampling adapter with sampling cassett connected to an IAQ sampling pump.

Fungal contamination in the indoor environment is a complex issue and can cause health hazards for the inhabitants. All fungi are potentially harmful when they are allowed to grow in the indoor environment. Fungal spores, whether dormant, viable, or nonviable, can be harmful when inhaled. Fungal contamination of the indoor environment has been linked to health problems, including headache, allergy, asthma, irritant effects, respiratory problems, mycoses (fungal diseases), and several other nonspecific health problems.[154] The longer fungi are allowed to grow indoors, the greater the chances are that fungal spores may become airborne and cause adverse health effects. If indoor fungal contamination is not effectively remediated, fungal problems can spread to other nonaffected areas and can cause health problems to the occupants. Inhalation of fungal spores is implicated as a contributing factor for organic dust toxic syndrome and noninfectious fungal indoor environmental syndrome.[155] In addition, concentrations of mycotoxins found in buildings have damaged cells of the central nervous system.[156–158]

The objective of Chakravarty and Kovar's[133] study was to evaluate the efficacy of five antifungal agents commonly used in remediation practices to eradicate and prevent future fungal growth.

ANTIFUNGAL AGENTS AND FUNGAL SPECIES

Antifungal agents used in Chakravarty and Kovar[133] study are Sanimaster (contains 5%–120% quaternary ammonium chloride compounds, 1%–5% ethanol, 1%–5% nonionic surfactant, and 1%–5% chelating agent); hydrogen peroxide (17%); isopropyl alcohol (70%); bleach (contains 6.15% sodium hypochlorite and <1% sodium hydroxide); and Sporicidin (contains total phenol 1.93% and glutaraldehyde 1.12%)

Six commonly occurring fungal species found in the indoor environment[140,159–161] were used in this study. These were *A. alternata* (Fr.) Keissl., *A. niger* van Tieghem, *C. globosum* Kunze ex Steus., *C. herbarum* (Pers.) Link ex Gray, *P. chrysogenum* Thom, and *S. chartarum* (Ehrenb. Ex Link) Hughes.

PREPARATION OF SPORE SUSPENSIONS

Spore suspensions were prepared by addition of 9 mL of peptone physiological salt solution (8.5 g of NaCl L^{-1} with 1 g of bacteriological peptone (oxoid) L^{-1}, supplemented with 0.1% Tween 80) to the culture. Suspensions were prepared from 25 tubes and filtered through a 17-μm pore-size nylon filter, reaching a final volume of 180 mL. Subsequently, the suspensions were centrifuged (4000g) for 3 minutes. Spores were resuspended in 2 mL of malt extract broth medium (CM57; Oxoid) and the suspension was adjusted to pH 4.0 with lactic acid. The spore suspensions were adjusted to densities of 10^8, 10^7, 10^6, and 10^5 spores mL^{-1}, and cells were counted in a hemocytometer.

EFFECT OF FIVE ANTIFUNGAL AGENTS ON SPORE GERMINATION

A. alternata, A. niger, C. globosum, and *C. herbarum* were grown on 2% malt extract agar (MEA) at 25°C in the dark for 1 week, whereas *S. chartarum* was grown on cellulose agar (CA) for 2 weeks.

The spore suspension was prepared by transferring from the fungal culture with a transfer loop into 9 mL sterile distilled water, and the concentration of the suspension was adjusted to approximately 10^5 spores/mL.

To test the effect of five antifungal agents (Sanimaster, 17% hydrogen peroxide, 70% isopropyl alcohol, bleach, and Sporicidin) on the spore germination of six fungi 10 uL of spore suspension was mixed with 10 μL of filter sterilized antifungal agents mentioned above. Slides with spores were kept moist by placing them on glass rods on the moistened filter paper in Petri dishes and sealed with parafilm. Spore germination was recorded after 12-hour incubation at 25°C in the dark and 100 spores were counted in each of four replicates.

Sensitivity of spores to five antifungal agents were prepared by Chakravarty and Kovar.[133] Nongerminated spores exposed to antifungal agents were washed with sterile distilled water and transferred to freshly prepared plates of water agar without antifungal agents. These were incubated as described above and the percentage of spore germination was recorded after 24 hours.

EFFECT OF ANTIFUNGAL AGENTS ON RADIAL GROWTH OF FUNGI

For this experiment, Chakravarty and Kovar[133] used 90-mm plastic Petri plates containing MEA (for *A. alternata*, *A. niger*, *C. globosum*, and *C. herbarum* and CA for *S. chartarum*) media and five antifungal agents described above were used. One milliliter of the filter sterilized antifungal agents was added separately to the Petri plates. There were five replicates for each antifungal agent. Following treatments resulted:

Sanimaster + *A. alternata*, hydrogen peroxide + *A. alternata*, 70% isopropyl alcohol + *A. alternata*, bleach + *A. alternata*, and sporicidin + *A. alternata*

Sanimaster + *A. niger*, hydrogen peroxide + *A. niger*, 70% isopropyl alcohol + *A. niger*, bleach + *A. niger*, and sporicidin + *A. niger*.

Sanimaster + *C. globosum*, hydrogen peroxide + *C. globosum*, 70% isopropyl alcohol + *C. globosum*, bleach + *C. globosum*, and sporicidin + *C. globosum*.

Sanimaster + *C. herbarum*, hydrogen peroxide + *C. herbarum*, 70% isopropyl alcohol + *C. herbarum*, bleach + *C. herbarum*, and sporicidin + *C. herbarum*.

Sanimaster + *S. chartarum*, hydrogen peroxide + *S. chartarum*, 70% isopropyl alcohol + *S. chartarum*, bleach + *S. chartarum*, and sporicidin + *S. chartarum*.

Control plates contained the above-mentioned fungal species and sterile distilled water was added instead of antifungal compounds.

The plates were incubated at 25°C in the dark for 2 weeks. The diameters of the colonies on the bottom layer were measured using a ruler.

IN VITRO TREATMENT OF ANTIFUNGAL AGENTS ON INOCULATED WOODS

Small blocks (16 × 8 cm) of pine wood free from decay and stain were cut from 2 × 4 pine wood boards (commercially purchased). All the blocks were autoclaved for 2 hours at 121°C. When cooled, blocks were separately inoculated with 5 mL spore suspension (10^5 spores/mL) of *A. alternata*, *A. niger*, *C. glovosum*, *C. herbarum*, *P. chrysogenum*, and *S. chartarum*. The control blocks received 5 mL of sterile distilled water. There were three replicates for each fungal treatment. The blocks were then placed in a plastic zippered bag, kept moist, and incubated at 25°C for 8 weeks. The blocks were examined periodically to observe the fungal growth. After 8 weeks, when the considerable fungal growth was observed, the wood blocks were separately treated with five antifungal agents Sanimaster, 17% hydrogen peroxide, 70% isopropyl alcohol, bleach, and Sporicidin. After 1 hour, the fungal growth was removed from the blocks. The blocks were allowed to air dry. For hydrogen peroxide, wood blocks were treated twice (6-hour intervals) and fungal colonies were removed by brushing (as recommended by the remediation company).

EFFECT OF ANTIFUNGAL TREATMENT ON FUNGAL GROWTH ON REMEDIATED WOOD BLOCKS

When fungal growth was cleaned with antifungal agents and growth was removed (as recommended by remediation companies), wood blocks were allowed to dry in ambient air for 5 weeks. After the blocks had dried, swab samples were taken from both treated and nontreated wood blocks. Swab samples were then aseptically inserted into culture tubes containing 10 mL of sterile distilled water. Culture tubes were vortexed for 10 seconds and 1 mL of the solution was poured into MEA medium for *A. alternata, A. niger, C. globosum,* and *C. herbarum* and CA medium for *S. chartrum* in the Petri plates for individual antifungal agent and fungal species. The plates were incubated at 25°C for 1 week with *A. niger* and *P. chrysogenum* (fast-growing fungi), and with *A. alternata, C. herbarum, C. globosum,* and *S. chartarum* (slow-growing fungi) for 2 weeks in the dark. Colony forming units (CFU) of each fungal species were recorded when fungal growth was observed. All the experiments were repeated three times. Data presented were means from one of the experiments, with three experiments showing similar results.

Data were subjected to analysis of variance.[162] The individual means were compared using the Scheffe's test for multiple comparisons using SAS software, version 9.0.[163]

Means followed by the same letters (a, b, c, etc.) in bars (in the graphs) for a particular fungal species against antifungal agents are not significantly ($P = 0.05$) different from each other by Scheffe's test for multiple comparison.

RESULTS

Effect of Five Antifungal Agents on Spore Germination

The spore germination of *A. alternata, A. niger, C. globosum, C. herbarum, P. chrysogenum, and S. chartarum* was significantly inhibited when treated with Sanimaster, hydrogen peroxide, isopropyl alcohol, bleach, and Sporicidin after 12 hours of treatment.

Sensitivity of Five Antifungal Agents on Spore Germination

These antifungal agents significantly inhibited the growth and spore germination within 24 hours of treatment. However, when the antifungal agents were washed off with distilled water, no significant differences were observed in spore germination after 24 hours of incubation period.

Effect of Five Antifungal Agents on Radial Growth

No significant differences in radial growth of the fungi were recorded between treated with antifungal agents and nontreated control plates after 2 weeks of incubation period.

Effect of Five Antifungal Agents on Colony Forming Units

Fungal growth was observed when swab samples were taken both from the treated and nontreated control wood blocks 5 weeks after treatment with antifungal agents.

DISCUSSION

Their results show that fungal growth including spore germination and CFUs were significantly inhibited one week after treatment. However, when treated spores were washed with distilled water and antifungal compounds were removed, these fungi recovered from the initial shock and spores became viable. All the antifungal compounds' treatments showed similar results. The toxic effects of these chemicals were reduced and most of these fungi become viable after a period of time. On the antifungal-treated wood blocks and after removing the fungal growth, small amounts of fungal inoculums were present and they remained in a dormant stage. When swab samples were taken from these treated wood blocks and inoculated onto suitable nutrient media, fungi came out of dormancy and became viable as indicated by their CFU onto the media.

Their results show that all the tested fungi showed effect of fungistasis or mycostasis, a phenomenon linked to exogenous dormancy where fungal growth is inhibited without any effect on viability[164–166] This inhibition is due to inhibitory effect of antifungal compounds when applied on the fungal contaminated surfaces. The inhibitory effect is reversible once the inhibitory substances are removed or become diluted; spores again become viable and mycelia can resume growth. Most of the fungicides are effective only on hard nonporous surfaces. Viable spores hiding in porous surfaces may be unaffected and can go dormant when fungicides are applied. The peak and valley terrain of porous substrates provide with viscid antimicrobial agents.

Correcting fungal contaminants requires understanding the extent of the problem and the underlying causes. In many cases this is quite simple, for example, when an obvious moisture source has affected only a small area, resulting in observable visible fungal growth. However, this can be difficult when the source(s) of moisture, their interaction with building conditions, or the location(s) of the growth are not readily apparent. When a complex fungal problem exists, it is wise to carefully assess the problem thoroughly and objectively before the beginning of remediation. To achieve a durable and effective solution, it is also imperative to understand the reason(s) for the moisture problem(s). Once pathways of moisture are known, then it becomes easy to locate hidden fungal growth. Knowing the source of the excess moisture is vital to correct it and prevent recurrence of the problem.

The success of remediating a large-scale fungal problem ultimately depends on how well the moisture and contamination problem is understood. If planning the remediation relies heavily on reports from past investigations, the accuracy and completeness of those efforts should be objectively assessed. It is essential to review the findings in the reports and evaluate how completely the important issues were assessed.

It is very important that fungal growth be physically removed and contained to prevent cross contamination of the living space. Attempts to kill or inactivate fungal growth and spores with products such as fungicides, heat, or fogging does not eliminate spores. The remediated area should be properly cleaned and dried. Even a small number of dormant fungal spores can grow vigorously when conditions become favorable for their growth and activities. Inhaling large number of dead or dormant fungal spores can be harmful and cause health hazards to building occupants. Also, the chemicals used to treat or limit fungal growth can be very harmful. If biocides are used, they must be registered with the state government pesticide control board and must be in accordance with state or federal government laws by a licensed pesticide applicator or licensed remediation companies.

Their findings indicate that the commonly used fungicides in the indoor environment cannot completely kill all the fungal inocula. Most of the fungi form dormant spores when exposed with fungicides. These dormant spores can germinate and resume growth when a favorable environment is available to them. The results provide further evidence that physical removal of indoor fungal contaminated material is necessary as a proper remediation practice when dealing with indoor air quality problems. Their study strengthens the evidence that effect of fungistasis or mycostasis, a phenomenon linked to exogenous dormancy where fungal growth is inhibited without any effect on viability.

AVOIDANCE OF FOOD AND CONTAMINANTS

NUTRITION

Avoidance of food pollutants, foods to which the patient is sensitive, caloric food reduce sickness and increased fasting are all foods which the clinician has in order to reduce total body pollutant load. It has been shown in our studies as well as animal studies that dietary dead or dying cellular elements and particular fasting is neuro protective. Fasting allows for more energy and sharpened brain function for improved normal activity. Fasting even 12 hours triggers autophagia, which will clean out cellular debris.

Although all cells in the body require energy to survive and function properly, excessive calorie intake over long time periods can compromise cell function and promote disorders such as cardiovascular disease, type-2 diabetes, cancers, chemical sensitivity, and chronic degenerative disease. Accordingly, dietary restriction (either caloric restriction or intermittent fasting, with maintained vitamin and mineral intake) can extend lifespan and can increase disease resistance.

Recent studies have shown that dietary restrictions can have profound effects on brain function and vulnerability to injury and disease (Table 6.6).

Dietary restriction can protect neurons against degeneration in animal models of Alzheimer's, Parkinson's, and Huntington's diseases and stroke. Moreover, dietary restriction can stimulate the production of new neurons from stem cells (neurogenesis) and can enhance synaptic plasticity, which may increase the ability of the brain to resist aging and restore function following injury (Table 6.7).

Interestingly, increasing the time interval between meals can have beneficial effects on the brain and overall health of mice that are independent of cumulative calorie intake. The beneficial effects of

TABLE 6.6
Effects of Dietary Restriction on the Nervous System

Effect	References
Mouse	
Enhanced learning in aged animals	Ingram et al.[167]
Enhanced motor function in aged animals	Ingram et al.[167]
Slows age-related loss of spiral ganglion neurons	Park et al.[168]
Reduces oxidative stress in brain cells of aged animals	Dubey et al.[53]
Protects against MPTP-induced damage to dopaminergic neurons and preserves motor function	Duan and Mattson[65]
Counteracts adverse effects of an Alzheimer's mutation in presenilin-1	Zhu et al.[169]
No benefit in Cu/Zn-SOD mutant ALS mice	Pedersen et al.[170]
Induces BDNF production and enhances neurogenesis	Lee et al.[171,172]
Suppresses injury-induced microglial activation	Lee et al.[173]
Rat	
Enhanced spatial learning in aged animals	Stewart et al.[174]
Attenuates age-related loss of cortical dendritic spines	Moroi-Fetters et al.[175]
Enhances dopamine overflow in striatum	Diao et al.[176]
Attenuates age-related increases in GFAP levels	Major et al.[54]
Attenuates age-related decrease in cardiac synaptic terminal norepinephrine uptake	Snyder et al.[177]
Protects against seizure-induced hippocampal damage and memory impairment	Bruce-Keller et al.[60]
Protects striatal neurons against mitochondrial toxins	Bruce-Keller et al.[60]
Protects against focal ischemic brain injury and improves functional outcome in a stroke model	Yu and Mattson[178]
Protects synapses against oxidative and metabolic stress	Guo and Mattson[179]
Protects thalamic neurons against thiamine deficiency	Calingasan and Gibson[180]
Prevents age-related deficit in hippocampal LTP	Eckles-Smith et al.[181]
Enhances hippocampal neurogenesis	Lee et al.[57]

Source: Mattson, M. P., Duan, W., Guo, Z. Meal size and frequency affect neuronal plasticity and vulnerability to disease: Cellular and molecular mechanisms. *Journal of Neurochemistry.* 417–431. Copyright Wiley-VCH Verlag GmbH & Co. KGaA. Reproduced with permission.

TABLE 6.7

Examples of the Effects of Dietary Restriction on Changes in Gene Expression in the Brain during Aging

Gene	Change During Aging	
	Usual Diet	**Dietary Restriction**
	Energy-Related	
Cytochrome oxidase	Decreased expression	Little or no change in expression
Glucose-6-phosphatase	Decreased expression	No change in expression
Fructose-1,6-bisphosphatase	Increased expression	No change in expression
Creatine kinase	Increased expression	Increased expression
	Stress-Related	
HSP-70	No change or decrease	No change or increase
GRP-78	No change or decrease	No change or increase
Gadd153	Increased expression	Increased expression
Proteasome z subunit	Decreased expression	Decreased expression
	Inflammation-Related	
GFAP	Increased expression	Little or no change in expression
Complement C1q	Increased expression	Little or no change in expression
Complement C4	Increased expression	Small increase in expression
	Plasticity-Related	
NMDA receptor NR1	Decreased expression	Little or no change in expression
BDNF	Decreased expression	Little or no change in expression
TrkB	Decreased expression	Not determined

Source: Mattson, M. P., Duan, W., Guo, Z. Meal size and frequency affect neuronal plasticity and vulnerability to disease: Cellular and molecular mechanisms. *Journal of Neurochemistry.* 417–431. Copyright Wiley-VCH Verlag GmbH & Co. KGaA. Reproduced with permission.

Note: Taken from data in, or cited in, Lee et al.[59,173] and Duan and Mattson.[65] In the study of Prolla and colleagues,[172] analyses were carried out on brain tissue samples from 24-month-old mice that had been maintained throughout their adult life on a diet with a 30% reduction in calories. In the studies of Mattson and colleagues,[65,173] analyses were carried out on brain tissue samples from young adult mice that had maintained on an every-other-day fasting regimen for 3 months.

dietary restriction, particularly those of intermittent fasting, appear to be the result of a cellular stress response that stimulates the production of proteins that enhance neuronal plasticity and resistance to oxidative and metabolic insults; they include neurotrophic factors such as brain-derived neurotrophic factor (BDNF), protein chaperones such as heat-shock proteins, and mitochondrial uncoupling proteins. Some beneficial effects of dietary restrictions can be achieved by administering hormones that *suppress* appetite (leptin and ciliary neurotrophic factor) or by supplementing the diet with 2-deoxy-D-glucose, which may act as a calorie restriction mimetic. However, fasting is preferred. The profound influences of the quantity and timing of food intake on neuronal function and vulnerability to disease have revealed novel molecular and cellular mechanisms, whereby diet affects the nervous system, and are leading to novel preventative and therapeutic approaches for neurodegenerative disorders.

Meal size and frequency affect neuronal plasticity and vulnerability to disease: cellular and molecular mechanism.[182] A 4–7 days diet appears adequate for the average chemically sensitive patient. The more severe the illness and inability to eat food with a reaction, the longer the rotation is needed. This is probably because the patient is following the law of nerve injury in the gastrointestinal and nasal tracts.

Autophagy

Humans are capable of eating parts of themselves in order to survive. This involves the degradation of cellular components, either because they are deleterious (e.g., damaged organelles and microbial invaders) or because the resulting breakdown products are needed to support metabolism. Fasting and autophogy has gained attention recently as essential contributors to human health and disease.

There are several forms of autophagy, each of which involves delivering intracellular cargo to lysosomes for degradation. The predominant form, macroautophagy (autophagy hereafter), produces vesicles (autophagosomes) that capture and deliver cytoplasmic material to lysosomes.[183] The autophagy-related genes (the *atg* genes) are conserved from yeast to mammals and regulate the cannibalism of intracellular cytoplasm, proteins, and organelles.

Autophagy is the only mechanism to degrade large structures such as organelles and protein aggregates. In the absence of stress, basal autophagy serves a housekeeping function. It provides a routine "garbage disposal" service to cells, eliminating damaged components that could otherwise become toxic. Such cellular refreshing is particularly important in quiescent and terminally differentiated cells, where damaged components are not diluted by cell replication. In starvation, autophagy provides a nutrient source, promoting survival. Autophagy is induced by a broad range of other stressors and can degrade protein aggregates, oxidized lipids, damaged organelles, and even intracellular pathogens. Although it is not always possible to resolve the metabolic and garbage disposal roles for autophagy, it is clear that autophagy prevents disease. Defects in autophagy are linked to liver disease, neurogeneration, Crohn's disease, aging, cancer, and metabolic syndrome.[184] It is estimated that autophagy eliminates 50–70 million dying or dead cells per day.

Overall Energetic Impact of Autophagy

To maintain homeostasis, tissue degradation by autophagy must be balanced by new macromolecule synthesis, which is energetically expensive. Each peptide bond in protein costs four high-energy phosphate bonds, two for tRNA charging and two for ribosome peptide bond formation. Assuming a free energy of ATP hydrolysis of -50 kJ/mol under physiological conditions, synthesizing 1 g of protein consumes 1.8 kJ of energy. For a typical human, this means that rebuilding 10% of the body's protein content would consume at least 2000 kJ, or 20% of daily dietary energy intake. In vitro estimates of autophagic rates have generally been at or above the 10% per day level, for example, 1% per hour for cultured hepatocytes.[185] Accordingly, although in vivo rates of autophagy are presumably lower, rebuilding the structures degraded by autophagy may be a major contributor to mammalian caloric requirements. Consistent with this possibility, knockout of p62, which brings cargo to autophagosomes, results in decreased calorie burning and eventually obesity.[186] During aging, both autophagy and total caloric expenditures decrease in tandem.[187] The possibility of a causative link, in which decreased autophagy leads to reduced energy burned for self-regeneration, is intriguing. Decreased autophagy in obesity may also contribute to the difficulty of losing weight.[188]

A subset of our obese chemically sensitive seen at the EHC-Dallas do have a problem of losing weight when fasting. These patients seem to need a strict rotary diet avoiding the foods to which they are sensitive. Thin chemically sensitive patients have just the opposite in that they have to conserve energy to survive.

Autophagy and Disease

Cellular garbage disposal by autophagy prevents the buildup of damaged proteins and organelles that cause chronic tissue damage and disease.

Most chemically sensitive patients thrive on fasting, which triggers the autophagic mechanism. Many of our patients will fast from one to four days a month in order to maintain their energy and health. Genetic inactivation of autophagy in mice revealed that the type of disease depends on the tissue type. In the brain, autophagy suppresses the accumulation of ubiquitinated proteins, disposes of aggregation-prone proteins and damaged organelles that cause Huntington's, chemical and Parkinson's diseases, and prevents neurodegeneration.[189,190] Most of the stable chemically sensitive patients maintain their health by using brain function as an indicator of overload or wellness. When the brain is dull, they do not eat until the sharpness returns; this may require 1–3 weeks or even 1–2 days.

In the liver, autophagy suppresses protein aggregate and lipid accumulation, oxidative stress, chronic cell death, inflammation, and cancer.[191,192] In intestinal Paneth cells, fasting preserves cellular function, prevents expression of damage and inflammatory markers, and prevents the development of Crohn's disease.[193]

Although the cell-refreshing role of autophagy functions in preventing the above diseases, autophagy's metabolic role may also contribute by ensuring consistent availability of internal nutrients and enabling cells to survive periods of poor external nutrition in good health. Some chemically sensitive patients are intolerant of most foods during this time autophagy can save their life, once the hypersensitivity for foods has been overcome. Regardless of the underlying mechanism, autophagy stimulation is under consideration for disease prevention. In support of this concept, autophagy mediates the protective effects of dietary restriction on aging-related diseases in model systems,[194] and autophagy suppression contributes to the deleterious consequences of obesity.[188] Induction of autophagy may result in the fasting rituals common in many religions as well as modern cleansing rituals, producing health benefits.

In contrast to normal cells in tissues, tumors often reside in an environment deprived of nutrients, growth factors, and oxygen as a result of insufficient or abnormal vascularization. Thus, the effects of autophagy in cancer are paradoxical: Although autophagy can prevent initiation of some cancers, it also may support tumor growth. Autophagy localizes to hypoxic tumor regions most distant from nutrient-supplying blood vessels, where it sustains tumor cell survival.[195] Whether the primary role of autophagy in tumors is to provide metabolic substrates or prevent buildup of damaged components is not yet known. But either way, inhibition of autophagy may suppress the growth of established tumors.[196]

Many of the pathways that control autophagy are deregulated in cancer (Figure 6.31), and cancer therapeutics targeting these pathways activate autophagy. Some do so directly by inhibiting mTOR, whereas others inhibit upstream nutrient or signaling pathways. Cytotoxic cancer therapies activate autophagy, presumably by inflicting damage. The functional role of autophagy in these settings needs to be established. A particularly interesting possibility is that autophagy favors tumor cell survival. If this proves correct, then inhibition of autophagy might synergize with existing cancer treatments.[196]

The institution of fasting triggers the process of autophagy.

This process of autophagy involves a series of protein complexes composed of *atg* gene products coordinate the formation of autophagosomes. The Atg1/ULK1 complex (Atg1 in yeast and ULK1 in mammals) is an essential positive regulator of autophagosome formation.[183] When nutrients are abundant, binding of the ULK1 complex by the mammalian target of rapamycin (mTOR) complex 1 (mTORC1) inhibits autophagy. mTORC1 is an important regulator of cell growth and metabolism. It is composed of five subunits that include Raptor, which binds ULK1, and mTOR, a serine-threonine kinase. By phosphorylating ULK1 and another complex member (the mammalian homolog of yeast Atg13), mTOR inhibits autophagy initiation. In starvation, mTORC1 dissociates from the ULK1 complex, freeing it to trigger autophagosome nucleation and elongation.

Autophagosome nucleation requires a complex containing Atg6 or its mammalian homolog, Beclin 1, that recruits the class III phosphatidylinositol 3-kinase VPS34 to generate phosphatidylinositol 3-phosphate.[197] Expansion of autophagosome membranes involves two ubiquitin-like molecules, Atg12 and Atg8 (called LC3 in mammals), and two associated conjugation systems. The E1-like Atg7 and E2-like Atg10 covalently link Atg12 with Atg5, which together bind Atg16L1 to form pre-autophagosomal structures. In the second ubiquitin-like reaction, LC3 is cleaved by the protease Atg4. Phosphatidylethanolamine is conjugated to cleaved LC3 by Atg7 and a second

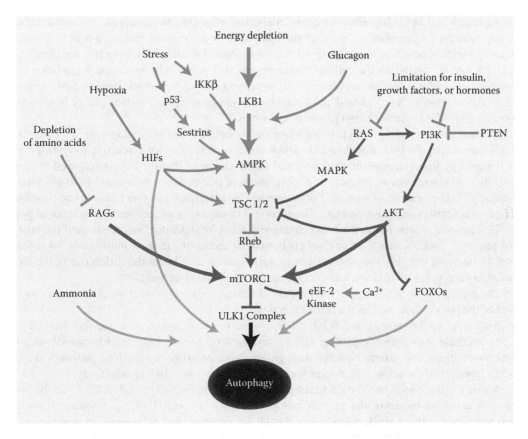

FIGURE 6.31 Signaling pathways that regulate autophagy. Common nutrient, growth factor, hormone, and stress signals that regulate autophagy. Dark lines depict events that positively regulate autophagy. Light lines depict those that negatively regulate autophagy.

E2-like enzyme, Atg3, and this lipidated LC3-II associates with newly forming autophagosome membranes. LC3-II remains on mature autophagosomes until after fusion with lysosomes and is commonly used to monitor autophagy.

The process beginning with the Beclin 1 complex gives rise to nascent autophagosome membranes. These membranes assemble around cargo, encapsulating the cargo in a vesicle that subsequently fuses with a lysosome, generating an auto-lysosome. The contents are then degraded by proteases, lipases, nucleases, and glycosidases. Lysosomal permeases release the breakdown products—amino acids, lipids, nucleosides, and carbohydrates—into the cytosol, where they are available for synthetic and metabolic pathways.

Substrates of Autophagy

According to Rabinowitz and White,[184] autophagy can be nonselective or selective. Nonselective, bulk degradation of cytoplasm and organelles by autophagy provides material to support metabolism during fasting. It also contributes to extensive tissue remodeling, as in *Drosophila* morphogenesis.[198] Whether mechanisms exist to prevent bulk autophagy from consuming essential components, such as a cell's final mitochondrion, remains unclear, and in some cases such consumption may lead to cell death.

However, to a point, fasting seems to restore optimum function and, thus, probably does not destroy the good tissue. Selective autophagy of proteins and of organelles such as mitochondria (mitophagy), ribosomes (ribophagy), endoplasmic reticulum (reticulophagy), peroxisomes (pexophagy), and lipids (lipophagy) occurs in specific situations. In mammals, the signal for targeting proteins for degradation by either the autophagy or proteasome pathways is ubiquitination. Many proteins accumulate in autophagy-defective mammalian cells, indicating that autophagy has a major role in controlling the cellular proteome and that proteasome-mediated degradation cannot compensate for defective autophagy.[191] To target proteins for autophagic degradation, ubiquitin on modified proteins is recognized and bound by autophagy receptors, such as p62 or Nbr1, which interact with LC3 to deliver cargo to autophagosomes.[183]

Mechanisms regulating selective autophagy of organelles are more elaborate. In mammals, autophagy of depolarized mitochondria, which protects cells from toxic reactive oxygen species, is initiated by Pink1-dependent mitochondrial translocation of Parkin. This is followed by ubiquitination of mitochondrial proteins and recruitment of p62 to direct mitochondria to autophagosomes.[199,200] The pruning of damaged mitochondria by autophagy has two homeostatic functions. The first is limiting oxidative damage. The second is maintaining a functional mitochondrial pool.

This process is seen in the food and chemically sensitive individual who fasts until the energy has returned. There is clearly a fine line between eating and fasting in these individuals. Some learn how to interpret this fine function extremely well because they know the difference of the signs between energy, loss of toxicity, and energy loss due to the need for food.

The regulation of autophagy in the process of fasting requires some clinical astuteness on the part of the physician as well as the learning patient.

According to Rabinowitz and White,[184] regulation of autophagy is now possibly worked out. Cells integrate information regarding nutrient availability, growth factor and hormonal receptor activation, stress, and internal energy through an elaborate array of signaling pathways (Figure 6.32). In mammals, insulin—the master hormone of the fed state—blocks autophagy.

A major intracellular hub for integrating autophagy-related signals is mTORC1.[201] In the presence of abundant nutrients and growth factors including insulin, TORC1 promotes cell growth and metabolic activity while suppressing the ULK1 complex and autophagy. In deprivation or stress, numerous signaling pathways inactivate mTORC1 kinase activity. These both suppress cell growth to reduce energy demand and induces autophagy to enable stress adaptation and survival. A second mTOR complex, mTORC2, positively regulates mTORC1. Upstream of mTORC1 is the cellular energy-sensing pathway controlled by adenosine monophosphate-activated protein kinase (AMPK).[202] High concentrations of AMP signal energy depletion, activate AMPK, and inhibit mTORC1, thus promoting autophagy (Figure 6.33).

Apparently, this occurs in chemically sensitive patients, who suddenly depletes themselves from food and pollutant overload. They then need to skip meals until they are cleared out and the energy comes back.

Regulation of autophagy also occurs through the forkhead box or FOXO transcription factors, whose activation leads to transcription of *atg* genes.[203] Similarly, hypoxia and activation of hypoxia-inducible factors, or HIFs, induces the transcription of mitophagy-specific genes and mitophagy (Figure 6.31). As shown previously, chemically sensitive patients have problems with oxygen extraction which may have to do with this process. Less well-characterized mTOR-independent regulators of autophagy also exist. One is ammonia, a by-product of amino acid catabolism, which stimulates autophagy, likely in poorly perfused tissues and tumors.[204] We do see chemically sensitive patients who actually smell like ammonia indicating demetabolism. Glucagon, a predominant hormone of the fasted state, also triggers autophagy in the liver. Adrenergic receptor activation, which like glucagon activates adenylate cyclase and cyclic adenosine monophosphate (cAMP) production, also stimulates liver autophagy.

According to Rabinowitz and White,[184] autophagy and starvation occur after 12 hours. All cells have internal nutrient stores for use during starvation. Glycogen and lipid droplets are overtly designed for this purpose. Their contents are accessed primarily through the actions of dedicated enzymes, such as glycogen phosphorylase and hormone-sensitive lipase. Many other cellular components have a dual function as nutrient stores. For example, ribosomes occupy approximately 50%

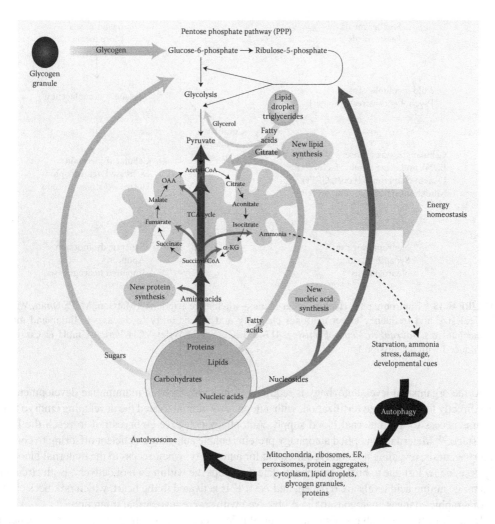

FIGURE 6.32 Use of the products of autophagy. Multiple forms of stress activate autophagy (bottom right). Degradation of proteins, lipids, carbohydrates, and nucleic acids liberates amino acids, fatty acids, sugars, and nucleosides that are released into the cytoplasm. (From Rabinowitz, J. D. and White, E. 2010. The American Association for the advancement of science. *Autophagy and Metabolism.* 330(6009): 1344–1348. Reprinted with permission from AAAS.)

of the dry weight of rapidly growing microbes. In addition to enabling rapid protein synthesis when nutrient conditions are favorable, this provides a store of amino acids for proteome remodeling when conditions turn for the worse. Autophagy has a key role in providing access to such undedicated nutrient stores.

Limitation of any of the major elemental nutrients triggers autophagy in yeast, with nitrogen limitation being the strongest stimulus.[205] When nitrogen is removed, yeast defective in autophagy become severely depleted of internal amino acids. This precludes the synthesis of proteins important for surviving nitrogen starvation and accelerates cell death.[206] Thus, autophagy provides the primary route to nitrogen during fasting.

Unlike microbes, mammalian cells benefit from a relatively constant nutrient environment. Nevertheless, autophagy can support mammalian cells through nutrient deprivation. For example, in lymphocytes, the ability to consume environmental nutrients is growth factor dependent. In the absence of growth factor stimulation, energy charge is maintained through autophagy, with cells shrinking approximately 50% in size over 3 months of self-cannibalization.[207]

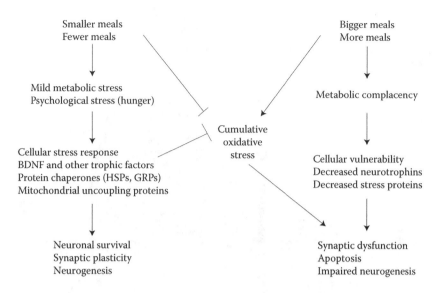

Smaller meals
Fewer meals

Bigger meals
More meals

Mild metabolic stress
Psychological stress (hunger)

Metabolic complacency

Cumulative
oxidative
stress

Cellular stress response
BDNF and other trophic factors
Protein chaperones (HSPs, GRPs)
Mitochondrial uncoupling proteins

Cellular vulnerability
Decreased neurotrophins
Decreased stress proteins

Neuronal survival
Synaptic plasticity
Neurogenesis

Synaptic dysfunction
Apoptosis
Impaired neurogenesis

FIGURE 6.33 Environmental Health Center-Dallas—dietary restrictions. (Mattson, M. P., Duan, W., Guo, Z. Meal size and frequency affect neuronal plasticity and vulnerability to disease: Cellular and molecular mechanisms. *Journal of Neurochemistry*. 417–431. Copyright Wiley-VCH Verlag GmbH & Co. KGaA. Reproduced with permission.)

At the organismal level, autophagy is required at multiple stages of mammalian development. The first directly follows oocyte fertilization, with autophagy essential to feed the developing embryo before it gains access to the maternal blood supply. Autophagy-defective embryos fail to reach the blastocyst stage.[208] Maternally supplied autophagy proteins enable autophagy-deficient offspring to complete embryogenesis, revealing a second requirement for autophagy: when access to the maternal blood supply is suddenly lost due to birth. Autophagy-defective pups die within 24 h of delivery. Both circulating and tissue amino acid levels are reduced, and AMPK is activated in the heart, which produces electrocardiographic changes analogous to those observed with severe myocardial infarction.[209]

In adult fasting, autophagy also has a central role, increasing within 24 h in the liver, pancreas, kidney, skeletal muscle, and the heart; the brain is spared.[210] Fortunately, with fasting for 12–48 h it appears that cleansing occurs in chemically sensitive patients and no harm is done. Pharmacological blockade of autophagy results in cardiac dysfunction early in starvation.[211] This dysfunction may be due to the buildup of toxins that are known to occur in the myocardium and failure to release them from the electrical conductions system. Although autophagy levels return to normal in the liver two days into fasting, Autophagy remains increased in both cardiac and skeletal muscle. Liver mass, however, persistently falls faster than muscle or total body mass. This decline is consistent with a failure of biosynthesis to balance basal consumption of liver by autophagy.[185] As liver mass falls, breakdown of muscle and adipose tissue feeds the liver, which exports glucose and ketone bodies required by the brain (Figure 6.34).

According to Rabinowitz and White,[184] the use of metabolites released by autophagy occurs. The breakdown products derived from autophagy have a dual role, providing substrate for both biosynthesis and energy generation (Figure 6.33). In terms of biosynthesis, the abundance of ribosomal (relative to messenger) RNA makes transcriptome remodeling straightforward. In contrast, proteome remodeling demands copious amino acids, and a major role of autophagy is to provide them.

In addition to providing anabolic substrates, nucleosides and amino acids can be catabolized for energy generation. RNA breakdown yields nucleosides, which are degraded to ribose-phosphate. Six ribose-phosphate molecules are energetically equivalent to five glucose phosphates, and, like glucose phosphate derived by glycogen breakdown, they can yield adenosine triphosphate (ATP)

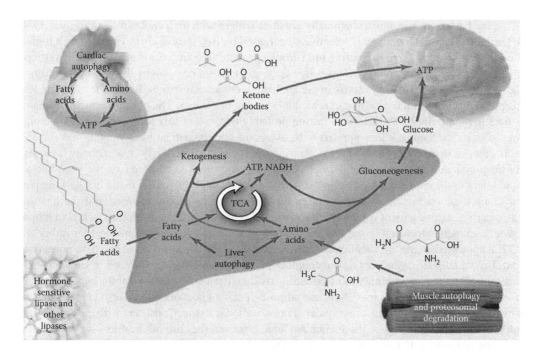

FIGURE 6.34 Role of autophagy in adult mammalian starvation. Depicted pathways predominate after depletion of glycogen stores, typically approximately 12 hours into starvation. Autophagy in the liver and heart (but not brain) generates fatty acids and amino acids, which are catabolized. (From Rabinowitz, J. D. and White, E. 2010. The American Association for the advancement of science. *Autophagy and Metabolism*. 330(6009):1344–1348. Reprinted with permission from AAAS.)

either aerobically or anaerobically. In contrast, amino acids, like lipids, yield ATP only through oxidative phosphorylation (Figure 6.31). The catastrophic effects of ischemia are a consequence of the relative paucity of nucleic acids and glycogen combined with the inefficiency of anaerobic glycolysis. Oxygen is the one nutrient that autophagy cannot provide.

In addition to being directly catabolized to yield energy, the liver can convert nucleosides, amino acids, and lipids into glucose and ketone bodies for distribution elsewhere in the body (Figure 6.32). Ribose-phosphate from nucleosides can be converted into glucose through the nonoxidative pentose phosphate pathway (PPP). Amino acids feed into central metabolism at multiple points, including pyruvate, tricarboxylic acid cycle (TCA) cycle intermediates, and acetyl–coenzyme A (CoA). Pyruvate and TCA cycle intermediates are substrates for gluconeogenesis. In contrast, mammals cannot convert acetyl-CoA into glucose. Because lipid degradation yields mostly acetyl-CoA, ketone bodies are essential for feeding the brain and other vital tissues during prolonged starvation.

According to Rabinowitz and White,[184] autophagy is a regulator of metabolism. Autophagy is important for regulating cellular metabolic capabilities for chemically sensitive patients who are sluggish and have lost energy. A striking example comes from yeast capable of living off of methanol or fatty acids, substrates that are burned in peroxisomes. When more appealing forms of carbon become available, the peroxisomes are no longer required and are cleared by autophagy.[212] The function of autophagy in removing unneeded peroxisomes is conserved in mammals. Peroxisomes are induced in the liver by various hydrophobic chemicals, known collectively as peroxisome proliferators. Removal of peroxisome proliferators leads to restoration of normal peroxisome abundance through autophagy.[212] Thus, chemically sensitive patients develop normal peroxisome levels.

Autophagy also regulates the abundance of liver lipid droplets by their constitutive degradation.[213] Defective autophagy in mice leads to larger and more plentiful lipid droplets, increased concentrations of hepatic triglycerides and cholesterol, and increased gross liver size. Therefore, one of the methods to re-regulate a chemically sensitive patient with high cholestrol and triglycerides is to periodically fast. Lipophagy is selectively decreased by free fatty acids in vitro and by a high-fat diet.[213] Thus, in addition to promoting lipid droplet growth, free fatty acids may impair lipid droplet breakdown. Because lipophagy releases free fatty acids, its suppression by them is a case of one of the most prevalent regulatory motifs in metabolism: feedback inhibition. But this feedback mechanism may backfire in the case of a chronic high-fat diet or obesity. The obese chemically sensitive patient may initially be refractory to fasting probably because of this feedback loop. However, as time goes by the feedback loop appears to be overcome and the patient loses weight.

In contrast to the role of autophagy in clearing lipid droplets from the liver, autophagy is required for the production of the large lipid droplets characteristic of white adipose tissue.[214,215] White adipose refers to the canonical fat storage tissue that expands in obesity. This tissue is a parking place for many toxic chemicals. When the fat is broken up, the toxics are released and the health of chemically sensitive patient is temporarily worsened. This white fat is in contrast to brown adipose tissue, a mitochondria-rich tissue that catabolizes glucose and lipids to generate heat rather than ATP. It appears damaged in chemically sensitive patients, who are always cold and have normal thyroid. Brown adipose tissue contains uncoupling protein 1, which allows protons to leak across the inner mitochondrial membrane, short-circuiting oxidative phosphorylation. Inhibition of autophagy blocks white adipocyte differentiation, and adipose-specific knockout of *atg7* results in mice whose white adipocytes manifest features typical of brown adipose tissue. Consistent with the rapid energy burning of brown adipocytes, these mice are lean; however, they are not healthy—when fed either a regular or high-fat diet, they are at increased risk of early death.[214]

Autophagy also contributes to both insulin secretion and physiological sensitivity to the hormone. It is essential for the health of pancreatic β cells and for the expansion of β-cell mass that occurs in response to a high-fat diet.[216,217] In the liver, defective autophagy leads to insulin resistance.[188] For reasons that are not yet fully clear, hepatic autophagy is decreased in obese mice, and its restoration through retroviral expression of *atg7* ameliorates their insulin resistance.

Chemically less contaminated foods, which contain a higher nutritive quality, must be used, thereby eliminating additives, preservatives, pesticides, and herbicides. The rotary diet (a form of a fast and dietary restriction) is a diet where one never eats the same food closer than one time in four days and as far apart as 7–30 days which is necessary for those with severe homeostatic dysfunction who are having difficulty getting rid of their total body toxic load. Fasting (from 1 to 7 days with total food abstinence) is often carried out periodically which will rapidly reduce the total body load. This procedure has been accomplished in over 10,000 patients at the EHC-Dallas and Buffalo. Two thousand of these patients were fasted under environmentally controlled conditions. Fasting has been shown to normalize pulse rate, blood pressure, respiratory rate (Tables 6.8 through 6.17), hormones, norepinephrine, renal leaks, immune dysfunction, pesticide and solvent levels, and edema in patients.

Fresh food should be used as much as possible with freezing or canning process carried out in glass or in wood-derived cellophane containers as a second best solution.

TABLE 6.8

Changes in Pulse, Blood Pressure, and Temperature After Fasting in the ECU for 2–7 Days (4000 Measurements)

Vital Signs	Before Fast	After Fast
Pulse	97.6 ± 3.6	78 ± 4.0
Blood pressure-normotensive	$130/85 \pm 5.0$	$110/80 \pm 5.0$
Hypertensive	$180/110 \pm 5.0$	$110/80 \pm 5.0$
Temperature	96.0 ± 0.5	98.6 ± 0.6

Source: Adapted from Environmental Health Center-Dallas.

TABLE 6.9

Twenty Moderate Chemically Sensitive and Chronic Fatigue Individuals

	Challenge (amount-ppm)	Threshold Limit Value[a] (ppm)
	Petroleum ethyl	
Alcohol	<0.5	1000
Phenol	<0.002	5
Formaldehyde	<0.2	2
Chlorine	<0.33	1
2, 4-DNP (pesticide)	<0.0034	No standard

Note: Ambient subthreshold dose double-blind challenges 15-minute exposure at a double environmentally controlled room after minimum 4 days of deadaptation with total load decreased including fasting.

[a] The time-weighted average concentration for a normal 8-hour work day or 40-hour work week.

TABLE 6.10

118 Double-Blind Challenges

33 Positive Challenges of Symptom Score 2 S.D. above Prechallenge Levels Ambient Subthreshold Doses		Negative Challenges of Symptoms Score 2 S.D. below Prechallenge Levels	
2	Saline	20	Saline
31	Chemicals-volatile	65	Chemicals
8	Insecticide (2,4-Dinitrophenol)	12	Insecticide
7	Chlorine	10	Chlorine
6	Formaldehyde	14	Formaldehyde
6	Phenol	13	Phenol
4	Petroleum alcohol	16	Petroleum alcohol

Source: Environmental Health Center-Dallas.

Avoidance of individual foods to which the patient is sensitive without using a rotary diet is discouraged because sensitivity has become the individual's problem and the patient will eventually become sensitive to more foods. These patients are rapid sensitizers at this stage of their illness. The rapid sensitization can occur from 1 week to 2 months of repeating the food too often in the diet. Once the spreading phenomenon has commenced in these patients, they will eventually show sensitivity to other foods and unless the rotary diet is instituted quickly they will have no safe foods. At this stage, these patients become rapid sensitizers.

AVOIDANCE OF POLLUTANTS IN CONTAMINATED WATER

Safe water is available in three forms: distilled, double filtered, and spring. Intake of each type will decrease the total body pollutant load.

DISTILLED WATER

Distillation in glass or steel only can be used. No plastic or rubber connectors can be used. Distilled water is the least safe of the clean water choices since it has some petroleum products that spill over

TABLE 6.11

Double-Blind Inhaled Challenges Ambient Doses of Toxic Chemicals Environmental Control Unit

Challenging Substance	Dose (ppm)	Clearly Positive Responses (Category I)	Intermediate Responses (Category II)	Total Responses	No. of Patients with Signs of Placebo Challenge (Category III)	No. of Patients with No Responses (Category IV)
Natural gas	–	4	1	5	0	45
Ethyl alcohol	<0.50	2	1	354	0	47
Phenol	<0.002	2	2	4	0	46
Formaldehyde	<0.20	5	2	2	0	43
Pesticide (2,4-Dinitrophenol)	<0.0034	1	1		0	48
Water #1			2[a]	2	0	48
Water #2			1[a]	1	0	49
Normal saline			1[a]	1	0	49
Total response		14[b]	15	29+	0	

Source: Adapted from Environmental Health Center-Dallas, 1986.

[a] For each of the four positive placebo responders, symptoms were reproduced (no signs) in only one of the three placebo challenges.

[b] Four patients responded to two chemicals.

TABLE 6.12

Chemical Sensitivity Double-Blind Inhaled Challenge after 4 Days Deadaptation in the ECU with Total Load Decreased

Chemical	Ambient Dose (ppm)	Sensitive	Not Sensitive
Natural gas	Ambient	16	4
Phenol	0.002	18	2
Formaldehyde	0.2	16	4
Insecticide (2, 4-DNP)	0.0034	18	2
Alcohol	0.5	17	3
Chlorine	0.33	19	14
Normal saline	–	4	16

Source: Adapted from Environmental Health Center-Dallas.

at the boiling point of water and the distillation process also takes out most of the minerals. Some patients who are extremely sensitive to the minerals are better off using distilled water. Distilled water should be contained in glass not plastic since liver and thyroid-damaging phthalates and female hormone-mimicking bis-phenols leach from the soft and hard plastic, respectively, into the water, thus, increasing the patients' total body load.

FILTERED WATER

Filtration using carbon and Millipore ceramic filters can also be used but the filters should be housed in stainless steel, and not phthalate-containing plastics for the reverse osmosis. Double

TABLE 6.13
Response to Double-Blind Inhaled Challenges Ambient Doses of Toxic Chemicals Environmental Control Unit

	Clearly Positive Group[a]	Intermediate Group[a]	Total[a]
No patients to responding chemicals	10	11	21 (18)
Responses to chemicals	14	11	25 (20)
Responses to placebos	0	4[b]	4[b]
Responses to chemicals (per chemical)	2.3 (2.0)	1.8 (2.09)	4.2 (4.0)
Responses to placebos (per placebo)	0	1.3	1.3
Chemical responders (% of total patients)	20% (16%)	22% (20%)	42% (36%)
Placebo responders (% of total patients)	0%	8%[b]	8%

Source: From Rea, W. J. et al. 1989. *Clin. Ecol.* 6 (3):113–118. With permission.
[a] Numbers in parentheses show data on double-blind challenges only, excluding natural gas.
[b] Four people reacted to one of the three placebos, with symptoms but no signs.

TABLE 6.14
Average Pulse Rates of 10 Clearly Responding Inhaled Double-Blind Challenged Patients to Ambient Doses of Toxic Chemicals, 1350 Measurements Environmental Control Unit (ECU)

	Pulse Rate Per Minute, 135 Measurements Per Patient	Difference between Positive and Negative Response (Standard Deviations)
Measured in room	79.2 ± 3.3	3.8
Measured in booth	78.7 ± 3.3	3.9
Negative placebo challenge	81.4 ± 2.9	3.5
Negative chemical challenge	80.6 ± 1.8	4.2
Positive chemical challenge	97.6 ± 3.6	

Source: Adapted from Environmental Health Center-Dallas, 1986.
Note: Primary signs and symptoms also reproduced.

TABLE 6.15
Ambient Subthreshold Chemical Challenge, 15-Minute Exposure Double-Blind, Double Environmentally Controlled Room

IgG	83% changed
EOS	95% changed
Total complement	68% changed

Source: Adapted from Environmental Health Center-Dallas, 1986.
Note: Forty patients in the ECU with total load reduced and at least 4 days of deadaptation. The change was over 20% from control during the course of the reaction. Serial levels of the above parameters measured before challenge, 5, 15, 30, 60, and 120 minutes after either oral or inhaled challenge.

TABLE 6.16
Hundred Chemically Sensitive Patients Inhaled Challenge after a Minimum of 4 Days Deadaptation (535 Separate Challenges) in the ECU

Chemical (ppm) Function	No. Patients	% Acute Symptoms	% Acute Signs	% BP Change	%Pulse Change	PFR Change	% Brain Change
Ethanol (<0.50)	72	+74	70	10	6	16	24
Phenol (<0.002)	78	+62	62	37	6	12	21
Chlorine (<0.33)	41	+79	75	13	5	15	27
Formaldehyde (<0.20)	82	+60	63	9	5	9	22
Pesticide (<0.0034)	39	+92	92	11	11	16	39
1,1,1-Trichloro-ethane (≤13)	10	+80	80	40	10	30	80
Saline placebo	213	15	15	9	2	2	3

Source: Adapted from Environmental Health Center-Dallas, 1986.
Note: Confirmed by intradermal tests.

TABLE 6.17
Inhaled Chemical Challenges, Double-Blind (Ambient Doses) after 4 Days Deadaptation in the ECU with Total Load Decreased

Patient Dose (ppm)	Saline	Gas Ambient	Chlorine <0.33	Petroleum Alcohol <0.5	Formaldehyde <0.2	Phenol <0.0002	Insecticides 2,4-DNP <0.0034
1	NR	+	NR	NR	NR	NR	NR
2	NR	+	NR	+	+	+	+
3	+	+	+	+	+	+	+
4	NR	NR	NR	+	+	+	+
5	NR	+	+	+	+	+	+
6	NR	+	+	+	+	+	+
7	NR	+	+	+	NR	NR	+
8	NR	NR	NR	NR	NR	NR	NR
9	NR	NR	NR	NR	NR	NR	NR
10	NR	+	+	+	+	+	+

Source: Adapted from Environmental Health Center-Dallas, 1986.

filtration using a whole house reverse osmosis filter followed by a second single steel, ceramic, and charcoal filter in the kitchen is recommended in order to get a double pass of the water through filtration. Plastic housing is not recommended for these filters because of the plasticizer leaching problem. Reverse osmosis will remove more chemicals but plastic membranes are used in this process; a ceramic, steel, and charcoal filter should be used after the reverse osmosis process in order to remove the plasticizers, which have leached into the water.

SPRING WATER

Spring water that is not usually contaminated with toxics, such as a natural substance like arsenic, sulfur, and phenol, is still the best choice if it is contained in glass bottle and has a high magnesium and calcium content. Water contained in glass bottles is essential to optimum health (Figure 6.35 and Table 6.18).

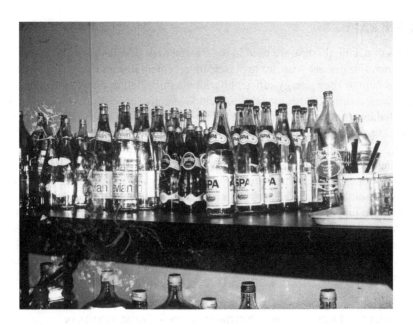

FIGURE 6.35   Spring water bottled in glass.

TABLE 6.18

**Volatile Organic Screening Test (VOST) for Selected EHC-Dallas Spring Water Samples:
Glass versus Plastic Containers**

VOST Component	Mountain Valley in Glass ppb	Mountain Valley in Plastic ppb	Spring House in Glass ppb	Spring House in Plastic ppb
Benzene	*0.01	0.03		0.04
Toluene	*0.03	0.09		0.12
Ethylbenzene				
Trimethylbenzene		0.03		
Xylene				
Styrene				
Dichloromethane	*0.33	0.05		0.92
Choroform				0.19
Carbon tetrachloride	*0.01	0.01	0.01	0.01
Bromoform			0.02	0.02
Bromodichloromethane		0.01		0.15
Dibromochloromethane				0.11
Trichlorethane				0.03
Tetrachloroethane				
Trichlorethylene		0.17		0.14
Tetrachloroethylene		0.11		0.07
Chlorobenzene				0.05
Dichlorobenzene				
Benzaldehyde				
Methylmercaptan				

Source: Adapted from Laseter, J. L. 1985. Personal communication. *2000 version—These items have been eliminated.

Note: Results are reported μg/L = ppb, and are based on GC/MS data. Clean H_2O is thus essential for health and should be used at all times.

NEEDLE THERAPY

Several types of needle therapy are used in the treatment of patients with chemical sensitivity and chronic degenerative disease who are hypersensitive, to help restore the dynamics of homeostasis. These entities help to keep energy-efficient harmonic information flow and feedback, thus restoring normal homeostasis. These modalities include specific dose (dilution) injection therapy for biological inhalants (pollen, dust, mold, algae), foods, some chemicals (including metals, solvents, etc.), viruses, bacteria, intestinal peptides, neurotransmitters, plant phenols (terpenes), nonspecific needling for acupuncture, light acupuncture, and neural therapy for removal of secondary disturbance fields or dyshomeostatic foci. Cold laser acupuncture has a specific place in our armamentarium since it can attack three areas using point acupuncture, neural therapy for scars, and maximum pain points, which release toxics and help to normalize the dynamics of homeostasis. None of these modalities will have a lasting effect if the total body load is not reduced and maintained constantly throughout life. The same is true for homeopathic, osteopathic, and cranial manipulation, chiropractic, reflex, and physical therapy treatment. On the other hand, if the hypersensitive state is not treated frequently, all environmental therapy will fail and the patient will remain unwell (Figure 6.36).

INJECTION THERAPY—PROVOCATION—NEUTRALIZATION—SERIAL DILUTION

The methods of injection treatment used in this treatment section have now been proven scientifically sound and clinically efficacious (5× less polluted environment for VOC, particulates, pesticides, molds, and mycotoxins). Hundreds of double-blind studies have been carried out.[218,219] Numerous clinical studies have been published showing the efficacy of the intradermal provocation, neutralization, and desensitization techniques for diagnosis and treatment of the hypersensitive state observed in chemically sensitive patients. These techniques can be used to aid the body in returning to homeostasis from the hypersensitive state. There are multiple studies showing the efficacy of sublingual therapy which works on a similar plane to injection therapy.[220] One can neutralize inhalants (pollens, dust, molds),[221] foods,[222,223] some chemicals,[221] bacteria, viruses, neurotransmitters, intestinal peptides, and metals by the sublingual or intradermal routes.

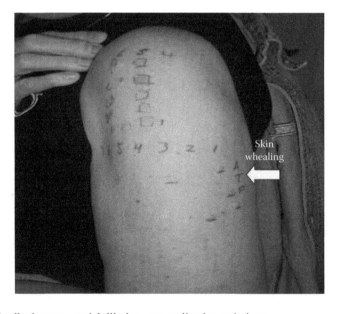

FIGURE 6.36 Needle therapy—serial dilution—neutralization technique.

In addition, autogenous vaccines can be made in order to deliver even more specific individuated antigens to the patients for therapy when stock vaccines will not work. Preservative-free antigens should be used.

There appears to be a discrepancy of 20% between the sublingual and the injection route of therapy in favor of the injection.

Evidence Base in Physics for Homeopathic and Intradermal Provocation Process, Products and Services

According to Smith,[224]

1. Homeopathy and serial dilution injection, neutralization, vaccines involve frequencies and their effects on living systems.
2. Clinical evidence comes from hypersensitive patients whose reactions can be treated with specially prepared homeopathic and provocation neutralization potencies.
3. Homeopathic and provocation neutralization potencies involve the memory of water for frequencies.
4. A theory and facts of these vaccines is based in quantum physics and is supported by experimental evidence.

Homeopathy and serial dilution neutralization vaccines are two of the branches of complementary and alternative medicine, which involves the therapeutic use of frequency. For at least the past 60 years, the promulgated and accepted wisdom is that the only biological effects of nonionizing electromagnetic fields are thermal and as such can be reliably predicted from "Classical Physics." One must conjecture that the motives for this have been military, commercial, and legal. The majority of healthy persons have regulatory systems well able to cope with the natural and manmade electromagnetic environment as with other environmental stresses so any frequency effects are not apparent.

Since the 1970s, Smith[225] has been involved with research into the ways that living systems make use of electric and magnetic fields and frequencies and has over 100 publications in this area. In 1982, he commenced an involvement with Monro[226] with the problems of chemically sensitive patients who had become hypersensitive to their electrical environment. This work quickly showed that once a threshold of intensity had been exceeded, the relevant factor was frequency. Initially, patients were challenged with frequencies from an oscillator at environmental field strengths. Their reactions to specific frequencies were the same as their reactions to the chemicals, volatiles, or particulates to which they happened to be sensitive.

The "Lee and Miller Technique"[218] used in the treatment of such patients involves successive serial dilutions of the allergen until one is found which turns off the patient's reaction. This needs to be more precise than the standard homeopathic and allopathic potencies. Here, dilutions take place by vortexing in the syringe. For the treatment of electrical sensitivities, a therapeutic frequency could be found, imprinted into water and used in the same way as an allergen dilution even though there was no chemical component present. This fitted conveniently into the existing facilities and practice of the hospital involved (Breakspear Hospital at Hemel Hempstead, England) and did not require an electrical oscillator for each patient. However, Rea et al.[219] carried out a double-blind trial at the Environmental Health Center, Dallas, Texas, using strict environmentally less polluted conditions. Selected patients with sensitivity to electricity could respond to a frequency to which they happened to be sensitive with 100% success and 0% response to placebos.

Examination of frequencies which had a clinical effect showed a correlation with the endogenous frequencies on the acupuncture meridians. When an acupuncture point is stressed either by pressure or with a needle, its endogenous frequency spreads throughout the body. Appropriate choice of meridians and points enables the acupuncturist to create a therapeutic frequency pattern from the patient's own body fields. Voll[227] showed that certain acupuncture meridians were linked to the ANS. Homeopathic potencies can be selected to stimulate specific acupuncture meridians and thence specific parts of the ANS.

The Physics of Homeopathy and Antigen, Intradermal Neutralization Provocation

Frequency, Coherence, and Fractality (Figure 6.37)

The importance of frequency in biological systems was recognized by Frohlich[225] who in the 1930s when told that the cell membrane potential was a fraction of a volt and existed across an extremely thin cell wall realized it represented an enormous electric field, strong enough to align molecules for assembly and resonating at about 100 GHz. By 1967, he had applied the theory of coherent modes of oscillation in nonlinear systems and long-range phase correlations to biological order. The subsequent development of his ideas and the work of his worldwide circle of collaborators were edited by him into two "Green Books": *Coherent Excitations in Biological Systems* and *Biological Coherence and Response to External Stimuli.*

In 1995, Preparata[228] with Del Giudice[229] and coworkers showed through quantum electrodynamics (QED) theory that water had phase coherence as a fundamental property arising from the exchange of radiation at the natural resonant frequencies of the water molecule. In a coherent system, the distance over which frequency coherence persists (coherence length) replaces velocity as the constant quantity making frequency proportional to velocity and a fractal quantity. Fractality enables the chemical, technological, and biological frequency bands to interact. Table 6.19 shows the frequency fractals for light from a mercury discharge lamp imprinted into water. If the chemical bond was not associated with frequency, spectroscopic analysis would be impossible. Chemistry therefore cannot be described by "Classical Physics." Solutions diluted to 1:05 and the 5th dilution or above are found in many chemically sensitive patients. These can be called homeopathic dilutions.

Fields

In mathematics, a field is a region of space containing mathematical objects, rather like the "field of view" seen with binoculars. In physics, a field is a region in which a mechanical force acts, for example, the gravitational field.

The "Classical Electromagnetic Field" is the basis of electronics and radio. "Classical Physics" describes a system for which the phase is well defined and the number of particles (quanta) is too large to matter. In contrast, a "Quantum Field" involves less particles and has a fundamental uncertainty described by the Heisenberg relation.[225]

These fields can be electric or magnetic. The magnetic field only exists in closed loops and a mathematical consequence is the magnetic vector potential explained theoretically by Aharanov and Bohm[230] and later found experimentally. This generates an electric field proportional to its frequency and in a coherent region this gives an oscillating potential which can be measured.

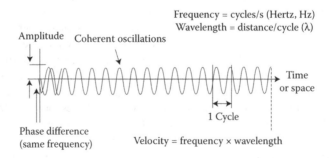

FIGURE 6.37 Diagram of the quantities associated with frequency. Smith (1982) shows the quantities associated with frequency irrespective of what is oscillating. If a frequency is propagating through space, there is a velocity and an associated wavelength.

TABLE 6.19

Multiple Frequencies Fractal Effect for the Mercury (Hg) Optical Spectrum Imprinted into Water

Hg Lines (Nm)	Optical (Hz)		Microwave (Hz)		Low Frequencies (Hz)
	$\times 10^{15}$	$\times 10^{6}$	$\times 10^{6}$	$\times 10^{6}$	$\times 1$
185	1.62		935		19.31
254	1.18		680		14.38
365/6	0.820		472		9.843
405	0.740		425		8.925
436	0.688		396		8.358
492	0.607		347		7.235
546	0.549		315		6.633
577/9	0.519		298		6.262
615	0.488		280		5.832
623	0.482		276		5.832
Ratio		1.7340		47.70	
Std. Dev.		±0.34%		±0.75%	

Source: Adapted from Smith, C. W. 2008. In *Herbert Fröhlich FRS: A Physicist ahead of His Time*, 2nd ed., G. J. Hyland, P. Rowlands, Eds., pp. 107–154. Liverpool: University of Liverpool; Preparata, G. 1995. *QED Coherence in Matter*. Singapore: World Scientific; Del Giudice, E., L. Giuliani. 1995. Coherence in water and the kT problem in living matter. http://www.icems.eu/papers/ramazzini_library5_part1.pdf.

The Physics of Water Memory

One important result from Smith and Monro[224] clinical work was the finding that the reactions of patients to environmental electromagnetic fields, chemicals, or potencies could be reproduced with frequency-imprinted water. Water in flame-sealed glass ampules could be imprinted with frequencies through the glass and without any possibility of chemical contact. This confirmed the basis of homeopathy, intradermal provocation neutralization, and coherence as frequencies in water.

In 1983, the laboratory of Smith (2008)[225] showed that living systems could respond to magnetic resonance conditions at geomagnetic field strengths. This is a quantum effect but following its publication a cyclotron theory attempted to keep the effects within "Classical Physics."

Later this suggested that a frequency might be retained in water if the precession of proton spin could be synchronized to an applied frequency to generate an internal magnetic field which exactly satisfied the proton magnetic resonance conditions locally within a coherence domain. This condition turned out to be independent of the frequency to be remembered and would be stable unless the domain is thermally broken up by removing the stabilizing geomagnetic field. The critical field for this is about 340 nT making the coherence domain 53 μm in diameter. The statistical fluctuation in the number of protons involved determines the bandwidth of the frequency imprint which can be parts per million in agreement with experiment.

Imprinting a frequency into water immobilizes free protons increasing the pH value. Figure 6.38 shows the pH of a solution of sodium hydroxide at pH 8.01 had increased to pH 8.05 at memory saturation after 377 separate frequencies had been imprinted. On erasure the pH returned to its initial value.

Writing Frequencies into Water

Frequency information can be imprinted into a glass vial of water by succussion. This is what creates a homeopathic potency. Frequency information from a patient's body also can be imprinted if the vial is held in a clenched fist while succussing the protruding end.

pH returns to original value after imprints have been erased

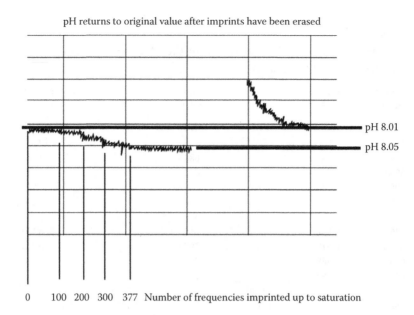

pH 8.01

pH 8.05

0   100 200 300 377 Number of frequencies imprinted up to saturation

FIGURE 6.38 Changes of pH on imprinting and erasing frequencies. (From Smith, C. W. 2008. In *Herbert Fröhlich FRS: A Physicist ahead of His Time*, 2nd ed., G. J. Hyland, P. Rowlands, Eds., pp. 107–154. Liverpool: University of Liverpool.)

Imprinting can take place through the glass of a vial containing water by immersing it in frequency-imprinted water. When water is placed near to a source of frequencies such as an oscillator and coil, a chemical or homeopathic potency can be imprinted by succussion or, with a strong permanent magnet or, by succussing a toroid (ring) of ferrite material. A sequence of 7-voltage pulses will effect an imprint; imprinting can also be done chemically.

Erasing Water Memory

A homeopathic potency or a water imprint for antigen serial dilutions provocation neutralization will be erased if the geomagnetic field is shielded by placing it briefly in a steel box. Erasure occurs when thermal energy becomes greater than the internal magnetic energy. This threshold, at about 1% of the Earth's magnetic field, is independent of the imprinted frequency over at least the 13 decades from 10^{-4} Hz to 10^9 Hz. Heating imprinted water alters the imprint so that it becomes "hidden" and living systems do not recognize it. It can be recovered by the application of certain frequencies including that of the heart acupuncture meridian. Certain combinations of frequencies will self-erase, that is, they are "nilpotent."

Reading Water Memory

Frequencies in water and living systems present a great measurement problem. Clinically, they may be anywhere in the electromagnetic spectrum from millihertz to gigahertz and the bioinformation is carried on the magnetic vector potential component of the field.

Several techniques have been applied to the objective measurement of frequencies in water and homeopathic potencies. They can be made to work over a limited range of frequencies.[225]

1. Electrodes immersed in water or a potency and connected to a low-noise high-gain amplifier have been used by Smith and Ludwig (Figure 6.39).[231]
2. Gairiaev[232] has used a special 2-beam laser interacting with a potency; this results in the emission of a radiofrequency modulated with the signature of the potency.

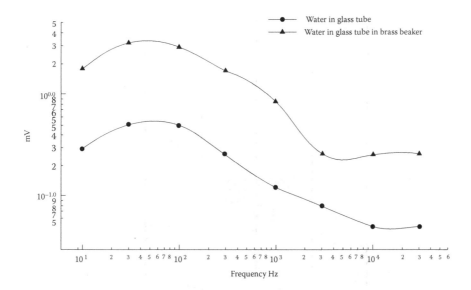

FIGURE 6.39 Measurement of frequencies imprinted into water using a low-noise amplifier and phase-sensitive detector (Brookdeal Electronics Ltd. LA350). Lower curve: Single electrode in water; upper curve; water in electroacupuncture beaker.

3. Elia[233] has used microcalorimetry to show a difference in heats of mixing between control water and a potency and in cooperation with Cardella has shown the same effect with water imprinted by placing in a microwave resonator.
4. Langer[234] has used both delayed luminescence and also the coupling between Tesla coils to demonstrate effects from potencies.
5. Rey[235] has irradiated samples with high energy ionizing radiation after freezing and on warming found differences in the thermoluminescence between potencies and controls.
6. Montagnier[236] has shown that some DNA sequences in pathogenic bacteria and viruses have a characteristic frequency signature even at high dilutions of agitated aqueous solutions.

The magnetic vector potential (**A**-field) component is in the direction of a current, that is, the proton precession and since $dA/dt\%-E$ an alternating **A**-field will generate an alternating **E**-field proportional to the frequency and an alternating potential in a coherent system. This is not a potential difference. It is in effect what electroacupuncture apparatus does without explaining the physics involved.

The frequency pattern of homeopathic phosphorous C6 tablets is shown in Table 6.20. Figure 6.40 shows this resonance measured with a low-noise amplifier and phase-sensitive detector (Brookdeal Electronics Ltd. LA350). The tablets were placed in an electroacupuncture brass beaker.

TABLE 6.20

Frequency Pattern of Homeopathic Phosphorous C6 Tablets

Phosphorous C6 Hz

2.113×10^{-1}
5.003×10^{0}
$5.000 \times 10^{+1}$
$3.003 \times 10^{+2}$
$6.005 \times 10^{+3}$ (± 1 Hz)

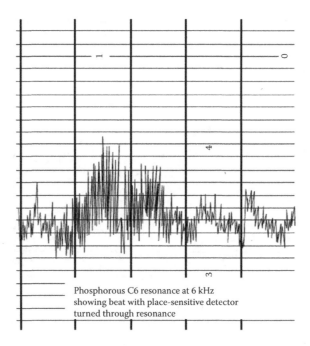

Phosphorous C6 resonance at 6 kHz
showing beat with place-sensitive detector
turned through resonance

FIGURE 6.40 Measurement of a frequency resonance in phosphorous C6. (From Smith, C. W. 2009. Can homeopathy ameliorate ongoing sickness? *J. Altern. Complement Med.* 15 (5):465–467.)

The frequency was stepped manually in 1 Hz intervals to show the beats between the potency resonance and the reference frequency. The chart speed was 20 mm/min.

CHEMICAL FREQUENCY SIGNATURES

Homeopathic and/or provocation–neutralization techniques potencies start from a concentrate which is usually of chemical or biological origin. Its chemical frequency signature is all that is needed for potentizing. A homeopathic repertory shows the wide range of frequency templates available for potentization.

Experiments with n-hexane showed that only 14 ppm of water is needed for a frequency signature to develop. Since the n-hexane spectrum is in the far infrared (FIR), water can only interact here. Of the many FIR water lines, a few (357 cm^{-1}, 213 cm^{-1}, and 128 cm^{-1}) are coherent enough for a water vapor laser and for "water memory." The chemical frequency signatures calculated for n-hexane were as measured. The same calculation applied to pairs of FIR water lines gave the measured frequency signatures of water. When a frequency is imprinted into water, the FIR frequencies develop two sidebands proportional to the imprinted frequency with corresponding fractal sidebands in other parts of the electromagnetic spectrum.

HOMEOPATHIC POTENCIES

When a single frequency is imprinted in water which is then serially diluted, the original frequency disappears to be replaced by the original frequency multiplied by the dilution ratio. Not all dilution ratios do this, some have no effect, others erase everything. Patterns developed from frequency signatures may be more complicated.

Figure 6.41 shows the frequency pattern for a set of potencies of thyroxin. It demonstrates the frequency basis for potentization of homeopathic remedies. Frequency-erased water was imprinted with the complete pattern of frequencies previously determined for thyroxin of potency D15. This was then potentized by conventional dilution and succussion. The frequencies measured for each

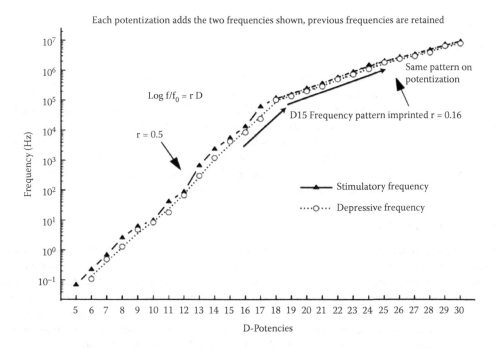

FIGURE 6.41 Frequency pattern for potencies of thyroxin. The potency D15 was synthesized from all constituent frequencies. On dilution and succession, this gave the frequencies as measured in potencies coming from the concentrate. (Adapted from Smith, C. W. 2008. *Herbert Fröhlich FRS: A Physicist ahead of His Time*, 2nd ed., G. J. Hyland, P. Rowlands, Eds., pp. 107–154. Liverpool: University of Liverpool.)

synthesized potency were exactly the same as those for the potencies prepared from the concentrate chemical thyroxin. Yet, the synthesized potencies had started from nothing but water. There is no discontinuity at potency D24, the dilution at which no molecule of an original substance should remain (Avogadro's number).

The frequency signature of chemicals must apply to pharmaceuticals which must also have a homeopathic activity. Table 6.21 compares aspirin and aconite; combined they would stimulate the Du Mai meridian.

TABLE 6.21
Frequency Signatures for Soluble Aspirin and Aconite C6

Soluble Aspirin	Aconite C6	Aspirin + Aconite C6
	↑4.911×10^{-4}	
↑3.032×10^{-1}	↓3.013×10^{-1}	
	↑7.712×10^{0}	↑4.133×10^{0}
	↓$5.513 \times 10^{+2}$	
↓$1.23 \times 10^{+6}$	↑$1.22 \times 10^{+6}$	
↑$7.10 \times 10^{+6}$	↓$7.10 \times 10^{+6}$	
	↑$3.35 \times 10^{+7}$	

Source: Adapted from Smith, C. W. 2008. *Herbert Fröhlich FRS: A Physicist ahead of His Time*, 2nd ed., G. J. Hyland, P. Rowlands, Eds., pp. 107–154. Liverpool: University of Liverpool.

Note: ↑ = Stimulatory (Hyperactive); ↓ = Depressive (Hypoactive)

CHAOS

Between the states of health and disease, there may be a state of mathematical chaos.[237] This is evident in some fragile chemically sensitive patients who have difficulty in getting and maintaining a stable dilution end point when attempts are made to modulate food and mold sensitivity for vaccine treatment. Chaos has been demonstrated in respect of the cardiac signal of a healthy human as well as in electroencephalograms, epidemics, fluid flow, and oscillatory chemical reactions. A chaotic system eventually settles down to its "attractor"—a stable condition that may be a point focus or a limit-cycle oscillation. However, some patients have to be stabilized by other means. From the clinical and homeopathic point of view, any experiment involving a patient in a chaotic domain is nonrepeatable from the same initial condition. Homeopathy can operate in the chaos region to switch a patient back from chaos to health. However, at times it cannot.

SIMILITERS AND PROVINGS

According to Hahnemann,[238] for the totality of symptoms to be cured, one must seek that medicine which has demonstrated the greatest propensity to produce either similar or opposite symptoms.

Frequency patterns are generally biphasic showing alternately stimulation and depression of biological activity. These are seen in the intradermal provocation neutralization process. Endogenous frequencies in biological systems fluctuate around their nominal value in a quasiperiodic manner which may be chaotic. Frequencies of acupuncture meridians can be entrained by dilutions, which may stimulate or depress biological activity and hence can be "therapeutic" or "proving." Chronic exposure to frequencies can result in "proving" symptoms which may become indistinguishable from a disease state. Eventually when the proper dilution is found, a neutralizing dose of the symptoms and signs is found.

In Table 6.22, the frequency pattern from a patient is compared with the frequency pattern of the dilution Lachesis C200 which may be the patient's similiter.

TABLE 6.22
Frequency Matching Indicates a Possible Similiter

Patient's Frequencies (Hz)	Nearby Meridians	Lachesis C200 (Hz)
↑1.514×10^{-2}	Small intestine	↑3.112×10^{-2}
↓7.611×10^{0}	Heart	↓6.142×10^{0}
$5.000 \times 10^{+1}$	50 Hz	↑$5.013 \times 10^{+1}$
↓$6.006 \times 10^{+1}$	Triple-Warmer (Sanjiao)	↓$6.114 \times 10^{+1}$
↑$2.95 \times 10^{+5}$	Skin degeneration	↑$2.25 \times 10^{+5}$
↓$1.23 \times 10^{+6}$	Small intestine	↓$1.32 \times 10^{+6}$
↑$3.45 \times 10^{+6}$	Organ degeneration	↑$3.15 \times 10^{+6}$
↓$7.70 \times 10^{+6}$		↓$7.30 \times 10^{+6}$
↑$3.18 \times 10^{+7}$	Fatty degeneration	↑$2.80 \times 10^{+7}$
↓$8.40 \times 10^{+7}$	Allergy	
↑$1.80 \times 10^{+8}$		

Source: Adapted from Smith, C. W. 2008. In *Herbert Fröhlich FRS: A Physicist ahead of His Time*, 2nd ed., G. J. Hyland, P. Rowlands, Eds., pp. 107–154. Liverpool: University of Liverpool.

Note: Paired-Values Correlation Coefficient 0.94.
↑ = Stimulatory (hyperactive); ↓ = Depressive or stressful (hypoactive). This dilution is per patient.

CONCLUSION

The theory of homeopathy and intradermal provocation neutralization has implications for both alternative and orthodox medicine and the chemical and electrical environments. It challenges convenient and comfortable paradigms.

SPECIFIC OPTIMUM DOSE ANTIGEN INJECTION TREATMENT: THE INTRADERMAL PROVOCATION–NEUTRALIZATION TECHNIQUE CONCENTRATE

Antigen dilution

1. 1 part of antigen concentrate to 4 saline—(1/5)
2. 4 parts of saline to 1 part of activated antigen—(1/25)
3. 1/25 parts of saline to 1 part antigen
4. 6/25 parts of saline to 1 part antigen
5. 3000 parts of saline to 1 part antigen

For desensitization and neutralization of molds, foods, viruses, bacteria, and chemicals, there are two injection techniques to reach the optimum dose therapy. One is the observed build-up doses that occur after the serial dilution testing while the other is the intradermal provocation neutralization technique where a strong dose provokes symptoms and outbreak while a lesser dose neutralizes them. After the number 5 dilution 1-3000, the doses become homeopathic.

Specific subcutaneous and sublingual antigen therapy appears to be information inducers attempting to alter physiology of the hypersensitive state so that the dynamics of homeostasis can be on an energy-efficient even keel. These functions appear to be through the ground regulation of nonimmune receptors (i.e., vanilloid) and the immune systems. Specific injection therapy with its rapid symptom provocation and optimum dose neutralization process appears to take advantage of both the specific and nonspecific information gathering process of the ECM and its neural sensitization and capsaicin receptor in the immune system. Their ground regulation system with its specific antigen optimum dose information is then rapidly disseminated to the target organ(s) and tissues throughout the body. Reciprocal effects can immediately occur (Figure 6.42). This process appears to be electromagnetic in nature. Of course at times serial dilution triggers are needed with build-up doses used to obtain the optimum treatment doses of desensitization. The neural sensitization and receptors (i.e., the GABA, muscarinic, vanilloids, NMDA, nitric oxide/peroxynitrate), immune changes such as gamma globulins G complement, and T and B cells make up the three great immune systems that cause hypersensitivity.

SPECIFIC ANTIGEN OPTIMUM DOSE INJECTION THERAPY AS AN INDUCER OF HOMEOSTASIS (DESENSITIZATION)

Normalization of immunological parameters (i.e., IgE, IgG, IgM, phagocytosis, etc.) appears to be a secondary response. Some can be primary involving the IgE mechanism (pollens, some foods), some molds, some chemical (IgE, IgG) haptens, diisocyanate; T-cell neutralization and desensitization can also occur with some intradermal treatment.

NONIMMUNOLOGICAL SENSITIZATION

Many other desensitizations can occur nonimmunologically which appears to be in the VR system and possibly in other receptor systems which can be involved in the ground regulation system. Therefore, this system would include peripheral sensory nerves, sensitization, dorsal root ganglion of the spinal cord, the trigeminal root ganglion (see sensitization of the small nerves with

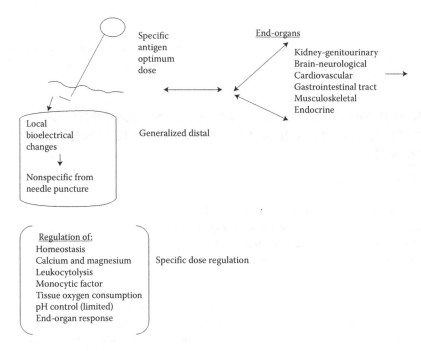

FIGURE 6.42 Specific optimum dose antigen injection therapy appears to be an inducer of homeostasis through the ground regulation system in chemically sensitive patients with local and distal reciprocal effects.

unmyelinated C fibers, large neurons with A as [A omega], mechano-heat-sensitive receptors). In other words, vanilloid-sensitive neurons are the regenerating morphologically, chemically, and functionally sensitive neurons. They encompass several subclasses of dorsal root ganglion and nerves.[239–242] As desensitization to vanilloids is the only trait that all these neurons seem to share, they are best described as vanilloid-sensitive neurons.[243–245]

These peripheral vanilloid-sensitive fibers enter the CNS central homeostatic mechanism that responds with the neutralizing adjustment to most of the mechanical changes. Some are placed along the line where the receptors develop a cortical number and condition of hypersensitivity comes into play, and this is where we see them. Peptidergic neurons express neurotrophin receptors txKA and p75, and nonpeptidergic neurons bind to the lectin B4 and express P2X3 receptors.[240,246] Vanilloid-sensitive neurons can combine with an incitant(s) in the protein kinase 1–3 system and when phosphorylated, increase sensitivity up to 1000 times. Thus, accounting for lower threshold triggering is seen in chemically sensitive patients. This phenomenon accounts for the ambient sensitivity of perfumes, volatile organic, hydrocarbons, molds, and foods found in chemically sensitive patients.

VANILLOID HYPERSENSITIVE AND INFLAMMATORY

Vanilloid-sensitive nerves may be stimulated to release prestored pro-inflammatory neuropeptides by both exogenous and endogenous stimuli. Some of these agents, such as bradykinin, have their own receptors; others may act on VRs. Protons are unique in that they have their own receptors (called acid-sensitive ion channels or ASICs) but they act also on VRs (Figure 6.43). The competitive VR antagonist capsazepine ameliorates carrageenan-induced inflammation *in vivo,* implying a role for an endogenous vanilloid in initiating the inflammatory cascade. Generally speaking, the tachykinin Substance P (SP) released from vanilloid-sensitive nerves causes smooth muscle cells to contract (e.g., bronchospasm, small vessel spasm) and opens endothelial gaps (plasma extravasation) by interacting at NK-1Rs. Also, SP can stimulate mucus secretion and activate various inflammatory cells. The patient will have phlegm in the throat, having to clear it several times. Also the

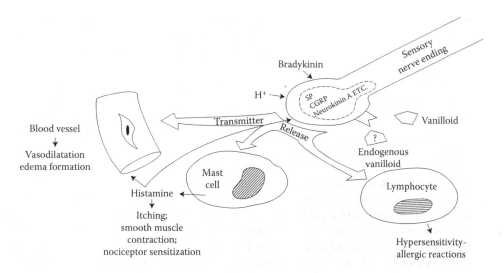

FIGURE 6.43   Schematic illustration of the role of peripheral vanilloid-sensitive nerve endings in evoking neurogenic inflammatory and allergic hypersensitivity reactions. (Reproduced with permission from Szallasi, A., P. M. Blumberg. 1993b. Mechanisms and therapeutic potential of vanilloids (capsaicin-like molecules). In *Advances in Pharmacology*, T. J. August, Anders, M. V., Murad, F. Eds., pp. 123–155. San Diego, CA: Academic Press; Permission granted Szallasi, A., P. M. Blumberg. 1999. Vanilloid (Capsaicin) receptors and mechanisms. *Pharmacol Rev.* 51(2):159–212.)

patient will have a blocking of vasodilation, accounting for the cold hands, feet, as well as the total body cold sensitivity. The predominant effect of calcitonin gene-related peptide (CGRP) is vasodilation. There are several important positive feedback mechanisms involved in neurogenic inflammation. For example, SP released from vanilloid-sensitive nerves activates mast cells. Mast cells liberate histamine, which, in turn, stimulates vanilloid-sensitive nerves to release more SP. It is easy to visualize how the defunctionalization of sensory nerves by vanilloids may prevent, or at least ameliorate, neurogenic inflammatory symptoms. Often incitant avoidance and/or injection neutralizing doses will turn off the incident dose reaction.

Among irritant compounds acting on primary sensory neurons, capsaicin and related vanilloids are unique in that initial stimulation by vanilloid triggers (i.e., solvents, pesticides, other toxics) is followed by a fasting refractory period traditionally termed desensitization.[247–251]

This refractory state in which neurons do not respond to vanilloid triggers are then resistant to various known temperature and mechanism sensitivities, to substances such as xylene and mustard oil, and endogenous substances such as histamine, capsaicin, bradykinin, and serotonin. It is clear that desensitization to vanilloid triggering mechanisms is a well-defined biochemical process, rather a cascade of events. The relative contributions of variability depending upon the dose of the triggering agent cause the injection neutralizing dose for symptoms and wheals seen in the injection provocation neutralizing technique used in this book.

DESENSITIZATION

For didactic reasons, we will distinguish below receptor "desensitization" and "tachyphylaxis" from "impairment of neuronal functions." Both desensitization and tachyphylaxis occur at the receptor level. By desensitization, we mean a rapid loss of activity of the receptor occupied by an agonist. For example, in the continuous presence of capsaicin, histamine- or serotonin-elicited currents quickly fade. However, the neutralization dose of capsaicin or the other two can be used to quell some cases of chemical sensitivity. We use these three as rescue antigens to immediately turn off a nonspecific reaction.

1. *Desensitization:* Desensitization of VRs probably reflects an agonist-induced conformational change in receptor protein, which ultimately leads to the closing of the channel pore. This condition occurs repeatedly in chemically sensitive patients. It is notable, however, that capsaicin may elicit not one but multiple currents that differ in desensitization kinetics.[252,253] It might also be relevant to desensitization that (3H)RTX (resiniferatoxin) binding shows an unusual dissociation kinetics that depends on fractional receptor occupancy.[254] If only a small percentage (10% or less) of specific RTX binding sites are occupied, dissociation follows first-order kinetics.[254] With increasing receptor occupancy, the release becomes multiphasic and progressively more receptors bind RTX in an irreversible manner.[254] This optimum dose neutralization therapy in chemically sensitive patients works rapidly but also leads to tachyphylaxis.

2. *Tachyphylaxis:* Tachyphylaxis represents gradually diminishing response to repeated agonist administrations over a period of time. This leads to permanent desensitization. As follows from the above definition, tachyphylaxis is selective to a subsequent vanilloid challenge and does not prevent neurons from responding to other stimuli. Impaired neurons do not respond to various stimuli regardless of whether or not those stimuli target VRs. Impairment of neuronal functions by vanilloids is often referred to as defunctionalization of vanilloid-sensitive neurons.[240] It is imperative to understand that both tachyphylaxis and impairment are reversible and thus should be clearly distinguished from gross neurotoxicity, an irreversible process. This process is often confused by some optimization physicians who do not understand this slow process (i.e., polio, end-stage neuroparalysis).

   According to a current electrophysiological model, VRs cycle between closed (resting) and open (active) states via numerous nonconducting intermediate states.[252] Consequently, tachyphylaxis can be viewed as the rate of recovery of VRs from the intermediate states to the resting state, when receptors can be activated again by agonist binding. This cycle probably occurs via conformational changes in the receptor protein. As we saw above, extracellular calcium may play a crucial role in regulating such conformational changes leading to tachyphylaxis or the lack of it. In chemically sensitive patient who has been taking a neutralizing dose of antigens, we have seen permanent immunity last for years or even a lifetime. However, in many patients, it has to be reinforced. After several years, it has to be reinforced by another series of injections.[253,255]

   Piperine (the active principle in black pepper) and zingerone (the pyrolytic product of ginger oleoresin) evoke similar, rapidly activating currents. Both piperine and zingerone are pungent.[256]. Piperine and zingerone differ, however, in tachyphylaxis. Piperine-evoked currents show little tachyphylaxis upon repeated applications.[257] By contrast, zingerone-induced ion fluxes dissipate rapidly.[257] Thus, vanilloids differ not only in their relative activation of rapid versus slow currents, but also in their ability to shift the activated conductances into a state of tachyphylaxis. This variability explains the clinical observation that some substances can be neutralized while others cannot.

3. *Is Lasting Tachyphylaxis Possible Without Prior Excitation?* Of great importance is the question whether it is possible to synthesize nonirritant vanilloids capable of *lasting* "desensitization" in the sense originally used by Nicholas Jancsó. Generally speaking, to find such a vanilloid (that is a ligand that does not evoke action potentials but desensitizes VRs) one requires a compound that will slowly activate VRs while relatively rapidly inactivating (via increasing intracellular calcium levels) voltage-dependent Na^1 and Ca^2 channels. Olvanil,[258,259] SDZ 249-482,[260,261] and low-dose RTX[262,263] represent prototypes. Many substances can have lasting desensitization.

4. *Impairment of Neuronal Functions after Vanilloid Treatment:* Vanilloid-sensitive nerves include polymodal nociceptors detecting noxious heat and pressure[264,265] and expressing receptors for algesic and pro-inflammatory agents such as hydrogen ions, bradykinin, histamine, and serotonin, just to name a few.[266–268] It is easy to visualize how the well-known

depletion by vanilloid treatment of neurotransmitters[240,246] prevents the actions of agents stimulating sensory nerves.

Vanilloids release sensory neuropeptides via exocytosis and maybe also via the axon reflex.[269] What is the mechanism by which vanilloids prevent the restoration of neuropeptides? Capsaicin was shown to block the intra-axonal transport of macromolecules, including nerve growth factor (NGF).[270–272] There is an NGF-responsive element in the pre-protachykinin gene encoding SP and neurokinin A (NKA).[273] Thus, it is easy to visualize how capsaicin treatment can downregulate SP and NKA expression by depleting NGF from the perikarya of sensory neurons. Less clear is the mechanism by which vanilloid treatment depletes neuropeptides whose expression does not depend on the presence of NGF.

5. *Downregulation of VRs as a Mechanism of Long-Term Desensitization to Vanilloids Occurs*: There is a complete, dose-dependent loss of specific RTX (RTX activates transient VR, a capsaicin analogue) binding sites in trigeminal and dorsal root ganglia, spinal cord, as well as urinary bladder of the rat following systemic RTX treatment. [274–276] This receptor loss occurred later (24 hours) than the loss of the biological responses (protective eye-wiping and xylene-induced neurogenic inflammation responses disappeared by 6 hours after treatment) and required higher RTX doses.[274] The receptor loss in the spinal cord was entirely due to a reduction in the B_{max}. In the bladder of rats pretreated with 30 mg/kg RTX, approximately at a concentration of the EC50 for the loss of binding sites in the spinal cord, both receptor binding and the neurogenic inflammatory responses recovered almost completely within 2 months after treatment.[275] By contrast, no recovery of specific [3H]RTX binding to spinal cord membranes was observed.[275] These findings suggest that VR loss after RTX treatment can be either reversible reflecting desensitization or irreversible (indicating neurotoxicity), and that peripheral and central terminals of vanilloid-sensitive neurons have a differential sensitivity to these long-term vanilloid actions.

These studies confirm the findings we see with the intradermal provocation neutralization treatment in our clinics in chemically sensitive patients. Thus, with the interdermal provocative neutralization technique, both immune and nonimmune treatment dose help chemically sensitive patients to recover.

According to Pischinger,[1] Perger and Heine[111] the injection needle puncture works in two ways (immune and nonimmune) by causing a lasting effect (5 days[111]). This can be the reason for the rotary diet used by environmental physicians for food. We have observed that the effects of treatment with specific subcutaneous neutralizing optimum dose injections for specific foods, chemicals, and biological inhalants last from 3 to 5 days on the average chemically sensitive patient. This time frame is usually our starting frequency for injection therapy as with the avoidance program to reduce total body load. Environmental treatment is very efficacious. According to Heine,[105] once the needle is plunged into the subcutaneous tissue, both specific, that is, perfumes, ethanol or phenol and nonspecific information stabilizing the neutralizing system and stabilizing homeostasis is perceived locally and distally (i.e., as we have observed, specifically, i.e., cane sugar, beef optimum neutralization dose information is sent locally and distally due to the needle injury [nonspecific acupuncture effect] itself and the specific "turn off" optimum dose of the sugar, beef, ethanol, phenol, etc. antigen [specific]). The body's propensity to normalize the dynamics of homeostasis recognizes that this specific dose of cane sugar, beef, ethanol, and so on, is appropriate or the cue for normalization, and thus, the body goes directly to the neutralization process both locally and distally. The responses to the optimum dose antigen are initially temporary lasting for several hours but at times with repeated injections (4–9 days) lasting desensitization usually occurs. These responses are initially nonimmunological through the ground regulation and VR system, though eventually secondary immunological and tachyphylaxis (long-term desensitization) effects probably occur. For example, Heine[105] has shown that the monocyte factor regulates the amount of leukocytolysis by increasing the amount of physiologic white cell lysis and downregulating receptors and the immune system. He has also shown that certain doses of the monocytic factor will stop the lysis of white blood cells and that monocytes and thus macrophages will then increase responding to the specific environmental stimuli. We have seen patients who had low lymphocytes before the specific food, biological inhalant, or chemical neutralization drops or shots were given, and these cells returned to normal after a period of these specific neutralizing (optimum dose) injections. It appears that the final immune modulation that occurs from injection therapy is a secondary process, with the electrical modulation of the ground regulation system being primary. One has to realize that the communication of the ECM and thus the ground regulation system into the cell is quite complicated but now understood.

Optimum-dose subcutaneous injection and sublingual therapy appear to be information inducers of the dynamics of homeostasis through the ground regulation system. Pischinger[40] demonstrated that a skin puncture affects the perimuscular tissue, the rest of the ECM, and the autonomic nerves. At the EHC-Dallas and Buffalo, we demonstrated this observation clinically in numerous chemically sensitive patients whose vascular responses to intradermal and subcutaneous neutralization treatment resulted in their extremities rapidly turning from blue to normal color. Their pain syndrome stopped instantly similar to the data on the desensitization dose in animals and at times depression and inability to talk was seen within a few minutes after the injection of the neutralizing dose of the specific offending antigen. Peak pulmonary flows usually return to control levels (Table 6.23).

According to Heine,[105] once the needle (i.e., containing the neutralizing dose of beef or cane sugar or ethanol/perfume, etc.) is plunged into the subcutaneous tissue, both specific and nonspecific responses to the information inserted occur. This information is gathered locally with a resulting response occurring in the area. The information is also sent distally to the central homeostatic mechanism where there is an acupuncture response (nonspecific) and a beef, cane sugar, phenol, ethanol, perfume newsprint, diesel, jet fuel neutralization optimum dose response (specific). The body's propensity to homeostasis recognizes that the specific neutralizing dose of the cane sugar, beef, perfume, and so on, is a "good treatment" for the malfunctioning connective tissue matrix and VRs. Therefore, normalization of the dynamics of homeostasis rapidly occurs. As one can see, these doses have to be electrically mediated because of their speed of response even though immunological and nonimmunological effects eventually occur. These electrical changes have been demonstrated by Wilson[277] using a skin galvanometer, and occur faster than biochemical or immunological reactions. It has been observed, at times, that the symptom and sign neutralization occurs instantly as the needle is being pulled out when the exact neutralizing dose of a specific antigen is used.

The intradermal provocation optimum dose neutralization procedure has proven very efficacious in the average chemically sensitive patient. However, initially 30% of the patients cannot wheal, apparently due to skin allergy to the specific antigen and specific receptor resistance or the weight of the total body pollutant load not only locally but also on the hypothalamus, reticular system, activating pineal gland, area postrema of the 4th ventricle, and limbic systems. These patients must have a longer period of avoidance of pollutants in air, food, and water as well as more sauna therapy and nutrition. Eventually as their load reduces, more than 90% will be able to be neutralized by the intradermal technique. Many that cannot, may have receptor heterogeny which will not allow desensitization.

Pischinger[13] and Heine[10] have shown that, at times, one can see a complete paralysis of the ground regulation system with an overreaction of one part of the immune system suggesting that one would not get skin whealing and neutralization response in these particular patients. This appears to be true in the CS patient who cannot wheal and therefore, cannot neutralize. It has also been shown that some vanilloids can desensitize some receptors but not others.

TABLE 6.23

A 55-Year-Old White Female Cortisone-Dependent (60 mg/day) for 2 Years Prior to Admission: Rapidly Deteriorating

	Optimum Dose Incitant	Preinjection	Peak Flow (L.P.M)	During Intradermal Challenge	Peak Flow after N.D.++	Amount cc/#	Signs and Symptoms that Cleared with N.D.
	Peak Flow with Injection Provocation and Neutralization						
+	(1) Fluogen® (8-31-87)	370	360	280	370	0.10/6	Extreme wheezing
+	(2) Fluogen® (10-22-87)	380	360		380	0.10/6	Cough, phlegm
+	(3) Fuogen® (10-28-87)	370	340	350	370	0.10/6	Cough, wheeze, sleep disorders
+	(1) Histamine (6-19-87)	310	260	290	310	0.10/7	Cough, wheeze
+	(2) Histamine (6-24-87)	360	330	340	350	0.20/7	Cough, wheeze
*	(3) Histamine (7-8-87)	200	160	160	140	non.d	Severe cough, wheezing, did not clear
**	Serotonin	260	280	360	380	0.10/4	Cough, throat itch, headache
+	Corn	330	260	380	300	0.10/4	Severe cough, wheeze
+	C. milk	400	360	380	410	0.05/1	Severe cough, wheeze
+	Eggs	390	340	350	380	0.05/1	Severe cough, wheeze
+	Mixed respiratory vaccine	400	370		410	0.10/4	
+	Wheat	330	300		350	0.20/3	Cough, wheeze, phlegm
+	Beef	350	320		330	0.10/3	Cough, scratch, headache, sleep
+	Turkey	360	320		370	0.15/2	Cough, scratch
+	Potato	350	330		350	0.02/2	Wheezing, cough, scratch, phlegm
+	Cauliflower	390		400	400	0.02/2	Cough, phlegm
XXX	Carbocaine	390		400	400	0.05/2	Throat tight
XXX	Banana	360	360	340	370	0.05/3	Throat itch
XXX	Orange	360	340		370	0.05/2	Throat itch
**	Onion	350	360		350	0.05/2	Throat itch
XXX	Turnip	340	330	310	320	0.10/2	Cough, throat itch
XXX	Spinach	360	340	320	340	0.05/1	Cough, throat itch
XXX	Green peas	350	330		349	0.05/1	Cough, throat itch
XXX	Peach	340	340	350	360	0.10/2	Cough, throat itch
XXX	Avocado	360	360	330	340	0.05/2	Throat itch
XXX	Grapefruit	370	350	330	360	0.05/4	Throat itch
XXX	Baker's yeast	340	350		360	0.05/4	Throat itch
XXX	Pork	390	390		400	0.10/2	Throat itch
XXX	Mold mix (1)	390	420		400	0.05/3	Phlegm, finger joint pain, throat itch
XXX	Mold mix (2)	350	350		360	0.05/.3	Throat itch, headache, eye itch

(*Continued*)

TABLE 6.23 (*Continued*)

A 55-Year-Old White Female Cortisone-Dependent (60 mg/day) for 2 Years Prior to Admission: Rapidly Deteriorating

	Optimum Dose Incitant	Preinjection	Peak Flow (L.P.M)	During Intradermal Challenge	Peak Flow after N.D.++	Amount cc/#	Signs and Symptoms that Cleared with N.D.
XXX	Mold mix (3)	360	350		370	0.05/3	Nose itch, throat scratches, burns
XXX	Mold mix (4)	350	350		400	0.05/3	Nose itch, throat scratches, burns
XXX	*Rhizopus*	350	400		400	0.05/3	Nose itch, throat scratches, burns
XXX	*Sporobolomyces*	400	400		400	0.05/3	Nose itch, throat scratch, burns
XXX	*Mycetes*		420		420	0.05/4	Nose itch, throat scratch, burns
XXX	Trichoderma	380	400		360	0.05/4	Nose itch, throat scratch, burns, headache
XXX	T.O.E.	410	430		420	0.05/4	Nose itch, throat scratch, burns, headache
XXX	Dust	370	340		360	0.05/3	Nose itch, throat scratch, burns, headache
XXX	Dust mite	360	350		330	0.05/3	Cough, phlegm, nose itch, throat scratch, burns, headache
–	Snow peas	360	360		360	No reaction	No reaction
–	Okra	390	400		400	No reaction	No reaction
–	Tylenol	400	400		360	No reaction	No reaction

Source: Adapted from Environmental Health Center-Dallas, 2015.

Note: Fasted in hospital for 5 days and total load decreased, bronchial peak flow increased from 0 on admission to 400 at the end of the fast.

Oral challenge showed patient sensitive to the above foods.

Blind injection challenge confirmed food sensitivities and showed other sensitivities. Note the varied response with change in peak flows upon intradermal provocation and neutralization.

Follow-up: Patient asymptomatic without medication using injections, rotary diet, and environmental control; totally symptom- and medication-free 4 years following treatment.

* Impossible to neutralize symptoms.

** Flow low before provocation from unknown cause; flow increased with N.D. signs cleared.

+ Significant drop in flow with increase with N.D. and signs cleared.

++N.D. Indicates neutralizing dose.

XXX Mild flow changes and sign reproduction or just symptom reproduction cleared with N.D.

CLINICAL STUDIES

The results of our provocation and neutralization studies are summarized in Tables 6.24 through 6.26 and Figure 6.44. In our first study Table 6.24, grossly obvious signs and symptoms such as tetany and severe muscle spasm were seen; the second double-blind study (Table 6.25) focused on

TABLE 6.24

Grossly Obvious Signs—Tetany (Food Triggered)

Short-term (unit)

    Signs and symptoms of patients neutralized:

      5 totally, 1 partially

    New food neutralized (6 patients initially) 175/251 (70%)

    Long-term (1 year)

      Same as above

Source: Adapted from Environmental Health Center-Dallas, 1986.

Note: ECU condition after 5 days deadaptation with the total load (burden) reduced. Intradermal neutralization following oral food challenge adds proof of neutralization with elimination of the tetany.

vasculitis and showed improvement of signs with neutralization. The third study (Table 6.26) identified pulmonary measures for a typical objective study.

As previously discussed, Pischinger[13] demonstrated that the peripheral sensory nerve, dorsal root ganglia of the sensory spinal, and so on, were sensitized, and also that a skin puncture affects the perivascular tissue, the ECM, and the autonomic nerves of the connective tissue. Jansco et al.[278] followed by Szallasi et al.[274] demonstrated in animals that the specific antigens will give short- and long-term desensitization. At the EHC-Dallas, we have confirmed this observation in numerous chemically sensitive patients whose vascular responses to intradermal and subcutaneous neutralization treatment resulted in their extremities rapidly turning from blue to normal color. We saw others, whose autonomic effects changed, for example, from sweating to nonsweating (vice versa), tachycardia to normal sinus rhythm, or vice versa. We were also able to measure the autonomic effect objectively by using the iris corder (pupillography for measurement of autonomic function) through the eyes (see Figure 6.30 and Chapter 27 of Rea, W. J., Chemical Sensitivity, Volume III[3]).

In addition, we often have observed the distal communication from the subcutaneous treatment injection site to distal organs. Similarly, we have provoked distal signs and symptoms after intradermal provocation injection (Figures 6.45 and 6.46).

We have shown after millions of injections that our patients respond similarly to those of Pischinger[13] and Heine,[27] and Jansco[278] who had ground regulation system and central homeostatic changes. The changes in the dynamics of the homeostatic mechanism respond generally, specifically, locally, and distally.

As our patients do, most of Pischinger's patients had local reactions in the form of wheals, followed by distal reactions, which could be triggered by many chemicals, food and biological inhalants. These patients were also, specifically, very sensitive to a few chemicals.

The ground regulation system also regulated edema,[274,279–281] and we have provoked and eliminated edema by both intradermal provocation and subcutaneous treatment.

Other needle injury phenomena that alter skin puncture reactions can occur. For example, numerous authors have shown that there is a difference between the needle and tissue, which causes tissue alterations resulting in electrical changes.[13,280,282,283] More importantly, Bethe[284] has measured an electrical potential difference between the needle and the tissue that several other investigators[285–290] suggest could cause informational changes both locally and distally once the ground regulation system is set in motion. Thus, subcutaneous neutralization (optimum doses) injections as used at the EHC-Dallas, Buffalo, and around the United States, would then send both specific and nonspecific information rapidly through the ground regulation system throughout the body. A photon emission from injured or dying cells reaches neighboring cells in 10^{-7} seconds and spreads throughout

TABLE 6.25

Elimination of Oral Food Challenge Reaction by Injections of the Appropriate Dilution of Food Extracts

Double Blind Using Saline Negatives (Placebos) Laboratory Data (Blood)

Patient No./ Age-yr./Sex	Admitting Chief N.D.[a] complaints	T-lymphocyte/ mm[e]	B-Cell Count/ mm^3	Complement -mg dL C3	C4	Total IgE IU/ mL	Food Tested	cc/1
1/27/F	Eczema, diarrhea	879	614	105	50	72	Chicken	0.20/1
2/39/M	Myalgia, arthralgia	994	795	145	20	241	Wheat	0.10/1
3/54/M	Rhinitis, fatigue	894	825	66	29	3	Wheat	0.10/1
4/46/M	Optic neuritis	841	308	50	24	2	Potato	0/10/3
5/27/F	Vasculitis optic neuritis	1688	9658	90	40	260	Beef	0.05/2
6/30/F	Dermatitis, arthritis	2707	1517	96	26	3	Corn	0.05/2
7/20/F	Headache, myalgia	743	726	154	38	5	Beef	0.25/1
8/69/F	Myalgia, fatigue	1026	595	66	36	63	Milk	0.06/3
9/24/F	Headache, mental dysfunction	1633	806	–	–	9	Beef	0.20/3
10/25/F	Asthma, headache	1522	680	78	36	64	Wheat	0.10/1
11/41/F	Headache, irritable bowel	522	696	48	70	4	Egg	0.10/1
12/49/F	Headache, myalgia	1169	662	112	50	0.7	Wheat	0.20/1
13/26/M	Fatigue, headache, Rhinitis	864	367	76	47	25	Milk	0.05/3
14/35/F	Myalgia, arthritis	401	366	16	81	633	White potato	0.25/1
15/42/M	Arthritis, diarrhea Mental dysfunction	531	307	164	37	16	Pork	0.15/2
16/25/F	Arthritis	414	175	78	26	28	Com	0.006/3
17/26/M	Irritable bowel	1012	792	–	–	264	Milk	0.05/2
18/44/F	Arthritis, psoriasis, Spogren's syndrome	2010	624	80	18	59	Chicken	0.25/1
19/33/M	Arthritis, myositis, Mental dysfunction	1004	469	–	–	264	Lamb	0.15/2
20/35/F	Seizure disorder, Irritable bowel	858	281	74	–	1	Beef	0.25/1

Source: Adapted from Environmental Health Center-Dallas, 1988.

[a] N.D. indicates neutralizing dose.

the entire organism with the speed of sound. Therefore, a rapid communication system is already available for dissemination of treatment information.[291] These observations explain the effect seen in literally thousands of patients at the EHC-Dallas and Buffalo: When the dose is correct, symptoms and signs neutralization begins the moment the needle is removed, and often all signs and symptoms disappear within 10–30 minutes. Pischinger[13] has actually shown that one can test the individual defense states of patients by doing a venous puncture and measuring cytolysis, venous O_2, skin polarization, thermoregulatory changes, and length of time the reaction symptoms occur after puncture. Figures 6.47 and 6.48 present data that demonstrate the presence of this phenomenon in different diseases, for example, asthma, which could be due to chemical sensitivity.

TABLE 6.26

Effective Rate of 30 Patients with Ragweed Booster Intradermal Neutralization

1978	Effective			Titration End Point (cc/##) for Year-Round Build-Up Dose									
Sex	Age	No.	%	0.05/1	0.05/2	0.05/3	0.05/4	0.05/5	0.05/6	0.05/7	0.05/8	0.05/9	0.05/10	0.05/11
M: 5	Range: 21	26	87	2(7)[a]	3(10)	6(20)	3(10)	4(13)	2(7)	5(17)	2(7)	1(3)	1(3)	1(3)
F: 25	to 70 yr.													
	Mean													
	48.7 yr.													

1979		Symptom and Sign Relieving		Neutralization Dose (cc/#) for In-Season Daily Multiple Doses				
0.10/1	**0.15/1**	**0.10/2**	**0.15/2**	**0.20/2**	**0.05/3**	**0.10/3**	**0.15/3**	**0.05/4**
1(3)	1(3)	1(3)	1(3)	1(3)	1(3)	1(3)	1(3)	1(3)
0.05/5	**0.10/5**	**0.15/5**	**0.05/6**	**0.05/7**	**0.15/7**	**0.05/8**	**0.05/9**	**0.15/10**
2(7)	1(3)	1(3)	2.(7)	4(13)	1(3)	2(7)	1(3)	1(3)

Symptoms Triggered

Nervous system:	5(17)
Gastrointestinal;	2(7)
Skin:	1(3)
Respiratory system:	2(7)
Musculoskeletal system:	2(7)

Period (Season)			Total Dose (cc)		
Range: 1- 10	Mean	4	Range : 10-1040	Mean	(per patient): 147

Source: Environmental Health Center-Dallas, 1995.

[a] Percentage in parentheses.

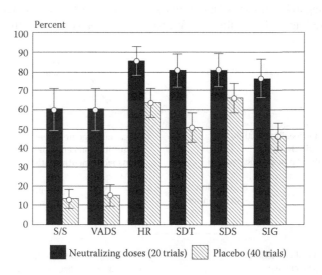

Neutralizing doses (20 trials)   Placebo (40 trials)

FIGURE 6.44 Elimination of reactions induced by oral food challenge and injection therapy. Neutralization is notably more effective than placebo in reducing the symptoms of food sensitivity after oral challenge. Double-blind injection. S/S signs and symptoms ($p < 0.001$); VADS, visual analog discomfort rating scale ($p < 0.001$); HR, heart rate ($p < 0.05$); SDT, Aaron Smith symbol digit modalities test ($p < 0.01$); SDS, symbol digit modalities subtest ($p < 0.05$); SIG, subjects' signature ($p < 0.001$).

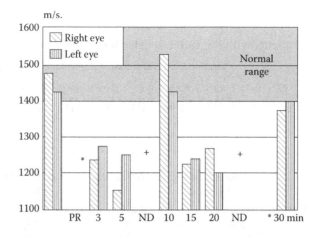

FIGURE 6.45 Cigarette smoke provocation (0.05 mL, #5). (Environmental Health Center-Dallas.)

The defense state reaction in healthy individuals corresponds to the alarm reaction Selye[292] identified in 1973 (Rea W. J., Chemical Sensitivity, Volume I, Chapter 3[293]). A stimulus of this needle puncture size is completely adjusted out within 3–4 hours. There are levels of response in chemically sensitive patients. The milder cases correspond to Selye's pattern.[292] However, the more severe chemically sensitive patients take up to 4 days to clear. We have refined Pischinger's[13] observations by taking a 25-gauge needle and creating a 7-mm wheal in the intradermis using the Lee[294] and Miller[223] provocation neutralization method. The normal individual will absorb this wheal in 10 minutes and have no distal reaction. Chemically sensitive patients will have a greater wheal in 10 minutes if he is particularly sensitive to that specific substance, that is, formaldehyde, phenol, but often the patient will also exhibit distal signs and symptoms, for example, headache, rhinitis, and/ or tachycardia. Many of the signs and symptoms can be cleared with the exact dilution neutralizing (optimum dose) dose of the incitant which will be a 1/5, 1/25, 1/125/625, and so on, of the specific substance according to Pischinger's[13] and Heine's[277] specific reaction and water memory principles. However, the more fragile chemically sensitive patient will not wheal but will give distal symptoms

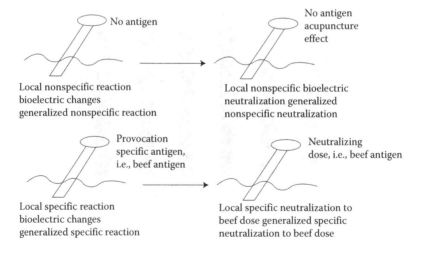

FIGURE 6.46 The local and generalized effects of nonspecific injection therapy by needle injury and specific antigen injection therapy by a specific incitant on chemically sensitive patients. (Environmental Health Center-Dallas.)

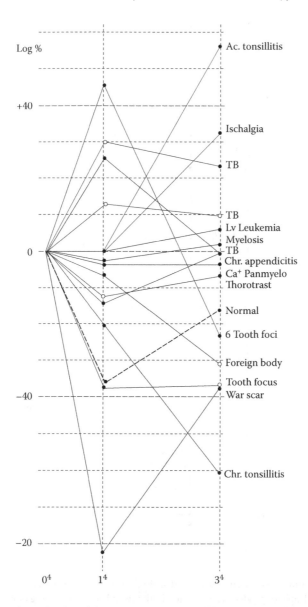

FIGURE 6.47 Types of reaction in a 3-hour stress test after taking 5 mL blood from the cubital vein. All initial values are entered as 0, and the deviations in the succeeding hours as + or − values in mg % iodine, utilization. Abscissa: time after taking blood in hours. (From Perger, F. 1991. *Matrix and Matrix Regulation: Basis for a Holistic Theory in Medicine*, A. Pischinger, Ed., H. Heiner, Eng. Trans. N. Mac Lean, p. 134, Brussels, Belgium: Editions Haug International. With permission.)

and signs that will not clear for hours to days. When this later phenomenon occurs, chemically sensitive patient's defense state is severely damaged with very retarded homeostasis. This patient cannot be neutralized and intravenous nutrient therapy with long periods of avoidance of pollutants and sauna therapy is often required before the whealing and neutralizing phenomenon is restored. In some cases, it is never restored.

Injection provocation neutralization and subcutaneous treatment exhibit bioelectrical changes similar to those shown by Pischinger.[1] Pischinger found that the bioelectrical phenomena occurring after a skin puncture were significant for the orientation of the defense state of the ground regulation system.[295] This orientation is certainly what appears to happen with the proper neutralization

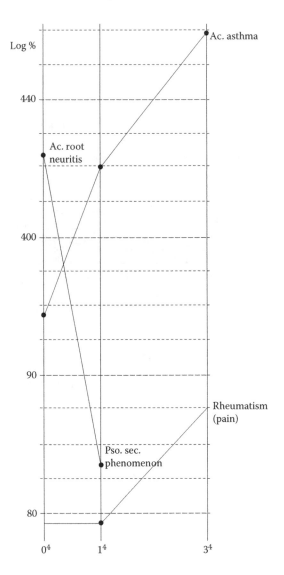

FIGURE 6.48 Puncture effect. Acute attacks of asthma or ischias are initiated with the increase in IUV. Scar infiltration with Impletol produces a reduction in the raised IUV and easing of pain in acute root neuritis (secondary phenomenon). (From Perger, F. 1991. *Matrix and Matrix Regulation: Basis for a Holistic Theory in Medicine*, A. Pischinger, Ed., H. Heine, Eng Trans. N. Mac Lean, p. 135. Brussels, Belgium: Editions Haug International. With permission.)

dose of a specific (i.e., corn or mycotoxin) or nonspecific (i.e., needle puncture such as histamine, capsaicin, or serotonin) to the VRs antigen, as seen in the chemically sensitive patients.

Many authors have measured and described the changes in skin polarization from injection.[285,295–297] Pischinger has also shown that every reaction in the ground regulation system takes place in a borderline area between alteration of biophysics and biochemistry. For example, changes in oxygen consumption, calcium, magnesium, and monocytic factor take their course more rapidly and with more sensitivity than enzyme-controlled, biochemical processes that occur.

These observations would correlate with ours and many other environmental medicine specialists such as Miller,[223] Waikman (Waikman, F. J. 1990, personal communication), Morris,[298] Brown (Brown, D. 1985, personal communication), and so on, who have found that intradermal or even sublingual provocation and neutralization occur more rapidly than biochemical or immunological reactions. Perger and Heine[297] also emphasize that each exogenous stimulus not only triggers a cellular and humoral reaction but also is always accompanied by alteration in the biopotential. This phenomenon appears to occur in chemically sensitive patients after an injection.

Injection therapy appears to regulate many substances caught in the ECM, and the matrix's unique molecular anatomy and physiology, which allows provocation neutralization therapy to be effective. The ground substance matrix is made up of PG and GAG (glucosamines, hexoseamines, D-glucosamine, D-galactosamine, hyaluronic acids, heparin, chondroitin sulfates, dermato-sulfates, and keratin sulfates). These substances are negatively charged linear carbohydrate chains that respond electrophysically and electrochemically. The PGs are sugar–protein biopolymers interspersed with water, which in itself experiences energy, have memory and bioelectric properties, and can thus be a vehicle to communicate with the rest of the body. Stabilization of this anatomical makeup of water interspersed between amino sugar molecules is through binding to a protein backbone that is bound to hyaluronic acid via binding proteins.[299] These PGs also bind to the glycocalyx of the cell membrane, allowing for communication from the extracellular fluid to the cell membrane and through it. Therefore, intradermal and subcutaneous neutralization injections not only may stabilize disordered water but also will rapidly communicate with cells via this ground regulation system.

Another fact that is essential in understanding injection neutralization therapy is that the extracellular fibroblast–macrophage system is an integral part of the ground regulation system. Thus, this system can be influenced by injection therapy by changing its configuration. Fibroblasts are able to react to a situation in seconds, with a quantitatively and qualitatively appropriate synthesis of PGs and structural glycoproteins. Macrophages in a normal situation can break down the ECM by phagocytosis, after the release of proteases, hydrolases, and so on, although they are slower when a chronic stimulus persists. However, since fibroblasts are unable to differentiate between the "good" and "bad" stimuli in a chronic stimulating noxious stimuli overload situation, such as in chemical or EMF sensitivity, they continue to produce PGs. Therefore, any stimuli will trigger the fibroblasts to turn out PGs until something, such as injection therapy with the proper neutralizing dose signal is given triggering an electrical switch, which will slow their production, allowing phagocytosis to eat up and thus, balance the system eventually turning the fibroblasts off completely. The phagocytes take out as many PGs as the fibroblasts put in, thus restoring the balance of the local homeodynamics of the area, as well as the distal tissues.

The result of chronic pollutant stimulation is chronic alteration of the ECM, whose structure then is not physiological but becomes pathological. When this pathological situation occurs, the extracellular fibroblast–macrophage system, due to its influence on all cellular elements, makes an important contribution to the development of chronic disease such as chemical sensitivity.[10]

MESSENGER PLASTICITY BY VANILLOIDS AS A NOVEL MECHANISM OF ANALGESIA

Early reports indicated a nondiscriminative depletion of sensory neuropeptides in the rat following systemic capsaicin treatment.[246] Most authorities agreed that this loss of neuropeptides might play a central role in desensitization to capsaicin.[240,246] Nevertheless, there has always been a lingering doubt as to what degree this depletion of neuropeptides reflects desensitization as opposed to possible neurotoxicity. Capsaicin activates a variety of autonomic reflexes.[246,300] Consequences include, but are not limited to, a severe depression of respiration, which was first noted by Toh and coworkers in 1955.[301] These acute responses severely limit the initial dose of capsaicin that can be given for desensitization. For instance, Gamse and coworkers noted in 1980 that rats given 50 mg/kg capsaicin subsequently needed manually assisted respiration for up to 5 minutes to survive the severe impairment in respiration. To circumvent this problem (and to achieve lasting desensitization), capsaicin needs to be given repeatedly in increasing doses, taking advantage of the tachyphylaxis as it develops. Although Jancsó and colleagues showed as early as 1961 that 4, 8, and finally 15 mg of capsaicin administered to adult rats (~80 mg/kg s.c.) over a period of 1–3 days is sufficient to render the animals fully insensitive to chemically evoked pain for 1–3 months, later studies adopted a more aggressive treatment protocol, which included 950 mg/kg capsaicin given s.c. over a period of 5 days.[302,303] Such high doses, of course, enhance the possibility for toxicity. In fact, using this protocol, a loss of dorsal root ganglion (DRG) neurons in adult rats was demonstrated.[304] We at the EHC-Dallas have used intradermal capsaicin neutralization for the nonspecific reactions especially pain syndrome for 10 years. The injections of the neutralizing dose in susceptible individuals can be given up to every 4 hours. These injections work with selected individuals.

Severing the peripheral fibers, for example, by axotomy, leads to dramatic changes in the expression of neuropeptides and their receptors in primary sensory neurons, including those sensitive to vanilloids.[305,306] Certain neuropeptides are upregulated, whereas other peptides, by contrast, are downregulated. It was suggested that those neuropeptides that are upregulated promote the survival and/or regeneration of neurons.[306] Coca et al.[307] advocated sympathectomy for some chemically sensitive patients. However, it was seen to have mixed unpredictable results and was abandoned. We actually have seen the onset of arrhythmia with chemical sensitivity in some postsympathectomy patients. These neuropeptides have been called injury peptides.[305] The best studied of these injury peptides is galanin. Galanin administered intrathecally has a clear analgesic effect in mice in both the tail-flick and hot-plate tests.[308] As first noted by Hökfelt and coworkers in 1987, galanin is upregulated in DRG neurons after their peripheral axons have been severed. In these axotomized animals, the galanin receptor antagonist M35 potentiates the facilitation of the flexor reflex, a neurophysiological equivalent of pain sensation.[309] Taken together, these findings suggest that galanin acts as an endogenous analgesic compound to counteract neuropathic pain evoked by nerve injury. Contrasting to this model, galanin was found to induce membrane depolarizations in DRG neurons in culture.[310] DRG neurons express both known classes of galanin receptors, referred to as GAL-R1[311] and GAL-R2,[312,313] respectively. However, the expression of both GAL-R1 and GAL-R2 is downregulated following axotomy,[313,314] which might protect DRG neurons from an exaggerated feedback response.

Most neuropeptides known to disappear from neurons with axotomy are thought to be involved in chemical neurotransmission. These changes in peptides and receptors are collectively referred to as messenger plasticity.[306] Messenger plasticity has attracted much publicity lately as a likely mechanism underlying the poor efficacy of opiates to relieve neuropathic pain: Cholecystokinin (CCK) upregulated by nerve injury is believed to act as an endogenous antiopiate.[315] Messenger plasticity also explains why SP antagonists are ineffective in axotomized animals (SP is downregulated), whereas vasointestinal polypeptide (VIP) antagonists gain therapeutic value (VIP is upregulated).[316]

Mechanisms underlying the upregulation of injury peptides are poorly understood; however, there is a striking parallel between the induction of c-Jun and the upregulation of galanin in rat DRG neurons following axotomy,[317] implying a role for immediate-early genes.[318-320]

By means of a single, well-tolerated injection of RTX, a complete, long-lasting desensitization against chemogenic pain,[262,321] noxious heat,[322] and neurogenic inflammation[275,321] can be achieved. Using this treatment protocol, RTX-treated rats show changes in neuropeptide, in neuropeptide receptor, and in nitric oxide synthase (NOS) expression very similar to those described in rats with axotomy.[245,322] For example, the expression of the neuropeptides galanin and VIP,[323,324] the neuropeptide receptor CCKB-R, as well as the enzyme NOS[323] are markedly enhanced. These changes are fully reversible. Other neuropeptides, for instance SP, are depleted.[245] This change in SP expression is also reversible and is due to a decrease in the steady-state levels of total mRNAs encoding SP.[325] Importantly, the number of DRG neurons showing an in situ hybridization signal for mRNAs encoding SP is not reduced.[325] Finally, there are neuropeptides that do not show changes in expression following RTX treatment. CGRP and somatostatin are notable examples of this phenomenon.[325] However, the regulation of neuropeptide expression by RTX seems to be very complex. For example, RTX dramatically upregulates CGRP expression in DRG neurons obtained from mouse embryos.[326]

However, RTX when given repeatedly in a capsaicin-like treatment protocol depletes CGRP-like immunoreactivity from DRG neurons.[327] The finding that single, moderate doses of RTX have a differential effect on neuropeptide expression compared with high, cumulative RTX doses represents a powerful argument that depletion of neuropeptides by high vanilloid doses reflects neurotoxicity rather than desensitization.

Despite the striking similarities between vanilloid and axotomy-induced changes in the expression of neuropeptides, there is an essential difference in the behavior of animals: Whereas mechanical nerve injury usually results in the development of neuropathic pain (as most dramatically demonstrated by autotomy behavior), vanilloids, by sharp contrast, have a clear analgesic action.[322] Spinal cord injury leads to allodynia-like behavior to cold stimuli.[328] RTX treatment abolishes this behavior.[329] Moreover, RTX induces a long-lasting analgesic action on the hot-plate test, as well as a transient hypoalgesia to mechanical stimuli.[328] This is surprising because capsaicin when given to adult rats fails to achieve similar changes.[330-332]

It has long been known that trains of equal stimuli to the sural nerve evoke contractions of increasing strength in the hamstring muscles.[306] This phenomenon is called facilitation of the flexor reflex (also known as the wind-up phenomenon) and is believed to reflect spinal hyperexcitability as a consequence of C-fiber activation.[333] A causal relationship between spinal hyperexcitability and neuropathic pain has been postulated.[306] The wind-up phenomenon is greatly reduced in RTX-treated rats.[334] These RTX-treated animals show enhanced galanin expression both at the mRNA and the peptide levels.[323] The galanin receptor antagonist M35 restored the C-fiber-mediated hyperexcitability in the RTX-treated rats.[334] Furthermore, the decrease in galanin expression with increasing time after RTX administration was accompanied by a gradual restoration of heat sensitivity.[334] Taken together, these observations imply that upregulation of the inhibitory neuropeptide, galanin, plays a central role in the prolonged analgesic action of RTX.

As already mentioned, CCKB receptor expression is markedly upregulated in RTX-treated animals. The level of mRNAs encoding CCKA receptors is moderately increased. This is surprising for two reasons. First, enhanced CCKB receptor expression in rats with nerve injury is believed to contribute to the persistent, morphine-resistant pain that develops in such animals.[315] RTX-treated animals, however, show marked analgesia and not chronic pain.[262,334] Second, capsaicin treatment results in a marked loss of CCK binding sites, suggesting the downregulation of CCK receptors.[335] A potentially important difference between the effects of mechanical nerve injury and RTX treatment is that CCK is elevated in axotomized[336] but not in RTX-treated rats.[337] Thus, probably there is no agonist to occupy the extra CCKB receptors following RTX treatment. Another vanilloid effect not mimicked by axotomy is the loss of VRs.[322]

The differential regulation of CCKB receptor expression in capsaicin- and RTX-treated animals is not unprecedented. The most likely explanation is a dominating nonspecific neurotoxicity by capsaicin.

Calcium in Modulating VR Functions

For capsaicin, desensitization has been shown to depend on a variety of factors, including concentration, the duration of application, and the presence or absence of extracellular calcium.[240,338] Mechanisms underlying desensitization will be discussed later; here, we concentrate on the role of calcium only. Numerous studies have shown that the removal of extracellular calcium diminished desensitization to capsaicin.[252,339-343] It was speculated that a rise in intracellular calcium served as an initial step only to activate biochemical pathways ultimately leading to VR desensitization. This model was reinforced by the findings that (1) specific inhibitors of protein phosphatase 2A (also known as calcineurin) reduced desensitization,[344] and (2) removal of ATP or GTP from the internal solution resulted in a nearly complete tachyphylaxis even in the presence of calcium.[255] Recent evidence implies an even more complex situation. In addition to the above calcium-activated indirect pathways of tachyphylaxis, a direct action of calcium on VRs leading to desensitization is also likely to exist. For example, the *Xenopus* oocytes require the presence of extracellular calcium.[345] In the absence of extracellular calcium, VR1 shows little or no tachyphylaxis in response to repeated capsaicin challenges. In the presence of calcium, capsaicin-evoked currents via VR1 have two distinct components, one desensitizing and one relatively constant upon repeated agonist applications.[345] Thus, the calcium dependence of vanilloid desensitization can be reproduced without a neuronal context.

To complicate matters even further, the role of calcium in modulating desensitization to vanilloids is also dependent on the agonist used. In contrast to observations with capsaicin, desensitization to olvanil is apparently not influenced by the removal of extracellular calcium.[253] Under resting conditions, the channel pore of C-type receptors is closed. Agonist binding is likely to induce a conformational change in receptor protein leading to an opening of the conductance. According to a recent model by Simon, vanilloidated conductances cycle between open and closed states via various transitional states reflecting desensitization.[252] Tachyphylaxis can be viewed as the time required for the receptors to recover from these transitional states to the closed state in which the receptor is capable of ligand binding again. For capsaicin, Simon argues that calcium may increase the probability of a transition from the open state into a transitional, desensitized state. Alternatively, calcium may inhibit the recovery of the receptor from the desensitized states to the closed state. Either mechanism may explain how the removal of extracellular calcium can reduce desensitization to capsaicin. Simon speculates[252] that olvanil utilizes a different mechanism (maybe receptor internalization) to achieve desensitization, hence the indifference of desensitization to olvanil for calcium (Figure 6.49). Two and a half cases of capsaicin neutralization.

OTHER MECHANISMS ARE INVOLVED IN THE TREATMENT OF CHEMICAL SENSITIVITY

Thus, in early chemical sensitivity, intradermal and subcutaneous injections or sublingual therapy of specific elements with their "turn off" dilutions will help regulate this process and allow homeostasis to occur. Since the sugar polymers of the ECM are thus suitable for information transmission and storage due to their high water binding action exchange capacity,[10] intradermal neutralization would tap into this system and then both chemically and electrically transmit the information of the homeostatic dose for that substance. Once this neutralization homeostatic dose is introduced, the cell sugar surface film mediates information between the cell interior and the extracellular fluid.[346] (See the Introduction to Volume IV, Rea, W. J., *Chemical Sensitivity*.)

This sugar film provides cell-specific and organ-specific receptor coating of the cell, yielding a significant influence on its function and integrity. The glycocalyx sugars consist of branched oligosaccharides with terminal N-acetylneuraminic acid and branch into proteins and lipid (glycoproteins and lipids) of the cell membrane.[346] If the lipid layer of the membrane is not damaged by lipophilic toxic chemicals, we have seen intradermal injection neutralization occurs repeatedly with rapid improvement of the patient. If the membranes are too overloaded or severely damaged by the toxic chemical, however, the neutralization does not work. This probably is a toxic effect that is reversible with decreasing the total body load over time.

Ground Regulation System

Picshinger[13] and Heine[347] have shown that, at times, one can see a complete paralysis of the ground regulation system with an overreaction of the immune system. This phenomenon apparently occurs in some hypersensitive patients. More severe responses were observed in approximately 30% of the patients we initially saw at the EHC-Dallas. At the EHC-Dallas, we have observed that when patients in the environmentally controlled unit are pollutant overloaded, intradermal injection will trigger symptoms and signs. In the more sensitive patient, the injections do not wheal the skin, nor will they neutralize a patient's symptoms and signs as do the injection procedure in the other two-thirds of the less sensitive patients. They only produce symptoms and signs. Once the total

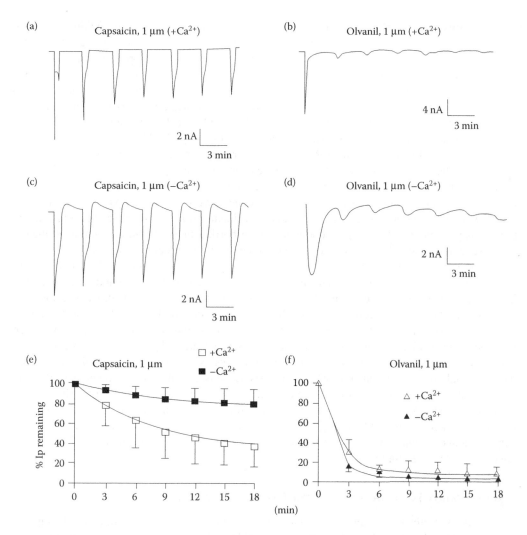

FIGURE 6.49   Tachyphylaxis of capsaicin- and olvanil-induced currents in rat trigeminal ganglion neurons in culture. Tachyphylaxis to olvanil is rapid (the second application evokes less than 20% of the control current) and does not require the presence of extracellular Ca^{2+}. By contrast, tachyphylaxis to capsaicin develops gradually (the 4th challenge still elicits a half-maximal response) and occurs in the presence of extracellular Ca^{2+} only. A possible interpretation of these findings is that capsaicin and olvanil employ different biochemical mechanisms to achieve tachyphylaxis. (Recordings are from Figures 1, 3, and 4 in Liu, L., S. A. Simon. 1998. The influence of removing extracellular Ca21 in the tachyphylaxis responses to capsaicin, zingerone, and olvanil in rat trigeminal ganglion neurons. *Brain Res.* 809:246–262. Reproduced with permission.)

body load is reduced by good environmental control, fasting, rotary diet, positive nutrition, and heat depuration/physical therapy, however, whealing usually returns and symptom neutralization occurs. There are some patients, however, who never can be neutralized. Homeostasis returns as the overload decreases. However, at times, homeopathic treatment will help the neutralization process. The response situations occur similar to that which occurs after a skin prick, as described by Pischinger[13] and Heine[347] and desensitization studies of Jancso[278] and Szallis[274] reviews. In addition, when rapid neutralization occurs, it is similar to the stable finite reaction described by Pischinger[13] which means that a more normal physiology will rapidly right a change in their electrical charge and will restore the dynamics of homeostasis.

Due to this anatomical configuration, important membrane functions (e.g., fluidity, the capacity for depolarization and repolarization), the activation of secondary messenger (e.g., cyclic AMP, GMP, inosite phosphate, and G-proteins) in the membrane, receptor properties, and many other factors occur.[346] These facts correlate with our observations that intradermal neutralization (desensitization) has rapid effects both intra- and extracellularly. We have seen patients repolarize rapidly once the proper neutralizing dose has been injected. Due to the negative charge, the glycocalyx has its own electrical potential, which differs from the ECM and the cell membrane, which reacts with its own change in potential after a certain charge alteration in the ECM (i.e., neutralization dose). The cell surface GAGs also bind to PGs and structural glycoproteins of the ECM, thus making contact with the cytoskeleton inside the cell via the membrane glycoproteins and lipids.[348] There are indications that the PGs and certain network proteins of the ECM (e.g., fibronectin) can penetrate the membrane directly and thus make immediate contact with the filamentous cytoskeleton.[349,350] In this way, an exceptionally precise and rapid extracellular–intracellular or vice versa information transfer is possible (similar to light conduction along fibrillar fibers).[351] Intradermal neutralization would send information to the cell interior to regulate the dynamics of homeostasis.

Disturbances of the ECM can lead to alterations of the glycocalyx sugars such that there are major changes in cell behavior. Some changes have been seen repeatedly with subcutaneous injection or intradermal neutralization treatment. After the loss of the terminal sialic acid, sugar components can be released that can be recognized from the construction of carbohydrate chains by foreign substances (e.g., bacteria, xenobiotics, or electromagnetic waves) and can bind them. However, plant, microbial, and host lectins can also bind to the glycocalyx sugars and provoke a wide variety of cell reactions (divisions and synthesis capacity). If these cause symptoms, intradermal neutralization injection could reset the points toward homeostasis. Lectins, mainly glycoproteins, have the function of recognizing sugar structures on the cell surface on insoluble glycoconjugates. Here, there is no relationship to the specific recognition mechanism of the immune system. These glycoproteins have no enzymatic activity. Obviously, they play a major role in immune modulation;[26,352–354] probably subcutaneous injection therapy with specific optimum dose neutralization does play into this area to modulate the immune system.

COMMUNICATION INSIDE THE CELL AND THE BASEMENT MEMBRANE

According to Pishinger,[13] Heine's,[347] and Jancso[278] studies, it is clear how injection therapy can communicate with the inside of the cell. On the inside of the cell membrane, there are filamented glycoproteins related to spectrin, vinculin, and actomyosin, and these glycoproteins bind to both the integral proteins (integrins of the cell membranes) and to the filaments of the cytoskeleton (Figure 6.50).

Basement Membrane

Injection provocation, neutralization for the proper antigen dose and subcutaneous specific antigen injection or sublingual treatment may also influence basement membranes. Basement membranes are a special form of ECM that form as a coproduct of epithelial cells and underlying connective tissue. An underlying basement membrane is needed for the growth of epithelium.[355] These membranes act like a molecular sieve. Many cell membranes (cardiac, muscle, axons) depolarize after appropriate stimuli (opening Na^+, K^+, Ca^{2+} channels). This membrane with its sugar polymers represents an important mobile calcium reservoir within and out of the cell. Thus, specific optimum dose neutralization injections may have direct access to ion flows; in addition needle puncture influences this particular function.[355] This phenomenon appears to be the case in the production and elimination of edema by injection optimum dose neutralization therapy. The same principle holds for mitochondrial membrane function.

Since the basement membrane (i.e., kidney, brain, lung, all blood vessels), of all epithelia, and endothelia are molecular sieves, every severe alteration in either membrane results in organ damage

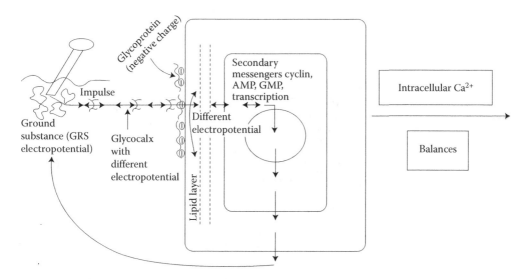

FIGURE 6.50   Communication of injection therapy with the cell. Ground substance is activated and the impulse goes to the glycocalyx which sends impulses into the cell for the final response.

(e.g., shock lung, renal autoimmune disease, oxygen and glucose deficiency in the brain). Certainly, intradermal optimum dose neutralization for food has helped heal kidney membranes (Rea, W. J., *Chemical Sensitivity* IV, Chapter 22[356]), and it appears that this technique heals basement membranes in other parts of the body if specific food and biological inhalant offenders are defined and eliminated.

Heine[357] has shown that there is a high concentration of vitamin C in the basement membrane of the epidermis, which scavenges free radicals and thus prevents inflammation from spreading from the connective tissue to the epidermis and vice versa. We have observed that intradermal optimum dose neutralization works better with higher levels of vitamin C probably resulting from its free radical scavenging ability. We have often observed that a patient could not be neutralized until vitamin C was administered intravenously. Our routine at the EHC-Dallas and Buffalo is to give any patient 15–25 g of intravenous vitamin C coupled with sodium bicarbonate after a severe skin test provocation reaction. This process allows for stabilization and the start-up of testing again. The reaction must be stopped before more testing can be done or inaccurate data will be obtained.

Water–Sugar–Polymer System

In all organisms, the water–sugar–polymer system experiences energy stabilization through binding to a protein backbone that is bound to hyaluronic acid via binding proteins. These PGs biopolymers of the ECM also acquire an increased electronegative charge through sulfation and amination as well as a terminal supply of acetyl neuraminic acid (sialic acid) (reviewed by Heine and Schaeg).[29] Injection optimum dose neutralization appears also to work at this level, as it has been observed to immediately stabilize some patients. Conversely, we have observed that if there is too high a pollutant load requiring excess sulfation and amination, neutralization does not work well until the pollutant load is reduced, thus taking the strain off these processes.

Molecular Construction

When trying to understand all aspects of the injection provocation and optimum dose neutralization and subcutaneous treatment process, one should study molecular construction. The molecular construction is important for understanding the functional relationships between water molecules and PG molecules, which influence electrical forces and memory and thus the neutralization process (Figure 6.51).

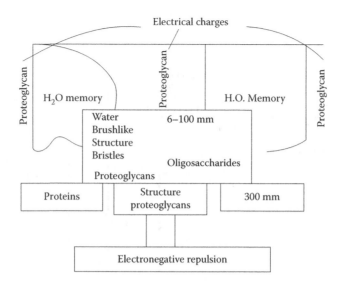

FIGURE 6.51 Functional relationships between water molecules and proteoglycans of the extracellular matrix that influence the injection neutralization process. (Modified from Pischinger, A. 1975. *Matrix and Matrix Regulation: Basis of a Holistic Theory in Medicine.* Karl F. Haug Verlag GmbH and Co., Heidelberg, Federal Republic of German. Brussels, Belgium: Editions Haug International.)

Functional Relationships between Water Molecules and Proteoglycans

PGs have a brush-like structure, with an approximately 300-mm long protein backbone as the "handle" of the brush; due to their mutually electronegative repulsion, the oligosaccharide chains form the stretched, approximately 60–100-nm long "bristles." The molecular weight of PGs lies between 10^6 and 10^9 Da.[358] This molecular form is obviously particularly suitable for binding water, and through this binding, a single PG molecule can take up a very large amount of space ("domain") compared to its molecular weight. The "domain" plays a significant role in determining the "molecular sieve character" as well as the viscoelastic (piezoelectric), shock-absorbing, and energy-absorbing behavior of the ECM.[346,358,359] One can see how the intradermal injections through the ordered water sequence might communicate to the basement membrane sieve to alter its nutrient and O_2 output in the tissues. We have observed that many patients who had blue feet and hands due to local tissue hypoxia suddenly became normal as the neutralization dose took effect and, conversely, their condition worsened with the administration of the wrong dose.

The molecular form of tissue water has been investigated in detail by Trincher.[360]

The special suitability of networks of water molecules for information conduction and storage between cells is, according to Trincher,[360] due to their molecular structure. This structure consists of approximately 50% fluid crystals of ordered water at body temperature. To maintain water in this condition, it should have its lowest energy requirement at 37.5°C.[360] False information stored in the liquid crystals could therefore be concealed by a temperature increase and thus by transfer to a more homogeneous fluid.[360] This false information could also be canceled by a specific neutralization antigen. The cell biophoton emission named by Popp[361] could also play a part in distant information reciprocal effects via these liquid–crystalline intercellular "bridges."

Smith (Smith, C. 1995, personal communication) feels that water is ordered without crystals and would have coherent resonance anyway. Smith (Smith, C. 1995, personal communication) appears to be correct after one studies the communication properties and histology of the matrix. He feels that crystals are not necessary for normal communication. Regardless of who is right, the appropriate intradermal neutralization dose could plug into this water and enforce the coherent resonance anyway (Figure 6.52).

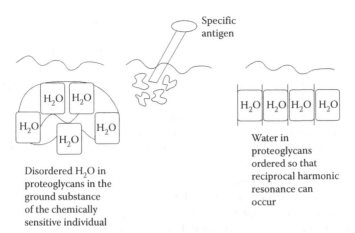

FIGURE 6.52 Injection neutralization therapy due to the needle skin puncture phenomenon appears to order water of the ground substance, thus allowing for an efficient, coherent resonance of the ground regulation system triggering homeostasis.

The mark of crystalline liquids is the formation of parallel swarms of molecules, arranged in two dimensions, which are limited to small areas and are not stable in time. They are in a state of constant formation and dissolution, and show statistically disordered positions related to one another. The size of these swarms lies approximately in the light-wave field. Even weak external powers are sufficient to bring about a greater state of order.[362] Injection provocation and neutralization could disorder and order water depending upon the dose communicating with ordered coherence.

The fact that water has memory emphasizes how the electromagnetic frequency of the optimum dose neutralization for a specific food, biological or chemical agent is stored. This electromagnetic frequency can then be activated when the property-specific dose enters the system via injections and electromagnetically matches the stored frequency, again reinforcing the tendency of the system toward homeostasis. The ground regulation system is an open-energy system and capable of removal and neutralization of the energy released in all metabolic processes by free radical reactions. From a certain size, the energy fluctuation that appears in this process can spread rapidly through the ECM via changes in the state of the ordered water, and these energy fluctuations can be used by the cell as information.

A minimal amount of energy is sufficient for this bioelectrical process, as shown by Pischinger puncture phenomenon[1] and Huneke's[363] second phenomenon of neural therapy. The energy displacements initiated in this way do not need to be biologically demonstrable. They can be measurable as biophysical fluctuation of the redox potential of the connective tissue, among other methods. It is therefore logical that, particularly in chronic diseases such as chemical sensitivity, tissue changes are obviously always accompanied by alteration in the PG/GAG pattern.[2,363] There is an altered redox potential in the ECM, which frequently cannot be regulated.[1,9] However, Wilson[275] clinically demonstrated this phenomenon when he showed that once intradermal provocation and neutralization showed voltage changes occurred on the skin, suggesting an ordering of the redox potential and thus the electrical potential. He also showed that if an individual consumed food to which he was sensitive and became ill, the intradermal neutralizing doses could be used to change the disordered voltage on the skin.

The ECM, therefore, present a labile system, the main components of which are sugar biopolymers, water, and the substances that dissolve in it. Here, system means "capacity," "standing in relationship" or "having a relationship to one another."[364] Thus, intradermal, subcutaneous, or sublingual specific optimum dose antigen neutralization can easily occur in this labile system, but can also disturb the system if the dose is not right.

Injection-specific antigen provocation, neutralization, and subcutaneous injection and sublingual treatment therapy appear to be dependent on the ground regulation system, extracellular ground matrix organization. Here, the system organization between water and the substances dissolved into it, namely, molecules (or ions) of dissolved solid bodies, liquids, and dissolved gases, is of special importance. Aqueous, hydrophilic substances, such as dissolved ions and generally hydrated molecules (e.g., sugar, urea, sialic acid, etc.), can be termed "structure breaker."[364] The sugar biopolymers of the ECM certainly condense the molecular swarms of water in their surroundings to individual molecular "domains." The arrangement is, however, significantly more noticeable as regards these changes than it would be in the sugar–water system in pure water. Thus, the water and ions are disordered which allows environmental disturbances to occur easily. Injection of specific antigen provocation and optimum dose neutralization, thus, can disrupt the system with provocation and reorder or balance it with the proper optimum dose neutralization.

In reverse, gases dissolved in water (e.g., O_2, N_2, CO_2) or other hydrophobic substances can be termed "structure makers" as regards stored water.[364] Gutman and Resch[364] point out that "structure makers" bring about a certain sort of ordered dynamism of the water structure. Radiological spectra of crystallized gaseous hydrates show that gas is necessary for their accommodation. Even if the water is ordered by PGs and not crystalline, gas molecules would have a certain freedom of movement. For example, on the inner surfaces of the spaces, the distance between oxygen molecules is less; this leads to internal surface tensions that make maintenance of the space possible. Gutmann and Resch[364] also point out that the limited rotary oscillation of gas molecules in the spaces can be turned to certain oscillation patterns and has to attune rhythmically to the oscillation behavior of the fluid. This, again, depends on the binding behavior of the "structure breakers," for example, the sugar biopolymers of the ECM. Basically, due to the alteration brought about by the alternating relationship between "structure breakers" and "structure makers," the entire ECM and cell system is affected, even if in different regional way. "Structure breakers" and "structure makers" thus exercise varying, mutually complementary "function" in the sense of retention of the dynamics of homeostasis. These structure breakers have greater hierarchical importance as regards structural character, and structure makers as regards structural information.[364] Intradermal neutralization injections appear to plug into and stabilize this process, allowing for the rhythmic coherence of normal molecular oscillation.

As stated previously in this chapter, since at the molecular level, open-ended systems such as the ground regulation system are compelled to oscillation due to their instability corresponding to their principle of activation and inhibition and their spring effect due to anatomical structure and their electrical (sugar) conduction (amino acids) insulation (water) properties, they can be influenced easily by external forces such as intradermal provocation and optimum dose neutralization and subcutaneous treatment injections.

Clinically, the injections of the optimum neutralizing dose clearly stabilize the patient, where in all probability they decrease the molecular oscillations, which thwarts a state of instability of the patient, and leads to homeostasis. The increased clinical lability, as seen in chemically sensitive patients, corresponds to Heine's finding of increased molecular lability with pollutant stress. Here, the individual would have a longer reaction time—4 hours to 5 days—after pollutant exposure due to the lability of the ground regulation system. Injection neutralization of the proper dose, usually corrects and stabilizes the mild-to-moderate food and biological inhalant chemically sensitive patient and decreases his exposure reactions, until they, eventually, disappear.

It is clear from Pischinger's,[13] Heine's,[347] and our studies that the injection neutralization process tends to regulate the dynamics of homeostasis with phagocytic–fibroblast balance, reduce inflammation, and increase the body's defense mechanisms.

Injection therapy in chemically sensitive patients is often necessary because the secondary biological (pollen, dust, and mold) inhalant, and food sensitivities created by chemical overload may start a vicious cycle of retriggering. This cycle results in worsening of the chemical sensitivity, even when chemical reexposure is not present. If not dealt with rapidly and efficiently, this nontoxic triggering often results in an increase in total body load, which then worsens the condition of the chemically sensitive patient. In addition, if these reactions are not brought under control, the spreading phenomenon may accelerate the disease process until end-organ involvement becomes fixed and the triggering of chemical sensitivity becomes an autonomous process that may become self-perpetuating and irreversible.

Our strategy in treating the chemically sensitive patient with both avoidance and injections has evolved from our treatment of 40,000 patients with chemical sensitivity and chronic degenerative disease, 80% of whom had primary or secondary food and biological inhalant problems.

Our goal in treatment is to use optimum dose injections to neutralize the effect of as many biologically as well as some chemically reactive substances as possible. We adopted this procedure when it became apparent for patients who did not receive injections or received a limited number recovered more slowly than those who rapidly improved with the use of multiple injections under less polluted environmentally controlled conditions. Originally, we use optimum dose injections to counter exposure to only a limited number of substances. Frequently, patients would develop exacerbations when pollen and pollution counts rose, or weather changed, or they were inadvertently exposed to food or other substances to which they were sensitive. In addition, we observed that many patients felt more energetic, had less mental and physical fatigue, and were much less vulnerable to small chemical exposures if they were given injections to cover a broad spectrum of substances to which they had become sensitive. Not only was injection therapy necessary but we also used chemically less contaminated vaccines to enhance precise avoidance.

The methods we use for optimum dose injection therapy at the EHC-Dallas and Buffalo are those that are the most scientifically sound and have been proven by other physicians to be clinically efficacious. Rinkel[221] and Hansel[220] have described the intradermal serial dilution titration technique, which has proven to be precise and efficacious. Lee[222] and Miller[223] originally detailed a variation on this technique called neutralization therapy. Twelve double-blind studies as well as other studies discussed throughout this book and over 100 basic scientific studies support the technique of provocation neutralization injection therapy.[365–379,498] In our hands, provocation by the intradermal route and long-term treatment by the subcutaneous or sublingual route have proven very efficacious in chemically sensitive patients. No negative studies have been reported in full-length scientific articles for the technique we use, although one alleged negative report by Jewett[379] has been published which really did not use our techniques. The optimum dose therapy used at the EHC-Dallas and Buffalo has produced few negative results; therefore, we have used it with over 10,000 patients who have received several million injections. Usually, we use subcutaneous treatment of the specific antigens, as well as sublingual treatment, which can be effective if the patients are unable to tolerate injections.[380–382] In some cases (e.g., hormone or specific estrogen/progesterone, luteinizing hormone, testosterone), the sublingual route is preferred. Pfeiffer,[383] Waikman (Waikman, F. J. 1990, personal communication), and Morris[298] have been the main proponents of this sublingual technique. Their observations and opinions have now been substantiated by several investigators around the world.[382,384–397] Both treatments are safe with no reported deaths from anaphylaxis.

Four principles govern our use of optimum dose injection and sublingual therapy at the EHC-Dallas and Buffalo. First, no harm should be done to the patient from the vaccine used for testing or treatment. Second, the vaccines must be efficacious and cost-effective. Third, they must produce enhanced results over avoidance treatment; and finally, all testing must be done under rigid environmental control in order to obtain the most precise diagnosis and subsequently, treatment antigen end points.

Our protocol for injection therapy in the moderately severe chemically sensitive or chronic degenerative disease patient is as follows:

1. Massive avoidance of pollutants in air, food, and water
2. Injection neutralization therapy of
   a. Foods
   b. Molds, pollens, dust
   c. Chemicals
      i. Natural gas, butane, propane
      ii. Ethanol
      iii. Phenol
      iv. Formaldehyde
      v. Car exhaust
      vi. Diesel
      vii. Gasoline
      viii. Men's cologne
      ix. Ladies cologne
      x. Orris root
      xi. Xylene
      xii. Toluene
      xiii. Benzene
      xiv. Terpenes
         A. Pine
         B. Juniper
         C. Creosol
         D. Cedar
         E. Hogwort
         F. Any of the other terpenes needed

TERPENES

Novel Vanilloids Lacking 3-Hydroxy-4-Methoxyphenyl (Vanillyl) Functionality
   Sesquiterpene Unsaturated 1,4-Dialdehydes and Related Bioactive Terpenoids. To date, approximately 80 terpenoids containing an a,b-unsaturated 1,4-dialdehyde (3-formyl 3-butenal) functionality have been isolated from natural sources.[398] The majority of these compounds are present in terrestrial plants and fungi. However, algae, liverworts, arthropods, sponges, and mollusks are included among the natural sources of unsaturated 1,4-dialdehydes. In general, these compounds are believed to form a multifaceted chemical defense system that protects the producing organism from parasites and predators.[399–404] Because these attacking organisms may range from bacteria to mammals, it is hardly surprising that most of these unsaturated dialdehydes exert a very broad spectrum of bioactivities.[398]
   A prominent representative of unsaturated dialdehydes is warburganal, isolated from the bark of *Warburgia ugandensis* and *W. stuhlmannii*, two tropical trees growing in East Africa.[399] Warburganal has antifungal, antibacterial, and phytotoxic activities.[405,406] Moreover, it is antifeedant to nematodes [407] and is spicy to humans.[400] Native tribes use the bark of warburgia trees as a spice to flavor food.[408] Along with warburganal, another unsaturated dialdehyde, polygodial, is also present in water pepper (*Polygonum hydropiper*).[408] At one time, water pepper was used as a pepper substitute in Europe and its sprout, called "mejiso" or "benitade" in Japanese, is still a popular relish for "sashimi" (raw fish).[409] The extract of *Cinnamosma fragrans*, a native plant of Madagascar, which contains several sesquiterpenes (e.g., cinnamolide, cinnamodial, and cinnamosmolide), was described as having a "distinct pepper-like taste."[410] The similarity between the pungent sensation

evoked in the human tongue by capsaicin and isovelleral-compared structures isolated from the hot mushroom *Lactarius vellereus* was also noted.[411] Despite these telling observations, it was not until 1996 that the possibility that unsaturated dialdehydes may be pungent by activating VRs was investigated.

Like capsaicin, the fungal terpenoid isovelleral causes protective eye-wiping movements in the rat upon intraocular instillation.[412] There is cross-tachyphylaxis between capsaicin and isovelleral actions both in the rat eye and the human tongue.[412] Isovelleral induces calcium uptake by rat DRG neurons in culture, which is fully inhibited by the competitive VR antagonist capsazepine.[412] Furthermore, isovelleral inhibits [3H]RTX binding by rat trigeminal ganglion or spinal cord membranes consistent with a competitive mechanism.[412] Taken together, these findings strongly suggest that isovelleral is pungent by activating VRs on sensory neurons. For a series of 14 terpenoids with an unsaturated 1,4-dialdehyde moiety, a good correlation was found between pungency on the human tongue and affinity for VRs in the rat spinal cord.[412]

However, as expected from their reactive nature, dialdehyde sesquiterpenes and other terpenoids possess additional sites of action, as reflected in the complex behavior of the calcium uptake responses induced by cinnamodial and cinnamosmolide.[412] At low concentrations, cinnamodial and cinnamosmolide evoke calcium uptake in a dose-dependent manner, which is superseded by a blockade of the response at higher concentrations. The separation between cinnamodial concentrations causing stimulation and block of the calcium influx, respectively, is incomplete, which makes cinnamodial only a partial agonist.[413] This observation may also explain the unexpectedly weak membrane polarization by cinnamodial compared with capsaicin under current clamp conditions.[413]

At the whole animal level, polygodial inhibits the pain response evoked by intradermal formalin or capsaicin injection in the mouse and it also blocks acetic acid-induced writhings.[414] Moreover, polygodial has antiallergic and anti-inflammatory activities.[415] Currently, the role played by vanilloid-sensitive neurons in these beneficial effects of polygodial is unclear. Polygodial has a supraspinal antinociceptive action mediated by opioid and/or serotoninergic mechanisms (J. B. Calixto, personal communication).

Furthermore, polygodial blocks tachykinin NK-2 receptors,[416] which might play a role in its antiallergic and anti-inflammatory actions. Polygodial appears to be an interesting new lead for drug development, inasmuch as it targets a variety of pathways involved in pain perception and inflammation.

Triprenyl Phenols as Vanilloids. The archetypal triprenyl phenol is scutigeral, isolated from *Albatrellus ovinus.*[417] Unlike terpenoid unsaturated dialdehydes, scutigeral is not pungent.[418] As a matter of fact, *A. ovinus* is a delicious mushroom often used by the food industry as a substitute for truffles. Scutigeral and related compounds were first isolated based on their affinity for dopamine D1 receptors.[417] Scutigeral induces calcium uptake by rat DRG neurons in culture and blocks RTX binding to rat spinal cord membranes. Calcium uptake by scutigeral is prevented by both capsazepine and ruthenium red.[419] Taken together, these observations are consistent with scutigeral being a vanilloid. The finding that scutigeral is nonpungent is surprising but hardly unprecedented. Olvanil is also considered nonpungent,[258,259] although it mimics most capsaicin responses.[258-260] Interestingly, pretreatment with scutigeral abolishes the first, rapidly activating current elicited by a subsequent capsaicin challenge, leaving the second, slowly activating current relatively intact.[419] This latter finding implies that scutigeral should be able to selectively block capsaicin responses mediated by the rapidly activating conductance. This hypothesis is currently being investigated.

Regardless of the mechanisms involved in the provocation optimum dose neutralization therapy, the treatment of chemically sensitive individual is efficacious and often necessary for recovery.

TRIGGER POINT INJECTIONS

Myofascial trigger point is a hyperirritable spot usually on a band of muscle that is painful on precise compression and can give rise to referred pain, tenderness, and autonomic and other epiphenomena.

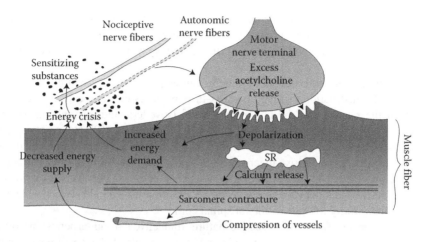

FIGURE 6.53 Illustration of a dysfunctional endplate region.

Twitch responses are usual. These points are found in areas with high concentration of the end-plate[420,421] (Figure 6.53).

Myofascial pain involves the sympathetic nervous system. Fibromyalgia involves central sensitization at the caudate nuclei of the thalamus in the midbrain. This central sensitization results in widespread allodynia (the perception of pain in response to a normally nonpainful stimulus). These patients also demonstrate numerous neuroendocrine abnormalities primarily involving the hypo-thalamo–pituitary–adrenal axis.

Neural Therapy Injection

Neural therapy was popularized in Europe by the brothers Ferdinand and Walter Huneke. Both these physicians knew about the efficacy of nerve blocks, which could serve as a diagnostic and therapeutic tool. In 1928, these German brothers developed their nerve block as a specific therapy for the treatment of broad range of medical infirmities. They based their therapy on the principles of the function of the ground regulation system for regulating the dynamics of homeostasis, and in their clinic they gained vast empirical knowledge as they used nerve blocks successfully on a large number of homeostatic dysfunctions and disease processes.[363] Lariche, the great French surgeon, whose specialty was the surgery of the sympathetic chain, used procaine injections liberally for severe autonomic dysfunction. (*Neural Therapy According to Huneke*, authors preface to the first English ed.) In Russia, the observation made by Spiess on the anti-inflammatory effects of local anesthetics were investigated more clearly. The pupils of Pavlov such as Sporansky, Virhneviski, Bykow, Wedenski, and others, confirmed that it is possible to influence the dynamics of homeostatic regulation of the ANS by injections of procaine.

The Huneke brothers[363] discovered the therapeutic potential of procaine by empirical means, independently of their predecessors. Once they were able to systematize their therapy, their work was aided by Fleckenstein's[422] studies, which showed that procaine will reseal a cell membrane leak when a cell has been traumatized by external or internal noxious stimuli. The potassium–sodium pump, thus, enables the process to displace the sodium that has penetrated into the cell and to replace this ion with potassium. By this means, the physiological potential of -60 to -90 V needed by the cell in order to function normally, is built up again.

This healing phenomenon enables the clinician, by using local anesthetics such as procaine or lido-caine, to repolarize cells and thus, to reactivate their functions where previous treatment had failed.

The injection treatment depends on correct positioning of the local anesthetic. The technique for using site injections in the area where the symptoms are located is shown as segmental therapy.

There are four methods of producing a segmental effect by the use of local anesthetics. The first is to inject directly into the site of the pain, the second is to inject the paravertebral area involved in the affected segment to which the pain refers. The third method is to inject into the sympathetic chain and ganglia (i.e., stellate, ciliary, sphenopalatine, etc.). Finally, the last method is to inject into and around arteries, veins, pleura, peritoneum, and afferent nerves.

In 1940, Ferdinand Huneke[363] also found that there might be interference fields active in the organism, which stand outside the segmental order and send out impulses via nerves, which can be pathogenic. He found that any focus of interference field is a permanent source of irritation because it burdens the dynamics of the homeostatic regulation process and continually forces the body to modify for additional stresses. As shown previously in this book, compensation for the additional stressors cost the body a greater expenditure of energy, which produces disequilibrium in the body's autonomic system. The homeostatic regulatory systems are made more labile and therefore, any small irritation may act as an additional stress, which can produce dyshomeostasis. Once the tolerance threshold has been exceeded, functional disturbances or pathological symptoms will manifest themselves. Huneke[363] showed how such interference fields can be eliminated by the lightening reactions by using sited injections of procaine and lidocaine. Normal cybernetic homeostatic regulation is restored instantly, and the pathological symptoms disappear, rapidly as this is anatomically possible. Gross organ changes can also provoke functional disturbances as a secondary effect of the interference field and these are therapeutically accessible. This type of pathophysiology can lead to feedback processes that form a vicious cycle and a rendering of neural therapy to be ineffective. At this stage of an illness, total body load reduction is necessary to reduce the load of pollutants on a specific organ in order for the neural therapy to hold.

In 1947, Scheidt[423] published the triest called the ANS (Das vegaetative system). He took the point of view that the nerve fibrils do not form a rigid network of conduits, but are mobile molecules, which continue to form new pathways, as required. This view went along with those who discovered that terminal reticulum of the ANS divides even more widely and more finely until the terminal network of the fibrils finally surrounds every single cell with a neuroplasmic reticulum and/or neurotransmitters are released. With this discovery, he supplied a secure anatomical foundation for the empirical and experimentally based findings of Huneke,[363] Ricker,[424] and Speransky.[425] All the fibers of the unimaginably fine synapses would if placed end to end make up three times the distance from the earth to the moon. Styehrs discovery was later extended by studies under the electron microscope, which showed that the nerve terminals do not in fact end directly in the cell membrane, but lie free in the extracellular fluid. These "nerve conductive fiber rings," as Scheidt[423] called them, compensate for differential, electrical voltages, which result from any stimulus. Scheidt suspected that these conductive fiber rings did not decompose completely after they had restored the balance of such differential voltages. The total quantity of these remnants of "old strata" picture has a different appearance for every individual. This old strata picture would, thus, form the material manifestation of the stimulus memory. This idea explains why a noxious stimulus insult many years old appears to fade away while in fact it remains in the background ready to act as a predisposition to an illness, when triggered by a new noxious stimuli. Huneke[363] coined the term "neural interference field" which applies to all primary and secondary disturbed autonomic tissues. Now neurotransmitters have been found that emphasize more heavily on these premises.

In 1951, Ratschow[426] tested neural therapy in 1011 cases, finding total inactivation of symptoms in 441, 427 had substantial improvement, and 143 were failures. When the injection was made in the hard zone, 70% had a lasting disappearance even when remote symptoms such as arthralgia occurred. In 1963, Pischinger[1] showed that there was no closed synapse for the parenchymatous cell in the autonomic periphery, but that the entire basic ANS acts practically as a ubiquitous synapse. Because of this phenomenon, one sees that numerous triggers of the ANS will evoke a response that may be local, regional, or generalized. According to Pischinger,[1] both the neural and humoral controls have their roots in the active cell-rich interstitial connective tissue. In this tissue, the autonomic regulation between the cell and the extracellular environment takes place.

The many day-to-day illnesses seen in medicine are a form of the vital element which is reversible if one addresses oneself early enough to its characteristic signs or if one changes the reaction of the organism (i.e., reversing polarity). By the means of injection therapy, it becomes possible to bring the pathologically modified living organism back to normality provided the organism is still capable of repair.

Studies in neural and humoral pathology have confirmed the theoretical foundation for all of the empirical findings made by the Huneke brothers. This disturbance in the autonomic equilibrium is soundly based on clear definable changes in the finished capability of the innervated blood vessels and nerve tissue from ganglia down to the last fibril arcing on the cell environment of the individual cell. The autonomic regulatory mechanism controls the breathing, circulation, metabolic, temperature, and hormone functions, and along the same ramified pathway, and acting together with all the cells and organs as a whole, makes life possible.

In neural therapy, one sends energy in the form of a neurotherapeutic agent (procaine) with a high electropotential of its own, selectively to a depolarized tissue, where it modifies the local cell environment and restores the cell to normal function. In other words, neural therapy is a medical application to correct the errored dynamics of homeostasis. Kellner[280] has shown that an interference field is like a chronic inflammatory area that cannot be removed or metabolized, and consists of lymphocytes, plasmocytes, and a disaggregation of the connective tissue matrix or data on neural therapy. A case report exemplifies the efficiency of certain types of neural therapy.

Case study: A 30-year-old white man had abdominal surgery for a bowel obstruction using a midline incision. He did well with correction of the food dysfunction and lesion. However, his incisional pain not only persisted but increased in severity. He had to control his pain with oral medication but this only seemed to exacerbate the problem. He gradually became incapacitated due to the unrelenting local pain, memory loss, headaches, and confusion. His wound was injected with 10 cc preservative-free 1% xylocaine without epinephrine. His condition improved immediately but after 5 days his symptoms returned. Another injection was given which totally eliminated all his symptoms permanently.

A second study illustrates how often one has to use multiple injections at one setting in order to accomplish success with treatment. A 41-year-old white woman had a severe exposure to formaldehyde. She developed severe bronchospasms with her peak pulmonary flow being 50 cc. She was doomed to be admitted to the intensive care unit and given bronchodilators and steroids. She was extremely sensitive to steroids and would collapse when exposed to them. Injection of preservative-free and epinephrine-free xylocaine was used in multiple areas of the upper back in the parascapular and paraspinitis areas. All trigger points with pain and spasm were injected. The peak flow rose to 200 cc/min and the patient was breathing easier. The patient was able to maintain this peak flow until the next day when another injection treatment was performed. Her peak flow rose to 410 cc/min and it was evident she was over the acute reaction to the formaldehyde which she then avoided meticulously.

Klinghardt[427] has shown that one can influence the ANS and in particular the heart with procaine injections. He likes to inject the right vagus behind the ear and jaw bone to relieve cavitations and cardiac arrhythmia. He also likes to inject the sphenopalatine ganglion of the trigeminal nerve which will access the VR system and reduce hypersensitivity. Injections will obscure and also help regulate energy flow and homeostasis.

ACUPUNCTURE

Recently, Gunn[428] has published data from a large series of patients with lumbar and cervical spondylosis which were improved by a form of needle therapy using stainless-steel needles. As shown in the neurological chapter (Chapter 2, Vol. 5), classical acupuncture and its modifications are demonstrated including Gunn's integrated muscle stimulation (IMS). In our center, a combination of treatments is used with tendency to use Gunn's techniques.

Light acupuncture can be used using prisms which emit different combinations of light. This treatment is reserved for the super sensitive patient who cannot tolerate needles.

Laser acupuncture appears to involve the principles of neural therapy and acupuncture in that due to the beam penetration one can treat both the small and large nerve. Two cases exemplify the efficiency of Gunn's IMS technique.[428]

The first case is a 50-year-old white woman who after exposure to mold in her house developed severe asthma. Her peak flow ranged from 50 to 150 cc/min. She was always in respiratory distress not responding to any medication treatment. All points of maximum tenderness and spasm were needled. Her peak flow increased to 250 cc/min. After using the needles four times in two weeks her peak flow rose to 400 cc/min and remained at that level for 3 months. At this time she was tested again and her peak flow which had dropped to 350 cc/min rose to 450 cc/min and persisted. By this time she had removed the mold from the house which proved to be the primary triggering agent.

The second case was a 52-year-old white woman who had been in a auto accident as a teenager. She had severe hand and neck injuries. She eventually developed bilateral thoracic outlet syndrome accompanied by a sequence of left eye pain, intractable left facial pain, shoulder and neck tightness bilaterally as well as a bilateral hand and arm weakness and tingling. She became sensitive to many foods and chemicals and was totally incapacitated being in bed 20 out of 24 hours/day. She had integrated muscle therapy at the base of the skull and in the maximum point tenderness in the trapezious, rhomboid, and parspinal muscle. She would get severe nausea and pain at times and had to lie on the floor after treatment. However, after 12 needle treatments she was able to stay up most of the day and she went on to college. Over the long term she has to take an occasional treatment.

These two cases are examples of Gunn's IMS treatment. We have found this treatment coupled with massage and intravenous magnesium to be a powerful technique on those who need needle treatment.

LOW DOSE ENZYME-ACTIVATED IMMUNOTHERAPY

Low dose enzyme-activated immunotherapy (LDA evolved from McEwen's EPD, enzyme-potentiated desensitization therapy).[429] This type of therapy can be given infrequently anywhere from 2 months to 1 year. The therapy consists of a mixture of antigens and the enzyme beta-glucuronidase. Its main proponent in this country is Shrader[430] and the mechanics of its action appear to be the induction of suppressor T-cells production in the regional lymph nodes through activation of the dendritic cells in the dermis in the presence of very low dosage of antigens by the enzyme beta-glucuronidase. The resultant T-cells suppress the inappropriate responses of the T-cells/per cells. Also other functions may occur. The connective tissue matrix among the PG/GAGs, the response elicited in this type of therapy are hormetic and not linear for dose responses. The response is a series of inverted "U" waves which McEwen[429] and Shrader[430] call the "W" effect. The response ranges from 10^{-20} (bad) to 10^{-16} (good) to 10^{17} (bad) and 10^{-6} (good) indicating a hormetic effect.

The component of EPD and LDA is protamine sulfate which potentiates beta-glucuronidase, 1,3 cyclohexanediol which controls the effect, and chrondroitin sulfate which stabilizes the various allergen mixes and beta-glucuronidase which potentiates the antigen. The mixes are used to prevent the spreading phenomena.

Conditions treated with LDA are hay fever and seasonal/perennial rhinitis, chronic sinusitis, sinus headaches, asthma, bronchitis, secretory otitis media, and other chronic ear infections, food allergies, intolerance, urticaria, angioedema, dermatitis, excema and migraines, brain fog, confusion, ulcerative colitis, Crohn's disease, irritable bowel syndrome, hyperactivity, chronic fatigue syndrome, and mold chemical sensitivity.

Greater than 90% of patients with seasonal hay fever, ear infections, and eczema cleared their symptoms. The mixes and doses used are the following:

Lx—low dose inhalants and foods: 10^{-13}–10^{-17}
Mx—medium dose inhalants and foods: 10^{-8}–10^{-12}
IC—high dose inhalants, no foods 10^{-16} to one
CF—chemical mix: 10^{-9}–10^{-17}
Bacteria mixes: 10^{-6}

There is no testing involved with this treatment and only clinical symptoms are used. Each of the four components is mixed with beta-glucuronidase. The dose after each enzyme is 10/cc and the combination of each component is 0.04_a. Therefore, the total dose is 0.054. The frequency is every 2–3 months for the first 6–8 treatments. The second treatment should be given 2 months after the first. After 6–8 months, the interval between shots can be extended.

Patients receiving LDA must follow certain guidelines. There is an initial critical 3-day diet consisting of any of the following: lamb, fish, rabbit, sweet potatoes, yams, potatoes, cooked celery, carrots, lettuce (outer leaves only unless cooked), cabbage, parsnips, rutabaga, taro root, filtered or bottled water, and rare meats.

Out of approximately 2500 patients, there is a small but significant complication rate that involves severe intractable asthma, refractory chemical sensitivity, and chronic malnutrition. These patients also developed a spreading phenomenon and were sensitive to all foods and most chemicals.

OXYGEN THERAPY

There are two types of oxygen therapy that at times appear to help the chemically sensitive. One type is the von Ardenne that helps the small vascular extract O_2 from the microcirculation. The other is the hyperbaric which pushes more O_2 across the lung membrane.

The von Ardenne type has been used quite successfully on the chemically sensitive patient in the last 15 years. A series of 100 patients is presented in Table 6.27 using the apparatus for the glass humidifier and cellophane bag as shown in Figure 6.54.

This therapy is done at 8 L/min for 2 h/day for 18–36 days. The therapy can be given after a patient gets an excess of exposure and is overloaded by a series of small exposures. Chemically sensitive patients must keep the antecubital brachial vein below 28 mmHg without a tourniquet. This means that sufficient oxygen is being extracted from the blood. We have completed this

TABLE 6.27
A Series of 100 Patients Who Have Been Administered Oxygen Therapy

Sex	Age	PVO$_2$ (mmHg) Before	PVO$_2$ (mmHg) After	Treatment Duration (day) 2 h at 8 L/min 18 days ≤ 10 No	%	$> 10 \leq 20$ No	%	$> 20 \leq 30$ No	%	$> 30 \leq 60$ No	%	> 60 No	%
M = 19	Range = 30–82	X = 42.02	X = 26.33	9	9	37	37	31	31	15	15	8	8
F = 81	years old	SD = 14.67	SD = 4.93										
	Mean = 52	Range = 29–75.4	Range= <20 to 39.2										

Source: Adapted from Environmental Health Center-Dallas, 2016.
Note: Symptom improvement 84/100 (84%).

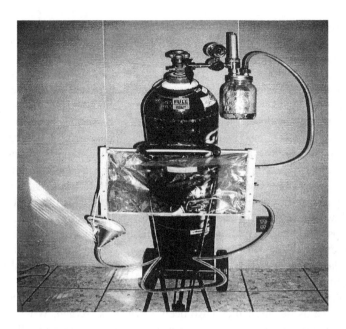

FIGURE 6.54   Glass humidifier and cellophane bag for oxygen therapy. (Adapted from Environmental Health Center-Dallas.)

procedure on over 2000 chemically sensitive patients at the EHC-Dallas under environmentally controlled conditions.

Hyperbaric Oxygen

The first use of hyperbaric oxygen (HBO) was in 1800s. During the 1930s, HBO became the treatment of choice for decompression sickness and gas embolism. By the 1960s, the therapy was also used to combat carbon monoxide poisoning. It is used as an adjunct in the treatment in wounds. Human physiology is oxygen-dependent and healing is rate-limited by oxygen availability. Inadequate oxygenation occurs in tissue compromised by infection, inflammation, hypoxia, traumatic injury, and edema seen in many chemically sensitive and chronic degenerative disease patients.

At normal atmospheric pressure, the oxygen needed for tissue metabolism is carried in the blood in chemical combination with hemoglobin in red blood cells. Only an insignificant amount is physically dissolved in the blood plasma. Because of increased diffusion distances caused by such factors as circulatory disruption and edema, the pressure-dependent gradient necessary for oxygen to diffuse from blood into the tissues may be inadequate to deliver sufficient amounts of oxygen to support basic metabolism. Physiologically significant amounts of oxygen are dissolved in the plasma at a pressure far in excess of the normal arterial PO_2 of 100 mmHg; however, this will cause the oxygen to diffuse over much greater distances and support both basic tissue metabolism and healing processes left in need of oxygen carried by hemoglobin. Under pressure, oxygen adheres to all the gas laws of physics; displaces all other gases in the body such as nitrogen in decompression illness, carbon monoxide, and cyanide.

HBO follows the law of mass action and completely saturates hemoglobin, increases plasma oxygen by 2000%. It dissolves in CSF, lymph, and urine. HBO perfuses all tissue spaces where all life takes place. It delivers metabolically available oxygen without chemical energy and transfers enough to sustain life without blood. It reduces CNS lactate peak in hypoxia. During HBO treatment, as ambient pressure in the chamber is increased, the amount of oxygen entering into solution in plasma also increases. At one atmosphere absolute (ATA) the volume of oxygen in solution is 0.3 mL/100 mL. When breathing oxygen at 3 ATA, the arterial PO_2 is increased to 2200 mmHg and the volume in solution rises 22 times to 6.6 mL/100 mL. It has been shown that under these circumstances, oxyhemoglobin passes unchanged through the capillaries since the volume of oxygen physically dissolved in solution at the pressure is sufficient to meet tissue demand without dissociation from hemoglobin.

The primary effect of administering oxygen at greater than normal atmospheric pressure is to dissolve it in physiologically significant amounts at much increased partial pressures in the blood plasma. The higher plasma oxygen tension increases the rate and distance that oxygen diffuses from patent capillaries across barriers created by edema and poor perfusion. Thus, oxygen becomes more readily available to tissues affected by disease like in chemical sensitivity or traumatic injury even when blood flow to those areas is impaired and red cells are not able to pass through restricted capillary beds. This facilitates healing through enhanced macrophage function, fibroblast proliferation and collagen synthesis, angiogenesis, and epithelialization. It also reduces tissue edema through reduced capillary pressure, seen in chemically sensitive patients, which facilitates reversal in transcapillary fluid flow so that the extravascular fluid is absorbed into circulation.

HBO also helps to protect and maintain the microcirculation by preventing neutrophil adherence to postcapillary endothelium which results in blockage, endothelial destruction, and chemically mediated arteriolar vasoconstriction. Thus, significant elevation of the arterial PO_2 on a periodic basis supports cellular metabolism and enhances healing processes.

HBOT prevents "reperfusion injury." That is severe tissue damage that happens when the blood supply returns to the tissues after they have been deprived of oxygen. When blood flow is interrupted by a crush injury, for instance, a series of events inside the damaged cells leads to the release of harmful oxygen radicals. These molecules can damage tissues that cannot be reversed and cause the blood vessels to clamp up and stop blood flow. HBOT encourages the body's oxygen radical scavengers to seek out the problem molecules and allow healing to continue. HBO-mediated inhibition of neutrophil β_2 integrin adhesion has been shown to ameliorate reperfusion injuries of brain, heart, lung, liver, skeletal muscle and intestine, as well as smoke-induced lung injury and encephalopathy due to carbon monoxide poisoning. HBOT helps block the action of harmful bacteria and strengthens the body's immune system. HBOT can disable the toxins of certain bacteria. It also increases oxygen concentration in the tissues. This helps them resist infection. In addition, the therapy improves the ability of white blood cells to find and destroy invaders.[431–433]

At low ATA of 1.3, it decreases inflammation. It is entirely possible that clinical benefits may arise from purely increasing the atmosphere pressure delivered, because increased pressure delivery without additional oxygen appears to decrease inflammation as measured by an inhibition of interferon-gamma release, and delivery of oxygen by mask without any increase in pressure may actually increase inflammation (as measured by an increase in interferon-gamma release). It has not appeared in our patients with O_2 therapy. HBOT possess strong anti-inflammatory properties and has been shown to improve immune function. There is evidence that oxidative stress can be reduced with HBOT through the upregulation of antioxidant enzymes. HBOT can also increase the function and production of mitochondria and improve neurotransmitter abnormalities.

In addition, HBOT upregulates enzymes that can help with detoxification problems specifically found in chemically sensitive individuals and autistic children. HBOT improves impaired production of porphyrins and the production of heme, thereby improving cytochrome oxidase function in mitochondrial electron transport chain. Thus, increased ATP production reduces fatigue in chemically sensitive patients. HBOT has been shown to mobilize stem cells from the bone marrow to the systemic circulation in humans. HBOT has shown that stem cells can enter the brain and form new neurons, astrocytes, and microglia. Thus, HBOT ameliorates underlying pathophysiological problems and leads to improvements of symptoms in chemically sensitive individuals and in autistics. HBOT ameliorates cerebral hypoperfusion, inflammation, mitochondrial dysfunction, and oxidative stress.[434]

Treatment with HBOT has been shown to possess potent anti-inflammatory properties in both animal and human studies. HBOT has been reported to decrease the production of pro-inflammatory cytokines (including TNF-alpha, interferon-gamma, IL-1, and IL-6) and neopterin levels in both animals and humans. The effect of HBOT on reducing inflammation may be mediated through a pressure-related effect and not necessarily by the oxygen delivered.[435,436]

Theoretically, HBOT might increase oxidative stress through the augmented production of reactive oxygen species (ROS) from the high concentration of oxygen.[437] This may occur because increased oxygen delivery to mitochondria can increase ROS production. However, HBOT has been shown to upregulate the production of antioxidant enzymes such as SOD,[438,439] glutathione peroxidase,[440] catalase,[441] paraoxonase,[442] and heme oxygenase-1.[443,444]

This increase in antioxidant enzyme levels has been termed "conditioning" and can protect against damage caused by ROS.[445,446] Interestingly, increasing ROS may be a potential mechanism of action of HBOT because ROS play an important role in cellular signaling and in triggering certain metabolic pathways.[447] Furthermore, as previously discussed, a slight increase in ROS produced by HBOT may be beneficial as these ROS appear to augment mitochondrial biogenesis.[448] Two studies have reported measurements of oxidative stress markers before and after HBOT in children with autism spectrum disorders (ASD).[449,450] In the first study, HBOT was administered daily at 1.3 atm to 48 children with ASD, and SOD, catalase, and glutathione peroxidase levels were measured before starting HBOT and after 1 day and 32 days of HBOT.[450] SOD was 4.5-fold and 4.7-fold higher at 1 and 32 days after starting HBOT, respectively. Mean catalase increased by 1.9-fold after 1 day and after 32 days was 90% of the initial level before beginning HBOT. Finally, mean glutathione peroxidase increased by 1.4-fold after 1 day and after 32 days was 1.2-fold higher than before beginning HBOT. The effects of HBOT on these antioxidant enzymes may be an example of conditioning as previously discussed.

In the second prospective study, 12 children with ASD received HBOT at 1.3 atm/24% oxygen and 6 children received HBOT at 1.5 atm/100% oxygen. Biomarkers were measured before and after 40 HBOT sessions.[449] Behavioral improvements were observed in these children and plasma oxidized glutathione levels did not significantly change at 1.3 atm ($p = 0.557$) or 1.5 atm ($p = 0.583$). Since oxidized glutathione is exported from cells when intracellular levels exceed the redox capacity,[451] this finding suggests that intracellular oxidative stress did not significantly worsen with HBOT at these two commonly used lower HBOT pressures in ASD.[449] Carbon monoxide poisoning, cyanide poisoning, crush injuries, gas gangrene (a form of gangrene in which gas collects in tissues), decompression sickness, acute or traumatic inadequate blood flow in the arteries, compromised skin grafts and flaps, infection in a bone (osteomyelitis), delayed radiation injury, flesh-eating disease (also called necrotizing soft-tissue infection), air or gas bubble trapped in a blood vessel (air or gas embolism), chronic infection called actinomycosis, diabetic wounds.

HBOT helps wound healing by bringing oxygen-rich plasma to tissue starved for oxygen. Wound injuries damage the body's blood vessels, which release fluid that leaks into the tissues and causes swelling. This swelling deprives the damaged cells of oxygen, and tissue starts to die. HBOT reduces swelling while flooding the tissues with oxygen. The elevated pressure in the chamber increases the amount of oxygen in the blood. HBOT aims to break the cycle of swelling, oxygen starvation, and tissue death. HBOT encourages the formation of new collagen (connective tissue) and new skin cells. It does so by encouraging new blood vessel formation. It also stimulates cells to produce certain substances, such as vascular endothelial growth factor. These attract and stimulate endothelial cells necessary for healing.

Injury and head trauma procedures were driven and developed by Harch[452] and Calabresse.[453] Later, the procedure was used by us at EHC-Dallas and Buffalo for chemically sensitive patients with head injury, which has proved effective in some. Johnson[454] and Sprague[455] have clinically shown that it has helped patients that are chemically sensitive who suffer from head and chemical injuries; however, they have not publicized on it but have a significant series of successful patients.

SAUNA AND PHYSICAL THERAPY UNDER LESS POLLUTED CONDITIONS

Thermal chamber depuration with exercise under environmentally controlled conditions, with massage and physical therapy, also helps reduce the total body load of toxics by mobilizing and

TABLE 6.28
Acute Heat Depuration Data in 100 Chemically Sensitive Patients

Procedure	Number	Range
Total time of heat per day	83 ± 10 min	10–40 min/session
Total exercise time per day	60 min	5–30 min/session
Total massage per day	45 min	15 min/session
Total average water intake	2100 cc	500–10,560 cc/day
Total weight loss	1.3 lb.	Decreased 1.5; decreased 5.8 lb/day
Average blood pressure		Systolic: decreased 28 ± 2.5
		Increased 58 ± 12.5
	2.2 ± 0.08 mm Hg	Diastolic: decreased 64 ± 0.9
		Increased 49 ± 10
Average temperature		Decreased 1.6, increased 5.2°F/day
Average pulse change	±0.8°F	Decreased 43; increased 50 beats/min
	3.8 ± beats/min	
	28 min after 5 min	

Source: Adapted from Environmental Health Center-Dallas, 1992.

eliminating toxics. A heat chamber depuration can be seen in Table 6.28 and Figure 6.55 exhibits a dry environmentally controlled sauna made out of glass, ceramic, and hardwood (no cedar, pines, or redwood), which helps mobilize toxics from fat cells and fat membrane layers of the cells, as well as sequestered toxics in the connective tissue matrix and muscle layers.

Chemically sensitive patients are usually sensitive to cold temperatures and have difficulty sweating. The first week in the sauna has to be carefully done using no more than 20 minutes per session. They frequently feel worse as the first toxics are neutralized. We have learned that most of the sick patients can tolerate three times per week for only 20 minutes. Usually 3 times a week is enough. As time goes on, they can tolerate much more time. The temperature really depends on whatever makes them sweat. Many of chemically sensitive patients cannot tolerate the infrared heat, so it must be

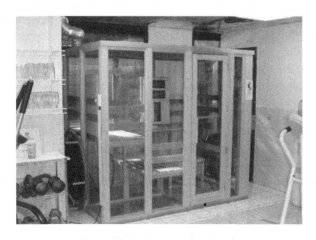

FIGURE 6.55 Wood and glass sauna. Saunas made from poplar, maple, and/or oak wood are acceptable. Those made from pine, cedar, or redwood are unacceptable under these polluted conditions. (Adapted from Environmental Health Center-Dallas.)

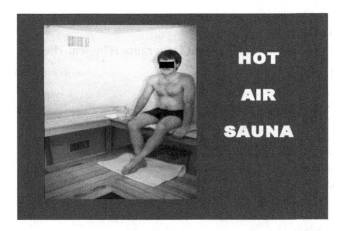

FIGURE 6.56   Ceramic sauna. (Adapted from Environmental Health Center-Dallas.)

turned off. Regular heat can be used instead without the infrared. One thousand patients have used sauna successfully in their treatment protocol (Figure 6.56).

The ANS then normalizes Table 6.29 allowing the patient to sweat easily, which helps the body to return to the dynamics of normal homeostasis.

Massage and exercise under environmentally controlled conditions help mobilize toxics sequestered in the fat cells and lipid layers of any cell but especially those that are in the connective tissue matrix and spastic muscle layers which are particularly prone to removal by these modalities (Table 6.30 and Figure 6.57).

All patients receive some form of exercise, but exercise with oxygen supplementation which aids oxygen extraction in the end organs is especially helpful (Tables 6.31 through 6.34 and Figure 6.58).

Heat depuration and physical therapy are clearly modalities and can decrease the total body load and improve the chemically sensitive patient with chronic degenerative disease.

Sauna should be made of nonsynthetic grout and ceramic tile or hard wood and glass. Heat generators should be constructed out of ceramic or steel coils or infrared heat. Patients stay in the sauna depending upon the severity of their illness, 20–40 minutes, 1–3 times a day. There is an ordering of chemicals depending on which detoxification system they have to go through. Some toxins release at a fast rate from the body than others (Table 6.35). Nutrients are necessary for heat depuration and are used for antioxidants and to help mobilize pollutants (Table 6.36).

TABLE 6.29

Change in the Autonomic Nervous System after Thermal Depuration/Physical Therapy under Environmentally Controlled Conditions (First and Last 1000 Patients)

	Autonomic Changes		Signs and Symptoms	
	# Patients	Percent	# Patients	Percent
Improved	61	50.8	76	78.6
Worse	11	9.2	7.0	7.1
No change	48	40	14	14.2

Source: Adapted from Environmental Health Center-Dallas.

TABLE 6.30
Complications of Thermal Depuration/Physical Therapy

Symptoms	Number of Patients
Fatigue	2
Dizzy	2
Headache	3
Nausea	4
Sleepy	2
Blurred vision	1
Dry throat	1
Leg, shoulder pain	2
Eye pain	1
Eyes burn	1
Leg shivers	1
Swelling hands	1
Hand shaky	1
Skin red and itching	1
Wheezing and tight chest	1
Elevated liver battery	7

Source: From Rea, W. J., Y. Pan, A. P. Johnson. 1987. *Clin. Ecol.* 5 (4):169–170. With permission.

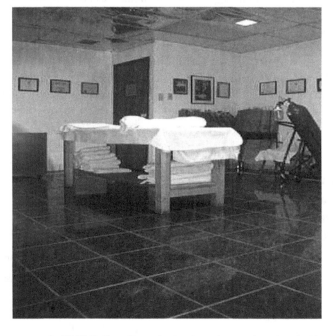

FIGURE 6.57   Massage at the EHC-Dallas. Ceramic, hardwood, organize chemically sensitive, metal ceiling, oxygen if needed. All under less polluted conditions. (Adapted from Environmental Health Center-Dallas, 2000.)

TABLE 6.31

Clearing of Toxic Chemicals: Mean Body Burden Reductions[a]

McCall Numbers[b]	Chemical	Treatment (%)		Control (%)	
		Pretreament	Follow-up	Pretreatment	Follow-up
Pesticides					
	Hexachlorobenzene	19	16	−11	−12
	Oxychlordane	5	37	15	6
	Heptachlor epoxide	6	26	3	−5
	Dichlorodiphenyl-Dichloroethylene	1	7	−8	−17
	Dieldrin	8	20	−3	7
	Mean	7.8	21.2	−0.8	−4.2
Polychlorinated Biphenyls					
146	2,2′4,4′5,5-Hexa	8	6	−10	−11
174	2,2′,3,4,4′-Hexa	5	4	−9	−10
203	Hexa	7	1	2	−1
244	2,3,3′,4,4′,5-Hexa	4	3	−7	−8
332	Hexa	8	−6	2	−8
360 + 372	Hepta	7	−2	−16	−18
448	Hepta	0	4	−53	−40
528	Hepta	3	−4	−5	−9
717	Hepta	2	2	−6	−11
	Mean	4.7	2.3	−10.8	−12.4

Source: From Shnare, D. W., P. C. Robinson. 1986. In *Hexachlorobenzene: Proc. Int. Symp. (IARD Scientific Publications No. 77)*, C. R. Morrisand, J. R. P. Lyonk, Eds. International Agency for Research on Cancer, pp. 597–603. With permission.

[a] Differences in body burden reduction between treatment and control groups at follow-up sampling (3 months pretreatment) are significant with f < 0.001 and <0.005 for pesticides and polychlorinated biphenyls, respectively. The difference at posttreatment was significant for all polychlorinated biphenyls with f < 0.001.

[b] McCall numbers are according to Sawyer (1977).

It is best if patients live in environmentally controlled living quarters, use safe water and eat an organic diet in order to continue the detoxification during the night.

Patients do clear toxins (Table 6.37) and they should have this therapy in a clinic under environmentally controlled conditions before home therapy is attempted. The course of treatment may be daily from 2 to 10 weeks with home sauna as needed after they have learned how to detox.

If sauna therapy is controlled properly, complications are minimal although we have had one patient develop seizures. Heart patients must be monitored carefully so they do not develop failure from the increased metabolism or arrhythmia from the electrolyte shifts (Table 6.36). However, most do well including those in heart failure (Japanese study).[409]

IMMUNE REPLACEMENT

Gamma Globulin

Besides avoidance of pollutants and injection therapy, which may or may not be immune mediated, replacement of IgG 1, 2, 3, 4 deficiency may be very efficacious. In some cases of deficiency,

TABLE 6.32

Clearing of Toxic Chemicals: Range of Adipose Tissue Concentration (ppm)

Chemical	Range	Level of Detection (ppm)
PCBs		
2,4,5,2',3',6'-hexa	0.01–0.37	0.005
2,4,5,2',4',6'-hexa	0.09–0.73	0.005
2,4,5,2',3',6'-hexa	0.07–0.67	0.005
2,3,4,5,2,4',5'hepta[a]	0.02–0.20	0.005
2,3,4,6,2',3',4'-hepta	0.007–0.23	0.005
2,3,4,5,3',4',5'-hepta[a]	0.08–0.59	0.01
2,3,5,6,3',4',5'-hepta[a]	0.05–0.35	0.01
PPBs		
2,4,5,3',4'-penta	ne–0.16	0.009
2,4,5,2',4',5'-hexa	0.01–2.72	0.004
2,3,4,2',4',5'-hexa	nd–0.22	0.001
2,4,5,3',4',5'-hexa	nd–0.09	0.002
2,3,5,2',4'5',6'-hepta	nd–0.26	0.002
2,3,4,5,2',4',5'-hepta	nd–0.01	0.002
DDE	0.30–1.58	0.05
Heptachlor epoxide	0.02–0.82	0.01
Deildrin	0.04–0.14	0.01

Source: Adapted from Schnare, D. W. et al. 1983. Reduction of human organohalide body burdens final research repot. 1–16 Foundation for Advancements in Science and Eduction, Los Angeles, CA. With permission.

[a] Chlorine configuration is estimated, based on gas chromatographic retention times.

it is very efficacious and in others, the replacement rarely boosts the chemically sensitive patient. Patients with isolated IgG 1, 2, 3, 4 deficiency usually do well with intravenous or replacement with intramuscular or subcutaneous injections in each hip 1 time per week for 4 weeks gamma globulin weekly. An occasional patient has to go 8 weeks and rare ones for 3–12 months. Patients get better and maintain their normal work if the triggering agents such as mycotoxin, natural gas, pesticides, EMF, and so on, can be eliminated. As one can see, the deficiencies can cause more than recurrent infections and replacement can clear recent infections (Table 6.38 and Figure 6.59a–d).

Autogenous Lymphocytic Factor

In this study, 315 individuals (25 controls, 290 chemically sensitive immunocompromised patients) were investigated at the EHC-Dallas. Each patient had been on a standard therapy of avoidance of pollutants, nutritional supplementation, and injections of antigens for foods, and biological inhalants, but did not attain their immunological competence. Peripheral lymphocytes were collected and DNA histograms were constructed. The flow cytometer was used to evaluate the cell cycle, hematological, and other immunological profiles. From the other portion of the blood specimen, lymphocytes were propagated *in vitro*, harvested, and a lysate, termed the ALF, was prepared. When treated with ALF, 88% of these individuals showed a significant ($p < 0.001$) clinical improvement which correlated with laboratory findings, involving regulation of abnormal cells cycles, increase in total lymphocytes and subsets T_4' T_8' ($p < 0.05$) and cell-mediated immunity (CMI) response

TABLE 6.33

Reductions in Adipose Tissue Concentrations (%)

Chemical	Post Treatment			4-Month Follow-up		
	%[b]	N	SD	%[b]	N	SD
2,4,5,2′,3′,6′-hexa[a]	32.83**	6	17.86	60.58**	6	24.93
2,4,5,2′,4′,6′-hexa	17.24	6	21.74	27.76*	6	27.68
2,4,5,2′,3′,6′-hexa[a]	20.36*	5	21.31	45.26**	5	25.08
2,3,4,5,2′,4′,5′-hepta[a]	34.89*	5	16.82	29.16	6	46.19
2,3,4,6,2′,3′,4′-hepta	26.21*	6	30.82	56.47	6	32.02
2,3,4,5,3′,4′,5′-hepta[a]	11.87	6	21.92	13.34	6	42.54
2,3,5,6,3′,4′,5′-hepta[a]	36.96*	6	27.99	58.95**	6	21.59
Total PCB (sum of peaks)	34.17**	6	24.41	38.44*	6	27.68
PBBs						
2,4,5,3′,4′-penta	34.0	4			4	34.2
2,4,5,2′,4′,5′-hexa	25.0*	5	39.7		5	37.3
2,3,4,2′,4′,5′-hexa	47.2*	3	12.4		3	35.4
2,4,5,3′,4′,5′-hexa	+4.2	4	84.3		5	50.5
2,3,5,3′,4′5′,6′-hepta	+8.0	2	96.2		4	27.1
2,3,4,5,2′,4′,5′-hepta	36.3	5	34.0		5	95.4
Total PBB (sum of peaks)	34.5**	6	209		5	33.0
DDE	3.5	7	26.1		6	22.9
Heptachlorepoxide	31.2	7	49.4		6	33.4
Dieldrin	+3.9	7	19.9		6	21.9

Source: From Schnare, D. W. et al. 1983. Reduction of human organohalide body burdens final research report. 1–16. Foundation for Advancements in Science and Education, Los Angeles, CA. With permission.

[a] Chlorine configuration is estimated, based on gas chromatographic retention times.

[b] *p < 0.05 and **p < 0.02 (Wilcoxon sign-rank test).

TABLE 6.34

Body Fat Mass Before and After Treatment

Participant		Body Weight (kg)	Percent Fat	Fat Weight (kg)
01	Pre-	83.9	15.2	12.8
	Post-	85.3	13.7	11.7
02	Pre-	74.0	13.6	10.1
	Post-	76.2	14.5	11.0
03	Pre-	87.4	25.9	22.6
	Post-	91.2	26.2	23.9
04	Pre-	91.9	34.2	31.4
	Post-	92.5	32.5	30.1
05	Pre-	51.9	15.3	7.9
	Post-	51.9	14.9	7.7
06	Pre-	85.0	24.1	20.5
	Post-	91.6	24.0	22.0

Source: From Schnare D. W. et al. 1983. Reduction of human organohalide body burdens final research report. 1–16. Foundation for Advancements in Science and Education, Los Angeles, CA. With permission.

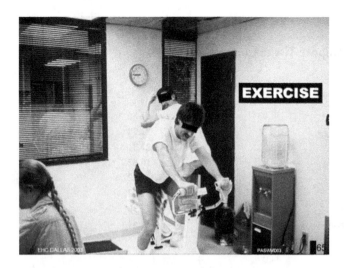

FIGURE 6.58 Environmentally controlled exercise room. Note aluminum ceiling and window blinds and hard floor. (Adapted from Environmental Health Center-Dallas, 1993, 2000.)

(p < 0.001). The ALF presumably acts as a biological response modifier. The cell cycle and ALF provide clinical tools for diagnosis and regulation of immunological incompetence.[456]

The cell cycle is the ordered and orderly events of biochemical and morphological sequences, leading from the formation of a daughter cell as a result of mitosis to the completion of the processes required for its own division into two daughter cells.[457] It is fundamental that following mitosis, two daughter cells are produced. These cells may initiate a new cycle (G_1 phase), some cells may become nonproliferative (G_0 phase) or progress to a restriction point where they are committed to the synthesis of cellular components (the S phase), and finally complete the cycle (the G_2M phase). The cell cycle then comprises the sum of the growth phases of a specific cell cycle. This cycle is repeated by continuously dividing cells. Even within the same organism, the specific cell cycle will vary with different classes of cells. The total time that is necessary to complete the S and G_2 phases is generally constant in different cell types. It seems reasonable then to assume that most of the time variation takes place in the G_1 phase. To establish homeostasis, it is imperative that the cell cycle be regulated. To this end, there are biological parameters which may be employed to ascertain the

TABLE 6.35

Mean Posttreatment Reductions for Some Chemicals (%)

Chemical	Adipose Tissue	Body Burden
2,4,5,2′,3′,6′-PCB	32.8**	32.3**
2,3,4,5,2′,4′,5′ hepta-PCB	34.9**	34.0**
Total PCB	34.2**	34.0**
2,4,5,2′,4′,5′ hexa-PBB	25.0*	27.2*
DDE	3.5	10.5
Heptachlor epoxide	31.2	38.1
Dieldrin	+3.9	2.5

Source: From Schnare, D. W. et al. 1983. Reduction of human organohalide body burdens final research report. 1–16. Foundation for Advancements in Science and Education, Los Angeles, CA. With permission.

*p < 0.05 and **p < 0.01.

TABLE 6.36

Nutrients Used in Heat Depuration Therapy for Chemically Sensitive Patients

Vitamins

Vitamin A in the form of β-carotene, 5000–10,000 IU daily

Vitamin B_1: 100 mg daily. These are needed for many detoxification reactions.

Vitamin B_2: 100 mg daily

Vitamin B_3: 0 to 3000 mg with an average of 1000 mg depending on tolerance. This tolerance usually increases as the patients improve during treatment. However, there are some patients who never tolerate niacin supplementation, though they can detoxify even if at a slower rate.

Vitamin B_5: 100 mg daily

Vitamin B_6: 100 mg daily

Vitamin B_{12}: 1000 μg 2×/week

Vitamin C: 4000–8000 mg/day

Vitamin E: 800 IU daily

Minerals

Magnesium: 242 mg (1000 to 1500 mg)

Manganese: 4.1 mg

Zinc: 30 mg

Chromium: 200 μg

Selenium: 4.9 μg

Potassium chloride: 1000 mg

Amino acids

α-Ketoglutaric: 75 mg 3×/day

Glutahione: 600 mg/day

Taurine: 2 g/day

Buffers

$CaCO_3$: 1 g/day

$KHCO_3$: 2 g/day

$NaHC_3$ 3 g/day

Source: Adapted from Environmental Health Center-Dallas, 1994.
Note: The chemically sensitive patient often needs B vitamins and frequently cannot tolerate them.

TABLE 6.37

Patients with At Least Two Blood Chemical Tests Before and After Treatment: Signs and Symptoms of Improvement

N:	1000
Sex:	39% male
	61% female
Age:	8–67 years old
Mean:	42.4
Course of treatment:	3.6–28 weeks
Mean percentage of sign and symptom improvement:	7.1 weeks
Improvement of levels of toxic chemicals in blood:	78.6%

Source: Adapted from Environmental Health Center-Dallas, 1992.

TABLE 6.38

Gamma Subset Deficiency in 30 Chemically Sensitive Patients

	Low Gamma Globulin	Controls (mg/dL)*
IgG1	10	382–929
IgG2	13	241–700
IgG3	10	22–178
IgG4	8	4–86

Source: Adapted from Environmental Health Center-Dallas, 2016.

* Replacement for injections weekly are 1 per week for 1 month at 70%; 26% for 2 months; 3% for 3 months; 1% for greater than four months.

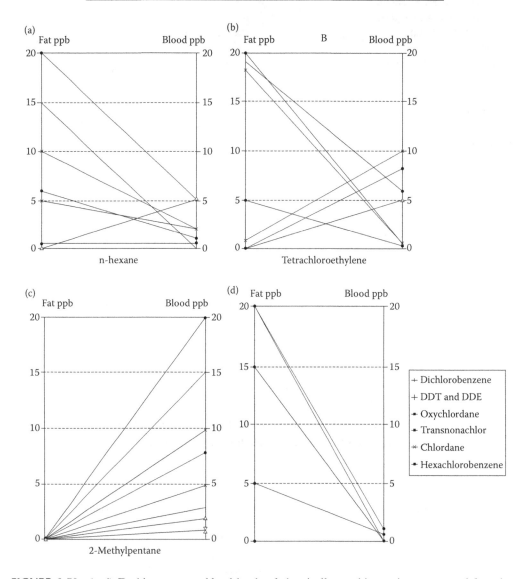

FIGURE 6.59 (a–d) Fat biopsy versus blood levels of chemically sensitive patients measured for n-hexane, tetrachloroethylene, 2-methylpentane, and chlorinated pesticides. (Adapted from Environmental Health Center-Dallas, 1991.)

normality of a particular cell cycle. The DNA content in the nucleus of a cell (2 N or diploid amount) is constant in all normal organisms.[458] There are only two exceptions where the DNA content is not constant; the amount of DNA will vary in cells which undergo meiosis in preparation for sexual reproduction, thus containing the 1 N or haploid amount of DNA. The other exception applies to those cells which undergo DNA synthesis in preparation for mitosis. These will contain between 2 N and 4 N amounts of DNA.

By employing the concept of DNA constancy in a particular organism, and the application of flow cytometric techniques, DNA flow histograms can be constructed depicting a normal cell cycle and the identification of abnormal cycles. The regulation of the cell cycle in eukaryotes seems to take place at two main transition points, prior to DNA replication at a point in the G_1 phase, termed the restriction point, and prior to cytokinesis at the G_2M phase boundary.[459] The progression of the cell cycle from one phase to the other is mediated by specialized proteins, cyclins, and the activation of enzymes called cyclin-dependent kinases (CDKs) and by a number of positive and negative feedback loops. To date seven CDKs have been identified and designated CDK 2 to 8.[460–466] Each CDK acts at different stages of the cell cycle and is differentially regulated by different cyclins.[467] The critical roles played by cyclins in the regulation of eukaryotic cell cycle is amply documented. These CDKs play very significant roles in the G_1S and G_2M transitions during the mammalian cell cycle. They regulate by phosphorylation, a number of key substrates which subsequently activate a transition from G_1 to S and from G_2 to M.[468] The catalytic subunits alone of these CDKs are not active and require the influence of positive regulatory subunits to ensure biochemically active protein kinase holoenzymes.[469] The positive regulatory subunits employed to this end are cyclins. The activity of CDKs is, therefore, regulated by both cyclins and specific phosphorylation and de-phosphorylation.[470–474] This process can regulate the state of hypersensitivity.

Cyclins were identified originally as proteins in the murine invertebrate cells. The concentration of these cyclins accumulate and are destroyed periodically at defined points during the cell cycle.[475] At present, eight cyclins have been identified; these are designated A, B, C, D, E, F, G_1, and H based on their amino acid sequences,[476,477] and in some instances, on genetic complementation experiments in yeast.[474,478–480] The influences of the cyclins are expressed differently; for example, cyclin A exhibits its influence through the S-M phase[481–486] of most cells, while cyclin B (which is conserved from yeasts to humans) propels cells into mitosis[459,475,487]. Both the A and B cyclins are degraded at the M phase by ubiquitin (Ub)-dependent proteolysis.[487] G_1 cyclins (CIN 1, CIN 2, CIN 3) are assumed to associate with a p34 CDC2 homologue, p34 CDC 28, driving yeast cells into S phase.[488–492,499] In the Environmental Health Center-Dallas (EHC-D), clinical cases are investigated varying from surgical to environmental illnesses. However, cases involving chemical sensitivity entail the principal aspect of our practice. Over a period of 22 years, our laboratory observations show that characteristically, a percentage of the chemically sensitive individuals portray a secondary deficit which is related to immune dysfunction, principally, depression of the suppressor T-cell.[493,494] Initial profiles of lymphocyte cell cycle progression, T and B lymphocytes, CMI, and hematograms of patients were compared with those taken subsequent to treatment with ALF.

Acting presumably as a biological response modifier, ALF was observed to modulate deregulated immune profiles. The focus of this investigation was first to observe the patterns of DNA histograms of the T lymphocyte cell cycles, especially in chemically sensitive individuals. The histograms provide a "snapshot" of the individual's present cell cycle. By comparing an individual's cell cycle with the classical normal cycle, very crucial information will be obtained to enable a scientific regulation of a patient's cell cycle. Second, the work was to prepare a lysate from the *in vitro* propagated peripheral T lymphocytes of an individual with an irregular T lymphocytic cell cycle, and observe the regulatory effect of this lysate, when injected subcutaneously into such an individual. Third, the intention was to establish a basis for the regulation of an individual's T lymphocytes which were observed to be irregular due to varied incitants, thus restoring normal T lymphocyte functions, and the enabling of a compromised individual to cope with multiple insults to his/her immune system. Fourth, we examined the responsiveness of T lymphocytes to ALF as measured by the CMI test, and to establish on an individual basis an index of T lymphocyte ability to respond. From our search of databases, and to the best of our knowledge, there is no documentation pertaining to the regulation of the T lymphocytic cell cycle by lysates of an individual's T lymphocytes, and its application to clinical medicine.

A total of 315 individuals were investigated and of these, 25 were controls. T lymphocyte cell cycle profiles, hematological, T and B profiles, and CMI tests were carried out on all candidates. Individuals with immune deregulation were treated with ALF. These individuals were chemically sensitive and chronically ill. The illnesses include dermatitis, vasculitis, asthma, organic brain syndrome, and Gulf war syndrome. In all cases, these illnesses were characterized with immune system suppression, dysfunction or deregulation. Major symptoms presented by these patients include one or more of the following symptoms: lacrimation, pruritus, swelling, and puffiness (ocular); fullness, noise, and dizziness (otic); congestion, sneezing, rhinorrhea, and blowing (nasal); lump, clearing, and postnasal drip (throat); hypersensitivity reactions (immune); arthritis and arthralgia, fatigue and muscle pain (musculoskeletal); pressure and cough (chest); weight loss and fatigue (constitutional); miliary, ethmoidal, and frontal (headache); insomnia, shortness of breath, and depression (neurological).

All 290 chemically sensitive individuals presented a history of being affected by environmental incitants found in categories such as food, biological inhalants, and chemicals. They presented histories of varied backgrounds, but common among them was that all showed irregular cell cycles and abnormal T lymphocyte profiles in both numbers and functions in T and B lymphocytes and subsets. DNA histograms showed over- or underaccumulation of various subtypes of lymphocytes in one or more phases of the cell cycle of each individual.

Delayed cutaneous hypersensitivity, or CMI responses were evaluated in 190 patients; the results were recorded before and after treatment with ALF. The multitest CMI test kit (Mèrieux Institute, Miami, Florida) was used. Each kit contained seven antigens: tetanus, diphtheria, candida, proteus, streptococcus, trichophyton, and tuberculin. The tests were evaluated and read at 48 hours. Evaluation involves scoring the size, and number of increase of the wheals. The diameter of each induration was measured in millimeters and averaged. A reaction was considered positive if the average diameter was 2 mm or more. T and B lymphocytes and subsets were evaluated flow cytometrically before and after treatment with ALF.

Results

Significant changes were observed within 1–6 weeks in patients treated with ALF. Changes were observed in immune regulation and overall clinical manifestations. With regard to clinical manifestations, there were noteworthy improvements (Table 6.39), although minimal symptoms continued after approximately 3 weeks of continued therapy. In a normal cell cycle, the highest percentage of lymphocytes should be in the G_0 to G_1 phase (Figure 6.60). This percentage will change dramatically when these lymphocytes are stimulated by various incitants (Figures 6.62 and 6.63). Consequently, different percentages will appear in the S and G_2M phases, producing a deregulated profile (Figures 6.60 through 6.64). Treatment with ALF regulates the T lymphocyte cell cycle profile. Immunologically, there were significant regulations of T lymphocyte cell cycles, especially from one phase of the cycle to another. Patients become less sensitive and more tolerant to specific incitants. As treatment continued, in general in about 6 weeks, a more drastic shift toward that of a normal profile was observed. Figures 6.60 through 6.64 summarize the regulatory changes of some of the cell cycles studied. Changes were observed in the profiles of the T and B cells where T and B lymphocytes and their subsets were evaluated before and after treatment. There was a significant ($p < 0.01$) change in the total lymphocyte count and subsets T_4, T_8 in 92 patients investigated. It should be noted that ALF seems to act as an immune modifier since the total lymphocytes, T_4, and T_8 were significantly elevated or reduced in order to maintain normalization (Tables 6.40 and 6.41).

TABLE 6.39

Representative Profile of Symptoms and Signs after Autogenous Lymphocytic Factor Treatment

Signs and Symptoms	Improvement: Number %		No change: Number %		Deterioration: Number %		Total Patients
Hypersensitive reaction	63	63	33	33	1	1	100
Recurrent infection	38	57	29	43	0	0	67
Fatigue	60	68	27	31	1	1	88
Lack of concentration	43	54	36	46	0	0	79
Arthritis	19	44	23	54	1	2	43
Gastrointestinal upset	29	40	43	60	0	0	72
Headache	28	44	33	53	2	3	64
Depression	42	58	30	42	0	0	72

Source: Adapted from Environmental Health Center-Dallas.

Patients showed significant improvement ($p < 0.001$) in their CMI scores (Tables 6.42 and 6.43). The regulatory effect of the immune system can be objectively assessed periodically after the initial treatment with ALF. The resourceful parameters are profiles of T lymphocyte cell cycle, T and B lymphocytes, and their subsets, CMI, signs and symptoms.

Side Effects of ALF

The side effects were minimal and occurred only in six adults (five women and one man) where the average age was 52 years. These patients were intolerant of ALF, their symptoms included pain and irritation in the throat, burning in the eyes, pain and irritation in the chest, heat palpitations, influenza-like symptoms, headache, fatigue, and chills.

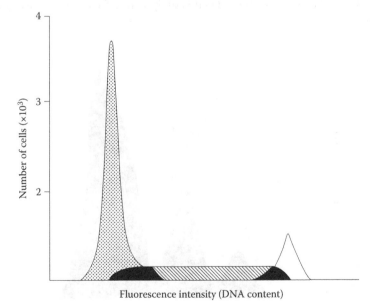

FIGURE 6.60 Diagrammatic representation of a normal mammalian cell cycle, showing the relative number of lymphocytes in each phase of the cycle, as displayed by the intensity of fluorescence of the fluorochrome-bound DNA in each lymphocyte.

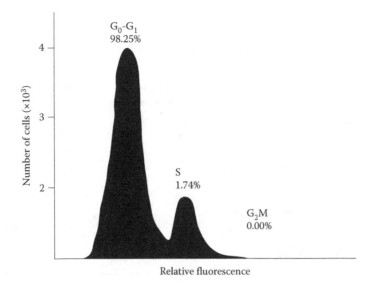

FIGURE 6.61 A representative DNA histogram of peripheral T lymphocytes from normal volunteers.

The flow cytometric profile of the T lymphocyte cell cycle as demonstrated by DNA histogram presents a reflection of the status of T lymphocytes in an individual. Of great importance is that its application is not limited to a certain category of individuals, but to normal subjects as well as individuals who are compromised by varied incitants. The essence of its clinico-biological importance, as detected in the present investigation, is that it is a reflection of T lymphocyte cell function, and may facilitate an in-depth approach to the treatment of some immunodeficient illnesses. The progression of T lymphocytes from one phase of the cell cycle to another is time-dependent, approximately 8–12 hours in the G_0-G_1 phase, 6–8 hours in the S phase, and 0.5–1 hour in the G_2M phase. The 290 individuals who were investigated in this study were affected principally by environmental

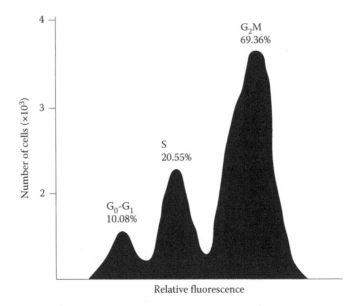

FIGURE 6.62 A representative irregular T lymphocyte cell cycle profile showing the effect(s) of stimulating the environmentally ill patients influence, primarily, the lymphocytes in the S phase.

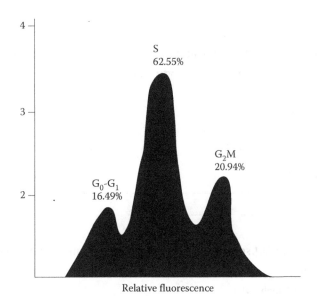

FIGURE 6.63 A representative irregular T lymphocyte cell cycle profile showing the effect(s) of the stimulating incitants on the lymphocytes in the G_2M phase. It seems that each incitant, or a mixture of incitants, affects lymphocytes in a particular phase(s) of the cell cycle, resulting in a variety of irregular cell cycle profiles and presumably dictates varied patterns of clinical manifestations. The abscissae in Figures 6.62 and 6.63 show the relative fluorescence of the fluorochrome-bound DNA in each cell.

incitants in categories such as foods, biological inhalants, and chemicals. They presented histories of varied backgrounds and different cell cycle profiles.

The DNA histogram cycles showed over- or underaccumulation of lymphocytes in one or more phases of the cell cycle of each individual (Figures 6.62 and 6.63). As shown in Figure 6.62, even the normal controls do not present an ideal DNA histogram profile of T lymphocytes. This is due to the fact that, in general, the ideal environment is seldom ever achieved, thus there is always some degree of immunological compromise to most individuals. It is reasonable then

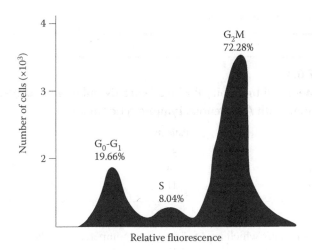

FIGURE 6.64 Initial T lymphocyte cell cycle profile of a patient on examination at the clinic. Note that the irregularity of the profile is emphasized in the G_2M phase.

TABLE 6.40

Representative Changes in T and B Cell Profiles after 92 Chemically Sensitive Patients Were Treated with Autogenous Lymphocytic Factor

Treatment	Total Lymphocytes	T_{11}	T_4	T_8	T_4/T_8	B_4
Before	2112 ± 632	1624 ± 457	930 ± 45	439 ± 58	2.3 ± 0.8	188 ± 102
After	$2232 \pm 678*$	1634 ± 544	$1027 \pm 297**$	$478 \pm 189**$	1.3 ± 7.4	171 ± 120

* $p < 0.05$; **$p < 0.01$; $n = 92$.

TABLE 6.41

Profile of T Lymphocyte Subsets Modulation after Treatment with Autogenous Lymphocytic Factor

After Treatment	Total lymphocytes: Number %		T_{11} Number %		T_4 Number %		T_8 Number %	
Increase	52	57	41	46	53	53	55	60
Decrease	40	43	51	54	39	42	37	40
Probability	<0.05		>0.05		<0.05		<0.01	

TABLE 6.42

Typical Cell-Mediated Response in (Number and Size) Chemically Sensitive Individuals with Autogenous Lymphocytic Factor

Patients	Before ALF	After ALF	P
190	5.46 ± 5.81	9.28 ± 7.25	<0.001

Results are given as mean $\pm$ SD.

TABLE 6.43

Cell-Mediated Immunity Positive Score (Number and Size) after Treatment with Autogenous Lymphocytic Factor

Score	Patients	%	P
Increase	58	74	<0.001
No change	9	12	
Decrease	11	14	

to assume that the incitants which lead to immunoincompetence of these individuals are capable of inactivating the particular enzyme(s), CDKs, or depleting specific cyclins whose combination with their specific kinases are instrumental in catalyzing the progression of T lymphocytes from one phase to another of the cell cycle. The T lymphocytes of the individual affected are locked in a particular phase, either resting, synthesizing, or multiplying too much in the G_0-G_1, S, G_2M phase, respectively. Thus, the subject manifests symptoms peculiar to the phase(s) affected. This hypothesis offers an opportunity to associate clinical manifestations with T lymphocyte cell cycle irregularity.

The treatment of lasting importance would be reasonably thought of as a biological response modifier, which would stimulate CDKs, regulate the cell cycle and the enzymes of purine and pyrimidine nucleotide synthesis. It is now generally accepted that these enzymes are elevated during the S phase.[495] It seems logical that ALF stimulates these regulatory functions. The ALF is a dialyzable mixture of the many effector substances which may be released from *in vitro* grown stimulated lymphocytes with the ability to invoke immunological influences *in vivo* or *in vitro*.[496] The expected biological activity(s) of ALF would be to act as a biological response modifier, with mechanisms of action as suppressor and regulator of the immune system, especially in the regulation of the T lymphocyte cell cycle.

Kamp et al.[468] showed that progression through the cell cycle requires the joint influence of positive regulator subunits, cyclins, and CDKs. These subunits regulate by phosphorylation a number of key substrates which subsequently activate a transition from G_1 to S, and G_2 to M phases of the cell cycle. Phosphate groups are transferred from ATP to a special amino acid in the target protein by protein kinases, while phosphatases remove the phosphate groups from the target proteins. The addition and removal of phosphate groups significantly affect the biochemical behavior of the target proteins. Many protein kinases and phosphatases have a specific affinity for their target proteins, and act as determinants for controlling the activity(s) of their target proteins. Indeed, ALF may possess these protein kinases which, acting as molecular switches, regulate an irregular T lymphocyte cell cycle to that of an ordered and orderly progression. Thus, helping the hypersensitivity being dampened or being thwarted.

As demonstrated (Figures 6.64 through 6.66), ALF regulates deregulated cell cycles, improves immunological profiles by increasing or decreasing the number of circulating lymphocytes and their subpopulations (Tables 6.39 and 6.40), and restores immune responses as demonstrated by enhanced cutaneous hypersensitivity (CMI) (Table 6.41). ALF also invoked immediate intradermal test response within 45 minutes of administration subsequent to the administration of antigen challenges, which were previously negative or delayed for at least 15 days. Responses were observed by the number and size of wheals to the antigens which were inoculated. It is noteworthy that some

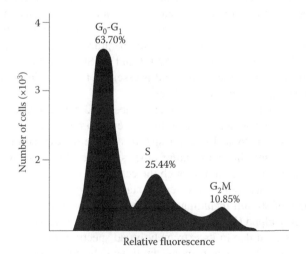

FIGURE 6.65 Cell cycle of the patient in Figure 6.64 after the subject was treated with autogenous lymphocytic factor (ALF) for 3 weeks. Note that the percentages of lymphocytes in each phase of the cell cycle are still irregular, but there has been a significant improvement. The highest percentage of lymphocytes now appears in the G_0-G_1 phase.

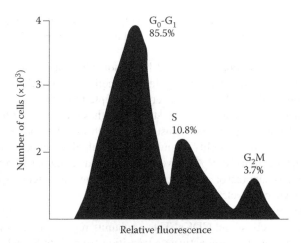

FIGURE 6.66 T lymphocyte cell cycle of a patient (Figures 6.64 and 6.65) subsequent to 3 months treatment with ALF. Note that the cell cycle has attained a relatively normal profile. ALF seems to act as a biological response modifier. The abscissae in Figures 6.64, 6.65, and 6.66 show the relative fluorescence of the fluorochrome-bound DNA in each cell.

chemically sensitive patients responded favorably, or completely recovered after environmental exposure to air, food, water, nutritional support, and exercise. Some patients responded but did not fully recover. The patients who recovered reacted profoundly to exposure of very minute environmental insults of ambient chemicals, biological inhalants, and foods. However, when these patients were treated with ALF, their hypersensitivity was markedly reduced or disappeared; there was also significant improvement in recurrent infection, fatigue, headaches, depression, concentration, and gastrointestinal upsets. Eight patients immediately improved on initial injection with ALF.

T-suppressor, T-helper cells, and total lymphocytes were increased as reflected in an increase in a low population, and a decrease in a too high population. This suggests that ALF is a modulator rather than a simulator. The mechanism(s) of action of ALF has not yet been ascertained. Indeed, the purification and determination of ALF from sorted T lymphocytes with or without helper phenotypes will be necessary to facilitate understanding the mechanism of action. However, it has been documented that the human cells contain a regulatory protein, cyclin dependent-kinase subunit (CKS) protein, which is a genetic suppressor of temperature-sensitive CDK mutations. There are two isoforms of this CKS protein, namely, CKSH1 and CKSH2. It is believed that CKSH2 protein binds to the catalytic subunit of the CDKs, and is essential for their biological function.[497] To this end, further investigations are being carried out.

The concept of a functional cell cycle is timely. Indeed, the profile of a cell cycle offers an insight into the immune status of a patient. However, the cell cycle profile does not indicate whether or not the lymphocytes are immunologically responsive or capable of responding to therapy. The influence of varied environmental incitants and/or other systemic illnesses may render these lymphocytes incapable of normal progression through the cell cycle, thus resulting in a nonfunctional cell cycle. *In vitro* lymphocyte activation represents a standard procedure for evaluating cell-mediated responses to a variety of stimuli including antibodies, polyclonal mitogens, specific antigens, and cytokines. Interleukin-1 alpha (IL_1 alpha) and ALF were used as activators in the present investigation. IL-1 alpha was used due to its extremely broad spectrum of bioactivity. ALF was used to observe its capability as a biological response modifier. The stipulatory process presented in this investigation offers a method of computing lymphocyte stipulatory response, and consequently an opportunity to establish an individual regime of treatment of illnesses associated with immunodeficiency. This investigation offers: (1) a vivid picture of the status of the immune profile of a patient as demonstrated by the DNA histogram of the T lymphocyte cell cycle, (2) an opportunity to regulate an irregular T lymphocyte cell cycle by treatment with ALF, and (3) a clinical tool for the regulation of abnormal cell cycles and/or hematological and immunological profiles in humans with immunological deregulation. We have used ALF in over 5000 chemically sensitive and immune-deregulated patients with a similar success rate and complications rate as the 290 patients.

NUTRITION

The clinician has to supplement the chemically sensitive patients with the appropriate nutrition to satisfy the detoxification mechanism of gluconation, methylation, sulfonation, acetylation, nitrozation, as well as other unknown and all deficiency entities. These nutrient mechanisms are separate but the clinician has to be sure whether oral or parenteral nutrition can be used, as well as when each is needed and how much of each will benefit the chemically sensitive patient. Excess at times can be a problem.

The following is the list of supplements essential for nutritional therapy: first intravenous then oral

- A series of IV type is usually presented to detoxify the chemically sensitive.
- Vitamin C, 15–25 g/day.
- Glutathione, 1000 ± 200 g.
- Multiple B vitamins, 1 ampule containing B1, B2, B3, B6, B12, and B-complex.
- Multimineral, containing 1 ampule (Ca^{2+}, Mg^{2+}, Zn^+, Cu^{2+}, and Cr^+)
- Extra magnesium glycinate 200–400 mg, other Mg^{2+} compounds.
- Extra taurine, 2 g.

These can be administered 1–3 times per week as needed until the patient feels better. Over 10,000 IVs have been given successfully over the years. However, 1000 have been aborted because the chemically sensitive patient could not tolerate them. These patients who cannot tolerate IVs also had a difficult time tolerating oral foods; until a rigid nonpolluted environment control was instituted.

A series of caloric intake of proteins and lipids can also be administered to sustain weight and the proper nutrition:

- Amino acid, 1000 cc in addition to the same amount of caloric intake daily
- Carbohydrate, 1000 calories/day
- Lipids, 500 cc and 1000 calories/day
- Multivitamin
- Multiminerals

The clinician needs a central venous line to administer these. Each chemically sensitive patient who can tolerate no food may be linked to how much of each they can process, because they are sensitive to the source. Although they are bypassing the gastrointestinal tract, they may have a limited volume of CHO, proteins, and lipids that they can tolerate. A classic case of a 41-year-old white woman with hyperalimentation for 1.5 years is a good example to further understand parenteral nutrition. This lasted until she finally was able to eat again. She had a central venous line with 2500 calories/day administered. Oral nutrition is the usual route. It is tailored to what the chemically sensitive can tolerate. What can be administered is 1000–5000 mg of vitamin C, glutathione 800–1200 mg, 1 capsule of multiminerals containing zinc, copper, chromium, magnesium, and manganese. Multivitamins B, in addition to vitamin D, E, and A, is individualized as well as other vitamins, nutrients, and minerals as needed.

A field of nutrition has grown up to treat the chemically sensitive and chronically ill patient which must be individualized. Some with extremely high and other extremely low sensitivities.

SURGERY AND NEUTRALIZATION OF IMPLANT MATERIAL

Implants can specifically act as incitant and or help create the total body pollutant load. It is preferrable that they can be removed but often the remains will have to be neutralized by injection for the remaining residual, which can still trigger the hypersensitivity response or, if the implants cannot be removed, aid in dampening the hypersensitivity response.

Teeth

1. The most common implants are dental fillings. Still some dark fillings have mercury in them. They need to be removed and replaced with gold or porcelain, which can be tested by the intradermal technique for compatability. There are several types of porcelain some of which some patients cannot tolerate. Acrylics, methyl methacrylate are used as a silicone. Many patients cannot tolerate in the long run as they can be the originators of the hypersensitivity phenomena.
2. Metals—stainless steel, titanium, titanium alloy containing chromium, colbalt, copper, zinc, lithium, and nickle.

SUMMARY

In summary, the environmentally compromised patient may be treated with:

1. Avoidance of pollutants in air, food, and water
2. Injection therapy for the hypersensitive stage
3. Sauna, physical therapy in environmentally controlled conditions in order to mobilize pollutants stuck in membranes
4. Immune modulation for immune modulators such as gamma globulin and autogenous lymphocytic factor
5. Nutrition to keep the detoxification and healing mechanisms optimum,
   a. Oral
   b. Intravenous
   c. Central venous for calories
6. Oxygen therapy
   a. Von Ardenne technique
   b. Hyperbaric
7. Surgery
   a. Removal of implants and fillings
   b. Removal of infected and affected incitants
   c. Replacement of O_2-starved vessels

REFERENCES

1. Pischinger, A. 1983. *Das System der Grundregulation, Grundlagen für eine ganzheitsbiologische Theorie der Medizin*. 4. Aufl. Karl. Heidelbert: Haug Verlag.
2. Heine, H. 1987. Die Grundregulation aus neuer Sicht. *Ärztezeitschr. F. Naturheilverf.* 28:909–914.
3. Seyle, H. 1946. The general adaptation syndrome and the diseases of adaptations. *J. Allergy* 17:23.
4. Rea, W. J. 1992. Chemical sensitivity. Vol I. *Mechanisms of Chemical Sensitivity*. p. 47. Boca Raton, FL: Lewis Publishers.
5. Rea, W. J. 1992. Chemical sensitivity. Vol I. *Mechanisms of Chemical Sensitivity*. p. 155. Boca Raton, FL: Lewis Publishers.
6. Rea, W. J. 1995. Chemical sensitivity. Vol III. *Clinical Manifestations of Pollutant Overload*. p. 1727. Boca Raton, FL: Lewis Publishers.

7. Levine, S. A, M. P. Kidd. 1985. *Antioxidant Adaption: Its Role in Free Radical Pathology.* San Leandro, CA: Biocurrents, Allergy Research Group.
8. Rea, W. J. 1992. Chemical sensitivity. Vol. 1. *Mechanisms of Chemical Sensitivity.* p. 221. Boca Raton, FL: Lewis Publishers.
9. Perger, F. 1987. *Die Vor-und Nachbehandlung von Herdsanierungen Natura-Heidelbert.*
10. Heine, H. 1991. The structure and function of the ground substance (extracellular matrix): Paradigms in medical thinking. In *Matrix and Matrix Regulation: Basis for a Holistic Theory in Medicine,* A. Pischinger. Ed., H. Heine, Eng. Trans. N. Mac Lean, p. 19. Brussels, Belgium: Editions Haug International.
11. Rea, W. J. 1997. Chemical sensitivity. Vol. IV. *Tools of Diagnosis and Methods of Treatment.* p. 2025. Boca Raton, FL: CRC Lewis Publishers.
12. Draczyski, G. 1991. Introduction. In *Matrix and Matrix Regulation: Basis for a Holistic Theory in Medicine,* A. Pischinger, Ed., H. Heine, Eng. Trans. N. Mac Lean, p. 7. Brussels, Belgium: Editions Haug International.
13. Pischinger, A. 1975. *Matrix and Matrix Regulation: Basis for a Holistic Theory in Medicine,* H. Heine, Ed., Eng. Trans. N. Mac Lean. Brussels, Belgium: Editions Haug International.
14. Bergsmann, O., G. Kellner, O. Maresch. 1971. Synopse zur Frage der biologischen Regulation. *Arzil Prasis* XXIII. 933, 1061, 1193, 1376.
15. Kellner, G. 1965. Nachweis der herderkrankung und ihre Grundlager. *Die Therapiewache* 15 (24):1267.
16. Perger, F. 1987. Das Zuysammenspiel zwischen den Regelsystemen der Abwehr und seine Storungen. *EHKd.* 36:566.
17. Hauss, W. H. 1961. Uber die Entstehung und Behandlung rheumatischer Erkrankungen. *Hippokrates* 32 (17):678.
18. Hauss, W. H., G. Junge-Hulsing. 1961. Uber die universelle unspezifishce Mesenchymreaktion. *Disch. Med. Wschr.* 86(16):763–768.
19. Bissell, M. J. 2003. Tissue architecture. The ultimate regulator of breast epithelial function. *Curr. Opin. Cell Biol.* 15(6).
20. Reichert, C. B. 1845. *Vergleichende Beobachtungen uber das Bindegewebe und die verwandten Gebilde.* Dorpat 1845, S. 168.
21. Bordeu, L. *Recherches sur le Tissu Muqueux ou L'organ Cellulaire.* Paris, 1767 1 und 2.
22. Pischinger, A. 1979. Die humoral-zellulare Reaktion des lympho-monozytaren Systems. *EHKd.* 28:317.
23. Heine, H. 1992. Biorthythmus und Strwktur der Grundsubstanz (Matrix) unter normalen und patholo-gischen Verhaltnissen. In *Normal Matrix ad Pathological Conditions,* H. Heine, P. Anastasiadis, Eds., p. 7. Stuttgart: Gustav Fischer Verlag.
24. Reicker, G. 1925. *Pathologie als Naurwissenschaft.* Berlin: Springer.
25. Eppinger, H. 1949. *Die Permeabilitatatspathologie als die Lehre vom Krankheitsbeginn.* Wien: Springer-Verlag.
26. Heine, H. 1988. Anatomische Strukur der Akupunkturpunkte. *Dtsch. Zschr. Akup* 31:26–30.
27. Heine, H. 1991. The structure and function of the ground substance (extracellular matrix): Paradigms in medical thinking. In *Matrix and Matrix Regulation: Basis for a Holistic Theory in Medicine,* A. Pischinger, Ed., H. Heine, Eng. Trans. N. Mac Lean, p. 17. Brussels, Belgium: Editions Haug International.
28. Hauss, W. H., G. Junge-Hülsing, G. Gerlach. 1968. *Die unsoezifische Mesenchymreaktion.* Stuttgart: Thieme.
29. Heine, H., G. Schaeg. 1979. *Informationssteuerung in der vegetativen Peripherie.* Z. f. Hautkrh.
30. Heine, H. 1991. The structure and function of the ground substance (extracellular matrix): Paradigms in medical thinking. *Matrix and Matric Regulation: Basis for a Holistic Theory in Medicine,* Pischinger A, ed. Heine H, Eng. Trans. N. Mac Lean, p. 20. Brussels, Belgium: Editions Haug International.
31. Rea, W. J. 1995. Chemical sensitivity. Vol. III. *Clinical Manesfestations of Pollutant Overload.* Boca Raton, FL: Lewis Publishers.
32. Heine, H. 1991. The structure and function of the ground substance (extracellular matrix): Paradigms in medical thinking. In *Matrix and Matric Regulation: Basis for a Holistic Theory in Medicine,* A. Pischinger, Ed., H. Heine, Eng. Trans. N. Mac Lean, pp. 21, 23. Brussels, Belgium: Editions Haug International.
33. Rea, W. J. 1992. Chemical sensitivity. Vol. I. *Mechanisms of Chemical Sensitivity.* p. 155. Boca Raton, FL: Lewis Publishers.
34. Rea, W. J. 1992. Chemical sensitivity. Vol. I. *Mechanisms of Chemical Sensitivity.* p. 47. Boca Raton, FL: Lewis Publishers.

35. Rea, W. J. 1995. Chemical sensitivity. Vol. III. *Clinical Manesfestations of Pollutant Overload*. 1727. Boca Raton, FL: Lewis Publishers.

36. Heine, H. 1991. The structure and function of the ground substance (extracellular matrix): Paradigms in medical thinking. In *Matrix and Matric Regulation: Basis for a Holistic Theory in Medicine*, A. Pischinger, Ed., H. Heine, Eng. Trans. N. Mac Lean, p. 23. Brussels, Belgium: Editions Haug International.

37. Heine, H. 1991. The structure and function of the ground substance (extracellular matrix): Paradigms in medical thinking. In *Matrix and Matric Regulation: Basis for a Holistic Theory in Medicine*, A. Pischinger, Ed., H. Heine, Eng. Trans. N. Mac Lean, p. 27. Brussels, Belgium: Editions Haug International.

38. Heine, H. 1991. The structure and function of the ground substance (extracellular matrix): Paradigms in medical thinking. In *Matrix and Matric Regulation: Basis for a Holistic Theory in Medicine*, A. Pischinger, Ed., H. Heine, Eng. Trans. N. Mac Lean, p. 28. Brussels, Belgium: Editions Haug International.

39. Pischinger, A. 1957. Die Bedeutung hochmolekularer ungesättigter Fettsäuren im Blut. *Therapiewoche* 7:397.

40. Pischinger, A. 1957. Das Scicksal der Leukozyten. *Blut. Z. mikr.-anat. Forsch.* 63:169–192.

41. Heine, H. 1991. The structure and function of the ground substance (extracellular matrix): Paradigms in medical thinking. In *Matrix and Matric Regulation: Basis for a Holistic Theory in Medicine*, A. Pischinger, Ed., H. Heine, Eng. Trans. N. Mac Lean, pp. 23–30. Brussels, Belgium: Editions Haug International.

42. Duan, W., Z. Zhang, D. M. Gash, M. P. Mattson. 1999. Participation of Par-4 in degeneration of dopaminergic neurons in models of Parkinson's disease. *Ann. Neurol.* 46:587–597.

43. Kruman, II, C. Culmsee, S. L. Chan, Y. Kruman, Z. Guo, L. Penix, M. P. Mattson. 2000. Homocysteine elicits a DNA damage response in neurons that promotes apoptosis and hypersensitivity to excitotoxicity. *J. Neurosci.* 20:6920–6926.

44. Seshadri, S., A. Beiser, J. Selhub, P. F. Jacques, I. H. Rosenberg, R. B. D'Agostino, P. W. Wilson, P. A. Wolf. 2002. Plasma homocysteine as a risk factor for dementia and Alzheimer's disease. *N. Engl. J. Med.* 346:476–483.

45. Fenech, M. 2001. The role of folic acid and Vitamin B12 in genomic stability of human cells. *Mutat. Res.* 475:57–67.

46. Kruman, II, T. S. Kumaravel, A. Lohani, R. G. Cutler, W. A. Pedersen, Y. Kruman, M. Evans, M. P. Mattson. 2002. Folic acid deficiency and homocysteine impair DNA repair and sensitize hippocampal neurons to death in experimental models of Alzheimer's disease. *J. Neurosci.* 22:1752–1762.

47. Halliwell, B. 2001. Role of free radicals in the neurodegenerative diseases: Therapeutic implications for antioxidant treatment. *Drugs Aging* 18:685–716.

48. Youdim, K. A, J. A. Joseph. 2001. A possible emerging role of phytochemicals in improving age-related neurological dysfunctions: A multiplicity of effects. *Free Radic. Biol. Med.* 30:583–594.

49. Mattson, M. P. 2000. Creatine: Prescription for bad genes and a hostile environment? *Trends Neurosci.* 23:511.

50. Weindruch, R., R. S. Sohal. 1997. Seminars in medicine of the Beth Israel Deaconess Medical Center. Caloric intake and aging. *N. Engl. J. Med.* 337:986–994.

51. Lin, S. J., P. A. Defossez, L. Guarente. 2000. Requirement of NAD and SIR2 for life-span extension by calorie restriction in *Saccharomyces cerevisiae*. *Science* 289:2126–2128.

52. Sze, J. Y., M. Victor, C. Loer, Y. Shi, G. Ruvkun. 2000. Food and metabolic signalling defects in a *Caenorhabditis elegans* serotonin synthesis mutant. *Nature* 403:560–564.

53. Dubey, A., M. J. Forster, H. Lal, R. S. Sohal. 1996. Effect of age and caloric intake on protein oxidation in different brain regions and on behavioral functions of the mouse. *Arch. Biochem. Biophys.* 333:189–197.

54. Major, D. E., J. P. Kesslak, C. W. Cotman, C. E. Finch, J. R. Day. 1997. Life-long dietary restriction attenuates age-related increases in hippocampal glial fibrillary acidic protein mRNA. *Neurobiol. Aging* 18:523–526.

55. Guo, Z., A. Ersoz, D. A. Butterfield, M. P. Mattson. 2000. Beneficial effects of dietary restriction on cerebral cortical synaptic terminals: Preservation of glucose transport and mitochondrial function after exposure to amyloid b-peptide and oxidative and metabolic insults. *J. Neurochem.* 75:314–320.

56. Yeung, J. M., E. Friedman. 1991. Effect of aging and diet restriction on monoamines and amino acids in cerebral cortex of Fischer-344 rats. *Growth Dev. Aging* 55:275–283.

57. Lee, J., W. Duan, J. M. Long, D. K. Ingram, M. P. Mattson. 2000. Dietary restriction increases survival of newly-generated neural cells and induces BDNF expression in the dentate gyrus of rats. *J. Mol. Neurosci.* 15:99–108.

58. Lee, J., J. P. Herman, M. P. Mattson. 2000. Dietary restriction selectively decreases glucocorticoid receptor expression in the hippocampus and cerebral cortex of rats. *Exp. Neurol.* 166:435–441.

59. Lee, C. K., R. Weindruch, T. A. Prolla. 2000. Gene-expression profile of the ageing brain in mice. *Nat. Genet.* 25:294–297.

60. Bruce-Keller, A. J., G. Umberger, R. McFall, M. P. Mattson. 1999. Food restriction reduces brain damage and improves behavioral outcome following excitotoxic and metabolic insults. *Ann. Neurol.* 45:8–15.

61. Mahoney, A. W., D. G. Hendricks, N. Bernhard, D. V. Sisson. 1983. Fasting and ketogenic diet effects on audiogenic seizures susceptibility of magnesium deficient rats. *Pharmacol. Biochem. Behav.* 18:683–687.

62. Greene, A. E., M. T. Todorova, R. McGowan, T. N. Seyfried. 2001. Caloric restriction inhibits seizure susceptibility in epileptic EL mice by reducing blood glucose. *Epilepsia* 42:1371–1378.

63. Yudkoff, M., Y. Daikhin, I. Nissim, A. Lazarow, I. Nissim. 2001. Ketogenic diet, amino acid metabolism, and seizure control. *J. Neurosci. Res.* 66:931–940.

64. Guo, Q., W. Fu, B. L. Sopher, M. W. Miller, C. B. Ware, G. M. Martin, M. P. Mattson. 1999. Increased vulnerability of hippocampal neurons to excitotoxic necrosis in presenilin-1 mutant knockin mice. *Nature Med.* 5:101–107.

65. Duan, W., M. P. Mattson. 1999. Dietary restriction and 2-deoxyglucose administration improve behavioral outcome and reduce degeneration of dopaminergic neurons in models of Parkinson's disease. *J. Neurosci. Res.* 57:195–206.

66. Rea, W. J. 1994. Chemical sensitivity. Vol. II. *Sources of Total Body Load.* p. 525. Boca Raton, FL: Lewis Publishers.

67. Heine, H. 1991. The structure and function of the ground substance (extracellular matrix): Paradigms in medical thinking. In *Matrix and Matrix Regulation: Basis for a Holistic Theory in Medicine*, A. Pischinger, Ed., H. Heine, Eng. Trans. N. Mac Lean, p. 31. Brussels, Belgium: Editions Haug International.

68. Stern und Wilhelm. 1937. *Z. Krebsforsch 46:379 zit. Bei Hinsberg*, Krebsrpoblem.

69. Heine, H. 1991. The structure and function of the ground substance (extracellular matrix): Paradigms in medical thinking. In *Matrix and Matrix Regulation: Basis for a Holistic Theory in Medicine*, A. Pischinger, Ed., H. Heine, Eng. Trans. N. Mac Lean, p. 41. Brussels, Belgium: Editions Haug International.

70. Rea, W.J. 1994. Chemical sensitivity. Vol. II. *Sources of Total Body Load.* p. 1011. Boca Raton, FL: Lewis Publishers.

71. Rutter, J., M. Reick, S. L. McKnight. 2002. Metabolism and the control of circadian rhythms. *Annu. Rev. Biochem.* 71:307–331.

72. Takahashi, J. S., H. K. Hong, C. H. Ko, E. L. McDearmon. 2008. The genetics of mammalian circadian order and disorder: Implications for physiology and disease. *Nat. Rev. Genet.* 9 (10):764–775.

73. Nakajima, M., K. Imai, H. Ito, T. Nishiwaki, Y. Murayama, H. Iwasaki, T. Oyama, T. Kondo. 2005. Reconstitution of circadian oscillation of cyanobacterial KaiC phosphorylation in vitro. *Science* 308 (5720):414–415.

74. O'Neill, J. S., E. S. Maywood, J. E. Chesham, J. S. Takahashi, M. H. Hastings. 2008. cAMP-dependent signaling as a core component of the mammalian circadian pacemaker. *Science* 320:949.

75. Ko, C. H., Y. R. Yamada, D. K. Welsh, E. D. Buhr, A. C. Liu, E. E. Zhang, M. R. Ralph, S. A. Kay, D. B. Forger, J. S. Takahashi. 2010. Emergence of noise-induced oscillations in the central circadian pacemaker. *PLoS Biol.* 8 (10):e1000513.

76. Zhang, E. E., A. C. Liu, T. Hirota, L. J. Miraglia, G. Welch, P. Y. Pongsawakul, X. Liu, A. Atwood, J. W. Huss 3rd, J. Janes, A. I. Su, J. B. Hogenesch, S. A. Kay. 2009. A genome-wide RNAi screen for modifiers of the circadian clock in human cells. *Cell* 139 (1):199–210.

77. Balsalobre, A., F. Damiola, U. Schibler. 1998. A serum shock induces circadian gene expression in mammalian tissue culture cells. *Cell* 93 (6):929–937.

78. Stokkan, K. A., S. Yamazaki, H. Tei, Y. Sakaki, M. Menaker. 2001. Entrainment of the circadian clock in the liver by feeding. *Science* 291 (5503):490–493.

79. Yang, X., M. Downes, R. T. Yu, A. L. Bookout, W. He, M. Straume, D. J. Mangelsdorf, R. M. Evans. 2006. Nuclear receptor expression links the circadian clock to metabolism. *Cell* 126 (4):801–810.

80. Le Martelot, G., T. Claudel, D. Gatfield, O. Schaad, B. Kornmann, G. Lo Sasso, A. Moschetta. 2009. REV-ERBalpha participates in circadian SREBP signaling and bile acid homeostasis. *PLoS Biol.* 7 (9):e1000181.

81. Arble, D. M., J. Bass, A. D. Laposky, M. H. Vitaterna, F. W. Turek. 2009. Circadian timing of food intake contributes to weight gain. *Obesity* 17 (11):2100–2102.

82. Schmutz, I., J. A. Ripperger, S. Baeriswyl-Aebischer, U. Albrecht. 2010. The mammalian clock component PERIOD2 coordinates circadian output by interaction with nuclear receptors. *Genes Dev.* 24:345.

83. Roesler, W. J., P. J. McFie, C. Dauvin. 1992. The liver-enriched transcription factor D-site-binding protein activates the promoter of the phosphoenolpyruvate carboxykinase gene in hepatoma cells. *J. Biol. Chem.* 267:21235.

84. Zhang, E. E., Y. Liu, R. Dentin, P. Y. Pongsawakul, A. C. Liu, T. Hirota, D. A. Nusinow, X. Sun, S. Landais, Y. Kodama, D. A. Brenner, M. Montminy, S. A. Kay. 2010. Cryptochrome mediates circadian regulation of cAMP signaling and hepatic gluconeogenesis. *Nat. Med.* 16 (10):1152–1156.

85. Dodd, A. N., N. Salathia, A. Hall, E. Kévei, R. Tóth, F. Nagy, J. M. Hibberd, A. J. Millar, A. A. Webb. 2005. Plant circadian clocks increase photosynthesis, growth, survival, and competitive advantage. *Science* 309 (5734):630–633.

86. Dioum, E. M., J. Rutter, J. R. Tuckerman, G. Gonzalez, M. A. Gilles-Gonzalez, S. L. McKnight. 2002. NPAS2: A gas-responsive transcription factor. *Science* 298(5602):2385–2387.

87. McNamara, P., S. B. Seo, R. D. Rudic, A. Sehgal, D. Chakravarti, G. A. FitzGerald. 2001. Regulation of CLOCK and MOP4 by nuclear hormone receptors in the vasculature: A humoral mechanism to reset a peripheral clock. *Cell* 105 (7):877–889.

88. Tasali, E., R. Leproult, D. A. Ehrmann, E. Van Cauter. 2008. Slow-wave sleep and the risk of type 2 diabetes in humans. *Proc. Natl. Acad. Sci. USA* 105 (3):1044–1049.

89. Saper, C. B., T. E. Scammell, J. Lu. 2005. Hypothalamic regulation of sleep and circadian rhythms. *Nature* 437 (7063):1257–1263.

90. Adamantidis, A., L. de Lecea. 2008. Sleep and metabolism: Shared circuits, new connections. *Trends Endocrinol. Metab.* 19 (10):362–370.

91. Funato, H., A. L. Tsai, J. T. Willie, Y. Kisanuki, S. C. Williams, T. Sakurai, M. Yanagisawa. 2009. Enhanced orexin receptor-2 signaling prevents diet-induced obesity and improves leptin sensitivity. *Cell Metab.* 9 (1):64–76.

92. Taheri, S., J. M. Zeitzer, E. Mignot. 2002. The role of hypocretins (orexins) in sleep regulation and narcolepsy. *Annu. Rev. Neurosci.* 25:283–313.

93. Laposky, A. D., M. A. Bradley, D. L. Williams, J. Bass, F. W. Turek. 2008. Sleep-wake regulation is altered in leptin-resistant (db/db) genetically obese and diabetic mice. *Am. J. Physiol. Regul. Integr. Comp. Physiol.* 295 (6):R2059–R2066.

94. Scheer, F. A., M. F. Hilton, C. S. Mantzoros, S. A. Shea. 2009. Adverse metabolic and cardiovascular consequences of circadian misalignment. *Proc. Natl. Acad. Sci. USA* 106 (11):4453–4458.

95. Kohsaka, A., A. D. Laposky, K. M. Ramsey, C. Estrada, C. Joshu, Y. Kobayashi, F. W. Turek, J. Bass. 2007. High-fat diet disrupts behavioral and molecular circadian rhythms in mice. *Cell Metab.* 6 (5):414–421.

96. Lamia, K. A., U. M. Sachdeva, L. DiTacchio, E. C. Williams, J. G. Alvarez, D. F. Egan, D. S. Vasquez, H. Juguilon, S. Panda, R. J. Shaw, C. B. Thompson, R. M. Evans. 2009. AMPK regulates the circadian clock by cryptochrome phosphorylation and degradation. *Science* 326 (5951):437–440.

97. Asher, G., D. Gatfield, M. Stratmann, H. Reinke, C. Dibner, F. Kreppel, R. Mostoslavsky, F. W. Alt, U. Schibler. 2008. SIRT1 regulates circadian clock gene expression through PER2 deacetylation. *Cell* 134 (2):317–328.

98. Nakahata, Y., M. Kaluzova, B. Grimaldi, S. Sahar, J. Hirayama, D. Chen, L. P. Guarente, P. Sassone-Corsi. 2008. The NAD$^+$-dependent deacetylase SIRT1 modulates CLOCK-mediated chromatin remodeling and circadian control. *Cell* 134 (2):329–340.

99. Ramsey, K. M., J. Yoshino, C. S. Brace, D. Abrassart, Y. Kobayashi, B. Marcheva, H. K. Hong, J. L. Chong, E. D. Buhr, C. Lee, J. S. Takahashi, S. Imai, J. Bass. 2009. *Science* 324 (5927):651–654. doi: 10.1126/science.1171641. Epub 2009 Mar 19.

100. Nakahata, Y., S. Sahar, G. Astarita, M. Kaluzova, P. Sassone-Corsi. 2009. Circadian control of the NAD$^+$ salvage pathway by CLOCK-SIRT1. *Science* 324 (5927):654–657.

101. Rodgers, J. T., P. Puigserver. 2007. Fasting-dependent glucose and lipid metabolic response through hepatic sirtuin 1. *Proc. Natl. Acad. Sci. USA* 104 (31):12861–12866.

102. Asher, G., H. Reinke, M. Altmeyer, M. Gutierrez-Arcelus, M. O. Hottiger, U. Schibler. 2010. Poly(ADP-ribose) polymerase 1 participates in the phase entrainment of circadian clocks to feeding. *Cell* 142 (6):943–953.

103. Heine, H. 1991. The structure and function of the ground substance (extracellular matrix): Paradigms in medical thinking. In *Matrix and Matrix Regulation: Basis for a Holistic Theory in Medicine*, A. Pischinger, Ed., *H. Heine, Eng. Trans. N. Mac Lean*, p. 43. Brussels, Belgium: Editions Haug International.

104. Rea, W. J. 1994. Chemical sensitivity. Vol. III. *Clinical Manifestations of Pollutant Overload*. p. 1299. Boca Raton, FL: Lewis Publishers.

105. Heine, H. Ed. 1991. *Matrix and Matrix Regulation: Basis for a Holistic Theory in Medicine*, A. Pischinger, Eng. Trans. N. Mac Lean. Brussels, Belgium: Editions Haug International.

106. Heine, H. 1991. The structure and function of the ground substance (extracellular matrix): Paradigms in medical thinking. In *Matrix and Matrix Regulation: Basis for a Holistic Theory in Medicine*, A. Pischinger, Ed., H. Heine, Eng. Trans. N. Mac Lean, p. 45. Brussels, Belgium: Editions Haug International.

107. Bergsmann, O. 1991. The ground system, regulation and regulatory disturbances in rehabilitation practice. In *Matrix and Matrix Regulation: Basis for a Holistic Theory in Medicine*, A. Pischinger, Ed., H. Heine, Eng. Trans. N. Mac Lean, p. 105. Brussels, Belgium: Editions Haug International.

108. Rea, W. J. 1995. Chemical sensitivity. Vol. III. *Clinical Manifestations of Pollutant Overload*. p. 1470. Boca Raton, FL: Lewis Publishers.

109. Popp, F. A. 1984. *Biophotonen. Schriftenreihe Krebsgeschehen Bd. 6, 2. Aufl.* VfM Dr. Ewald Fischer, Heidelberg.

110. Bergsmann, O. 1991. The ground system, regulation and regulatory disturbances in rehabilitation practice. In *Matrix and Matrix Regulation: Basis for a Holistic Theory in Medicine*, A. Pischinger, Ed., H. Heine, Eng. Trans. N. Mac Lean, p. 106. Brussels, Belgium: Editions Haug International.

111. Perger, F. 1991. Therapeutic consequences of ground regulation research. In *Matrix and Matrix Regulation: Basis for a Holistic Theory in Medicine*, A. Pischinger, Ed., H. Heine, Eng. Trans. N. Mac Lean, p. 200. Brussels, Belgium: Editions Haug International.

112. Thompson, A. J. S., C. C. Patterson. 2001. Acute asthma exacerbations and air pollutants in children living in Belfast, Northern Ireland. *Arch. Environ. Health* 56:234–241.

113. Tolbert, P. E., J. A. Mulholland, D. L. MacIntosh, F. Xu, D. Daniels, O. J. Devine, B. P. Carlin, M. Klein, J. Dorley, A. J. Butler, D. F. Nordenberg, H. Frumkin, P. Barry Ryan, M. C. White. 2000. Air quality and pediatric emergency room visits for asthma in Atlanta, Georgia, USA. *Am. J. Epidemiol.* 151:798–810.

114. Wong, G. W., F. W. Ko, T. S. Lau, S. T. Li, D. Hui, S. W. Pang, R. Leung, T. F. Fok, C. K. Lai. 2001. Temporal relationship between air pollution and hospital admissions for asthmatic children in Hong Kong. *Clin. Exp. Allergy* 31:565–569.

115. Peters, A., D. D. Dockery, J. F. Miller, M. A. Mittelman. 2001. Increased particular matter and the triggering of myocardial infarction. *Circulation* 103:2810–2815.

116. Zanobetti, A., J. Schwartz. 2005. The effect of particulates on emergency admissions for myocardial infarction: A multicity case-crossover analysis. *Environ. Health. Perspect.* 113:978–982.

117. Hong, Y. C., J. T. Lee, H. Kim, H. J. Kwon. 2002. Air pollution: A new risk for stroke mortality. *Stroke* 33:2165–2169.

118. Maheswaran, R., R. P. Haining, P. Brindley, J. Law, T. Pearson, P. R. Fryers, S. Wise, M. J. Campbell. 2005. Outdoor air pollution and stroke in Sheffield, United Kingdom. A small-area level geographic study. *Stroke* 36:239–243.

119. Long, C. M., H. H. Suh, P. J. Catalano, P. Koutrakis. 2001. Using time- and size-resolved particulate data to quantify indoor penetration and deposition behavior. *Environ. Sci. Technol.* 35 (10):2089–2099.

120. Chaloulakou, A., I. Mavroidis, A. Duci. 2003. Indoor and outdoor carbon monoxide concentration relationships at different microenvironments in the Athens area. *Chemosphere* 52 (6):1007–1019.

121. Rea, W. J. 1996. *Chemical Sensitivity: Clinical Manifestations of Pollutant Overload*. Boca Raton, Florida: Lewis Publishers; 1996.

122. Koutrakis, S., S. N. Sax, J. A. Sarnat, J. A. Coull, P. Demokritou, P. Oyola, J. Carcia, E. Gramsch. 2005. Analysis of PM_{10}, $PM_{2.5-10}$ concentrations in Santiago, Chile, from 1989 to 2001. *J. Air Waste Manag. Assoc.* 55 (3):342–351.

123. Motallebi, N., C. A. Taylor, B. E. Croes. 2003. Particulate matter in California: Part 2-spatial, temporal and compositional patterns of $PM_{2.5}$, $PM_{120-2.5}$ and PM_{10}. *J. Air Waste Manag. Assoc.* 53 (12):1517–1530.

124. Duci, A., A. Chaloulakou, N. Spyrellis. 2003. Exposure to carbon monoxide in the Athens area during commuting. *Sci. Total Environ.* 309 (1–3):47–58.

125. Jo, W. K., I. H. Yoon, C. W. Nam. 2000. Analysis of air pollution in 2 major Korean cities: Trends seasonal variations, daily 1-hour maximum versus other hour-based concentrations and standard exceedances. *Environ. Pollut.* 110:11–18.

126. Linn, W. S., Y. Szlachcic, H. Gong, P. O. Kinney, K. T. Berhane. 2000. Air pollution and daily hospital admissions in metropolitan Los Angeles. *Environ. Health Perspect.* 108 (5):427–434.

127. Aneja, V. P., A. Agarwal, P. A. Roelle, S. B. Phillips, Q. Tong, N. Watkins, R. Yablonsky. 2001. Measurements and analysis of criteria air pollutants in New Delhi, India. *Environ. Int.* 27 (1):35–42.

128. Cernushi, S., M. Giugliano, G. Lonati, F. Marzolo. 1998. Development and application of statistical models for CO concentration and duration in the Milan urban area. *Sci. Total Environ.* 220 (2–3):147–156.

129. Chuersuwan, N., B. J. Turpin, C. Peetarinen. 2000. Evaluation of time-resolved $PM_{2.5}$ data in urban/suburban areas of New Jersey. *J Air Waste Manag Assoc.* 50 (10):1780–1789.

130. Petroeschevsky, A., R. W. Simpson, L. Thalib, S. Rutherford. 2001. Associations between outdoor air pollution and hospital admissions in Brisbane Australia. *Arch. Environ. Health* 56 (1):37–52.

131. Rea, W. J. 2002. Optimum Environments for Optimum Health and Creativity, Designing and Building a HealthyHomeandOffice.http://www.amazon.com/Optimum-Environments-Health-Creativity-Designing/dp/0972129901.

132. Rousseau, D., W. J. Rea, J. Enwright. 1988. Your Home, Your Health and Well Being. http://www.amazon.com/Your-Home-Health-Well-Being/dp/0898152232. Accessed September 26, 2017.

133. Chakravarty, P., B. Kovar. 2013. Evaluation of five antifungal agents used in remediation practices against six common indoor fungal species. *J. Occup. Environ. Hyg.* 10 (1):D11–D16. doi: 10.1080/15459624.2012.740987.

134. Fernandez, D., R. M. Valencia, T. Molnar, A. Vega, E. Sagues. 1998. Daily and seasonal variations of *Alternaria* and *Cladosporium* airborne spores in Leon (North-West Spain). *Aerobiologia* 14:215–220.

135. Gregory, P. H. 1961. *The Microbiology of the Atmosphere.* New York: Interscience Publishers, Inc.

136. Grinn-Gofron, A., P. Rapiejko. 2009. Occurrence of *Cladosporium* spp. and *Alternaria* spp. spores in Western, Northern and Central-Eastern Poland in 2004–2006 and relations to some meterological factors. *Atmospheric Res.* 93 (4):747–758.

137. Horner, W. E., A. Helbling, J. E. Salvaggio, S. B. Lehrer. 1995. Fungal allergens. *Clin. Microbiol. Rev.* 40:161–179.

138. Henriquez, V. I., G. R. Villegas, J. M. R. Nolla. 2001. Airborne fungi monitoring in Santiago, Chile. *Aerobiologia* 17:137–142.

139. Kasprzyk, I. 2008. Aeromycology—Main research fields of interest during the last 25 years. *Ann. Agri. Environ. Med.* 15:1–7.

140. Lacey, M. E., J. S. West. 2006. *The Air Spora.* Dordrecht, The Netherlands: Springer.

141. Simmon-Nobbe, B., U. Denk, V. Pöll, R. Rid, M. Breitenbach. 2008. The spectrum of fungal allergy. *Int. Arch. Allergy Immunol.* 145:58–86.

142. Andrae, S., O. Axelson, B. Bjorksten, M. Fredriksson, N. I. Kjellman. 1988. Symptoms of bronchial hyper-reactivity and asthma in relation to environmental factors. *Arch. Dis. Child.* 63:473–478.

143. Strachan, D. P., C. H. Sanders. 1989. Damphousing and childhood asthma; respiratory effects of indoor air temperature and humidity. *J. Epidemiol. Community Health* 43:7–14.

144. Dales, R. E., H. Zwanenburg, R. Burnett, C. A. Frenklin. 1991. Respiratory health effects of home dampness and molds among Canadian children. *Am. J. Epidemiol.* 134:196–203.

145. Brunekreff, B. 1992. Associations between questionnaire reports of home dampness and childhood respiratory symptoms. *Sci. Total Environ.* 127:79–89.

146. Jaakkola, J. J., N. Jaakkola, R. Ruotsalainen. 1993. Home dampness and molds as determinants of respiratory symptoms and asthma in preschool children. *J. Expo. Anal. Environ. Epidemiol.* 3 (suppl. 1):129–142.

147. Yang, C. Y., J. F. Chu, M. F. Cheng, M. C. Lin. 1997. Effects of indoor environmental factors on respiratory health of children in subtropical climate. *Environ. Res.* 75:49–55.

148. Pirasts, R., C. Nellu, P. Greco, U. Pelosi. 2009. Indoor exposure to environmental tobacco smoke and dampness: Respiratory symptoms in Sardinian children—DRIAS study. *Environ. Res.* 109:59–65.

149. Hwang, B. F., I. P. Liu, T. P. Huang. 2011. Molds, parental atopy and pediatric incident asthma. *Indoor Air* 2:472–478.

150. Shelton, B. G., K. H. Kirkland, W. D. Flanders, G. K. Morris. 2002. Profiles of airborne fungi in buildings and outdoor environments in the United States. *Appl. Environ. Microbiol.* 68:1743–1753.

151. Kirk, P. M., P. F. Cannon, J. C. David, J. A. Stalpers (Eds.). 2001. *Ainsworth and Bisby's Dictionary of the Fungi,* 9th ed. Egham, UK: CABI Bioscience.

152. Barnet, H. L., B. B. Hunter. 1987. *Illustrated Genera of Imperfect Fungi*, 4th ed. New York: MacMillan Publishing Co.

153. Ellis, M. B. 1983. *Dematiaceous Hyphomycetes*. Slough, UK: Commonwealth Agricultural Bureau.

154. Burge, P. S. 2004. Sick building syndrome. *Occup. Environ. Med.* 61:185–190.

155. Nielsen, K. F. 2003. Mycotoxin production by indoor moulds. *Fungal Gen. Biol.* 39:103–117.

156. Gorny, R. L., T. Reponen, K. Willeke, D. Schmechel, E. Robine, M. Boissier, S. A. Grinshpun. 2002. Fungal fragments as indoor air biocontaminants. *Appl. Environ. Microbiol.* 68:3522–3531.

157. Brasel, T. L., J. M. Martin, C. G. Wilson, D. C. Straus. 2005. Detection of airborne *Stachybotrys chartarum* macrocylic trichothecene mycotoxins in the indoor environment. *Appl. Environ. Microbiol.* 71:7376–7388.

158. Karunasena, E., M. D. Larranaga, J. S. Simoni, D. R. Douglas, D. C. Straus. 2010. Building-associated neurological damage modeled in human cells: A mechanism of neurotoxic effects by exposure to mycotoxins in the indoor environment. *Mycopathologia* 170:377–390.

159. Hoog, de G. S., J. Guarro, M. J. Figueras. 2000. *Atlas of Clinical Fungi. Centraalbureau voor Schimmelcultures*, Utrecht, The Netherlands: Centraalbureau voor Schimmelcultures.

160. Larone, D. A. 2002. *Medically Important Fungi—A Guide to Identification*, 4th ed., Washington, DC: ASM Press.

161. Burge, H. A., J. A. Otten. 1999. Fungi. In *Bioaerosols: Assessment and Control*. Cincinnati, Ohio: ACGIHR.

162. Zar, J. H. 1984. *Biostatistical Analysis*, 2nd ed. Englewood Cliffs, NJ: Prentice-Hall, Inc.

163. SAS Institute Inc. 2011. *SAS User's Guide*. Cary, NC: SAS Institute Inc.

164. Chakravarty, P., R. L. Peterson, B. E. Ellis. 1990. Integrated control of *Fusarium* damping off in red pine seedlings with *Paxillus involutus* and fungicides. *Can. J. Forest Res.* 20:1282–1288.

165. Chakravarty, P., P. F. Jackobs, R. L. Peterson. 1990. Effect of fungicides benomyl and oxine benzoate on the mycelial growth of four isolates of E-strain fungi *in vitro*. *Eur. J. Forest Pathol.* 20:381–385.

166. Unestam, T., P. Chakravarty, E. Damm. 1991. Fungicides: *In vitro* tests not useful for evaluating effects on ectomycorrhizae. *Agric. Ecosyst Environ.* 28:535–538.

167. Ingram, D. K., R. Weindruch, E. L. Spangler, J. R. Freeman, R. L. Walford. 1987. Dietary restriction benefits learning and motor performance of aged mice. *J. Gerontol.* 42:78–81.

168. Park, J. C., K. C. Cook, E. A. Verde. 1990. Dietary restriction slows the abnormally rapid loss of spiral ganglion neurons in C57BL/6 mice. *Hear Res.* 48:275–279.

169. Zhu, H., Q. Guo, M. P. Mattson. 1999. Dietary restriction protects hippocampal neurons against the death-promoting action of a presenilin-1 mutation. *Brain Res.* 842:224–229.

170. Pedersen, W. A., M. P. Mattson. 1999. No benefit of dietary restriction on disease onset or progression in amyotrophic lateral sclerosis Cu/Zn-superoxide dismutase mutant mice. *Brain Res.* 833:117–120.

171. Lee, J., W. W. Auyeung, M. P. Mattson. 2002. Kainate-induced seizures increase microgliosis, but not neurogenesis in adult mice: Modification by dietary restriction. *Neuromol. Med.* 4 (3):179–195.

172. Lee, J., C. Lu., S. L. Chan, M. A. Lane, M. P. Mattson. 2002. Phenformin suppresses calcium responses to glutamate and protects hippocampal neurons against excitotoxicity. *Exp. Neurol.* 175:161–167.

173. Lee, J., K. B. Seroogy, M. P. Mattson. 2002. Dietary restriction enhances neurotrophin expression and neurogenesis in the hippocampus of adult mice. *J. Neurochem.* 80:539–547.

174. Stewart J., J. Mitchell, N. Kalant. 1989. The effects of life-long food restriction on spatial memory in young and aged Fischer 344 rats measured in the eight-arm radial and the Morris water mazes. *Neurobiol. Aging* 10:669–675.

175. Moroi-Fetters, S. E., R. F. Mervis, E. D. London, D. K. Ingram. 1989. Dietary restriction suppresses age-related changes in dendritic spines. *Neurobiol. Aging* 10:317–322.

176. Diao, L. H., P. C. Bickford, J. O. Stevens, E. J. Cline, G. A. Gerhardt. 1997. Caloric restriction enhances evoked DA overflow in striatum and nucleus accumbens of aged Fischer 344 rats. *Brain Res.* 763:276–280.

177. Snyder, D. L., V. J. Aloyo, W. Wang, J. Roberts. 1998. Influence of age and dietary restriction on norepinephrine uptake into cardiac synaptosomes. *J. Cardiovasc. Pharmacol.* 32:896–901.

178. Yu, Z. F., M. P. Mattson. 1999. Dietary restriction and 2-deoxyglucose administration reduce focal ischemic brain damage and improve behavioral outcome: evidence for a preconditioning mechanism. *J. Neurosci. Res.* 57:830–839.

179. Guo, Z. H., M. P. Mattson. 1999. Neurotrophic factors protect synaptic terminals against amyloid- and oxidative stress-induced impairment of glucose transport, glutamate transport and mitochondrial function. *Cereb. Cortex* 10:50–57.

180. Calingasan, N. Y., G. E. Gibson. 2000. Dietary restriction attenuates the neuronal loss, induction of heme oxygenase-1 and blood–brain barrier breakdown induced by impaired oxidative metabolism. *Brain Res.* 885:62–69.

181. Eckles-Smith, K., D. Clayton, P. Bickford, M. D. Browning. 2000. Caloric restriction prevents age-related deficits in LTP and in NMDA receptor expression. *Mol. Brain Res.* 78:154–162.

182. Mattson, M. P., W. Duan, Z. Guo. 2003. Meal size and frequency affect neuronal plasticity and vulnerability to disease: Cellular and molecular mechanisms. *J. Neurosci.* 84:417–431.

183. Kuma, A., N. Mizushima. 2010. Physiological role of autophagy as an intracellular recycling system: With an emphasis on nutrient metabolism. *Semin. Cell Dev. Biol.* 21 (7):683–690.

184. Rabinowitz, J. D., R. E. White. 2010. Autophagy and metabolism. *Science* 330 (6009): 1344–1348. doi: 10.1126/science.1193497.

185. Komatsu, M., S. Waguri, T. Ueno, J. Iwata, S. Murata, I. Tanida, J. Ezaki, N. Mizushima, Y. Ohsumi, Y. Uchiyama, E. Kominami, K. Tanaka, T. Chiba. 2005. Impairment of starvation-induced and constitutive autophagy in Atg7-deficient mice. *J. Cell Biol.* 169 (3):425–434.

186. Rodriguez, A., A. Durán, M. Selloum, M. F. Champy, F. J. Diez-Guerra, J. M. Flores, M. Serrano, J. Auwerx, M. T. Diaz-Meco, J. Moscat. 2006. Mature-onset obesity and insulin resistance in mice deficient in the signaling adapter p62. *Cell Metab.* 3 (3):211–222.

187. Cuervo, A. M., J. F. Dice. 2000. Age-related decline in chaperone-mediated autophagy. *J. Biol. Chem.* 275 (40):31505–31513.

188. Yang, L., P. Li, S. Fu, E. S. Calay, G. S. Hotamisligil. 2010. Defective hepatic autophagy in obesity promotes ER stress and causes insulin resistance. *Cell Metab.* 11 (6):467–478.

189. Hara, T., K. Nakamura, M. Matsui, A. Yamamoto, Y. Nakahara, R. Suzuki-Migishima, M. Yokoyama, K. Mishima, I. Saito, H. Okano, N. Mizushima. 2006. Suppression of basal autophagy in neural cells causes neurodegenerative disease in mice. *Nature* 441 (7095):885–889.

190. Komatsu, M., S. Waguri, T. Chiba, S. Murata, J. Iwata, I. Tanida, T. Ueno, M. Koike, Y. Uchiyama, E. Kominami, K. Tanaka. 2006. Loss of autophagy in the central nervous system causes neurodegeneration in mice. *Nature* 441 (7095):880–884.

191. Mathew, R., C. M. Karp, B. Beaudoin, N. Vuong, G. Chen, H. Y. Chen, K. Bray, A. Reddy, G. Bhanot, C. Gelinas, R. S. Dipaola, V. Karantza-Wadsworth, E. White. 2009. Autophagy suppresses tumorigenesis through elimination of p62. *Cell* 137 (6):1062–1075.

192. Komatsu, M., S. Waguri, M. Koike, Y. S. Sou, T. Ueno, T. Hara, N. Mizushima, J. Iwata, J. Ezaki, S. Murata, J. Hamazaki, Y. Nishito, S. Iemura, T. Natsume, T. Yanagawa, J. Uwayama, E. Warabi, H. Yoshida, T. Ishii, A. Kobayashi, M. Yamamoto, Z. Yue, Y. Uchiyama, E. Kominami, K. Tanaka. 2007. Homeostatic levels of p62 control cytoplasmic inclusion body formation in autophagy-deficient mice. *Cell* 131 (6):1149–1163.

193. Cadwell, K., J. Y. Liu, S. L. Brown, H. Miyoshi, J. Loh, J. K. Lennerz, C. Kishi, W. Kc, J. A. Carrero, S. Hunt, C. D. Stone, E. M. Brunt, R. J. Xavier, B. P. Sleckman, E. Li, N. Mizushima, T. S. Stappenbeck, H. W. Virgin 4th. 2008. A key role for autophagy and the autophagy gene Atg16l1 in mouse and human intestinal Paneth cells. *Nature* 456 (7219):259–263.

194. Kapahi, P., D. Chen, A. N. Rogers, S. D. Katewa, P. W. Li, E. L. Thomas, L. Kockel. 2010. Review with TOR, less is more: A key role for the conserved nutrient-sensing TOR pathway in aging. *Cell Metab.* 11 (6):453–465.

195. Degenhardt, K., R. Mathew, B. Beaudoin, K. Bray, D. Anderson, G. Chen, C. Mukherjee, Y. Shi, C. Gélinas, Y. Fan, D. A. Nelson, S. Jin, E. White. 2006. Autophagy promotes tumor cell survival and restricts necrosis, inflammation, and tumorigenesis. *Cancer Cell* 10 (1):51–64.

196. White, E., R. S. DiPaola. 2009. The double-edged sword of autophagy modulation in cancer. *Clin. Cancer Res.* 15 (17):5308–5316.

197. Funderburk, S. F., Q. J. Wang, Z. Yue. 2010. The Beclin 1-VPS34 complex—At the crossroads of autophagy and beyond. *Trends Cell Biol.* 20 (6):355–362.

198. Berry, D. L., E. H. Baehrecke. 2007. Growth arrest and autophagy are required for salivary gland cell degradation in Drosophila. *Cell* 131 (6):1137–1148.

199. Geisler, S., K. M. Holmström, D. Skujat, F. C. Fiesel, O. C. Rothfuss, P. J. Kahle, W. Springer. 2010. PINK1/Parkin-mediated mitophagy is dependent on VDAC1 and p62/SQSTM1. *Nat. Cell Biol.* 12 (2):119–131.

200. Narendra, D., A. Tanaka, D. F. Suen, R. J. Youle. 2008. Parkin is recruited selectively to impaired mitochondria and promotes their autophagy. *J. Cell Biol.* 183 (5):795–803.

201. Efeyan, A., D. M. Sabatini. 2010. mTOR and cancer: Many loops in one pathway. *Curr. Opin. Cell Biol.* 22 (2):169–176.

202. Shackelford, D. B., R. J. Shaw. 2009. The LKB1-AMPK pathway: Metabolism and growth control in tumour suppression. *Nat. Rev. Cancer* 9 (8):563–575.

203. Zhao, J., J. Brault, A. Schild, P. Cao, M. Sandri, S. Schiaffino, S. H. Lecker, A. L. Goldberg. 2007. FoxO3 coordinately activates protein degradation by the autophagic/lysosomal and proteasomal pathways in atrophying muscle cells. *Cell Metab.* 6 (6):472–483.

204. Eng, C. H., K. Yu, J. Lucas, E. White, R. T. Abraham. 2010. Ammonia derived from glutaminolysis is a diffusible regulator of autophagy. *Sci. Signal.* 3 (119):ra31.

205. Takeshige, K., M. Baba, S. Tsuboi, T. Noda, Y. Ohsumi. 1992. Autophagy in yeast demonstrated with proteinase-deficient mutants and conditions for its induction. *J. Cell Biol.* 119 (2):301–311.

206. Onodera, J., Y. Ohsumi. 2005. Autophagy is required for maintenance of amino acid levels and protein synthesis under nitrogen starvation. *J. Biol Chem.* 280 (36):31582–31586.

207. Lum, J. J., D. E. Bauer, M. Kong, M. H. Harris, C. Li, T. Lindsten, C. B. Thompson. 2005. Growth factor regulation of autophagy and cell survival in the absence of apoptosis. *Cell* 120 (2):237–248.

208. Tsukamoto, S., A. Kuma, M. Murakami, C. Kishi, A. Yamamoto, N. Mizushima. 2008. Autophagy is essential for preimplantation development of mouse embryos. *Science* 321 (5885):117–120.

209. Kuma, A., M. Hatano, M. Matsui, A. Yamamoto, H. Nakaya, T. Yoshimori, Y. Ohsumi, T. Tokuhisa, N. Mizushima. 2004. The role of autophagy during the early neonatal starvation period. *Nature* 432 (7020):1032–1036.

210. Mizushima, N., A. Yamamoto, M. Matsui, T. Yoshimori, Y. Ohsumi. 2004. In vivo analysis of autophagy in response to nutrient starvation using transgenic mice expressing a fluorescent autophagosome marker. *Mol. Biol. Cell* 15 (3):1101–1111.

211. Kanamori, H., G. Takemura, R. Maruyama, K. Goto, A. Tsujimoto, A. Ogino, L. Li, I. Kawamura, T. Takeyama, T. Kawaguchi, K. Nagashima, T. Fujiwara, H. Fujiwara, M. Seishima, S. Minatoguchi. Functional significance and morphological characterization of starvation-induced autophagy in the adult heart. *Am. J. Pathol.* 174 (5):1705–1714.

212. Oku, M., Y. Sakai. 2010. Peroxisomes as dynamic organelles: Autophagic degradation. *FEBS J.* 277 (16):3289–3294.

213. Singh, R., S. Kaushik, Y. Wang, Y. Xiang, I. Novak, M. Komatsu, K. Tanaka, A. M. Cuervo, M. J. Czaja. 2009. Autophagy regulates lipid metabolism. *Nature* 458 (7242):1131–1135.

214. Singh, R., Y. Xiang, Y. Wang, K. Baikati, A. M. Cuervo, Y. K. Luu, Y. Tang, J. E. Pessin, G. J. Schwartz, M. J. Czaja. 2009. Autophagy regulates adipose mass and differentiation in mice. *J. Clin. Invest.* 119 (11):3329–3339.

215. Zhang, Y., S. Goldman, R. Baerga, Y. Zhao, M. Komatsu, S. Jin. 2009. Adipose-specific deletion of autophagy-related gene 7 (atg7) in mice reveals a role in adipogenesis. *Proc. Natl. Acad. Sci. U. S. A.* 106 (47):19860–19865.

216. Ebato, C., T. Uchida, M. Arakawa, M. Komatsu, T. Ueno, K. Komiya, K. Azuma, T. Hirose, K. Tanaka, E. Kominami, R. Kawamori, Y. Fujitani, H. Watada. 2008. Autophagy is important in islet homeostasis and compensatory increase of beta cell mass in response to high-fat diet. *Cell Metab.* 8 (4):325–332.

217. Jung, H. S., K. W. Chung, J. Won Kim, J. Kim, M. Komatsu, K. Tanaka, Y. H. Nguyen, T. M. Kang, K. H. Yoon, J. W. Kim, Y. T. Jeong, M. S, Han, M. K. Lee, K. W. Kim, J. Shin, M. S. Lee. 2008. Loss of autophagy diminishes pancreatic beta cell mass and function with resultant hyperglycemia. *Cell Metab.* 8 (4):318–324.

218. Miller, J., C. Lee. 1972. *Food Allergy: Provocative Testing and Injection Therapy.* Springfield, IL: Charles C. Thomas.

219. Rea, W. J., Y. Pan, E. J. Fenyves, I. Sujisawa, H. Suyama, N. Samadid, G. H. Ross. 1991. Electromagnetic field sensitivity. *J. Bioelectr.* 10 (1&2):241–256.

220. Hansel, F. K. 1957. Optimal dosage therapy in allergy and immunity. *Ann. Otol. Phino.* 66:729–742.

221. Rinkel, H. J. 1949. Inhalant allergy. I. Whealing response of skin to serial dilution testing. *Ann. Allergy* 7:625–650.

222. Lee, C. H., R. I. Williams, E. L. Binkley. 1969. Provocative testing and treatment for foods. *Arch. Otolaryngol.* 90:113.

223. Miller, J. B. 1972. *Food Allergy: Provocative Testing and Injection Therapy.* Springfield, IL: Charles C. Thomas.

224. Smith, C. 2010. Evidence Base in Physics for Homeopathic Products and Services. Submission to the Science and Technology Committee in respect of Evidence Check 2: Homeopathy.

225. Smith, C. W. 2008. Fröhlich's interpretation of biology through theoretical physics. In *Herbert Fröhlich FRS: A Physicist ahead of His Time,* 2nd ed., G. J. Hyland, P. Rowlands, Eds., pp. 107–154. Liverpool: University of Liverpool.

226. Monro, J. 1982. Electrical Sensitivities and the Electrical Environment, Breakspear Hospital, London.
227. Voll, R. "EAV" Electro Acupuncture According to Voll. http://www.biontologyarizona.com/dr-rein-hard-voll/. Accessed September 26, 2017.
228. Preparata, G. 1995. *QED Coherence in Matter.* Singapore: World Scientific.
229. Del Giudice, E., L. Giuliani. 1995. Coherence in water and the kT problem in living matter. http://www.icems.eu/papers/ramazzini_library5_part1.pdf.
230. Aharonov, Y., D. Bohm. 1959. Significance of electromagnetic potentials in quantum theory. *Phys. Rev.* 115:485–491.
231. Smith, C., W. Ludwig. 2009–2010. Evidence check 2: Homeopathy, fourth report of session 2009–10, report. By Great Britain: Parliament: House of Commons: Science and Technology Committee.
232. Gairiaev, P. 2009–2010. Evidence check 2: Homeopathy, fourth report of session 2009–10, report. By Great Britain: Parliament: House of Commons: Science and Technology Committee.
233. Elia, V. 2009–2010. Evidence check 2: Homeopathy, fourth report of session 2009–10, report. By Great Britain: Parliament: House of Commons: Science and Technology Committee.
234. Lenger K, R. P. Bajpai, M. Spielmann. 2014. Identification of unknown homeopathic remedies by delayed luminescence. *Cell Biochem. Biophys.* 68 (2):321–334. doi: 10.1007/s12013-013-9712-7.
235. Rey, L. 2007. Can low-temperature thermoluminescence cast light on the nature of ultra-high dilutions? *Homeopathy* 96 (3):170–174.
236. Montagnier, L. 2009. Luc Montagnier, Nobel Prize Winner, Takes Homeopathy Seriously. http://www.huffingtonpost.com/dana-ullman/luc-montagnier-homeopathy-taken-seriously_b_814619.html.
237. Smith, C. W. 2009. Can homeopathy ameliorate ongoing sickness? *J. Altern. Complement Med.* 15 (5):465–467.
238. Hahnemann, S. 1982. *Organon of Medicine.* Los Angeles: J. P. Tarcher.
239. Holzer, P. 1988. Local effector functions of capsaicin-sensitive sensory nerve endings: Involvement of tachykinins, calcitonin gene-related peptide and other neuropeptides. *Neuroscience* 24:739–768.
240. Holzer, P. 1991. Capsaicin: Cellular targets, mechanisms of action, and selectivity for thin sensory neurons. *Pharmacol. Rev.* 43:143–201.
241. Szolcsányi, J. 1996. Capsaicin-sensitive sensory nerve terminals with local and systemic efferent functions: Facts and scopes of an unorthodox neuroregulatory mechanism. In *Progress in Brain Research: The Polymodal Receptor—A Gateway to Pathological Pain*, T. Kumazawa, L. Kruger, Eds., pp. 343–359. Amsterdam: Elsevier.
242. Holzer, P., C. A. Maggi. 1998. Dissociation of dorsal root ganglion neurons into afferent and efferent-like neurons. *Neuroscience* 86:389–398.
243. Szallasi, A., P. M. Blumberg. 1990. Minireview. Resiniferatoxin and analogs provide novel insights into the pharmacology of the vanilloid (capsaicin) receptor. *Life Sci.* 47:1399–1408.
244. Szallasi, A., P. M. Blumberg. 1990. Specific binding of resiniferatoxin, an ultrapotent capsaicin analog, by dorsal root ganglion membranes. *Brain Res.* 524:106–111.
245. Szallasi, A. 1996. Vanilloid-sensitive neurons: A fundamental subdivision of the peripheral nervous system. *J. Periph. Nerv. Syst.* 1:6–18.
246. Buck, S. H., T. F. Burks. 1986. The neuropharmacology of capsaicin: A review of some recent observations. *Pharmacol. Rev.* 38:179–226.
247. Jancsó, N., A. Jancsó. 1949. Desensitization of sensory nerve endings (in Hungarian). *Kísérletes Orvostudomány* 2(Suppl):15.
248. Jancsó, N. 1955. Speicherung. Stoffanreicherung im Retikuloendothel und in der Niere. Budapest: Akadᵤmiai Kiadó.
249. Jancsó, N. 1968. Desensitization with capsaicin and related acylamides as a tool for studying the function of pain receptors. In *Pharmacology of Pain*, K. Lin, D. Armstrong and E. D. Pardo, Eds., pp. 33–55. Oxford, UK: Pergamon.
250. Szolcsányi, J. 1984. Capsaicin and neurogenic inflammation: History and early findings. In *Antidromic Vasodilatation and Neurogenic Inflammation*, L. A. Chahl, J. Szolcsányi and F. Lembeck, Eds., pp. 2–25. Budapest: Akadémiai Kiadó.
251. Jancsó, G. 1994. Histamine, capsaicin and neurogenic inflammation. A historical note on the contribution of Miklós (Nicholas) Jancsó (1903–1966) to sensory pharmacology. In *Advances in Psychoneuroimmunology*, I. Bérczi, J. Szelényi, Eds., pp. 17–23. New York: Plenum Press.
252. Liu, L., S. A. Simon. 1996. Capsaicin-induced currents with distinct desensitization and Ca21 dependence in rat trigeminal ganglion cells. *J. Neurophysiol* 75:1503–1514.
253. Liu, L., S. A. Simon. 1998. The influence of removing extracellular Ca21 in the tachyphylaxis responses to capsaicin, zingerone and olvanil in rat trigeminal ganglion neurons. *Brain Res.* 809:246–262.

254. Szallasi, A., P. M. Blumberg. 1993. [3 H]Resiniferatoxin binding by the vanilloid receptor: Species-related differences, effects of temperature and sulfhydryl reagents. *Naunyn-Schmiedeberg's Arch. Pharmacol.* 347:84–91.

255. Koplas, P. A., R. L. Rosenberg, G. S. Oxford. 1997. The role of calcium in the desensitization of capsaicin responses in rat dorsal root ganglion neurons. *J. Neurosci.* 17:3525–3537.

256. Szolcsányi, J. 1982. Capsaicin type pungent agents producing pyrexia. In *Handbook of Experimental Pharmacology*, A. S. Milton, Ed., pp. 437–478. Berlin: Springer.

257. Liu, L., S. A. Simon. 1996. Similarities and differences in the currents activated by capsaicin, piperine and zingerone in rat trigeminal ganglion cells. *J. Neurophysiol.* 76:1858–1869.

258. Brand, L., E. Berman, R. Schwen, M. Loomans, J. Janusz, R. Bohne, C. Maddin, J. Gardner, T. LaHann, R. Farmer, L. Jones, C. Chiabrando, R. Fanelli. 1987. NE-19550: A novel, orally active antiinflammatory analgesic. *Drugs Expl. Clin. Res.* 13:259–265.

259. Dray, A., J. Bettaney, C. Reuff, C. S. J. Walpole, R. Wrigglesworth. 1990. NE-19550 and NE-21610, antinociceptive capsaicin analogues: Studies on nociceptive fibers of the neonatal rat tail in vitro. *Eur. J. Pharmacol.* 181:289–293.

260. Bevan, S., R. J. Docherty, H. P. Rang, L. Urbán. 1995. Membrane actions of SDZ 249–482, an analgesic capsaicin analogue with reduced excitatory actions. *Am. Pain. Soc. Abstr.* A–33.

261. Wrigglesworth, R., C. S. J. Walpole, S. Bevan, E. A. Campbell, A. Dray, G. A. Hughes, I. F. James, K. J. Masdin, J. Winter. 1996. Analogues of capsaicin with agonist activity as novel analgesic agents: Structure-activity studies. 4. Potent, orally active analgesics. *J. Med. Chem.* 39:4942–4951.

262. Szallasi, A., P. M. Blumberg. 1989. Resiniferatoxin, a phorbol-related diterpene, acts as an ultrapotent analog of capsaicin, the irritant constituent in red pepper. *Neuroscience* 30:515–520.

263. Cruz, F., M. Guimarães, C. Silva, M. Reis. 1997. Suppression of bladder hyperreflexia by intravesical resiniferatoxin. *Lancet* 350:640–641.

264. Szolcsányi, J. 1989. Capsaicin, irritation, and desensitization. Neurophysiological basis and future perspectives. In *Chemical Senses Vol. 2, Irritation*, B. G. Green, J. R. Mason, M. R. Kare, Eds. pp. 141–168. New York: Marcel Dekker.

265. Meyer, R. A., J. N. Campbell, S. N. Raja. 1994. Peripheral neural mechanisms of nociception. In *Textbook of Pain*, P. D. Wall, R. Melzack, Eds., pp. 13–43. London: Churchill Livingstone.

266. Maggi, C. A. 1991. The pharmacology of the efferent function of sensory nerves. *J. Auton. Pharmacol.* 11:173–208.

267. Lundberg, J. M. 1993. Capsaicin-sensitive sensory nerves in the airways—Implications for protective reflexes and disease. In *Capsaicin in the Study of Pain*, J. N. Wood, Ed., pp. 219–238. San Diego, CA: Academic Press.

268. Rang, H. P., S. Bevan, A. Dray. 1994. Nociceptive peripheral neurons: Cellular properties. In *Textbook of Pain*, P. D. Wall, R. Melzack, Eds., pp. 57–78. Edinburgh: Churchill Livingstone.

269. Lundberg, J. M. 1996. Pharmacology of cotransmission in the autonomic nervous system: Integrative aspects on amines, neuropeptides, adenosine triphosphate, amino acids, and nitric oxide. *Pharmacol. Rev.* 48:113–177.

270. Gamse, R., U. Petsche, F. Lembeck, G. Jancsó. 1982. Capsaicin applied to the peripheral nerve inhibits axoplasmic transport of substance P and somatostatin. *Brain Res.* 238:447–462.

271. Miller, M. S., S. H. Buck, I. G. Sipes, H. I. Yamamura, T. F. Burks. 1982. Regulation of substance P by nerve growth factor: Disruption by capsaicin. *Brain Res.* 250:193–196.

272. Taylor, D. C. M., Fr-K. Pierau, J. Szolcsányi. 1984. Long-lasting inhibition of horseradish peroxidase (HRP) transport in sensory nerves induced by capsaicin pretreatment of the receptive field. *Brain Res.* 298:45–49.

273. Gilchrist, C. A., C. F. Morrison, K. E. Chapman, A. J. Harmar. 1991. Identification of nerve growth factor-responsive sequences within the 59 region of the bovine preprotachykinin gene. *DNA Cell Biol.* 10:743–749.

274. Szallasi, A., P. M. Blumberg. 1992. Vanilloid receptor loss in rat sensory neurons associated with long term desensitization to resiniferatoxin. *Neurosci. Lett.* 136:51–54.

275. Goso, C., G. Piovacari, A. Szallasi. 1993. Resiniferatoxin-induced loss of vanilloid receptors is reversible in the urinary bladder but not in the spinal cord of the rat. *Neurosci. Lett.* 162:197–200.

276. Szallasi, A., S. Nilsson, T. Farkas-Szallasi, P. M. Blumberg, T. Hökfelt, J. M. Lundberg. 1995. Vanilloid (capsaicin) receptors in the rat: Distribution in the brain, regional differences in the spinal cord, axonal transport to the periphery, and depletion by systemic vanilloid treatment. *Brain Res.* 703:175–183.

277. Wilson, C. 1989. Joint conference of American-British Society of Allergy and Environmental Medicine.

278. Jancsó-Gábor, A., J. Szolcsányi, N. Jancsó. 1970. Stimulation and desensitization of the hypothalamic heat-sensitive structure by capsaicin in rats. *J. Physiol.* 208:449–459.

279. Kellner, G. 1969. Probleme der Wundsetzung und der beeinflußten Wundheilung Osterr. *Zschr. F. Stomatol.* 66:122.

280. Kellner, G. 1971. Herdgeschelen und Herdnachweis. ZWR 1; Bergsmann, O. 1965. Asymmetrische Leukozytenbefunde bei Lungentuberkulose. *Wr. Klin. Wschr.* 77(37):618.

281. Perger, F. 1991. Therapeutic consequences of ground regulation research. In *Matrix and Matrix Regulation: Basis for a Holistic Theory in Medicine*, A. Pischinger, Ed., H. Heine, Eng. Trans. N. Mac Lean, p. 136. Brussels, Belgium: Editions Haug International.

282. Bergsmann, O. 1965. Herdwirkung in der Pulmologie. *Die Therapiewoche* 15 (24):1284.

283. Perger, F. 1991. Therapeutic consequences of ground regulation research. In *Matrix and Matrix Regulation: Basis for a Holistic Theory in Medicine*, A. Pischinger, Ed., H. Heine, Eng. Trans. N. Mac Lean, p. 138. Brussels, Belgium: Editions Haug International.

284. Bethe, A. 1952. *Allgemeine Physiologie*. Berlin-Heidelberg: Springer-Verlag.

285. Gildemeister, F. 1928. Uber elekrischen Widerstand, Kapazitat und Polarisation der Haut. *II Mitt. Pflugers Arch. F. Ges. Phys.* 219:98–110.

286. Hauswirth, O. 1953. Vegetative Konstitutiionstherapie. Wien: Springer-Verlag.

287. Kracmar, F. 1961. Vegetative Konstitution un elektrischer Unfall. *Electromed* 6:169–174.

288. Neuberger, F. 1960. Zur Objektivierung endo-und exogerner Einflusse auf den Tonus der akustischen und/oder vestibularen Sensorik. *Monatsschr. F. Ohrenheilkunde and Laryngo-Rhinologie* 94:262–274.

289. Croon, R. 1976. Elektroneural-Diagnostik un d Therapie nach Cron. *Physik. Med. Rehabil.* Jg 17/44:81.

290. Maresch, O. May 1970. *Physikalische Beuteilung der Heilwasser. Vortag Symposium uber Badertherapie*. Baden-Wein.

291. Popp, F. A. 1984. *Biophotonen 2., verb. U. Erw. Aufl. Verlag fur medizin Dr.* Ewald Fischer GmbH. Heidelberg.

292. Selye, H. 1946. The general adaptation syndrome and the diseases of adaptation. *J. Allergy* 17:23.

293. Rea, W. J. 1992. *Chemical Sensitivity*. Vol. 1. p. 17. Boca Raton, FL: Lewis Publishers.

294. Lee, C. 1961. A new test for diagnosis and treatment of food allergies. *Buchanan County Med. Bull.* 25:9.

295. Kracmar, F. 1971. Zur iophysik des vegetativen Grundsystems. *Physik. Medizin und Rehabilitation Z. allg. Med.* 12:120–122 Dort weitere Literatur.

296. Diehl, F. 1937. Studien zur Permeabilitat der menschilichen Haut unter verschiedenen Bedingungen. *Z. f. exp. Med.* 100:145–191.

297. Perger, F. 1991. Therapeutic consequences of ground regulation research. In *Matrix and Matrix Regulation: Basis for a Holistic Theory in Medicine*. A. Pischinger, Ed., H. Heine, Eng. Trans. N. Mac Lean, p. 140. Brussels, Belgium: Editions Haug International.

298. Morris, D. L. 1988. Treatment of respiratory disease with ultra-small doses of antigens. *Ann. Allergy* 28:494–500.

299. Heine, H. 1991. The structure and function of the ground substance (extracellular matrix): Paradigms in medical thinking. In *Matrix and Matrix Regulation: Basis for a Holistic Theory in Medicine*, A. Pischinger, Ed., H. Heine, Eng. Trans. N. Mac Lean, p. 52. Brussels, Belgium: Editions Haug International.

300. Monsereenusorn, Y., S. Kongsamut, P. D. Pezalla. 1982. Capsaicin—A literature survey. *CRC Crit Rev Toxicol* 10:321–339.

301. Toh, C. C., T. S. Lee, A. K. Kiang. 1955. The pharmacological actions of capsaicin and analogues. *Br. J. Pharmacol.* 10:175–181.

302. Jancsó, G., E. Khinyár. 1975. Functional linkage between nociception and fluorideresistant acid phosphatase activity in the Rolando substance. *Neurobiology* 5:42–43.

303. Jessell, T. M., L. L. Iversen, A. C. Cuello. 1978. Capsaicin-induced depletion of substance from primary sensory neurones. *Brain Res.* 152:183–188.

304. Jancsó, G., E. Király, F. Joó, G. Such, A. Nagy. 1985. Selective degeneration by capsaicin of a subpopulation of primary sensory neurones in the adult rat. *Neurosci. Lett.* 59:209–214.

305. Jancsó, G. 1992. Pathobiological reactions of C-fibre primary sensory neurones to peripheral nerve injury. *Exp. Physiol.* 77:405–431.

306. Hökfelt, T., X. Zhang, Z. Wiesenfeld-Hallin. 1994. Messenger plasticity in primary sensory neurons following axotomy and its functional implications. *Trends Neurosci.* 17:22–30.

307. Coca, A. F. 1949. Anti-allergic action of sympathetomy. *Ann. N. Y. Acad. Sci.* 50:807.

308. Post, C., L. Alari, T. Hökfelt. 1988. Intrathecal galanin increases the latency in the tail flick and hot plate tests in the mouse. *Acta Physiol. Scand.* 132:583–584.

309. Wiesenfeld-Hallin, Z., X-J. Xu, Ü. Langel, E. Bedecs, T. Hökfelt, T. Bártfai. 1992. Galanin-mediated control of pain: Enhanced role after nerve injury. *Proc. Natl. Acad. Sci. USA* 89:3334–3337.

310. Puttick, R. M., R. D. Pinnock, G. N. Woodruff. 1994. Galanin-induced membrane depolarization of neonatal rat cultured dorsal root ganglion cells. *Eur. J. Pharmacol.* 254:303–306.

311. Burgevin, M-C., I. Loquet, D. Quarteronet, E. Habert-Ortoli. 1995. Cloning, pharmacological characterization, and anatomical distribution of a rat cDNA encoding for a galanin receptor. *J. Mol. Neurosci.* 6:33–41.

312. Ahmad, S., S. H. Shen, P. Walker, C. Wahlestedt. 1996. Molecular cloning of a novel widely distributed galanin receptor subtype (GALR2). In *Abstracts of the 8th World Congress on Pain*, p. 131, Vancouver, Canada.

313. Shi, T. J. S., X. Zhang, K. Holmberg, Z. Q. D. Xu, T. Hökfelt. 1997. Expression and regulation of galanin-R2 receptors in rat primary sensory neurons: Effect of axotomy and inflammation. *Neurosci. Lett.* 237:57–60.

314. Xu, Z-Q., T-J. Shi, M. Landry, T. Hökfelt. 1996. Evidence for galanin receptors in primary sensory neurons and effect of axotomy and inflammation. *Neuroreport* 8:237–242.

315. Stanfa, L., A. Dickenson, X-J. Xu, Z. Wiesenfeld-Hallin. 1994. Cholecystokinin and morphine analgesia: Variations on a theme. *Trends Pharmacol. Sci.* 15:65–66.

316. Wiesenfeld-Hallin, Z., X-J. Xu, R. Håkanson, D-M. Feng, K. Folkers. 1990. Plasticity of the peptidergic mediation of spinal reflex facilitation after peripheral nerve section in the rat. *Neurosci. Lett.* 116:293–298.

317. Herdegen, T., C. E. Fiallos-Estrada, R. Bravo, M. Zimmermann. 1993. Colocalization and covariation of c-JUN transcription factor with galanin in primary afferent neurons and with CGRP in spinal motoneurons following transection of rat sciatic nerve. *Mol. Brain Res.* 17:147–154.

318. Jenkins, R., S. P. Hunt. 1991. Long-term increase in the levels of c-jun mRNA and Jun protein-like immunoreactivity in motor and sensory neurons following axon damage. *Neurosci. Lett.* 129:107–110.

319. Leah, J. D., T. Herdegen, R. Bravo. 1991. Selective expression of Jun protein following axotomy and axonal transport block in peripheral nerves in the rat: Evidence for a role in the regeneration process. *Brain Res.* 566:198–207.

320. Herdegen, T., C. E. Fiallos-Estrada, W. Schmid, R. Bravo, M. Zimmermann. 1992. The transcription factors c-JUN, JUN D and CREB, but not FOS and KROX-24, are differentially regulated in axotomized neurons following transection of rat sciatic nerve. *Mol. Brain Res.* 14:155–165.

321. Szallasi, A., F. Joó, P. M. Blumberg. 1989. Duration of desensitization and ultrastructural changes in dorsal root ganglia in rats treated with resiniferatoxin, an ultrapotent capsaicin analog. *Brain Res.* 503:68–72.

322. Szallasi, A., P. M. Blumberg. 1996. Vanilloid receptors: New insights enhance potential as a therapeutic target. *Pain* 68:195–208.

323. Farkas-Szallasi, T., J. M. Lundberg, Z. Wiesenfeld-Hallin, T. Hökfelt, A. Szallasi. 1995. Increased levels of GMAP, VIP and nitric oxide synthase, and their mRNAs, in lumbar dorsal root ganglia of the rat following systemic resiniferatoxin treatment. *Neuroreport* 6:2220–2234.

324. Xu, X-J., T. Farkas-Szallasi, J. M. Lundberg, T. Hökfelt, Z. Wiesenfeld-Hallin, A. Szallasi. 1997. Effects of the capsaicin analogue resiniferatoxin on spinal nociceptive mechanisms in the rat: Behavioral, electrophysiological and in situ hybridization studies. *Brain Res.* 752:52–60.

325. Szallasi, A., T. Farkas-Szallasi, J. B. Tucker, J. M. Lundberg, T. Hökfelt, J. E. Krause. 1999b. Effects of systemic resiniferatoxin treatment on substance P (SP) mRNA in rat dorsal root ganglia and SP receptor mRNA in the spinal dorsal horn. *Brain Res.* 815:177–184.

326. Jakab, G, A. Szallasi, D.V. Agoston. 1994. The calcitonin gene-related peptide (CGRP) phenotype is expressed early and up-regulated by resiniferatoxin (RTX) in mouse sensory neurons. *Dev. Brain Res.* 80:290–294.

327. Szolcsányi, J., A. Szallasi, Z. Szallasi, F. Joó, P. M. Blumberg. 1990. Resiniferatoxin: An ultrapotent selective modulator of capsaicin-sensitive primary afferent neurons. *J. Pharmacol. Exp. Ther.* 255:923–928.

328. Xu, X-J., J-X. Hao, H. Aldskogius, Å. Seiger, Z. Wiesenfeld-Hallin. 1992. Chronic pain-related syndrome in rats after ischemic spinal cord lesion: A possible animal model for pain in patients with spinal cord injury. *Pain* 48:279–290.

329. Hao, J-X., W. Yu, X-J. Xu, Z. Wiesenfeld-Hallin. 1996. Capsaicin-sensitive afferents mediate chronic cold, but not mechanical, allodynia-like behavior in spinally injured rats. *Brain Res.* 722:177–180.

330. Obál, F. Jr., G. Benedek, A. Jancsó-Gábor, F. Obál. 1979. Salivary cooling, escape reaction, and heat pain in capsaicin-desensitized rats. *Pflüger's Arch.* 382:249–254.

331. Hayes, A. G., M. B. Tyers. 1980. Effects of capsaicin on nociceptive heat, pressure and chemical threshold and on substance P levels in the rat. *Brain Res.* 189:561–564.

332. Jancsó, G., A. Jancsó-Gábor. 1980. Effect of capsaicin on morphine analgesia—Possible involvement of hypothalamic structures. *Naunyn-Schmiedeberg's Arch. Pharmacol.* 311:285–288.

333. Wall, P. D., C. Woolf. 1984. Muscle, but not cutaneous C-afferent input produced prolonged increases in the excitability of the flexion reflex in the rat. *J. Physiol.* 356:443–458.

334. Xu, X-J., T. Farkas-Szallasi, J. M. Lundberg, T. Hökfelt, Z. Wiesenfeld-Hallin, A. Szallasi. 1997. Effects of the capsaicin analogue resiniferatoxin on spinal nociceptive mechanisms in the rat: Behavioral, electrophysiological and in situ hybridization studies. *Brain Res.* 752:52–60.

335. Ghilardi, J. R., C. J. Allen, S. R. Vigna, D. C. McVey, P. W. Mantyh. 1992. Trigeminal and dorsal root ganglion neurons express CCK receptor binding sites in rat, rabbit, and monkey: Possible site of opiate-CCK analgesic interactions. *J. Neurosci.* 12:4854–4866.

336. Verge, V. M. K., Z. Wiesenfeld-Hallin, T. Hökfelt. 1993. Cholecystokinin in mammalian primary sensory neurons and spinal cord: In situ hybridization studies in rat and monkey. *Eur J Neurosci* 5:240–250.

337. Wu, J., Q. Lin, D. J. McAdoo, W. D. Willis. 1998. Nitric oxide contributes to central sensitization following intradermal injection of capsaicin. *Neuroreport* 9:589–592.

338. Szolcsányi, J. 1993. Actions of capsaicin on sensory receptors. In *Capsaicin in the Study of Pain*, J. N. Wood, Ed., pp. 1–26. San Diego: Academic Press.

339. Santicioli, P., R. Patacchini, C. A. Maggi, A. Meli. 1987. Exposure to calcium-free medium protects sensory fibers from capsaicin desensitization. *Neurosci. Lett.* 80:167–172.

340. Amann, R. 1990. Desensitization of capsaicin-evoked neuropeptide release—Influence of Ca21 and temperature. *Naunyn-Schmiedeberg's Arch. Pharmacol.* 342:671–676.

341. Craft, R. M., F. Porreca. 1992. Treatment parameters of desensitization to capsaicin. *Life Sci.* 51:1767–1775.

342. Cholewinski, A., G. M. Burgess, S. Bevan. 1993. The role of calcium in capsaicin induced desensitization in rat cultured dorsal root ganglion neurons. *Neuroscience* 55:1015–1023.

343. Garcia-Hirschfeld, J., L. G. López-Briones, C. Belmonte, M. Valdeolmillos. 1995. Intracellular free calcium responses to protons and capsaicin in cultured trigeminal neurons. *Neuroscience* 67:235–243.

344. Docherty, R. J., J. C. Yeats, S. Bevan, H. W. G. M. Boddeke. 1996. Inhibition of calcineurin inhibits the desensitization of capsaicin-evoked currents in cultured dorsal root ganglion neurones from adult rats. *Pflügers Arch. Eur. J. Physiol.* 431:828–837.

345. Caterina, M. J., M. A. Schumacher, M. Tominaga, T. A. Rosen, J. D. Levine, D. Julius. 1997. The capsaicin receptor: A heat-activated ion channel in the pain pathway. *Nature* 389:816–824.

346. Hay, E. D. 1983. Collagen and embryonic development. In *Cell Biology of Extracellular Matrix*, 2nd ed, E. D. Hay, Ed., pp. 379–410. New York: Plenum Press.

347. Heine, H. 1991. The structure and function of the ground substance (extracellular matrix): Paradigms in medical thinking. In *Matrix and Matrix Regulation. Basis for a Holistic Theory in Medicine*, A. Pischinger, Ed., H. Heine, Eng. Trans. N. Mac Lean, p. 36. Brussels, Belgium: Editions Haug International.

348. Perger, F. 1991. Therapeutic consequences of ground regulation research. 1991. *In Matrix and Matrix Regulation: Basis for a Holistic Theory in Medicine*, A. Pischinger, Ed., H. Heine, Eng. Trans. N. Mac Lean, p. 148. Brussels, Belgium: Editions Haug International.

349. Yanada, K. M. 1983. Fibronectin and other structural proteins. In *Cell Biology of Extracellular Matrix*, 2nd ed., E. D. Hay, Ed., pp. 95–114. New York: Plenum Press.

350. Iozzo, R. V. 1985. Biology of disease. Proteoglycans: Structure, function, and role in neoplasia. *Lab. Invest.* 53:337–396.

351. Heine, H. 1986. Basalmembranen als. Regulations system zwixchen epithelialen Zellvrbaden. *Gegenbaurs morph. Jahrb.* 132:325–331.

352. Uhlenbruck, G., H. J. Beuth, K. Oette, T. Schotten, H. L. Ko, K. Roszkow, W. Roskowsk, W. Roskowski, R. L. Utticken, G. Pulverer. 1986. Kektine und die Organotropie der Metastasierung. *Disch. Med. Wschr.* 111:991–995.

353. Heine, H. 1988. Akupunkturtherapie-perforationen der oberflachlichen Korperfaszie durch kutane Gefap-Nervenbundel. *Therapeutikon* 4:238–244.

354. Heine, H. 1988. Markjerung von Blutzellen mit enem Lektin-KarbohydratKomplex. Erweiterite Funktionsdiagnostik an Blutausstrichen. *A. Mikroskanat. Forsch* 102:54–62.

355. Toole, B. P. 1983. Glycosaminioglycans in morpohogenesis. In *Cell Biology of Extracellular Matrix*, 2nd ed., E. D. Hay, Ed. 259–294. New York: Plenum Press.

356. Rea, W. J. 1995. Chemical Sensitivity. Vol. III: *Clinical Manifestations of Pollutant Overload*. p. 1495. Boca Raton, FL: Lewis Publishers.

357. Heine, H. 1987. Regulations phanomene der Tumorgrundsubstanz. *Ditsch. Zschr. Onkol.* 19:67–72.

358. Hascall, V. C., G. K. Hascall. 1991. Proteoglycans. In *Cell Biology of Extracellular Matrix*, 2nd ed., E. D. Hay, Ed., pp. 39–64. New York: Plenum Press.

359. Balasz, E. A., P. A. Gibbs. 1970. The rheological properties and biological function of yaluronic acid. *Chemistry and Molecular Biology of the Intercellular Matrix*, Vol. 3, E. A. Balasz, Ed., pp. 1241–1254. New York: Academic Press.

360. Trincher, K. 1981. *Gesetze der biologischen Thermodynamik. Urban u. Schwarzenberg Wien.* Munchen, Baltimore.

361. Popp, F. A. 1983. *New Horizonte in der Medzin.* Heidelberg: Karl F. Haug Verlag.

362. Hollemann, A. F., F. Richter. 1964. *Lehrbuch der organischen Chemie,* S:37–41. Berlin: W. de Gruyter.

363. Huneke, F. 1975. *Das Sekundenphanomen. 4. Aufl.* Heidelberg: Karl F. Haug Verlag Dosch, *Manual of Neural Therapy According to Huneke* (ISBN 9783131406026) 2007 Georg Thieme Verlag KG.

364. Gutmann, V., G. Resch. 1988. Hochpotenz und Molekularkonzept. *Therapeutikon* 4:245–252.

365. Miller, J. B. 1977. A double-blind study of food extract injection therapy: A preliminary report. *Ann. Allergy* 38 (3):185–0.

366. Miller, J. B. 1976. Food allergy: Technique of intradermal testing and subcutaneous injection therapy. *Trans. Am. Soc. Ophthalmol. Otolaryngol. Allergy* 16:154–168.

367. Rapp, D. J. 1978. Double-blind confirmation and treatment of milk sensitivity. *Med. J. Aust.* 1:571.

368. Rapp, D. J. 1979. Food allergy treatment for hyperkinesis. *J. Learn. Disabil.* 12:42–50.

369. Rapp, D. J. 1978. Weeping eyes in wheat allergy. *Trans. Am. Soc. Ophthalmol. Otolaryngol. Allergy* 18:149–150.

370. Boris, M., M. Schiff, S. Midorf, L. Inselman. 1983. Bronchoprovocation blocked by neutralizing therapy (Abstract). *J. Allergy Clin. Immunol.* 71:92.

371. McGovern, J. J. 1980. Correlation of clinical food allergy symptoms with serial pharmacologic and immunologic changes in the patient's plasma (Abstract). *Ann. Allergy* 44:57–58.

372. O'Shea, J. A., S. F. Porter. 1981. Double-blind study of children with hyperkinetic syndrome treated by multi-allergen extract sublingually. *J. Learn. Disabil.* 14:189–190.

373. Darlington, L. G. 1983. Food allergy and rheumatoid disease. *Ann. Rheum. Dis.* 42:219–220.

374. Monro, J. 1983. Food allergy in migraine. *Proc. Nutr. Soc.* 42:241–0.

375. Rea, W. J., R. N. Podell, M. L. Williams, E. J. Fenyves, D. E. Sprague, A. R. Johnson. 1984. Elimination of oral food challenge reaction by injection of food extracts. *Arch. Otolaryngol.* 110:248–252.

376. King, W. P., W. A. Rubin, R. G. Fadal, W. A. Ward, R. J. Trevino, W. B. Pierce, J. A. Stewart, J. H. Boyles. 1988. Provocation-neutralization: A two-part study. Part I. The intracutaneous provocative food test: A multi-center comparison study. *Otolaryngol. Head Neck Surg.* 99 (3):263–271.

377. King, W. P., R. G. Fadal, W. A. Ward, R. J. Trevino, W. B. Pierce, J. A. Stewart, J. H. Boyles. 1988. Provocation-neutralization: A two part study. Part II. Subcutaneous neutralization therapy: A multi-center study. *Otolaryngol. Head Neck Surg.* 99 (3):272–277.

378. Gerdes, K. 1989. Provocative-neutralization testing: A look at the controversy. *Clin. Ecol.* 6:21–29.

379. Jewett, D. L., G. Fein, M. H. Greenberg. 1990. A double-blind study of symptom provocation to determine food sensitivity. *N. Engl. J. Med.* 323 (7):429–433.

380. Podell, R. N. 1983. Intracutaneous and sublingual provocation and neutralization. *Clin. Ecol.* 2:13–20.

381. Forman, R. A. 1981. Critique of evaluation studies of sublingual and intracutaneous provocative tests for food allergy. *Med. Hypothesis* 7:1019–1027.

382. Scadding, G. K., J. Brostoff. 1986. Low-dose sublingual therapy in patients with allergic rhinitis due to house-dust mite. *Clin. Allergy* 16:483–491.

383. Pfeiffer, G. O. 1970. Sublingual procedures. *Trans. Soc. Ophthalmol. Otolaryngol. Allergy* 11:104.

384. Bjorksten, B., J. M. Dewdney. 1987. Oral immunotherapy in allergy—Is it effective? *Clin. Allergy* 17:91–94.

385. Leng, X., Y. X. Fu, S. T. Ye, S. Q. Duan. 1990. A double-blind trial of oral immunotherapy for *Artemisia* pollen asthma with evaluation of bronchial response to the pollen allergen and serum-specific IgE antibody. *Ann. Allergy* 64:27–31.

386. Morris, D. L. 1970. Treatment of respiratory disease with ultra-small doses of antigens. *Ann. Allergy* 28:494–500.

387. Taudorf, E., L. C. Laursen, A. Lanner, B. Bjorksten, S. Dreborg, M. Soborg, B. Weeke. 1987. Oral immunotherapy in birch pollen hayfever. *J. Allergy Clin. Immunol.* 80:153–161.

388. Van Nierkerk, C. H., J. I. De Wet. 1987. Efficacy of grass-maize pollen oral immunotherapy in patients with seasonal hay-fever; A double-blind study. *Clin. Allergy* 17:507–513.

389. Taudorf, E., L. Laursen, A. lanner, B. Bjorksten, S. Dreborg, A. Weeke. 1989. Specific IgE, IgG and IgA antibody response to oral immunotherapy in birch pollinosis. *J. Allergy Clin. Immunol.* 83 (3):589–594.

390. Tari, M. G., M. Mancino, G. Monti. 1990. Efficacy of sublingual immunotherapy in patients with rhinitis and asthma due to house dust mite—A double-blind study. *Allergol. Immunopathol.* 18 (4):277–284.

391. Moller, C., S. Dreborg, A. Lanner. B. Bjorksten. 1986. Oral immunotherapy of children with rhinoconjuctivitis due to birch pollen allergy. *Allergy* 41:271–279.

392. Wortman, F. 1977. Oral hyposensitization of children with pollinosis of house-dust asthma. *Allergol. Immunopathol.* 5 (15):15–26.

393. Holt, P. G., J. Vines, D. Britten. 1988. Sublingual allergen administration. I. Selective suppression of IgE production in rats by high allergen doses. *Clin. Allergy* 18:229–234.

394. Giovane, A. L., M. Bardare, G. Passalacqua, S. Ruffoni, A. Scordamaglia, E. Ghezzi, G. W. Canonica. 1994. A three-year double-blind placebo-controlled study with specific oral immunotherapy to Dermatophagiodes: Evidence of safety and efficacy in pediatric patients. *Clin. Exp. Allergy* 24 (1):53–59.

395. Felziani, V., R. M. Marfisi, S. Parmiani. 1993. Rush immunotherapy with sublingual administration of grass allergen extract. *Allergol. Immunopathol.* 21 (5):173–178.

396. Sabbah, A., S. Hassoun, J. Le Sellin, C. Andre, H. Sicard. 1994. A double-blind placebo-controlled trial by the sublingual route of immunotherapy with a standardized grass pollen extract. *Allergy* 49 (5):309–313.

397. Troise, C., S. Voltolini, A. Canessa, S. Pecora, A.C. Negrini. 1995. Sublingual immunotherapy in Parietaria pollen-induced rhinitis. A double-blind study. *J. Investig. Allergol. Clin. Immunol.* 5 (1):25–30.

398. Jonassohn, M., O. Sterner. 1997. Terpenoid unsaturated 1,4-dialdehydes, occurrence and biological activities. *Trends Org. Chem.* 6:23–43.

399. Kubo, I., K. Nakanishi. 1979. Some terpenoid insect antifeedants from tropical plants. In *Advances in Pesticide Science*, H. Geissbühler, Ed. pp. 284–294. Oxford: Pergamon.

400. Kubo, I., I. Ganjian. 1981. Insect antifeedant terpenes, hot-tasting to humans. *Experientia* 37:1063–1064.

401. Camazine, S., J. Resch, T. Eisner, J. Meinwald. 1983. Mushroom chemical defence: Pungent sesquiterpenoid dialdehyde antifeedant to opossum. *J. Chem. Ecol.* 9:1439–1447.

402. Cimino, G., S. De Rosa, S. De Stefano, G. Sodano, G. Villani. 1983. Dorid nudibranch elaborates its own chemical defence. *Science* 219:1237–1238.

403. Caprioli, V., G. Cimino, R. Colle, M. Gavagnini, G. Sodano, A. Spinella. 1987. Insect antifeedant activity and hot taste for humans of selected natural and synthetic 1,4-dialdehydes. *J. Nat. Prod.* 50:146–151.

404. Vidari, G., P. Vita-Finzi, S. Abdo, C. Jativa, X. Chiriboga, M. E. Maldonato. 1997. Phytochemical studies on Ecuadorian plants. In *Virtual Activity, Real Pharmacology, Different Approaches to the Search for Bioactive Natural Compounds*, L. Verotta, Ed., pp. 227–237. Trivandrum, India: Research Signpost.

405. Anke, H., O. Sterner. 1991. Comparison of the antimicrobial and cytotoxic activities of twenty unsaturated dialdehydes from plants and mushrooms. *Planta Med.* 57:344–356.

406. Jonassohn, M. 1996. *Sesquiterpenoid unsaturated dialdehydes. Structural properties that affect reactivity and bioactivity*. PhD thesis. Lund University, Lund.

407. Kubo, I., Y-W. Lee, M. Pettei, F. Pilkiewicz, K. Nakanishi. 1976. Potent army worm antifeedants from the East African Warburgia plants. *J. Chem. Soc. Chem. Commun.* 3:1013–1014.

408. Watt, J. M., M. G. Breyer-Brandwijk. 1962. *Medicinal and Poisonous Plants of Southern and Eastern Africa*. Edinburgh: E. S. Livingstone Ltd.

409. Fukuyama, Y., T. Sato, Y. Asakawa, T. Takemoto. 1982. A potent warburganal and related drimane-type sesquiterpenoid from polygonum hydropiper. *Phytochemistry* 21:2895–2898.

410. Canonica, L., P. Corbella, G. Gariboldi, G. Jommi, J. Krepinsky, G. Ferrari, C. Casagrande. 1969. Sesquiterpenoids of *Cinnamoma fragrans* Baillon. Structure of cinnamolide, cinnamosmolide and cinnamodial. *Tetrahedron* 25:3895–3902.

411. List, P. H., H. Hackenberger. 1973. Die scharf schmeckenden Stoffe von Lactarius vellereus Fries. *Z Pilzkd* 39:97–102.

412. Szallasi, A., M. Jonassohn, G. Ács, T. Bíró, P. Ács, P.M. Blumberg, O. Sterner. 1996. The stimulation of capsaicin-sensitive neurones in a vanilloid receptor-mediated fashion by pungent terpenoids possessing an unsaturated 1,4-dialdehyde moiety. *Br. J. Pharmacol.* 119:283–290.

413. Szallasi, A., T. Bíró, S. Modarres, P. M. Blumberg, J. E. Krause, G. Appendino. 1998. Phorboid ligands that distinguish between R- and C-type vanilloid receptors (VRs). *Soc Neurosci Abstr* 24:641–645.

414. Mendes, G. L., A. R. S. Santos, M. M. Campos, K. S. Tratsk, R. A. Yunes, V. C. Filho, J. B. Calixto. 1998. Anti-hyperalgesic properties of the extract and of the main sesquiterpene polygodial isolated from the barks of *Drymis winteri* (Winteraceae). *Life Sci.* 63:369–381.

415. Tratsk, K. S., M. M. Campos, Z. R. Vaz, V. C. Filho, V. Schlemper, R. A. Yunes, J. B. Calixto. 1997. Anti-allergic effects and oedema inhibition caused by the extract of *Drymis winteri*. *Inflamm. Res.* 46:509–514.

416. El Sayah, M., V. C. Filho, R. A. Yunes, T. R. Pinheiro, J. B. Calixto. 1998. Action of polygodial, a sesquiterpene isolated from *Drymis winteri*, in the guinea-pig ileum and trachea "in vitro". *Eur. J. Pharmacol.* 344:215–221.

417. Dekermendjian, K., R. Shan, M. Nielsen, M. Stadler, O. Sterner, M. R. Witt. 1997. The finity of the brain dopamine D1 receptor in vitro for triprenyl phenols isolated from fruit bodies of *Albatrellus ovinus*. *Eur. J. Med. Chem.* 32:351–356.

418. Szallasi, A., T. Bíró, S. Modarres, L. Garlaschelli, M. Petersen, A. Klusch, G. Vidari, M. Jonassohn, S. De Rosa, O. Sterner, J. M. Blumberg, J. E. Krause. 1998. Dialdehyde sesquiterpenes and other terpenoids as vanilloids. *Eur. J. Pharmacol.* 356:81–89.

419. Szallasi, A., T. Bíró, T. Szabó, S. Modarres, M. Petersen, A. Klusch, P. M. Blumberg, J. E. Krause, O. Sterner. 1999. A non-pungent triprenyl phenol of fungal origin, scutigeral, stimulates rat dorsal root ganglion neurons via interaction at vanilloid receptors. *Br. J. Pharmacol.* 126:1351–1358.

420. Travell, J. G., D. G. Simons. 1983. *Myofascial Pain and Dysfunction: The Trigger Point Manual.* Volume 1, 1st ed. Baltimore: Williams & Wilkins.

421. Simons, D. G., J. G. Travell, L. Simons. 1999. *Travell and Simons' Myofascial pain and Dysfunction. The Trigger Point Manual.* Vol. 1, 2nd ed. Baltimore: Williams & Wilkins.

422. Fleckenstein, A., C. Van Breeman, E. Hoffmeister, A. Fleckenstein. 1985. Calcium antagonists and calcium agonists: Fundamental criteria and classification, *Bayer Symposium IX: Cardiovascular Effects of Dihydropyridine-type Calcium Agonists and Agonists*, A. Fleckenstein, C. Van Breeman, E. Hoffmeister, Eds., pp. 3–31. Berlin: Springer-Verlag.

423. Scheidt, W. 1946. *Das Vegetative System.* Hamburg: Hermes.

424. Ricker, W. E. 1975. Computation and interpretation of biological statistics of fish populations. *Bulletin of the Fisheries Research Board of Canada*, No. 191.

425. Speransky, A. D. 1937. *Elements of the Theory of Medicine.* Moscow: Meditsina.

426. Ratschow, M. 1951. Criticism of the effectiveness of neural-therapy (healing anesthesia). *Dtsch Med. Wochenschr.* 76 (10):308–311.

427. Klinghardt, D. K. 2002. Neural therapy. Vol. 11, No. 2, pp. 25–29.

428. Gunn, C. C. 1980. Dry needling of muscle motor points for chronic low back pain. *Spine* 5:279–291.

429. McEwen, L. Enzyme Potentiated Desensitisation (EPD)—A promising low-dose method of immunotherapy. Downloaded from www.feingold.org/Research/PDFstudies/McEwen-summary.pdf. Accessed September 26, 2017.

430. Shrader, W. A. Jr. 2000. The use of bacterial antigen EPD immunotherapy for the treatment of rheumatoid arthritis and reactive arthritis: The role of molecular mimicry (unpublished), 1996, revised 1998, 2000.

431. Zamboni, W. A., A. C. Roth, R. C. Russell, B. Graham, H. Suchy, J. O. Kucan. 1993. Morphologic analysis of the microcirculation during reperfusion of ischemic skeletal muscle and the effect of hyperbaric oxygen. *Plast. Reconstr. Surg.* 91:1110–1123.

432. Atochin, D., D. Fisher, I. Demchenko, S. R. Thom. 2000. Neutrophil sequestration and the effect of hyperbaric oxygen in a rat model of temporary middle cerebral artery occlusion. *Undersea Hyperbaric Med.* 27:185–190.

433. Kihara, K., S. Ueno, M. Sakoda, T. Aikou. 2005. Effects of hyperbaric oxygen exposure on experimental hepatic ischemia reperfusion injury: Relationship between its timing and neutrophil sequestration. *Liver Transpl.* 11:1574–1580.

434. Rossignol, D. A., J. J. Bradstreet, K. Van Dyke, C. Schneider, S. H. Freedenfeld, N. O'Hara, S. Cave, J. A. Buckley, E. A. Mumper, R. E. Frye. 2012. Hyperbaric oxygen treatment in autism spectrum disorders. *Med. Gas Res.* 2 (1):16.

435. Sumen, G., M. Cimsit, L. Eroglu. 2001. Hyperbaric oxygen treatment reduces carrageenan-induced acute inflammation in rats. *Eur. J. Pharmacol.* 431 (2):265–268.

436. Takeshima, F., K. Makiyama, T. Doi. 1999. Hyperbaric oxygen as adjunct therapy for Crohn's intractable enteric ulcer. *Am. J. Gastroenterol.* 94 (11):3374–3375.

437. Alleva, R., E. Nasole, F. Di Donato, B. Borghi, J. Neuzil, M. Tomasetti. 2005. alphaLipoic acid supplementation inhibits oxidative damage, accelerating chronic wound healing in patients undergoing hyperbaric oxygen therapy. *Biochem. Biophys. Res. Commun.* 333 (2):404–410.

438. Ozden, T. A., H. Uzun, M. Bohloli, A. S. Toklu, M. Paksoy, G. Simsek, H. Durak, H. Issever, T. Ipek. 2004. The effects of hyperbaric oxygen treatment on oxidant and antioxidants levels during liver regeneration in rats. *Tohoku J. Exp. Med.* 203 (4):253–265.

439. Gregorevic, P., G. S. Lynch, D. A. Williams. 2001. Hyperbaric oxygen modulates antioxidant enzyme activity in rat skeletal muscles. *Eur. J. Appl. Physiol.* 86 (1):24–27.

440. Gulec, B., M. Yasar, S. Yildiz, S. Oter, C. Akay, S. Deveci, D. Sen. 2004. Effect of hyperbaric oxygen on experimental acute distal colitis. *Physiol. Res.* 53 (5):493–499.

441. Nie, H., L. Xiong, N. Lao, S. Chen, N. Xu, Z. Zhu. 2006. Hyperbaric oxygen preconditioning induces tolerance against spinal cord ischemia by upregulation of antioxidant enzymes in rabbits. *J. Cereb. Blood Flow Metab.* 26 (5):666–674.

442. Sharifi, M., W. Fares, I. Abdel-Karim, J. M. Koch, J. Sopko, D. Adler. 2004. Usefulness of hyperbaric oxygen therapy to inhibit restenosis after percutaneous coronary intervention for acute myocardial infarction or unstable angina pectoris. *Am. J. Cardiol.* 93 (12):1533–1535.

443. Speit, G., C. Dennog, U. Eichhorn, A. Rothfuss, B. Kaina. 2000. Induction of heme oxygenase-1 and adaptive protection against the induction of DNA damage after hyperbaric oxygen treatment. *Carcinogenesis* 21 (10):1795–1799.

444. Rothfuss, A., P. Radermacher, G. Speit. 2001. Involvement of heme oxygenase-1 (HO-1) in the adaptive protection of human lymphocytes after hyperbaric oxygen (HBO) treatment. *Carcinogenesis* 22 (12):1979–1985.

445. Rossignol, D. A. 2007. Hyperbaric oxygen therapy might improve certain pathophysiological findings in autism. *Med. Hypotheses* 68 (6):1208–1227.

446. Rothfuss, A., G. Speit. 2002. Investigations on the mechanism of hyperbaric oxygen (HBO)-induced adaptive protection against oxidative stress. *Mutat. Res.* 508 (1–2):157–165.

447. Thom, S. R. 2009. Oxidative stress is fundamental to hyperbaric oxygen therapy. *J. Appl. Physiol.* 106 (3):988–995.

448. Gutsaeva, D. R., H. B. Suliman, M. S. Carraway, I. T. Demchenko, C. A. Piantadosi. 2006. Oxygen-induced mitochondrial biogenesis in the rat hippocampus. *Neuroscience* 137 (2):493–504.

449. Rossignol, D. A., L. W. Rossignol, S. J. James, S. Melnyk, E. Mumper. 2007. The effects of hyperbaric oxygen therapy on oxidative stress, inflammation, and symptoms in children with autism: An open-label pilot study. *BMC Pediatr.* 7 (1):36.

450. Audhya, T. 2007. Autism Research Institute Garden Grove Think Tank Meeting, 2007. In *Adjustment of SOD, GPO & Catalase Activity in RBC of Normal and Autistic Children during Hyperoxia.* Garden Grove, CA.

451. Dickinson, D. A., H. J. Forman. 2002. Glutathione in defense and signaling: Lessons from a small thiol. *Ann. N. Y. Acad. Sci.* 973:488–504.

452. Harch, P. G. 2015. Hyperbaric oxygen in chronic traumatic brain injury: Oxygen, pressure, and gene therapy. *Med. Gas Res.* 5 (1):9.

453. Calabrese, E. J. 1984. *Ecogenetics: Genetic Variation in Susceptibility to Environmental Agents.* New York: Wiley.

454. Phelps, G. 2016. Hyperbaric Centers of Texas Is Hidden Secret for Athletes—Dr. Alfred Johnson's Richardson Practice Helps Pros Heal Injuries. Richardson Living. November 17, 2013. Accessed August 29, 2016. http://richardsonliving.com/contributed/hyperbaric-centers-texas-hidden-secret-athletes-0.

455. Sprague, D. 1987. The concept of an environmental unit. In *Food Allergy and Intolerance*, J. Brostoff, S. Challacombe, Eds., pp. 947–960. Philadelphia: Bailliere Tindall/W.B. Saunders.

456. Griffiths, B. B., W. J. Rea, B. Griffiths, Y. Pan. 1998. The role of the T lymphocytic cell cycle and an autogenous lymphocytic factor in clinical medicine. *Cytobios* 93 (372):49–66.

457. Lee, W. M., C. V. Dang. 1995. Control of cell growth, differentiation and death. In *Hematology, Basic Principles and Practice*, R. Hoffman, E. KaBenz Jr., S. J. Shattil, B. Furie, H. J. Cohen, L. E. Silberstain, Eds., pp 69–84. New York: Churchill Livingstone.

458. Givan, A. L. 1992. Cell from within. In *Flow Cytometry: First principles*, A. L. Givan, Ed., pp. 103–133. New York: Wiley-Liss.

459. Nurse, P., Y. Bissett. 1981. Gene required in G_1 for commitment to cell cycle and in G_2 for control of mitosis in fission yeast. *Nature* 292:558–560.

460. Meyerson, M., G. H. Enders, C. L. Wie, L. Su, C. Gorka, C. Nelson, E. Harlow, L. Tsai. 1992. A family of human CDC2 related protein kinases. *EMBO J.* 11:2909–2917.

461. Lorinez, A. T., S. I. Reed. 1984. Primary structure homology between the product of yeast cell division control gene BBC-28 and vertebrate oncogenes. *Nature* 307:183–185.

462. Nurse, P. 1994. Ordering S phase and M phase in the cell cycle. *Cell* 79:547–550.

463. Sherr, C. J. 1994. G$_1$ phase progression: Cycling on cue. *Cell* 79:551–555.
464. Helchman, K. A., J. M. Roberts. 1994. Rules to replicate by. *Cell* 79:557–562.
465. King, R. W., P. K. Jackson, M. W. Kirschner. 1994. Mitosis in transition. *Cell* 79:557–562.
466. Hunter, T., J. Pines. 1994. Cyclins and cancer 11: Cyclin D and CDK inhibitors come to age. *Cell* 79:573–582.
467. Meyerson, M., E. Harlow. 1994. Identification of G$_1$ kinase activity of CDK$_6$, a novel cyclin D partner. *Mol. Cell. Biol.* 14:2077–2086.
468. Kamp, A., N. A. Gruis, J. Weaver-Feldhaus, Q. Liu, K. Harshman, S. V. Tavitigian, E. Stockert, R. S. Day III, B. E. Johnson, M. J. Skolnick. 1994. A cell cycle regulator potentially involved in genesis of many tumor types. *Science* 264:436–440.
469. Desai, D., Y. Gu, D. O. Morgan. 1992. Activation of human cyclin-dependent kinases in vitro. *Mol. Cell. Biol.* 3:571–582.
470. Gold, K. L., P. Nurse. 1989. Tyrosine phosphorylation of the fission yeast CDC2$^+$ protein kinase regulated entry into mitosis. *Nature* 324:39–45.
471. Draetca, G., D. Beach. 1988. Activation of CDC2 protein kinase during mitosis in human cells: Cell cycle-dependent phosphorylation and subunit rearrangement. *Cell* 3:17–26.
472. Solomon, M. J., M. Glotzer, T. H. Lee, M. Philippe, M. W. Krischner. 1990. Cyclin activation of p34 CDC2. *Cell* 63:1013–1024.
473. Gutier, J., M. J. Solomon, R. N. Booher, J. F. Bazan, M. W. Krischner. 1991. CDC25 is specific tyrosine phosphatase that directly activates p34 CDC2. *Cell* 67:197–211.
474. Murray, A. W., M. W. Krischner. 1989. Cyclin synthesis drives the early embryonic cell cycle. *Nature* 339:275–280.
475. Evans, T. E., E. T. Rosenthal, J. Youngblom, D. Distel, T. Hunt. 1983. Cyclin: A protein specified by maternal mRNA in sea urchin eggs that is destroyed at each cleavage division. *Cell* 33:389–396.
476. Pines, J., T. Hunter. 1989. Isolation of human cyclin C DNA: Evidence for cyclin M-RNA and protein regulation in the cell cycle and for interaction with P34 CDC2. *Cell* 58:833–846.
477. Xiong, Y., T. Connolly, B. Futcher, D. Beach. 1991. Human D-type cyclin. *Cell* 65:691–699.
478. Nurse, P. 1990. Universal control mechanism regulating onset of M-phase. *Nature* 344:503–508.
479. Lewin, B. 1990. Driving the cell cycle: M phase kinase, its partners, and substrates. *Cell* 61:743–752.
480. Sherr, C. J. 1993. Mammalian G$_1$ cyclins. *Cell* 73:1059–1065.
481. Wang, J., X. Chenevesse, B. Hanglein, C. Brechot. 1990. Hepatitis B virus integration in a cyclin A gene in a hepatocellular carcinoma. *Nature* 343:555–557.
482. Fang, F., J. W. Newport. 1991. Evidence that the G$_1$-S and G$_2$-M transitions are controlled by different CDC2 proteins in higher eukaryotes. *Cell* 66:731–742.
483. Walker, D. H., J. L. Maller. 1991. Role of cyclin A in the dependence of mitosis on completion of DNA replication. *Nature* 354:314–317.
484. Lehner, C., P. O'Farrell. 1990. The roles of Drosophila cyclins A and B in mitotic control. *Cell* 61:535–547.
485. Pagano, M., P. Pepperkok, F. Verde, W. Ansorge, G. Draetta. 1992. Cyclin A is required at two points in the human cell cycle. *EMBO J.* 11:961–971.
486. Zindy, F., E. Lamas, X. Chenevesse, J. Sobezak, J. Wang, D. Fesquet, B. Hanglein, C. Brechot. 1992. Cyclin A is required in S phase in normal epithelial cells. *Biochem. Biophys. Res. Commun.* 182:1144–1154.
487. Glotzer, M., W. A. Murray, M. W. Kirshner. 1991. Cyclin is degraded by the ubiquitin pathway. *Nature* 349:132–138.
488. Reed, S.I. 1992. G$_1$ specific cyclins in search of an S-phase-promoting factor. *Trends Genet.* 7:95–99.
489. Cross, F. R. 1988. DAF 1 a mutant affecting size control, pheromone arrest, and cell kinetics of *Saccharomyces cerevisiae. Mol. Cell. Biol.* 8:4675–4684.
490. Richardson, H. E., C. Wittenberg, F. Cross, S. I. Reed. 1989. An essential G$_1$ function for cyclin-like proteins in yeast. *Cell* 59:1127–1133.
491. Hadwiger, J. A., C. Wittenberg, H. E. Richardson, M. Lopes, S. I. Reed. 1989. A family of cyclin homology that control the G phase in yeast. *Proc. Natl. Acad. Sci. USA* 86:6255–6259.
492. Wittenberg, C., K. Sugimoto, S. I. Reed. 1990. G$_1$-specific cyclins of *S. cerevisiae*: Cell cycle periodicity, regulation by mating pheromone, and association with the p34 CDC28 protein kinase. *Cell* 62:225–237.
493. Rea, W. J., Y. Pan, A. R. Johnson, E. J. Fenyves, N. Smadi. 1986. T and B lymphocytes parameters measured in chemically sensitive patients and controls. *Clin. Ecol.* 4:11–14.
494. Rea, W. J., Y. Pan, A. R. Johnson, E. J. Fenyves. 1987. T and B lymphocytes in chemically sensitive patients with toxic volatile organic hydrocarbons in their blood. *Clin. Ecol.* 5:171–175.

495. Cory, J. G. 1993. Purine and pyrimidine nucleotide metabolism. In *Biochemistry with Clinical Correlation*, T. M. Devlin, Ed., pp. 529–573. New York: Wiley-Liss.
496. Griffiths, B. B., W. J. Rea. 1995. Pending U.S. patent number 08/380,063.
497. Parge, H. E., A. S. Arvai, D. T. Murtari, S. I. Reed, J. A. Tainer. 1993. Human CksHs2 atomic structure: A role for its hexameric assembly in cell cycle control. *Science* 262:387–395.
498. King, D. S. 1981. Can allergic exposure provoke psychological symptoms? A double-blind test. *Biol. Psychiatry* 16 (1):3–19.
499. Nasmyth, K. A. 1990. Far-reaching discoveries about the regulation of START. *Cell* 63:1117–1120.

Index

Note: The letter 't' and 'f' followed by the numbers represents 'tables' and 'figures' respectively.